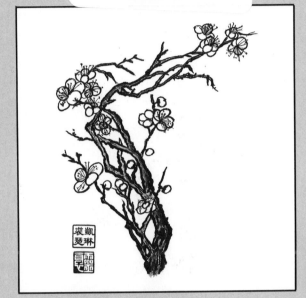

PLUM

The plum tree and its blossoms symbolize a person's inner knowledge, and the reemergence and continuity of the life cycle. The plum tree is the winter essence, hardy, and bursting forth in cold months with perfect delicate blossoms announcing the return of spring, hope, and endurance. Its gnarled trunk and branches represent the wisdom of old age, and nature's law of everlasting eternal wisdom.

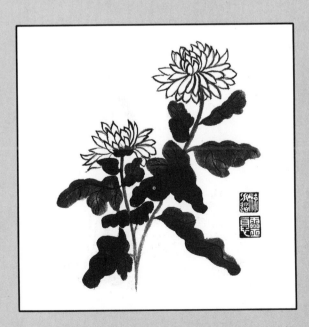

CHRYSANTHEMUM

The chrysanthemum and its many petals symbolize a person's place in the greater totality of the universe. It represents the autumn, with its fortitude and patience. It exemplifies the holistic principle that the whole is greater than the sum of its parts. Each petal joins, overlaps, and radiates outward, creating the form of the flower.

Critical Care Nursing
Body–Mind–Spirit

Critical Care
Body–Mind–Spirit
THIRD EDITION

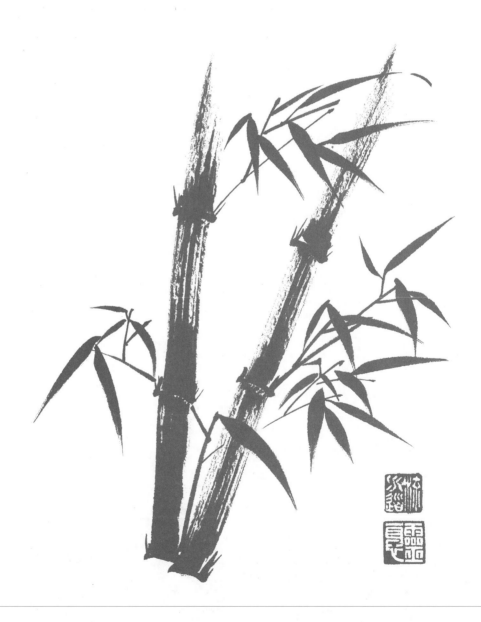

Nursing

Barbara Montgomery Dossey, R.N., M.S.

Director, Holistic Nursing Consultants
Santa Fe, New Mexico
Director, Bodymind Systems
Temple, Texas

Cathie E. Guzzetta, R.N., Ph.D., FAAN

Director, Holistic Nursing Consultants
Bethesda, Maryland
Formerly, Associate Professor and Chairperson, Cardiovascular Nursing
The Catholic University of America
Washington, D.C.

Cornelia Vanderstaay Kenner, R.N., M.D.

Internal Medicine Residency Program
University of Illinois
Urbana, Illinois

J. B. Lippincott Company   *Philadelphia*
New York   London   Hagerstown

Sponsoring Editor: *David Carroll*
Coordinating Editorial Assistant: *Amy Stonehouse*
Project Editor: *Dina K. Rubin*
Indexer: *Sandi Schroeder*
Designer: *Holly Reid McLaughlin*
Design Coordinator: *Doug Smock*
Cover: *Patti Maddaloni*
Production Manager: *Caren Erlichman*
Production Coordinator: *William F. Hallman*
Compositor: *Tapsco, Incorporated*
Printer/Binder: *Courier Book Company/Westford*

3rd Edition

6   5   4   3   2   1

Library of Congress Cataloging in Publications Data

Dossey, Barbara Montgomery.
    Critical care nursing: body-mind-spirit/Barbara Montgomery
Dossey, Cathie E. Guzzetta, Cornelia Vanderstaay Kenner.—3rd ed.
    p. cm.
    Kenner's name appears first on the second edition.
    Includes bibliographical references and index.
    ISBN 0-397-54871-0
    1. Intensive care nursing.   2. Holistic medicine.   3. Mind and
body.   I. Guzzetta, Cathie E.   II. Kenner, Cornelia Vanderstaay.
III. Title.
    [DNLM: 1. Critical Care—nurses' instruction.   2. Holistic
Health—nurses' instruction.   WY 154 L34c]
    RT120.I5K46   1992
    610.73'61—dc20
    DNLM/DLC
    for Library of Congress   91-18392
                                                                  CIP

Any procedure or practice described in this book should be applied
by the health-care practitioner under appropriate supervision in accordance with professional standards of care used with regard to the
unique circumstances that apply in each practice situation. Care has
been taken to confirm the accuracy of information presented and to
describe generally accepted practices. However, the authors, editors,
and publisher cannot accept any responsibility for errors or omissions
or for any consequences from application of the information in this
book and make no warranty, express or implied, with respect to the
contents of the book.

Every effort has been made to ensure drug selections and dosages are
in accordance with current recommendations and practice. Because
of ongoing research, changes in government regulations and the constant flow of information on drug therapy, reactions and interactions,
the reader is cautioned to check the package insert for each drug for
indications, dosages, warnings and precautions, particularly if the drug
is new or infrequently used.

To our critical care nursing colleagues
    Who are exploring new meanings of healing in their work
    Who are facilitating healing in their own lives and at the bedside
    Who are becoming nurse healers

Contributors

Carolyn Rea Atkins, R.N., B.S., CCTC
Director of Clinical Operations
Dallas Nephrology Associates
Dallas Transplant Institute
Dallas, Texas
CHAPTER 46

R. Jack Ayres, Jr., J.D.
Assistant Professor of Hospital Administration and
    Lecturer in Medical Jurisprudence
Southwestern Medical School
The University of Texas Health Science Center at
    Dallas
Director of Emergency Legal Assistant Program
Parkland Memorial Hospital
Dallas, Texas
CHAPTER 9

Paula Shiroma Bender, R.N., M.S.N.
Clinical Nurse Specialist/Heart Transplant
    Coordinator
Heart Center
Methodist Medical Center
Dallas, Texas
CHAPTER 46

Donald A. Bille, R.N., Ph.D.
Clinical Training Specialist
Kaiser Permanente, Mid-Atlantic States Region
Washington, D.C.
CHAPTER 11

Dora Headrick Bradley, R.N., M.S., Ph.C.
Doctoral Candidate
College of Nursing
University of South Carolina
Columbia, South Carolina
CHAPTER 8

Shelia Bunton, R.N., M.S.N.
United States Army Nurse Corps—
    Lieutenant Colonel
Clinical Headnurse
Surgical Intensive Care Unit
Tripler Army Medical Center
Honolulu, Hawaii
CHAPTER 5

Patricia E. Casey, R.N., M.S.N.
Education Coordinator, Cardiovascular Nursing
Department of Nursing Education and Research
Fairfax Hospital
Falls Church, Virginia
Clinical Educator
The Catholic University of America
Washington, D.C.
CHAPTER 24, Appendix I, Appendix II

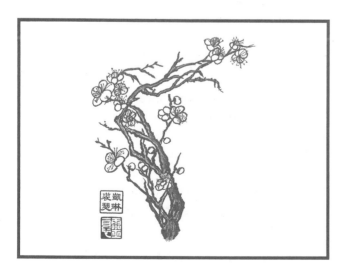

Marilyn B. Chassie, R.N., Ph.D., CNAA
Associate Dean for Academic Affairs
Associate Professor
College of Nursing
University of South Carolina
Columbia, South Carolina
CHAPTER 8

Marianne Chulay, R.N., DNSc, CCRN, FCCM
Clinical Nurse Specialist, Critical Care
Clinical Center, National Institutes of Health
Bethesda, Maryland
CHAPTER 16

Angela P. Clark, R.N., Ph.D.
Assistant Professor
School of Nursing
University of Texas, Austin
Clinical Nurse Specialist in Diabetes Care
Formerly, Clinical Nurse Specialist and Consultant to
    the Diabetes Center
St. David's Hospital
Austin, Texas
CHAPTER 37, 38

Elaine Keiss Daily, R.N., B.S.
Clinical Cardiac Research Nurse
University of California at San Diego Medical Center
San Diego, California
CHAPTER 17, 23

Barbara Montgomery Dossey, R.N., M.S.
Director, Holistic Nursing Consultants
Santa Fe, New Mexico
Director, Bodymind Systems
Temple, Texas
CHAPTER 1, 2, 3, 23, 25, 27, 32

Mary Elizabeth Egloff, R.N., M.S.N., CCRN
Pulmonary Clinical Nurse Specialist
Pulmonary Services
Sharp Memorial Hospital
San Diego, California
CHAPTER 19

James A. Fain, R.N., Ph.D.
Assistant Professor and Chairperson
Master's Program for Non-Nurse College Graduates
School of Nursing
Yale University
New Haven, Connecticut
CHAPTER 34

Loretta Forlaw, R.N., M.S.N., CNSN
United States Army Nurse Corps—
    Lieutenant Colonel
Quality Assurance Coordinator/Research Consultant
    and Nutritional Support Consultant
Fitzsimmons Army Medical Center
Aurora, Colorado
CHAPTER 35, 36

Linda C. Gary, R.N., M.N.
Clinical Nurse Specialist
Cardiovascular Critical Care Educator–
    "The Cardiology Connection"
Clifton, Texas
CHAPTER 12

Barbara Giordano, R.N., M.S.
Administrative Nursing Supervisor
J. Weiler Hospital of the Albert Einstein College of
    Medicine
New York, New York
CHAPTER 33, 45

Cathie E. Guzzetta, R.N., Ph.D., FAAN
Director
Holistic Nursing Consultants
Bethesda, Maryland
Formerly, Associate Professor and Chairperson
Cardiovascular Nursing
The Catholic University of America
Washington, D.C.
CHAPTER 1, 5, 6, 7, 12, 24, 26, 28, 39, 47

Elizabeth I. Helvig, R.N., M.S.
Burn Clinical Specialist
Harborview Medical Center
Seattle, Washington
CHAPTER 43

Carolyn D. Henson, R.N., B.S., M.A.
President
Wellness Communications, Incorporated
Editor, "RX: Live Well"
Dallas, Texas
Case Study—Ch. 47

Cornelia Vanderstaay Kenner, R.N., M.S., M.D.
Internal Medicine Residency Program
University of Illinois
Urbana, Illinois
CHAPTER 1, 15, 17, 22, 29, 30, 35, 36, 40–44

Christine Ashley Kessler, R.N., M.N., C.S.
Clinical Nurse Specialist
Critical Care
Mount Vernon Hospital
Alexandria, Virginia
CHAPTER 39

Linette Klevan, R.N., B.S.
Coordinator
Department of Electrophysiology
Sentara Norfolk General Hospital
Norfolk, Virginia
CHAPTER 13

Doris A. McGirt, R.N., M.S.N.
Cardiovascular Clinical Nurse Specialist
Representing Intermedics, Incorporated
Pacemaker Division
Angleton, Texas
CHAPTER 13, 15

Susan K. Mitchell, R.N., B.S.N., CCRN
Regional Quality Management Consultant
Aetna Health Plans
Irving, Texas
CHAPTER 30, 31

Linda A. Prinkey, R.N., M.S.N., CCRN
Cardiovascular Program Coordinator
Prince George's Hospital Center
Cheverly, Maryland
CHAPTER 14

Barbara Riegel, R.N., M.N., DNSc(C), C.S.
Clinical Nurse Researcher
Critical Care
Sharp Memorial Hospital
San Diego, California
CHAPTER 25

Lori Rippert, R.N., B.S.N., CCTC
Clinical Manager
Senior Transplant Coordinator
Baylor University
Dallas, Texas
CHAPTER 46

Sarah E. Shannon, R.N., Ph.C., CCRN
Doctoral Candidate
School of Nursing
University of Washington
Seattle, Washington
CHAPTER 10

Linda M. Sulzbach, R.N., M.S.N., CCRN
Unit-based Critical Care Clinical Nurse Specialist
Cardiac Care Unit
Hospital of the University of Pennsylvania
Philadelphia, Pennsylvania
CHAPTER 27

Miranda Toups, R.N., B.S.N.
Private Practice of Jin Shin Jyutsu and Therapeutic
  Touch
P.R.N. Charge and Staff Nurse
Oncology Unit
St. Paul Medical Center
Dallas, Texas
CHAPTER 32

Martha L. Tyler, R.N., M.N., R.R.T.
Assistant Professor, Physiological Nursing and
  Adjunct Assistant Professor, Medicine
University of Washington, Seattle
Respiratory Disease Division
Harborview Medical Center
Seattle, Washington
CHAPTER 21

Diann B. Uustal, R.N., M.S., Ed.D.
President
Educational Resources in Nursing and Wholistic
  Health
East Greenwich, Rhode Island
CHAPTER 4

Connie A. Walleck, R.N., M.S., CNRN, FCCM
Senior Associate Director of Nursing
Adjunct Assistant Professor of Nursing
University Hospital
State University of New York at Syracuse
Syracuse, New York
CHAPTER 42, 44

Kathleen M. White, R.N., M.S.
Lecturer and Consultant
Critical Care and Trauma Nursing
Mobile, Alabama
CHAPTER 22, 41

Gayle Whitman, R.N., M.S.N., CCRN
Director, Cardiothoracic Nursing
Cleveland Clinic Foundation
Cleveland, Ohio
CHAPTER 18, 26

Susan Fickertt Wilson, R.N., Ph.D.
Associate Professor
Harris College of Nursing
Texas Christian University
Fort Worth, Texas
CHAPTER 20

Rowena R. Yates, R.N., B.S.N.
Account Supervisor, Health Care Marketing Division
MDK Advertising
Los Angeles, California
CHAPTER 30, 31

Reviewers

We gratefully acknowledge the expertise, interest, and assistance of the following individuals who reviewed sections of the text.

Judy Accrocco, R.N.
Manager, Educational Services
Intermedics, Incorporated
Pacemaker Division
Angleton, Texas

Thomas Ahrens, R.N., DNSc, CCRN
Clinical Nurse Specialist
Barnes Hospital
St. Louis, Missouri

Judythe Alston, R.N.C., M.A., Ed.M.
Staff Development Instructor
Weiler/Einstein-Montifore Medical Center
Bronx, New York

Patricia E. Casey, R.N., M.S.N.
Education Coordinator, Cardiovascular Nursing
Department of Nursing Education and Research
Fairfax Hospital
Falls Church, Virginia
Clinical Educator
The Catholic University of America
Washington, D.C.

Nicholas A. Cossa, M.D.
Cardiologist
Fairfax Hospital
Falls Church, Virginia

Claire Day, R.N., B.S., CCTC
Senior Transplant Coordinator
Shands Hospital
University of Florida
Gainesville, Florida

Robert DiBianco, M.D.
Director Cardiology Research
Washington Adventist Hospital
Takoma Park, Maryland
Associate Clinical Professor of Medicine
Georgetown University
Washington, D.C.

Mildred J. Eberlin, R.N., B.S.N.
Graduate Assistant
Office of Academic Affairs
College of Nursing
University of South Carolina
Columbia, South Carolina

Barbara Elick, R.N., B.S.N., CCRN, CCTC, CPTC
Chief Transplant Coordinator
Surgery Department
University of Minnesota Transplant Center
Minneapolis, Minnesota

Christine Fletcher, R.N., M.S.
Staff Nurse, Critical Care Units
National Naval Medical Center
Bethesda, Maryland

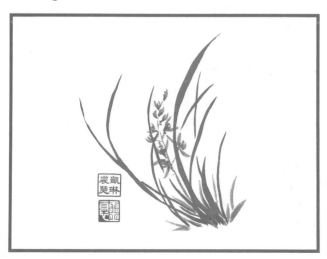

Dorrie Fontaine, R.N., DNSc
Assistant Professor, Trauma Critical Care Program
University of Maryland School of Nursing
Baltimore, Maryland

Ted D. Friehling, M.D.
Clinical Associate Professor
Georgetown University, Washington, D.C.
and Medical College of Pennsylvania
Pittsburgh, Pennsylvania

Michael Jastremski, M.D., FACEP, FCCM
Chairman, Division of Critical Care and
   Emergency Medicine
University Hospital
State University of New York at Syracuse
Syracuse, New York

Lynn Keegan, R.N., Ph.D.
Director
Bodymind Systems
Temple, Texas
Nursing Faculty
McLennan Community College
Waco, Texas

Leslie Kolkmeier, R.N., B.S., R.R.T.
Private Practice
Applied Psychophysiology and Biofeedback
Plano, Texas

Melva Kravitz, R.N., Ph.D.
Director of Nursing
Shriners Burns Institute
Galveston, Texas

Barbara J. Loveys, R.N., Ph.C.
Doctoral Candidate
School of Nursing
University of Washington
Seattle, Washington

Margaret Nield, R.N., Ph.D.
Pulmonary Clinical Nurse Researcher
Pulmonary Services
Sharp Memorial Hospital
San Diego, California

Mary Elizabeth O'Brien, R.N., Ph.D., FAAN
Director of Nursing Research
School of Nursing
The Catholic University of America
Washington, D.C.

Linda Ohler, R.N., M.S.N., CCRN
Transplant Coordinator
Fairfax Hospital
Falls Church, Virginia

Eric A. Orzeck, M.D., FACP
Private Practice
Endocrinology and Internal Medicine
Houston, Texas

Linda A. Prinkey, R.N., M.S.N., CCRN
Cardiovascular Program Coordinator
Prince George's Hospital Center
Cheverly, Maryland

Diane Sager, R.N., M.S.N.
Consultant
Cardiac Pacemakers
Olney, Maryland

Tory Schmitz, R.N., M.S.N., CCRN
Assistant Head Nurse
Medical Intensive Care Unit
Methodist Hospital
Houston, Texas

Patricia C. Seifert, R.N., M.S.N., CNOR
Operating Room Coordinator
Cardiac Surgery
The Arlington Hospital
Arlington, Virginia

Anita P. Sherer, R.N., M.S.N., CCRN
Clinical Nurse Specialist–Cardiology
The Moses H. Cone Memorial Hospital
Greensboro, North Carolina

Carol A. Stephenson, R.N., Ed.D.
Associate Professor
Harris College of Nursing
Texas Christian University
Fort Worth, Texas

Debra Tribett, R.N., M.S., CCRN
Clinical Nurse Specialist, Critical Care Nursing
Clinical Center, National Institutes of Health
Bethesda, Maryland

Mary M. Wagner, R.N., M.S.
Clinical Assistant Professor
Psychophysiological Nursing Department
College of Nursing
University of South Carolina
Columbia, South Carolina

Madeline Musante Wake, R.N., Ph.D.
Assistant Professor
College of Nursing
Marquette University
Milwaukee, Wisconsin

Arthur F. Whereat, M.D.
Associate Professor of Medicine
University of Pennsylvania School of Medicine
Philadelphia, Pennsylvania

Foreword

The third edition of *Critical Care Nursing: Body–Mind–Spirit* continues the legacy established by Dossey, Guzzetta, and Kenner and their award winning earlier editions. Not only do these authors and their expert contributors build on the solid foundation they established previously, but they expand the legacy by synthesizing the latest scientific thinking and breakthroughs in medical and nursing practice.

As we approach the 21st century, there is an inordinate amount of knowledge, technology, and attention placed on learning and practicing in acute, highly specialized critical care settings. Indeed, due to the rising acuity level of hospitalized patients, many general hospitals have become one big critical care unit. Thus, the emphasis is on nurses having to acquire, learn, and relearn how to manipulate and coordinate the latest techniques, equipment, and procedures, rather than on how to integrate technology, scientific knowledge, and clinical judgment into the caring and healing practices of nursing.

Critical Care Nursing: Body–Mind–Spirit provides the advanced knowledge that moves professional critical care nursing beyond fundamental techniques and specialized knowledge, toward a higher level: professional caring and healing processes and practices that potentiate health and healing. These dimensions of critical care nursing bring together the latest advances in technology with the latest thinking about "Era III Medicine."

These Era III advances have the potential to transform our views of body–mind–spirit wholes, and the dynamic unity of unbroken wholeness among individuals, nature, and environment. These breakthroughs include notions of an expanding human consciousness that can transcend time and space, and affect health and healing outcomes.

These authors, experts in critical care nursing, are committed to higher dimensions of nursing, caring, and healing that translate and integrate the most recent scientific data into concrete nursing actions. In doing so, they bring new meaning to the concept of body–mind–spirit interaction, while helping us to understand the "critical" nature of critical care nursing. This combination of skills enables nurses to become agents for change within the health care system. These experts demonstrate and help fill the need for an expanded scientific and moral and ethical approach to critical care nursing that truly embraces the body–mind–spirit whole of the one caring and the one being cared for.

Because critical care nursing is an intense human caring experience, nursing becomes transpersonal and even metaphysical.* When these aspects of nursing are acknowledged and incorporated into our practices, then nursing cultivates access to the intuitive, aesthetic, personal, and ethical modes of thought, feeling, and action. Thus, there can be greater use of higher self and expanded states of consciousness when engaging in the caring and healing demands of patients and families in a critical care setting.

Dossey, Guzzetta, and Kenner guide and challenge students, educators, practitioners, and researchers toward more integrative, meaningful practices:

practices that establish critical care nursing as a model for caring and healing practices;
practices that demonstrate caring and healing as special ways of knowing-doing-being; and
professional nursing practices that apply and generate nursing knowledge and theory.

Thus, these experts create new pathways whereby competencies of "being" and human caring and healing interac-

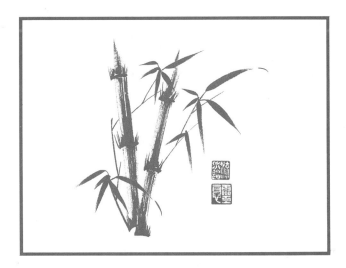

* Watson, J. Watson's Philosophy and Theory of Human Caring in Nursing. In J. Riehl-Sisca (ed.), *Conceptual Models for Nursing Practice* (3rd ed.). N.J.: Appleton and Lange, 1989.

tions are balanced with competencies of technological and scientific knowledge. The blending of the knowing-doing-being of nursing helps to reestablish the expert caring and healing practices intrinsic to nursing's moral and historical underpinnings.

Perhaps the most important aspect of this work is that it provides substance and form for the ancient caring and healing practices that can now be reclaimed and made visible in critical care nursing, the most modern and demanding setting of today and the future—practices that have relevance to all of nursing.

Jean Watson, R.N., Ph.D., FAAN
Professor of Nursing
Director, Center for Human Caring
University of Colorado Health Sciences Center
Denver, Colorado

Preface

Over the past 11 years *Critical Care Nursing: Body–Mind–Spirit* has set a standard in critical care by translating from theory into practice what is meant by the psychophysiology of body-mind healing. This book demonstrates that even in the midst of acute sickness, catastrophic illness, or death, healing can take place.

The focus of this book is on adult patients with critical illness. From this perspective, the content of this book is traditional. It presents a thorough discussion of how the body functions and what causes bodily disturbances. It addresses how nurses assess and diagnose these disturbances, and how the latest technologies, therapies, and drugs can be used to treat the dysfunctions. Simultaneously, this book examines the impact of critical illness on patients' and families' minds and spirits. It is at this point that our book departs from the traditional content of most critical care books. Throughout this edition, we integrate scientific knowledge and research that support the assertion that emotions, attitudes, and thoughts are intimately connected with human illness. Therefore, we assert that bodily illness can no longer be treated exclusively with body-oriented therapies. Thus, the central theme is that the practice of contemporary critical care nursing must combine science and holism in order to facilitate healing in patients and families as well as ourselves.

Healing is not just curing symptoms. Rather, healing is the exquisite blending of technology with caring, love, compassion,

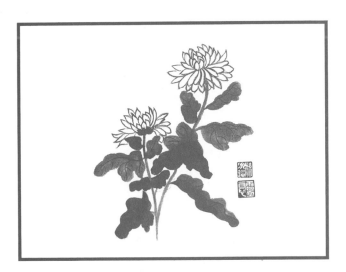

and creativity. Healing is a lifelong journey into understanding the wholeness of human existence. Along this journey, our lives mesh with those of our patients and their families where moments of new meaning and insight emerge in the midst of crisis. Healing occurs when we help patients, families, and ourselves embrace what is feared most. It occurs when we seek harmony and balance. Healing is learning how to open what has been closed so that we can expand our inner human potentials. It is the fullest expression of oneself that is demonstrated by the light and shadow and the male and the female principles that reside within each of us. It is accessing what we have forgotten about connections, unity, and interdependence. With a new awareness of these interrelationships, healing becomes possible.

In the third edition of this book we have translated healing into action—or the *knowing-doing-being* of healing. We challenge critical care nurses to undertake their own translation of healing by asking three significant questions:

What do you *know* about the meaning of healing?
What can you *do* each day to facilitate healing in yourself and at the bedside?
How can you *be* a nurse healer?

Unit I deals with the knowing-doing-being of healing. It presents concepts of psychophysiologic unity and provides the framework and philosophy of the text. It explains the relationships among body–mind–spirit and assists readers in understanding these crucial concepts. This unit translates what you need to *know* in understanding the meaning of healing. Because the healer must simultaneously undergo healing, the chapter on holistic caring for the caregiver explores, guides, and translates into action what you might *do* each day to facilitate healing in yourself and others. In order to heal and be healed, the chapters on body–mind–spirit, psychophysiology of bodymind healing, and psychophysiologic self-regulation interventions were developed to address how you can *be* a nurse healer.

Because the framework for understanding the rest of the book is contained in Unit I, we recommend that it be read first. The knowing-doing-being of healing is integrated throughout the book and developed in the Visions of Healing, which introduce each chapter, as well as in the Reflections which accompany each case study. This information transforms the theoretical notions of healing into understandable nursing actions.

Unit II builds on the foundation presented in Unit I. The threads of psychophysiologic unity are integrated in the chapters on nursing assessment and nursing diagnosis. A prototype critical care assessment tool, based on the nine human response patterns of the North American Nursing Diagnosis Association's Taxonomy I, is presented to enhance the identification of nursing diagnoses in practice. The current status and use of nursing diagnoses also are presented. The conflicts plaguing nursing diagnoses in critical care are addressed clearly. The chapter on research in critical care delineates how to implement research at the bedside and enhance the role of critical care nurses as researchers. The psychosocial assessment and intervention chapter provides the knowledge base for assessing and treating the psychologic sequelae of illness experienced by most critically ill patients. Within this unit, crucial legal issues of daily bedside critical care practice also are addressed. The chapter on ethics presents a fresh and unique approach because it introduces a nursing ethic of bedside practice rather than the traditional ethics of the biomedical model. Practical approaches to patient and family teaching also are developed to enhance clinical teaching skills when time is short and acuity is high.

Due to the increased technologic advances in critical care, Unit III is new to this edition. It explores current developments in critical care technology, cardiac monitoring and dysrhythmias, electrical safety, pacemakers and the automatic implantable cardioverter-defibrillators, cardioversion and defibrillation, airway and ventilatory management, hemodynamic monitoring, and mechanical assistance for patients with a failing heart. The latest information is provided to update your critical care knowledge base.

Units IV through IX concentrate on the nursing care of patients with specific dysfunctions including respiratory, cardiovascular, neurologic, renal and gastrointestinal, metabolic, and trauma problems. Unit X also is new to this edition. It discusses the selected problems of patients with immunosuppression, transplantation, and near-death experiences. The book concludes with two appendices that outline cardiopulmonary resuscitation procedures and drugs used for advanced cardiac life support. An outstanding feature of this book is the numerous chapters that have been written by well-known experts in the field.

The organization of the chapters is intended to be flexible and vary according to the learners' needs. Each chapter begins with learning objectives that can be used to guide informal or formal teaching and to gauge the learners' progress. A patient case study is presented within each clinical chapter in Units IV through X. Case studies can be read before proceeding with the chapter to obtain the overall picture of the problem, or as a review and summary after finishing the chapter. They also can be used as a teaching tool in clinical conferences.

Each clinical chapter in Units IV through X begins with a thorough discussion of normal physiology, as well as the etiology and pathophysiology of the dysfunction. The remainder of the chapter is devoted to the nursing process. The nursing framework is integrated more distinctly in this edition. The assessment section of each clinical chapter builds on the assessment chapter presented at the beginning of each unit. Nursing diagnoses, a fundamental component of clinical patient care, are presented based on the nine human response patterns of Taxonomy I. Each clinical chapter also has a new section called the Nursing Care Plan Summary which incorporates nursing diagnoses, patient outcomes, and nursing orders, and is followed by a discussion of implementation and evaluation of care. The clinical chapters conclude with suggested research questions to stimulate thinking and encourage future research.

We believe that *Critical Care Nursing: Body–Mind–Spirit* continues its dynamic exploration of the psychophysiology of body–mind–spirit healing and provides a rich traditional and nontraditional source of advanced knowledge for critical care nurses. Our book is intended for all students, practitioners, educators, and researchers who are interested in updating and expanding their critical care knowledge within a holistic or body–mind–spirit framework. As we continue to combine scientific discovery with visions of healing, we will arm ourselves with the supplemental forces to counter indifference, depersonalization, and inhumanity. We will chart a new course for the 21st century, as we unleash our power to heal and be healed, that is certain to change the knowing-doing-being of nursing.

Barbara Montgomery Dossey, R.N., M.S.
Cathie E. Guzzetta, R.N., Ph.D., FAAN
Cornelia Vanderstaay Kenner, R.N., M.S., M.D.

Acknowledgments

To our current contributors; to Pam Davis and Kim Tierney, who have shared their healing stories; to Ann West, Nursing Editor, second edition; and those involved in the second edition, specifically Carolyn Bascom Bilodeau, Diane T. Ender, Patricia M. Faulhaber, Cindy Festge, Mary Jordheim Gokey, Anna Belle Kinney, Martha Dowling Reiman, and Yvonne Wagner, who have documented their expertise and wisdom in order to advance the art and science of critical care nursing.

To David P. Carroll, Senior Nursing Editor, J.B. Lippincott, for sharing with us his magnificent insights and visions of critical care nursing and for his intuitive understanding of what is meant by healing and being a nurse healer.

To our families—Larry Dossey; Philip, Angela, and P.C. Guzzetta; and Paul, Andrew, and John Kenner—who, through their love, caring, and patience, are a part of the healing unity and relatedness that this book is all about.

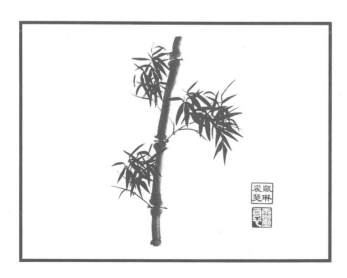

Contents

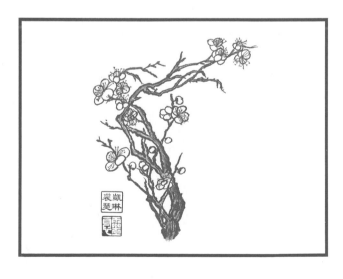

Unit III
Technology in Critical Care Nursing   155

Unit V

The Critically Ill Adult With Cardiovascular Problems 387

Unit VIII

The Critically Ill Adult With Metabolic Problems   653

Unit X
The Critically Ill Adult With Selected Problems   877

Contents
Visions of Healing

Guide to Nursing Diagnoses

The following nursing diagnoses and related factors (or risk factors) are discussed throughout the book. This guide is organized according to the nine response patterns of NANDA's Taxonomy I. Nursing diagnoses approved by NANDA are in blue. Diagnoses not yet approved by NANDA are in black. Nurses who find these non-approved critical care nursing diagnoses useful in their practice should consider submitting them to NANDA for approval.

PATTERN 1: EXCHANGING

Altered Nutrition: Less Than Body Requirements

- (Discussion, Chap. 36, Altered Nutrition, p. 674)
- Related to inadequate intake secondary to hypoxia and fatigue (Chap. 20, Adult Respiratory Distress Syndrome, p. 322)
- Related to catabolic response to injury (Chap. 30, Head Injury. p. 577)
- Related to catabolic response to injury (Chap. 31, Cerebral Vascular Disease, p. 602)
- Related to uremic syndrome (Chap. 33, Acute Renal Failure, p. 633)
- Related to inadequate dietary intake and impaired pancreatic secretions (Chap. 34, Gastrointestinal Disorders, p. 649)
- Related to decreased intake or increased nutrient requirements (Chap. 35, Metabolic Assessment, p. 656)

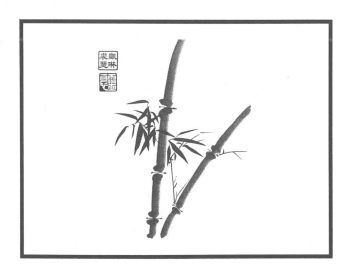

- Related to anorexia, malabsorption, or hypermetabolism (Chap. 36, Altered Nutrition, p. 682)
- Related to increased gastric motility, protein catabolism, and hypermetabolism of tissues (Chap. 39, Thyroid Crisis, p. 731)
- Related to the metabolic response after burn injury (Chap. 43, Burn Injury, p. 832)

High Risk for Infection

- Related to invasive monitoring (Chap. 17, Hemodynamic Monitoring, p. 248 and Table 17–9)
- Related to catheter insertion site, invasive lines, procedures, and possible debilitated state (for patient on the intra-aortic balloon pump) (Chap. 18, Mechanical Assistance for the Patient With a Failing Heart, p. 267)
- Related to ventricular assist device insertion, presence of multiple invasive lines, and debilitated state (Chap. 18, Mechanical Assistance for the Patient With a Failing Heart, p. 276)
- Related to total artificial heart insertion, immobility, presence of multiple invasive lines, and debilitated state (Chap. 18, Mechanical Assistance for the Patient With a Failing Heart, p. 283)
- Related to decreased pulmonary function, possible steroid therapy, and ineffective airway clearance (Chap. 20, Adult Respiratory Distress Syndrome, p. 321)
- Related to invasive lines, surgical incisions, immunologic derangements, or inadequate preoperative nutritional status: postoperative period (Chap. 26, Cardiac Surgery, p. 492)
- Related to (include name of organism responsible for cardiac valve infection) (Chap. 28, Infective Endocarditis, p. 524)
- Related to intravenous therapy (Chap. 28, Infective Endocarditis, p. 529)
- Related to invasive procedures or meningitis (Chap. 31, Cerebral Vascular Disease, p. 602)
- Related to destruction of tissue and altered host defense mechanism (Chap. 43, Burn Injury, p. 832)
- Related to immunosuppression and invasion of microorganisms (Chap. 44, Multisystem Organ Failure, p. 868)

Hypothermia

- Related to liver dysfunction, exposure of the bowel to low ambient temperature in the operating room, or a hypother-

Fluid Volume Deficit

- (Discussion, Chap. 35, Metabolic Assessment, p. 660)
- Related to third-space loss during shock and incomplete replacement of isotonic fluid and blood loss (Chap. 22, Chest Trauma, p. 354)
- Related to bleeding due to anticoagulation and thrombolytic therapy (Chap. 23, Pulmonary Embolism, p. 376)
- Related to vomiting, decreased fluid intake, fever, and diaphoresis (Chap. 34, Gastrointestinal Disorders, p. 648)
- Related to inadequate delivery of fluid, patient's inability to report thirst, or excessive fluid losses (Chap. 35, Metabolic Assessment, p. 661)
- Related to osmotic diuresis (Chap. 37, Diabetic Ketoacidosis, p. 700)
- Related to diaphoresis, vomiting, diarrhea, or gastric suctioning (Chap. 39, Thyroid Crisis, p. 732)
- Related to injury and loss of blood (Chap. 41, Abdominal Trauma, p. 778)
- Related to injury and loss of blood (Chap. 42, Extremity Trauma, p. 799)
- Related to the combination of uremic osmotic diuresis and a newly functioning transplanted kidney (for renal transplantation patients) (Chap. 46, Transplantation, p. 951)

Altered Fluid and Electrolyte Balance

- (Discussion, Chap. 35, Metabolic Assessment, p. 660)
- Related to closed head injury (Chap. 30, Head Injury, p. 577)
- Related to cerebrovascular insults (Chap. 31, Cerebral Vascular Disease, p. 600)
- Related to renal dysfunction and massive muscle destruction (Chap. 33, Acute Renal Failure, p. 633)
- Related to altered tissue perfusion and sepsis (Chap. 44, Multisystem Organ Failure, p. 863)
- Related to end-stage renal failure (for renal transplantation patients) (Chap. 46, Transplantation, p. 950)

Altered Electrolyte Balance

- (Discussion, Chap. 35, Metabolic Assessment, p. 660)
- Related to insufficient or excessive delivery of specific electrolyte or insufficient or excessive delivery of free water, or renal failure (hyponatremia, hypernatremia, hypokalemia, hyperkalemia) (Chap. 35, Metabolic Assessment, p. 662)
- Related to osmotic diuresis (Chap. 37, Diabetic Ketoacidosis, p. 700)
- Related to hypernatremia and hypokalemia (Chap. 38, Hyperosmolar Coma, p. 712)
- Related to vomiting, diarrhea, nasogastric suctioning, and bone demineralization (Chap. 39, Thyroid Crisis, p. 732)

Altered Mineral Balance

- (Discussion, Chap. 35, Metabolic Assessment, p. 660)
- Related to excessive or inadequate delivery of minerals or renal failure or specific etiology (hypocalcemia, hypercalcemia, hypomagnesemia, hypermagnesemia, hypophosphatemia) (Chap. 35, Metabolic Assessment, p. 664)

Altered Metabolic Processes

- (Discussion, Chap. 35, Metabolic Assessment, p. 655)
- Related to inadequate nutrient intake or altered biochemical activity (hyperglycemia, hypoglycemia), hyperosmolar nonketotic dehydration, essential fatty acid deficiency, or excessive intravenous fat emulsion (Chap. 35, Metabolic Assessment, p. 656)
- Related to insufficient insulin to meet metabolic needs (hyperglycemia) (Chap. 37, Diabetic Ketoacidosis, p. 699)
- Related to decreased use of glucose (hyperglycemia) (Chap. 38, Hyperosmolar Coma, p. 712)

Altered Acid-Base Balance

- (Discussion, Chap. 35, Metabolic Assessment, p. 665)
- Related to excessive metabolic acids or renal failure (metabolic acidosis) (Chap. 35, Metabolic Assessment, p. 669)
- Related to hypokalemia, vomiting, or diuretic effect (metabolic alkalosis) (Chap. 35, Metabolic Assessment, p. 669)
- Related to retention of carbon dioxide (respiratory acidosis) (Chap. 35, Metabolic Assessment, p. 670)
- Related to increased excretion of carbon dioxide (respiratory alkalosis) (Chap. 35, Metabolic Assessment, p. 670)
- Related to acidic metabolic byproducts (Chap. 37, Diabetic Ketoacidosis, p. 701)

High Risk for Complications of Diabetic Ketoacidosis

- Related to other body systems (Chap. 37, Diabetic Ketoacidosis, p. 701)

High Risk for Complications of Hyperosmolar Coma

- Related to other body systems and age (Chap. 38, Hyperosmolar Coma, p. 714)

Acute Hyperosmolality

- Related to hyperglycemia and hypernatremia (Chap. 38, Hyperosmolar Coma, p. 711)

Decreased Cardiac Output

- (Discussion, Chap. 17, Hemodynamic Monitoring, p. 236)
- Related to left ventricular failure (for the patient on the intra-aortic balloon pump) (Chap. 18, Mechanical Assistance for the Patient With a Failing Heart, p. 268)
- Related to ventricular failure (for the patient with a ventricular assist device) (Chap. 18, Mechanical Assistance for the Patient With a Failing Heart, p. 277)
- Related to mechanical dysfunction (for a patient with a total artificial heart) (Chap. 18, Mechanical Assistance for the Patient With a Failing Heart, p. 282)
- Related to myocardial compromise (Chap. 22, Chest Trauma, p. 355)
- Related to increased pulmonary vascular resistance due to embolism, tachycardia, and dysrhythmias (Chap. 23, Pulmonary Embolism, p. 375)
- Related to recurrent pulmonary embolism (Chap. 23, Pulmonary Embolism, p. 376)

- Related to electrical factors (dysrhythmias), mechanical factors (preload, afterload, inotropic factors), and structural factors (papillary muscle dysfunction or tear and aneurysm) (Chap. 25, Acute Myocardial Infarction, p. 426)
- Related to vasoconstriction: postoperative period (Chap. 26, Cardiac Surgery, p. 470)
- Related to a decrease in mechanical factors (contractility from myocardial depression): postoperative period (Chap. 26, Cardiac Surgery, p. 473)
- Related to mechanical factors (cardiac tamponade): postoperative period (Chap. 26, Cardiac Surgery, p. 476)
- Related to electrical factors (dysrhythmias): postoperative period (Chap. 26, Cardiac Surgery, p. 478)
- Related to inappropriate volume status: postoperative period (Chap. 26, Cardiac Surgery, p. 481)
- Related to fluid in pericardial sac from pericardial effusion (or high risk for cardiac tamponade related to pericardial effusion) (Chap. 27, Acute Pericarditis, p. 511)
- Related to complications of infected heart valve (Chap. 28, Infective Endocarditis, p. 528)
- Related to hemorrhage, shock, or traumatic conditions (Chap. 40, Trauma Assessment, p. 746)
- Related to blood loss and hemorrhagic shock (Chap. 41, Abdominal Trauma, p. 777)
- Related to shock and blood loss (Chap. 42, Extremity Trauma, p. 799)
- Related to fluid changes and shock syndrome (Chap. 43, Burn Injury, p. 829)
- Related to mechanical factors (impaired myocardial contractility, increased preload, increased afterload) and electrical factors (dysrhythmias) (for pretransplant cardiac transplantation patients) (Chap. 46, Transplantation, p. 953)

Altered Cardiac Output

- Related to hypermetabolic responses that may result in low blood pressure, heart failure, and dysrhythmias (Chap. 39, Thyroid Crisis, p. 727)

Impaired Gas Exchange

- (Discussion, Chap. 16, Airway and Ventilatory Management, p. 226 and Chap. 19, Respiratory Assessment, p. 305)
- Related to atelectasis, anesthesia, and ventilation-perfusion mismatch (for the patient with a ventricular assist device) (Chap. 18, Mechanical Assistance for the Patient With a Failing Heart, p. 279)
- Related to alveolar-capillary membrane changes (from ARDS or fat emboli from fractures) (Chap. 20, Adult Respiratory Distress Syndrome, p. 320)
- Related to hypoventilation or absence of ventilation (hypoxemia) (Chap. 21, Chronic Obstructive Lung Disease, p. 331)
- Related to ventilation-perfusion mismatch or intrapulmonary shunt (hypoxemia) (Chap. 21, Chronic Obstructive Lung Disease, p. 332)
- Related to hemopneumothorax (Chap. 22, Chest Trauma, p. 355)
- Related to ventilation-perfusion mismatch or pulmonary edema as a result of pulmonary embolus (Chap. 23, Pulmonary Embolism, p. 375)
- Related to anesthesia and sedation, volume overloading, hemothorax/pneumothorax, or noncardiac permeability edema: postoperative period (Chap. 26, Cardiac Surgery, p. 485)
- Related to altered respiratory drive and cerebral dysfunction (Chap. 30, Head Injury, p. 574)
- Related to decreased level of consciousness and/or immobility (Chap. 31, Cerebral Vascular Disease, p. 600)
- Related to obstructed airway (Chap. 40, Trauma Assessment, p. 746)
- Related to atelectasis (Chap. 41, Abdominal Trauma, p. 780)
- Related to fat embolism (Chap. 42, Extremity Trauma, p. 804)
- Related to carbon monoxide poisoning, upper airway obstruction, or smoke inhalation (Chap. 43, Burn Injury, p. 830)
- Related to altered circulatory volume, pulmonary interstitial edema, atelectasis, and decreased lung compliance (Chap. 44, Multisystem Organ Failure, p. 860)

Ineffective Airway Clearance

- (Discussion, Chap. 16, Airway and Ventilatory Management, p. 220)
- Related to pulmonary and interstitial edema (Chap. 20, Adult Respiratory Distress Syndrome, p. 321)
- Related to retained secretions (Chap. 22, Chest Trauma, p. 358)

Ineffective Breathing Pattern

- (Discussion, Chap. 19, Respiratory Assessment, p. 300)
- Related to decreased compliance (Chap. 20, Adult Respiratory Distress Syndrome, p. 320)
- Related to pulmonary contusions (Chap. 22, Chest Trauma, p. 357)
- Related to abdominal pain with guarding and retroperitoneal inflammation (Chap. 34, Gastrointestinal Disorders, p. 649)
- Related to anesthesia-induced neuromuscular impairment (for organ transplantation patients) (Chap. 46, Transplantation, p. 948)

High Risk for Complications of Artificial Airways

- Related to artificial airway movement, altered cuff pressure, and infection (Chap. 16, Airway and Ventilatory Management, p. 222)

High Risk for Complications Associated With Mechanical Ventilation

- Related to altered ventilator settings or altered physiology (Chap. 16, Airway and Ventilatory Management, p. 226)

High Risk for Injury

- Related to hemorrhage, thromboemboli, venous air embolism, pulmonary infarction or hemorrhage, cardiac dysrhythmias, or conduction disturbances (Chap. 17, Hemodynamic Monitoring, p. 248)
- Related to excessive hemorrhage (for the patient with a ventricular assist device) (Chap. 18, Mechanical Assistance for the Patient With a Failing Heart, p. 276)

- Related to hemorrhage (for a patient with a total artificial heart) (Chap. 18, Mechanical Assistance for the Patient With a Failing Heart, p. 282)
- Related to traumatic fracture of the cervical vertebra and cervical traction (Chap. 30, Head Injury, p. 579)
- Related to rebleeding and additional episodes of cerebral vascular disease (Chap. 31, Cerebral Vascular Disease, p. 598)
- Related to fatigue, tremors, osteoporosis, and exophthalmus (Chap. 39, Thyroid Crisis, p. 730)
- Related to forces exerted during hyperflexion, hyperextension, or compression injury (cervical spinal fracture) (Chap. 40, Trauma Assessment, p. 748)
- Related to coagulopathy (Chap. 44, Multisystem Organ Failure, p. 865)

High Risk for Vascular Injury

- Related to intra-ortic balloon catheter trauma (for the patient on the intra-aortic balloon pump) (Chap. 18, Mechanical Assistance for the Patient With a Failing Heart, p. 266)

High Risk for Development of Postpericardiotomy Syndrome

- Related to trauma or residual blood in the pericardial sac: postoperative period (Chap. 26, Cardiac Surgery, p. 493)

Altered Protection

- Related to immunosuppressed state (and development of opportunistic infection) (Chap. 45, Immunosuppressed Patients, p. 899)
- Related to organ failure preoperatively and immunosuppressive medications or therapy postoperatively (for organ transplantation patients) (Chap. 46, Transplantation, p. 946)

Impaired Skin Integrity

- Related to traction and immobilization after extremity trauma (Chap. 42, Extremity Trauma, p. 801)
- Related to burn trauma and the open wound (Chap. 43, Burn Injury, p. 835)
- Related to disease process and neutropenia (Chap. 45, Immunosuppressed Patients, p. 898)

PATTERN 2: COMMUNICATING

Impaired Verbal Communication

- Related to intubation, depressed cerebration, or loss of physical strength coupled with fear and anxiety (Chap. 8, Psychosocial Assessment, p. 115 and Chap. 16, Airway and Ventilatory Management, p. 222)

PATTERN 3: RELATING

Altered Role Performance

- (Discussion, Chap. 8, Psychosocial Assessment, p. 102)

Altered Sexuality Patterns (Sexual Aggressiveness)

- Related to maladaptation to psychologic stress (Chap. 8, Psychosocial Assessment, p. 114)

PATTERN 4: VALUING

Spiritual Distress (Distress of the Human Spirit)

- (Discussion, Chap. 1, Body-Mind-Spirit, p. 11 and Tables 1–1 to 1–4)

PATTERN 5: CHOOSING

Ineffective Individual Coping

- Related to feelings of a depressive nature or acute illness (Chap. 8, Psychosocial Assessment, p. 112)
- Related to unanticipated need for ventricular assist device (Chap. 18, Mechanical Assistance for the Patient With a Failing Heart, p. 279)
- Related to total artificial heart implantation (Chap. 18, Mechanical Assistance for the Patient With a Failing Heart, p. 284)
- Related to deficit and possible alterations in life-style (Chap. 31, Cerebral Vascular Disease, p. 603)
- Related to excessive anxiety and decompensation of interpersonal relationships (Chap. 39, Thyroid Crisis, p. 730)
- Related to acute illness and critical care unit (Chap. 41, Abdominal Trauma, p. 785 and Chap. 44, Multisystem Organ Failure, p. 870)
- Related to fear and anxiety (Chap. 43, Burn Injury, p. 834)
- Related to forced dependency, immobility, and social isolation (Chap. 45, Immunosuppressed Patients, p. 900)
- Related to possible cancellation of surgery due to abnormal laboratory or physical findings (for preoperative organ transplantation patients) (Chap. 46, Transplantation, p. 947)
- Related to stress (rejection episodes, isolation from family) or adverse effects of medical therapy (for postoperative organ transplantation patients) (Chap. 46, Transplantation, p. 948)
- Related to near-death experience (or potential for enhanced adaptive/effective coping) (Chap. 47, Near-Death Experiences, p. 966)

Ineffective Denial

- Related to inability to cope with fear and anxiety (Chap. 8, Psychosocial Assessment, p. 109)

Ineffective Family Coping: Compromised

- Related to feelings of a depressive nature or acute illness (Chap. 8, Psychosocial Assessment, p. 112 and Table 8-1)
- Related to unanticipated need for patient's ventricular assist device (Chap. 18, Mechanical Assistance for the Patient With a Failing Heart, p. 279)
- Related to patient's total artificial heart implantation (Chap. 18, Mechanical Assistance for the Patient With a Failing Heart, p. 284)
- Related to deficit and possible alterations in life-style (Chap. 31, Cerebral Vascular Disease, p. 603)

- Related to acute illness and critical care unit (Chap. 41, Abdominal Trauma, p. 785)
- Related to ineffective communication patterns between them and those involved in the patient care delivery system (for organ transplantation patients) (Chap. 46, Transplantation, p. 949)

High Risk for Noncompliance

- Related to inadequate knowledge about illness and future care (Chap. 27, Acute Pericarditis, p. 512)
- Related to inadequate knowledge of illness and future prophylactic care (Chap. 28, Infective Endocarditis, p. 531)
- Related to inadequate knowledge of acute illness (Chap. 33, Acute Renal Failure, p. 634)
- Related to lack of knowledge of follow-up care (for organ transplantation patients) (Chap. 46, Transplantation, p. 949)

PATTERN 6: MOVING

Impaired Physical Mobility

- Related to ventricular assist device and severity of illness (Chap. 18, Mechanical Assistance for the Patient With a Failing Heart, p. 279)
- Related to total artificial heart device and severity of illness (Chap. 18, Mechanical Assistance for the Patient With a Failing Heart, p. 284)
- Related to chest injury (Chap. 22, Chest Trauma, p. 359)
- Related to cerebral insult and alterations in lifestyle (Chap. 31, Cerebral Vascular Disease, p. 599)
- Related to extremity trauma and fracture (Chap. 42, Extremity Trauma, p. 802)
- Related to burn wound edema, pain, and contracture formation (Chap. 43, Burn Injury, p. 838)

Activity Intolerance

- Related to myocardial ischemia, illness, and physical deconditioning from bed rest (Chap. 25, Acute Myocardial Infarction, p. 432)
- Related to end-stage cardiomyopathy (for pretransplant cardiac transplantation patients) (Chap. 46, Transplantation, p. 954)

Altered Activities of Daily Living

- Related to acute renal failure processes (Chap. 33, Acute Renal Failure, p. 634)

Sleep Pattern Disturbance

- Related to invasive monitoring procedures (Chap. 17, Hemodynamic Monitoring, p. 250)
- Related to multi-environmental stimuli and acute care environment (Chap. 44, Multisystem Organ Failure, p. 867)

Self-Care Deficit

- Related to dyspnea and hypoxemia (Chap. 21, Chronic Obstructive Lung Disease, p. 333)

PATTERN 7: PERCEIVING

Self-Esteem Disturbance

- Related to maladaptation to psychologic stress (manifested by sexual aggressiveness) (Chap. 8, Psychosocial Assessment, p. 114)
- Related to cardiac transplantation (Chap. 46, Transplantation, p. 955)

Sensory/Perceptual Alterations

- Related to decreased level of consciousness (Chap. 8, Psychosocial Assessment, p. 114)
- Related to interrupted sleep/rest cycles and sensory deprivation (auditory and visual, for the patient on the intra-aortic balloon pump) (Chap. 18, Mechanical Assistance for the Patient With a Failing Heart, p. 269)
- Related to confinement in a small area with inadequate stimulation (Chap. 22, Chest Trauma, p. 359)
- Related to closed head injury (Chap. 30, Head Injury, p. 578)

Hopelessness

- Related to perceived change in quality of life and impending death (Chap. 8, Psychosocial Assessment, p. 118)

Powerlessness

- Related to chronicity (for pretransplant cardiac transplantation patients) (Chap. 46, Transplantation, p. 954)

PATTERN 8: KNOWING

Knowledge Deficit

- Related to follow-up and home care (Chap. 20, Adult Respiratory Distress Syndrome, p. 322)
- Related to limited understanding of therapy (Chap. 22, Chest Trauma, p. 359)
- Related to long-term anticoagulation therapy for prevention of recurrent pulmonary embolism (Chap. 23, Pulmonary Embolism, p. 377)
- Related to acute or chronic illness (Chap. 25, Acute Myocardial Infarction, p. 433)
- Related to impending surgery and inadequate knowledge of preoperative and postoperative management: preoperative period (Chap. 26, Cardiac Surgery, p. 460)
- Related to the immediate rehabilitation period: postoperative period (Chap. 26, Cardiac Surgery, p. 494)
- Related to prevention of further episodes of diabetic ketoacidosis and to health maintenance (Chap. 37, Diabetic Ketoacidosis, p. 702)
- Related to acute onset of illness (regarding hyperosmolar coma, dehydration, and prevention) (Chap. 38, Hyperosmolar Coma, p. 713)
- Related to insufficient knowledge about thyroid illness (Chap. 39, Thyroid Crisis, p. 733)
- Related to immunosuppressive medications, rejection, and rejection therapy (for organ transplantation patients) (Chap. 46, Transplantation, p. 945)
- Related to cardiac transplantation and associated implications for post-transplant health maintenance (Chap. 46, Transplantation, p. 954)

Altered Thought Processes

- Related to cerebral dysfunction (Chap. 30, Head Injury, p. 578)
- Related to hyperosmolality (Chap. 38, Hyperosmolar Coma, p. 712)

PATTERN 9: FEELING

Pain (Altered Comfort)

- Related to chest trauma (Chap. 22, Chest Trauma, p. 358)
- Related to inadequate myocardial tissue perfusion, inflammation, or irritation (Chap. 25, Acute Myocardial Infarction, p. 426)
- Related to pericardial inflammation (Chap. 27, Acute Pericarditis, p. 510)
- Related to inflamed pancreas (Chap. 34, Gastrointestinal Disorders, p. 648)
- Related to trauma (Chap. 41, Abdominal Trauma, p. 781)
- Related to anxiety and extremity trauma (Chap. 42, Extremity Trauma, p. 803)
- Related to burn injury and anxiety (Chap. 43, Burn Injury, p. 830)
- Related to genital herpes (Chap. 45, Immunosuppressed Patients, p. 898)

Anticipatory Grieving

- Related to the terminal nature of the patient's critical illness (Chap. 8, Psychosocial Assessment, p. 116)

High Risk for Violence: Self-Directed

- Related to act of suicidal ideation or aggressive suicidal behaviors (Chap. 8, Psychosocial Assessment, p. 117)

Anxiety

- (Discussion, Chap. 3, Psychophysiologic Self-Regulation Interventions for relaxation, imagery, and music, p. 34)
- Related to acute illness, life threatening illness, and unknown resolution of illness (Chap. 8, Psychosocial Assessment, p. 111)
- Related to fear of technologic equipment and procedures associated with hemodynamic monitoring (Chap. 17, Hemodynamic Monitoring, p. 250)
- Related to difficulty in breathing and possibility of dying (Chap. 22, Chest Trauma, p. 359)
- Related to CCU regimen, acute illness, or fear of death (Chap. 25, Acute Myocardial Infarction, p. 431)
- Related to lack of knowledge of disease process or to chest-wall pain (Chap. 27, Acute Pericarditis, p. 511)
- Related to diagnostic testing, acute illness, and prolonged treatment (Chap. 28, Infective Endocarditis, p. 531)
- Related to the threat of further neurologic damage (Chap. 30, Head Injury, p. 579)
- Related to length of time in unit and continuing unknown prognosis (Chap. 41, Abdominal Trauma, p. 784)
- Related to hospitalization and upcoming surgery (for organ transplantation patients) (Chap. 46, Transplantation, p. 944)

Fear

- Related to suffocation, being on mechanical ventilation, uncertainty of prognosis, and inability to verbally communicate (Chap. 20, Adult Respiratory Distress Syndrome, p. 322)

Critical Care Nursing
Body–Mind–Spirit

I

Concepts of Psychobiologic Unity

NURSE-PATIENT INTERACTIONS

For the critical care nurse to know and feel that patient experiences are *always*, in some measure, nurse experiences is to also understand the opposite: nurse experiences are always patient experiences.

When this is keenly felt, critical care nurses know that they can transmit more to the patient than mere drugs and bed baths.

Words, glances, and touches become powerful tools of therapy. The nurse-patient interaction is never a neutral event.

As we live, we are transmitters of life.
And when we fail to transmit life, life fails to flow through us.

And if, as we work, we can transmit life into our work, life, still more life, rushes into us to compensate, to be ready and we ripple with life through the days.

Give, and it shall be given unto you
Is still the truth about life.
But giving life is not so easy.
It doesn't mean handing it out to some mean fool, or letting the living dead eat you up.
It means kindling the life-quality where it was not, even if it's only in the whiteness of a
washed pocket-handkerchief.

D. H. Lawrence
"We Are Transmitters"

1

Body—Mind—Spirit

Barbara Montgomery Dossey   *Cathie E. Guzzetta*
Cornelia Vanderstaay Kenner

OUR MISSION

Body-Mind-Spirit is a bold title for any book. It is perhaps more suggestive of an essay on mysticism than a textbook on critical care nursing.

Some readers of this book may view the mixture of professionalism and concern with body, mind, and spirit as inappropriate; they may regard the introduction of these concerns as a retreat from today's scientific position to a past era of superstition, quackery, and witchcraft. To others, however, a body-mind-spirit approach to critical care nursing suggests that "at last someone feels the way I do."

Throughout this book, we hope to illuminate those concepts in a way that will prove useful to both the skeptics and the believers.

LEARNING OBJECTIVES

After reading this chapter, the nurse should be able to do the following:

1. Define psychobiologic unity.
2. Describe components of the healing process.
3. State practical steps the nurse can take to promote patient healing and patient self-healing.
4. State four ways to distinguish technique from technology.
5. List characteristics of a nurse healer.
6. Define Era I, Era II, and Era III Medicine.
7. List ten steps for helping patients experience their spirituality.
8. Discuss what is involved in developing one's inward journey.

BODY—MIND—SPIRIT

Bodymind is the simultaneous connections of body-mind-spirit. The concept of body-mind-spirit must include a proper idea of body—not as something static or unchanging but as an entity that is dynamic and everchanging. Mind, too, must be properly envisioned—not as something derivative of matter or subservient to it but as something that, although interacting with matter, has a fundamental status all its own. Spirit is a broad concept in which a person turns inward to the human traits of honesty, love, caring, wisdom, imagination, compassion, and belief systems. It may or may not involve organized religion. It is this quality of a higher authority, guiding spirit, or transcendence that is mystical and beyond defining. It frequently means experiencing the flowing, dynamic balance that allows and creates the unfolding of healing between mind and body. It is the unknown, undefined quality of human resilience. To further develop these ideas, healing is now explored.

What does healing mean? What does a healer do in healing? Is there anything that you do in a day that constitutes healing and being a healer? What is healing in the modern sense? Let us develop the root of these words and incorporate their true meaning into our daily nursing practice.

The root word of healing and healer is *hale*, which means to facilitate movement toward wholeness or to make whole on all levels—physical, mental, emotional, social, and spiritual. Healing is a lifelong journey into wholeness. It is seeking harmony and balance in one's life. It is learning to embrace what is feared most. It also involves opening what has closed, and expanding our creativity, compassion, and love. The healing journey involves remembering what has been forgotten about our connections. It is seeking and expressing our self in its fullness—the light and shadow of human experience—and learning to trust life.[1]

As sophisticated as our modern medical system is, there are

no criteria for what constitutes healing. In fact, it often seems that there are two different sets of criteria for the evaluation of healing. One set of criteria looks at "the numbers" of biologic data; the other set is more subjective and assesses the experience of the patient "feeling stronger" or "feeling better."

If we use the root word in the true sense, healing incorporates both sets of criteria. The either/or—either a body problem or an emotional problem—is a false dichotomy. There is no such thing for "bodymind" is a single integrated entity. To change body or mind is to change the other simultaneously.

What does a healer recognize about healing and interactions with others? A healer is aware of the importance of a ritual and of understanding the other person's belief system. A healer enlists the consciousness of the other person during the interaction. A healer recognizes that consciousness operates not only within a person, but it also operates between and among individuals—between nurse and patient, and among nurse, patient, family, and colleagues.

Contemporary nurses are broadening their experience of themselves as healers. By paying increased attention to their philosophy, values, and beliefs about the profession, nurses empower themselves to recognize their unique qualities. As this recognition of their unique qualities evolves, caring grows and the true philosophy and science of caring emerges in their nursing practice. Refer to Chapters 2 through 4 for details. The concepts of psychobiologic unity are developed in the following paragraphs.

PSYCHOBIOLOGIC UNITY

The suggestion that mind and body are connected should strike no one in nursing as offensive. After all, today the concept of psychosomatic disease is hardly disputed. However, what is suggested in this book goes far beyond this concept. What is suggested is that the patient is a human being who in the words of Frank, is a *psychobiologic unit.*[8] As Frank has pointed out, the Cartesian view of the human being as divisible into two parts, mind and body, has been enormously beneficial for science. It has allowed scientists to investigate the human organism impartially, without having to consider the soul.

The primary assumption guiding current technologic health care is that it is the patient's body that becomes sick (Fig. 1–1). The patient's mind may, of course, be secondarily involved, but the mind is the prime cause of disease only in rather special cases. Technologic therapies, therefore, are body-oriented. Antibiotics are administered to infected bodies, hearts are defibrillated, and appendixes are removed. These methods of therapy, compared with the methods of a century ago, are enormously successful and are rightly viewed as monumental achievements. Unfortunately, however, what is obvious to anyone who has worked in a critical care setting for any length of time is that although illnesses may be eradicated with body-oriented therapy, patients' psychological responses to disease may impair their ability to return to full health. Psychologic forces may actually interfere with healing.[8,15] Conversely, patients with positive psychologic attitudes may respond more positively than others to therapy.[11]

The interrelatedness of mind and body, the need for laughter, and the importance of positive emotions in health care are crucial.[4] (Refer to p. 905 for details of laughter). Lifesaving procedures may be administered with the person's whole being

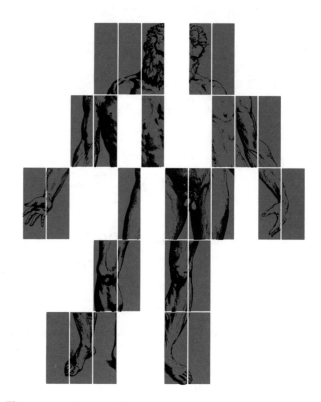

Figure 1–1

Lack of total-person concept. Separation of the person's body from his or her mind and spirit and subsequent division into a number of parts.

in mind so that panic is prevented and the fear-and-anxiety cycle broken. Often there seems to be a mind-body interaction affecting (positively or negatively) patients' responses to what is done for them in the critical care setting.

The eventual impact of this knowledge on the traditional forms of critical care therapy cannot be predicted with certainty. What is certain is that concepts of body-mind unity will continue to affect critical care therapy in ways that are even now astonishing.

CRITICAL CARE NURSING PRACTICE

Critical care nursing is the *key element* in the patient care delivery system of critical care units across the country. Nursing today is involved in every issue in critical care and in every level of the critical care unit. It is a time of renaissance, a time for looking at and evaluating current practice and making modifications and improvements. It is a time when the roles of physician and nurse are recognized as interdependent, *i.e.*, dependent on one another but separate. No longer is the nurse-physician relationship vertical; now it is seen as horizontal, as a partnership. In other words, the nurse-physician relationship is one of collaboration, both disciplines intent on the patient's welfare.[9]

Today's nurse is assuming the role of patient care coordinator. Coordination has become even more difficult with the multitude of technologic advances: monitors, transducers, infusion devices, ventilators, mechanical assist devices, and the seemingly endless number of special catheters. With this proliferation and the subsequent requirement of proficiency, it is important for the nurse to retain the focus for nursing: the patient, the whole patient, the body-mind-spirit of the patient. Swamped by machines and tubes, the patient may be lost. However, it is this patient, this individual, for whom the practice of nursing exists, and it is the coordination of this patient's care for which the nurse and, ultimately, nursing are responsible and accountable.

There is general agreement that nursing is centered on health. Regaining and maintaining health are positive goals, and nurses can help patients and their families attain them. Critical care nurses cannot provide assistance in every area of a patient's life, but they can communicate with other nurses and health team members so that the combined effort will be of even more benefit to the patient.

A focus on health and well-being means focusing on the whole person. Learning about the body-mind-spirit of the patient means that the nurse will use the nursing process in creative ways that evoke the experience of sharing. "Sharing" is not something nurses "decide" to do in caring for critically ill patients. It is not something that can stop or start at will. Sharing is something that *occurs* at a fundamental level, even though one may not be aware of the occurrence. *Even the simplest nursing act can never be a neutral event* (Fig. 1–2).

When nurses focus on the patient's body-mind-spirit, they view each patient as an individual, realizing that no one therapy will work equally well for all patients. Also, the patient becomes a participant in achieving the goal of health, a partner in the healing process. A human being is a remarkable being whose body, mind, and spirit interrelate so that self-healing occurs.

To help patients learn about themselves and not to let the situation that brought them to the critical care unit be repeated is the duty of the critical care nurse. *Rehabilitation starts on the day of admission.* Patients need help in learning to use psychophysiologic self-regulating techniques that will assist them in healing, and the critical care nurse acts as the patient's coach. It is only by using the concept of the whole person that the nurse will be able to lend support, assistance, and guidance for regaining health.

CRISIS, HEALING, AND TECHNOLOGY

Two major challenges confront the critical care nurse: combining technology with more human contact, and developing an awareness of our human potential. The outcomes will be a rehumanizing of the acute care setting and a renewal of the commitment to healing and caring as well as to curing.

Over the last 25 years, technology has proliferated at such a fast pace that it has threatened to overwhelm the healing and caring component. Critical care nurses must not only continue to learn about the high technology required in critical care but also actively participate in learning new skills for developing their inner knowledge, intuition, and wisdom and the discipline to integrate such skills into daily practice. In the best of cases, this knowledge can forestall the negative effects of an increasingly cold and remote technology.

Critical care nurses have the potential to turn around the painful dissonance that abounds in critical care, where "high tech" and "high touch" are out of balance.

Distinguishing Technique From Technology

Zwolski proposes four principles that describe a technical system:[18]

1. Technique is distinguishable from technology.
2. A technique cannot produce the philosophy that directs it.
3. Technology at its incomplete and imperfect stages creates new problems.
4. Technology produces fragmentation.

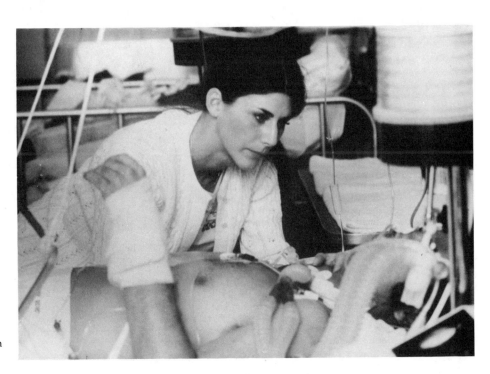

Figure 1–2
Even the simplest nursing act can never be a neutral event.

Healing takes place in critical care when the critical care nurse distinguishes technique from technology. A technique is simply a standard method that can be taught, a recipe that can be duplicated and, if followed, will always lead to an end result. An example of technique is the nursing process. However, a technique reaches its limit at precisely the point where the individual nurse's creativity and intuition enter. Although steps in recognizing creativity and intuition can be taught, what emerges for each nurse is unique. Technology in the broadest sense is the application of science.[12] Examples of technology are endless, such as arterial monitoring, ultrasound, intra-aortic balloon counterpulsation, heart valves, and pharmaceuticals.

Patients or nurses may view techniques and technology as separate entities, but in actuality they cannot be separated. Table 1–1 gives some patient situations illustrating relationships between technique and technology. Both physical and psychologic responses are seen in the first two examples. The third example demonstrates a common occurrence of how patients often develop their own techniques as a response to another technique with which they interact. The last two ex- amples demonstrate the nurse's independent techniques for healing interventions and clinical decision making.

In the technologic environment, the critical care nurse's mission is defined clearly as the diagnosis and treatment of human responses to actual or potential health problems (refer to Chap. 5). This definition must also be expanded to include the human responses to techniques and technologies. Frequently, what happens in critical care is that the patient gets lost. The distinction between the means (the technique) and the ends (the philosophy or vision that directs it) becomes blurred, so that the technique is the end in itself. Think about the technique of keeping a patient alive by using technology of ventilatory support, intravenous fluids, and hyperalimentation at all cost. Before complications, this patient's personal request (vision) was not to be attached to life support, but the health care team has become so engaged in the illusion of technique that the patient's personal request has become lost or denied, which presents an unethical situation.

The question that the critical care nurse must ask continuously is if the technique or the technology is good for the patient and under what conditions should it be used. Critical

Table 1–1
Examples of Technique—Technology Analysis

EXAMPLE	ANALYSIS
Mr. A. is told that he is about to be transferred out of the CCU. Almost immediately his blood pressure and pulse destabilize, and there is an increase in the frequency of PVCs. He says to the nurse, "I am afraid of being disconnected from these monitors."	Mr. A has developed a psychologic reliance on monitoring devices. This has caused him to respond to this technology in a physiologic manner.
Mrs. B. is an asthmatic who refuses to take the medicine prescribed for her. Upon questioning by the nurse, she says, "This medicine won't help me. I need something that is warm."	Mrs. B is responding to her prescribed regimen (pharmacologic technology). She has a belief that is more valid for her than any scientifically proven facts. Her faith and trust in her own belief system and her distrust of the scientific facts are truly potent variables to be considered in terms of compliance and eventual health outcomes.
Mr. C. is on hemodialysis. Before every session he binges on junk food. Even though he has been warned against doing this, he continues the practice. He has told the nurses, "I need to do this." He seems to look forward to the confrontation this always causes.	Mr. C. is responding to a technique (hemodialysis) with his own technique (ritual) for coping.
Mrs. D., who has terminal cancer, is suffering from intractable pain. Working with the nurses on various visualization and imagery techniques, Mrs. D. experiences relief from her pain and the dosage of prescribed medication is able to be reduced.	The use of a technique (visualization and imagery) as a therapeutic treatment
Mr. E., who has had a recent MI, is restless. His vital signs and other cardiac parameters are within normal limits. Nonetheless, the nurse caring for Mr. E. senses that he is about to go into cardiogenic shock. Accordingly, she initiates appropriate interventions.	The use of a technique (intuition) as part of clinical decision making

MI: myocardial infarction; PVC: premature ventricular contraction.

(Zwolski, K. Professional nursing in a technological system. *Image* 2:238, 1989; with permission.)

care nurses must always protect the patient's visions and values. This is the philosophy of nurse as patient advocate, the core of what it means to practice the art, science, and spirit of nursing.

Much has been accomplished with technology, but it has also resulted in complex problems with which both patient and professionals are not prepared to cope.[12] We so frequently get fooled by technology, which is imperfect and incomplete. The term *halfway technologies* has been used to describe our current situation.[18] An example is iatrogenic illnesses, which are illnesses related to technologic development of sophisticated diagnostic procedures and therapeutic procedures. Over the last 30 years, improvement has been seen with infectious disease and acute illness. Yes, we live longer, but we are increasingly faced with the "failure of success," the phenomenon whereby some diseases are more prevalent as a result of medical advances. For example, because we live longer, we are now faced with more chronic and degenerative illness. For some people, this also brings about a decline in general well-being and meaning for living. Fragmentation is also brought about with technology. There is more specialization with more competition in the bureaucratic structure for available personnel and resources.

As we enter the 21st century, techniques and technology will increase; both can be intimidating. The theory is that technology frees the nurse to spend more time with the patient, but often nurses end up "nursing" the machines and forgetting the patient. However, much of the technology frees the nurse to nurture the patient. Data can be gathered more quickly; thus, the nurse has more time to stop and be fully present with the patient. For example, what is the impact on the patient when the nurse makes it a point to hold a patient's hand when calibrating a Swan-Ganz catheter? What is the outcome when the nurse speaks calmly to the patient and touches the patient before taking any kind of pressure readings, *i.e.*, intracranial pressure monitoring or pulmonary capillary wedge pressures? What happens when the nurse touches the patient's arm when taking a blood pressure, as compared with placing the cuff on without touch? Nurses must look beyond the machines and rehumanize the care of critically ill patients. Nurses will continue to assume the role of unifier because they represent the profession of caring as compared with the profession of medicine as curing. They are the bridge between the technologic environment and the acutely ill patients and their families.

Zwolski suggests that as we consider the four principles of technique and technology, nurses must broaden their horizons, knowledge, and skills to elicit healing in self and others. A holistic approach to patient care is mandatory. Nurses must gain new behaviors through education in the following areas:[18]

- Ongoing and thorough assessment of the patient's response to the techniques and technology they encounter in the health care system, including the ability to appraise critically and evaluate the effect on patients
- Decisions about when to use alternate health-promoting techniques and the power to implement these decisions
- Patient advocacy
- Involvement in health care policy decisions
- Conducting research relevant to these concerns

FOUNDATIONS FOR HEALING*
Nurse-Patient Relationships

The traditional nurse-patient relationship is familiar to most people. Traditionally, nurses are seen as standing apart from the patient. They help the patient in familiar ways and occasionally in sophisticated, perhaps even heroic, ways. But whether nurses are giving simple care (such as a bed bath) or sophisticated care (such as resuscitative measures), they stand apart from the patient, who is an *object* being treated, a person having things done *for* or *to* the body. The patient has become, basically, an object of nursing care.

This way of viewing the patient is so common-sensical that we wonder why we should look for another way. And we wonder whether there are other ways of viewing the nurse-patient relationship. We wonder why some nurses are better healers than others. Do they differ in personality, intuition, calming influences, or just in the way they relate to patients?

The "patient-as-object" is more correctly a state of unrelatedness, although it seems accurate because it is the way patients see themselves in relation to the nurse. They see themselves as recipients: as people *to* whom and *for* whom things are done, *e.g.*, as people *into* whom medication is injected. They also view themselves as objects of critical care nursing. Indeed, they are objectified in many ways. They are given a specific room with a number. They are given an arm band with another number. And, in change-of-shift jargon, they may be referred to impersonally as "the inferior MI in 4 with Mobitz I and rare PVCs."

If there were no more to the nurse-patient relationship than practicality, nurses might as well be replaced by machines. Obviously, however, the nurse-patient relationship is much more subtle. It has been said that each time a nurse *encounters* a patient, *something happens*. The meeting is never a *neutral event*. It is the power of the nurse-patient relationship that makes nursing an exciting blend of emotions and sophisticated skills, not a series of automatic performances. The blends are as varied as the nurses and patients themselves. The critical care nurse must understand that every patient encounter is meaningful, that it always has an impact, that it always affects both the patient and the nurse. The effect may be dramatic or subtle, but something—either positive or negative—always occurs. In the next section, ways in which the nurse-patient relationship can take on new meaning are considered.

A Human Science

We have a human science when we evoke states of healing and healer. In Weber's eloquent framework for foundations of healing, the universal healing power, not the healer's personal energy, accomplishes the healing. The healer is like a channel, passively yet, paradoxically, with discernment permitting the cosmic energy to flow unobstructedly through his or her own energy fields into those of the healee. The healer must be aware of the disturbances in the healee's wholeness at the higher levels. It is the healer who constitutes the link between the universal and the particular; his or her role is

* Source: Used with permission from Dossey, B., Keegan, L., Guzzetta, C. and Kolkmeier, L. *Holistic Nursing: A Handbook for Practice.* Rockville, Maryland: Aspen Publishers, Inc., 1988.

analogous to an electrical transformer capable of stepping down the source—in this case, the prodigious cosmic energy—into a form used by our bodymind systems.[17]

A human science is based on the following principles:[16]

• A philosophy of human freedom, choices, and responsibility
• A biology and psychology of holism (nonreducible persons connected with others and nature)
• A theory of origins, methods, and limits of knowledge (epistemology) that allows not only for practical experience (empirics) but also for advancement of esthetics, ethical values, intuition, and process discovery
• A branch of metaphysics that deals with nature of being/ reality (ontology) of space and time
• A context of interhuman events, processes, and relationships
• A scientific world view that is open

If we are to operationalize nursing as a human science, we must understand the idea of the person, nursing, and human care. Three areas to focus on are being-in-the-world (Fig. 1–3), the self, and a phenomenal field.[16] The person is viewed as being-in-the-world, possessing the spheres of body-mind-spirit. These spheres influence one's concept of self. The self indicates the perceptions of ''I'' and relationships to others. Another level of self is the higher self, the spiritual self that rises above ordinary waking consciousness. A phenomenal field is the individual's frame of reference, which can be known only to the person. This phenomenal field (a person's subjective reality) influences how a person responds in any given situation. It involves many levels of consciousness, such as awareness, perceptions of self, self to others, body sensations, thoughts, values, feelings, beliefs, and hopes. So when nurse and patient come together, two phenomenal fields come together. Both are in a process of being, becoming, and developing transpersonal understanding.

Transpersonal Human Care and Caring Transactions

We can speak of transpersonal human care and caring transactions as the professional, ethical, scientific, aesthetic, caring, and personalized giving-receiving behaviors and responses between two people (nurse and other) that allow for contact between the subjective world of persons (through physical, mental, and spiritual routes).[16] The nurse and patient come together and share a phenomenal field of their individual uniqueness, which creates an event of caring as seen in Figure 1–3.

The dynamics of the human caring process involve nurse, patient, and the phenomenal field of each person. The human caring process thus has a transpersonal dimension. That transpersonal dimension is an intersubjective human-to-human relationship in which the person of the nurse affects and is affected by the person of the other. Both are fully present in the moment and feel a union with the other. They share a phenomenal field that becomes part of the life history of both and are coparticipants in becoming in the now and the future. Such an ideal of caring entails an ideal of intersubjectivity, in which both persons are involved.

This coming together can be done in a mechanical manner in which the nurse or patient responds without acknowledging the other or recognizing each other's potentials. On the other hand, the nurse and patient can come together with a presence of caring that involves actions and choices by both.

Nurse-Healer as a Guide

Reflect for a moment on the characteristics of a nurse that facilitate healing in self, patients, and others. Table 1–2 lists these qualities. The clearer we become about knowing ourselves, the clearer we will be in relating to other people, with the outcome being more meaningful relationships. The highest form of knowing is loving,[4,14] so as we learn to love ourselves, the more closely we are attuned to our intuition and self-healing.

A nurse-healer is a guide who uses the art of guiding to help others discover and recognize new health behaviors, make choices, and discover insights about how to cope effectively. A guide helps a person explore purpose and meaning in life. Guiding is a special art and intervention that nurses may use at all times. The purpose of guiding is to bring to the present moment a patient's fullest potential. This process helps the patient be in congruence with his or her inner resources, decrease stress, and enhance self-direction toward balance and harmony.

A nurse-healer guides the patient in developing all areas of human potential. The patient is offered the knowledge of the inner journey of self-discovery, but the nurse as guide does not assume to know what is the best course for the patient. Patients must make their own choices. As patients seek guidance and help with life possibilities and dilemmas, the nurse as a guide knows some of the hazards and precautions that occur with lifestyle changes and can only suggest new options. The nurse has no way of knowing what each experience holds for a person, for moment by moment, the contrast of polarities, such as health and illness, joy and sadness, are always present in one's life.

The Light and Shadow

The dance of human life is a matter of polarity, the light and the shadow.[10] Polarity implies difference, like the North and South poles. Just as a magnet cannot be a magnet without opposites, so does human existence require polarities. Without the shadow, we have no concept of the light. Contrast is essential in every aspect of our life. Think of a few of the polarities of daily experience with which we are familiar: happiness and sadness, strengths and weaknesses, resolution and conflict, elation and depression. Another example of this contrast is wellness and illness. The only way we have a concept of personal wellness is to have at some point in our life a firsthand experience with illness or major life stressors.

Particularly in Western culture, emphasis is placed throughout our lives on the high peaks, and the dark side—the shadow—is ignored. One of the major obstacles to understanding our wholeness is this inability to recognize our dark side. The human psyche does not cope well with the polarity, for the ego loves clarity.[6] Yet, it is when we repress the polarity that it is taken into our unconscious and causes psychophysiologic disturbances.[6]

When a major stressor, disaster, or illness occurs, the easiest course is to repress the meaning of the darkness. Over time, the failure to understand this meaning becomes a futile spiral. At some point, one must address the shadow side of life be-

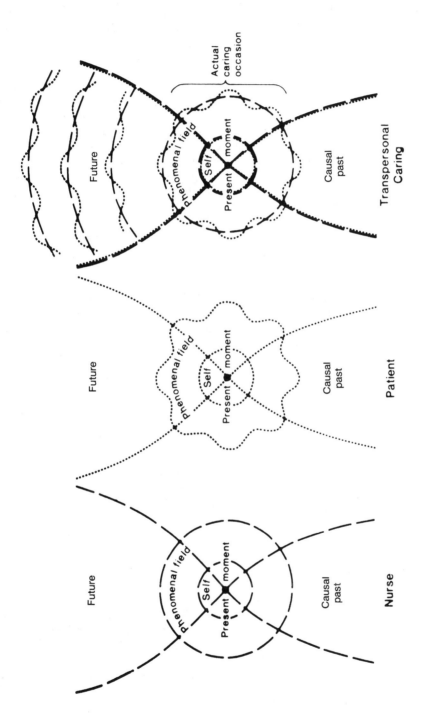

Figure 1-3
Dynamics of the human caring process. Illustration by Melvin L. Gabel, University of Colorado Health Sciences Center, Biomedical Communications Department. (Watson J. *Nursing: Human Science and Human Care—A Theory of Nursing.* New York: Appleton & Lange, 1985:59; with permission.)

Table 1–2
Characteristics of a Nurse-Healer

Aware that self-healing is a continual process
Familiar with the terrain of self-development
Open to self-discovery
Continues to develop clarity about life's purposes to keep from acting mechanical and bored
Aware of present and future steps in personal growth
Models self-care in order to help self and patients with the inward process
Aware that his or her presence is equally important as technical skills
Respects and loves patients regardless of who or how they are
Offers the patient methods for working on life issues
Guides the patient in discovering creative options
Presumes that the patient knows the best life choices
Listens actively
Empowers patients to recognize that they can cope with life processes
Shares insights without imposing personal values and beliefs
Accepts what patients say without judging
Sees time with patients as being there for them to serve and share

(Dossey, B., Keegan, L., Guzzetta, C., *et al. Holistic Nursing: A Handbook for Practice.* Rockville, MD: Aspen Publishers, 1988; with permission.)

cause it is always present. There is a part of us that always needs healing (the wounded healer), yet we find it easy to ignore this woundedness. We must learn to sense our limitations, as well as to recognize our strengths. All great healers acknowledge their inherent weakness and fallibilities.

When a patient and nurse come together and both deny their woundedness, the outcome of care is mechanical at best. Neither the patient nor the nurse is able to use inner wisdom on his or her own behalf to activate self-healing. Both have devalued this innate potential. Inner healing does not flow from the nurse to the patient. The nurse cannot give inner healing to the patient, for it already exists within the patient. Rather, the nurse acts as a facilitator to evoke the patient's process of inner healing. Healing occurs when the patient and the nurse both acknowledge the polarity of light and shadow and use it to move toward balance and harmony.

As the best of both traditional and holistic practices merge, much of the work that remains to be done will be to learn the art of healing and being a healer, and to work on the self, our imperfect, fallible self.[13] We must recognize our polarity, our weaknesses and strengths, and acknowledge our inadequacies. It is only then that we know a powerful part of our being and allow new strengths to be born. It is the use of self, in a loving and compassionate way, that provides us with our most powerful instrument for healing.[13]

Implication for Healing: Era III Medicine

With the increase in technology and the discontentment with the current health care system, it often seems that healing, particularly in the critical care setting, is impossible. If we review the history of medicine and look to the future, there seems to be hope on the horizon. All therapies since the age of science fall into certain eras, as seen in Table 1–3.[7]

Table 1–3
Medical Eras

	ERA I	**ERA II**	**ERA III**
Space-time characteristic	Local	Local	Nonlocal
Synonym	Mechanical or "modern" medicine	Mind-body, complementary, or alternative medicine	Nonlocal medicine
Description	Causal, deterministic, describable by classical concepts of space-time and matter-energy; mind not a factor; "mind" a result of brain mechanisms	Mind a major factor in healing *within* the single person; mind has causal power and, thus is not fully explainable by classical concepts in physics; includes but goes beyond Era I.	Mind a factor in healing both *within* and *between* persons; mind not completely localized to points in space (brains or bodies) or time (present moment or single lifetimes); mind unbounded in space and time and thus ultimately unitary or One; healing at a distance is permitted; not describable by classical concepts of space-time or matter-energy
Examples	Any form of therapy focusing solely on effects of *things* on the body are Era I approaches including techniques such as acupuncture and homeopathy, the use of herbs, etc. Includes almost all forms of "modern" medicine—drugs, surgery, irradiation, CPR, etc.	Any therapy emphasizing the effects of consciousness *solely* within the individual body is an Era II approach. Psychoneuroimmunology, counseling, hypnosis, biofeedback, relaxation therapies, and most types of imagery-based "alternative" therapies are included.	Any therapy in which effects of consciousness bridge between different persons is an Era III approach. All forms of distant healing, intercessory prayer, "psychic" and shamanic healing, so-called "miracles," diagnosis at a distance, and noncontact therapeutic touch are included. Certain emotions—love, compassion, empathy—may exert nonlocal effects. When they enter Era I and II therapies, these may take on Era III characteristics. Any time a therapist is involved, this possibility holds.

For a detailed description of the three medical eras, *see* Dossey, L. *Meaning and Medicine: A Doctor's Stories of Breakthrough and Healing.* New York: Bantam, 1991.

According to Dossey, Era I can be called *materialistic medicine*. It was a magnificent step forward in healing. Wonder cures such as antibiotics, cures of certain infectious diseases and acute illnesses occurred. As he states:[7]

In Era I, which has existed for most of the past one-hundred years in the West, the emphasis is on the material body, which is viewed largely as a complex machine. Era I medicine is guided by the laws of energy and matter laid down by Newton three hundred years ago. According to this perspective, the Universe and all in it—including the body—are a vast clockwork functioning according to deterministic laws. The effects of mind and consciousness are absent, and all forms of therapy must be physical in nature—drugs, surgery, irradiation, etc.

In the last two decades, Era II, or *mind-body medicine,* has brought about another era of healing. In this period, scientific studies demonstrated the powerful role of consciousness—of emotions, perceived meaning, attitudes, perceptions—in changing physiology of all major diseases. These influences were so dramatic that in some situations it meant life or death. These therapies do not conflict with Era I therapies, but are complementary. New disciplines in medicine have been developed, such as the field of psychoneuroimmunology, which studies the interrelationships of the autonomic, neurologic, endocrine, and immune systems. Some of the therapies in this era are biofeedback, meditation, imagery, and various forms of relaxation therapies. The major difference between Era I and Era II is the role of consciousness, which was lacking in Era I. Era I and Era II do have much in common in that they are both local in nature. Era I emphasizes a brain-bound mind and the concept that the individual occupies a specific location in space and a certain span of time. Era II also has a local approach, emphasizing the mind and consciousness of an individual operating on the individual body within the local space-time framework. Local means the here and now. In psychologic terms, it is the description of the self, or the experience of "I," that lets us know that we exist and that we are set apart from others in the world by being here and not somewhere else.

As exciting as both of these eras of medicine have been, they are limited and incomplete; however, we can look toward an advanced era, Era III medicine, or a *nonlocal medicine.* Era III has arisen out of science and is nonlocal in nature. In Era II, the emphasis is on the role of mind and consciousness on the individual body of a single person and a single lifetime. In Era III, minds of individuals are spread through space and time, are omnipresent, infinite, immortal, and, ultimately, one. The impact of this on healing is that health and healing are not just an individual or personal experience as seen in Era I and Era II. Health and healing become a collective affair.

This is a fundamental shift in our thinking because it says that minds of people not only matter but influence each other in close proximity as well as distances (*i.e.,* the nonlocal nature of mind). A number of challenging scientific studies were conducted that are examples of the nonlocal therapeutic phenomenon. One such study is the "prayer study" done by Randolf Byrd, a cardiologist.[2] This 10-month study met the rigid scientific criteria of clinical medical studies, with its randomized, prospective, and double-blind design in which neither doctors, nurses, or patients knew to which group the patients belonged. Protestant and Roman Catholic groups across the United States made up the prayer groups. The prayer groups were given the names of sick patients, were told something of their conditions, and were asked to pray for the patients daily. No instructions on how to pray were given. Each person prayed for many patients. Between five and seven people prayed for each patient daily. Byrd computer-assigned 393 patients admitted to a coronary care unit at San Francisco General Hospital either to a group that was prayed for by home prayer groups (192 patients) or to a group that was not remembered in prayer (201 patients). The study results were significant in that the prayed-for patients differed from the non–prayed-for patients in the following areas:

- They were five times less likely than the unremembered group to require antibiotics (3 patients compared with 16 patients).
- They were three times less likely to develop pulmonary edema (6 compared with 18 patients).
- None of the prayed-for group required endotracheal intubation (12 in the unremembered group required mechanical ventilatory support).
- Fewer patients in the prayed-for group died (although the difference was not significant).

We might pass off the results of this study as a coincidence, but if this were a drug or a new technology being studied, it would be heralded as a "breakthrough," and more money would be alloted for further studies and refinement of the technology. What is being suggested by this study is the power of the mind and its ability to send information when people are in close proximity or on the opposite coast. Byrd did not find that prayer groups in San Francisco were any more effective than those in the same city or thousands of miles away.

Era III includes the important contributions of Era I and II that are complementary, not antagonistic. We do have minds that affect our bodies, and we have bodies that respond to the physical effects of drugs, radiation, surgery, and other interventions. With Era III, however, we have another dimension: "the medicine of nonlocality" that goes beyond our limitations as humans.[7] When the health care professional understands the therapeutic potential of the mind, therapy for them then has a transcendent quality in which one has an ability to raise one's ordinary state of consciousness above control at a lower level. There is more of a sense of becoming "all minds"—the minds of all people on the health care team, the patient, and the families and friends in close proximity as well as those at a distance.

The Path Toward Spirituality

During critical illness and recovery, patients frequently search for how to create new perceptions for their life as well as to find wholeness and spirituality; they need guidance in their transformation. In order to deal with the spiritual dimension more effectively with critically ill patients, the nurse should be aware of the following complex factors that shape one's world view and influence the nurse's ability to help patients with spiritual issues:[3]

- Pluralism: Nurses and patients each have a vast array of beliefs, values, meaning, and purpose.

- Fear: The nurse may exhibit confusion about his or her own beliefs and values, lack of confidence in his or her ability to handle situations, and invasion of patient's privacy.
- Awareness of own spiritual quest: The nurse may be contemplating meaning, purpose, hope, and presence of love in his or her own life.
- Confusion: The nurse's conflict between religious and spiritual concepts.
- Basic attitudes: These comprise the nurse's belief system about illness, aging, and suffering.

As the nurse becomes more aware of the areas that affect the spiritual dimension, the nurse and patient can be in dialogue without using traditional religious language to share and express their spiritual dimension. The nurse can encourage the patient to explore his or her spirituality as seen in Table 1–4.

Many variables determine the dialogue between the nurse and patient, such as where the nurse and patient are on their healing journey, each one's ability to listen actively and reflect, and the level of trusting relationship that has been established to help the patient understand the transpersonal self (see Table 1–4).[3]

BECOMING MORE FULLY HUMAN

Strategies to enhance healing of the critical care nurse, such as how to become more fully human, how to recognize the inward healing journey, healing awareness, and the quality of centeredness, are now explored. In order for nurses to teach the patient self-regulation interventions, it is essential that they know the relaxation response from experience. With self-regulation interventions, a quality of love and caring evolves within the technologic environment. There is less superficial conversation. The nurse is able to guide the patient with self-regulation interventions to become open to inner wisdom when reflective states are achieved. When a nurse truly understands the role of being a guide to facilitate the healing process in the patient and self, there is an experience that transcends the individual identities of two separate people. For brief periods of time, the energy fields of nurse and patient blend and are not bound by space and time.

It is easy in daily life to view the workday routine as dull and boring ("same old stuff day in and day out"). We see the ordinary as uninspiring and long for another holiday that perhaps will be filled with peak experiences such as a magic sunset with orange, red, and gold clouds and a special person. However, if we just look around us and marvel at the ordinary, if we look with new eyes, take a deep breath, and feel as we exhale, we will see colors and textures, notice smells, and feel our bodies as we do so.

Watson states that caring is based on one's philosophy and values and is a guiding force that affects every nurse-patient encounter.[16] Nurses must be in touch with their feelings, giving them a foundation for empathy with themselves, their patients, and their support systems. The extent to which nurses are able to develop fully their self-potential is related to their sensitivity to self. As nurses continue to develop their sensitivity, they more actively listen to the perceptions and world views of their patients and others. They not only increase their own self-growth but also encourage self-growth in others. Professionals need to protect their sense of meaning in life against the daily erosion of burnout. They must not only protect it but nourish it. Preservation of the meaning of life in the practice of nursing is not a causal function but a daily discipline.[3] Nurses must continuously search for self-meaning and meaning in others, and they must be open to supporting patients as they seek meaning in their own experience. In doing so, they can help patients repattern their life experiences toward healing.

When nurses take full advantage of their own strengths and resources as well as those of their patients, what evolves is a shared responsibility, a collaboration toward a mutual goal. Each nurse and each patient engages in a dynamic process. As nurses collaborate with patients, a relationship occurs on many levels. This collaboration is based on the nurses' attitude toward sensitivity and their receptivity to another's resources and potential.

Nurses cannot humanize critical care until they learn how to be more fully human themselves. They do not have to leave parts of themselves at home and assume certain maladaptive behaviors that are rampant in critical care, such as blaming problems on the hospital system, administrators, other staff members, or patients and families.

Table 1–4

Guidelines for Helping Persons Experience Their Own Spirituality

1. Know yourself as a spiritual being. What gives your life meaning? What is especially frightening?
2. Remember that being aware of the presence of God does not depend on being able to define or describe God.
3. Remember that each person is the expert about one's own path. It is then that we can explore their uniqueness.
4. Understand spiritual assessment as an ongoing process within the context of a relationship.
5. Be aware that the need to be with and to bear painful feelings is as significant and important as the need to do and to do for persons experiencing spiritual distress.
6. Help the person and yourself find goals, hope, and pleasure for the present moment.
7. Encourage reminiscing and share in life review, a process during which persons remember and often resolve or understand old pain and conflicts from a new perspective.
8. Allow persons to grieve for themselves and those around them.
9. Know that by being present we can decrease the separation and aloneness which persons often fear.
10. Remember and know that you are helping a person toward wholeness–in the moment—now—even when pain and limitation are part of the moment.

(Burkhardt, M., and Nagai-Jacobson, M. G. Dealing with spiritual concerns of clients in the community. American Holistic Nurses Association Annual Conference. June, 1987; with permission.)

Only we can take care of ourselves properly. Only we can identify our individual humanity and have a clear understanding of our beliefs and values. Our values form our philosophy and determine how we participate in nursing. When we continue to strive for clarity, we rediscover our wholeness because our course of action is in accordance with our belief system. In other words, we become what we believe. We give up all internal contradictions. As we discover within ourselves the integrity of our own body-mind-spirit nexus, we are then in a position to deliver humanistic nursing care. We must be responsible for learning a sense of balance and a sense of calm in critical care. We must take the responsibility of learning different skills that evoke the relaxation response. By doing so, our calm becomes contagious. These ideas are basic, and they can be used at any time. We do not have to be in a quiet room to evoke the relaxation response. Practicing the following relaxation and imagery techniques allows us to bring about the response at will:

- We should focus on rhythmic breathing. As we inhale and exhale, we should just "be" with our breathing, mindful of the experience of air moving in and out. It is so simple. Another variation is breath counting. With each exhale, we count one.
- While charting or taking a break, we should imagine that we have an imaginary skyhook coming out of the top of our head. We attach the imaginary skyhook to our imaginary skyline. We allow our shoulders to drop, and we feel the relaxation filling our total body as we float freely up into the sky.
- We should assess our bodies many times during the day for good postural alignment, scanning it to feel areas of tension and imagining that tense muscle fibers are smoothing out.
- We should be aware of special images we can clearly bring to mind to help us feel peaceful and quiet, to gain an inner calm, such as an ocean, a special place in nature, a meadow, or even a place in our own home.
- We should sit quietly, close our eyes, relax our face muscles, and breathe with our abdomen, being aware of focusing our attention. There are several ways of focusing. We can watch our flow of consciousness—all those thoughts that come and go—not trying to hang onto any particular thought. We can focus on one thing, such as a symbol or our breath. Any time our mind wanders, we just bring our attention back to the object. This exercise is also helpful when we start to become angry. Just for a moment, we shift our awareness away from the anger and think of a relaxing image or bathe in a calming color. After focusing on it for a few seconds, we mentally rehearse a way to deal with the anger in the least stressful way.
- We should use the quieting response, perhaps imagining that we have breathing holes in the bottom of our feet. (There are no rules in the imagination!) Whenever we start to feel tense, we smile and say, "I can help calm myself," and we focus on the breathing holes in our feet. We then take a deep breath through our feet and feel the relaxation move all the way to the top of our head. As we exhale, we feel the tension moving all the way down our body and out our feet. This exercise takes only a few seconds and is very helpful during the most difficult situations in critical care (e.g., during a cardiac arrest or while caring for a patient in cardiogenic shock).

The Inward Arc

When a nurse reflects on the inner dimension of self, a process referred to as the *inward arc*, this conscious journey toward wholeness evolves toward self-transcendence.

In Figure 1–4, the outward arc of personal ego development precedes the inward arc of transpersonal spiritual awakening. Self-consciousness arises during healthy human development. As the self continues to develop and mature, different self-concepts, identities, and life experiences are understood that lead toward the conscious journey of the inward arc, the inner understanding. The psyche has many layers of consciousness. As one moves more inward, seeking inner knowledge along with personal understanding, one experiences the Absolute that is composed of higher-ordered wholes and integrations. Basic structures of the psyche are not replaced, but become part of the larger unity. The ultimate part of the journey is awakening, or enlightenment to the knowledge that one is part of the whole.

Healing Awareness

This transpersonal model helps us understand healing awareness, our ability to discipline ourselves to be present in the moment and understand the meaning of the moment. Several ways to acquire this ability are by developing our skills through relaxation and imagery practice and various meditative disciplines that allow inner silence and the presence of inward focusing. These skills can be practiced in any place and at any time. What surfaces with this state of being present in the moment is a noninterfering intention that allows natural healing to flow.[4]

Healing awareness requires authenticity. Authenticity implies consistency between *inner experience* and *outer expression* and *congruence between beliefs* and *behaviors*.[4] Perception and beliefs tend to be mutually reinforcing (*i.e.*, if a person believes

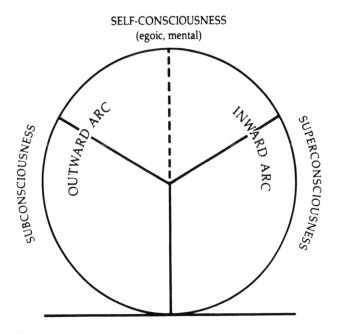

Figure 1–4

The general life cycle. (Vaughan F. *The Inward Arc.* Boston: Shambhala Publications. 1985; with permission.)

something to be true, then the perception will selectively reinforce it). Much unhealthy living occurs because people do not operate from a state of *authenticity.*

When we operate from authenticity, there is harmony in our behaviors, thoughts, and feelings. When nurses model healing awareness, consciously or unconsciously, the experience is translated and is evoked in patients and others. Patients learn more from what nurses do and their persona than what nurses teach or say. When operating from authenticity, we are in a better position to act with intention and clear purpose and to have the freedom for creating choices that can empower our lives. If authenticity is not present, a perceptual internal conflict exists that manifests as anxiety, burnout, and confusion about living and may result in symptoms that can lead to illness.

Centering

Centering is the state achieved when one moves within oneself to an inner reference of stability. It is a sense of self-relatedness that can be thought of as a place of inner being, a place of quietude within which one can feel truly integrated, unified, and focused. Centering has been described as the source of our conscious awareness of our involvement in life. It is a personal space apart from either involvement or the consequent reaction to that involvement.

To be *centered* implies a quality and essence of being present in the moment. Centering is a skill that is learned by *daily practice* of at least 15 to 20 minutes of solitude to quiet the inner dialogue and body simultaneously. This can be achieved through practice of the relaxation response and other relaxation interventions (imagery and music) and of various meditative disciplines.

When we develop the skills and awareness of centering, our ability to become more sensitive to our life patterns and processes increases. We act more frequently with purposeful *intention.* We have a greater ability to be with our state of *resolution (i.e.,* we are more willing to experience and face our fears and worries). Centering allows us to devote more time to be silent within. This quality of inner silence lets us understand more of the wisdom that we gain access to when we acknowledge our polarities in life. Our *love* flows naturally, for we are open to the expressions of nonjudgmental love. When this quality is integrated in our life, we are more consistently available for meaningful *relationships.*

Working With Others*

The following guidelines are helpful as we engage in helping ourselves and our patients experience wholeness:

- What we communicate by word, act, attitude, and setting will affect our potential for change. Everything affects our patients—our choice of words, our presence with silence, our greetings, and our personal surroundings.
- What we believe is important. Our beliefs affect our self-image, which in turn affects our actions. They also influence

* Source: Adapted from *Spiritual Aspects of the Healing Arts* by E. Peper and C. Kushel pp 132–137, with permission of Theosophical Publishing House, 1985.

our capacity for self-healing. Our beliefs are conveyed to our patients.
- Perceive yourself and your patient as whole. You and the patient are whole and not a portion of disturbance or pathology. Perceive the cancer patient as a person with cancer. Release the label. We encourage pathology when we focus primarily on disease and not on the patient's healing potential.
- The practitioner needs to be self-experienced. We cannot guide patients down new paths to new experiences if we do not know the path from experience. The more we know from experience, the more we know that change is possible.
- Every part is connected to every other part, and every part in the system affects every other part. We form a network in which everyone participates. There is no such thing as an independent observer. Nurse and patient are always creating change in one another.
- Consider the whole setting. Patients are asked to consider changing life patterns. Look at all the patient's life potentials—physical, mental, emotional, spiritual, relationships, and choices. It is only when we consider the whole patient and the significant others that we have a chance at directing the patient toward wholeness.
- Teaching competence is the basis for change. Teach in such a manner that the patient cannot fail. Help the patient with realistic goals that can be measured. Attaining success directly affects beliefs.
- Develop and support a positive self-image. One must accept and like oneself if change is to occur.
- Encourage learning without judgment. To develop skills that are necessary for change, it is helpful to allow all learning experiences to occur without judgment. For example, a person with chest pain should be encouraged to tend to the chest pain. Give pain medication and encourage the patient to be with the chest pain by knowing that the pain medication is in his or her body and working. Teach the patient how to use relaxation, imagery, and music to help manage the pain.
- Acknowledge all changes, however slight. Each change leads to another. Each slight change is progress.
- Reframe experiences positively. Our internal thoughts are very changeable. Instead of saying "I'll never get well," reframe it by saying "I'm getting stronger moment by moment." The reframing allows bodymind to respond with new possibilities.
- New skills must be practiced. Learning is an ongoing process. Involve friends and family in the learning. The new skills must be integrated into all aspects of life.
- Fear of failure leads to failure. Fears become our prophesies. Negative anticipation creates tension and leads to failure.
- Be oriented to the present. Consciously stay in the present moment. Change takes place in the present, not in the past or the future.

HELPING COLLEAGUES MANAGE STRESS

As nurses care for critically ill patients, they should be able to identify stressors, recognize personal responses to stress, and know the strategies of stress management. They need to be able to analyze accurately and to help nurses cope with their colleagues' responses to stress. A humanistic approach means that nurses have compassion for their colleagues as well as their patients. The humanistic approach requires the *coping* nurse to recognize *maladaptive coping* in colleagues and help them with their coping strategies. In addition to the anxiety- and tension-relieving techniques previously described, nurses can help by assessing attitudinal changes, accepting (and not feeling threatened by) the values of others, using appropriate resources, and developing a system to improve the coping strategies of the staff of the critical care unit.

Nurses can recognize negative attitudes and maladaptive responses in their colleagues by behaviors and feelings such as excessive criticism, procrastination, anger, hostility, denial, overprotectiveness, complaints, depression, transference of blame, deficits in or lack of social skills, self-justification, fatigue, blunting of sensitivities, psychologic numbness, profound guilt, and inability to resume meaningful activities or make optimal decisions. Nurses must also intuitively perceive without condemnation the feelings that lie beneath some attitude or statement of a fellow nurse.

For the staff to provide the best possible nursing care, the process must consist of determining what is producing the anxiety and tension in the critical care unit, group planning of ways to reduce anxiety and tension, awareness of and involvement in the staff's responses, analyzing personal stress and discussing that stress with other nurses, consulting with other professionals, identifying short- and long-term outcomes, establishing evaluation tools and feedback mechanisms to help in the adaptation to change, and planning the content of the system to reduce anxiety and tension. Anticipated results of the systems approach just outlined are reduction in nursing turnover, decrease in absenteeism, reduction in the number of accidents and poor judgments (documented, it is hoped, by incident reports), increase in skill, increased speed in decision making, and, equally important, improvement in the staff's attitude. A positive subjective response is important and should not be discounted. More objective measures that can be sampled include a decrease in the number of complaints, criticisms, procrastinations, and hostile reactions, and an increase in warm, receptive attitudes, responsible self-direction, positive attitudes despite upsetting routines, sense of pride about work accomplished, and a feeling of confidence.

To incorporate the content of the systems approach to stress management, the following should be done:

- Formal group sessions should be held at which qualified people discuss the systems content.
- Informal group sessions should be held that allow open participation and discussion of stressors and responses to stressors under the direction of a qualified counselor.
- Techniques of constructive peer evaluation should be taught to the critical care personnel.
- Self-evaluation and awareness of stressors and feelings should be encouraged. People may be encouraged to keep a private record of their own stress cues and responses.
- Professional counseling or support should be readily available to the critical care personnel.
- Communication between all staff levels should be improved, lines of communication should be defined, and friendly conversations in places other than the critical care unit (*e.g.,* the cafeteria and social gatherings) should be encouraged.
- Recognition conferences should be held at which the successes of the critical care unit staff (and not their failures)

are pointed out and at which other types of positive reinforcement are given to the staff.

Chapter 4 gives specific guidelines and experiential exercises to enhance caring for self and others. In order to become more fully human, spend time assessing your human potentials in the areas of physical, emotional, intellectual, social, and spiritual dimensions. In Chapter 10, you can further expand these ideas by living your ethics.

SUMMARY

This chapter has focused on a new sense of consciousness that is emerging in nursing today. Consciousness is the process through which people know themselves in the world. As nurses continue to enlarge their awareness and skills of processing information by both the right and left hemispheres, they will continue to facilitate growth toward centeredness, health, and wholeness. This growth will help them to continue to be alert to nursing knowledge and therapeutic skills and will help them to use self-healing at the highest level. One of the most consistent and basic human strengths is the ability to gain insight from experience. Experience is a great teacher. We may suffer with experience, but we also learn. As we continue to balance the "high tech" with "high touch," we will continue to see therapeutic skills, the nursing process, as having equal relevance with all aspects of our own humanity— our insight, caring, and compassion. For nurses to use self-regulation interventions in the most effective manner and at a deep level, they must know the interventions from personal experience. The theory can be learned from textbooks, but experience comes from the daily integration of the interventions into one's personal and professional life. Nurses who are experienced with self-regulation skills know how to modulate their voices, listen, and touch with care and know how to be fully present to activate and facilitate others through these very special healing interventions.

Finally, it is the feeling of the authors that this awareness has never faded from view in nursing. In the entire domain of health care, nursing has remained a repository of an inner awareness of the unity of body, mind, and spirit. Such awareness has set nurses apart from other providers of health care. We demonstrate this quality, this awareness, to those we care for, and they sense it when they are ill. This inner quality must be acknowledged and nourished just as purposefully as we develop our technical skills. Without it, nursing is not nursing, but rather a sterile exercise in technique, technology, and data.

Thus, when we speak throughout this book of oneness of body, mind, and spirit, we are introducing nothing new. Awareness of this essential oneness is part of nursing and has always been. Let us celebrate our wisdom!

It should be emphasized that what is being suggested is that the "either/or" approach to understanding human illness—that disease is *either* physical *or* psychologic—is no longer an accurate model for nurses to follow. In practice, it is sometimes admittedly convenient to focus on the "physical" or "the psychologic" needs of the patient, but we should always remind ourselves that mind and body are too closely interwoven to be described as separate processes. Today we know that emotion, thought, attitude, and feeling states are intimately connected with the expression of human illness and that disease states themselves generate changes in our mental lives that in turn, affect the disease states—an endless, reverberating chain of events that defies any ultimate distinction between body and mind. If we find ourselves in any given patient's illness trying to decide "which came first, the physical abnormality or the psychologic malfunction," we should understand that we have fallen into an inaccurate way of thinking about our patients, for ultimately *there are not two separate categories* into which they can be divided—the mental and the physical. True, we can proceed *as if* there were two categories, but we should always exert great caution to not transform this "as if" way of thinking into an assumed reality.

DIRECTIONS FOR FUTURE RESEARCH

A coherent framework for body-mind-spirit has been formulated. It is mandatory that critical care nurses document some of the positive roles of human consciousness in health and illness. As nurses investigate ideas of psychobiologic unity, this will not only enlarge our understanding of oneness but also that of the patients for whom we care.

Research questions to be considered are as follows:

1. What techniques in critical care can facilitate healing, how are they evaluated, and what are the patients' responses to these techniques?
2. What value do patients and families in critical care attach to healing modalities, and what value does nursing attach to them?
3. What are the anticipated or actual solutions or complications that result from healing techniques?
4. What type of fragmentation in critical care is being produced by techniques and technology, and what effect does it have on the patient, family, and the nurse?
5. What are holistic guidelines and therapies to help patients and families tap their spiritual dimension when faced with critical illness?
6. Evaluate if patient outcomes differ when patients interact with nurses who practice self-regulation interventions as opposed to nurses who do not use self-regulation interventions.
7. Evaluate if nurses who use self-regulation interventions have more empathy, caring, and job satisfaction.
8. Evaluate tools that guide the nurse in use of self-regulation interventions in clinical practice.

REFERENCES

1. Achterberg, J., Dossey, B., and Kolkmeier, L. *Rituals of Healing.* New York: Bantam, 1992.
2. Byrd, R. Positive therapeutic effects of intercessory prayer in a coronary care unit population. *South. Med. J.* 81:826, 1988.
3. Burkhardt, M., and Nagai-Jacobson, M. Dealing with spiritual concerns of clients in the community. *J. Commun. Health Nurs.* 2: 193, 1985.
4. Dossey, B. Nurse as Healer: Toward the Inward Journey. In B. Dossey, L. Keegan, C. Guzzetta, and L. Kolkmeier. *Holistic Nursing: A Handbook for Practice.* Rockville, MD: Aspen, 1988.
5. Dossey, L. *Space, Time and Medicine.* Boston: Shambhala Publications, 1982.
6. Dossey, L. *Beyond Illness: Discovering the Experience of Health.* Boston: Shambhala, 1984.
7. Dossey, L. *Recovering the Soul: A Scientific and Spiritual Search.* New York: Bantam, 1989.
8. Frank, J. D. Mind-body relationships in illness and healing. *J. Int. Acad. Prev. Med.* 2:46, 1975.
9. Guzzetta, C. Nursing process and standards of care. In B. Dossey, L. Keegan, C. Guzzetta, and L. Kolkmeier. *Holistic Nursing: A Handbook for Practice.* Rockville, MD: Aspen, 1988.
10. Huang, C. *Quantum Soup.* Berkeley, CA: Celestial Arts, 1991.
11. Lown, B., Temte, J. V., and Reich, P. Basis for recurring ventricular fibrillation in the absence of coronary heart disease and its management. *N. Engl. J. Med.* 294:623, 1975.
12. Pillar, B., Jacox, A., and Redman, B. Technology, its assessment, and nursing. *Nurs. Res.* 38:16, 1990.
13. Quinn, J. The Healing Arts in Modern Health Care. In D. Kunz (Ed.), *Spiritual Aspects of the Healing Arts.* Wheaton, IL: The Theosophical Publishing House, 1985.
14. Remen, N. *The Human Patient.* Garden City, NY: Anchor Press/Doubleday, 1980.
15. Stone, R. A., and DeLeo, J. Psychotherapeutic control of hypertension. *N. Engl. J. Med.* 294:80, 1976.
16. Watson, S. *Nursing: Human Science and Human Care* Norwalk, CT: Appleton-Lange, 1985.
17. Weber, R., Philosophical Foundations and Frameworks for Healing. In D. Kunz (Ed.), *Spiritual Aspects of the Healing Arts.* Wheaton, IL: The Theosophical Publishing House, 1985.
18. Zwolski, K. Professional nursing in a technical system. *Image* 21: 239, 1989.

2

The Psychophysiology of Bodymind Healing*

Barbara Montgomery Dossey

MIND MODULATION

The holistic model acknowledges the interconnectedness of the bodymind, which is capable of producing reciprocal changes in physiology and emotions. Thus, any physiologic event is capable of producing corresponding psychologic alterations and, conversely, any psychologic event can produce corresponding physiologic alterations. From this model, we know that the psychophysiologic stress associated with an acute illness, for example, is capable of producing mind modulation of major body functions, resulting in adverse psychophysiologic effects. Mind modulation is the natural process by which thoughts, feelings, attitudes, and emotions (or neural messages) are converted in the brain to neurohormonal messenger molecules and sent to all body systems. Such mind modulation is capable of producing changes in the autonomic, endocrine, immune, and neuropeptide systems.

We are observing an increasing number of methodologically sound and scientifically convincing research studies that support the notion that a person's psychologic state can actually produce body illness. Impressive evidence documents, for example, that emotions such as anxiety, fear, and social isolation are associated with coronary artery disease, hypertension, dysrhythmias, myocardial ischemia, and sudden cardiac death. Furthermore, we know that disease states themselves generate changes in our mental lives that, in turn, affect the disease state, producing a cyclic chain of events that defies any ultimate distinction between body-mind-spirit.

Such studies lend support to the holistic model by providing evidence of bodymind communication and the negative role that consciousness can play in matters of illness. As we approach the 21st century, however, it is time to ask the next logical question. If our minds can produce body illnesses, can our minds also be used to prevent illness, diminish complications, and promote healing? From the holistic perspective, the answer is yes. It is possible that mind therapies to reduce emotional stressors may be as important to patient outcomes as are the traditional body-oriented technomedical therapies that have been used exclusively for centuries.

LEARNING OBJECTIVES

After reading this chapter, the nurse should be able to do the following:

1. Define natural systems theory.
2. Discuss the placebo effect.
3. Define state-dependent learning.
4. Discuss mind modulation and the autonomic, endocrine, immune, and neuropeptide systems.

* (Modified from Dossey, B. The Psychophysiology of Bodymind Healing. In B. Dossey, L. Keegan, C. Guzzetta, *et al. Holistic Nursing: A Handbook for Practice.* Rockville, MD: Aspen Publishers, 1988; with permission.)

NATURAL SYSTEMS THEORY

Natural systems theory, which is derived primarily from the work of von Bertalanffy,[5,21] provides us with a model of psychobiologic unity. It provides a way of visualizing the interconnectedness of natural structures in the universe. The theory is complex, but it has relevance to the health care professions as seen in Figure 2–1.

In brief, natural structures of vastly different sizes, from the level of subatomic particles all the way to the biosphere, possess definite characteristics at each level and are governed by similar principles of organization. The components of the hierarchy of natural systems also share similar characteristics.[6,7] Therefore, if one knows about the behavior of one component,

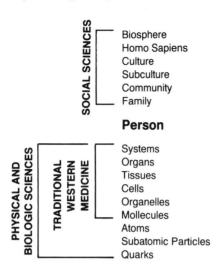

Figure 2–1
The pattern of natural systems components that make up human beings. (Dossey, B., Keegan, L., Guzzetta, C., *et al. Holistic Nursing: A Handbook for Practice.* Rockville, MD: Aspen Publishers, 1988; with permission.)

one automatically knows about the behavior of all the others. Knowledge about molecules provides knowledge about tissues, organ systems, families, species, as well as all the other components that compose the hierarchy of natural systems.

A key characteristic of the hierarchy of natural systems is information flow. Information flows everywhere and is omnidirectional. Regardless of where the information originates, it spreads up and down the hierarchy. Each level can be involved, or the information flow can involve giant feedback loops that may bypass whole levels. Either way, information flow has a domino effect, as the whole system is affected by information originating at any point in the system. This concept has important implications for our views of health and disease.

The traditional view of disease usually stops at the level of the organ, although it may proceed to the level of the person, as shown in Figure 2–1. However, the natural systems approach gives us a more accurate way of viewing disease. Disease can result from a disturbance in any level from the subatomic to the suprapersonal. Health can be seen as the harmonious interaction of all the components of the natural systems hierarchy, whereas disease results when a force disturbs or disrupts the structure of the natural systems themselves.

Let us now explore how thoughts at the level of person impact on body systems.

STATES OF CONSCIOUSNESS

In order to know how nurse-patients interactions can consistently promote healing, we must consider states of consciousness. This discussion focuses on exploring consciousness and the state of totality, which is an awareness of one's own feelings and thoughts, and attention to stimuli in the immediate surroundings.

Altered States and Usual States of Consciousness

In the past, nurses have used the term *states of consciousness* to describe pathologic or altered states of consciousness (ASC) resulting from drug manipulation, metabolic derangements, psychotic states, posttraumatic head injuries or anoxia. However, when we speak of ASC, we must include not only those aforementioned states but also daydreaming, dream states, deep relaxation, and meditative practices. In other words, ASC involve healthy natural states as well as the traditionally recognized pathologic states. Usual states of consciousness (USC) are the ordinary states of waking consciousness in which people spend most of their working hours.

Left and Right Hemispheric Function

Consciousness involves left and right hemispheric functioning. It is important to understand that one hemisphere is not more important than the other and that hemispheric differentiation has been oversimplified. It is inaccurate to say that someone is either right or left brain, because all activities involve both hemispheres simultaneously. It is true, however, that the left and right hemispheres do have specialized functions. The left hemisphere is more involved in logical, analytic thought processing than the right hemisphere. The right hemisphere is more adept at nonlogical, nonanalytical thought processing and spatial tasks than the left hemisphere.

The hemispheres work together at all times. When we say that a person is "being very intuitive," most of us are implying that the person is really "right brain." This is not the whole picture. When a person has a hunch or a flash of insight, it is the left hemisphere that processes and synthesizes the activities that precede the intuition. Nurses must not deny their intuition and just focus on scientific principles but consciously use both ways of knowing in order to practice the art and science of nursing.

Additionally, the right hemisphere is not entirely nonanalytical. Think of some of the spatial activities in which the right hemisphere specializes, such as pattern recognition; analysis of mazes, maps, and diagrams; and handling of geometric forms. Left hemisphere reasoning skills also use spatial activities. For example, nurses use visual-spatial skills when solving the problem of malfunctioning intravenous lines. Visually and spatially, they see the line setup while thinking through the normal line flow in relation to stopcocks and then to the insertion site. If no external malfunctions are found, they then visualize the line from the insertion point under the skin to the catheter position and think about possible internal blocked sites.

Another example of the right and left hemispheres working together occurs when a nurse walks down the hall after leaving a person's bedside and intuitively feels that something is not right. While continuing to walk away from the room, the nurse thinks about objective data, such as no change in physical assessment findings and vital signs within the normal range, but a strong intuitive sense draws the nurse back to the bedside now to see this person in a state of cardiac arrest.

We think of emotions as right brain, but any nurse has seen how a patient in emotional pain can logically explain the character and etiology of pain. Another example is the nurse who is in pain explaining the pain logically to another person. Emotions have components of both right and left hemispheres. We go back and forth with both hemispheres in all activities, and we must learn to honor both ways of knowing. Let's now explore state-dependent learning.

STATE-DEPENDENT LEARNING

What is learned and remembered is dependent on one's psychophysiologic state at the time of the experience and is referred to as *state-dependent learning*. Our memories are state-dependent because they are dependent on and limited to the state in which they were acquired.[18] Thoughts that we experience in our daily routines are habitual patterns of state-dependent memories joined together by associative connections.

State-dependent learning plays a major role in mind-body healing and hypnosis, although most learning theories do not integrate memory and bodymind relationships. However, in his review of the state-dependent learning literature from 1855 to 1987, Rossi does connect it with discoveries of molecular biology and psychoneuroimmunology. Four integrated hypotheses can be made about the relationship of memory to bodymind relationships:[15]

1. The limbic-hypothalamic system is the major anatomic connecting link between mind and body.
2. State-dependent memory, learning, and behavior processes encoded in the limbic-hypothalamic and closely related systems are the major information transducers between mind and body.
3. All methods of mind-body healing and therapeutic hypnosis operate by gaining access to and reframing the state-dependent memory and learning systems that encode symptoms and problems.
4. The state-dependent encoding of mind-body symptoms and problems can be reached by psychologic as well as physiologic approaches—and the placebo response is a synergistic interaction of both.

Within the limbic-hypothalamic system are patterns of both positive and negative emotions. The fundamental task for each nurse is to help activate a person's psychophysiologic resources to evoke painful memories that need to be healed, along with effective coping patterns, joyful experiences, memories of health and general well-being and creative work. In gaining access to the raw material of one's inner resources, these imagery patterns can be reframed into patterns that may modulate positive changes at the biochemical levels within the cells. Let us now explore the placebo effect.

PLACEBO EFFECT

The word *placebo* is derived from the Latin word meaning "I will please." A placebo may be an inert substance that is taken in the form of medication, or it can also be a treatment, technique, or ritual. The placebo response occurs if the person improves or symptoms lessen. A person experiences a change (physical, mental, psychologic, or spiritual), although medical science cannot explain scientifically the results, other than "the natural course of the disease or symptoms."

The placebo response also is affected by one's positive or negative attitudes and emotions toward wellness and healing. Attitudes and emotions move us toward healing or in the opposite direction to the extreme of death. For example, a person may believe that touching or breathing a certain substance will cause a bad response, and indeed the "bad response" occurs. On the other hand, a person might believe that touching something before an event will cause a good response, and indeed the "good response" occurs.

Placebo medications are supposedly unable to cause electrochemical changes in the body. However, when a person gets better or symptoms disappear or lessen after a placebo medication, electrochemical changes *have* occurred within the body. When the patient receives a placebo medication or treatments with the belief that they will help, the psychoneuroimmunologic responses and the way the medication is metabolized within the body are different than if the person dreads the medication or treatment. The placebo response is evidence that a suggestion can be translated into changes at the cellular level. Each person has remarkable power and wisdom to effect bodymind changes; the challenge is to enhance this ability. One can think of the placebo as the healer that resides within. However, this innate wisdom can become blocked by negative stress, denial, or depression.

The nurse's attitude has a marked influence on drug, treatment, and expectation effectiveness. Therefore, the nurse should perform all nursing interventions with awareness of eliciting the placebo response in patients. Placebos provide pain relief and can serve as a bodymind healing factor because patients' beliefs and expectations directly influence treatments, procedures, and recovery from illness. They need to be informed about how medications work, not only for correct use and safety but also to enhance the drug effect by the placebo response. Although not clearly understood, patient faith in the medication directly influences the placebo response.

To elicit the placebo response in patients, the nurse should follow these guidelines:

- Avoid using placebos to determine if a person's pain is real or "in the person's imagination."
- Avoid using placebos to determine pain severity.
- Avoid using placebos to judge a person's personality, suggestibility, or psychopathology.
- Avoid assuming that the psychologic reactions occurring after a drug is given must be due to the drug. Side effects may be due to the placebo response.
- Avoid dispensing medication as though it were a mundane chore.

MIND MODULATION OF THE AUTONOMIC NERVOUS SYSTEM

To further understand the new information of mind modulation, the channels of bodymind communication by way of the autonomic, endocrine, immune, and neuropeptide systems are now discussed. Credit is given to Rossi for the title of mind modulation as it relates to these systems.

Mind modulates the biochemical functions within the major organ systems through the autonomic nervous system, as shown in Figure 2–2. The process of mind modulation of cel-

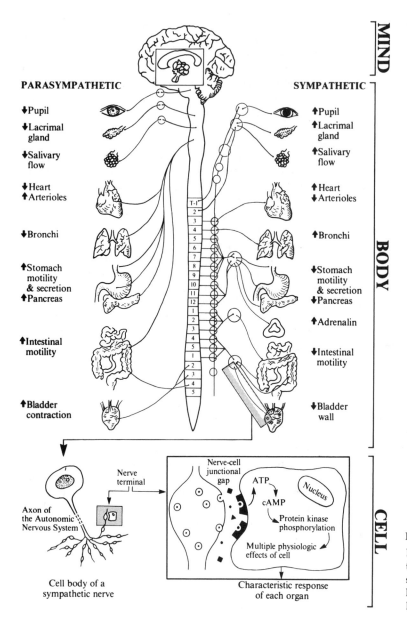

Figure 2–2

Bodymind communication. Mind modulation of the autonomic nervous system and its two approaches—the sympathetic and the parasympathetic, down to the cellular level. Rossi E. L. *The Psychobiology of Mind-Body Healing.* New York: W. W. Norton, 1986; with permission.)

lular activities by the autonomic nervous system has three stages:[17]

1. Images and thoughts are generated in the frontal cortex.
2. Images and thoughts are transmitted through the state-dependent memory learning and emotional areas of the limbic-hypothalamic system to the neurotransmitters that regulate the organs of the autonomic nervous system branches.
3. The neurotransmitters—norepinephrine (sympathetic branch) and acetylcholine (parasympathetic branch)—initiate the information transduction that activates the biochemical changes within the different tissues down to the cellular level. Neurotransmitters act as messenger molecules. They cross the nerve cell junctional gap and fit into receptors found in the cell walls, thus changing the receptor molecular structure. This causes a change in cell wall permeability and a shift of such ions as sodium, potassium, and calcium. The basic metabolism of each cell is also

changed by a series of hundreds of complex activations of cell enzymes that are the second messenger system.

These three stages give us a better understanding of how different behavioral therapies work. When patients are taught to use relaxation, imagery, music therapy, or hypnosis, their sympathetic response to stress is reduced and the calming effects of the parasympathetic systems take over.

MIND MODULATION OF THE ENDOCRINE SYSTEM

The endocrine system is responsible for the secretion of hormones and the regulation of these hormones throughout the body, as seen in Figure 2–3. Stimulation of the senses results in activation of specific hormones. Research into how hormones, sensation, and perception are integrated with thought and behavior has found that hormones released by sensory stimulation act to modulate the strength of memory of the

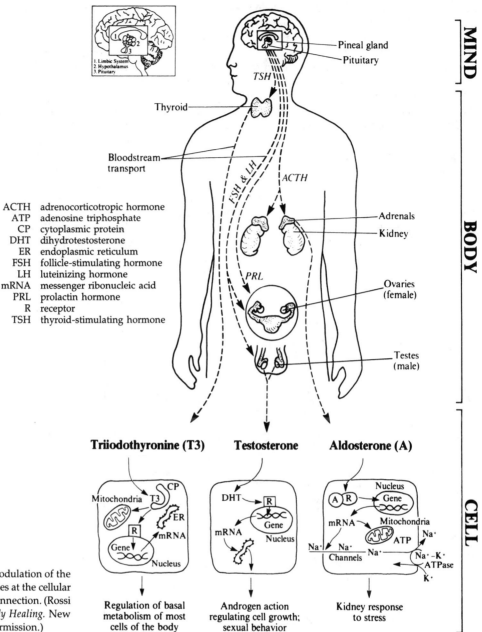

Figure 2-3
Bodymind communication. Mind modulation of the endocrine system, with three examples at the cellular level of the mind/gene/molecule connection. (Rossi E. L. *The Psychobiology of Mind-Body Healing.* New York: W. W. Norton, 1986; with permission.)

sensory experience. In addition, central modulating influences on memory in the limbic system interact with influences of the peripheral hormones.[8]

The central concept of neuroendocrinology is neurosecretion: the transduction of information of the limbic-hypothalamic system into somatic processes of the body through the pituitary and endocrine system.[16] Thoughts from the limbic system excite or inhibit the neural impulses of the cerebral cortex and are converted into pituitary regulation by the influence of the hypothalamus. This understanding is the basis for the inclusion of psychobiology as a branch of information theory.[16] This information gives scientific support to the importance of right brain hemisphere exercises that help a person tap into self-healing.

The most recent discoveries in the field of endocrinology are the pituitary hormones—endorphins and enkephalins—

that influence modulation of stress, pain, perception, addictions, appetite, learning and memory, and work and sports performance, to name a few areas.[4]

The endorphins are so new that they do not yet have a physiologic classification. The endorphin system may represent a new division of the autonomic nervous system.[10] Endorphins have been discovered throughout the body—in the brain, spinal cord, and the enteric system (gastrointestinal tract). The enteric tract, which is responsible for the internal regulation of the stomach and intestines, is considered by some researchers to be a third branch of the autonomic nervous system.[12] This may explain why people feel their emotions in their gut.

Other scientists feel that endorphins are not a branch of the autonomic system but are definitely part of the endocrine system. In support of this stance, they note that the major biosynthesis of one of the major endorphins (beta-endorphin) and enkephalins (meta-enkephalin) occurs in the same mother molecule as the adrenocorticotropic hormone (ACTH) in the anterior pituitary.[12] They are both released in response to stress and circadian and ultradian rhythms.

All of the body's major systems—the autonomic, endocrine, immune, and neuropeptide systems—are communication channels whereby the person's thoughts and images activate the genetic material and cellular structures to reorganize according to new information to help a person toward healing.

MIND MODULATION OF THE IMMUNE SYSTEM

The immune system is the third major regulatory system of the body. In the new discipline of psychoneuroimmunology, researchers investigate how the brain affects the body's immune cells. The brain sends signals along nerves to enhance defenses against infection and make the body fight more aggressively against disease. Figure 2–4 illustrates mind modulation of the immune system.

Researchers have identified actual psychophysiologic mechanisms whereby the hypothalamus can change both cellular and humoral immune activity in its anterior and posterior nuclei. Receptor sites, located on the surfaces of the T and B lymphocytes, have the ability to activate, direct, and modify immune function. They are described as being like locks (the receptors) and keys (neurotransmitters) that open and turn on the activity of each system.

None of the body systems is separate from the other, for images and stressors perceived by the person's mind are transduced to the messenger molecules—the neurotransmitters of the autonomic nervous system and the hormones of the endocrine system. Recent evidence from researchers in psychoneuroimmunology shows that there is a bidirectional in-

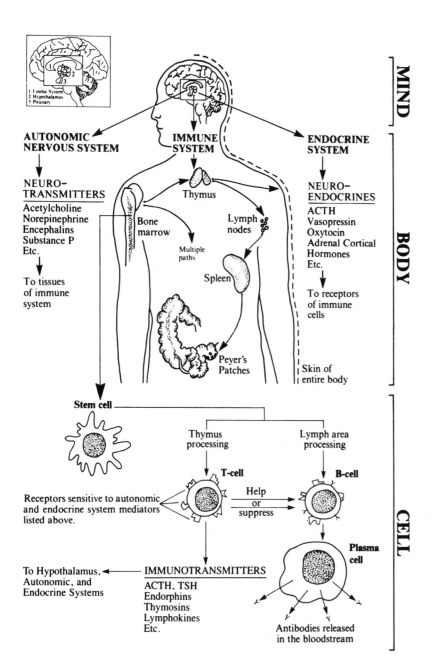

Figure 2–4

Bodymind communications. Mind modulation of the immune system by neurotransmitters of the autonomic nervous system and hormones of the endocrine system that communicate with the immune system. The immunotransmitters that communicate with these systems are shown. (Rossi E. L. *The Psychobiology of Mind-Body Healing* New York: W. W. Norton, 1986; with permission.)

formation circuitry operating between the immune system and the autonomic and endocrine systems. It is also known that the three systems can modulate the activity of each other.[12]

Six types of experimental data provide support for mind-modulating influences of the immune system:[18]

1. The neuroanatomic and neurochemical evidence for the innervation of lymphoid tissue (bone marrow, thymus, spleen, tonsils, Peyer's patches, lymph nodes, and so forth) by the central nervous system. This means that mind by way of the central nervous system has direct neural access for modulating all these organs of the immune system.
2. The observations that inhibiting or stimulating the hypothalamus changes immunologic reactivity and, conversely, that activation of an immune response in the body results in measurable changes within the hypothalamus. Because the hypothalamus is regulated by higher brain centers (through connections with the limbic cortex), these intercommunications between the immune system and hypothalamus may be open to mind modulation.
3. The finding that lymphocytes bear receptors for hormones of the endocrine system and neurotransmitters of the autonomic nervous system. Therefore, all the mind-modulating effects of the autonomic and endocrine systems may be communicated to the immune system as well. This conclusion is also supported by the next point.
4. Evidence that alterations in hormone and neurotransmitter function modify immunologic reactivity and, conversely, that elicitation of an immune response is accompanied by changes in hormonal and neurotransmitter levels.
5. Data documenting the effect of behavioral interventions, including conditioning on various parameters of immune function.
6. Experimental and clinical studies in which psychologic factors, such as stress and depression, have been found to influence the onset of disease processes.

Researchers are able to demonstrate that people can be taught to modulate the immune system with certain biobehavioral interventions. For example, persons with cancer can be taught to reframe how they imagine their cancer cells. Instead of imaging the cancer cells as strong and invading healthy body structures, they are taught to image them as weak and confused. These relaxation and imagery interventions seem to work, because they facilitate the inner healer, the innate wisdom that resides within a person. In Chapter 3, references and a detailed discussion of the imagery process are provided.

MIND MODULATION OF THE NEUROPEPTIDE SYSTEM

Neuropeptides and their receptors are one key to understanding the bodymind interconnections and how emotions are experienced throughout the body. Figure 2–5 shows focal areas of the neuropeptide communicating system.

Neuropeptides are amino acids produced in the brain, and when they lock into their receptor sites (distinct classes of recognition molecules), they can facilitate or block a response.[1] Beta-endorphin was the first neuropeptide discovered. It is called a neuropeptide because it is produced in brain nerve cells and consists of peptides. Beta-endorphins also have been found recently in the pituitary and the gonads.[12] Approximately 50 to 60 additional neuropeptides have been discovered that are as specific as beta-endorphin. These neuropeptides come directly from the body's DNA. It is now known that neuropeptides are located and circulate throughout the body. The information transfer occurs as a result of the specificity of the receptor sites found in the body.

Pert refers to the communication of the neuropeptide system as the "informational substrate."[12] The autonomic, endocrine, and immune systems, which form a complex bidirectional network of communication, are the channel carriers for the neuropeptides, the messenger molecules responsible for connecting body and emotions. The neuropeptides integrate all of these systems.

The receptor sites for the neuropeptides can be seen as the keys to the biochemistry of emotions. The limbic system regulates the emotions and the body physiology. When Pert and her team began mapping opiate receptor sites with radioactive molecules, they found that the limbic system had 40 times the number of opiate receptor sites than any other area of the brain.[10]

Traditionally, hormones were thought to be produced only by glands and not nerve cells. New mapping techniques, which locate the site of action of neuropeptides through radioactive labeling, have recently detected hormones in the brain.[19]

These new data have changed our view of the neuropeptides. Insulin was thought to be produced by the pancreas and to flow from the pancreas to specific receptor sites. Now it is known that it is also produced and stored in the brain and that insulin receptor sites are present in the brain. Angiotensin receptors are found not only in the kidney but also in the brain. The release of the neuropeptide angiotensin leads to behaviors that increase water consumption and water conservation.

Other receptor sites, called *nodal* points, have been found outside of the brain.[20] Nodal points are located in places that receive significant emotional modulation (*e.g.*, the dorsal (back) horn of the spinal cord). The dorsal horn is where sensory information comes in and is transmitted to and processed by the brain.

The cells of the immune system travel around and interact with the neuropeptides. Monocytes, the scavenger cells that ingest foreign substances, are also responsible for wound healing and tissue repair mechanisms.[2] In addition, monocytes have receptor sites for opiates and other neuropeptides. Every neuropeptide receptor located by mapping has been found on human monocytes.[12] Monocytes circulate in the body, communicating with T and B cells, identifying foreign substances, and locating areas needing repair. These monocytes not only have receptor sites but they can also make neuropeptides. This means that these monocytes make the chemicals that control mood and tissue integrity. Thus, we see the anatomy and physiology of bodymind connections.

The gut is another example of bodymind connection. The enteric nervous system operates the gastrointestinal system in a semi-independent manner. The entire tract from the esophagus to the anus is lined with cells containing neuropeptides and receptor sites. When people say that they have a "gut feeling," it can now be demonstrated that this emotion indeed resides in the gut.[12]

Currently, neuropeptide research is focused in the following six areas:[20]

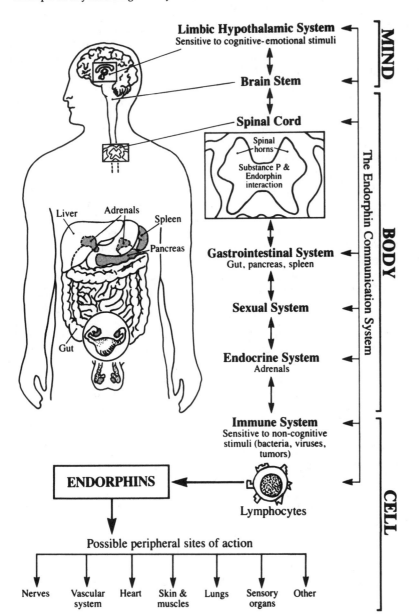

Figure 2–5

Bodymind communication. The nodal or focal areas of the neuropeptide communication system, with the endorphin neuropeptide in bodymind regulation indicated. (Rossi E. L. *The Psychobiology of Mind-Body Healing.* New York: W. W. Norton, 1986; with permission.)

1. Limbic-hypothalamic locus of neuropeptide activity
2. Brain-stem and spinal cord locus of neuropeptide activity
3. Immune integration by the neuropeptides
4. Endocrine system integration by the neuropeptides
5. Enteric nervous system and neuropeptide activity
6. Sexual system and neuropeptide activity

SUMMARY

This chapter has explored the scientific data on the psychophysiology of bodymind healing. The ideas of natural systems theory and information theory were developed as a theoretical basis for bodymind healing. Mind modulation of the autonomic, endocrine, immune, and neuropeptide systems was also developed to support the use of psychophysiologic self-regulation as nursing interventions.

DIRECTIONS FOR FUTURE RESEARCH

1. Examine the scientific basis for study of patient behavior and evaluation of nursing care specific to the stress response.
2. Investigate effective ways for nurses and patients to learn to modulate stress.
3. Evaluate learning strategies in order to teach patients how to gain access to, reframe, and use their own unique inner repertoire of psychophysiologic resources that can ultimately lead to bodymind healing.

REFERENCES

1. Achterberg, J. *Imagery in Healing.* Boston: Shambhala, 1985:48–87.

2. Achterberg, J. *Imagery in Healing.* 161–172.
3. Brody, H. The systems view of man: Implications for medicine, science, and ethics. *Perspect. Biol. Med.* 17:71–92, 1973.
4. Davis, J. *Endorphins.* New York: Dial Press, 1983:26–31.
5. Dossey, L. *Space, Time, and Medicine.* Boston: Shambhala, 1982: 98–101.
6. Dossey, L. Ancient messages in modern science. *Am. Theosophist* 70:10, 1982.
7. Lazlo, E. *The Systems View of the World.* New York: George Braziller, 1972:42–37.
8. McGaugh, Preserving the presence of the past: Hormonal influences on memory storage. *Am. Psychologist* 3:163–165, 1983.
9. Pert, C. The wisdom of the receptors: Neuropeptides, the emotions, and bodymind. *Advances* 3:8–16, 1986.
10. Pert, C. The wisdom of the receptors: Neuropeptides, the emotions, and bodymind. *Advances* 3:11, 1986.
11. Pert, C. The wisdom of the receptors: Neuropeptides, the emotions, and bodymind. *Advances* 3:12, 1986.
12. Pert, C. The wisdom of the receptors: Neuropeptides, the emotions, and bodymind. *Advances* 3:14, 1986.
13. Pert, C. The wisdom of the receptors: Neuropeptides, the emotions, and bodymind. *Advances* 3:16, 1986.
14. Rossi, E. *The Psychobiology of Mind-Body Healing.* New York: W. W. Norton, 1986:36–37.
15. Rossi, E. *The Psychophysiology of Mind-Body Healing.* New York: W.W. Norton, 1986:55.
16. Rossi, E. *The Psychobiology of Mind-Body Healing.* New York: W.W. Norton, 1986:104.
17. Rossi, E. *The Psychobiology of Mind-Body Healing.* New York: W.W. Norton, 1986:107.
18. Rossi, E. *The Psychobiology of Mind-Body Healing.* New York: W.W. Norton, 1986:153–154.
19. Rossi, E. *The Psychobiology of Mind-Body Healing.* New York: W.W. Norton, 1986:182.
20. Rossi, E. *The Psychobiology of Mind-Body Healing.* New York: W.W. Norton, 1986:183–189.

3

Psychophysiologic Self-Regulation Interventions

Barbara Montgomery Dossey

BODY-ORIENTED THERAPIES ARE NOT ENOUGH

A rapidly accumulating body of knowledge supports the link between emotions and illness and points away from a purely mechanistic model of how human beings function. The mind not only can play a negative role but also has the potential to affect our health, illness, and healing in a positive and powerful manner.

If we are finally ready to look at the "facts" that have become abundant in the literature, we collide with the implications. We are struck with the realization that body illnesses can no longer be treated exclusively by body-oriented therapies. We must begin to emphasize mind-oriented therapies if we hope to facilitate complete and effective healing in our patients. It must be emphasized that the holistic focus insists that we supplement—but not supplant—modern technomedical therapies with something more.

Incorporating relaxation techniques, music therapy, imagery, and biofeedback into practice provides the nurse with interventions needed to care for the whole patient. Such self-regulation techniques enlarge the nurse's options for effective therapy and can produce results as real as those produced by traditional forms of therapy. Holistic self-regulation therapies are used to treat the anxiety, stress, and pain inherent in acute and chronic body illnesses. They are used to establish a sense of balance and control in one's emotional status, which in turn directly affects the physiologic status.

Yet, patients frequently do not know how to activate the healing potential within their own body-mind-spirit. Nurses have the ability, however, to assist patients in activating this process. Our challenge is to help them understand that body and mind are connected and that mind therapies, used in conjunction with traditional medical therapies, can intensify the healing process.

LEARNING OBJECTIVES

After reading this chapter, the nurse should be able to do the following:

1. Define three psychophysiologic self-regulation strategies—relaxation, imagery, and music therapy.
2. Identify patient outcome, outcome criteria, and evaluation for use of self-regulation strategies in critical care.
3. List the steps for establishing an audiocassette library in critical care.

CONNECTING BODY-MIND-SPIRIT

Anxiety, fear, the phenomenon of pain, and matters of life and death in critical care are complex experiences for critically ill patients and their families. Events that occur with acute illness and within the highly technologic critical care environment can evoke every possible emotion. Often patients in critical care have difficulty communicating their fear and pain, which aggravates their already compromised state. Although there is a wealth of literature about anxiety, fear, and pain mechanisms of the critically ill patient, there has been limited use of self-regulation interventions for the critically ill patient and their families.

Self-regulation strategies can evoke a positive psychophysiologic response that enhances the mind's modulation of all body systems—autonomic, endocrine, immune, and neuropeptide.[8,11,16] These interventions, which can be used in all phases of critical care and with all patients, can be reinforced on all shifts, allowing patients to be involved actively in the healing process. These skills can also be taught to families and friends to break their tension and anxiety cycle, particularly for those who keep long hours in the family waiting rooms. The result is a feeling of being more in control along with relief of pain, anxiety, and fear.

Frequently, in critical care situations, patients and families want specific answers about the course of events. However, there may be no exact answers but rather a "wait and see" situation, which may contribute to already high levels of anxiety, fear, powerlessness, or pain. Critical care nurses can help patients and families significantly reduce these states by teaching and integrating self-regulation interventions into clinical practice. Critical care nurses have the unique opportunity of being present to guide patients and families through major life stressors and emotional upheaval.

The specific knowledge base for self-regulation interventions such as relaxation, imagery, and music therapy for use with critically ill patients and their families will be explored. As discussed in Chapter 2, anxiety, fear, and the patient's perceived meaning about an illness are potent stimulators of the sympathetic nervous system. Thus, self-regulation interventions are *to be used in conjunction* with technologic modalities after assessment. To treat a patient who has decreased blood flow to an injured extremity with just a relaxation exercise or to treat a patient with severe pain accompanying an evolving acute infarction with only an imagery exercise is unacceptable, dangerous, and unethical.

There is much confusion about self-regulation interventions. Health and illness involves the mind as well as the body. It is not uncommon to hear a person say, "If I had the right image, knew the right relaxation exercise, or had the right relationship, I would not have become ill." This attitude is not desirable. Such thinking allows a sense of shame and guilt to occur and leaves a person with a feeling of hopelessness. What is most needed is a balanced approach when illness arises.

RELAXATION

Relaxation is a psychophysiologic state characterized by parasympathetic dominance that is achieved by specific strategies to evoke the relaxation response (RR). The relaxation response is an alert hypometabolic state of decrease sympathetic nervous system arousal in which one feels a sense of calmness.[4] Visual cues to relaxation are seen in Table 3–1.

The process of psychophysiologic self-regulation (PPSR) has three parts: body and inner self-awareness, relaxation and imagery skills, and making effective choices.

When these skills are learned, they allow one to experience the following:[12]

- An inward focus of attention
- Awareness of altered perceptions of linear time—past, present, and future
- Ability to cease judging events as good or bad
- Control of one's state of awareness
- A relaxed inner calmness that may or may not be goal-directed
- A merging of awareness and conscious activity as a unit

Relaxation training allows one to achieve the relaxation response, which has the following benefits[12]:

- Decreases the anxiety associated with strange environments and stressful or painful situations
- Increases the effect of pain medications
- Helps the patient dissociate from pain
- Decreases fatigue by interrupting the fight-or-flight response
- Eases the muscle tension of skeletal contractions
- Increases relaxed breathing to replace shallow breaths that result from anxiety and fear
- Provides periods of rest that are as beneficial as a nap
- Decreases heart rate, blood pressure, and respirations
- Sends healing messages to the autonomic, endocrine, immune, and neuropeptide systems

In critical care, the nurse can provide time for the patient to experience relaxation. The patient can be guided individually by the nurse in relaxation exercises, or a tape recorder and earphones can be provided with specific relaxation tapes for the patient to listen to throughout the day or night. Specific guidelines for use of relaxation tapes are seen in Table 3–2.

The relaxation interventions that can be used successfully in critical care are as follows:

- *Autogenic training:* The repetitive use of phrases to bring about desired states in the body (*e.g.*, "Heaviness and warmth are flowing through my body")
- *Biofeedback:* Specific instrumentation to mirror psychophysiologic processes of which the patient is not normally aware; may be helpful for weaning patients from ventilators[3]
- *Body scanning:* Focusing on various body parts to detect levels of accumulated tension
- *Progressive muscle relaxation:* The process of alternately tensing and releasing different muscle groups to become aware of subtle muscle tension

---

Table 3–1

Visual Cues to Relaxation

A change in breathing pattern: slower, deeper breaths progressing to slow, somewhat shallower
     breathing as relaxation deepens
More audible breathing
Fluttering of eyelids
Blanching of the skin around the nose and mouth
Easing of jaw tightness, sometimes to the extent that the lips part and jaw drops slightly
If patient is supine, toes point outward, rather than straight up
Complete lack of muscle holding—ask patient's permission to lift arm gently by the wrist: you should
     feel no resistance, and arm should move as easily as any other object of similar weight.

(Dossey, B., Keegan, L., Guzzetta, C., *et al. Holistic Nursing: A Handbook for Practice.* Rockville, MD: Aspen, 1988; with permission.)

Table 3–2
Guidelines for the Use of Relaxation Tapes

Listen to an exercise at least once a day and preferably twice a day.
Never listen to a tape when you are driving or doing any other activity.
Arrange to have uninterrupted privacy while you listen to your tape.
Listen with headphones to help block out distracting noises from the environment.
Listen to your tape in a relaxing position, one in which you will not have to support your body.

(Dossey, B., Keegan, L., Guzzetta, C., *et al. Holistic Nursing: A Handbook for Practice.* Rockville, MD: Aspen, 1988; with permission.)

- *Relaxation response:* Repeating a chosen word (mantra), phrase, or prayer silently or aloud as a focusing device to decrease pain, tension, anxiety, or fear
- *Self-hypnosis:* Self-talk that voluntarily places a person in control to change the perception of time, memory, or sensations
- *Deep-breathing relaxation exercises:* Focusing on the breath to release tension, pain, and anxiety

Relaxation strategies empower patients to be in control of a situation. Miller reported on use of deep breathing with patients in the immediate postoperative period after cardiac surgery. As a result of relaxation, significant decreases were demonstrated in blood pressure, heart rate, respiratory rate, and report of pain on the visual descriptor scale. All the experimental subjects stated that the relaxation technique was simple to perform and that they would recommend it to others who have postoperative pain.[14]

IMAGERY

Imagery can be defined as the internal experiences of memories, dreams, fantasies, and visions. It may involve all of the senses and be thought of as the hypothetical bridge between the conscious processing of information and physiologic change.[1,8] Images can exert influence over the voluntary (peripheral) as well as the involuntary (autonomic) nervous system. The goal of the imagery process is for the patient to create concrete, symbolic, process, end-state, and general healing images, which are discussed in the next section, and to reach one's potential, which directly evokes positive psychophysiologic responses.

What frequently occurs in the imagination of the critical care patient is negative imagery. It seems that the more critically ill a patient is, the more negative the imagery, and often the images contain erroneous information. By using imagery, the nurse can help patients change their perceptions about their disease, treatment, and healing abilities. Thus, the patient is able to decrease the stress, anxiety, and fear that can lead to a devastating spiral of hopelessness.

A person can have only one conscious thought at any one time. As the nurse educates the patient about the healing process, erroneous or weak images can be redirected, strengthening the patient's own body systems and normal mechanisms. To individualize the imagery process for a particular patient, the nurse must have a fundamental knowledge of the physiology involved in the disease or disability; know the interaction of all treatments, such as medication, tests, and surgery, that affect the patient's psychophysiologic state; and understand the patient's belief systems. When teaching occurs, the imagery process can be incorporated with useful teaching sheets, as seen in Case Studies 1 and 2 at the end of this chapter.

Types of Imagery

Each patient's imagery process is unique. In order to achieve the most effective results with this intervention, it is helpful to focus on the types of images and the process that evolve with each type as seen in Table 3–3. First of all, a patient can be helped to use the imagination to evoke positive psychophysiologic outcomes. It also helps to combine general relaxation interventions and music to enhance the imagery process. Patients are becoming increasingly aware that they can be taught to use their own healing resources to aid in recovery from illness.

The nurse can guide the patient with the following format:[2]

Table 3–3
Types of Imagery

RECEPTIVE VERSUS ACTIVE IMAGERY	
Receptive	"Bubbles up": "as if" one received images Go inward: Listen to bodymind
Active	Conscious formation of image Direct image: body area or activity that requires attention

CONCRETE VERSUS SYMBOLIC IMAGERY	
Concrete	Real life: under the microscope Biologic correctness
Symbolic	Metamorphosis: personal energy of a person Can't be forced

PROCESS, END-STATE, AND GENERAL HEALING IMAGES	
Process	Step-by-step goal to be achieved Mechanics of biologic correct images
End State	Image final healed state to follow process imagery
General Healing	An event, healing light, forgiveness, inner guide/advisor

PACKAGED VERSUS CUSTOMIZED IMAGERY	
Packaged	Commercial tapes that have general images
Customized	Images that bubble up Become personalized by a person

(Achterberg, J., Dossey, B., and Kolkmeier, L. *Rituals of Healing.* New York: Bantam, 1992; with permission.)

- Identify the problem or disease or goal of imagery.
- Begin with several minutes of relaxing by attention to rhythmic breathing or general relaxation interventions discussed under relaxation.
- Develop images of the following:
  The problem or disease
  Inner healing resources
  External healing resources (treatments)
- End with images of final, desired state of well-being.

For best results when dealing with life-threatening disease, the patient should be encouraged to use imagery skills 20 minutes two to three times a day. As simple as the following format appears, it requires focused concentration. Thus, the nurse must assess each patient to determine to what degree the imagery process can be understood and integrated with varying levels of consciousness due to physiologic/trauma alterations, anxiety, and pain medication. Table 3–3 lists the different types of imagery.

Receptive Versus Active Imagery

In *receptive imagery*, images seem to "bubble up" into conscious thought.[2] The experience with these images is as if they have been received. This type of imagery is common when daydreaming and falling asleep. A simple example is to let images come as you think about frequent areas of body tension such as the back of the neck or shoulders. Let an experience just "bubble up." Which of your senses is dominant? Common feelings in this area are tingling, tightness, or warmth. Remember that imagery involves all the senses and provides remarkable messages about the state of the bodymind frequently throughout the day.

Active imagery is the conscious formation of an image.[2] Attend to the image as it comes from the area of the neck or shoulders. As you focus or concentrate on these areas, common images are knots in muscles, or grinding or popping of muscles. Whatever images or feelings emerge, you can consciously send a message (*i.e.*, "literally speak to a body part") by responding with images that come from your senses, such as seeing smooth muscles or feeling the release of tension.

Concrete Versus Symbolic Imagery

Concrete images are analogous to viewing images as they appear under a microscope.[2] In the last example, if one focused long enough on tight muscles, images of tight muscles might appear. In working with imagery, it is important to help patients image with correct biologic images. For example, when cancer is present, the immune system is underactive, and when autoimmune problems (rheumatoid arthritis or allergies) are present, the immune system is overactive. Thus, when teaching these two groups of patients about biologic correctness, the patient education and teaching sheets about the healing imagery process are vastly different. Emphasis on correct use of our natural imagery process cannot be over emphasized. As discussed in Chapter 2, we communicate with the body by our images. Our images and their associated thoughts get transduced by state-dependent memory to the body through the neurotransmitters of our body systems. There are many ways to teach about biologic correctness such as from drug ads, anatomy coloring books, or education information pamplets from professional organizations about specific diseases, (American Heart Association, American Lung Association, and so forth).

Symbolic imagery is an evolving process that cannot be forced.[2] As a patient becomes involved in the process, his or her inner wisdom releases symbolic images that have healing qualities. These images come from a patient's attitudes, belief systems, and cultural experiences. Each patient's symbolic images are unique. An example of symbolic imagery is a man with cancer who lets images unique to him and his life emerge. He saw his mind as a huge computer, his bodymind communication center, with files containing programs to turn on his immune system. He chose his different computer programs to turn on his T cells and B cells to fight against his cancer.

The nurse is present to help guide the patient in deepening the relaxation response, which allows the patient to free up this inner knowledge. Both concrete and symbolic images are helpful. Symbolic images are more powerful because a person is more involved in the process and, thus, more symbolism.

Process, End-State, and General Healing Images

Process imagery is the step-by-step biologic healing process.[2] For example, in teaching a patient about bone healing after a traumatic fracture, it would be the evolution of the bone-healing process from hematoma formation to redeposition of bone over weeks. This is developed in Case Study I (p. 37) along with a teaching sheet to help patients with the imagery process.

End-state images involve imaging the final, healed state in whatever way is appropriate.[2] To use the preceding example, an end-state image after a fracture would be for a person to image walking strong, returning to running, and feeling the leg strong and being free of pain.

General healing images involve an event rather than a process.[2] An example would be to experience being bathed with relaxation, warmth, or coolness. Another example might be for sound or color to penetrate one's being. General healing images also may come in experiences of God, or an inner guide—a wise person, animal, or totem, or rhythmic images such as an old man or lady walking toward the person. The best general images are those that emerge for each person that have the personal healing significance. As the patient invests time in the imagery process, the power of the process increases.

Packaged Versus Customized Imagery

Packaged imagery involves listening to or using someone else's images from books.[2] All purchased tapes on self-hypnosis, relaxation, and imagery are in this category. These tapes can be very helpful as general guides to begin the learning process. Nurses must begin to establish an audiocassette library on each nursing unit, because patients can be guided in this experience when a nurse cannot be present (see Table 3-6).

Customized imagery are images that are unique to a person, those images that seem to have "bubbled up."[2] For example, a patient evolving images to aid in cancer therapy might see white blood cells as thousands of strong angels full of energy, whereas another patient might see white blood cells as large barbed hooks that attack the cancer cells.

The most important message is that each patient must be the interpreter of the images. It is very important for the nurse to investigate patient's feelings and perceptions about the illness and hospitalization. These factors create each patient's unique images. The nurse must recognize when the patient's disease is more powerful than the patient's own internal and external healing resources. When patients recognize the negative imagery process that is invading their life, it frequently is the turning point for mobilizing their innate healing ability.

Even when the patient will not return to health and chooses to move toward death, the same process is used. Imagery can have profound power by assisting in the peaceful release of this life at the appropriate time. Patients then can begin to move toward death. What seems to happen is that the patient releases the ego; there is a stepping aside and participation in the pure experience of fear and release. There is no "ego" or "observer." There is only the present reality of pure experience.[2]

Empowering Relaxation, Imagery, and Music Scripts*

For more effective delivery of the spoken word in different imagery scripts, consider the following techniques. The reader can refer to this section when reading Case Studies 1 and 2, because examples of these techniques are given in the Case Study scripts. When used correctly, these techniques satisfy both brain hemispheres[15]:

- Truism
- Embedded commands
- Linkage
- Reframing
- Metaphor
- Therapeutic double-bind
- Synesthesia
- Interspersal technique

A *truism* is a statement that the patient believes or accepts to be true. It may precede a suggestion and be connected to another truism. When this occurs, the analytic left hemisphere is satisfied that a fact is logical. It does not analyze or negate, and it leaves the right hemisphere free to accept the suggestion.

Consider this example for use with a person learning relaxation and imagery for hypertension:

As you take your next breath in, become aware of the fact that you are breathing air into your lungs (truism) and the oxygen from that breath moves from your lungs into your bloodstream (truism), . . . You can let yourself imagine that your blood vessels are very relaxed at this time as you continue into this deep state of relaxation.

The suggestion "to let yourself imagine" is preceded by two truisms: that you are breathing air into your lungs, and that the breath moves from your lungs into your bloodstream. The truisms are followed by suggestions of hoped-for physiologic changes of relaxed blood vessels while the person is in a deep state of relaxation. The left hemisphere is occupied with the truism and leaves the right hemisphere free to go with the suggestions of deep relaxation and to feel what is present when the blood vessels relax.

* (Peterson, G. and Mehl, L. *Pregnancy as Healing: A Holistic Philosophy for Prenatal Care.* Berkeley, CA: Mindbody Communications, 1984)

Embedded commands are separate messages for the right hemisphere. They are usually in short phrases that stand out because of pauses. The guide also uses a change in intonation, such as pitch, volume, speed, and textural quality of the voice, and a change in normal grammatical structure. This confuses the left hemisphere and causes the embedded command to stand out. When a person's name is also used, the right hemisphere may comprehend the short message much easier.

An example would be: "You don't have to . . . Susan, cry, . . . if you don't want to." When using (1) changes in the quality of the voice, (2) pauses, and (3) calling the person by name, the right hemisphere will hear the suggestion, "Susan, cry," in one or all three of the ways listed.

Linkages are conditional statements that connect behaviors or actions with a suggestion. Linkages are best used with a truism as a distraction to satisfy the left hemisphere.

A linkage could be used with a person lying flat on a stretcher who is about to undergo a cardiac catheterization. The nurse would say, "Let yourself relax into the surface under your body. As you are moving down the hall, you will see overhead lights on the ceiling. Each time you pass under a light, let it remind you to take a deep breath and relax more deeply."

Reframing is a technique to help a person contact the part of a behavior that is keeping him or her stuck or that is preventing a certain behavior from occurring. Reframing suspends a person from the old or current belief systems. It allows the opportunity to reassociate and reorganize a problem or experience in a manner that resolves it toward a healthier state. Instead of "I'll never get well" reframe it to "I'm stronger moment by moment."

A *metaphor* is a figure of speech containing an implied comparison, in which a word or phrase ordinarily and primarily used for one thing is applied to another. Metaphor is used in imagery scripts for healing and teaching purposes. Metaphor works because the right brain can deepen the experience to the spoken word. For example, "Imagine the relaxation flowing down through your body like a gentle warm waterfall." Such words as warming, cooling, releasing, and sinking can be expanded on to enhance right-brain activity.

The *therapeutic double-bind* is effective because the left hemisphere is occupied and involved in making several different choices that lead to participation in the given suggestion. For example, "As you are stretched out in the chair, you might find that you could change your position even more to go deeper into relaxation, and get more comfortable until you find just the right position."

Synesthesia is the technique of cross-sensing several of the senses simultaneously so that the person becomes more aware of the different sense modalities that are present. For example, "Can you hear the color of the wind." or "Can you see the sounds around you?"

Interspersal is a technique of making specific words or phrases within a script stand out as a separate suggestion. This is accomplished by changing the volume or tone of the voice more dramatically than with embedded commands. An example might be, "Allow yourself to . . . relax into the pain with the next breath . . . feel . . . as you . . . breathe into the pain.

Drawing Images

Drawing is also an intervention that can be used in critical care. After a relaxation and guided imagery exercise, the nurse can provide paper and crayons. When using drawing as an intervention, the nurse can suggest to the patient the following:

- Allow yourself to draw ideas that have realistic or symbolic meaning to you about your healing.
- Choose colors that reflect the healing process.
- Do not judge the drawing but let it be an expression of the present moment and your insight about healing.
- Notice your self-talk because it is constant.

Often what is revealed is negative imaging or how one blocks one's natural ability to move toward healing. The nurse can help the patient become aware that the drawing should reflect process or end-state images of healing.

The nurse should identify the following elements:

- *Disease or disability:* the vividness of the patient's views of disease, illness, or disability
- *Internal healing resources:* the vividness of how the patient perceives the healing ability and its effectiveness in combating the disease
- *External healing resources:* the vividness of the treatment description and the effectiveness of some positive mechanism of action

MUSIC THERAPY

Music therapy is defined as a behavioral science that uses specific types of music to affect physiology, emotions, and behavior to lead toward healing.[9] Music can be an important nursing intervention that enhances the relaxation response and positive imagery states. A recent experimental study has demonstrated the effectiveness of music therapy and relaxation interventions in reducing the psychophysiologic stress of patients in a coronary care unit.[10] The relaxation and music groups participated in three sessions over a 2-day period and were compared with controls. Patients' stress was evaluated by apical heart rate, peripheral temperatures, cardiac complications, and qualitative patient evaluation data. Those patients in the relaxation and music therapy group had decreased apical heart rates and increased peripheral skin temperatures as well as a lowered incidence of cardiac complications. The results of this study indicated that relaxation and music therapy are effective modalities to reduce stress in coronary care unit patients.

Table 3–4 lists ways to evaluate your response to music. Table 3–5 gives guidelines for evaluation of the patient's subjective experience with music therapy.

In theory, music vibrations can help restore regulatory function to the body and mind of the patient under stress and help maintain and enhance the modulation of autonomic, endocrine, immune, and neuropeptide systems.

When the patient chooses music that has individual appeal, it is a vehicle to transcend ordinary states of awareness and attain a shifting perception of time. People perceive time in two ways: virtual and experiential.[9] Virtual time is the left-brain mode of logically processing hours, minutes, and seconds. Experiential time is perceived by the memory and has the potential of transcending ordinary states of awareness.

Music brings about experiential time because a state of tension and resolution occurs. Tension and resolution are perceived by memory in a linear sequence expressed as an event or resolution. The perception of time is influenced by the speed of these linear sequences. Slow, relaxing music lengthens the perception of time because memory has more time to experience the events (tension and resolution) and the spaces between the events. With increased relaxation, sensory thresholds are lowered, and the patient has an expanded awareness state that is dominant.[9] This dominant state allows time for relaxation states and creates an end-result image of healing that enhances positive psychophysiologic responses.

Music will enhance different mood and physiologic responses, depending on one's state at the time the music is heard. It is important to be aware of the isoprinciple when using music.[5,6] The *isoprinciple* means that music is matched to the person's mood. In critical care, however the aim is not to match the mood, for it is often one of anxiety, fear, or hopelessness. What is to be matched is a vision of what is to be achieved, such as increased relaxation, healing, or peaceful death. With the therapeutic use of music different anxiety

Table 3-4
Evaluating Your Response to Music

1. Set aside 20 minutes of relaxation time.
2. Find a comfortable position.
3. Find a quiet place where you will not be interrupted.
4. Check your pulse rate.
5. Observe your breathing pattern (fast, slow, normal).
6. Assess your muscular tension (pain, muscle tightness, shoulder stiffness, jaw and neck tension). Are you loose, limp, sleepy?
7. Evaluate your mood state (angry, happy, sad).
8. Listen to the music for 20 minutes. Let your body respond to the music as it wishes: loosen muscles, lie down, dance, clap, hum.
9. Following the session, assess your breathing pattern.
10. Assess your muscular tension (more relaxed? more stimulated? tighter? tenser? calm?).
11. Evaluate your mood state.
12. Record the name of the music selection and your before-and-after responses in a music notebook for use when developing your own therapeutic tapes.
13. On a separate page in your notebook, recall and write down the many ways that music has empowered your life psychologically, physically, and spiritually. Include your most dramatic, intimate, and emotional memories associated with music. You will begin to realize the importance of sound in your life and recognize its healing potential.

(Dossey, B., Keegan, L., Guzzetta, C., *et al. Holistic Nursing: A Handbook for Practice.* Rockville, MD: Aspen, 1988; with permission.)

Table 3-5
Evaluation of the Patient's Subjective Experience with Music Therapy

Was this a new kind of music listening experience for you? Can you describe it?
Did you have any visual experiences? Of people, places, or objects? Can you describe them?
Did you see any colors while listening? Did the color change as the music changed?
Were you less aware of your surroundings? Were you able to concentrate on the music?
Did you like the music?
Did the music produce any feelings or emotions?
Did you notice any textures, smells, movements, or taste while experiencing the music?
Was the experience pleasant?
Did you feel relaxed and refreshed after the experience?
Would you like to try this again?
What would be helpful to make this a better experience for you?

(Dossey, B., Keegan, L., Guzzetta, C., *et al. Holistic Nursing: A Handbook for Practice.* Rockville, MD: Aspen, 1988; with permission.)

states shift because the music allows the body and mind to resonate with the vibrations of the music, thus releasing the psychophysiologic tension.

Patients should choose their music. Table 3–6 gives steps for establishing an audiocassette library. Selection is important, and a variety of music should be available. What one person will find relaxing may make another tense. A variety of musical selections might include easy listening, jazz, semiclassical, classical, operatic, folk, choral, new age, and popular. It is better to have music without words so that people can concentrate on the flow of the music rather than the message of the words.[9]

NURSING PROCESS

ASSESSMENT

In using relaxation, imagery, and music, nurses should assess the following patient parameters:

- Anxiety and tension levels, fear, boredom, pain, and the need to relax
- Knowledge, presence of relaxation skills, or past experience with the interventions
- Interest in learning ways to decrease anxiety states
- Comfort level—empty bladder and relaxed position, comfortable room temperature, indirect lights, and quiet environment when possible
- Patient's perceptions about reality and locus of control; beliefs about healing ability
- Ability of patient to work with eyes closed to help establish states of internal awareness and achieve relaxation and imagery states faster. If patients are reluctant or resistant to close their eyes, have them gaze at a fixed point about 3 or 4 feet in front of them. Their peripheral vision will blur, and their eyelids will usually get heavy, which allows them to experience this natural phenomenon of relaxation.
- Possibility of 15 to 20 minutes of uninterrupted time; note on door stating "Relaxation session in progress"
- The dominant imagery patterns (positive and negative im-

Table 3-6
Establishing an Audiocassette Library

TAPES AND RECORDERS	TAPE/RECORDER/HEADSET CHECK-OUT PROCEDURE
Have several tape recorders with comfortable headsets per unit. Place all equipment in a safe and convenient location. Have a variety of music tapes available. Commercial tapes are relatively inexpensive and readily available. A complete tape library will include music, relaxation, imagery, stress management tapes, and specific tapes for smoking cessation, pre- and postsurgery, weight reduction, pain management, insomnia, self-esteem, subliminal learning, etc. Consider different types of music, such as easy listening, light and heavy classical, popular, jazz, hymns, choral, and nontraditional selections. Ask staff members to donate one favorite tape to the library. Write the different tape companies listed in the Resource list, and request their tape selections and descriptions. Encourage nurses to develop tapes for specific client/patient problems that can help with procedures, tests, and treatments. The tapes may or may not have soothing background music. Have brochures and catalogues of recording companies available upon request from the patient. Encourage use of different tapes for further relaxation, imagery, and stress management training.	If tapes are checked out by the patient's family, have the person make a deposit for the tape. It is suggested that the deposit cover the cost of the tape in case it is not returned. Establish who will have authority to check out the tapes and recorder. If in the hospital, a volunteer could assist in checking out the equipment for the patient after the nurse has assessed the patient's needs and selected the appropriate tape. Prepare a sign-out log that records the patient's name, room, date, and check-out time. Instruct the patient in the use of the recorder and specific tapes if required. Allow 20 to 30 minutes of listening without interruption twice a day. Place a sign on the patient's door stating, "Session in Progress—Do Not Disturb." Following the listening session, evaluate the patient's response to the tape and answer any questions. Chart the patient's specific response to tape(s). For example, were the desired outcomes achieved, *e.g.,* lowered respiratory rate, decreased heart rate and blood pressure, decreased muscle tension and anxiety? Identify the patient's subjective evaluation, *e.g.,* found the experience relaxing, helped with sleep, assisted in coping with pain, assisted with painful procedure, etc. Return the tape/recorder/headset to the library, and record the check-in information in the log.

(Dossey, B., Keegan, L., Guzzetta, C., *et al. Holistic Nursing: A Handbook for Practice.* Rockville, MD: Aspen, 1988; with permission.)

ages about healing) surrounding the acute situation; recognition of negative images and how positive images direct psychophysiologic energy toward healing
- Patient's understanding that it is not necessary to hear, see, feel, touch, and taste literally when working with guided imagery, only to experience what the image might be like
- Patient's understanding that imagery is basically a way we talk to ourselves and make friends with our body systems; a safe, normal phenomenon that varies with each person
- Patient's awareness of imagery to enhance healing
- Patient's primary sensory modality to be used in the guided imagery process. If the dominant modality is seeing, the nurse uses such phrases as "In your mind's eye see the healing occur."
- Imagery to be used in scripts as related to desires, wants, needs, and current events
- Patient's experience with the imagery process. If the patient is a beginner, it is best to start with beginning images such as a relaxed scene or feeling. Creative cues help patients release and tap into internal information that is not normally accessible in ordinary states of consciousness.
- Music history and types of music preferred; music that evokes joy, excitement, sadness, or relaxation. If the patient is unconscious, the family should be asked about the patient's musical preference.
- Past history of using music to evoke relaxation and imagery
- Patient's mood (isoprinciple), which may determine the type of music selected

NURSING DIAGNOSES

After the assessment, the nurse should establish diagnoses that are related to the nine human response patterns described in Chapter 5. Frequent nursing diagnoses compatible with relaxation, imagery, and music interventions in critical care are as follows:

- *Exchanging:* All interventions can be used with all diagnoses in this category.
- *Communicating:* impaired verbal communication pattern
- *Relating:* social isolation
- *Valuing:* spiritual distress
- *Choosing:* ineffective coping, impaired adjustment; noncompliance, ineffective denial, decisional conflict
- *Moving:* activity intolerance, diversional activity deficit, sleep pattern disturbance, fatigue
- *Perceiving:* body image disturbance, self-esteem disturbance, hopelessness, powerlessness, sensory/perceptual alteration
- *Knowing:* altered thought process, knowledge deficit
- *Feeling:* pain, grieving, anxiety

PATIENT OUTCOMES

Patient outcomes, outcome criteria, and evaluation for relaxation, imagery, and music interventions are listed in Tables 3–7, 3–8, and 3–9.

PLAN AND INTERVENTION

- Explain briefly the benefits of each intervention that is to be used: relaxation, imagery, or music.
- Establish the goals to be accomplished with the interventions.
- Explain the "letting go" feeling that will be experienced: total body/muscle relaxation; change in breathing patterns; increased warmth or heaviness or lightness of different body parts; change in perception of time.

Table 3-7
Nursing Intervention: Relaxation

PATIENT OUTCOMES	OUTCOME CRITERIA	EVALUATION
1. The patient will demonstrate a decrease in anxiety, tension, and other manifestations of the stress response as a result of the relaxation intervention.	1. The patient will exhibit decreased anxiety, tension, and other manifestations of the stress response as evidenced by the following: a. Heart rate within normal limits b. Decreased respiratory rate c. Increased tidal volume d. Return of blood pressure toward normal e. Resolution of anxious behaviors, such as anxious facial expressions and mannerisms, repetitious talking or behavior, inability to sleep, restlessness, or expressed anxiety	1. The patient exhibited decreased anxiety, tension, and other manifestations of the stress response as evidenced by normal vital signs; a slow, deep breathing pattern; and decreased anxious behaviors.
2. The patient will demonstrate a stabilization or decrease in pain as a result of the relaxation intervention.	2. The patient will demonstrate a decrease in pain as evidenced by the following: a. Reduction or elimination of pain control medication b. Increase in activities or mobility	2. Patient intake of pain medication stabilized and then decreased with relaxation skills practice. Patient began to participate in activities previously limited by pain.
3. The patient will link breathing awareness to a commonly occurring cue and use this combination to reduce tension.	3. The patient will become aware of breathing patterns and habitually link relaxing breathing to a cue in the environment.	3. Patient uses turning in bed as a cue to take a slow, deep breath and relax jaw muscles.

(Dossey, B., Keegan, L., Guzzetta, C., *et al. Holistic Nursing: A Handbook for Practice.* Rockville, MD: Aspen, 1988; with permission.)

Table 3-8
Nursing Intervention: Imagery

PATIENT OUTCOME	OUTCOME CRITERIA	EVALUATION
The patient will demonstrate skills in imagery.	1. The patient will participate in imagery to learn basic skills.	1. The patient practiced imagery and reported learning basic skills.
	2. Following the imagery experience the patient will do the following: a. Exhibit decreased anxiety and fear b. Demonstrate increased effective individual coping c. Demonstrate increased personal power over daily events d. Image strengths that move toward an effective life-style e. Change image of self-defeating life-style habits f. Recognize images that are created by self-talk g. Create end-state images of desired health, habits, feelings, wants, and needs in daily living	2. The patient did the following: a. Reported a decrease in anxiety and fear b. Demonstrated increased effective individual coping with life events c. Demonstrated increased personal power over daily events d. Imaged strengths that moved toward an effective life-style e. Changed image of self-defeating life-style behavior f. Recognized images that were created by self-talk g. Created end-state images of desired habits, feelings, wants, and needs for daily living
	3. The patient will participate in drawing of symptoms and free drawing as appropriate.	3. The patient participated in drawing of symptoms and free drawing as appropriate.
	4. The patient will do the following: a. Demonstrate understanding of drawing as a form of communication with self and symptoms b. Choose colors that have personal meaning c. Express imagery drawing that has special meaning d. Allow drawing to be done in a nonjudgmental manner	4. The patient did the following: a. Demonstrated understanding of drawing as a form of communicating with self and symptoms b. Chose colors that had personal meaning c. Expressed images that had special meaning d. Allowed drawing to be done in a nonjudgmental manner

(Dossey, B., Keegan, L., Guzzetta, C., *et al. Holistic Nursing: A Handbook for Practice. Rockville, MD: Aspen, 1988; with permission.*)

- Record baseline vital signs and any physiologic parameters for comparison after intervention.
- Start with basic relaxation/breathing exercise; lengthen the exercise as needed; include appropriate imagery scripts. (See the case studies for examples of relaxation and imagery scripts.)
- Watch for cues of relaxation such as change in breathing patterns; fluttering of eyelids; easing of jaws with lips apart; change in skin color, particularly around mouth and nose; and toes pointing outward.
- Modify relaxation, imagery, and music depending on the situation. For example, the intubated patient, who cannot control respiratory volume or rate, can be encouraged to drop the jaw to allow the rhythm of the ventilator to soothe tight muscles, and to feel the flow of relaxation throughout the body.
- Intersperse suggestions to enhance relaxation such as "let go," "tension melting away," "smooth out," "throw tension away."
- Be alert to signs of emotional release indicated by a shift in breathing patterns (faster, deeper, or slower), tears, or total release of tension.
- Let session be a few minutes to 15 to 20 minutes. Close session by gradually bringing patients back to a wakeful state; or, if patients are listening to a recorded tape, suggest that they return to a wakeful state whenever they wish.

- Record the psychophysiologic response to interventions in the patient's chart. Record subjective statements of the patient along with physiologic parameters.

Specifics for Imagery

- Establish with the patient that positive imagery enhances healing.
- Choose specific imagery scripts following the assessment. (For details of scripts, the reader is referred to references 2, 8, 9, and 12.)
- Have the patient choose images that have special meaning.
- Reinforce that good imagery provides a focus and organizes energy to facilitate healing.
- Tell the patient to allow spontaneous images to emerge from one's inner self that focus on what one wants to happen.
- Tell the patient that whenever unpleasant images occur to shift them to positive healing images.
- It is not necessary to know the patient's imagery while guiding; the discussion of images follows the guiding.
- Have crayons and paper available for patients to draw their imagery process.

Specifics for Music

- Tell the patient to concentrate on the music. If distracting thoughts occur, suggest that the patient once again return and focus attention on the music.

Table 3-9
Nursing Intervention: Music

PATIENT OUTCOME	OUTCOME CRITERIA	EVALUATION
The patient will demonstrate positive physical and psychologic effects in response to music therapy.	1. The patient will participate with music therapy in the healing process.	1. The patient utilized music one to two times a day to facilitate healing.
	2. The patient will select music of choice for listening.	2. The patient chose music of choice for listening.
	3. The patient will demonstrate positive physical and psychologic effects.	3. The patient demonstrated positive physical and psychologic effects.
	Physical effects: a. Decreased respiratory rate b. Decreased heart rate c. Decreased blood pressure d. Decreased muscle tension e. Decreased fatigue	Physical effects: a. Decreased respiratory rate from 28 to 18/minute b. Decreased heart rate from 120 to 90 beats/minute c. Decreased blood pressure from 160/100 to 130/70 d. Decreased muscle tension e. Decreased fatigue
	Psychologic effects: a. Positive emotions b. Decreased restlessness and agitation c. Decreased anxiety and depression d. Increased motivation e. Increased nonverbal expression of feelings f. Increased positive imagery g. Decreased isolation	Psychologic effects: a. Positive emotions b. Decreased restlessness and agitation c. Decreased anxiety and depression d. Increased motivation e. Increased nonverbal expression of feelings f. Increased positive imagery g. Decreased isolation

(Dossey, B., Keegan, L., Guzzetta, C., *et al. Holistic Nursing: A Handbook for Practice.* Rockville, MD: Aspen, 1988; with permission.)

- Tell the patient to allow the music to flow within and all around the body.
- Let the music suggest new ways to feel, to relax, and to create new healing messages. Consult the resource list at the end of this chapter for relaxation, imagery, and music tapes for use in the critical care setting.

CASE STUDY 1

Three days after a motorcycle accident resulting in a compound fracture of the right femur, Mr. R.T. was taught relaxation and imagery. During the assessment, the nurse learned that the patient feared a permanent disability like that of his uncle, who was in a similar accident. The uncle has suffered from osteomyelitis and nonunion. To engage the patient more in the healing process, he was given imagery teaching sheets that helped him experience the natural healing process (Fig. 3–1). The nurse also made him an audiotape, which follows:

This tape is designed to help you understand what happens when your bones heal. Before I begin to talk about it, however, I would like you to get very relaxed so that your body will feel a little better and you will be more able to concentrate on what I am saying. First, I would like you to begin concentrating on your breathing: inhaling, exhaling completely; thinking to yourself, relax, inhale, exhale. Again. And again. Whenever you feel tension or anxiety or pain during this tape, I would like you to breathe deeply and say to yourself, relax. Inhale, exhale. Now gently close your eyes and as I count downward from ten think of yourself getting more and more relaxed, letting all the tension and the pain flow out. Ten. Nine. Eight. Seven. Six. Five. Four. Three. Two. One. Very good. Now let's take a mental trip through your body, so that we can identify any

remaining tension or anxiety, beginning with your feet, thinking of them getting very heavy, relaxing, sinking down. Mentally imagine all the tension flowing out of your feet, allowing the muscles to become very loose and very smooth. Think for a moment about your legs and your calves particularly. Think of them, too, becoming very heavy. All the tension leaving them. Upper legs, abdomen, and your hips. Now at the count of three I want you to concentrate on making the lower half of your body feel twice as relaxed as it is now. Just let it happen. One. Two. Three. Think of all the muscles up and down your back and let them relax. The muscles in your neck and in your shoulders, and see the knots unwinding, anxiety and fear flowing out. The muscles in the upper part of your arm, the lower part of your arm, and your hands. Let them go; let the tension dissolve. Now think for a moment about your head, remembering there are a lot of muscles and a tendency to store tension in your head; see that relaxing, the muscles around your eyes, around your jaw, your mouth. Let them go and become very, very loose. Just let that happen. Remember that when your body is relaxed, like it should be now, the pain is less and you are better able to participate in the healing process. Now, in your imaginary journey, go to the area where your bone has been broken. I want you particularly to think about the healing of your body's bone, forming a mental picture of the process as I describe it to you. Remember, whenever you feel anxious or are in pain, take a deep breath and say to yourself, relax.

Okay, now I am going to tell you about the first weeks as your bone is healing, and I want you to try and listen very carefully to see and feel this process happening—remembering all the while that the body is a magnificent machine and has built-in means for healing and for returning to health. Almost

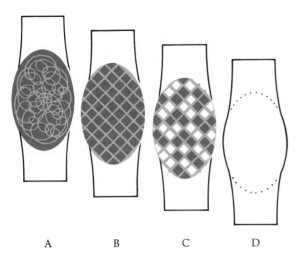

Figure 3–1

The patient learns to visualize the process of bone healing. (*A*) Cellular proliferation. Within the hematoma surrounding the fracture, cells and tissues proliferate and are arranged in a random structure. (*B*) Callus formation. At about 10 to 14 days after the fracture, the cells within the hematoma become organized in a fibrous lattice. With sufficient organization, the callus becomes clinically stable. The callus obliterates the medullary canal and surrounds the two ends of bone by irregularly surrounding the fracture defect. (*C*) New bone formation at about 25 to 40 days after the fracture; calcium is laid down within the fibrous lattice. The early bone of the callus is fiber bone that has spicules perpendicular to the corical surface. Fiber bone is gradually replaced and remodeled by osteonal bone. (*D*) Healed bone. The fracture has been bridged over by new bone. Conversion and remodeling continue up to 3 years following an acute fracture.

on the first day, I want you to imagine the body secreting a kind of paste that will eventually become like an epoxy glue. This glue is very important because it latches onto both ends of the bone and helps them to stick, to become one again. Let me tell you how this glue is formed.

Blood will collect about the ends of your broken bone. More cells will form within this collection of blood. At first there will not be any pattern to the way the cells grow. Gradually, at about ten to fourteen days after the bone has been broken, there will come some order to the way the new cells are arranged. The pattern will look like a lattice arranged in neat rows up and down. Please spend some time thinking about this and letting it happen. Now I want you to imagine your body sending nutrients into this area of cells. Let's call the area a callus; it's a bridge between and around the two ends of bone. Soon new bone begins to form in the callus. Your body will lay down calcium within this framework and grow strong. More and more calcium will be laid down and the bone will become stronger and stronger. The bone will gradually heal. The old broken area will be no more; it will be bridged over by new bone. Now, continuing to stay very relaxed and very calm, and mentally alert, begin to open your eyes whenever you feel ready.

CASE STUDY 2

Mr. S.L. was admitted to the burn unit with a 65% total body surface area (TBSA) burn. To help the patient through the painful wound care, an audiotape was made for him to listen to several times a day so that he could focus on positive images and use relaxation and desensitization skills to dissociate from the pain. Figure 3–2 shows the nurse placing the audio headset on the patient, and Figure 3–3 shows the pictures of the wound-healing process. The script of the audiotape follows:

I want you to get comfortable on your bed. Put all of your thoughts away . . . get comfortable and close your eyes and just relax and listen . . . relax and listen. You might even let yourself get a little sleepy—just feel good for a little while.

Close your eyes. Take a deep breath—let it all out. Let yourself sink back . . . feeling good . . . feeling better all the time.

As I count down from ten to one, let each count be a signal to get more and more relaxed—ten—nine—eight—seven—six—five.

More and more comfortable now—four—three—two—one.

Relax your feet now, letting them get warm and comfortable. Relax your legs and let them get soothed and calm. Feeling heavier now. Relax, letting all the tension out of your stomach. Relax your hips, deeper and deeper, more and more.

Take another deep breath, exhale. Let all the tension go out. Now relax your back. All up and down your back.

Your neck, your shoulders. Your right arm is now relaxing and your right hand.

Feeling more and more peaceful, your left arm and your left hand are relaxed. Deeper and deeper—it feels good to relax—to get calm—a little more and more, and your face, your head, relaxing, deeper and deeper; your head may be feeling heavy, warm.

At the count of three, let go of any tension you may still have—one, two, three.

Feeling comfortable now, maybe a little drowsy, eyes closed.

While I talk now about your treatment, just relax and remember whenever you feel tense or fearful, just take a deep breath and say, "relax, peace, calm."

Just let the fear go. Image now as the time approaches for you to get your dressings taken off and go to the bath—picture this in your imagination. Just relax, feeling deeper and deeper, breathing deeply whenever you feel uncomfortable. The nurse comes in now and starts to cut your bandages off. Imagine this happening. Whenever you feel uncomfortable, breathe, relax. Imagine this happening, feeling the nurse cut the bandages off and your skin feeling the coolness. Take a deep breath and let any discomfort go, feeling relaxed and calm now. As she unwraps the bandages and takes them off, you become aware of a feeling of coolness. Let this happen. All discomfort passes. Take a deep breath. Let any discomfort go. Staying very relaxed

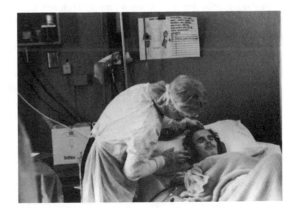

Figure 3–2

Relaxation and imagery. The procedure consists of audiotaped relaxation instructions followed by a guided imagery experience or imaginary trip through the wound care experience.

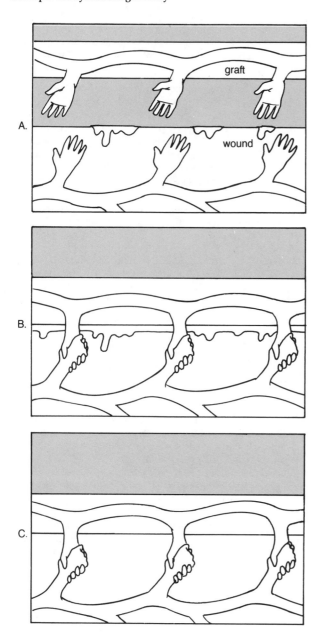

Figure 3–3

Guided imagery technique to facilitate wound healing and to give the patient something on which to concentrate in the days immediately after grafting. Preoperatively, the patient learns to image the daily progression of wound healing. Postoperatively, after completing a relaxation exercise, the patient forms a mental picture of what is transpiring in the wound, the adhesion of surfaces, and the bridging of the space between the graft bed and graft. The vessels from the patient grow into the graft and establish vascular continuity. (Adapted from Achterberg J., and Lawlis, F. *Bridges of the BodyMind.* Champaign, IL: Institute for Personality and Ability Testing, 1985; with permission.)

and calm now. You begin to get out of your bed, relaxed and calm and feeling very good.

Moving now toward the door. As you move down the hall toward your bath—feeling rather cool, but no pain—breathing deeply and deeply, exercising your muscles—longer and stronger—keep breathing.

Exercise your lungs with each breath—remember to exhale completely, relaxing. At the count of three, I want you to let

go of any tension you might have anyplace in your body. One, two, three.

See yourself moving now as you approach the bath. You see the person there who will be helping you when you need help.

As you move into the bath, you feel the water—it feels strong at first—and gradually more and more comfortable. Your skin will begin to feel good under the water—very clean and soothed. The burned skin that is no longer alive needs to be taken off so that your new skin can grow. When this becomes uncomfortable, remember to take a deep breath and let the moment pass—staying very relaxed and calm—letting the good feeling of the warm water take your attention.

Continue to relax now deeper and deeper, looking forward to your return to your bed, and perhaps a nap.

You see yourself getting out of the bath now, drying off gently, and covering yourself now as you return to your bed or your chair, staying very calm and very relaxed.

Letting the discomfort pass. If you must wait for a while, use this time to continue to relax—like you are now, dozing just a little. You may feel chilled but that's natural and will go away when your bandages are put back on.

Feeling very good now, relax more and more. The nurse now comes in with your new bandages.

First, white soothing cream is put over your burns. This feels very good, very soothing and smooth. As soon as it touches your skin, it feels very good.

Now, fine mesh gauze is placed over the cream and any remaining discomfort begins to leave.

New bandages are put on. You feel warmer and warmer each minute. All discomfort fades now. Remember to work with your treatment by letting your body stay relaxed like this, feeling good, breathing deeply, whenever you feel discomfort. Inhaling, exhaling completely. Now, for the next few minutes, imagine yourself well, healthy, in the most beautiful place imaginable. Continue to breathe deeply, inhale, and exhale, relax, relax, relax.

The script is followed by a 10-minute period of rhythmic ocean sounds.

The imagery component then helps the patient relax and form some mental picture about what is going to happen. It acts in the same way as desensitization because potentially anxiety-producing events are introduced while the patient is relaxed. The physiologic state of relaxation, not fear, is therefore associated with the wound-care information.

The procedure works in the same way as sensory education because the sensations as well as the procedural steps the patient will experience are described while the patient is in a relaxed state. In essence, the patient's interpretation of the imminent wound-care procedure is benign, and the pain is decreased. Thus, there are no surprises between the expected and experienced sensations.

SUMMARY

This chapter has focused on psychophysiologic self-regulation and the self-regulation interventions (relaxation, imagery, and music) and their application in the critical care environment. These interventions help reduce the anxiety and fear that patients feel in critical care. The critical care nurse who is experienced with self-regulation interventions has an increased opportunity to help activate and facilitate healing.

DIRECTIONS FOR FUTURE RESEARCH

1. Conduct studies with critically ill that use control groups to validate changes brought about by relaxation, imagery,

and music interventions as single interventions or as combined interventions.

2. Determine the relationship of scripts, physiologic response, and healing in critical care.

3. Develop valid and reliable tools to measure the effects of relaxation, imagery, and music as nursing interventions.

4. Determine the effectiveness of a patient's specific images and if these images simultaneously alter the patient's condition toward decreased or increased psychophysiologic healing.

5. Evaluate the effect of music versus other self-regulation interventions with various patient groups to determine which interventions are the most effective with which groups.

6. Evaluate the attitudes and stress level of nurses who routinely use music as a nursing intervention as compared with nurses who do not use self-regulation interventions.

RESOURCES

Relaxation, Imagery, and Music Tapes

The following is a list of sources for relaxation, imagery, and music tapes for use in the critical care setting:

Awakening Productions, 4132 Tuller Avenue, Culver, CA 90230.

Bodymind Systems, 910 Dakota Drive, Temple, TX 76504, (817) 773–2337.

Health Horizons, 3919 N. Twin Oaks Road, San Marcos, CA 92069, (619) 471–9349.

Institute for Music, Health, and Education, P.O. Box 1244, Boulder, CO 80306, (303) 443–8484.

Mind/Body Health Sciences, 22 Lawson Terrace, Scituate, MA 02066, (617) 545–6890.

New Era Media, P.O. Box 410685-BT, San Francisco, CA 94141 (415) 863–3555

Narada Distributing, 207 East Buffalo, Milwaukee, WI 53202

Windham Hill Productions, P.O. Box 9388, Stanford, CA 94305

Sources Cassette, Department 99, P.O. Box W, Stanford, CA 94305, (415) 328–7171.

REFERENCES

1. Achterberg, J. *Imagery in Healing.* Boston: Shambhala, 1985.

2. Achterberg, J., Dossey, B., Kolkmeier, L. *Rituals of Healing.* New York: Bantam, 1992.

3. Acosta, F. Biofeedback and progressive relaxation in weaning the anxious patient from the ventilator: a brief report. *Heart and Lung* 19:299, 1988.

4. Benson, H. *The Relaxation Response.* New York: William Morrow, 1975.

5. Bonny, H., and Savary, L. *Music and Your Mind.* New York: Harper & Row, 1978.

6. Campbell, D. *Introduction to the Musical Brain.* St Louis: MMB Music, 1986.

7. Campbell, D. *The Roar of Silence.* Wheaton, IL: Theosophical Publishing Company, 1990.

8. Dossey, B. Imagery: Awakening the Inner Healer. In Dossey, B., Keegan, L., Guzzetta, C., and Kolkmeier, L. *Holistic Nursing Practice: A Handbook for Practice.* Rockville, MD: Aspen, 1988.

9. Guzzetta, C. Music Therapy: Hearing the Melody of the Soul. In Dossey, B., Keegan, L., Guzzetta, C., and Kolkmeier, L. *Holistic Nursing: A Handbook for Practice.* Rockville, MD: Aspen, 1988.

10. Guzzetta, C. Effects of relaxation and music therapy on patients in a coronary care unit with presumptive acute myocardial infarction. *Heart Lung* 18:609–616, 1989.

11. Horowitz, B., Fitzpatrick, J., and Flaherty, G. Relaxation techniques for pain relief after open heart surgery. *DCCN* 3:364–71, 1984.

12. Kolkmeier, L. Relaxation: Opening the Door to Change. In Dossey, B., Keegan, L., Guzzetta, C., and Kolkmeier, L. *Holistic Nursing Practice: A Handbook for Practice.* Rockville, MD: Aspen, 1988.

13. McClellan, R. Music and Altered States. *Dromenon* 2:7, 1979.

14. Miller, K., Perry, P. Relaxation technique and postoperative pain in patients undergoing cardiac surgery, *Heart Lung* 19:136–146, 1990.

15. Peterson, G., and Mehl, L. *Pregnancy as Healing: A Philosophy for Prenatal Care.* Berkley, California: Mind body Communication, 1984.

16. Puntillo, K. The phenomenon of pain and critical care nursing. *Heart Lung* 17:262–271, 1988.

4

Rx: Holistic Caring for the Caregiver

Diann B. Uustal

ENHANCING YOUR HEALING WORK

Can healing take place in critical care when daily you and your colleagues are rattled by crises and unexpected events. Do you work on a unit where there is unconditional love for each other? What is your comfort level in sharing your gentleness, your sensitivity, your strengths, and your vulnerable side with your colleagues? What would it take for you and your colleagues to recognize the healing work that is done each day? How often is healing work acknowledged or even recognized by you or your colleagues? Do you think that most of the work in critical care is just curing of symptoms?

Here are a few ideas for enhancing the recognition and validation of the healing work that is done each day in critical care:

- After the beginning of shift report each day, you and your colleagues take a few minutes to share with each other different personal aspects that are in need of healing. For example, one person might say "When you think of me today, send me energy because my mother is ill and I'm worried about her," or "I'm grieving over John's death last week and my heart is aching."
- Once a week set aside time to tell each other about healing moments in your practice or your life so that more awareness is developed about facilitating the healing process in self and others. For example, you teach a patient a relaxation exercise and the patient's pain is significantly reduced.
- Each month you are given a paid resource day to use in any way you wish to promote your own body-mind healing.
- Request inservice education to include classes on self-nurturing, learning ways to increase skills of being present to serve and share with intention, to facilitate healing and empowerment, and to learn new healing skills.
- When healing work is done each day, you finish work with a sense of being spirit-filled rather than spirit-drained. This occurs because support and love have been shared freely among all team members.

LEARNING OBJECTIVES

After reading and interacting with the exercises in this chapter, the nurse should be able to do the following:

1. Describe at least one strategy that can be used for balancing caring for self and caring for others.
2. Compare and contrast the focus of the traditional ethic of caring and the contemporary ethic of caring.
3. Identify at least one tool that can be used to enhance one's wellness and self-esteem.
4. Describe at least one strategy for facilitating collegiality in nursing.

RX: HOLISTIC CARING FOR THE CAREGIVER

The ethic of caring is the cornerstone of nursing's moral art and science. Understandably, this ethic of caring has been appropriately directed toward the patient or client. However, this concept of caring needs to be expanded in a way that is consistent with the values and visions of holistic nursing as we quickly approach the 21st century.

I believe that the caring ethic must include the traditional focus of the nurse who cares for a patient or client as well as concentrate on caring for the caregiver, or the individual nurse. To extend this concept even further, caring among nurses, or collegiality, is yet another aspect of the ethic of caring in nursing that must be included and strengthened.

This chapter is an invitation to take some time for yourself and time for personal and professional reflection on what is of value to you. It is a chance to reflect on the "fundamentals" of nursing and to re-examine your philosophy of caring as a holistic nursing practitioner, educator, manager, or researcher. The chapter's spotlight is on who you are as a person and what you can do to enhance your self-esteem and professional development and on what can be done to encourage collegiality among nurses. There are a number of creative exercises designed specifically to help you examine and consider ways of caring for the caregiver and of staying healthy and in balance as you continue to focus on other's needs as a professional. Other strategies offer unique ideas on how collegiality can be encouraged and maintained in nursing.

You will find that this chapter is an invitation to participate with the material actively and to give yourself an opportunity to consider who you are personally and professionally. So don't merely read this chapter, interact with it. Take out a pencil and some paper and respond to the questions and exercises. Your responses will provide you with food for thought, and the strategies will serve as a mirror for personal reflection and a springboard for professional action and increased satisfaction in nursing.

TIME OUT FOR THE CAREGIVER

The primary thesis of the first portion of this chapter is deceptively simple. Caring for the caregiver is essential to caring therapeutically for others. In other words, even nurses need to take time out to care for themselves! I believe that this is a fundamental and first step toward the contemporary ethic of caring.

Nurses are caring people whose focus, understandably, is on helping others. There is a deep and rewarding joy in caring for people; however, in order to care for others effectively, you must first know how to care for yourself. It seems to be a simple enough truth. Maybe you would be comfortable calling it "common sense," but you know what is often said about common sense. It isn't all that common! There is a delicate balance between caring too much at your own expense or, on the other end of the continuum, not caring enough because you don't want to get too emotionally involved.

Too few of us as caregivers take the time to care for ourselves. Caring for yourself in order to be able to care for others more effectively is not only common sense but a psychological principle that is even found in scripture. You are encouraged to ". . . love your neighbor as yourself." (Matthew 19:19)[1] The preposition *as* is important and gives us insight. *As* does not mean "more than" or "less than" ourselves, it means "the same as" or "like" we care for ourselves. This verse urges us to love and care for ourselves, not just for our own pleasure, but so that we can care for and minister to others. Too many of us as professional caregivers run a hard pace and frequently do not take the time for the refreshment and revitalization necessary for us to continue to share all that we are. If you do not take time to care for yourself, you will simply have far less to give to family, friends, patients, and other colleagues, and you will burn out. In his book, *The Secret of Staying in Love*, John Powell said, ". . . It's a package deal. You have two people you must love: yourself and your neighbor."[3]

Nurses are a significant part of the healing process and relationship. They are less effective, however, with patients and families if they are in need of intensive care themselves. The intensity of caring is sometimes costly and potentially exhausting for the caregiver. An increasing amount of evidence indicates that nurses are in need of special care themselves because of the impact of ethical and professional practice issues as well as the nursing shortage. Many experienced nurses are leaving the profession, and there are fewer people choosing nursing as a career. Hospitals report increasing difficulty in both the retention and recruitment of talented, insightful, competent nursing practitioners. As a result, there is an ever-increasing risk to safe patient care as the shortage of nurses escalates nationwide. Combine this with the fact that nurses have been conditioned for years to have low self-esteem and to neglect their own concerns in favor of meeting the needs of others and you are faced with one of the most troublesome concerns in health care.

Many nurses will nod in agreement as they read that caring for the caregiver is important, but will they make the changes required for an effective balance between meeting one's needs and other's needs? Some people will interpret caring for one's self as selfishness, whereas others will acknowledge self-care as an attitude of self-respect. Unfortunately, caring for the caregiver is a deceptively simple notion that is often elusive and less imperative in our demanding personal and professional lives. To complicate matters, it is rarely taught or discussed in nursing curricula as we prepare men and women for the demands of a profession that specializes in the art and science of caring.

CARING FOR YOURSELF SHOULD BE AT LEAST AS EQUALLY IMPORTANT AS CARING FOR OTHERS

So how do you take care of yourself? Stop for a minute and reflect on this question. Don't just quickly read on. Get a pen and piece of paper and jot down what you do to care for the caregiver—you. Write as many things down as you can think of. Don't edit or censor your thinking.

Now look back on your responses. What can you learn from this simple strategy about how you care for yourself? By asking some additional questions, you can gain more insight. For example, how many things on your list are things you do to care for yourself from a physical perspective. Put a "P" next to those. Maybe you swim a mile, bicycle, or fast walk three times a week.

Look over your list again. How many things indicate what you do for yourself emotionally. Put an "E" next to these. Perhaps when you're feeling down you call a good friend or buy yourself a little something special to cheer yourself up.

What do you do to enhance your wellness that's primarily intellectual in nature? Put an "I" next to those responses on your list. Keeping your mind in shape by pursuing areas of interest is another way to care for the caregiver. You need not engage in a demanding scholarly activity. You can take a course in something you've wanted to learn about for a while—perhaps photography.

Look at your list again. What are you doing to take some time out for the caregiver that is social? Identify those items on your list with an "S." What have you done lately that was for pure fun and relaxation.

Lastly, put an "Sp" next to those things you're doing that are spiritual in nature. Each of us has a spiritual dimension, and how you express this is unique to you. To neglect this area of self-care is to neglect an essential aspect of the person you are.[7]

As you look at how you've categorized your list, what can you learn about your patterns of self-care? Perhaps you notice that you do lots of things socially but not as much physically. Maybe you care for yourself well emotionally but do less than you could from a spiritual perspective. What could you be doing more of or less of to enhance self-caring in each of these five areas?

What is one thing you could do for yourself in the next couple of days to refresh or revitalize in each of these areas? Look at your patterns of recreation, and look at the word *recreation* closely. It says "re-creation." After caring for others at the pace and intensity that you do, what do you do to help yourself stay healthy from a holistic perspective and to "re-create".[7] You can't minister to people out of an empty well. How do you replenish your well when it starts to run dry?

In holistic nursing, we state that we care for the whole person and focus on the patient's needs from a holistic perspective—physically, emotionally, intellectually, socially, and spiritually. Are you caring for your whole self as conscientiously as you do for others? Taking responsibility for your health is more than jargon in a holistic health textbook. It is one way to focus creatively on your own needs and to achieve a better balance in caring for your self. As a result, you will be better prepared to meet other's needs effectively.

If you are a member of a support group in nursing or have some occasion to talk with other nurses, take some time to ask what other people do to enhance their wellness and share your ideas. After all, two heads are better than one, and you just might find some new strategies that you'd be willing to try.

Enhancing Personal Wellness and Self-Esteem

Here's another strategy you can use to enhance your wellness and self-esteem, and improve your self-caring. If you were asked to write a list of all the things you do frequently to keep yourself healthy, you would probably generate many of the ideas that are listed in the following exercise. Read the following ideas and circle the numbers of the sentences that appeal to you as possibilities for strengthening your wellness and strategies for caring for yourself.[7]

1. Remind yourself and validate yourself for your positive qualities.
2. Clarify the difference between "self-respect" (taking time for yourself, so that you can care for others, too) and "selfishness" (the value judgment you or others level on yourself when you take time for yourself).
3. Maximize your assets. Minimize your liabilities.
4. Expect the best from yourself and others, but remember that if you, or others, could be doing any better, you, or they, would be.
5. Don't put yourself down. When you're feeling down, focus on the positive aspects of yourself rather than on negative judgments.

6. Assess a mistake you've made, and concentrate on what you can do differently rather than putting yourself down and concentrating on what you've done wrong.
7. Set realistic goals and reward yourself for the progress you make, no matter how small.
8. Learn to ask for what you need and want.
9. Be gentle on yourself, in thought, word, and deed.
10. Give the gift of encouragement, support, and praise to family and colleagues, and learn to receive it yourself.
11. Establish a quiet time. Find a quiet spot, and use it daily for prayer, meditation, and renewing.
12. Think and say positive things to yourself. Stop negative thoughts that are recurring messages.
13. Take time for "laugh therapy" and time for fun. Both release endorphins.
14. Say no. Withdrawal and anger are far more harmful than admitting an inability to do more. (What part of "no" don't you understand?)
15. Examine your complaining. Is it complaining that relieves stress or complaining that reinforces stress?
16. Learn to take mental health breaks and mini-vacations.
17. Focus on anything but work during your breaks and lunches.
18. Take control of your mouth. What goes into it, and what comes out!
19. Recall the dreams and goals that you had for yourself as a child or younger person, or that you have as a nurse, and reflect on what has happened to those dreams.
20. Be content with who you are. Change what you can, prevent what's preventable, and enjoy the rest.
21. If you can't say something nice, don't say it at all (to yourself and others)!
22. Recall what you do well and what you have done well in the past.
23. Examine your attitudes toward change.
24. Identify the stressors in your life, or career, and examine positive coping strategies to eliminate or reduce them.
25. Mentally inventory all the good things that have happened during the day and the thing you are thankful for.

Now be creative and add some wellness, self-esteem ideas of your own.

Discuss these ideas with your colleagues in a nursing team conference (one that is focused on nurse's needs and not on the patient's needs). Challenge each other to do a "homework assignment." Try one of the wellness or self-esteem ideas, and use it as a way of caring for yourself. Use these ideas as practical strategies to facilitate the change(s) you want.

Let me give you an example. Look at sentence number 8. It says, "Ask for what you need and want." With a person you consider to be a significant other, take some time to explore what you need or want in the relationship or from each other. Sit with each other and decide how much time you'll spend talking. Then agree to share the time and decide who will talk first. The other person will do two things. She or he will repeatedly ask you the question, "What do you need or want more of in this relationship or from me?" Your partner will briefly record what you say each time the question is asked. After the agreed upon time is up, switch roles and give your partner the chance to respond to the same question and you record his or her responses.

You will find that after the first few responses, which are often light-hearted or superficial, you will be more comfortable sharing what you really want, expect, or hope for in the relationship or from each other. It takes effort and energy to maintain a positive alliance, and it is powerful to have the freedom to ask for what you need and want. Good relationships don't just happen. They are created, and they are worth it! This exercise is bound to reveal a lot that can enhance the quality of your relationship whether it be a friendship, colleagueship, or marriage.

Here's another example of how you can reflect more closely on another two of the wellness ideas from this strategy. Look at the sentences numbered 1 and 5. They read, "Remind yourself and validate yourself for your positive qualities"; "Don't put yourself down," and "When you're feeling down, focus on the positive aspects of yourself rather than on negative judgments." All of us can fall into the habit of putting ourselves down or saying negative things that limit our potential. Psychologists tell us that we are our own best self-put-down artists and that we know ourselves and our own imperfections better than anyone else. It is much more difficult for us to focus on the positive aspects of who we are than it is to be critical of ourselves. They also say our minds are never silent and that we should listen and pay attention to our own self-talk.

Self-esteem is formed by two simple things. What people say to us and about us and what we say to ourselves. So why put yourself down or talk negatively to yourself or about yourself? (There are always other people who are too willing to do it for you!) Negative self-talk only limits your full potential,[5] and hampers your self actualization.[2] Talk positively to yourself; you'll really appreciate it!

Monitor your self-talk. Take the time to jot down some of the put downs you say silently or out loud to yourself. What do you notice? All too often many of us find that we are much more critical of ourselves than is necessary, and this significantly colors our attitude about ourselves and, thus, our self-esteem. We are what we think, and what we think influences what we will try. In turn, this influences what we dare to accomplish or can achieve.

Unfortunately, it isn't always enough to monitor your own self-talk. Sometimes people with whom you live or work can be negative unnecessarily. Sometimes this "constructive criticism," which is always "offered for your own good," is unsolicited, poorly timed, and not always in your best interest. This type of constructive criticism has been termed *constrictive criticism*. Evaluate the content of the message. If it is negative criticism, more for criticism's sake and not yours, speak up and stop the put down.[6]

Easier said than done, I agree. But if you don't take responsibility for yourself and stop the put downs, you will pay too high a price with your self-esteem. I'd be willing to bet that you have sung the jingle "sticks 'n stones will break my bones, but names will never hurt me!" Well, you've grown up now, and you know that names can hurt—some names more than others. You might also have been raised on the advice to "turn the other cheek," which is a powerful strategy, but not appropriate for all situations. For many of us, these value messages are not enough to deal with the put downs or to stop certain people from dumping on us. (And you thought the "dumping syndrome" occurred after a patient had a gastrectomy!) There are some people in each of our lives who are very difficult to confront, and it seems almost easier to take it than to deal with the toxic person directly.

Addressing this issue of "toxic waste" and its effect on your self-esteem is one aspect of caring for the caregiver and taking responsibility for your health. It is also assertiveness training in action. In a way that is comfortable and genuine for you, you need to say, "Stop, that bothers me!" or "That hurt my feelings. I don't like it when you put me down in front of the group. If you have something to say that will help me improve, say it in a positive way and privately."

I know, it's easy to talk about but much more difficult to take action and change behavior. If you don't start cleaning up the toxic waste somewhere, a little at a time, one person at a time, your mind's environment (or self-esteem) will be polluted! Of course, there are some people you may never be able to confront in this manner for a myriad of reasons. Don't start with the most negative person in your life who is the most emotionally provoking. Take care of yourself by stopping the unwanted, and often uninvited, put-downs one at a time because you value yourself.

The point of this whole exercise is to offer you some additional ideas for caring for the caregiver. Use any of the ideas as food for thought or personal prescriptions for your wellness. They can be the beginning of effective, practical strategies for facilitating the changes you value.

My "Mental Garden"

The analogy of a gardener in relation to the cultivation of one's self-esteem might be useful as you think about your own self-esteem. When you plant a vegetable or flower garden, you are careful to select the best seeds, plant them carefully, and water them. You weed your garden so the seedlings are not choked out by the weeds.

Now use this example to think about your mental garden. What kind of mental garden are you cultivating? Validating or positive thoughts are the "flowers" you or others plant and cultivate. The "weeds" are the put-downs you say to yourself or those that are said by others. So think about the kind of gardener you are, and jot down your responses to the following questions:

What are the thoughts you say to yourself that are positive and are like flower seedlings?

What thoughts are like weeds (or self put-downs) that you need to stop saying to yourself and pluck out of your garden? Write them down so you will recognize them more easily and can take steps to eliminate them.

What weeds (put-downs) are sown by others that you need to pluck? Be specific. (Remember, sometimes put-downs are sown in the guise of humor or as a joke. But a joke isn't funny if it's at the expense of who you are.)

Do you have a mental garden that has more flowers or more weeds?

How effective of a gardener are you? What could you do to be more effective? Think critically and creatively, and be specific.

You wouldn't intentionally sow weeds among your flowers or a vegetable garden, so why do the same thing to your mental garden by sowing negative critical thoughts or allowing others to do the same? Take responsibility for your own mental health—one thought at a time!

THE IMPORTANCE OF CULTIVATING SELF-ESTEEM

It is important to examine, cultivate, and nourish one's self-esteem. Self-esteem is simply described as all the beliefs and attitudes you have about yourself. It is shaped by what you do, how you think, and your successes and failures. It is just plain feeling good about yourself. A healthy self-esteem is built on feelings of confidence, acceptance, achievement, and healthy self-talk.

Two major influences affect the development of your self-esteem: what others say to you and what you say to yourself. Stop reading for a moment and reflect on what you've just read. Get a piece of paper again, and write your responses to the following questions. You'll learn more about yourself by doing than by just reading!

Thought Conditioners: Enhancing Your Self-Esteem

Your self-esteem is built on feelings of confidence. What do you think—say—to yourself that fosters an attitude of confidence in yourself? Examine your responses.

What builds your feelings of self-esteem and confidence?
What do you say and think to yourself that increases your self-esteem, confidence, and acceptance of yourself?
What are three messages you've heard from significant others that have influenced your self-esteem positively?
What achievements have you accomplished that have enhanced your feelings of self-esteem? Don't edit your thinking.
Identify two things you'd like to achieve that would enhance your self-esteem.

How do you feel when you focus on yourself? Is it uncomfortable to take the time for introspection? Does it feel embarassing to look closely at who you are and what you really think about yourself?

Next, read and reflect on this poem, which is entitled "Life's Prizes":

Most of us	Behind the ear.
Miss out	A four pound bass.
On life's	A full moon.
Big prizes.	An empty parking space.
The Pulitzer.	A crackling fire.
The Nobel.	A great meal.
Oscars.	A glorious sunset.
Tonys.	Hot soup.
Emmys.	Cold beer.
But we're	Don't fret about
All eligible	Copping life's
For life's	Grand awards,
Small pleasures.	Enjoy its
A pat	Tiny delights.
On the back.	
A kiss	*Author Unknown*

Be creative and re-write the poem so that it has more meaning for you! In addition, here are some questions for you to think about:

What are some of the "big prizes" or "grand awards" you've missed out on in your life?
What are some "small pleasures" in your life that too often you forget to celebrate?
What are some of the "tiny delights" that bring you happiness?
Is the last sentence of the poem good advice for you? What do you need to do to enjoy more of life's "tiny delights"?

Things I Appreciate Most About Myself

Here is another specific strategy you can use to examine and enhance your self-esteem and, in turn, influence your ability to care for others more effectively. Think about the things you like best about yourself, and record your thoughts. Perhaps it is easier to get in touch with what you don't like, but that doesn't build self-esteem—it erodes it. Concentrate on what you like best, and don't stop writing until you run out of things you like.

Good! Now reflect on what you've written from a holistic perspective as well as from the whole-person perspective Carl Rogers alludes to in his writings. Each of us as a whole person is made up of five components: physical, emotional, intellectual, social, and spiritual qualities. What are those physical, emotional, intellectual, social, and spiritual qualities you like best about yourself? "Code" or examine your list more carefully in order to learn as much as possible from what you have identified. Classify your list in the following way:

1. Put the letter "P" next to any entry on your list that is a physical quality.
2. Place an "E" next to any item on your list that is an emotional quality.
3. Put an "I" next to any item that is an intellectual quality.
4. Put an "S" next to any entry that is social in nature.
5. Place an "Sp" next to any quality that is a spiritual quality.
6. Use a "W" to indicate any quality you work at to maintain.
7. Put an asterisk (*) next to an entry to indicate that someone with whom you work or live has recently told you that it is a quality they like in you.
8. Write two additional qualities you would like to have as characteristics describing yourself.
9. Number the top three qualities you want to be known or remembered for the most.
10. Make up your own way to code your list.

The first five ways to "code" your list are an attempt to help you look at yourself from a whole-person perspective. It makes sense to care for ourselves in each of these areas before we attempt to meet our patients' and clients' needs holistically.

What else did you notice, and what can you learn from this exercise? Maybe you observed that there isn't much you've written about your physical qualities and that this is an area in which you're critical of yourself. This is not an uncommon issue, and many of us, especially women, are particularly critical of ourselves from a physical perspective. Perhaps you need to focus more on stopping your own negative criticism and negative self-talk about your physical self. You are what you think, and if you think poorly about yourself, it will influence your view of yourself, your perceptions of others, and your ability to care for yourself and others. People who have a low self-concept are often critical of themselves as well as others. The way you judge yourself is often the way you criticize and judge others, and this can affect your caring of yourself and others.

Finally, look carefully at your list and how you've "coded" it one more time. Complete the following unfinished sentences as you reflect on what you've written:

"I found out that I _____."

"I can appreciate that I _____."

"I learned that I _____."

"I discovered that I _____."

"I am pleased that I _____."

Generate some of your own statements based on what you learned from the strategy.

It's true that you're not always going to feel good about all aspects of yourself. We all have days when we're down on ourselves for many different reasons. Sometimes an attitude of critical self-evaluation is an incentive for self-improvement, but a steady attitude of self put-downs can erode anyone's self-esteem. Consciously cultivate a positive attitude about yourself. Consciously recall your skills and talents, and remember that this affects not only your attitudes about yourself, but also your personal relationships with others and your professional caregiving. Hugh Prather wrote, "The more you know about yourself, and the more positive your self-image, the better chance you have of increasing your self-esteem and of enjoying a meaningful, happy life."[4]

COLLEGIALITY AND CARING IN THE WORKPLACE

It's something to be able to paint a picture, or to carve a statue, and so to make a few objects beautiful. But it is far more glorious to carve and paint the atmosphere in which we work, to effect the quality of the day. This is the highest of the arts.

Henry David Thoreau

Colleagueship and collegiality have numerous definitions, ranging from the simple to the profoundly complex. The purpose of this section is to offer some practical strategies for building and strengthening colleagueship among nurses. Many nurses complain that the lack of collegiality in nursing is a serious problem that affects morale, retention, recruitment, and satisfaction in nursing.

Colleagueship, or good relationships of any kind, don't just "happen"; they are created. A sense of team spirit and cooperation are fine attitudes, but if they are valued, there must be behavioral change and action that goes beyond the rhetoric and demonstrates commitment to these values. I believe that collegiality is the ethic of caring shared among nurses and is a natural extension of the ethic of caring that also focuses on patient care and self-care for the caregiver. Collegiality is an expression of fidelity, or promise keeping, from an ethical perspective, that ideally ought to be shared among nurses no matter what their expertise or practice arena. What are you doing to shape the quality of the atmosphere in which you practice nursing and to enhance collegial relationships among nurses?

Enhancing collegiality and fidelity among nurses is an essential component of image building and professionalism. Remember the game you played in the schoolyard called Red Rover? You would all stand in a line hanging on to one another's hands, and a member of the other team would run full speed and try to break through your line. The object was to support each other, hang on tight, and act as a team. The "strength in numbers" when you stick together is the moral of the game we played.

It seems as if some nurses need to remember how to play Red Rover. Have they forgotten that nurse-nurse fidelity and backing each other up in tough situations is an essential part of colleagueship? Have you ever noticed how well physicians play this colleagueship game? They often back each other up even when they're wrong! In nursing, it is too often the case that nurses don't stick together even when they're right! I have found that nurses all over the country adamantly discuss the lack of colleagueship in nursing as one of the most stressful professional practice issues they encounter.

What specifically can be done to change this situation? How can we strengthen the ties that bind (not gag) nurses? Are there some practical, cost-, and time-effective ways for nurses to extend the ethic of caring to each other? I'd like to offer some practical strategies that are cost-effective, do not require any special consulting skills, and that nurses all over the country are using and finding effective.

THE GIFT OF ENCOURAGEMENT

The following are two of my favorite scriptures that help me focus on the concept of validation, or positive regard, as Carl Rogers[5] would call it: "Kind words are like honey, enjoyable and healthful." (Proverbs 16:24); "A word fitly spoken is like apples of gold in pictures of silver" (Proverbs 25:11).[1] The gift of encouraging words can be one of the most special intangible gifts nurses can give to each other.

We all want to feel good about ourselves, but as we get older, we receive praise less frequently and spontaneously from others, such as parents and teachers. When we were younger, many of us got "warm fuzzies" in school, or we watched our children receive them. The idea originally blossomed in the sixties and early seventies with the popularity of values clarification in the schools. The point is, none of us is ever too old for sincere praise or too confident that we don't enjoy the positive regard or validation from others. Everyone needs and appreciates a compliment now and then! Unfortunately, though, and as a result of our socialization, we actually learn to be more comfortable with put-downs than praise. Watch what happens when someone compliments or praises you. Often we refuse to accept the compliment, or worse, we get suspicious of what the other person wants.

Validation or praise is like a gift. It's a gift that will encourage you to think positively about yourself or see something positive about yourself through someone else's eyes. Psychologists say that if we notice that we are not receiving very much validation, it's often because we do not psychologically "hear" it when it is shared, or we simply refuse to truly acknowledge it and open ourselves up to it. After a while, people stop sharing the gifts that are not acknowledged.

One effective way to enhance collegiality is to give the gift of encouragement and to learn to receive it graciously as well. Of course, the validation or praise must be sincere. It is the spirit or attitude of seeing something positive in your colleague and calling it to his or her attention. It's the attitude of "catching others smiling" or "doing something right" and reflecting this back to the person. There is something important about validation that is essential to understand. There is a significant difference between validating the character of the individual and validating what the person does. A child may earn good grades and receive validation, but what happens when the grade is not as good? A nurse may usually be very effective and pleasant to work with in a demanding situation, but in another circumstance, may be unbearable to work with. Even an Olympic athlete can have a bad day. Therefore, the "secret" of validation is that the praise should focus on the person and not just on the performance.

Most of us have very little difficulty praising someone we care for and enjoy working with; however, the people we do not care for as much need your validation too. It's an understatement to say that it's more difficult to validate someone you don't like as much; however, it is possible to find something good in everyone and to praise that goodness. This is the litmus test of how committed we are to affecting positive attitudes and fostering colleagueship.

Notes of Praise

Here's the most simple, cost-effective strategy you can use with your colleagues that will enhance wellness and positive regard in the workplace and foster collegial relationships. Bring in some business envelopes and have each person put his/her first name on the outside of the envelope. Encourage your colleagues to decorate the envelopes in any way they wish. Post all the envelopes on a bulletin board on the unit, or put them on your lockers.

The purpose is simple. When you see one of your colleagues do something well or recognize a special quality in them, jot them a validating or positive note and put it in their envelope. In other words, catch them doing something right, and then give them the gift of encouragement. Explain that this isn't a popularity contest. It's a way of stimulating each other to share what we often notice in one another, yet less frequently share out loud. Remember, every person wants to feel good about herself or himself, so this strategy will be effective if your colleagues will give it a try!

The gift of encouragement does not need to be a dissertation, just a simple one-liner designed to praise someone and enhance a sense of self-esteem and team spirit. Here are some examples of ways in which you could begin your one-liners:

I really like the way you . . .
Way to go!
I'm proud of you for . . .
Remarkable job!
Thanks for your extra effort!
You're special!
Just want you to know . . .
I knew you could do it!
Creative thinking—keep it up!
Super!
Hurray for you!
You're on target!
Your caring counts!

The secret of these one-liners are simple. Keep them short and sincere. Focus on the individual's personal qualities as well as the behavior you're praising. Make it a policy on your unit to validate each other more frequently than you criticize. Look for and expect the best in each other, and when you see it, acknowledge it.

Try this strategy where you work. It will enhance wellness in the workplace. An encouraging word is a gift that is inexpensive, yet priceless, and it can help build a team's morale and increase satisfaction in nursing. Do you want to enjoy a level of collegiality that's often elusive in busy nursing units? Would you like to increase the delivery of quality care for patients? Would you like to help others feel better about themselves and, at the same time, enjoy your own work atmosphere more? Then look for the best in your colleagues, validate them, and send them some one-liners that are sure to boost their spirits individually and collectively. Attitudes are contagious. Are yours worth catching?

A Common-Sense Approach to Enhancing Collegiality

What else can nurses do to enhance collaboration and collegiality? Here are some more practical ideas that can make a significant difference. Some of them are so unpretentious that they're often overlooked and are not used as effectively as they could be.

"No put downs"! Help establish this ground rule for your workplace environment. It is simple, but don't be fooled into thinking it's simplistic. Ask each person to censor and stop the put-downs that can occur. Remind your colleagues that put-downs, or negative criticism, can be what one says to oneself as well as what is said to others. The "no put-downs policy" will do a lot to improve the atmosphere as well as the morale among nursing colleagues. Invite other disciplines and departments to join you, and watch what is created beyond your own unit. "No put-downs" does not mean that constructive appraisal of our own or our colleagues' behavior is not done. Peer review is one way to strengthen personal and professional growth. Establish guidelines for constructive appraisal of each other's professional performance and for peer review that are based on validating people for what they do well as well as offering constructive criticism.

Expect the best from yourself and those with whom you work. Encourage people to practice nursing, management, or teaching based on the goals, values, and ethics that are inherently important and bring satisfaction to professional nurses. Have regular discussions on the values that are relevant and precious and bring satisfaction to both professionals and patients in your area. Discuss openly how you can get closer to actualizing these values as individuals and as a team.

State the expectations you have of each other clearly, and make your implicit expectations explicit. This is an invitation for each nurse, not only those in management, to be involved in shaping the values and atmosphere out of which nursing care is delivered. When expectations are based on ethical values, and they are a shared direction, you will find the group's morale, direction, and pride in their accomplishments will be greater.

Model the values you believe in. Encourage each other to practice professionally and make decisions based on nursing's commitment to ethical values. Don't let the system in which you find yourself diminish the importance of these values and visions for professional nursing. Back each other up in ethical conflict.

Discuss conflicts in values openly and provide for "safe gripe sessions." Keep conflicts that can occur out in the open by using good communication patterns and management techniques. Issues that are discussed early, not allowed to brew, and presented in an atmosphere of active listening and respect for each person's opinion can be resolved more directly.

Validate and celebrate risk-taking behavior that demonstrates a value that is "costly" to implement (in terms of energy and risk taking, not just monetarily). During a team conference, it could be a "regular feature" to call to the team's attention a "moment to celebrate" or a "new and good accomplishment." The validation counts, and the behavior that is valued will be reinforced. After a while, you will find that the group will volunteer spontaneously to talk about a "victory" they've won collectively or individually.

Be patient with one another, and be willing to be less critical, more positive, more forgiving, and tolerant of each other's shortcomings and mistakes. Examine how each person typically behaves under pressure and how this might affect the team as a whole. Encourage each member to take responsibility for her own actions and the impact her attitudes could have on collegiality.

Establish, reward, and recognize standards of excellence. Recognition is important to each of us. Unfortunately, nurse's and nursing's contribution too often goes unnoticed and uncelebrated. Once a year, on Nurse's Day, is not enough to encourage and recognize the behaviors that are outstanding all year long. Applaud achievement and excellence publicly, creatively, and at frequent intervals. For example, one unit has Special Person Days. One team member is selected and her efforts are applauded and appreciated for the week by other colleagues. The person's picture is posted in a prominent place on the unit where colleagues from other departments and families and visitors can see. The successes, achievements, or reasons the person was chosen by her peers are noted also. Other nursing units have added to the validation by submitting the person's picture and description of her contributions to the hospital newspaper's section called "Extra-Ordinary People." Colleagues enjoy the sincere recognition and appreciation from their peers.

Recognize nurses for their professional expertise. Find out an individual's assets, and create ways to help an individual use them. Ask each member of the team to identify her areas of expertise. Schedule routine brown-bag lunches during which information and expertise are shared in short time frames. You could also have team members identify what they think a particular colleague's area of expertise is and what they would like to know more about from that colleague. There are some times when a colleague will be able to identify an asset more easily (and with less embarrassment) than an individual. Use each other as consultants.

Reward and recognize collaboration and colleagueship. Make it the team's winning style, and place a premium on collaboration and cooperation and its positive effects on morale, patient care, career satisfaction, and personal and professional development.

Encourage a mentoring, networking, or buddy system. This can be formal or informal based on your group's needs, expertise, retention, and recruitment variables. New graduates and

nurses who are "floated" to your unit should be welcomed and assisted to perform as capably as they can. No one likes to feel unappreciated, unfamiliar with the environment, or incapable because of inexperience.

Encourage individual caregivers to take responsibility for their own health from a holistic perspective, which includes physical, emotional, intellectual, social, and spiritual components, so that each caregiver's motivation remains high in his or her performance is effective and valued professionally.

Establish and maintain a support group to deal with feelings that arise in the context of nurse-patient relationships. If possible, choose a facilitator who has organizational development or group counseling skills. Be supportive of each other's issues and pressures, but be sure to refer people for additional professional assistance.

Plan time for discussions that focus on how to keep morale high and on identifying and addressing changes that need to be implemented. Not compromising on this type of nursing care conference, which is not centered on patient's needs, is important. Many managers and nurses allow themselves to become too busy to focus on the needs of nurses and the nursing profession. Investing in each other's satisfaction, welfare, concerns, and professional development is critical. If the individual members of the group are healthier, the group's ability to meet the health care needs of individual patients and their families will be more effective.

These ideas, when used consistently, can affect the quality of the day and the atmosphere out of which we care for ourselves, each other as colleagues, and our patients more effectively. I challenge you to use them to establish an undeniable camaraderie and to establish the kind of collegial ties that bind professional nurses nationwide.

The following poem is one that is familiar to most of us, although it has been adapted from "Children Learn What They Live." Post it in a place where you can all profit from the ethical implications of something that is often regarded as advice only for parents caring for their children. Remember, all we ever needed to know about colleagueship we probably already learned in the sandbox.

If colleagues live with criticism,
  they learn to condemn.
If colleagues live with hostility,
  they learn to fight.
If colleagues live with ridicule,
  they learn to be shy.
If colleagues live with shame,
  they learn to feel guilty.
If colleagues live with tolerance,
  they learn to be patient.
If colleagues live with encouragement,
  they learn confidence.
If colleagues live with praise,
  they learn to appreciate.
If colleagues live with fairness,
  they learn justice.
If colleagues live with security,
  they learn to have faith.
If colleagues live with approval,
  they learn to like themselves.
If colleagues live with acceptance and friendship,
  they learn to find satisfaction in professional nursing.[7]

```
┌─────────────────────────────────────────────────────────────────────────┐
│                              Self-Contract                                │
│                                                                           │
│     1. One thing I especially want to change is:                          │
│                                                                           │
│     2. My specific plans and steps for accomplishing this goal are:        │
│           (Make sure your plans are measurable, manageable, and meaningful to you!) │
│                                                                           │
│     3. Indications that I am meeting my goal are:                          │
│           (Celebrate these successes on the way to your goal—they help you persevere!) │
│                                                                           │
│     4. Ways in which I might sabotage myself and prevent myself from reaching this goal are: │
│           (This will take a lot of honesty and insight. You might even want to consult with a friend │
│           who knows you well.)                                             │
│                                                                           │
│     5. Ways in which I can reduce and eliminate my self-sabotaging patterns are: │
│                                                                           │
│     6. I plan to reach my goal by:_____ .          │
│                                                                           │
│     A COPY OF THIS CONTRACT IS SHARED WITH _____ , WHO WILL    │
│     ENCOURAGE ME TO KEEP MY CONTRACT WITH MYSELF IN THE FOLLOWING WAYS:    │
│                                                                           │
│                                                                           │
│     Signed:_____         │
│     Witnessed by: _____         │
└─────────────────────────────────────────────────────────────────────────┘
```

Figure 4-1

Self-contract.

It is hoped that you have been challenged to care for yourself and your colleagues as well as your clients and patients in new ways. However, all the insight you've gained is meaningless if you do not use it to effect the behavioral change that you value. Here's one last strategy for closing the gap between your intent and your action.

Identify one area in yourself that you think needs changing, and commit to this change in writing. Take responsibility for your own holistic health in action as well as in words. Fill in the self-contract presented in Figure 4–1, or make up your own version. Have someone with whom you are comfortable witness your intent at the bottom of your contract. Everyone needs a little help from a "balcony" friend to cheer one on and upward.

SUMMARY

The concept of caring traditionally has directed the nurse toward focusing on and caring for a patients' needs. The ethic of caring, a cornerstone of nursing's moral art, was expanded to include the ethic of self-care for the caregiver as well as collegiality, or caring among nurses.

This chapter and its exercises were designed as a mirror for personal reflection to help you examine and enhance your wellness and self-esteem so that you can continue to be the caring, professional person you are. Caring for the caregiver is one way you can care more effectively for others. My hope is that you participated in the exercises and found them thought provoking and useful as tools for helping you take responsibility for caring for yourself and enhancing collegiality.

This chapter has offered you a unique, interactive educational experience. It's purpose was to broaden your perspective on the traditional ethic of caring provided to clients to include a more contemporary concept of caring that involves caring for yourself as well as caring among nursing professionals. I hope that you are a step closer to actualizing your goals in relation to your personal and professional development, competency, and satisfaction in holistic nursing. Take pride in your role as a professional nurse, and know that your caring counts!

DIRECTIONS FOR FUTURE RESEARCH

1. Determine the effects of daily use of personal wellness and daily affirmations on the nurse's self-esteem.
2. Evaluate changes in behavior and perceived quality of life when nurses are guided in learning skills to enhance their own human potentials.
3. Develop tools that help nurses recognize, enhance, and facilitate their own intuition.
4. Determine the changes in collegiality and caring in the workplace when nurses use personal wellness strategies.

REFERENCES

1. *Harper Study Bible.* Revised Standard Version. Grand Rapids, MI: Zondervan Bible Publishers, 1962.
2. Maslow, A. *Toward a Psychology of Being.* New York: Van Nostrand Reinhold, 1961.
3. Powell, J. *The Secret of Staying in Love.* Niles, IL: Argus, 1970.
4. Prather, H. *Notes to Myself.* New York: Bantam, 1971.
5. Rogers, C. *On Becoming a Person.* Boston: Houghton Mifflin, 1961.
6. Simon, S. *Negative Criticism.* Niles, IL: Argus, 1978.
7. Uustal, D. *Values and Ethics in Nursing: From Theory to Practice.* Providence, RI: Herald Press, 1985. (Available for $21.95 [includes postage and handling] from Educational Resources in Nursing, 880 Division St., East Greenwich, RI 02818.)

SUGGESTED READINGS

Branden, N. *If You Could Hear What I Cannot Say.* New York: Bantam, 1983.

Fulghum, R. *All I Really Needed to Know I Learned in Kindergarten.* New York: Villard Books, 1989.

Helmstetter, S. *What to Say When You Talk to Yourself.* New York: Simon & Schuster, 1986.

Jongeward, D., and Scott, D. *Women as Winners.* Reading, MA: Addison-Wesley, 1976.

Landorf, J. *Balcony People.* Waco, TX: Word Books, 1984.

Leininger, M. (Ed.). *Care: Discovery and Uses in Clinical and Community Nursing.* Detroit: Wayne State University Press, 1988.

Massey, M. *The People Puzzle: Understanding Yourself and Others.* Reston, VA: Reston Publishing Co., 1979.

McKay, M., and Fanning, P. *Self-Esteem.* Oakland, CA.: New Harbinger Publications, 1987.

Peck, M. S. *The Road Less Traveled.* New York: Simon & Schuster, 1978.

Sheehy, G. *Passages.* New York: Bantam, 1976.

Siegel, B. *Love, Medicine and Miracles.* New York: Harper & Row, 1986.

Siegel, B. *Peace, Love and Healing.* New York: Harper & Row, 1989.

Simon, S. *Getting Unstuck.* New York: Warner Communications, 1988.

Watson, J. *Nursing: Human Science and Human Care. A Theory of Nursing.* Publication no. 15-2236. New York: National League for Nursing, 1988.

Watson, J. *Nursing: The Philosophy and Science of Caring.* Boulder, CO: Colorado Associated University, 1985.

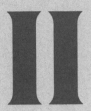

II

Critical Care Nursing Practice

THE HEALING ROOM

What would it take for you to be healed at work rather than physically and emotionally drained? As you read the following list of possibilities, stay open to the ideas. If you say they cannot happen, they will not. However, if you and your colleagues create your visions of healing and present them to administration in the context of "This is what we need to facilitate healing in ourselves and our patients" and "This is how we see creating a Healing Room," then it will become a reality. Here are a list of possibilities that can enhance your healing as the demands of critical care nursing practice increase:

- Is it possible for a room near the unit to be emptied and converted into a room to nourish the staff called the Healing Room?
- Can you imagine signing up each day to go to the Healing Room on or near the unit for 20 to 30 minutes to nourish yourself with a period of relaxation and rest?
- Is it possible to imagine that you have the support of your colleagues and administration to go to the Healing Room? This rest period is valued and honored, and you are encouraged to nourish yourself.
- Can you imagine the Healing Room with comfortable pillows on a carpeted floor, beautiful pictures hanging on the wall, a few healing objects placed on several low tables for easy viewing, and an audio cassette library with a wide range of music, relaxation, and imagery tapes, headphones, and tape recorders? There might also a sign on the door that reads "This Healing Room is for your relaxation and rest. Please enjoy." (For details of establishing an audio cassette library, refer to Chapter 3.)

What were your experiences as you read the characteristics of the Healing Room? What else would you add to your room? It is also important to create a similar kind of space for yourself where you live so that you allow time each day for inner reflection and healing to renew your body-mind-spirit.

5

Nursing Assessment

Cathie E. Guzzetta   *Shelia Bunton*

ALLOWING HEALING TO MANIFEST

Being a nurse places you in a unique position to explore your personal and transpersonal growth. True healing requires attention to your woundedness and the polarities, the purpose, and meaning in life. This attention can be enhanced by learning to move to a place of centeredness in order to be present with intention. Practicing and learning skills to quiet the mind create space to develop skills of active listening. Learning about the inward journey affords many unique opportunities to be with self, patients, and others. You can facilitate healing for the patient in the midst of acute illness to increase inner awareness and self-understanding and to learn new skills that provide opportunities for reaching your potentials. Awareness of healing and being a nurse-healer allows nurse-patient interactions to take on new dimensions. Reflect on the following questions and answer them in your own way:

- How do I feel within when I use the word *healer* to describe myself?
- Do I acknowledge my strengths and weaknesses?
- Do I recognize that self-healing is a continual process?
- What do I experience when I become centered?
- Do I listen actively?
- Do I acknowledge my intuition?
- What are my strategies for moving forward on my healing journey?

LEARNING OBJECTIVES

After reading this chapter, the nurse should be able to do the following:

1. Discuss the purposes of the nursing process.
2. Critically examine the major problems encountered when using a medical data base during a nursing assessment.
3. Discuss the steps involved in developing a Critical Care Response Pattern Assessment Tool based on NANDA's Unitary Person Framework, Taxonomy I, and specific Standards of Care.
4. Examine the general focus questions and parameters that can be used to elicit the appropriate data when assessing a patient using the Critical Care Response Pattern Assessment Tool.
5. Using the Critical Care Response Pattern Assessment Tool, assess a critically ill patient, formulate nursing diagnoses, and develop the plan of care.
6. Evaluate and revise the Critical Care Response Pattern Assessment Tool based on the needs and requirements of your clinical practice.

NURSING PROCESS IN THE 1990s

In 1967, Yura and Walsh[40] first identified the phases of the nursing process as assessment, planning, implementation, and evaluation. Since 1967, nursing has undergone many changes. Advances in standards of care, quality-assurance programs, nursing audits, and the revision of nurse-practice acts have impacted on the nursing process.[5,19,20,34] Thus, in the 1990s, the nursing process specifies two additional steps that serve to enhance the quality of patient care and expand the scope of nursing practice. The six steps included in the nursing process are assessment, formulation of nursing diagnoses, identification of patient outcomes, planning, implementation, and evaluation (Fig. 5–1).[7]

When the nursing process is used, it fulfills the purposes of nursing,[40] which are as follows:

- Maintain the patient's health.
- Provide nursing care that will return patients to a state of health or help them achieve a peaceful death.
- Prevent, detect, and treat illness and the complications of illness.

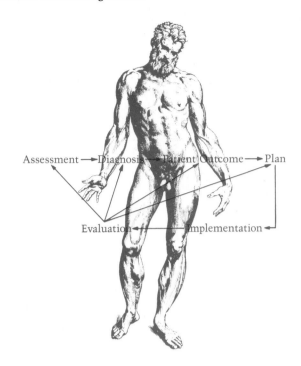

Assessment → Diagnosis → Patient Outcome → Plan

Evaluation   Implementation

Figure 5–1

Components of the nursing process.

- Provide care and treatment necessary to promote comfort.
- Maximize the quality of life by improving patients' resources and making the appropriate referrals for community help.

The nursing process incorporates a patient-centered framework. Much emphasis has been focused in the past two decades, however, on advancing the practice of nursing by using a conceptual model of nursing to guide the steps of the nursing process. Such models include King's systems model,[22] Orem's self-care model,[29] Newman's health-as-expanding-consciousness model,[28] and Yura and Walsh's needs model.[39] Roy's adaptation model,[32] Rogers' unitary man model,[31] and Christman and Fowler's systems-in-change model[6] appear to lend themselves well to use in critical care. Such models are used to develop the nursing data base for assessment, to formulate nursing diagnoses, to identify patient outcomes, and to guide the planning, implementation, and evaluation steps of the nursing process. All allege to be grounded in a holistic framework.[12] They all offer the potential for advancing nursing practice because they provide a frame of reference, centered around the patient and family, to describe, explain, predict, and control the outcomes of patient care. Moreover, they provide the foundation for future research and theory development in nursing.

Unfortunately, because the theoretical concepts are so different in each of the models, nurses are guided to widely divergent categories for assessment.[13] Thus, it has not been possible to standardize a nursing data base within the profession such as physicians have done with their standardized medical data base. Furthermore, none of these models of nursing were designed specifically to enhance the identification of nursing diagnoses.

The following sections discuss the purpose of assessment and the need to incorporate a holistic nursing data base into

practice. A new Critical Care Response Pattern Assessment Tool prototype, based on a nursing framework, is then presented. The discussion focuses on how the tool provides the necessary data to validate the existence of nursing diagnoses and guide the remaining steps of the nursing process.

PURPOSE OF THE NURSING ASSESSMENT

A nursing assessment is a logical, systematic, and ordered collection of data used to evaluate the health status of a patient in order to identify problems of the body-mind-spirit. Nurses must integrate logic, disciplined thinking, deliberate action, and methodology with a clear understanding of holism. They must know the anatomic, physiologic, pathophysiologic, and etiologic elements of the disease process, as well as their psychologic and clinical sequelae. Assessment demands that nurses have insight into human behavior, relationships, developmental processes, and reactions to stressors and that they be sensitive and open to human interactions. Frequently, assessment demands that nurses learn new techniques, approaches, and procedures.

Data are collected by means of communication, observation, interviewing, and physical assessment skills. Pertinent biopsychosocial data are obtained from the patient, family, significant others, members of the health team, previous patient records, and the results of diagnostic and laboratory testing.[34] These areas are discussed in further detail in the next sections and in Chapters 11, 12, 16, 17, 19, 24, 29, 32, 35, 40, and 45.

After the assessment, the data are synthesized and analyzed so that nursing diagnoses can be identified. Assessment provides the baseline data for formulating nursing diagnoses, patient outcomes, and the plan of care. Assessment is a continuing process, never a completed one. A comprehensive, holistic assessment provides information that enables nurses to deliver quality patient care. It establishes the foundation for comparison and the basis for interpreting future observations, plans, and evaluation. The findings from the initial and ongoing assessment assist nurses in making decisions about whether to alter, expand, or discontinue the current treatment plans.

Overlooking things that are, or appear to be, insignificant is a common human failing.[25] Because critically ill patients tend to have multiple and complex problems, it is quite possible to misinterpret or fail to identify cues to those problems. A subtle change in a physical or psychologic sign or symptom could be the first indication of a serious problem. Thus, any change in the patient's condition must not be ignored. The cause of the change must be carefully explored. Every clue must be analyzed. Every unexpected sign must be fully understood before it is dismissed as unimportant. Subtle yet significant findings must be carefully observed or appropriately reported and treated.

The patient's status is reassessed as often as necessary after the initial assessment has been completed and after the patient's nursing diagnoses, patient outcomes, and nursing orders have been formulated. Reassessment can help to determine the acuteness and severity of the problem by comparing the findings to the baseline data.

A holistic assessment consists of more than just collecting biopsychosocial data about the patient. Both nurses and patients are open systems. They exchange information and energy. Their energy fields overlap and are affected by one another. Nurses must learn to use their therapeutic healing resources. They must be open to subtle cues, environmental changes, and intuitive feelings that can have an enormous impact on the data collected and the conclusions drawn during a patient assessment. When nurses are aware of collecting data with purposeful intention, they become receptive to the encounter, thus allowing the free flow of information to occur at many levels.

ASSESSMENT IN THE 1990s: THE NEED TO CHANGE FROM A MEDICAL TO A HOLISTIC ASSESSMENT

The kind of assessment tool format used by many nurses in the United States usually includes information related to demographic data, patient's chief complaint, current illness, past medical history, family history, review of systems, and a physical examination. Psychosocial questions also are generally included at the beginning or the end of the tool. This type of format is popular and comfortably used in critical care units throughout the country. In the first edition of this book (1981), the authors presented two types of assessment formats similar to the one just described. One was based on a head-to-toe assessment (which begins with the patient's head and continues to the feet), and the other focused on an assessment of major-body-systems (in which individual body systems, *e.g.,* the respiratory, cardiovascular, and neurologic systems, are appraised).

Unfortunately, if such assessment formats are analyzed, it would be discovered that they are nothing more than medical assessment tools (data base) with some randomly selected psychosocial questions tacked on.[12,13] The head-to-toe and the major-body-systems approaches, in fact, guide the collection of physiologic data only. They do not guide data collection in the psychosocial realm. They do not provide the nurse with a framework for what psychosocial parameters should be assessed, what questions should be asked, or how the psychosocial data should be interrelated to the physiologic realm.

Because the medical data base is guided by the biomedical model, it views the patient from a different perspective than nursing.[7,14] Moreover, it asks questions and organizes its information differently from that found in a nursing data base. Most important, when using a medical data base in practice, nurses do not collect all of the necessary data to assess their patients holistically.[12] Although a complete physical assessment is generally accomplished, the psychosocial assessment is haphazard and produces fragmented and incomplete data. Thus, major obstacles are created when trying to identify all of the patient's body-mind-spirit problems because all the necessary data are not obtained during the assessment. Therefore, it is impossible to support the existence of nursing diagnoses.[12] Nurses who are having difficulty in using nursing diagnoses should carefully examine whether they are using a medical rather than a nursing data base in their practice.[17]

Because of the need to shift from a biomedical to a holistic approach to patient care, nursing leaders have stressed the importance of using nursing models or frameworks to guide clinical practice.[10] The following pages discuss development of a Critical Care Response Pattern Assessment Tool prototype based on the Unitary Person Framework developed by the North American Nursing Diagnosis Association (NANDA).

UNITARY PERSON FRAMEWORK

The Unitary Person Framework was created by NANDA to guide the development and identification of nursing diagnoses. (*Note:* This is not Martha Roger's Unitary Man Model. Although it uses some of Roger's concepts, the Unitary Person Framework incorporates and synthesizes the ideas of 14 theorists involved with its development.)

The Unitary Person Framework focuses on the health of the person—the area of most relevance to nursing. The person is conceptualized as an open system in mutual interaction with the environment. Within this framework, concern for the mind is seen as equivalent to concern for the body.[7] The person is in a process of continuous development moving toward increasing complexity and diversity involving roles, function, structure, and services.[33] This continuous process of development occurs in persons progressing through the life span and from generation to generation.

The Unitary Person Framework asserts that each person is characterized by a unique pattern and organization. This unique pattern and organization, in turn, describe the person's state of health as manifested by the nine human response patterns described in Table 5–1.[33] Health is viewed as a pattern of energy exchange that enhances the integrity of the person to move toward life's fullest potential.

The patterns defined in Table 5–1 reflect all parts of the whole person. If nurses evaluate all nine patterns, they will achieve a holistic assessment. These nine patterns provide the working categories for developing a holistic nursing data base. They have also been used as the classification schema for organizing the list of nursing diagnoses as discussed below.

TAXONOMY I

Taxonomy I (Table 5–2) was developed recently by NANDA from the Unitary Person Framework to enhance the development of nursing diagnoses.[2,5,24] In the past, the accepted list of nursing diagnoses was organized alphabetically. Currently, the alphabetical list has been replaced by Taxonomy I, which is organized according to the nine human response patterns.

Table 5-1

Nine Human Response Patterns of the Unitary Person Framework

Exchanging: a human response pattern involving mutual giving and receiving
Communicating: a human response pattern involving sending messages
Relating: a human response pattern involving establishing bonds
Valuing: a human response pattern involving the assigning of relative worth
Choosing: a human response pattern involving the selection of alternatives
Moving: a human response pattern involving activity
Perceiving: a human response pattern involving the reception of information
Knowing: a human response pattern involving the meaning associated with information
Feeling: a human response pattern involving the subjective awareness of information

(The North American Nursing Diagnosis Association, St. Louis, 1989.)

Table 5-2

Taxonomy I Revised (1990)

PATTERN 1:   EXCHANGING

1.1.2.1	Altered nutrition: more than body requirements
1.1.2.2	Altered nutrition: less than body requirements
1.1.2.3	Altered nutrition: potential for more than body requirements
1.2.1.1	Potential for infection
1.2.2.1	Potential altered body temperature
1.2.2.2	Hypothermia
1.2.2.3	Hyperthermia
1.2.2.4	Ineffective thermoregulation
1.2.3.1	Dysreflexia
1.3.1.1	Constipation*
1.3.1.1.1	Perceived constipation
1.3.1.1.2	Colonic constipation
1.3.1.2	Diarrhea*
1.3.1.3	Bowel incontinence*
1.3.2	Altered urinary elimination
1.3.2.1.1	Stress incontinence
1.3.2.1.2	Reflex incontinence
1.3.2.1.3	Urge incontinence
1.3.2.1.4	Functional incontinence
1.3.2.1.5	Total incontinence
1.3.2.2	Urinary retention
1.4.1.1	Altered (specify type) tissue perfusion (renal, cerebral, cardiopulmonary, gastrointestinal, peripheral)*
1.4.1.2.1	Fluid volume excess
1.4.1.2.2.1	Fluid volume deficit
1.4.1.2.2.2	Potential fluid volume deficit
1.4.2.1	Decreased cardiac output*
1.5.1.1	Impaired gas exchange
1.5.1.2	Ineffective airway clearance
1.5.1.3	Ineffective breathing pattern
1.6.1	Potential for injury
1.6.1.1	Potential for suffocation
1.6.1.2	Potential for poisoning
1.6.1.3	Potential for trauma
1.6.1.4	Potential for aspiration
1.6.1.5	Potential for disuse syndrome
1.6.2	Altered protection†
1.6.2.1	Impaired tissue integrity
1.6.2.1.1	Altered oral mucous membrane*
1.6.2.1.2.1	Impaired skin integrity
1.6.2.1.2.2	Potential impaired skin integrity

PATTERN 2:   COMMUNICATING

2.1.1.1	Impaired verbal communication

PATTERN 3:   RELATING

3.1.1	Impaired social interaction
3.1.2	Social isolation
3.2.1	Altered role performance*
3.2.1.1.1	Altered parenting
3.2.1.1.2	Potential altered parenting
3.2.1.2.1	Sexual dysfunction
3.2.2	Altered family processes
3.2.3.1	Parental role conflict
3.3	Altered sexuality patterns

PATTERN 4:   VALUING

4.1.1	Spiritual distress (distress of the human spirit)

PATTERN 5:   CHOOSING

5.1.1.1	Ineffective individual coping
5.1.1.1.1	Impaired adjustment
5.1.1.1.2	Defensive coping
5.1.1.1.3	Ineffective denial
5.1.2.1.1	Ineffective family coping: disabling
5.1.2.1.2	Ineffective family coping: compromised
5.1.2.2	Family coping: potential for growth
5.2.1.1	Noncompliance (specify)
5.3.1.1	Decisional conflict (specify)
5.4	Health seeking behaviors (specify)

PATTERN 6:   MOVING

6.1.1.1	Impaired physical mobility
6.1.1.2	Activity intolerance
6.1.1.2.1	Fatigue
6.1.1.3	Potential activity intolerance
6.2.1	Sleep pattern disturbance
6.3.1.1	Diversional activity deficit
6.4.1.1	Impaired home maintenance management
6.4.2	Altered health maintenance
6.5.1	Feeding self care deficit*
6.5.1.1	Impaired swallowing
6.5.1.2	Ineffective breastfeeding
6.5.1.3	Effective breastfeeding†
6.5.2	Bathing/hygiene self care deficit*
6.5.3	Dressing/grooming self care deficit*
6.5.4	Toileting self care deficit*
6.6	Altered growth and development

PATTERN 7:   PERCEIVING

7.1.1	Body image disturbance*
7.1.2	Self esteem disturbance*
7.1.2.1	Chronic low self esteem
7.1.2.2	Situational low self esteem
7.1.3	Personal identity disturbance*
7.2	Sensory/perceptual alterations (specify) (visual, auditory, kinesthetic, gustatory, tactile, olfactory)
7.2.1.1	Unilateral neglect
7.3.1	Hopelessness
7.3.2	Powerlessness

PATTERN 8:   KNOWING

8.1.1	Knowledge deficit (specify)
8.3	Altered thought processes

PATTERN 9:   FEELING

9.1.1	Pain*
9.1.1.1	Chronic pain
9.2.1.1	Dysfunctional grieving
9.2.1.2	Anticipatory grieving
9.2.2	Potential for violence: self-directed or directed at others
9.2.3	Post-trauma response
9.2.3.1	Rape-trauma syndrome
9.2.3.1.1	Rape-trauma syndrome: compound reaction
9.2.3.1.2	Rape-trauma syndrome: silent reaction
9.3.1	Anxiety
9.3.2	Fear

* Categories with modified label terminology.
† New diagnostic categories approved 1990.
Note: NANDA approved diagnoses currently designated as ''Potential'' will be labeled ''High Risk for'' in 1992.
(The North American Nursing Diagnosis Association, St. Louis, 1990.)

A taxonomy is used to arrange entities systematically into categories according to relevant features. Taxonomies help one to understand the entities by identifying how they are different and similar. They also are used to identify relationships and conceptual gaps among the entities. Taxonomies are useful because they facilitate communication, information retrieval, and computer access. For these reasons, NANDA has approved Taxonomy I as the current classification system for nursing diagnoses. All approved nursing diagnoses have been placed within various lower-level response patterns categories within the Taxonomy. First-level categories define the pattern of concern (*e.g.,* exchanging pattern), whereas second-level categories include "altered" response patterns such as altered nutrition. An alteration is defined as the "process or state of becoming or being made different without changing into something else."[24] Third-level categories define the specific areas to be assessed (*e.g.,* systemic, immunologic, bowel, role performance, or individual versus family). Fourth- and fifth-level categories tend to be more specific in defining the particular problem (*e.g.,* a fourth-level category is altered systemic nutrition: more than body requirements, whereas a fifth-level category is fatigue under the moving pattern). The numbering system does not reflect priorities of the patterns but merely represents how the entities are related and fit together.

Definitions for diagnostic qualifiers also were approved to provide a standardized terminology for developing new and revising old diagnoses (Table 5–3). As Taxonomy I is tested in clinical practice, it is expected to be revised.[5,24]

CRITICAL CARE RESPONSE PATTERN ASSESSMENT TOOL PROTOTYPE

The development of the Critical Care Response Pattern Assessment Tool emerged as a logical extension of the work accomplished by two of our leading nursing organizations. In 1981, the American Nurses' Association published the Social Policy Statement, which was of monumental significance to nursing practice. Within this publication, nursing was defined as the "diagnosis and treatment of human responses to actual or potential health problems."[1] Several years later, NANDA defined a nursing diagnosis (within the context of the Unitary Person Framework) as "a judgment about the health of the

unitary person based on the data collected from the nine human response patterns."[33] The central idea that arose from these definitions was very basic yet critical regarding the implication for nursing assessment:

If nurses are to make judgments about the health of an individual based on the data collected from the nine human response patterns, then construction of a nursing data base that incorporates the signs and symptoms necessary to evaluate the nine human response patterns is fundamental.[12]

From this central idea, the Critical Care Response Pattern Assessment Tool was developed based on NANDA's Unitary Person Framework and Taxonomy I.[13,30] The first stage of the tool's development incorporated the nine human response patterns as the foundation or skeleton of the tool. The order of the response patterns (as they appear in Taxonomy I), however, was rearranged to permit historical and interview data to emerge before physiologic data were collected. Therefore, the "exchanging pattern" normally found first in Taxonomy I and primarily involving physiologic parameters, was moved to a latter part of the tool. During the second stage of the tool's development, the process Standards for Nursing Care of the Critically Ill[34] were included into the tool's skeleton. These standards of practice provide model statements that guide the nurse in delivering and evaluating the quality of patient care.

In the last stage of the tool's development, specific assessment parameters (signs and symptoms) related to most critical care nursing diagnoses within each of the nine human response patterns were included.[12,13] When available, NANDA's defining characteristics were used.[5] The case study reported in the following box (Case Study Box 5-1) describes a patient admitted to the intensive care unit with total bowel obstruction. The Critical Care Response Pattern Assessment Tool[30] (Fig. 5–2) illustrates the data that were collected to assess the patient's body-mind-spirit problems.

The tool clusters assessment parameters for a particular patient problem so a judgment can be made about whether the problem actually exists in the patient being assessed.[13] Subjective variables followed by objectives variables are included for each major category of the tool. To reduce the tool's length and because varying levels of abstractness are found in the tool, not all possible assessment parameters related to each diagnosis are included. Instead, summary assessment parameters are provided (*e.g.,* barriers to communication under the communicating pattern is an example of a summary assessment parameter used to assess alterations in verbal communication). If the nurse is unsure of what data are to be extracted from such summary assessment parameters, the focus questions and parameters discussed on pages 68 to 80 outline recommended questions and physical assessment data that can be used.

Assessment parameters necessary to evaluate the critically ill patient fully were included. The exchanging pattern, for example, includes detailed, complex physiologic variables. A holistic assessment includes the collection of data from all the human response patterns; thus, the thorough assessment of the exchanging pattern is as important to a holistic assessment as is a complete assessment of the other eight response patterns.[13]

Within the exchanging pattern, lower-level categories were rearranged to permit a logical physical assessment. In addition,

---

Table 5-3
NANDA Diagnosis Qualifiers

Altered: A change from baseline
Impaired: Made worse, weakened; damaged, reduced; deteriorated
Depleted: Emptied wholly or partially; exhausted of
Deficient: Inadequate in amount, quality, or degree; defective; not sufficient; incomplete
Excessive: Characterized by an amount or quantity that is greater than is necessary, desirable, or useful
Dysfunction: Abnormal; incomplete functioning
Disturbed: Agitated; interrupted, interfered with
Ineffective: Not producing the desired effect
Decreased: Lessened, lesser in size, amount or degree
Increased: Greater in size, amount or degree
Acute: Severe but of short duration
Chronic: Lasting a long time; recurring; habitual; constant
Intermittent: Stopping and starting again at intervals; periodic; cyclic

(The North American Nursing Diagnosis Association, St. Louis, 1990.)

assessment parameters were grouped to prevent repetition of information. Some of the categories were combined (*e.g.*, gastrointestinal and bowel), others were added because they were highly relevant to critically ill patients (*e.g.*, leakage of spinal fluid was added under physical integrity in the exchanging pattern), and some were deleted because they were not relevant (*e.g.*, altered breastfeeding). After the Critical Care Response Pattern Assessment Tool was developed, it was tested and refined on critically ill patients by nurse experts.[13,30]

Following refinement of this tool, many questions were received about how the tool might be changed for use with other patient populations (*e.g.*, neurosurgical, neonatal, perioperative, transplant, trauma, rehabilitation patients, and so forth). This work has recently been accomplished in a new text. Twenty-three assessment tools, all based on the Unitary Person Framework and Taxonomy I, have been developed for use with diverse patient populations.[13] Although the tools incorporate different assessment parameters because they were designed to assess the unique problems of various patient groups, the theory, process, structure, and outcome of the tools are the same, thereby offering a model for standardizing nursing data bases across the country.[13]

Using the Critical Care Response Pattern Assessment Tool

The Critical Care Response Pattern Assessment Tool is different from the assessment formats conventionally used by most nurses. It does not follow the traditional organization of a typical medical data base. The tool was developed to elicit data about holistic responses rather than to elicit information that exclusively reflects medical patterns. It provides a new method of collecting, synthesizing, and interrelating the data to understand patterns and processes that form the whole rather than identifying unrelated and fragmented signs and symptoms. Because the tool represents a nursing data base developed from a nursing framework, it permits a holistic assessment to take place so that nursing diagnoses can be easily identified.[13]

Although changing traditional assessment methods is not an easy task, nurses will become familiar with the tool's organization after it is used several times in clinical practice. With experience, nurses will become accustomed to new ways of clustering and synthesizing data. With continued use, the time necessary to complete the tool will be reduced and the ability to identify the appropriate signs and symptoms for each category will be enhanced.[13]

Nurses should collect assessment data within a time period that reflects the gravity of the patient's problems. Priority sections can be identified during the initial assessment. Other sections can be completed later, usually within 24 hours of the patient's admission. If the patient is unstable, for example, timing is often crucial. The patient is rapidly evaluated using the ABCs of basic life support and a rapid head-to-toe assessment. Data for this rapid evaluation are found under the exchanging pattern beginning with oxygenation and circulation (and disregarding the sequential ordering of the variables in this section). The other response patterns are then assessed after the patient has stabilized.[13]

As a learning technique, the nursing diagnoses that are associated with a cluster of assessment parameters are listed in the right-hand column of the tool to facilitate the process of formulating the appropriate nursing diagnoses. Some of these

diagnoses are repeated several times for the convenience of identifying certain data directly with a corresponding diagnosis. These diagnoses are neither absolute nor static but are intended to focus thinking and to direct more detailed attention to a possible problem.[13]

When specific signs and symptoms are identified that indicate the existence of a particular diagnosis, the nurse circles the diagnosis in the right-hand column of the tool. Although a circled diagnosis alerts the nurse to a possible problem, it does not confirm its existence. Should a particular problem be suspected, a more complete evaluation is necessary based on the critical defining characteristics of the specific nursing diagnosis. If the patient is at high risk for developing the problem, write high risk or HR next to the diagnosis before circling it. Although some signs and symptoms can indicate a number of diagnoses (*e.g.*, mental confusion can indicate altered oxygenation, altered cardiac output, altered thought processes, and so forth), assessment variables have been arranged with the diagnosis most likely to result from the data assessed. Thus, data to support one diagnosis may occasionally be found in other patterns or arranged with other diagnoses (*e.g.*, tachycardia identified in the exchanging pattern may support the diagnosis of severe anxiety in the feeling pattern). Therefore, synthesis of all data is essential.[13]

It is also important to realize that other diagnoses not listed in the right-hand column may exist related to the data collected. Moreover, many patient problems that nurses encounter are not yet found in Taxonomy I because this classification

---

CASE STUDY BOX 5-1

Mr. L. H. is a 45-year-old airplane mechanic who lives in American Samoa. In October, he was seen in a Samoan hospital for a mild head injury incurred while he was repairing a helicopter propeller blade. During his hospitalization, routine laboratory tests, x-rays, and examinations revealed an obstruction of the large bowel and a perforated colon. An exploratory laparotomy was performed, with the result that Mr. L. H. underwent a colectomy with jejunostomy tube placement. Over the first month, Mr. L. H.'s condition deteriorated and his obstruction returned. At this time, he was transferred to a large medical center in Hawaii.

The patient arrived on the unit in obviously poor health and excruciating pain. Although he was receiving 50% oxygen per face mask, his respiratory rate of 52 bore arterial blood gases with pH of 7.28, PO_2 of 58, PCO_2 of 47, and a saturation of 89%. Crackles were heard on auscultation.

Once undressed, jaundiced, dry skin was found to be reddened, raw, and bleeding from Mr. L. H.'s nipples to his hips. The removal of an abdominal dressing revealed leakage of pancreatic fluid from a jejunostomy tube and three drains that protruded from the sides of his open exploratory laparotomy incision. The diagnosis of large bowel obstruction was confirmed by x-ray and computed tomographic (CT) scan.

Shortly after admission, the patient was intubated and taken to surgery for re-exploration. He currently has a tracheostomy and is slowly healing on a medical regimen of antibiotics, hyperalimentation, and bed rest.

Mr. L. H.'s assessment was completed in two sessions. During the initial session, the patient became too short of breath and fatigued from his respiratory efforts to continue. His son, John, assisted the next day in completing the assessment data.

system is still in the stage of development. Because the list of nursing diagnoses is incomplete, there will be times that the patient exhibits signs and symptoms that support the existence of a new diagnosis. In such a case, synthesize the data, label the new problem, and write the new diagnosis in the right-hand column.[13]

Following the assessment, the nurse scans the circled problems, synthesizes the data to determine if other clusters of signs and symptoms also support the existence of a specific problem, and then makes a decision regarding whether the diagnosis actually exists. When synthesizing the data, it may be discovered that all of the circled diagnoses do not actually exist and that the data collected indicate a more global nursing diagnosis. For example, the data identified for fear and social isolation, when synthesized, may actually support the diagnoses of altered self-esteem related to the effects of cardiac transplantation surgery. Thus, there will be times when all of the circled diagnoses will not appear on the problem list at the end of the tool.[13]

When the nursing diagnoses have been formulated, they are prioritized and written on the problem list at the end of the tool. Patient outcomes, a plan for intervention, and a method of evaluation are identified for the most critical diagnoses. The diagnoses that are judged not to be as critical can be considered at a later date or can be referred to other health team members for assistance as appropriate.[13]

CRITICAL CARE RESPONSE PATTERN ASSESSMENT TOOL*

Name _Mr. L.H._ Age _45_ Sex _male_

Address _American Samoa_ Telephone _555-1122_

Significant other _son – John_ Telephone _555-9988_

Date of admission _2 Nov_ Medical diagnosis _Total bowel obstruction_

Allergies _None known_

Nursing Diagnosis

COMMUNICATING—A pattern involving sending messages
(Read,) (write,) (understand English) (circle) _____
Other language _Samoan_
Barriers to communication _possible comprehension of English_
Alternate form of communication _if intubated, will need sign board & pen/paper_

Altered communication
Verbal
Impaired

KNOWING—A pattern involving the meaning associated with information
Current health problems _Total bowel obstruction c̄ possible colonic mass, liver failure second to ETOH abuse_

Previous illnesses/hospitalizations/surgeries _Oct – exploratory laparotomy, colectomy, jejunostomy tube placement for large bowel obstruction at another hospital. Transferred to this hospital one month later with reobstruction._

History of the following problems:
Heart _Ø_

Peripheral vascular _Ø_

Lung _Ø_

Liver _failure, hepatitis_ Kidney _Ø_

Cerebrovascular _Ø_ Rheumatic fever _Ø_

Thyroid _Ø_

Drug abuse _Ø_

Other _Pancreatitis, ETOH abuse_

Knowledge deficit

Recent history of the following:
Blood transfusion _yes_ Trauma _Ø_ CO poisoning _Ø_
Heat stroke _Ø_ Sepsis _yes_ Muscle injury _Ø_
Nephrotoxic medications _____

* (Modified from Prinkey, L. A., and Bunton, S. D. Critical Care Assessment Tool. In C. E. Guzzetta, S. D. Bunton, L. A. Prinkey, *et al, Clinical Assessment Tools for Use with Nursing Diagnoses.* St. Louis: C.V. Mosby: 184–190; 1989; with permission.)

Figure 5-2

Critical Care Response Pattern Assessment Tool.

(continued)

CRITICAL CARE RESPONSE PATTERN ASSESSMENT TOOL   *(Continued)*

Current medications _Multiple vitamin = 1 qd; Valium = 5 mg IV q̄ 8 hr.;_   Knowledge deficit
Haldol 2 mg IV prn q̄ 4 hrs; Ampicillin 500 mg IVPB q̄ 6 hr.
_____

Risk factors	Present	Perceptions/Knowledge of
1. Hypertension	_____	_____
2. Hyperlipidemia	_____	_____
3. Smoking	_√_	_Aware that smoking can cause cancers_
4. Obesity	_____	_____
5. Diabetes	_____	_____
6. Sedentary living	_____	_____
7. Stress	_____	_____
8. Alcohol use	_√_	_Enjoys the feeling, therefore drinks_
9. Oral contraceptives	_____	_____
10. Family history	_unremarkable_	

Perception/knowledge of illness/test/surgery _(son) "He knows he drank too_
much. Hopes surgery will fix him."

Expectations of therapy _"To repair my stomach so I can eat."_

Misconceptions _⁓_____

Readiness to learn _⁓_____

   Requests information concerning _N/A_____

   Educational level _High school_____

   Learning impeded by _Current physical condition and pain_

Orientation

Level of alertness _awake, oriented; mentation decreases c̄ removal of oxygen_   Altered thought processes

Orientation: Person _√_   Place _√_   Time _√_

Appropriate behavior/communication _yes, if oxygen is on_

Memory

Memory intact: Yes _√_   No _____   Recent _√_   Remote _√_

VALUING—A pattern involving the assessment of relative worth

Religious preference _none_

Important religious practices _does not practice_   Spiritual distress

Spiritual concerns _⁓_

Cultural orientation _Samoan_

Cultural practices _centers around family togetherness_

RELATING—A pattern involving establishing bonds

Role

Marital status _divorced 5 years_   Altered role performance

Age and health of significant other _16 y.o. son in good health_   Parenting
  Sexual dysfunction

Number of children _3_   Ages _16, 11, 9 (one here, two at home)_

Role in home _"Live alone, son stays sometimes."_

Financial support _Sole support to children living with mother_

Occupation _airplane mechanic_   Altered family processes

   Job satisfaction/concerns _"I hope they hold my spot & not hire someone else."_   Parental role conflict

   Physical/mental energy expenditures _high physical, moderate mental_

Sexual relationships (satisfactory/unsatisfactory) _____   Altered sexuality patterns

   Sexual partner(s) _girlfriend_

   Physical difficulties/effects of illness related to sex _none_

Socialization   Altered socialization

Quality of relationships with others:

Patient's description _I get along OK with other people & my children_   Impaired social interaction

Significant others' description _(son) "He is a loner."_

Staff observations _Visits with son & sister, no observable stress noted_

Verbalizes feelings of being alone _no_   Social isolation

Attributed to _—_

FEELING—A pattern involving the subjective awareness of information

Comfort

Pain/discomfort: Yes ✓ No ____   Altered comfort

Onset _—_   Duration _constant_   (Pain/chronic)

Location _abdomen_ Quality _intense_   Radiation _∅_   Pain/acute

Associated factors _numerous abdominal tubes/drains_

Aggravating factors _dressing changes_

Alleviating factors _Increased pain medications_

Objective manifestations _Has "watchful eye" over those about him,_
particularly when discussing his wound.

Emotional Integrity/States

Recent stressful life events _Was hit in head by propeller at work, this lead_
to hospitalization, testing, & resultant surgery.

Verbalizes feelings of _anxiety_   (Anxiety)

  Source ① _"Where money for bills will come from?"_   Fear

  ② _"How long will I have to stay here?"_   Grieving

Physical manifestations _lackluster eyes, frequently has beaten look_   Dysfunctional

                                                               Anticipatory

---

MOVING—A pattern involving activity

Self-care

Ability to perform self-care (Specify level) _Level 4—cannot perform self-care_ (Self-care deficit)

  0 = Completely independent

  1 = Requires use of equipment or devices

  2 = Requires help from another person for assistance, supervision, or teaching

  3 = Requires help from another person and equipment devices

  4 = Dependent, does not participate in activity   (Feeding)

Specify deficits _unable to meet self requirements_   Impaired swallowing

Discharge planning needs _inabilities should be restored at discharge_ (Bathing/hygiene)

                                                               (Dressing/grooming)

                                                               (Toileting)

(continued)

CRITICAL CARE RESPONSE PATTERN ASSESSMENT TOOL *(Continued)*

Activity

Limitations of movement (Specify level) *Level 2—requires assistance with*   ⟨Impaired physical mobility⟩

turning side to side

Limitations in activities *bedrest by medical recommendations*   Activity intolerance

_____   ⟨Fatigue⟩

Braces/casts/splints/traction (circle) _____

Fracture(s) _____   Extensive burns _____

Paralysis _____   Amputation(s) _____

Verbal report of fatigue *complains of weakness* _____

Exercise habits *none* _____

Rest

Sleep/rest pattern *"only a few hours a night"* _____   Sleep pattern disturbance

Sleep aids (pillows, meds, food) *alcohol* _____

Difficulty falling/remaining asleep *"not usually"* _____

Recreation

Leisure activities *none* _____   Diversional activity deficit

Social activities *none* _____

Activities of Daily Living

Home Maintenance Management

   Size & arrangement of home (stairs, bathroom) *single story, small*   Impaired home maintenance management

   _____ Safety needs _____

   Home responsibilities *"Bring home paycheck."* _____

   _____

Health Maintenance

   Health insurance *"Aviators Mutual Life Insurance" —job related*   Altered health maintenance

   Regular physical check-ups *"Only when I feel bad"* _____

PERCEIVING—A pattern involving the reception of information

Self-esteem/Body Image

Perception of self and situation *unable to evaluate* _____   Altered self-concept

   _____   Self-esteem disturbance

   _____   Chronic low

Description of body structure/functioning _____   Situational low

   _____   Body image disturbance

Effects of illness/surgery on self-concept _____

   _____

Meaningfulness

Verbalizes hopelessness *no* _____   Hopelessness

Verbalizes loss of control *no* _____   Powerlessness

Sensory/Perception

History of restricted environment *bedrest* _____   Altered sensory/perception

Vision impaired *Ø*   Glasses *Ø* _____   Visual

Auditory impaired *Ø*   Hearing aid *Ø* _____   Auditory

Kinesthetics impaired *unable to evaluate* _____   Kinesthetic

Gustatory impaired *Ø* _____   Gustatory

Figure 5-2 *(Continued)*

Tactile impaired ___*decreased between nipples & hips, numbness*___   Tactile

Olfactory impaired ___*Ø*___   Olfactory

Reflexes: Biceps   R _*2+*_ L _*2+*_   Triceps R _*2+*_ L _*2+*_

Brachioradialis R _*2+*_ L _*2+*_   Knee   R _*1+*_ L _*1+*_

Ankle   R _*1+*_ L _*1+*_   Plantar R _*1+*_ L _*1+*_

EXCHANGING—A pattern involving mutual giving and receiving

Circulation

Cerebral

Neurologic changes/symptoms ___*decreased mentation when without O₂*___   Altered cerebral tissue perfusion

Seizure activity ___*none*___   Dysreflexia

Pupils   Eye Opening
L 2 ③ 4 5 6 mm   None (1)
R 2 ③ 4 5 6 mm   To pain (2)
Reaction: Brisk _____   To speech (3)   Fluid volume
Sluggish _✓_ Non reactive _____ (Spontaneous (4))   Deficit

Excess

Best Verbal   Best Motor
Mute (1)   Flaccid (1)
Incomprehensible sound (2)   Extensor response (2)   Decreased cardiac output
Inappropriate words (3)   Flexor response (3)
Confused conversation (4)   Semipurposeful (4)
(Oriented (5))   Localized to pain (5)
                                (Obeys commands (6))

Glasgow coma scale total ___*15*___   Altered cerebral tissue perfusion

Intracranial pressure ___—___

Peripheral   Altered peripheral tissue perfusion
Pulses: A = absent   B = bruits   D = doppler
+3 = bounding   +2 = palpable   +1 = faintly palpable

Carotid   R _*2+*_ L _*2+*_   Popliteal   R _*2+*_ L _*2+*_   Fluid volume
Brachial R _*2+*_ L _*2+*_   Posterior tibial R _*2+*_ L _*2+*_   Deficit
Radial   R _*2+*_ L _*2+*_   Dorsalis pedis   R _*2+*_ L _*2+*_   Excess
Femoral   R _*2+*_ L _*2+*_

Blood pressure:
    Sitting   Lying   Standing   Excess
R _____ L _____   R _*78/60*_ L _*80/60*_   R _____ L _____
A-Line reading ___*82/62 (left radial)*___
Jugular venous distention R _*no*_ L _*no*_ CVP ___*Ø*___
Skin temp _*hot, dry*_ Color _*reddened skin*_
Capillary refill ___*<3 seconds*___ Clubbing ___—___   Decreased cardiac output
Edema _*bilateral, feet, 1+*_

Cardiac
PMI _*4th intercostal space*_ Pacemaker ___—___   Altered cardiopulmonary tissue perfusion
Apical rate & rhythm _*110 & regular*_
Heart sounds/murmurs _*nml S₁ - S₂, muffled*_
Dysrhythmias ___—___ *sinus tachycardia*

(continued)

CRITICAL CARE RESPONSE PATTERN ASSESSMENT TOOL *(Continued)*

Cardiac output _8.2_ Cardiac index _——_ ⟨Decreased cardiac output⟩

PAP _22/7_ PCWP _5_

IV fluids _D₅1/2, D₅RL + 20 mEq KCl @ total 100 cc/hr_

IV medications _Ampicillin IVPB_ Dysreflexia

Serum enzymes _pending_

Physical Integrity

Tissue integrity _generally poor, turgor poor_

Skin rashes _jaundice_ Lesions _——_ Decubitus ulcers _sacral, 3 mm_ ⟨Impaired skin integrity⟩

Petechiae _——_ Bruises _see below*_ Impaired tissue integrity

Abrasions _see below*_ Surgical incision _exp. lap. scar, six drains_

Bleeding: massive/moderate/⟨minimal⟩(circle) _through middle, right drain_ Disuse syndrome

*Left flank from nipples to mid-thigh raw, red, bleeding. Most likely from leaking peritoneal drainage.

Extravasation from burns _∅_

Burns: Degree _∅_ Type _____ Location _____ Fluid volume

Degree _____ Type _____ Location _____ Deficit

Degree _____ Type _____ Location _____ Excess

Percentage of body surface area _____ High risk for infection

Leakage of spinal fluid from ears/nose/other (circle) _____ Altered protection

Dialysis access: Yes _____ No _✓_

Fistula _____ A-V shunt _____ PD catheter _____

Central line _____

Current condition of access _____

Oxygenation

Complaints of dyspnea _Yes_ Precipitated by _movement, dressing change_

Orthopnea _——_ ⟨Ineffective breathing patterns⟩

Rate _52_ Rhythm _regular_ Depth _shallow_

⟨Labored⟩/unlabored (circle) Use of accessory muscles _Yes_ Ineffective airway clearance

Chest expansion _minimal_ Splinting _Yes_

Cough: Productive/nonproductive _absent_ ⟨Impaired gas exchange⟩

Sputum: Color _——_ Amount _——_ Consistency _——_ High risk for aspiration

Breath sounds _severely decreased, crackles throughout_

Arterial blood gases _pH = 7.28, PO₂ = 58, PCO₂ = 47, sat = 89,_

bicarb = 22, BE = −3

Oxygen percent and device _50% face mask_

Ventilator _(probable)_

Physical Regulation

Immune High risk for infection

Lymph nodes enlarged _no_ Location _——_ Hypothermia

Hyperthermia

WBC count _12_ Differential _pending_ Altered body temperature

HIV testing results _negative_ Ineffective thermoregulation

Altered protection

Temperature _99.8_ Route _oral_

Figure 5-2 *(Continued)*

Nutrition

Eating patterns *(son = informant)*

  Number of meals per day *"only picks—eats very little, drinks a lot"*

Special diet *none*

Where eaten *home, & at work*

Food preferences/intolerances _____

Food allergies *none known*

Caffeine intake (coffee, tea, soft drinks)

  "A couple cups of coffee a day"

Appetite changes _____

Presence of nausea/vomiting *"only after large amounts of alcohol"*

Condition of mouth/throat *Teeth in poor repair, tongue coated with whitish substance*

Height *5'8"* Weight *120 #* Ideal body weight *154 #*

Current therapy

  NPO *✓* NG suction *none*

Tube feeding _____

TPN *Hyperalimentation*

Labs

  Na *143 mEq/L* K *3.6 mEq/L* CL *101 mEq/L*

CO_2 *21 mM* Glucose *146 mg/dl*

Cholesterol _____ Triglycerides _____ Fasting _____

Albumin *3.1 g/dl* Total protein _____ Total lymphocyte count _____

PT *pending* PTT *pending* Platelets *65* Hct *35.7* Hgb *14.3*

Total bilirubin = 25.5 mg/dl

Elimination

Gastrointestinal/Bowel

  Usual bowel habits *"once a day"*

Use of laxatives, enemas, and/or suppositories *none*

Alterations from norm _____

Abdominal physical exam *unable to assess due to drains, retaining sutures*

Liver: Enlarged *yes* Ascites *none*

Bleeding: Gastric *yes* frank *✓* occult _____

    Intestinal *yes* frank *✓* occult _____

    Esophageal tube _____

Renal/Urinary

  Possible kidney contusion/other injury *none*

Usual urinary pattern *frequent, small amounts*

Alteration from norm _____

Urostomy _____ Dialysis _____

Bladder distention *none stated or palpated*

Color *yellow/dark* Catheter *in place, #24F, how long questionable*

Urine output: 24 hour _____ Average hourly *40 cc/hr*

BUN *28 mg/dl* Creatinine *2.8 mg/dl* Specific gravity *1.004*

Urine studies _____

Altered nutrition

  More than body requirements

  Less than body requirements

Impaired oral mucous membranes

(Altered nutrition)

  More than body requirements

  (Less than body requirements)

  High risk for aspiration

Altered bowel elimination

  Constipation

    Perceived

    Colonic

  Diarrhea

  Incontinence

(Altered GI tissue perfusion)

Altered urinary elimination

  Incontinence

  Retention

Altered renal tissue perfusion

Fluid volume

  Deficit

  Excess

Decreased cardiac output

(continued)

CRITICAL CARE RESPONSE PATTERN ASSESSMENT TOOL *(Continued)*

CHOOSING—A pattern involving the selection of alternatives

Coping

Patient's ability to cope *seems accepting of current status, no evidence of ineffective coping, believes he possesses ability to solve problems.*

Family's ability to cope/give support *son, sister supportive, but state feeling hopeless to assist in ways other than visiting.*

Patient's acceptance of illness *"I guess I brought this on myself—no one made me drink."*

Patient's adjustment to illness *No evidence of angry feelings, states he wishes to do whatever is best to bring about healing.*

Ineffective individual coping

    Defensive coping

    Ineffective denial

    Impaired adjustment

Ineffective family coping

    Disabled

    Compromised

Judgment

Decision-making ability:

  Patient's perspective *"I try to do what's right."*

  Family's perspective *(son) Usually his decisions are sound.*

Ability to choose from alternatives ———

Decisional conflict

Participation

Compliance with past/current health care regimen *Poor, does not seek routine health care.*

Willingness to comply with future health care regimen *Unable to assess at this time, question compliance in light of past health care regimen.*

Noncompliance

Health-Seeking Behaviors

Expression of desire to seek higher level of wellness *not at this time*

Health seeking behaviors

Prioritized nursing diagnoses/problem list:

1. *Ineffective breathing patterns/impaired gas exchange related to splinted breathing & pain.*
2. *Decreased cardiac output related to altered preload.*
3. *Impaired skin integrity related to leakage of gastric secretions.*
4. *Altered GI tissue perfusion/altered nutrition related to extent of abdominal wound/drains.*
5. *Pain/chronic related to deep abdominal wound.*
6. *Impaired physical mobility related to complete bedrest.*
7. *Fatigue related to prolonged hospitalization and lack of exercise/rest.*
8. *Self-care deficit related to decreased strength & endurance.*
9. *Anxiety related to unknown length of hospitalization & unemployment.*

Signature *Shelia Bunton, RN, MSN*   Date *3 Nov*

Figure 5-2 *(Continued)*

In the past, nurses were inadequately prepared, both in attitude and by lack of knowledge, to perform a primary patient assessment. When physical assessment skills were added as a logical extension of the nursing role, significant advances were made in delivery of health care. However, the time has come to realize that mastery of physical assessment skills alone no longer constitutes the criteria necessary for performing a comprehensive and holistic nursing assessment. In the 1990s, current state-of-the-art knowledge dictates that nurses use a nursing model or framework to guide the assessment so that physical problems can be identified and mind and spirit problems can be evaluated thoroughly.

The following sections discuss the techniques used to perform a thorough nursing assessment.

Assessment Techniques

Techniques used in doing a nursing assessment include interviewing, inspection, palpation, percussion, and auscultation.

The Interview

The patient interview is conducted to gather specific information about the patient's nine human response patterns that can be used to formulate nursing diagnoses and to develop a plan of patient care. The patient interview is also conducted to establish a trusting relationship between the patient and the nurse. The interview can help the professional nurse gain insight into patients' ability to function, their behavior, and the severity of their illness.

Interviewing involves communication and energy exchange between two individuals. Communication is the act of transmitting facts, feelings, and meanings by words, gestures, or other actions; thus, communication may be verbal or nonverbal. Facilitating communication, as well as providing emotional support, involves actively listening to patients to determine their perceptions of the acute event. Close attention must be paid to the patient's facial expression, voice quality, body language, and other subjective and objective data.

Obtaining an informative interview depends on the nurse's approach as well as the patient's response. The patient may be more motivated to respond if the nurse has an interested, accepting, and empathetic approach. A nonjudgmental attitude toward the philosophy, attitudes, and behaviors of patients is needed. A calm, unhurried approach can convey a feeling of interest in the patient, and it is essential in facilitating the communication process. A pleasant, private, and unstressful setting for the interview is also essential. Guidelines for successful interviewing follow.

Structure of the Interview
- Use an organized approach.
- Begin the interview relatively slowly and allow time to put the patient at ease.
- Progress from the general to the specific and from the nonpersonal to the personal.
- Make careful transitions between topics.
- Structure the conversation to help patients direct their thoughts.
- Listen attentively so that questions are not repeated needlessly.
- Before discussing emotional or embarrassing topics (*e.g.,*

sexual activities, alcohol, mental illness or use of illegal drugs), gain the patient's confidence and cooperation.

Data Collection During the Interview
- Investigate important clues the patient gives.
- Ask important questions pertinent to the subject being discussed.
- Let patients tell their own story.
- Recognize time relationships between signs and symptoms and patterns.
- Identify pertinent negative signs and symptoms.

Validation of Data During the Interview
- Use terms the patient understands (*e.g.*, heart attack, stomach pain) and adjust to the patient's vocabulary.
- Give the patient time to complete the answers to questions.
- Determine the patient's expectations and understanding of the illness.
- Consider various interpretations of the patient's symptoms.
- Do not overwhelm the patient with numerous, complicated, or long questions.

Because one purpose of the interview is to obtain as much information as possible, it is essential that nurses learn techniques to both control the interview and facilitate communication. Patients do not have a systematic, overall knowledge of their illness and therefore cannot be expected to give an organized history. Some patients need help in expressing their ideas, and others need help in directing their thoughts. Several types of statements and questions can be of help. Depending on the patient and the situation, the skilled interviewer may use some or all of the following statements and questions to gather, identify, explore, and clarify information.

Neutral questions are questions that are structurally unbiased and do not prompt the patient to give a more acceptable or pleasing answer. Neutral questions should be used whenever possible. They may be either open or closed. "Tell me more about your chest pain" is an open neutral question. The closed neutral question is one that is structured to include several choices: "Would you say that your last episode of chest pain lasted for 5 minutes, 15 minutes, 30 minutes, or more?"

Simple direct questions are questions that require a direct answer, such as yes or no. These are important in gaining specific facts, such as statistical data, and they help the patient focus on a particular point of interest. Because the simple direct question demands a direct response, it is closed and generally tends to discourage verbalization. "Do you ever wake up at night with chest pain?" "Have any of your relatives had diabetes?"

Supplementary statements may encourage an open, neutral interview. Statements such as "Yes," "Go on," or "Umm" and pauses allow patients to verbalize as they wish and help them remember what they want to say.

Leading questions generate a bias and may put words in the patient's mouth. However, leading questions may be useful for testing the validity of the patient's answers: "Would you say that your chest pain only develops several hours after eating a large meal?"

Open-ended questions may also help to generate free-flowing communication. Transitional phrases, such as "You were saying?" and "And after that, you . . . ?" are often effective.

Reflecting content is a common communication technique. The nurse repeats the patient's feeling or interpretation of a particular subject:

Patient: I was pretty scared when I came to the hospital.
Nurse: You were pretty scared?
Patient: Yes, I thought I was going to die.

Although a thorough, well-conducted interview is fundamental to an accurate assessment, the interview must be combined with the physical assessment techniques of inspection, palpation, percussion, and auscultation.

Inspection

Inspection (or *observation*) refers to the visual examination of the patient in which normal, unusual, and abnormal features are noted. One must learn not only to see but also to observe.[26,35] The nurse observes for size, appearance, symmetry, normalcy, anatomic landmarks, color, movement, temperature, and abnormalities.

Palpation

After inspection, palpation is generally done. *Palpation* involves the use of the hands and fingers to determine texture, temperature, moisture, elasticity, position, pulsations, vibrations, consistency, and shape. It is also done to identify pain, tenderness, swelling, organ enlargement, muscular spasm, rigidity, or crepitus. In most situations, the nurse uses a light pressure technique and presses down on the area being examined several times. The fingertips are the most sensitive areas used for palpation for general purposes, with the back of the hands or fingers used for temperature sense and the palmar surface of the metacarpal joints used for vibratory sense. (Deep palpation and the bimanual technique are explained in Chap. 32.)

Percussion

Percussion is usually done after palpation. It involves striking the body surface with a finger or fingers to produce a sound. Percussion may be direct (the body surface is struck directly with the fingers) or indirect (the index or middle finger is placed firmly on the skin, and the distal third of that finger is struck with the middle finger of the other hand). Percussion is used to determine size, density, organ boundaries, and location. The sounds heard on percussion may be tympanic, resonant, dull, or flat.

Auscultation

Auscultation, listening to sounds produced by various organs and tissues, generally involves the use of a stethoscope (see Chap. 19 and 24). The frequency, intensity, quality, and duration of each sound are considered.

To achieve a holistic assessment, interviewing and physical assessment skills must be combined with the appropriate assessment format. In order to elicit meaningful data from the Critical Care Response Pattern Assessment Tool, the following focus questions and parameters are presented.

FOCUS QUESTIONS AND PARAMETERS FOR ELICITING APPROPRIATE DATA WHEN USING THE CRITICAL CARE RESPONSE PATTERN ASSESSMENT TOOL*

Focus questions and parameters were developed and refined to assist the nurse in directing the line of questioning when using the Critical Care Response Pattern Assessment Tool.[11] The questions and parameters were developed to clarify summary assessment variables in the tool and provide the nurse with suggestions on how to gather the necessary data to assess a particular pattern of concern. If the nurse is not sure what data should be collected from the variables "ability to cope" or "acceptance of illness" (under the choosing pattern), for example, then the focus questions and parameters will help to elicit the necessary data.

The following sections present suggested focus question and parameters when assessing the patient's nine human response patterns using the Critical Care Response Pattern Assessment Tool. These questions and parameters follow the content of the tool. The sequence of the data collection will depend on the type and condition of the patient.

COMMUNICATING PATTERN

The purpose of assessing the communicating pattern is to determine the patient's ability to communicate both verbally and nonverbally. Basic information about the ability to communicate will be revealed immediately during the assessment by collecting the patient's identifying information (*e.g.*, name, age, address, telephone, medical diagnosis, and allergies). This pattern is evaluated first because the rest of the assessment depends on the ability and reliability of the patient to communicate the appropriate information. Thus, it may be necessary initially to obtain the information from the patient's family (significant other) or to validate the data with them.

Read, Write, and Understand English

"Do you have any difficulty reading or writing English? Speaking English? How well?" Does the patient have any physiologic reason for not understanding English (*i.e.*, reduced circulation to the brain, stroke, brain tumor)? Does the patient have a psychologic reason (*i.e.*, psychosis, lack of stimuli)?

---

* Material in this section adapted from Guzzetta, C. E. General Focus Question and Parameters for Eliciting Appropriate Data. In C. E. Guzzetta, S. D. Bunton, L. A. Prinkey, et al. *Clinical Assessment Tools for Use with Nursing Diagnoses.* St. Louis: Mosby-Year Book, 1989: 23–39; with permission.

Other Languages

"What language do you speak at home? Most of the day? Do you speak any other languages?" Is anyone available to act as the patient's interpreter or provide flash cards?

Barriers to Communication

Is the patient able to speak? Is the patient intubated? How long? Does the patient have a tracheostomy or laryngectomy? A talking tracheostomy? Use esophageal talking? Does the patient stutter or have slurred speech? Have difficulty speaking because of shortness of breath? Have facial paralysis or a mandibular fracture? Lacerations or burns of the face or mouth that affect the ability to speak? Is the patient able to modulate speech, find words, identify objects, and speak sentences?[4,21]

Alternate Form of Communication

Does the patient have difficulty with phonation? What other forms of communication does the patient use (*i.e.*, sign language, sign board, writing, typewriter, or computer)?[21]

KNOWING PATTERN

The purpose of assessing the knowing pattern is to determine what the patient knows about the current and past health status. Assessment guides the collection of data regarding knowledge and perception of risk factors, illness, tests, surgery, medications, readiness to learn, misconceptions, and level of orientation.

Current Health Problems

"What brought you to the hospital?" (This line of questioning should include a description of the patient's current problems.) Attempt to elicit the signs, symptoms, and problems in the order in which they occurred. This information will provide a focus for collecting more specific data in the associated pattern of concern (*e.g.*, for a patient who was admitted to a critical care unit for syncope, the nurse performs a comprehensive assessment of the neurologic and cardiac categories under the exchanging pattern). For each sign and symptom identified in the pattern of concern, determine when, where, and under what circumstances the sign and symptom occurred. Also determine its location, quality, quantity, duration, and aggravating, alleviating, and associated factors. Within each pattern, also state pertinent "negatives" or absences of certain signs or symptoms that might generally be involved with the problem (*e.g.*, absence of pedal edema, sudden weight gain, or dyspnea in a patient suspected of having decreased cardiac output).

Previous Illnesses, Hospitalizations, or Surgeries

Summarize all the patient's major and minor health and illness problems. Summarize past hospitalizations (chronologic dates and, if appropriate, attending physicians). Summarize past surgical procedures (chronologic dates, attending physicians, and complications, if appropriate).

History of the Following Problems

Heart.   "Have you had any history of heart disease, heart attack, heart murmur, heart infection, chest pain, or palpitations?"

Peripheral Vascular.   "Have you had any leg problems?" Does the patient complain of intermittent claudication?

Lung.   "Have you had a history of lung disease, tuberculosis, lung infections, asthma, bronchitis, or asbestos exposure?"

Liver.   "Have you had any liver problems or liver enlargement? Have you ever had infectious mononucleosis? Hepatitis?"

Kidney.   "Have you had any kidney problems, kidney infections, or kidney stones?"

Cerebrovascular.   "Have you had any dizziness, blackouts, strokes, or high blood pressure?"

Rheumatic Fever.   "Have you ever had rheumatic fever?"

Thyroid.   "Have you ever had any thyroid problems (*i.e.*, hyperthyroid or hypothyroid problems)?"

Drug Abuse.   Does the patient have a history of drug abuse? If so, what kind? How long? Any treatment?

Other.   "Have you ever had any gallbladder, gastrointestinal, or genitourinary problems?"

Recent History of the Following
(Assessing for Risk of Acute Renal Failure)[30]

Blood Transfusions.   "Have you ever had a blood transfusion? How many? How long ago? Any adverse reactions?"

Trauma.   "Have you had a traumatic injury (*e.g.*, crushing injury or car accident)?"

Carbon Monoxide Poisoning.   "Did you have any prolonged exposure to smoke or car exhaust? How long? What signs and symptoms? How treated thus far?"

Heat Stroke.   "Have you had prolonged exposure to heat? How long? What signs and symptoms? How treated thus far?"

Sepsis.   "Have you recently had a severe infection? How long? What signs and symptoms? How treated thus far?"

Muscle Injury.   "Have you recently performed any prolonged or strenuous activities? What kind? How long?"

Nephrotoxic Medications.   "Have you recently received any of the following: anesthesia, neomycin, gentamicin, tobramycin, amikacin, or cyclosporine?"

Current Medications

"What medications are you taking? How long have you been taking this medication?" (Determine the name of the medication, dosage, frequency, and side effects.) "What medications did you take yesterday before you came to the hospital?" Determine if the patient is taking any over-the-counter medications such as aspirin, acetaminophen, ibuprofen, laxatives, sleeping pills, or diet pills. Also determine if the patient is taking narcotics, insulin, digitalis, estrogen, or steroid hormone replacement.[15,26]

Risk Factors

Determine whether the patient has any of the subsequent coronary artery disease risk factors, and determine the patient's perception and level of knowledge about each. Is the patient aware of how the risk factors (if present) affect the heart? Does the patient consider the risk factor to be a true risk to health (see Chap. 24)?[15,38]

- Hypertension
- Hyperlipidemia
- Smoking
- Obesity
- Diabetes
- Sedentary living
- Stress
- Alcohol use
- Oral contraceptives
- Family history: Determine the age, sex, and health status of living family members, including parents, siblings, children, and spouse. Determine the age, sex, and cause of death of deceased family members. Determine any family history associated with the aforementioned risk factors. Also determine any familial disease history related to cancer, heart disease, peripheral vascular disease, cerebrovascular disease, stroke, migraine headaches, respiratory disease, tuberculosis, nervous or mental conditions, epilepsy, kidney or liver disease, arthritic conditions, hematologic abnormalities, rheumatic fever, sickle cell anemia, or thyroid disease.

Perception and Knowledge of Illness, Tests, or Surgery

"What is your biggest health problem? Can you tell me what you know about this problem? What do you think caused this problem? Can you tell me about the tests you are about to undergo? Can you tell me what you know about the surgery you are about to have?"

Expectations of Therapy

"How do you expect your health problem to be treated while you are here? What has been planned to help you while you are here? What do you think will be the results of this therapy?"

Misconceptions

"Have you heard anything about your illness that puzzles you? Have you received any especially disturbing information from staff, family, or friends? Do you have any questions about your illness and treatment?"

Readiness to Learn

Does the patient ask questions about the therapy, treatment, illness, or prognosis? Does the patient deny that a problem exists? Does the patient demonstrate readiness to learn by good eye contact, body language, and motivation to listen?[15]

Requests Information.   Indicates readiness to learn; specify what information is requested.

Educational Level.   "How many years of education do you have?"

Learning Impeded.   Does the patient's current physical condition permit or prohibit learning to take place (i.e., barriers such as pain, distractions, and confusion)? Does the patient's emotional and psychologic status permit or prohibit learning to take place?

Orientation

Level of Alertness.   Is the patient alert? Lethargic? Comatose? Does the patient attend to events occurring in the room or in close proximity to the bed?

Orientation.   Is the patient oriented to person, place, and time?

Appropriate Behavior and Communication.   Is the patient confused? Is the patient's behavior appropriate for the situation? Is the patient's verbal and nonverbal form of communication appropriate for the situation?

Memory

Memory Intact.   (Circle yes or no.)

Recent.   "What day, month, and year is it? Where do you live? What is your telephone number? What kind of clothes did you wear to the hospital? What did you eat for dinner last night? Breakfast this morning?"

Remote.   "Can you recall the holidays we celebrated last month? In the month of _____? Tell me about your childhood (i.e., where did you live? go to school?)."

VALUING PATTERN

The valuing pattern is assessed to determine spiritual and cultural values and beliefs that may affect the patient's perception of the illness and ability to accept specific kinds of therapy.

Religious Preference

"What is your religion? Do you practice your religion? Is religion important to you? Do your religious practices provide support for you?"

Important Religious Practices

"Is it important for you to be able to attend your church or synagogue services? Would you like to talk to a priest, rabbi, or minister? What religious items are important for you to have while you are here (*e.g.*, Bible, rosary)? Do your religious beliefs and practices affect how you will be treated for your illness? Are there any treatments that are forbidden by your religion? During your hospitalization, how can we assist you to maintain religious practices important to you?"

Spiritual Concerns

Does the patient show excessive concern for the meaning of life or death? Does the patient express anger toward God? Inner conflicts about beliefs? Concern about relationship with God? Inability to decide whether to participate in regular religious practices? Does the patient question the meaning of suffering or existence? Does the patient displace anger toward a religious representative? Does the patient regard illness as a form of punishment?

Cultural Orientation

"What is your cultural background or heritage? Were you born in another country? When did you come to the United States? Is your family from another country? Do you have strong ties to the customs of your country? Are you a member of any particular cultural or ethnic group?"

Cultural Practices

"Do you practice any special customs? How closely are you tied to them? How does your family usually react when a family member becomes sick? Are family members usually with you when you are sick? Are there any foods you are not permitted to eat? Are there any medical or surgical treatments you will not accept because of your beliefs? How does your illness (or desire for health) affect your ability to participate in your usual customs?"

RELATING PATTERN

The purpose of assessing the relating pattern is to determine how well the patient relates to others. The assessment focuses on the areas of role performance at home and at work, and on sexual and social relationships.

Role

Marital Status. Is the patient married, divorced, widowed, single, separated, or have a nonmarital or common-law partner?

Role in Home. "Are you the major decision maker in your home? Major provider of child care? Provider of discipline for children? Person responsible for other siblings or parents?" (Also refer to home responsibilities under the moving pattern for other questions.) "How has this illness changed your responsibilities in your home and your role as a spouse or parent? Do you feel you are able to carry out the tasks normally expected of you at home? How do you feel about these changes?"

Financial Support. "Are you the major breadwinner in the family? Do you have enough money to meet your expenses? Do you need assistance with your finances?"

Occupation. "What kind of work do you do? How many hours do you work per week? Do you take work home with you? Are you retired? Are you involved in volunteer work? How do you think this illness will affect your ability to return to work?"

Job Satisfactions and Concerns. "Do you like your job? Do you have any major concerns or problems related to your job?"

Physical and Mental Energy Expenditures. "Do your job, activities at home, or volunteer work involve strenuous physical activity? Do they involve intense concentration or mental energy? Do you feel that your work is very stressful? Does it require most of your energy and efforts? Do your job and activities leave you feeling physically and emotionally exhausted?"

Sexual Relationships

(Circle satisfactory or unsatisfactory.) If unsatisfactory, does the patient report difficulties, limitations, or changes in sexual behaviors or activities? Does the patient verbalize a change of interest in self or others? An inability to achieve desired satisfaction?

Sexual Partners. Is the patient a known homosexual or prostitute? Does the patient have more than one sexual partner? If so, how many? Has the patient had sexual contact with a person who has a positive human immunodeficiency virus (HIV) test? (Also identify any history of blood transfusions or intravenous drug use to assess for the risk of HIV infection.)

Physical Difficulties and Effects of Illness Related to Sex. Does the patient describe an actual or perceived limitation in sexual activity imposed by disease, illness, or therapy? Does the patient verbalize some form of altered body structure or function such as pregnancy, recent childbirth, drugs, surgery, physical anomalies, paralysis, disease processes, trauma, or radiation that might interfere with sexual functioning?[4,21]

Socialization
(Quality of Relationship With Others)

Patient's Description. "How do you and _____ get along? Any problems? In general, how do you get along with other people? Do you feel comfortable in social situations? Talking to family, friends, and peers? In most situations, do you feel a sense of belonging? Interest? Caring? Do you feel that your family is supportive of the things you do and the things about which you think and care?"

Significant Others' Description. Ask the family or significant others the preceding questions and look for major discrepancies in perceptions.

Staff Observations. Do the patient and significant other appear to get along? Are they supportive of each other? Do they constantly fight or upset each other? How does the patient interact with the staff? Are social interactions successful and comfortable?[18]

Verbalizes Feelings of Being Alone. "Do you prefer to be alone most of the time? Do you feel that your physical, psychologic, or emotional state isolates you from people? Do you feel alone? Rejected? Different from others? Why? Do you feel that you are able to do what people expect you to do?"[21]

Does the patient have supportive significant others available? Is the patient uncommunicative, sad, or withdrawn? Is the patient preoccupied with his or her own thoughts? (Also refer to social activities under the moving pattern.)

FEELING PATTERN

The purpose of assessing the feeling pattern is to determine how the patient physically and psychologically feels and to evaluate how such feelings impact on the patient's current health status.

Comfort

Pain and Discomfort. "Do you have any pain or discomfort?" (Circle yes or no.) For each source of pain or discomfort, determine the following:[15]

Onset. "When did the pain begin? How long have you had the pain?" (Chronic pain is defined as verbal report or observed evidence of pain experienced for more than 6 months.) "Was the pain gradual or sudden? Have you ever had the pain before?"

Duration. "How long did it last?"

Location. "Where is the pain or discomfort? Please point to the area or areas."

Quality. "Is the pain sharp, dull, continuous, or intermittent? Is it mild or severe?"

Radiation. "Does the pain go to other areas of the body? Does it travel?"

Associated Factors. "Because of the pain, have you noticed any other problems (i.e., nausea or vomiting, shortness of breath, sweating, or dizziness)?"

Aggravating Factors. "What makes the pain worse (e.g., deep breathing, moving, or eating)?"

Alleviating Factors. "What makes the pain better (e.g., antacids, medication, eating, changing positions, or shallow breathing)?"

Objective Manifestations. Observe the patient for guarding or protective behavior; self-focusing (altered time perception, withdrawal from social contact, impaired thought processes); moaning, crying, restlessness; facial mask of pain (e.g., eyes lack luster, "beaten look," fixed or scattered movement, grimace); alteration in muscle tone; and autonomic alterations

in response to pain (not seen in chronic stable pain) such as diaphoresis, blood pressure and pulse changes, pupillary changes, increased or decreased respiratory rate. For chronic pain, also observe for fear of reinjury, physical and social withdrawal, anorexia, and changes in weight and sleep pattern.[5]

Emotional Integrity and States

Recent Stressful Life Events. "Within the last year, have you experienced any stressful events (e.g., family, financial, or work-related problems such as death or serious illness of a parent, spouse, or child, loss or change of job, retirement, loss or change of home, major financial burdens)? Has anything upset you recently?"

Verbalizes Feelings and Source. "How are you feeling about yourself? Your situation? Do you have any uneasy feelings or feelings of anxiety, fear, or anger? Are you experiencing any grief or personal loss?"

Anxiety. Does the patient verbalize an unconscious conflict about values and goals in life? A feeling of increased tension, apprehension, uncertainty, inadequacy, or shakiness? Does the patient verbalize feeling jittery, distressed, rattled, overexcited, or scared?[5]

Fear. Does the patient have a feeling of dread to an identifiable source that can be validated?[5]

For Grieving. Does the patient express distress or guilt over a loss or an anticipated loss? Denial of loss? Difficulty in expressing loss? Does the patient express altered eating, activity, or sleep patterns? A labile affect or alterations in concentration?[5]

Physical Manifestations. Does the patient exhibit symptoms and behavior consistent with anxiety (e.g., elevated heart rate or blood pressure above normal; cool extremities; restlessness; facial tension; darting eye movements; continuous nonpurposeful activity [such as picking at sheets, nails, hair, or constant leg motion]; verbose, nondirected conversation; startle reflex to normal sounds)? Does the patient exhibit symptoms and behavior consistent with other feelings such as depression (e.g., lack of eye contact, withdrawn behavior, constant weeping or crying, loss of appetite, interrupted sleep patterns, unusually long sleep patterns, nonengagement, or sad facial expressions)?[5,9,21]

MOVING PATTERN

The purpose of assessing the moving pattern is to evaluate the patient's ability to move, perform activities of daily living, maintain self-care, sleep and play, and sustain environmental and health maintenance.

Self-Care

Ability to Perform Self-Care. Assess the patient's functional ability to perform self-care. The following suggested code can be used to define the level of functional ability.[5] It is used to classify the nursing diagnoses listed under self-care deficits as well as the diagnosis of impaired physical mobility (see next section).

0 Completely independent
1 Requires use of equipment or devices
2 Requires help from another person for assistance, supervision, or teaching
3 Requires help from another person and equipment devices
4 Dependent, does not participate in activity

Feeding. Is the patient able to feed self and drink without assistance? Is the patient able to bring food from a receptacle to the mouth?

Swallowing. Is the patient able to voluntarily pass fluids or solids from the mouth to the stomach? Observe if the patient is having difficulty swallowing (*e.g.*, assess for stasis of food in the oral cavity, observe for coughing or choking while swallowing). Does the patient have neurologic impairment (*e.g.*, absent gag reflex, decreased muscle strength needed for mastication, perceptual impairment, or facial paralysis)? (See throat under exchanging pattern.) Does the patient have a mechanical obstruction (*e.g.*, edema, tracheostomy tube, tumor)? Is the patient too fatigued to swallow, have a limited awareness of surroundings, or have a reddened, irritated oropharyngeal cavity?[5]

Bathing and Hygiene. "What is your usual form of bathing? When? How often? Are you able to wash your body, get in and out of the bath or shower, and regulate the water flow and temperature? Do you require a special rail or stool in the tub? Are you able to wash your hair and brush your teeth?"[5]

Dressing and Grooming. Is the patient able to put on and take off necessary items of clothing? Is the patient able to fasten clothing? Is the patient able to maintain a satisfactory appearance (*e.g.*, brush hair or apply makeup)?[5]

Toileting. "Are you able to get to the toilet or commode? Are you able to sit on and rise from the toilet or commode? Are you able to manipulate your clothing for toileting? Are you able to carry out proper toilet hygiene? Are you able to flush the toilet or empty the commode?"[5]

Specify Deficits. From above list.

Discharge Planning Needs. Based on the preceding list, do any of the self-care deficits indicate a need for a home referral for assistance (*i.e.*, visiting nurse or companion)? Will the patient need special training or assistive devices to be independent (or less dependent) at home?

Activity

Limitations of Movement. (Specify level. See suggested code for functional level classification in Moving Pattern section.)

"Do you have any difficulty moving or walking? Are you able to move in bed and get up to a chair? Do you have any limitations in your movement (*e.g.*, unable to raise your arm above your head)? Have you noticed any decrease in muscle strength, muscle control, or muscle size? Have restrictions been imposed on your activities or movement because of medical recommendations?"[5]

Is the patient reluctant to move? Demonstrate a limited range of motion? Impaired coordination? Does the patient have any perceptual, cognitive, neuromuscular, or musculoskeletal impairments? Does the patient need assistance to ambulate or transfer? Does the patient use crutches or a cane, walker, or wheelchair?

Limitations in Activities. "Have you noticed any pain, discomfort, or shortness of breath when you perform your normal daily activities? Have you noticed any decreased strength or endurance in your normal daily activities? Are there any activities you once did that you cannot do any more or at present? Why?" What is the patient's response to activity (*i.e.*, do heart rate and blood pressure return to preactivity levels within 3 minutes after the activity)? Can the patient ambulate without symptoms (*i.e.*, pain or shortness of breath)? Are there any electrocardiographic changes reflecting dysrhythmias or myocardial ischemia during activities?

Braces, Casts, Splints, and Traction. Does the patient have any braces, casts, splints, or traction that limit movement and activities? What kind? Why? For how long?

Fracture, Extensive Burns, Paralysis, and Amputations. Does the patient have fractures, extensive burns, paralysis, or amputations that limit movement and activities? What kind? Why? For how long?

Verbal Report of Fatigue. "Have you found yourself feeling constantly tired, weak, having no energy, or feeling too weak to accomplish daily activities?"

Does the patient verbalize feelings of exhaustion, irritability, lethargy, or listlessness; lack of energy; inability to concentrate; disinterest in surroundings; inability to maintain usual routines?[5]

Exercise Habits. "Are you involved in any type of exercise program?" (Determine type, duration, and frequency.) "Can you tell me what kind of exercise is involved in your job, outside activities, sports, and during your household activities?"

Rest

Sleep and Rest Pattern. "When do you usually sleep (*i.e.*, during the day, evening, or night)? Can you tell me how many hours you generally sleep at a time (not necessarily at night)? Do you take any rest periods during the day for naps, relaxation, or meditation? What is the length, time, and reason for these rest periods?"

Sleep Aids. "Do you use any aids to help you to sleep (*e.g.*, pillows, tranquilizers, hypnotics, alcohol, hot milk, warm bath or shower, music, or food)?"[27]

Difficulties Falling or Remaining Asleep. "Do you have any difficulties falling asleep? Staying asleep? Going back to sleep once you are awake? Do you have frequent or recurrent nightmares that awaken you? Do you usually feel rested after sleeping?"

Does the patient verbalize changes in behavior or performance (*i.e.*, irritability, restlessness, disorientation, lethargy, or listlessness)? Does the patient exhibit physical signs of sleep pattern disturbance (*i.e.*, mild fleeting nystagmus, light hand tremor, ptosis of eyelid, expressionless face, dark circles under eyes, frequent yawning, changes in posture)?[5]

Recreation

Leisure Activities.   "What fun or relaxing things do you do in your leisure time? Do you have any hobbies? Do you enjoy any sports? Do you enjoy reading, listening to music, painting, playing cards, sewing, and so forth?"

Does the patient verbalize boredom? Does the environment, patient's condition, or lengthy treatments prohibit involvement in diversional activities? Does the patient wish to engage in diversional activities or is there a lack of interest? Is it possible for the patient to engage in any of his or her usual hobbies or diversional activities while in the hospital?[5]

Social Activities.   "Are you involved in any social activities (*e.g.*, church groups, clubs, or organizations)? Were social activities important to you before this hospitalization?"

Activities of Daily Living

Home Management

Size and Arrangement of Home (Stairs, Bathroom).   "Do you have any difficulties in your home regarding the location of your bedroom or bathroom, or do you have any stairs to climb? Do you have the necessary cooking equipment, linens, cloths, and hygienic aids? Are you familiar with your neighborhood resources (*e.g.*, neighbors, grocery store, laundry, and pharmacy)?"

Safety Needs.   "Can you describe any safety devices that you may need (*e.g.*, railing in bathtub) or safety hazards (*e.g.*, torn carpet or frayed electrical cords) in your home?"[5]

Home Responsibilities.   "Tell me what your typical day is like concerning meal planning and preparation, shopping, cleaning, child care, bill paying, and household chores?"

Health Maintenance

Health Insurance.   "Do you have health insurance? Do you receive any financial medical assistance (*i.e.*, Medicare? Medicaid)? Do you need any assistance with filing health insurance claims?"

Regular Physical Checkups.   "Do you see a physician for regular checkups? Do you see other physicians or nurse practitioners for any other reason? How often do you visit a dentist?"

Does the patient demonstrate a lack of knowledge about basic health practices? Does the patient indicate a lack of responsibility for meeting basic health practices? Does the patient report a lack of equipment or financial or personal resources?[5]

PERCEIVING PATTERN

The perceiving pattern is assessed to evaluate the patient's self-perceptions. The assessment focuses on self-concept as manifested by self-esteem and body image. The perceiving pattern also includes an assessment of perceived hopelessness and powerlessness as well as an assessment of the patient's sensory perception.

Self-Esteem and Body Image

Perception of Self and Situation.   "If you could describe what kind of person you are, what would you say? How do you feel about yourself as a person? Are you comfortable about the way you look, feel, and function? What does this illness or surgery mean to you? And your family? How serious do you think your condition is?"

When assessing for self-esteem, observe whether the patient demonstrates negative talk or verbalizes expressions of shame or guilt. Does the patient believe that he or she is unable to deal with events, project blame to others, rationalize positive and exaggerate negative feedback about self? Distinguish whether such negative verbalization about self is of a long-standing (or chronic) nature or is situational in response to the current illness.[5]

Description of Body Structure and Functioning.   When assessing for body image disturbances, observe the patient for verbal or nonverbal expressions of an actual or perceived change in body structure or functioning. For example, if the patient has a missing body part, does the patient refuse to look at the body part? Hide or overexpose a body part? Ignore, neglect, or traumatize a body part? Refuse to discuss the illness, injury, or surgery? Have negative feelings about the body, or a preoccupation with a change or loss of a body part? Does the patient demonstrate responsibility for self-care or demonstrate self-neglect?[5]

Meaningfulness

Verbalizes Hopelessness.   "What are your attitudes and feelings about the future? Do you believe there is a possible solution to your problem? What are your plans for the future?" Does the patient demonstrate negative feelings, passivity, decreased verbalization, flat affect, a lack of initiative, decreased response to stimuli, decreased appetite, increased sleep, lack of involvement in care, and sighing and verbal cues such as "I can't?"[5] (Also see emotional integrity states under the feeling pattern.) Has the patient attempted or considered suicide?

Verbalizes Lack of Control (Powerlessness).   "What do you think that you can do to change, improve, or help your current situation or problem?" Does the patient perceive a loss of control regarding the outcomes of care? Or over self-care? Is the patient depressed or apathetic about physical deterioration despite compliance with the medical regimen? Does the patient choose not to participate in decision making even when opportunities are provided? Does the patient express dissatisfaction or frustration over an inability to perform previous tasks or activities?[5]

Sensory Perception

History of Restricted Environment. Has the patient experienced any restricted environments (*e.g.*, isolation, intensive care, bed rest, traction, confining illness, or incubator)? Has the patient experienced any socially restricted environments (*e.g.*, institutionalization, home-bound, chronic illness, dying, or infant deprivation)?[5]

Vision Impaired. "Do you have difficulty seeing? How is your near vision? Far vision?" Can the patient see the nurse, newsprint, or objects across the room? Does the patient have cataracts or a false eye?

Glasses. "Do you wear glasses or contact lenses? How well do they correct your vision?"

Auditory Impaired. "Do you have any difficulty hearing?" Can the patient hear normal conversation?

Hearing Aid. Does the patient use a hearing aid? Which ear? Does the patient like to use it? Does it improve hearing?

Kinesthetics Impaired. Can the patient walk across the room appropriately? Can the patient maintain a sense of balance? Does the patient complain of dizziness? Does the patient demonstrate a lack of coordination?

Gustatory Impaired. Does the patient complain of loss of taste? Does the patient complain of metallic or unusual tastes?

Tactile Impaired. Does the patient complain of any loss in the sense of touch? Is the patient able to distinguish between dull, sharp, and light touches? Does the patient complain of numbness, tingling, decreased sensation, hypersensitivity, or a prickly feeling?

Olfactory Impaired. Does the patient complain of a loss of smell? Can the patient recognize the smell of rubbing alcohol after closing the eyes?

Reflexes. Test each deep tendon reflex (Table 5-4); compare the responses on corresponding sides, and grade the responses using the following scale[26,35]:

0	No response
1+	Sluggish or diminished
2+	Active or expected response
3+	More brisk than usual
4+	Brisk or hyperactive

EXCHANGING PATTERN

The purpose of assessing the exchanging pattern is to evaluate the patient's physical condition. The assessment focuses on cerebral, peripheral, cardiovascular, respiratory, nutritional, gastrointestinal, and renal variables, as well as laboratory values.

Cerebral Circulation

Neurologic Changes and Symptoms. Does the patient complain of difficulty walking, vertigo, dizziness, loss of bal-

Table 5-4
Testing for Deep Tendon Reflexes

Biceps: The patient's arm is flexed at a 45° angle at the elbow. Palpate the biceps tendon in the antecubital fossa. Place your fingers over the biceps muscle and your thumb over the tendon. With the reflex hammer, strike your thumb. Flexion of the elbow should occur.

Brachioradialis: The patient's arm is flexed up to a 45° angle and rests on your arm with the hand slightly pronated. With the reflex hammer, directly strike the brachioradialis tendon. Observe for flexion and supination of the forearm.

Triceps: The patient's arm is flexed up to a 90° angle, with the patient's hand resting against the side of your body. Palpate the triceps tendon and strike it directly with the reflex hammer just above the elbow. Contraction of the triceps muscle causes extension of the elbow.

Knee: The patient's knee is flexed up to a 90° angle, with the lower leg loosely hung. Support the patient's upper leg with your hand without allowing it to rest against the side of the table. With the reflex hammer, strike the patellar tendon just below the patella. The lower leg will extend when the quadriceps contract.

Ankle: With the patient sitting, flex the knee and dorsiflex the ankle up to a 90° angle while holding the heel of the foot in your hands. Strike the Achilles tendon at the level of the ankle malleoli. Contraction of the gastrocnemius muscle causes plantar flexion of the foot at the ankle. Note also the speed of relaxation after muscular contraction.

Plantar: The patient's ankle is held in one hand while a sharp object is stroked from the lateral surface of the sole, starting at the heel of the foot and going to the base of the foot, curving medially across the ball and ending beneath the great toe. The normal response is flexion of all toes (negative Babinski's reflex). Extension or dorsiflexion of the great toe and fanning of the others represents a positive Babinski's reflex, which may reflect upper motor neuron disease.[42,57]

---

ance, falls, weakness or numbness, development of tremors, confusion, or forgetfulness? Does the family or patient report any changes in personality? (See Chap. 29.)

Does the patient exhibit any neurologic signs or symptoms of *dysreflexia* (*e.g.*, a patient with a spinal cord injury at T7 or above who experiences uninhibited sympathetic nervous system responses such as paroxysmal hypertension, bradycardia or tachycardia, diaphoresis, red splotches on the skin above the injury, pallor of skin below the injury, and a diffuse headache).

Seizure Activity. Does the patient have seizure activity?[30] (Check yes or no.)

Type. Determine if the seizure was grand mal, petit mal, Jacksonian, or psychomotor.

Aura. Determine whether prior to the seizure the patient experienced any weakness, dizziness, numbness, strange sensations in the arms or legs, odors, or other pertinent sensations.

Pupils. Assess pupillary size, shape, and equality. Determine reactions to light (*i.e.*, brisk, sluggish, or nonreactive). When determining reaction to light, determine direct-light pupillary reflex (constriction of lighted eye) and consensual pupillary reflex (constriction of unlighted eye).

Glasgow Coma Scale. Determine the patient's level of consciousness using the Glasgow Coma Scale, which consists of three categories (eye opening, best verbal response, and best motor response). Each category is scored, and the total is the Glasgow Coma score. The highest possible score is 15. (See Chap. 29.)

Intracranial Pressure. Is the patient being monitored for intracranial pressure? What is the pressure? (Normal is 1 to 15 mm Hg.)

Peripheral Circulation

Pulses. Each set of pulses should be evaluated for its quality, symmetry, and the presence of an audible bruit.[26,35] (See Chap. 24.)

Blood Pressure. What is the patient's blood pressure in the right and left arm while sitting, lying, and standing? Are the bilateral pressures equal? (See Chap. 24.)

A-line Reading. What is the arterial blood pressure as measured by the arterial line? Is there a palpable femoral or carotid pulse?

Jugular Venous Distention. Does the patient have distended venous neck veins? (Increased jugular venous pressure is observed during inspiration in congestive heart failure, cardiac tamponade, and restrictive cardiomyopathies.[15] (See Chap. 24.)

Central Venous Pressure. What is the patient's central venous pressure? (Normal is 4 to 15 cm H_2O or 3 to 11 mm Hg.)

Skin Temperature. Is the patient's skin temperature normal, warm, hot, cool, clammy, or moist?

Color. Does the patient exhibit pink, pale, or red coloring? Does the patient exhibit pallor, jaundice, mottling, increased pigmentation, blanching, or cyanosis (note degree and location of cyanosis: eyes, ears, nose, mouth, tongue, neck, chest, legs, extremities, hands, fingers, and toes)?[3]

Capillary Refill. Does the patient have normal capillary refill? Capillary refill is assessed by pressing the nail bed, earlobe, or forehead so it blanches, releasing the pressure, and observing whether the skin color returns to normal within 2 seconds.[23]

Clubbing. Does the patient exhibit clubbing of the nail beds?[15] (See Chap. 24.)

Edema. Does the patient have edema? Is the edema pitting, nonpitting, or dependent?

Cardiac Circulation

Point of Maximum Impulse. Determine the point of maximum impulse, which is normally found near the fifth intercostal space midclavicular line. (See Chap. 24.)

Pacemaker. Observe for an external or internal pacemaker. If internal, record the type and how it is functioning. If external,

record the type, settings, and how it is functioning. (See Chap. 13.)

Apical Rate and Rhythm. What is the patient's apical heart rate? Is the rhythm regular or irregular? If irregular, is it regularly irregular or totally irregular? Does an apical-radial pulse deficit exist?

Heart Sounds and Murmurs. Listen for the first and second heart sounds, and determine whether there is a third or fourth heart sound or whether the patient has any ejection sounds, midsystolic clicks, opening snaps, or murmurs. (See Chap. 24.)

Dysrhythmias. Does the patient have dysrhythmias (*i.e.,* tachydysrhythmias, bradydysrhythmias; atrial, junctional, or ventricular dysrhythmias; first-, second-, or third-degree heart blocks; premature atrial, junctional, or ventricular beats? Note any hemodynamic symptoms associated with the dysrhythmia (*i.e.,* hypotension, dizziness, confusion, low urinary output, or decreased cardiac output). (See Chap. 12.)

Cardiac Output/Cardiac Index. What is the cardiac output? (Normal is 5 L/minute.[15])
  What is the patient's cardiac index? (Normal is 3.5 L/minute/m²; it ranges from 2.5 to 4.5 L/minute/m². The cardiac index is derived by dividing the cardiac output by the body surface area[38]). (See Chap. 17.)

Pulmonary Artery Pressure. What is the patient's pulmonary artery pressure (PAP)? (Normal is less than 25 mm Hg systolic and 5 to 10 mm Hg diastolic, with a mean pulmonary artery pressure of less than 13 mm Hg.[15]) (See Chap. 17.)

Pulmonary Capillary Wedge Pressure. What is the patient's pulmonary capillary wedge pressure? (Normal ranges from 4 to 12 mm Hg.)

Intravenous Fluids. What type of intravenous fluids is the patient receiving? What is the amount and rate of administration?

Intravenous Medications. Is the patient receiving any vasoactive intravenous medications? What is the name, dosage, and rate of administration?

Serum Enzymes. What are the levels of the patient's serum cardiac enzymes? (See Chap. 25.)

Physical Integrity

Tissue Integrity. Does the patient have any corneal, mucous membrane, integumentary, or subcutaneous tissue damage (*e.g.,* a crushing injury or intravenous infiltration)?

Skin Integrity. What is the general assessment of the skin in terms of hydration, vascularity, elasticity, texture, turgor, mobility, and thickness?
  Does the patient have any disruption of skin surfaces or skin layers (*e.g.,* rashes, lesions, petechiae, bruises, abrasions, moles, tumors, bullae, papules, blisters, pustules, vesicles, ulcerations, erosions, nodules, cysts, scales, crusts, fissures, cal-

luses, bites, scars, keloids, hives, excoriations, plaques, bleeding, pruritus, dermatitis, or intravenous drug "track" marks)?

Does the patient have any invasion of body structures (*e.g.,* surgical incisions, invasive hemodynamic lines, intravenous lines, stomas, tracheostomy tube, or gastric tube)?[26,35]

What is the condition, shape, texture, color, and thickness of the nails? What is the color of the nail beds? Does the patient have any nail lesions or splinter hemorrhages?

What is the color, distribution, quantity, and texture of the hair? What is the pattern of hair loss?

Is the patient at risk for *disuse syndrome* (*e.g.,* is the patient at risk for body system deteriorization because of musculoskeletal inactivity due to paralysis, mechanical or prescribed immobilization, severe pain, or an altered level of consciousness). Observe for complications of immobility such as decubitus ulcers.

Bleeding. Is the patient actively bleeding externally? If so, is the bleeding minimal, moderate, or massive in amount (circle). Note the presence and extent of hematomas.

Extravasation From Burns. Is there serosanguineous or serous fluid draining from burned areas?

Burns. If the patient has been burned, determine the degree, type, and location of the burn and estimate the percentage of body surface area burned.[30] (See Chap. 43.)

Leakage of Spinal Fluid. Is there any spinal fluid leakage from the ears, nose, or elsewhere (circle)?

Dialysis Access and Condition. Determine if the patient has a dialysis access (check yes or no). What type of access does the patient have (*e.g.,* hemodialysis via a fistula, arteriovenous shunt, or central line or peritoneal dialysis via a trochar catheter)? Determine the condition of the access (*e.g.,* skin erosion or clots or kinks in the catheter).

Oxygenation

Complaints of Dyspnea. Does the patient complain of dyspnea? When does it occur? What precipitates the feeling? What alleviates it? What is the body position associated with it?[15] (See Chap. 24.)

Orthopnea. Does the patient complain of orthopnea (*i.e.,* the patient is unable to breathe normally in the recumbent position and usually sleeps with two to three pillows to improve breathing?[15]

Rate, Rhythm, and Depth. What is the patient's rate, rhythm, and depth of respirations? Is the patient's breathing regular? Is the depth shallow, moderate, or deep? Does the patient exhibit abnormal breathing patterns (*i.e.,* asymmetric, obstructive, or restrictive)?

Labored or Unlabored. Does the patient appear to be using a great deal of energy during breathing? Does the patient perceive that it takes a lot of work to breathe?

Use of Accessory Muscles. Does the patient use accessory muscles (*i.e.,* costal or abdominal) for respiration? (List group used.)

Chest Expansion. Does the patient's chest expand normally and symmetrically? (Describe abnormal movements.)

Splinting. Does the patient minimize coughing or avoid deep breathing to reduce pain (*i.e.,* from a surgical incision)?

Cough and Sputum. Does the patient have a productive or nonproductive cough? Is the patient's cough effort effective or ineffective? Weak or strong? What is the color, amount, odor, and consistency of the sputum?

Breath Sounds. Does the patient have normal vesicular, bronchovesicular, and bronchial breath sounds? Does the patient have adventitious sounds (*i.e.,* rhonchi, crackles, wheezes, or pleural friction rubs)? Does the patient have vocal resonance (*i.e.,* bronchophony, egophony, or whispered pectoriloquy)? (See Chap. 19.)

Arterial Blood Gases. Does the patient have normal arterial blood gases?

Oxygen Percent and Device. If the patient is receiving oxygen, what is the percentage of oxygen delivered? What type of device is used to deliver it (*i.e.,* nasal cannula, face mask, or catheter)?

Ventilator. What type of ventilator is used? What are the settings? How does the patient react to it (*i.e.,* permitting the ventilator to do the work or fighting it)?

Physical Regulation
Immune

Lymph Nodes Enlarged. Determine the size, shape, mobility, tenderness, and enlargement of the lymph nodes.

Location. Assess lymph nodes in the head, neck, axillae, and inguinal and pelvic areas.

White Blood Cell Count and Differential. Elevation of the total white blood cell count (leukocytes) usually indicates infection. The differential count is performed to determine the percentage of the types of leukocytes (*i.e.,* neutrophils, lymphocytes, monocytes, eosinophils, and basophils) in the blood. Elevation of the neutrophils commonly indicates bacterial infections. Elevation of lymphocytes can indicate bacterial or viral infections or lymphocytic leukemia, elevations of monocytes can indicate bacterial or viral infections, and elevations of eosinophils can indicate allergic disorders or parasitic disease. Elevations of basophils are rare but can indicate some kind of myeloproliferative disease such as myelofibrosis or polycythemia vera.[23] The normal values for the white blood cell count and differential vary from institution to institution. Refer to your institution's designated normal values.

HIV Testing Results.   Has the patient tested positive for HIV? Is the patient aware of the test results?

Temperature.   Normal rectal temperature is 36.1° C (97° F) to 37.0° C (99.6° F).

Route.   Was the temperature taken orally, rectally, or axillary? The rectal route is 2° F higher than the axillary route and 1° F higher than the oral route. The rectal temperature is considered the most accurate.

Nutrition
Eating Patterns

Number of Meals Per Day.   "How many meals do you usually eat each day? Can you tell me what you eat and drink in a typical day?" (Prompt by naming food groups, specific meals, time of day, and probe regarding snacks.)

Special Diet.   "Do you have any fluid or dietary needs or restrictions (*e.g.,* low-sodium, low-fat, low-calorie, low-sugar, or low-protein diet)?"

Where Eaten.   "Do you eat most of your meals at home or out?"

Food Preferences or Intolerances.   "What kinds of food do you prefer? Are there any foods that do not agree with you (*i.e.,* that you do not tolerate)?"

Food Allergies.   "Do you have any food allergies (*i.e.,* dairy products, seafood, or fruits), or are you allergic to monosodium glutamate?"

Caffeine Intake.   "Can you tell me how many caffeinated beverages you drink each day (*i.e.,* caffeinated coffee, tea, or soft drinks)? Do you eat a lot of chocolate?"

Appetite Changes.   "Have you noticed any change in your appetite lately (*i.e.,* have you found yourself eating more, eating less, or drinking more or less)?"[8] (*Note:* Ask the patient specifically what was consumed the day before coming to the hospital. The patient may have been quite ill before admission, and the oral intake the day before admission may not reflect usual dietary and fluid habits. Also, the information may be helpful in determining specific nutritional and hydration problems that may have been precipitated by the acute illness.)

Condition of Mouth and Throat.   Assess the condition and function of the patient's mouth, lips, buccal mucosa, teeth, tongue, hard and soft palate, and throat.[26,35]

General Assessment.   Is the patient able to bite, chew, and taste? Does the patient have any oral pain or odor?

Lips.   What is the color, symmetry, and hydration of the lips? Does the patient have any crusting, fever blisters (herpes simplex), cracking, swelling, numbness, drooling, or ulcerations?

Buccal Mucosa.   What is the color, hydration, and pigmentation of the buccal mucosa? Does the patient have any ul-

cerations, nodules, white patches, plaques, dryness, excess saliva, or hemorrhage? What is the color and condition of the gums? Does the patient have any inflammation, edema, bleeding, lesions, retraction, discoloration, or pain?

Teeth.   What is the condition of the teeth? Does the patient have any missing, dark, or loose teeth; caries; pain; or sensitivity to heat or cold? Does the patient have a bridge or dentures (should be removed for examination)?

Tongue.   What is the symmetry, color, mobility, size, hydration, and marking of the tongue? Does the patient have pain, soreness, ulcerations, burning, edema, fasciculations, nodules, abnormal smoothness, midline protrusion, or tumors under the tongue?

Hard Palate.   Does the patient have lesions, ulcers, or cysts?

Soft Palate.   What is the color and symmetry of the uvula, anterior and posterior pillars, tonsils, and posterior pharynx? Is there edema, exudate, inflammation, ulceration, tonsillar enlargement, pain, or tenderness? When patient says "ah," note the rise of the soft palate and uvula.

Throat.   Is the patient at risk for aspiration (*e.g.,* risk for entry of gastrointestinal secretions, oropharyngeal secretions, or solids or fluids into the tracheobronchial passages?[5] Does the patient complain of difficulty swallowing? (See impaired swallowing under moving pattern.) Does the patient have a reduced level of consciousness or a depressed cough or gag reflex? Does the patient have a tracheostomy or endotracheal or gastrointestinal tube? Are the patient's jaws wired, or does the patient have facial, oral, or neck edema, tumor, or injury?

Ideal Body Weight.   Calculate ideal body weight. For men, 5 ft equals 106 lb; for each additional inch, add 6 lb (*e.g.,* for a man 5 feet 2 inches, the ideal weight is 118 lb). For women, 5 ft equals 100 lb; for each additional inch, add 5 lb (*e.g.,* for a woman 5 feet 5 inches, the ideal weight is 125 lb).

Current Therapy.   Is the patient receiving nothing by mouth? Is the patient receiving nasogastric suctioning? Tube feedings (what type, amount, and frequency)? Total parenteral nutrition (what type, additives, and rate)?

Laboratory Information.   Assess the patient's blood sodium, potassium, chloride, hemoglobin, hematocrit, glucose, cholesterol, and triglyceride test results. (Were glucose, cholesterol and triglyceride tests performed when the patient was fasting? Circle yes or no.) (Refer to your institution's designated normal values.)

Elimination
Gastrointestinal and Bowel

Usual Bowel Habits and Bowel Regulation.   What are the patient's usual bowel habits? Does the patient use any laxatives, enemas, suppositories, bran, fruits, or fruit juices to regulate bowel movements?

Alterations From Normal.   Does the patient have any difficulty with constipation, bowel cramping, diarrhea, or bowel incontinence? Does the patient strain or have pain or rectal bleeding with defecation? Does the patient have a colostomy or ileostomy? For how long? Why?

Abdominal Physical Examination.   Observe the abdominal surface for rashes, scars, lesions, striae, or dilated veins. Note the size, shape, contour, and symmetry of the abdomen. With the diaphragm of the stethoscope, determine the frequency, quality, and pitch of bowel sounds. (Do auscultation before palpation or percussion so bowel sounds will not be altered.) Percuss the abdomen to determine liver borders, gastric air bubbles (in left upper quadrant), splenic dullness, air, fluid, or masses. Palpate the abdomen to determine organ enlargement, muscle spasm or rigidity, masses (note the location, size, shape, mobility, tenderness, consistency, pulsations), involuntary guarding, rebound tenderness, and pain. (See Chap. 32.)

Liver and Ascites.   Is the liver enlarged? Does the patient have ascites (*i.e.*, edema of the abdominal cavity)?

Bleeding and Esophageal Tube.   Does the patient have gastric or intestinal bleeding? Is it frank or occult? Does the patient have any type of esophageal tube to control bleeding from esophageal varicies?

Renal and Urinary

Possible Kidney Contusion and Other Injury.   Did the patient receive a forceable blow near the kidneys? Did the patient sustain a stab wound or gunshot wound near the kidneys?

Usual Urinary Pattern and Alterations.   How many times per day does the patient urinate? Does the patient have any alterations from normal such as incontinence or retention of urine? Does the patient describe any frequency, burning, pain, dribbling, urgency, hematuria, nocturia, oliguria, or polyuria? Does the patient have a urostomy? Is the patient receiving dialysis? What kind and how often? (See Chap. 33).

Bladder Distention.   Is the bladder distended? Does the patient complain of bladder discomfort?

Color.   What is the color of the urine? Is there any blood?

Catheter.   Does the patient have a urinary catheter? What type? How long? Any problems?

Urine Output: 24 Hour and Average Hourly.   What is the patient's 24-hour urinary output? Hourly output?

Blood Urea Nitrogen, Creatinine, and Specific Gravity. What are the patient's blood urea nitrogen and creatinine levels? What is the specific gravity of the urine?

Urine Studies.   Assess the results of any urine studies (renal scan or urine culture) or other urine values (*i.e.*, acetone, glucose, blood, or protein is abnormal), and pH.

CHOOSING PATTERN

The purpose of assessing the choosing pattern is to determine the patient's ability to choose alternatives consistent with health-promoting behaviors. Data are collected in the areas of coping and problem solving related to illness and surgery, as well as the patient's willingness to comply with the past and future health care regimen.

Coping

Patient's Ability to Cope

For Ineffective Individual Coping.   "Do you believe that you solve problems well? Is it easy or hard for you to accept help from others even if you might need it? When you have a really big problem, how do you deal with it? Do you get depressed? Cry? Become nervous? Eat food? Drink alcohol? Take drugs? What kinds of activities help you to reduce stress (*e.g.*, listen to music, exercise, use relaxation techniques, go for a walk)?"[5]

Does the patient or family verbalize an inability to meet basic needs? Does the family report that the patient is unable to ask others for help? Does the patient believe that he or she is able to meet the role expectations of the family? (Also see self-concept under the perceiving pattern.)

For Defensive Coping.   Does the patient deny obvious problems or weaknesses? Place blame or responsibility for health or functions on others? Rationalize failures? Repeatedly project a falsely positive self-evaluation? Overreact to slight criticism?[5]

Family's Ability to Cope and Give Support

For Disabling Family Coping.   Is the family member or primary significant other neglectful of the patient regarding basic human needs or illness treatment? Distort reality regarding the patient's health problem, including denial about its existence or severity? Demonstrate behaviors such as rejection, intolerance, abandonment, or desertion? Does the family member demonstrate prolonged overconcern for the patient? Take on illness symptomatology of the patient? Make decisions or take actions that are detrimental to the psychologic, social, or economic well-being of the patient?[5]

For Compromised Family Coping.   Does the patient verbalize concerns regarding the family member's (or supportive primary person's) response to the illness? Does the family member verbalize inadequate understanding or knowledge regarding the patient's illness (treatment, prognosis, rehabilitation, and so forth) that interferes with their effective assistance or supportive behaviors? Does the family member attempt supportive behaviors with less than supportive outcomes?[5]

Acceptance and Adjustment to Illness

For Ineffective Denial.   Has the patient delayed in seeking health care assistance? Does the patient perceive the relevance of symptoms and danger? Minimize the symptoms? Displace the source of symptoms to other organs (*e.g.*, chest pain displaced as indigestion)? Displace fear regarding the condition?

Dismiss distressing events? Unconsciously or consciously deny knowledge or meaning of the illness?[5]

For Impaired Adjustment.   Does the patient verbalize that he or she does not accept the change in health status brought upon by the illness? Has the patient demonstrated an inability or unwillingness to become involved in problem solving or goal planning for the future, taking into consideration the current health status? Does the patient demonstrate an extended period of shock, disbelief, or anger regarding the current change in health status? A lack of movement toward independence or future-oriented planning?[5]

Judgment and Decision-Making Ability

Patient's Perspective.   "Do you believe you usually make sound judgments? Under what circumstances would you say you have difficulty making decisions? When faced with a big decision, do you ever find it difficult to make up your mind as to what to do?"

Family's Perspectives.   Does the family or significant other verbalize that the patient tends to make timely and sound decisions?

Ability to Choose From Alternatives.   If the patient is facing a decision regarding care or treatment, does he or she verbalize uncertainty about possible choices? Vacillate between possible alternatives? Verbalize a feeling of distress in making the decision? Demonstrate a serious delay in the decision-making process?[5]

Participation

Compliance With Past or Current Health Care Regimen. "In the past, have you had difficulty remembering to take your medications? Do you usually take all the medications the physician prescribes for you? Have you had any problems following your diet? Exercise program? Other activities or treatments prescribed by your physician? What problems have you had? Why do you think you have had problems with these areas?" Does the family or physician report that the patient has missed medical appointments or has deviated from previous health care instructions?

Willingness to Comply With Future Health Care Regimen. "In the future, do you think you will have problems following your diet? Exercise program? Taking your medications? Following other prescribed activities or treatments? Do you plan to follow the physician's instructions? Do you foresee any problems with following these instructions? Is there anything that is particularly unpleasant or difficult for you regarding these instructions? Can you think of anything that will interfere with your ability to _____?"[21]

Does the patient have any disturbances in memory, problem-solving ability, concentration, or psychopathology that could interfere with performance of the prescribed regimen? Does the patient have the motivation to comply with the regimen?

What are the family's or significant others' predictions about the patient's future compliance? Do the significant others understand the illness and treatment? Believe in the treatment? Have the time, energy, and resources to help the patient comply with the regimen? View their support and assistance as part of their role and responsibilities?

Health-Seeking Behaviors

Desire to Seek Higher Level of Wellness.   Evaluate the patient's level of health-seeking behaviors. Explore whether the patient is interested in finding ways to alter personal health habits or the environment to move toward a higher level of wellness. Does the patient express a need to change unhealthy habits (*e.g.*, smoking, overeating, lack of exercise, stress), and is the patient motivated to change such behaviors? Is the patient familiar with programs or resources that can be used for health promotion?[5]

ASSESSING THE PATIENT'S ENVIRONMENT

Assess the critical care environment and the patient's perceptions of the environment related to temperature, light, touch, noise, sounds, sights, colors, and odors.[6,37] Environmental safety should be systematically evaluated regarding electrical, mechanical, chemical, pathogenic, and thermal factors.

Be aware of how the critical care environment affects the patient. The response is extremely individual. Table 5–5 documents a patient interview and how the environment was perceived by one patient.

DIAGNOSTIC TESTS

Diagnostic tests are used to corroborate the information gathered in the assessment process. Tests are only as good as the person interpreting the results. The results of a single test are not definitive. If an accurate picture of a patient's condition is to emerge, all the observations must be considered in the clinical evaluation.

THE CHALLENGE OF NURSING ASSESSMENT

The Critical Care Response Pattern Assessment Tool (see Fig. 5–2) is a working demonstration tool.[30] Nurses considering using this tool should feel free to change and revise it based on their needs in clinical practice. Nurses can evaluate the tool's adequacy for collecting appropriate data and its organization, clarity, and length. From this evaluation, the ordering of the tool can be rearranged, and additions, deletions, or clarification of assessment variables can be made. For example, if it is judged that the data under the choosing pattern should be assessed earlier, then this pattern could be moved to an earlier place in the tool. If it is decided that the tool is too long, variables or sections can be deleted (*e.g.*, delete section on environmental maintenance under moving pattern or delete reflexes under the perceiving pattern if this information is judged not to be critical to the assessment). Thus, nurses are encouraged to try out the tool and to change and revise it as they deem appropriate.[30]

For those nurses willing to accept the challenge and com-

Table 5-5
Sensory Perceptions of a Critically Ill Patient: Patient Interview

Sounds
"I didn't like the breathing machine, so when I figured out that's what was making that airy sound, I didn't like that sound either."
"The voices of the staff were loud."
"The beep of the heart monitor was constant; I felt reassured once I realized what the sound was."

Sights
"Everything was cloudy until the nurses used a cotton swab to clean one part of one eye. Then I could see clearly through that part, but the other part of that eye—and the other eye—still had some damage from the accident. It was like I was looking through a smoky haze."
"The light from the windows varied a lot. I actually thought I was in four or five different rooms, but it was just different times of the day or cloudy days."
"I had some hallucinations, and I saw all sorts of things outside the window that I know weren't really there."

Tactile sensations
"I was cold a lot. Then I'd spike a temperature and be hot."
"The air hurt whenever it touched me, so I wanted the nurses to wrap me up completely in bandages, and I didn't even want the tips of my fingers to be out."
"My heels hung off the edge of the mattress a lot, especially when the nurses raised my head up. I'm 6 feet 4 inches tall."

Taste
"I was thirsty. That's all I can remember, how much I wanted something to drink. Finally, the nurses gave me something on a stick to suck on. I was kind of out of it, and the first one tasted like a Dr. Pepper. I knew I had to figure out how to get another one of those. I was more aware of things when I got the second one. It tasted kind of like a lemon and honey taste; I guess that's the best way to describe it. I'm not sure, but I think maybe it gets rid of the saliva. But it makes your mouth—the inside of your mouth—pucker up like if you ate a plum."

Trip to tank room
"The nurses brought that steel frame with the canvas webbing up to my room. There was a plastic bag over it, and it was cold and hard when I got on it. In the tank room, the nurses put a light on over me and it was warm, which felt good, but it was also awfully bright. My eyes were real sensitive to the light. The nurses attached some hooks to the frame I was on, and if one of them bumped against my skin, they were cold and it hurt. There was a black rubber cord attached to the winch. The sound of the winch was like an old barn door closing or like rollers in a sliding track."
"The tank was stainless steel, and I think there also were some stainless steel cabinets. It looked real technological or clinical. There might have been two tanks in the room, but I was always in the same one. There were three people. They put me into just where my back touched the water and the rest of me was above water. There was a lot of water sound. The water below in the tank was flowing, and the spray splattered the water against the sides of the metal tub. The room was echoey."
"Two people each washed one arm, and the third person worked on my chest. They used those Betadine sponges, mostly the sponge side, but sometimes they used the bristles on my fingernails. They talked to each other, but not much to me. They had very passive faces, like they were deep in thought."

Smells
"I could smell okay, but I can remember very few smells. I don't pay much attention to that. I don't think men really do. When the floors were cleaned, there was an antiseptic smell."
"The bandages we had had a smell to them, but it was not strong. I don't even know how to describe it, maybe like iodine; no, I guess that's what it looks like. I can't describe the smell."

mitment of refining and perfecting their assessment skills, the following suggestions are offered:

- For several days, make it a goal to evaluate and improve your interviewing techniques. Become aware of your deficiencies, especially those that block communication.
- Based on the information discussed under the section on general focus questions and parameters for eliciting appropriate data, perform a nursing assessment using the Critical Care Response Pattern Assessment Tool. Then reread the information on the general focus questions and parameters to see whether you missed anything. Did you organize your objectives, thoughts, and observations? Was your approach systematic and complete? What areas need more study and practice? Do you believe you have assessed the body-mind-spirit problems of this patient?
- Write down your observations and findings, and formulate your nursing diagnoses and problem list. Does this list reflect the body-mind-spirit problems of this patient? Can you express your thoughts and findings adequately and logically?
- Make a resolution to look at machines and tubes only after assessing the patient.
- Be more aware of everything in the patient's environment.

Listen to your patient. While assessing the patient, try not to overlook even one minor point. Be sensitive to the patient and surroundings. Pay attention to and trust your intuitive thoughts. Smell, feel, hear, touch, and look at everything.

SUMMARY

The nursing process is a systematic way of assessing and diagnosing priority patient problems, establishing patient outcomes, developing a patient care plan, implementing the plan, and evaluating to what degree the outcomes were achieved. When a conceptual model or framework of nursing is used to guide the nursing assessment and the remaining steps of the nursing process, nurses focus on patients and families as whole beings, thereby transforming complex technical skills into humanistic nursing care.

REFERENCES

1. American Nurses' Association Congress for Nursing Practice. *Nursing: A Social Policy Statement.* Kansas City, MO: 1980.
2. Aydelotte, M. K., and Peterson, K. H. Keynote Address: Nursing Taxonomics—State of the Art. In A. M. McLane (Ed.), *Classification*

of Nursing Diagnoses: Proceedings of the Seventh Conference. St. Louis: Mosby-Year Book, 1987.

3. Bates, B. *A Guide to Physical Examination.* Philadelphia: JB Lippincott, 1983.

4. Carpenito, L. J. *Nursing Diagnoses: Application to Clinical Practice.* Philadelphia: JB Lippincott, 1987.

5. Carroll-Johnson, R. M. (Ed.). *Classification of Nursing Diagnoses: Proceedings of the Eighth Conference.* Philadelphia: JB Lippincott, 1989.

6. Christman, M. K., and Fowler, M. D. The Systems-in-Change Model for Nursing Practice. In J. Riehl and C. Roy (Eds.), *Conceptual Models for Nursing Practice.* New York: Appleton-Century-Crofts, 1980.

7. Dossey, B. M., and Guzzetta, C. E. Person-Centered Caring and the Nursing Process. In C. E. Guzzetta and B. M. Dossey, *Cardiovascular Nursing: Bodymind Tapestry.* St. Louis: Mosby-Year Book, 1984.

8. Fields, W. L., and McGinn-Campbell, L. M. *Introduction to Health Assessment.* Reston, VA: Reston Publishing Co., 1983.

9. Gordon, M. *Manual of Nursing Diagnosis.* New York: McGraw-Hill, 1987.

10. Guzzetta, C. E. Nursing diagnoses: Effect on the profession. *Heart Lung* 16:629, 1987.

11. Guzzetta, C. E. General Focus Question and Parameters for Eliciting Appropriate Data. In C. E. Guzzetta, S. D. Bunton, L. A. Prinkey, *et al* (Eds.), *Clinical Assessment Tools for Use with Nursing Diagnoses.* St. Louis: Mosby-Year Book, 1989: 23–39.

12. Guzzetta, C. E., Bunton, S. D., Prinkey, L. A., *et al.* Unitary person assessment tool: Easing problems with nursing diagnoses. *Focus Crit. Care* 15:12, 1988.

13. Guzzetta, C. E., Bunton, S. D., Prinkey, L. A., *et al* (Eds.). *Clinical Assessment Tools for Use with Nursing Diagnoses.* St. Louis: Mosby-Year Book, 1989.

14. Guzzetta, C. E., and Dossey, B. M. Nursing diagnosis: Framework-process-problems. *Heart Lung* 12:281, 1983.

15. Guzzetta, C. E., and Dossey, B. M. *Cardiovascular Nursing: Biobehavioral Interventions.* St. Louis: Mosby-Year Book, 1992 (in press).

16. Guzzetta, C. E., and Sherer, A. P. Holistic Approach to Nursing Diagnosis. In C. E. Guzzetta and B. M. Dossey, *Cardiovascular Nursing: Biobehavioral Interventions.* St. Louis: Mosby-Year Book, 1992 (in press).

17. Guzzetta, C. E., and Kinney, M. R. Mastering the transition from medical to nursing diagnosis. *Prog. Cardiovasc. Nurs.* 1:41, 1986.

18. Haak, S., and Huether, S. Person with Acute Myocardial Infarction. In C. E. Guzzetta and B. M. Dossey, *Cardiovascular Nursing: Biobehavioral Interventions.* St. Louis: Mosby-Year Book, 1992 (in press).

19. Kim, M. J., and Moritz, D. A. (Eds.). *Classification of Nursing Diagnoses: Proceeding of the Third and Fourth National Conferences.* New York: McGraw-Hill, 1982.

20. Kim, M. J., McFarland, G. K., and McLane, A. M. *Classification of Nursing Diagnoses: Proceedings of the Fifth National Conference.* St. Louis: Mosby-Year Book, 1984.

21. Kim, M. J., McFarland, G. K., and McLane, A. M. *Pocket Guide to Nursing Diagnoses* (3rd ed.). St. Louis: Mosby-Year Book, 1989.

22. King, I. *Towards a Theory of Nursing.* Boston: Little, Brown, 1981.

23. Kinney, M. K., Packa, D. R., and Dunbar, S. B. (Eds.). *AACN's Clinical Reference for Critical Care Nursing* (2nd ed.). St. Louis: Mosby-Year Book, 1988.

24. Kritek, P. B. Development of a Taxonomic Structure for Nursing Diagnoses: A Review and Update. In M. Hurley (Ed.), *Classification of Nursing Diagnoses: Proceedings of the Sixth Conference.* St. Louis: Mosby-Year Book, 1986.

25. Lee, J. Y. *Sokdam: Capsules of Eastern Wisdom.* Korea: Folklore Research Institute, 1977.

26. Malasanos, L., Barkanskas, V., Moss, M., *et al.* *Health Assessment* (3rd ed.). St. Louis: Mosby-Year Book, 1986.

27. McFarland, G. K., and McFarlane, E. A. *Nursing Diagnoses and Intervention: Planning for Care.* St. Louis: Mosby-Year Book, 1989.

28. Newman, M. A. *Health as Expanding Consciousness.* St. Louis: Mosby-Year Book, 1986.

29. Orem, D. E. *Nursing: Concepts of Practice.* New York: McGraw-Hill, 1985.

30. Prinkey, L. A., and Bunton, S. D. Critical Care Assessment Tool. In C. E. Guzzetta, S. D. Bunton, L. A. Prinkey, *et al* (Eds.). *Clinical Assessment Tools for Use with Nursing Diagnoses.* St. Louis: Mosby-Year Book, 1989: 170–197.

31. Rogers, M. *Introduction to the Theoretical Basis of Nursing.* Philadelphia: FA Davis, 1969.

32. Roy, C. *Introduction to Nursing: An Adaptation Model.* Englewood Cliffs, NJ: Prentice-Hall, 1976.

33. Roy, C. Framework for Classification Systems Development: Progress and Issues. In M. J. Kim, G. K. McFarland, and A. M. McLane (Eds.), *Classification of Nursing Diagnoses: Proceedings of the Fifth Conference.* St. Louis: Mosby-Year Book, 1984.

34. Sanford, S. J., and Disch, J. M. *American Association of Critical-Care Nurses Standards for Nursing Care of the Critically Ill.* Norwalk, CT: Appleton & Lange, 1989.

35. Seidel, H. M., Ball, F. W., Dains, J. E., *et al.* *Mosby's Guide to Physical Examination.* St. Louis: Mosby-Year Book, 1987.

36. Thompson, J., McFarland, G., Hirsh, J., *et al.* *Clinical Nursing.* St. Louis: Mosby-Year Book, 1986.

37. Topf, M. A framework for research on the aversive physical aspects of the environment. *Res. Nurs. Health* 7:35, 1984.

38. Underhill, S. L., Woods, S. L., Sivarajan, E., *et al.* *Cardiac Nursing.* Philadelphia: JB Lippincott, 1989.

39. Yura, H., and Walsh, M. B. *Human Needs and the Nursing Process.* New York: Appleton-Century-Crofts, 1984.

40. Yura, H., and Walsh, M. B. *The Nursing Process: Assessing, Planning, Implementing, Evaluating.* Norwalk, CT: Appleton & Lange, 1985.

6

Nursing Diagnoses, Patient Outcomes, Implementation, and Evaluation

Cathie E. Guzzetta

COMMENCING YOUR HEALING JOURNEY

You are the spiritual expert about your life and must continue to develop your spiritual understanding. If spirituality is a given and is the essence of your being, it is useful to acknowledge your innate qualities. When you give these qualities names and tend to them, you begin to use them as healing tools. The following is a list of ways in which you may open to your healing potential:

- Connecting—connecting with self, others, higher power, universe; allows you to experience being grounded
- Disconnecting—opening yourself to new creative endeavors (*e.g.,* relaxation, imagery, dance, and laughter)
- Skillpower—challenging your mind to learn things other than nursing; exploring your inner wisdom (*e.g.,* taking a class of a new interest; consulting a therapist if you feel stuck)
- Purifying—washing away, not necessarily with water (*e.g.,* sitting quietly by a roaring fire or out in nature in the sunshine; "playing in the dirt" without transforming the garden; taking a long bath or shower)
- Journeying—traveling in your imagination (*e.g.,* reading a good book; walking or taking a leisurely drive; writing in a journal)
- Transforming—using raw materials to restore order and create something new (*e.g.,* painting, weaving, needlepoint, or other craft; gardening or creative cooking; cleaning a closet, drawers, or desk)*

LEARNING OBJECTIVES

After reading this chapter, the nurse should be able to do the following:

1. Compare and contrast a medical versus a nursing diagnosis.
2. Discuss the benefits of standardizing nursing diagnostic terminology within the profession.
3. Compare and contrast the components of an actual nursing diagnosis, a high-risk nursing diagnosis, and a wellness diagnosis.
4. Discuss the guidelines suggested for writing the diagnostic statement for each of the three types of nursing diagnoses.

5. Identify problems in using nursing diagnosis that are unique to critical care.
6. Discuss the need to develop a comprehensive system to classify all of nursing practice.
7. Outline the criteria to use when developing expected patient outcomes for an actual versus a high-risk nursing diagnosis.
8. Outline the criteria to use when selecting appropriate nursing interventions for a specific nursing diagnosis.
9. Discuss which components of the nursing process are evaluated during the evaluation phase.

DEFINITION OF NURSING DIAGNOSIS

The term *diagnosis* is derived from the Greek word *diagignoskein,* which means "to distinguish" or "to discriminate."[42] The

* Modified from Burkhardt, M., and Nagai-Jacobson, M. G. Spirituality: Cornerstone of Holistic Nursing Practice. In B. Dossey, Spirituality and healing. *Holistic Nurs. Pract.* 3(3):21, 1989.

literal meaning of *diagnosis* is the act of gathering information or data about what is preventing a return to normal functioning, what is causing some difficulty, or what needs to be corrected and distinguishing the *what* by its characteristics. Although the term *nursing diagnosis* has been defined in multiple ways, a currently accepted definition is a "cluster of signs and symptoms describing an actual or potential health problem (state-of-the-patient) which nurses, because of their education and experience, are licensed and able to treat."[14] After the Ninth Conference on Classification of Nursing Diagnoses (March 1990), sponsored by the North American Nursing Diagnosis Association, the definition of nursing diagnosis was revised as "a clinical judgment about individual, family, or community responses to actual or potential health problems/life processes. Nursing diagnoses provide the basis for selection of nursing interventions to achieve outcomes for which the nurse is accountable."[34]

Despite the momentum and the work accomplished by the North American Nursing Diagnosis Association (NANDA), the term *nursing diagnosis* has been associated with some strong negative reactions from various nursing and medical groups. Some believe that only physicians are educated and licensed to diagnose. This belief has arisen because the distinction between a medical and a nursing diagnosis is not clear.

The distinction between a medical and a nursing diagnosis can be appreciated by examining the models that guide nursing and medical practice. Medical practice is guided by the biomedical or molecular model of disease causation. The major tenet of this model asserts that all disease is caused by a malfunction of specific molecules or organs.[12] Medicine, therefore, has been involved traditionally with the pathology, diagnosis, and cure of disease. In other words, most medical specialties have been involved primarily with the physical or biological aspects of patient care. As a result, medical diagnoses are involved with identifying the etiology of disease, and treatment is directed toward this etiology.[22]

In contrast, nursing practice is guided by a holistic model that reflects the interrelationship of body–mind–spirit and focuses on maintaining, regaining, and promoting health.[23] Caring is held with the same regard as curing.[41] The major tenets of the holistic model are that human beings and their environment are open systems continually interacting, exchanging, and creating unique patterns, processes, and organizations within the energy field; that signs and symptoms are viewed as part of the ongoing, complex, and interlocking system and not as isolated findings; that human consciousness is a coequal factor in any interpretation of the cause and response of health or illness; and that the patient is an active participant in health and illness. The holistic model conveys the oneness and unity of the individual. It allows the nurse to understand that any change in the physiologic state is always accompanied by an appropriate change in the psychologic state and, conversely, that any change in the psychologic state is always accompanied by an appropriate change in the physiologic state.[17,21] Thus, nursing diagnoses are involved with human responses to stressors or other factors that adversely affect achievement of optimal health.[8,26] Treatment is directed toward causes of the response or factors influencing it.

Because nurses administer accepted modes of therapy for each nursing diagnosis that they are licensed and able to treat, a health problem is not considered a nursing diagnosis if it is treated with modalities that are legally defined by the practice of medicine (e.g., prescription drugs, radiation, surgery). However, some health problems (*e.g.*, pain) are treated by both nursing and medicine. Moreover, many nurses have the knowledge, education, experience, and skills to make medical diagnoses. In critical care, for example, nurses frequently diagnose ventricular fibrillation, cardiac arrest, acute heart failure, pulmonary edema, cardiac tamponade, and other medical problems. In many critical care settings, nurses initiate treatment for such problems because of standing orders or medically approved protocols. Medical problems treated with standing orders or protocols, however, are not called nursing diagnoses because they do not reflect problems that nurses can treat independently.

STANDARDIZING NURSING TERMINOLOGY

Although nurses have always been involved in identifying patient problems, there has never been a consistent method by which to standardize and communicate the terminology.[10] NANDA has made a monumental impact in this area with its work in defining, explaining, classifying, and validating summary statements about health problems.[26,27] This work has led to standardized labels for patient problems that nurses encounter. A consistent terminology and a formalized approach to the diagnostic process have increased communication and clarification about health problems to all members of the health team.[24]

To enhance the standardization and development of nursing diagnoses, NANDA created the Unitary Person Framework that focuses on the patterns and organization of individuals as a way of describing their state of health (see Chap. 5, p. 55). Within this framework, the individual's health is evaluated by assessing the nine human response patterns (*e.g.*, communicating, knowing, valuing, relating, feeling, moving, perceiving, exchanging, and choosing [see Table 5–1]). From this framework, the old alphabetical list of nursing diagnoses has been reorganized by Taxonomy I, which categorizes the accepted nursing diagnoses according to the nine human response patterns[36] (see Chap. 5, Table 5–2).

Based on NANDA's Unitary Person Framework and Taxonomy I, a new Critical Care Response Pattern Assessment Tool was developed to assess the patient's nine response patterns reflecting all parts of the whole person.[20] Nursing diagnoses flow easily from the assessment when using this tool[19] (see Chap. 5, Fig. 5-2).

Nursing diagnoses are formulated by analyzing, synthesizing, and interpreting the data collected from the nine human response patterns. Nursing diagnoses are used to identify the patient's actual or high-risk health problems or wellness diagnosis.[11,34] Nursing diagnoses help to designate priorities in patient problems and to provide the direction for developing the remaining steps of the nursing process. They may address an actual health problem or, just as likely, a high-risk health problem that appropriate nursing intervention can prevent, alleviate, or at least reduce. Based on the nursing diagnoses, the nurse prescribes treatments or therapies.[16]

It is important to remember that the accepted list of nursing diagnoses presented in Taxonomy I (Table 5–2) has not been fully developed yet. The term *accepted list* means that the nursing diagnoses identified in Taxonomy I have been accepted for clinical testing but have not all been validated by research. As a result, it is not known yet whether all these diagnoses are useful in describing patient problems or whether some even exist in clinical practice.[21] Taxonomy I will be modified, revised, and expanded as each of the diagnostic categories is validated by research.[32]

Research also is being conducted so that specific patient outcomes and nursing interventions can be developed for each diagnosis.[8,26,27,31] The results of such work will augment the scientific knowledge needed to predict and control the outcomes of nursing practice. A major goal of the American Nurses' Association (ANA) is to develop a uniform classification system for describing nursing practice. The classification system is to include assessment, diagnosis, interventions, and outcomes as the broad categories that would be identified, defined, and classified in the future.[1,29] While NANDA has been recognized as the official body to develop nursing diagnoses, the ANA will direct its efforts towards classifying the areas of assessment, outcomes, and interventions.

The ANA also has been working jointly with NANDA in efforts to develop a coding translation of the nursing diagnoses in Taxonomy I. Their work has resulted in a revised taxonomy that has been submitted for possible inclusion in the next edition of the World Health Organization's International Classification of Diseases (WHO ICD-10) as conditions that necessitate nursing care.[29] Acceptance of the taxonomy into ICD-10 would be a monumental accomplishment for nursing and would promote the use of the taxonomy internationally and in collaboration with other groups.[13] The International Council of Nurses (ICN) also has expressed interest in discussing nursing diagnoses from an international perspective. Thus, national and international progress is being made towards developing a uniform nomenclature for nursing.

TYPES OF NURSING DIAGNOSES

NANDA has identified three types of nursing diagnoses: actual nursing diagnoses, high-risk nursing diagnoses, and wellness diagnoses. These are discussed in the following paragraphs.

Actual Nursing Diagnoses

An actual nursing diagnosis is a problem identified from the patient assessment that represents a pattern of related cues. The name of the actual nursing diagnosis (diagnostic label) is identified from NANDA's accepted list of nursing diagnoses found in Taxonomy I (see Table 5–2). Diagnostic labels for an actual nursing diagnosis may include (but are not limited to) the diagnostic qualifiers outlined in Table 5–3. Because the problem identifies what needs to be changed for a healthier state, it is used to guide the nurse in identifying patient outcomes in the plan of care.[21,26]

It should be emphasized that the accepted list of nursing diagnoses does not include all possible problems encountered and dealt with by nurses. After assessing the patient, it may be found that one or more of the patient's problems are not on the accepted list. If it is determined that the patient exhibits observable signs and symptoms supporting a new nursing diagnosis, then word the problem concisely, identify the probable etiology (or related factor), and write the diagnostic statement.[23]

For each actual nursing diagnosis, *related factors* are identified. Related factors are "conditions or circumstances that can cause or contribute to the development of a diagnosis."[34] Related factors are antecedent to, associated with, related to, contributing to, or abetting the actual nursing diagnosis.[34] Related factors help to identify what is maintaining the problem and preventing an improvement in health. This category guides the nurse in selecting the appropriate nursing interventions and in developing the plan of care, because it conveys what must change in order to achieve a state of health.[26] In the past, related factors were termed the "etiology" of the diagnosis. Because the cause-and-effect relationship between most nursing diagnoses and their etiologies has not been established yet by research, the term *related factor* (which can incorporate the etiology but is not limited to it) is a more accurate description.

The actual nursing diagnosis is written as a *two-part diagnostic statement* formed by connecting the problem and the related factor with the phrase *related to* (*e.g.*, anxiety related to impending pacemaker surgery). Refer to Table 6–1 for guidelines in writing the diagnostic statement. The connecting phrase *related to* is legally recommended rather than due to or caused by because, again, the cause of most nursing diagnoses have not been supported scientifically.[21,33] The actual nursing diagnosis also can be written as a *three-part diagnostic statement* if the signs and symptoms (defining characteristics) are included (*e.g.*, anxiety related to impending pacemaker surgery demonstrated by expressed feelings of uncertainty, distress, concern about the future, trembling hands, and con-

---

Table 6–1

Guidelines for Writing the Diagnostic Statement

Consider the following guidelines when writing the diagnostic statement[21,23]:

1. The first main clause should reflect an actual or high-risk health problem and not an environmental problem. Environmental factors are stated in the second main clause.

   Wrong: Excessive environmental stimuli related to monitoring equipment.
   Right: Sensory perceptual alterations (auditory and visual) related to excessive environmental stimuli.

2. Several unrelated problems should not be written in the first main clause even though the etiology (or related factors) of the problems may be the same. Problems may be judged as unrelated when the nursing plan requires separate interventions for each problem.

   Wrong: Anxiety and activity intolerance related to frequent episodes of chest pain.
   Right: Anxiety related to frequent episodes of chest pain.
   Right: Activity intolerance related to frequent episodes of chest pain.

3. The diagnostic statement should be written so that both the problem and related factors refer to different findings.

   Wrong: Self-feeding deficit related to inability to feed self.
   Right: Self-feeding deficit (level 2) related to muscle weakness.

4. The diagnostic statement should be written to avoid legal ramifications.

   Wrong: High risk for (physical) injury related to lack of safety precautions.
   Right: High risk for (physical) injury related to mental confusion.

5. The nursing diagnosis should not be written as a patient need.

   Wrong: Need for maintenance of nutritional intake.
   Right: Altered nutrition (less than body requirements) related to nausea/vomiting.

stant nonpurposeful activity of extremities). This format is recommended when teaching students or when initially implementing nursing diagnoses in the clinical setting, because it provides on-the-spot documentation to support and link the findings from the clinical assessment to the diagnosis formulated.[23]

Before formulating a judgment about whether an actual nursing diagnosis exists, it must be determined, from an assessment of the patient's nine human response patterns, whether the patient exhibits the clinical defining characteristics of the diagnosis. *Clinical defining characteristics* are the diagnostic cues that cluster as manifestations of a nursing diagnosis. They provide the concrete and measurable clinical evidence obtained from the assessment that identify the signs, symptoms, or behaviors representing the diagnostic label.[34] They are used to discriminate and differentiate among various nursing diagnoses. Defining characteristics are divided into major and minor categories.

Major defining characteristics are the critical indicators that are present in 80% to 100% of the patients experiencing the diagnosis.[34] *Minor defining characteristics* are supporting indicators that are present in 50% to 79% of the patients experiencing the diagnosis. Although they are not always present, minor defining characteristics complete the clinical picture and assist the nurse in making the diagnosis.[34]

Many of the defining characteristics for each nursing diagnosis are still being defined, developed, and validated by research. Many are not yet classified into the major and minor categories. When nurses formulate their tentative diagnosis, they should refer to the currently published defining characteristics[8,15,26–28,30] to determine if such characteristics actually were observed in their patients to support the existence of the diagnosis being considered. When the published list of defining characteristics is incomplete, nurses should use their education and experience to determine whether the signs, symptoms, and behaviors observed in their patient demonstrate the actual health problem identified.[21]

High-Risk Nursing Diagnoses

High-risk nursing diagnoses have been introduced recently by NANDA. As of 1992, all "NANDA approved diagnoses currently designated as Potential will be labeled 'High-Risk For'."[34] A high-risk nursing diagnosis is a "clinical judgment that an individual, family, or community is more vulnerable to develop the problem than others in the same or similar situation."[34] Any of the nursing diagnoses found in Taxonomy I (see Table 5–2) can be used as the diagnostic label for high-risk nursing diagnoses. The diagnostic qualifiers used are the same as for the actual nursing diagnoses (see Table 5–3).

For high-risk nursing diagnoses, risk factors rather than related factors are identified. *A risk factor* is a "behavior, condition, or circumstance that renders an individual, family, or community more vulnerable to a particular problem than others in the same or similar situation. High-risk nursing diagnoses are supported by risk factors that guide nursing interventions to reduce or prevent the occurrence of the problem."[34]

There are no signs and symptoms for high-risk nursing diagnoses. A *two-part diagnostic statement* is written (*e.g.*, high risk for infection related to temporary pacemaker lead).

The decision to change potential diagnoses to that of high-risk diagnoses is a major breakthrough for critical care nurses.

All patients may have the potential for infection, for example, but patients with a temporary pacemaker lead, those on hemodynamic monitoring, or those who are immunosuppressed can be judged to be at high risk for infection. Much of critical care nursing involves preventing or reducing major complications of critically ill patients. When a critically ill patient is identified at high risk for infection, the nurse implements specific nursing care aimed at its prevention. When infection is found not to occur in this high-risk patient, the nursing contribution in achieving the desired patient outcome can be demonstrated and documented. This high-risk category is beneficial in justifying allocation of resources and personnel, in directing third-party payment, and in validating that appropriate standards of nursing practice were used successfully to prevent or reduce problems in susceptible patients.[23]

Wellness Nursing Diagnoses

NANDA recently has identified the category of wellness diagnoses. A wellness diagnosis is a "clinical judgment about an individual, family, or community in transition from a specific level of wellness to a higher level of wellness."[34] The diagnostic qualifier for wellness nursing diagnoses is the phrase "potential for enhanced," which is used together with one of the diagnostic labels found in Taxonomy I (see Table 5–2). *Enhanced* is defined as "made greater, to increase in quality, or more desired."[34] A *one-part diagnostic statement* is written for wellness diagnoses (*e.g.*, potential for enhanced adjustment to illness).[23]

In the past, the nursing diagnosis movement was criticized for ignoring the wellness movement. Wellness and health promotion are national priorities aimed at maintaining and promoting wellness behaviors in patients. Inclusion of wellness nursing diagnoses broadens our perspective from an illness-dominated framework to one that incorporates a positive wellness orientation. It permits us to demonstrate and document our contribution to maintaining and promoting wellness.[23]

USING NURSING DIAGNOSES IN CRITICAL CARE

Nurses who wish to use nursing diagnoses in their clinical practice should consider the guidelines presented in Table 6–2.[21]

In critical care there are many problems that exist when using nursing diagnoses.[21,23,35,39,40] For example, what is the best way to implement nursing diagnoses in critical care? Why are there so few physiologic diagnoses in Taxonomy I? Can nursing diagnoses be used effectively in critical care because many of the patient's problems are physiologic? Why is there a lack of physiologic defining characteristics for many nursing diagnoses? Are there important specific, critical care nursing diagnoses that are missing from the accepted list of nursing diagnoses? Which nursing diagnoses occur commonly in critically ill patients? Conferences and discussions led by critical care nurses are addressing some of these issues.[38–40]

Perhaps one of the most serious problems found in using nursing diagnoses in critical care is one that is created by the restricting definition of a nursing diagnosis. If a nursing diagnosis is defined to include only those problems that nurses identify and treat independently, it excludes dependent prob-

Table 6–2
Guidelines for Using Nursing Diagnoses

Consider the following guidelines when using nursing diagnoses[10,21,33]:

1. Carry a list of the accepted nursing diagnoses in your pocket.
2. Refer to the accepted list when writing each nursing diagnoses.
3. Early in the shift, establish the habit of doing a complete biopsychosocial patient assessment using a standardized nursing data base. Be sure to assess the nine human response patterns and review the previous 24 to 48 hours of nurses' notes, progress notes, and medical and nursing orders.
4. After establishing a baseline assessment, write down the diagnostic statements in the patient's care plan.
5. Identify patient outcomes and nursing orders, implement nursing orders, and evaluate patient outcomes for each nursing diagnosis.
6. Continue to reassess and reevaluate throughout the shift.
7. Refer back to each nursing diagnosis when giving nursing care and when holding patient/health team conferences.
8. When charting on a patient, use each nursing diagnosis as a guide.
9. Use the nursing diagnosis list as the outline for the end-of-shift report. Make sure the nurse on the next shift understands each diagnosis.

lems and those controlled by protocols and standing orders. If nursing practice is composed of the independent and dependent/interdependent role of the nurse, then nursing diagnoses reflect only part of the problems encountered by nurses in practice.[21,23]

To deal with this issue, Carpenito has suggested that nursing interventions address two types of problems: nursing diagnoses and collaborative problems.[7] Collaborative problems are defined as "physiologic complications for which nurses use monitoring skills to detect onset or status so that nurses can collaborate with medicine to provide definitive therapy."[7] Rather than making up new titles for such problems, she suggests that collaborative problems be called "potential complication: (specify)." Examples of collaborative problems are "potential complications: hemorrhage, dysrhythmias, or allergic reactions." Because collaborative problems require intervention by both medicine and nursing, Carpenito believes that it is not appropriate to develop outcome criteria for such problems.[7]

Even if collaborative problems are used together with nursing diagnoses, the list of nursing diagnoses will still reflect only part of the problems that nurses encounter. This situation has prompted critical care nurses to ask several questions: Can a nursing diagnostic classification system be useful in advancing nursing practice if it reflects only part of what nursing does? Why must nursing diagnoses reflect only the independent role of the nurse? Can nursing diagnoses be developed to reflect all problems identified and dealt with by nurses?[21,23]

To answer these questions, it is necessary to reexamine some of the traditional definitions that differentiate the independent from the dependent/interdependent role of the nurse. Although these roles can be at least theoretically differentiated, nurses, particularly those practicing in critical care, realize that such a division is artificial and frequently impossible to define at the bedside. Consider one example of many found daily in critical care, which reflects the dependent/interdependent role of the nurse:

Mr. G. is a newly admitted patient with a presumptive diagnosis of acute myocardial infarction. While Mr. G.'s nurse was administering care to another patient in the next room, the monitoring technician alerted her that Mr. G. was having 20 to 25 PVCs per minute. On her way to assess Mr. G., the nurse reached for a bolus of lidocaine. She immediately assessed that Mr. G. was restless, pale, and hypotensive. She further determined that he had a sinus bradycardia of 48 with ventricular escape beats (an acute change from his normal sinus rhythm of 90 without ectopy 1 hour before) and a peripheral pulse of 40. She put the lidocaine back in the drawer and initiated the intensive care unit's protocol for a patient with symptomatic bradycardia. She administered intravenous atropine while she continued to assess the patient and his cardiac rhythm, explained her actions to him, and reassured him. Simultaneously, she called in a colleague, reported her assessment findings and her interventions, and asked that an immediate ECG be ordered and the physician be called. Within 5 minutes the patient was normotensive, no longer restless and pale, and in a sinus rhythm with a rate of 74.

Does the preceding example reflect the dependent role of the nurse as traditionally defined? *Dependent* can be defined as those actions which are determined by another. Are any nursing actions in critical care totally "dependent" in the 1990s? In departing from traditional thinking, the preceding example illustrates the interdependent role of the nurse and physician as the nurse coparticipates with the patient and the physician in treating illness.[21,23]

Conversely, consider the independent role of the nurse. *Independence* is defined as "not subject to control by others" or "not affiliated with a larger unit." From this viewpoint, can any nursing actions be totally independent?[21,23] Furthermore, how much of nursing practice, particularly in critical care, is totally independent?[26] One must also ask independent of whom or what—the patient, the physician, the health team, the hospital?

The confusion surrounding the dependent versus independent roles of the nurse perhaps arises from the logical deduction that in practice these roles have never existed as traditionally defined. Perhaps it is time that we begin to accept what we say we believe regarding the holistic framework of nursing, the interrelatedness of all individuals, and the potential for joint practice. Perhaps it is time to define the nurse's role as one of *interdependence, coparticipation,* and *collaboration* with the patient, family, physician, and health team.[21,23] It is time that we go beyond the either/or issue of roles to a definition that is consistent with the framework we claim guides our practice.[9,21,22]

Accepting the interdependent role of the nurse eliminates the artificial divisions that have created many problems and it clarifies much of the confusion. It clarifies a role that reflects the current level and direction of our practice adequately. It is consistent with a holistic focus in caring for our patients. It permits us to describe all that we do, because we are not restricted by artificially induced divisions in our role.

We know that the nursing diagnosis movement has had a greater impact on nursing than originally anticipated.[18] Some believe that Taxonomy I's classification of nursing diagnoses may actually become "nothing less than the systematic description of the entire domain of nursing."[25] Currently educators are using the classification system of nursing diagnoses to design their curriculum, identify educational objectives, and assist students to learn nursing content. Nursing administrators are using the classification system to classify patient needs, document the intensity of the services required, and allocate personnel resources.[25] Researchers use the classification system as a major focus for developing descriptive, exploratory, and experimental studies for investigation. Major textbooks are incorporating nursing diagnoses as a central framework. Computer software programs are being developed to incorporate nursing diagnoses as a foundational element of a nursing data base system. However, if we continue to define nursing diagnoses to reflect only the independent role of the nurse, then the classification system will never have the potential to define comprehensively what it is that nursing does. Moreover, a scientific body of knowledge can never be developed, tested, and validated for predicting and controlling patient outcomes when only part of nursing practice is addressed.

On a typical day in critical care, for example, nurses may find that 90% of what they do involves the dependent/interdependent role, whereas only 10% involves the so-called independent role of the nurse. If most of our day involves dependent/interdependent functioning, then it is clear that nursing diagnoses do not capture the essence of critical care nursing practice. The current list of accepted nursing diagnoses poorly describes the scope of responsibilities and the major contributions of the critical care nurse in changing or improving patient outcomes.[37] If a large part of our role is associated with the medical diagnoses, then we will not be able to develop labels and standardize nursing interventions for most of what we do. Likewise, if the physiologic problems we deal with are termed collaborative problems, for which no outcome criteria are developed, then we will not be able to evaluate the effects of our care or document our role in detecting and preventing the devastating complications of injury and disease.[37]

Physiologic problems do not belong solely to the medical domain. Because holistic nursing care implies an approach that deals with the whole patient, a list of nursing diagnoses that describes primarily psychosocial problems but disregards important physiologic problems is not one that has been developed holistically. Furthermore, because most patient care plans will be placed on computers for the purposes of documentation, evaluation, and hospital billing, labels that omit or incompletely identify problems that nurses deal with or those that reflect medical diagnoses will be counterproductive to advancing nursing practice.

We must develop a comprehensive system to classify all of nursing practice. The labels need to include all problems encountered and dealt with by nurses.[18] The patient problems that we encounter and the things that we do related to the medical diagnosis must be clearly defined and labeled. The reasons for doing so are compelling. We need to label all that we do for the purposes of documentation and communication. Such labels will provide strong support for justifying staffing patterns, directing third-party payment, and establishing prospective reimbursement fees.[7] Only when nurses can label clearly, concisely, and accurately what it is they do will they be recognized consistently for their actions and reimbursed for their services. The labels will permit information to be easily retrievable from computers for quality assurance programs and research purposes, so that effective nursing interventions can be identified and investigated. Labels that reflect all that we do will permit us to demonstrate our contribution to patient outcomes. They will provide us with the evidence to document the complex responsibilities and skills needed in caring for patients with multifaceted physiologic problems.[37] Thus, if nursing diagnoses are to measure nursing productivity

and effectiveness, there must be an all-inclusive system to classify nursing practice.

The case studies and nursing diagnoses in Units 4 to 10 of this text demonstrate various methods of establishing nursing diagnoses. Some of the nursing diagnoses in these chapters violate traditional definitions because they do not represent only health problems that nurses treat independently. Rather, they represent health problems that are interdependently treated by the nurse. For example, the authors believe that the nursing diagnosis of "decreased cardiac output related to disturbances in electrical, mechanical, or structural factors" is a specific nursing diagnostic label that describes the specific physiologic problems or complications that a patient with acute myocardial infarction (or other patients) may develop and which nurses identify and treat.[21,23] The approach used in formulating these nursing diagnoses is not necessarily consistent with current guidelines and therefore may create some controversy. Such controversy can be beneficial, however, when it is involved in questioning, examining, and expanding the nursing diagnosis movement and in discovering practical and realistic guidelines for using nursing diagnoses in practice.

FUTURE CHALLENGE IN NURSING DIAGNOSIS

It is not easy to accept that there is no one "right" approach to using nursing diagnoses. Accepting this fact can produce discomfort. However, we believe that there are many useful approaches. Nurses must examine such approaches and adapt, refine, and change them based on the beliefs, needs, and requirements of their particular nursing staff or institution.[23]

As critical care nurses, we are confronted with unique problems in our clinical settings. We need to assume responsibility for confronting such problems and developing the solutions. We need to examine the assumptions underlying the use of nursing diagnoses. We need to ask why nursing diagnoses currently reflect only part of our practice. We need to reevaluate traditional beliefs associated with the "dependent, independent, and interdependent" roles of the nurse.[21,23] We must question why nursing diagnoses do not include all problems with which we deal. We must identify and label problems we encounter as critical care nurses that are not on the list.

We encourage nurses to continue to question, develop, and refine various approaches to using nursing diagnoses. Although the guidelines governing nursing diagnoses have not been fully developed, it is suggested that the following criteria be used to evaluate the product of any approach being considered[23]:

- The approach should be holistic.
- The approach should permit all the patient's body–mind–spirit problems to be identified and documented in the care plan.
- The approach should reflect all problems encountered and dealt with by nurses.

Nurses also have a responsibility to communicate their successes and problems to others who have a similar framework of practice. As various approaches are chosen, implemented, validated, and refined in practice, it is likely that a more comprehensive and yet very different approach to nursing diagnoses will emerge.

PATIENT OUTCOMES

Identifying patient outcomes is the third step in the nursing process. After nursing diagnoses have been established and prioritized for the patient, specific and concise patient outcomes are written. Specific patient outcomes provide a standard, or the desired goal or objective, that the patient can achieve realistically as a result of nursing care.[2] The patient outcomes (sometimes developed more specifically as outcome criteria) are measurable statements developed for each diagnosis that serve as the tools or tests to evaluate whether the patient has attained the desired state.

One or more patient outcomes may be written for each nursing diagnosis. These outcomes should identify one or more of the following[3,4]:

1. What specifically should or should not occur in the patient's status.
2. The level and time at which some change should occur.
3. What patients should verbalize about what they know, understand, or feel about the situation.
4. Specific patient behaviors or signs/symptoms that are expected to occur as a result of the intervention.
5. Specific patient behaviors that are expected to occur as a result of adequate management of the environment.

Using such guidelines, short-, intermediate-, or long-range goals are developed appropriately as patient outcomes. These outcomes then later serve as the criteria to evaluate the effectiveness of the nursing care.

When developing patient outcomes for each patient problem, the authors have found it helpful to remember the four *P*'s for patient outcomes: *p*hysiologic outcomes, *p*sychosocial outcomes, *p*revention outcomes, and *p*atient teaching outcomes. Frequently, patient outcomes from each of the four *P*'s can be written for each of the patient's nursing diagnoses.

Preventing health problems is an important consideration when *high-risk nursing diagnoses* are identified. When writing expected patient outcomes for high-risk diagnoses, the following criteria should be considered[6]:

- A pattern of risk factors will be reduced or eliminated.
- The high-risk diagnosis will not progress to an actual state.
- There will be a delay in time before the actual diagnosis appears.
- The severity of the actual diagnosis will be reduced.

PLANNING

The fourth step in the nursing process is planning. The plan of care involves selecting the appropriate nursing interventions and writing the nursing orders. A nursing intervention (also called nursing treatments, nursing therapies or therapeutics, nursing prescriptions) can be defined as any direct care that the nurse performs for the patient. Such care can include nurse-initiated treatments, physician-initiated treatments, and performing daily essential functions for patients who are unable to perform those themselves.[6]

Patient outcomes are the guide for selecting nursing interventions. There should be a logical flow between the diagnosis, patient outcome, and plan of care. The nursing interventions selected focus on activities that nurses do to assist the patient in achieving the desired outcomes to resolve the patient problem.

When selecting a nursing intervention the following criteria should be kept in mind[4–6]:

- Identify the type of nursing diagnosis being considered. Usually, nursing interventions are aimed at altering the etiologic or related factors associated with the diagnosis. If the etiology is altered successfully, then the patient's status should improve. At other times, however, the etiology cannot be altered, and it is appropriate to treat the signs and symptoms of the problem. When high-risk diagnoses are identified, nursing interventions are aimed at altering or eliminating the risk factors involved.
- Evaluate the research base that validates the effectiveness of the intervention, its clinical significance, and the nursing control associated with the intervention (see Chap. 7).
- Assess the feasibility of implementing the intervention successfully. Consider which nursing diagnoses need to be treated first, how a specific nursing intervention fits into the total plan of care, its cost, the time it will take, and whether the nurse and the patient/family are able to implement the intervention.
- Investigate the acceptability of the intervention to the patient in terms of their own goals and priorities related to the plan of care.
- Evaluate the nursing competency necessary to implement the intervention successfully.

It is essential that the nurse involve the patient closely in the planning phase when appropriate. Problems, however, must be given a priority—high, medium, or low—and there will be times when the critical care nurse cannot involve the patient in the initial phases. If the patient is in a critical state—for example, with an obstructed airway—a high-priority problem exists and the nurse must first intervene to correct the problem. When communication is possible, the patient should be involved in the plan and in decisions about prioritizing problems. Many problems are multifaceted, and solutions must be decided on with the help of the patient and family. If the patient understands the reasons for actions and becomes an active member of the health team, success in achieving the desired patient outcomes is more probable.

For each patient outcome, the plan of care can be written in terms of nursing orders. A *nursing order* is a specific written directive for a nursing intervention. It lists three elements: what action is to be performed (a detailed description may be necessary), who performs the action, and when the action is to occur (*e.g.,* Staff Nurse: Assist patient with drinking high-calorie protein supplement, 240 ml at 2:30 P.M.). Nursing orders are the written directives for nursing interventions and flow directly from the patient outcomes. They are developed to ensure that the probability of achieving the desired patient outcome is high. Nursing orders are written and discussed with everyone involved in the patient's care, and they are revised as necessary according to the nursing diagnoses.

A written patient care plan is the source of information about patients and about the nursing interventions that are appropriate for solving their problems. A clearly stated care plan provides all the nurses involved in the patient's care with a written list of the patient's nursing diagnoses. It allows all the nurses to know the high-, medium-, and low-priority problems, what the short- and long-range patient outcomes are, how problems can be resolved, and how the patient can be assisted to achieve the desired outcomes. It clearly communicates to the nursing staff and other health team members which patient outcomes and what nursing interventions are associated with which diagnosis. It serves as a vehicle for enhancing and coordinating the delivery of patient care.

With some critical care problems, certain nursing interventions must be implemented before the patient care plan and the nursing orders can be written. As soon as these problems are stabilized or solved, the nurse puts the plan in writing and updates it as often as necessary, because in the critical care setting, the patient's problems may change rapidly.

At the New England Medical Center Hospitals, a dramatic restructuring of traditional health care delivery has been implemented called Nursing Case Management. Nursing Case Management is a model and set of technologies for the strategic management of cost and quality outcomes.[43,44] A component of this model involves *case management plans*, which are detailed documents that identify the nursing diagnoses, clinical outcomes for each diagnosis that are achievable within the Diagnosis Related Group (DRG)—allotted length of stay, intermediate goals and estimated dates for each outcome, and nursing and physician interventions that facilitate movement toward each goal. *Critical paths*, also used within this system, are shorthand versions of case management plans that identify the critical incidents that must occur in a predictable and timely manner to achieve an appropriate length of stay. They are used in the Kardex, medication book, or at the bedside for shift reports, nurse–physician rounds, and case consultation to plan and monitor care. Nursing Case Management offers great potential not only for changing traditional approaches to care planning but also for transforming task-oriented nursing to an outcome-based practice.[43,44]

IMPLEMENTING

The fifth step in the nursing process is implementation. Implementation involves carrying out the nursing orders for each nursing diagnosis. Nursing interventions are needed to carry out the physician's orders; the physician writes the orders, and the nurse is responsible for performing the appropriate nursing actions. It is the nurse's responsibility to use critical thinking in carrying out medical and nursing orders. In making decisions, the nurse must use sound judgment based on knowledge before deciding what action is to occur, when it is to occur, and how it is to occur.

The nursing interventions performed during the implementation phase involve the nurse's intellectual, interpersonal, and technical skills. Data are continually collected during this phase, because each nursing intervention and each patient encounter have the potential to alter the patient's physiology, psychology, and health status. When the patient's care plan establishes the priority of the problems and patient outcomes, nursing care will have meaning and purpose. Frequently, highly technical skills are required to solve problems in the critical care setting and nurses must work together to perform such tasks. Thus, a clearly communicated plan of care is fundamental.

The focus of such complex care, however, must center on the patient and all body–mind–spirit problems. Nurses must

realize that body-oriented interventions are only part of the essential therapy that critically ill patients require. There is a rapidly accumulating body of knowledge that is supporting the link between emotions and illness and pointing away from a purely biomedical model of how human beings function.[22] This knowledge takes into account not only the profoundly devastating effects but also the enormous healing effects of the mind in changing psychophysiology. Thus, therapies to reduce the emotional stressors experienced by critically ill patients may be as important to achieving successful patient outcomes as are the traditional and highly technical physiologic therapies. Nurses need to incorporate holistic modalities such as imagery, music therapy, meditation, and other forms of relaxation techniques along with traditional forms of therapies (see Chap. 3). Including such modalities as part of critical care nursing practice demonstrates a movement toward a more holistic approach, which recognizes the tremendous impact of consciousness in matters of illness and recovery. Patients are helped to realize that they possess powerful healing potential within themselves. They are guided in learning techniques that give them some level of control over the situation and permit them to influence their psychophysiology positively. Such therapies encourage patients to become active participants in their recovery and provide them with a sense of involvement in their care. Such an approach actualizes holistic nursing care, wherein the patient and nurse are viewed as a unit, exchanging and interacting, in the healing process.

EVALUATING

The last step in the nursing process is evaluation. Nurses and their patients are the agents of evaluation. Other members of the health team, as well as the patient's family, also may be involved. The evaluation phase of the nursing process looks at immediate, intermediate, and long-range patient outcomes. The purpose of evaluation is not to determine whether the nursing orders have been carried out, but rather to determine if successful patient outcomes have been achieved as a result of patient care, and to what extent.[11] Evaluation also should include the behavioral expectations of the patient relative to the established patient outcomes.

Documentation is an important part of this process. Data are collected and recorded about the effects of the nursing interventions on patient outcomes. The information recorded should be related to the identified problem, the results of the nursing intervention, and the patient's response in achieving the desired outcome. When relevant information is recorded concisely and logically, all members of the health team have a clear understanding of the patient's progress.

The patient care plan is periodically evaluated and reevaluated because of the dynamic nature of human beings as well as the frequent changes that occur during an acute illness. The establishment of new patient outcomes and the need for alterations in the current diagnoses are also assessed. An effective evaluation must be based on a set of standards or criteria that set up an ideal to be achieved. Evaluation also identifies any omissions in the previous phases of the nursing process, as well as what was effective in each phase. Moreover, it serves as the basis for identifying clinical research questions. By looking critically at the effect that bedside nursing has on the patient, important questions and trends will surface. Collation of these questions will help nursing research maintain a clinically relevant impetus.

During the evaluation process, nurses must ask themselves what the expected patient behaviors were and what behaviors actually occurred. The subjective and objective data that are collected must be evaluated. Factors preventing solutions to problems, as well as factors helping attain outcomes, are evaluated. The nurse looks at the nursing diagnoses, care plans, and nursing orders to decide whether they were realistic or unrealistic for the patient. Once the evaluation is done, a new direction for the nurse and patient is established. Problems are either solved or they take on a new priority that requires the formulation of new outcomes and interventions for specific patient care and teaching.

During all phases of patient education, it is most important that a written record be kept to document the communication between the patient, family, and health team. The nurse then is able to make judgments about what patients need to know, what they are capable of learning, how they can best be taught, and what they have learned. Nurses must be aware of the principles involved in the teaching–learning process (see Chap. 11).

SUMMARY

The nursing diagnoses movement is continuing to grow rapidly and is having a major impact on national and international nursing practice. Although implementing nursing diagnoses in critical care presents many challenging problems for clinicians, several approaches have been suggested as possible solutions to such problems. When clear and concise nursing diagnoses are identified and prioritized, they provide the direction for carrying out the remaining steps of the nursing process to achieve quality patient care.

REFERENCES

1. American Nurses' Association. *Classification Systems for Describing Nursing Practice.* Kansas City, MO: ANA, 1989.
2. Alfaro, R. *Application of Nursing Process: A Step-by-Step Guide.* Philadelphia: J. B. Lippincott, 1986.
3. Block, D. Interrelated issues in evaluation and evaluation research. *Nurs. Res.* 29:69, 1980.
4. Bulechek, G. M., and McCloskey, J. C. *Nursing Interventions: Treatments for Nursing Diagnoses.* Philadelphia: W. B. Saunders, 1985.
5. Bulechek, G. M., and McCloskey, J. C. Nursing interventions: What they are and how to choose them. *Holistic Nurs. Prac.* 1: 43, 1987.
6. Bulechek, G. M., and McCloskey, J. C. Nursing interventions: Treatments for potential nursing diagnoses. In R. M. Carroll-Johnson (ed.), *Classification of Nursing Diagnoses: Proceedings of the Eighth Conference.* Philadelphia: J. B. Lippincott, 1989, pp. 23–30.
7. Carpenito, L. J. Nursing diagnoses in critical care: Impact on practice and outcomes. *Heart Lung* 16:595, 1987.
8. Carroll-Johnson, R. M. (ed.). *Classification of Nursing Diagnoses: Proceedings of the Eighth Conference.* Philadelphia: J. B. Lippincott, 1989.
9. Christman, M. K., and Fowler, M. D. The systems-in-change model for nursing practice. In J. Riehl and C. Roy (eds.), *Conceptual Models for Nursing Practice.* New York: Appleton-Century-Crofts, 1980.
10. Dossey, B. M., and Guzzetta, C. E. Nursing diagnosis. *Nurs. 81* 11:34, 1981.
11. Dossey, B. M., and Guzzetta, C. E. Person-centered caring and the nursing process. In C. E. Guzzetta and B. M. Dossey (eds.), *Cardiovascular Nursing: Bodymind Tapestry.* St. Louis: C. V. Mosby, 1984.
12. Dossey, L. *Space, Time, and Medicine.* Boulder, CO: Shambhala, 1982.
13. Fitzpatrick, J. J., Kerr, M. K., Saba, V. K., et al. Translating nursing diagnosis into ICD code. *Am. J. Nurs.* 89:493, 1989.
14. Gordon, M. Nursing diagnoses and the diagnostic process. *Am. J. Nurs.* 76:1298, 1976.
15. Gordon, M. *Manual of Nursing Diagnosis.* New York: McGraw-Hill, 1987.
16. Gordon, M. *Nursing Diagnosis: Process and Application.* New York: McGraw-Hill, 1987.
17. Green, E., and Green, A. *Beyond Biofeedback.* New York: Delta Books, 1977.
18. Guzzetta, C. E. Nursing diagnoses: Effect on the profession. *Heart Lung* 16:629, 1987.
19. Guzzetta, C. E., Bunton, S. D., Prinkey, L. A., Sherer, A. P., and Seifert, P. C. Unitary person assessment tool: Easing problems with nursing diagnoses. *Focus Crit. Care* 15:12, 1988.
20. Guzzetta, C. E., Bunton, S. D., Prinkey, L. A., Sherer, A. P., and Seifert, P. C. *Clinical Assessment Tools for Use with Nursing Diagnoses.* St. Louis: C. V. Mosby, 1989.
21. Guzzetta, C. E., and Dossey, B. M. Nursing diagnosis: Framework-process-problems. *Heart Lung* 12:281, 1983.
22. Guzzetta, C. E., and Dossey, B. M. *Cardiovascular Nursing: Biobehavioral Interventions.* St. Louis: Mosby Year Book, 1992.
23. Guzzetta, C. E., and Dossey, B. M. Holistic approach to nursing diagnosis. In C. E. Guzzetta and B. M. Dossey. *Cardiovascular Nursing: Biobehavioral Interventions.* St. Louis: Mosby Year Book, 1992.
24. Guzzetta, C. E., and Kinney, M. R. Mastering the transition from medical to nursing diagnosis. *Prog. Cardiovasc. Nurs.* 1:41, 1986.
25. Jenny, J. Classifying nursing diagnoses: A self-care approach. *Nurs. Health Care.* 10:83, 1989.
26. Kim, M. J., and Moritz, D. A. (eds.). *Classification of Nursing Diagnoses: Proceeding of the Third and Fourth National Conferences.* New York: McGraw-Hill, 1982.
27. Kim, M. J., McFarland, G. K., and McLane, A. M. *Classification of Nursing Diagnoses: Proceedings of the Fifth National Conference.* St. Louis: C. V. Mosby, 1984.
28. Kim, M. J., McFarland, G. K., and McLane, A. M. *Pocket Guide to Nursing Diagnoses.* (3rd ed.). St. Louis: C. V. Mosby, 1989.
29. Lang, N. M., and Gebbie, K. Nursing taxonomy: NANDA and ANA joint venture toward ICD-10. In R. M. Carroll-Johnson, (ed.), *Classification of Nursing Diagnoses: Proceedings of the Eighth Conference.* Philadelphia: J. B. Lippincott, 1989, pp. 11–17.
30. Lengel, N. L. *Handbook of Nursing Diagnosis.* Bowie, MD: Robert J. Brady, 1982.
31. McFarland, G. K., and McFarlane, E. A. *Nursing Diagnoses and Intervention: Planning for Care.* St. Louis: C. V. Mosby, 1989.
32. McLane, A. M. Measurement and validation of diagnostic concepts: A decade of progress. *Heart Lung* 16:616, 1987.
33. Mundinger, M., and Jauron, G. Developing a nursing diagnosis. *Nurs. Outlook* 23:97, 1975.
34. North American Nursing Diagnosis Association. *Taxonomy I, Revised 1990.* St. Louis: NANDA, 1990.
35. Price, M. R. Nursing diagnosis: Making a concept come alive. *Am. J. Nurs.* 80:668, 1980.
36. Roy, C. Framework for classification systems development: Progress and issues. In M. J. Kim, G. K. McFarland, and A. M. McLane (eds.), *Classification of Nursing Diagnoses: Proceedings of the Fifth Conference.* St. Louis: C. V. Mosby, 1984.
37. Steele, D., and Whalen, J. A. A proposal for two new nursing

diagnoses: Potential for organ failure and potential for tissue destruction. *Heart Lung* 14:426, 1985.

38. Tanner, C. A. Symposium on nursing diagnoses in critical care: Overview. *Heart Lung* 14:423, 1985.

39. Wake, M. Special Interest Groups Report: Nursing diagnosis in critical care. In M. J. Kim, G. K. McFarland, and A. M. McLane (eds.), *Classification of Nursing Diagnoses: Proceeding from the Fifth National Conference*. St. Louis: C. V. Mosby, 1984.

40. Wake, M. Symposium: Nursing diagnosis in critical care: Overview. *Heart Lung* 16:593, 1987.

41. Watson, J. *Nursing: Human Science and Human Care*. Norwalk, CT: Appleton-Century-Crofts, 1985.

42. *Webster's New Universal Unabridged Dictionary* (2nd ed.). New York: New World Dictionaries/Simon & Schuster, 1983.

43. Zander, K. Nursing case management: Strategic management of cost and quality outcomes. *J. Nurs. Admin.* 18:23, 1988.

44. Zander, K. Managed care and nursing case management. In G. G. Mayer, M. J. Madden, and E. Lawrenz (eds.), *Patient Care Delivery Models*. Rockville, MD: Aspen, 1990.

7

Research in Critical Care Nursing

Cathie E. Guzzetta

OBJECTIVITY VERSUS PARTICIPATION

A universal belief embraced as a "research rule" by investigators is that objectivity must govern the scientific process. This belief has been shaken, however, by Werner Heisenberg, the Nobel Prize winner who studied information obtained from an electron. The Heisenberg Uncertainty Principle, which subsequently evolved, contends that one cannot look at a physical object without changing it. Thus, physical objects and people are changed when we observe them. The implications of this principle to research are clear. Researchers do not stand apart from their research or their research subjects. Because researchers are a part of nature and not separate from it, researchers are a part of the research that they study. Researchers are not objective observers in the world they study; rather, they are participants in that world. The researcher's participation may be a word, an action, a touch, an observation, or simply his or her presence. In short, the researcher becomes an integral part of the experiment, and this participation affects the results of the research. The term *nonparticipant observer* in research is no longer meaningful.

The outcomes of any research study also are affected because patients are changed when they enter into a research study. Related to this principle is the *placebo effect*. In various investigations, the effects of a treatment, drug, or therapy are tested against the effects of a placebo. Placebos are expected to have no effect on patients or their outcomes. Placebos can activate the production of endorphins in the brain, however, and stimulate the endocrine system to alter body chemistry and, for example, activate the individual's defense mechanisms to fight illness. The placebo's effect also is dependent on the patient's relationship with and confidence in the healer. Thus, with a trusting relationship, the researcher's direct participation with the patient may trigger the placebo effect and change the individual and the outcomes of the research. In this situation, the changes that occur somehow activate the healer potential within the individual, thereby transforming belief into psychophysiologic healing and providing further evidence of bodymind connectedness.*

LEARNING OBJECTIVES

After reading this chapter, the nurse should be able to do the following:

1. Discuss why research is a critical mandate for advancing nursing practice.
2. Define the term *intuition,* and discuss how it can be cultivated in nursing.
3. Define the term *curiosity,* and discuss its link to intuition.
4. Discuss how curiosity can be cultivated in nursing.
5. Discuss several top-priority areas for critical care nursing research identified by the American Association of Critical-Care Nurses.
6. Compare and contrast quantitative versus qualitative research methods.
7. Read and evaluate a qualitative and a quantitative research report in one of the nursing journals.
8. Discuss the steps necessary when implementing the results of clinical research into practice.
9. Assess his or her current level of involvement in research, and explore ways to expand this role.

* Modified from Guzzetta, C. E. Research and Holistic Implications. In B. Dossey, L. Keegan, C. Guzzetta, *et al. Holistic Nursing: A Handbook for Practice.* Rockville, MD: Aspen Publishers, 1988: 147–155.

IDENTIFYING PROBLEMS FROM CLINICAL PRACTICE

Think about some nursing procedure you have done lately (*e.g.,* changing an abdominal dressing, unclotting an intravenous line, measuring a cardiac output, suctioning a patient on PEEP). Now ask yourself a few important questions[22]:

- Why did you perform the procedure the way you did?
- Did you perform it that way because someone told you that is the way it always has been done?
- Did you learn it that way in school? Or during your hospital orientation? Or by trial and error?
- Do you know whether the procedure you used was the best for the patient?
- Do you know whether your actions were based on the results of scientific investigation?

In reality, too much of clinical nursing practice is still based on tradition, rituals, and trial and error. In the 1990s, however, professional nurses must demand that nursing practice be based on sound, scientific principles to guide assessments, diagnoses, patient outcomes, and nursing interventions. Research must be viewed as both a basic tool of practice and a professional imperative to the progress of nursing.

Research in practice evolves from clinical problems. Have you ever experienced a serious problem in practice? Have you ever had a hunch about how it might be solved? Did you ever have an intuitive feeling that the way you were performing a certain procedure was not necessarily the best for the patient? Have you ever had questions about the soundness of a particular nursing intervention? Have you ever been curious about looking for the answer?[22]

These kinds of conflicts evoke curiosity in nurses and are the stimulus for clinical research. Any thinking, reflective critical care nurse runs into dozens of problems daily that would lend themselves to research. Problems are identified by intuition, hunches, conflicts, and questions that arise from procedures, techniques, and delivery of patient care. The research process begins every time you ask, "I wonder what would happen if . . . ?" or "Why am I doing it this way?" or "It might be better for the patient if I . . . ."[22]

Intuition and Curiosity

How can all nurses become more involved in research? Curiosity and listening to one's intuition may be the first steps. Although these concepts traditionally have not been valued in nursing, they are important tools for the discovery of new knowledge. They also have the potential to stimulate individual involvement in research. The following discussion focuses on the role of intuition and curiosity in research.

Daily at the bedside, nurses observe and evaluate patients. Such activities involve a rational, analytic, and verbal (or left brain) way of thinking. Most nurses, however, are not aware of the importance of a nonverbal and intuitive (right brain) way of thinking. In nursing, unfortunately, we have not placed much value on this intuitive "soft data."

Historically in nursing, intuitive perceptions have been seen as opposing the empirical, factual knowledge base of practice.[40] Intuitive feelings have been assigned only minimal value and have elicited negative reactions. I admit that I have been among the many to hold such an opinion. During a critical care course I taught a number of years ago, I stated, "We can no longer allow intuition to guide our practice. We need to develop the technical expertise to care for critically ill patients, and we must be able to justify our conclusions based on quantifiable data."[12]

The idea that only quantifiable data are important in science is no longer justifiable. Scientific exploration involves not only analytic thinking but also a qualitative yet undefinable process that scientists use to organize fragmented findings into meaningful wholes.[30] This undefinable process is called *intuition*, or the tacit dimension, which is fundamental to all knowing.[31] It is a process whereby we know more than we can explain.

Clinical intuition has been described as a "process by which the nurse knows something about the patient which cannot be verbalized, or for which the source of the knowledge cannot be determined."[40] It is a "gut feeling" about something even when there are no "hard data" to support that feeling. It allows one to know immediately about something without consciously using reason.[34] Intuitive perceptions, however, do not conflict with analytic reasoning.[20] Rather, intuition is simply another dimension of knowing. When analytic and intuitive thinking are used together, whole-brain thinking emerges.

Some exciting "hard data" have been published recently in the nursing literature to support the notion that intuitive processes are a valid means of conscious knowing and are necessary and desirable perceptions in nursing practice.[34,40] From these studies, certain factors, conditions, or attributes that facilitate intuitive thinking have been identified. Intuitive thinking generally is found to occur in the more experienced and technically proficient nurse, particularly when a caring relationship is developed with the patient and day-to-day, ongoing care is provided.[40] Another factor involves self-receptivity or the ability to be open and vulnerable. The nurse must be able emotionally to receive information and have a desire to "tune in." Personal and emotional problems reduce this receptivity. Thus, the nurse's energy level influences his or her readiness to receive, perceive, and interpret information and cues. When the nurse is open and receptive to subtle cues and feelings that are communicated between two human beings, intuitive thinking is enhanced. It is diminished, on the other hand, when energy levels are low, such as during times of stress or illness. Self-confidence is another facilitating factor that enables nurses to believe in their intuitive experience. It involves the ability to acknowledge and act on new levels of (intuitive) knowledge without feeling any discomfort about a lack of objective data.[40]

If intuitive thinking can be cultivated in nursing, the potential for identifying patient problems and finding solutions might be enhanced to an astonishing degree. Although intuitive thinking cannot be taught directly, we can emphasize the value of such thinking in our nursing curricula and continuing education courses.[10] We can teach the skills necessary to recognize subjective data and to verbalize feelings, cues, and decisions.[40] Intuitive experiences can be shared with colleagues and students. We can support nurses who have experienced intuitive events and encourage them to review and analyze the process. The usefulness of the cues in identifying problems and in making correct decisions can be evaluated systematically. Finally, inexperienced nurses can be provided with subtle and repeated cue patterns that will assist them in recognizing intuitive information to increase their confidence about interpreting the cues and acting on their decisions.[40]

It is likely that the benefits of intuitive thinking will not flourish unless such thinking is cultivated along with the concept of *curiosity*—or the yen to discover.[37] Curiosity, like intuition, is an elusive concept. Whereas intuition involves a way of thinking or feeling, curiosity suggests a behavior. Thus, even if intuitive feelings reveal a possible problem, without curiosity, the behavior involving the search for the answer will not occur.

The dictionary describes curiosity as a desire to learn about things, particularly things that are novel, rare, or extraordinary.[38] When a conflict arises, it causes an arousal in the individual, followed by a drive or motivation to do something resulting in the behavior necessary to try to resolve the problem.[2] When the conflict is strange or incongruous, it is more likely to initiate curious behavior.[37]

If conflict is a condition necessary to produce curious behavior,[2] then certainly critical care units, which are filled with complexity, uncertainty, unexpectedness, and change, provide nurses with a variety of reasons for which to be curious. Likewise, if curiosity is a necessary prerequisite for the discovery of new knowledge, then educators, head nurses, supervisors, and clinical nurse specialists must find ways to enhance each nurse's potential to become a curious, questioning, inquisitive practitioner.[37]

There are many ways to foster curiosity. Cultivating intuitive thinking, as discussed previously, is an important factor. Students in critical care courses, for example, might be assigned the weekly task of reporting conflicts, problems, or intuitive hunches that they find to be novel, complex, or incongruous—issues that excite them because they desire to seek new knowledge.[37] Curiosity is stimulated by employing as many of the senses as possible in the process of discovery.[37] Thus, when identifying conflicts, nurses should be prompted to identify them during hands-on bedside care while consciously and deliberately employing all of their senses. During the assignment, students are directed to observe, inspect, touch, manipulate, smell, and hear everything in the environment to enhance information flow for every possible subtle cue.[37]

Students can be asked to report these experiences and discuss them with their fellow students on a weekly basis to help define the problem, obtain feedback, and clarify the issues. For example, if a nurse expresses an intuitive feeling derived from a recent bedside experience that there must be a better way to prevent infections from invasive lines, then the yen for discovery has begun and must be encouraged. The instructor might help the student to ask questions such as "What research has already been done on this problem? What is the best treatment for this problem? What is the best way to implement the treatment?" Critical care educators and inservice instructors could encourage this student to consult with appropriate resource individuals, such as infection control nurses, call other critical care units to discover if they have encountered a similar problem and find out what procedures they are using, be given time to look up and read articles on the subject, and perhaps call the Centers for Disease Control in Atlanta for more information.

In a follow-up conference, students would then be encouraged to present a small report of their findings to colleagues and be assisted in synthesizing the information so that the results might be formulated into a recommendation for changing bedside practice or a question that might lend itself to further investigation.[37]

Staff nurses might be stimulated to follow a similar approach at a weekly or biweekly "research think-tank meeting." A core of nurses who have verbalized a yen for discovery might be brought together to discuss some of the problems, conflicts, and intuitive feelings they have encountered at the bedside. The brainstorming session might result in a list of problems that could be given priorities and a list of individuals who are interested in working on the problems. These nurses might be given the opportunity to consult with resource personnel

in other departments, hospitals, or universities. They might be given release time, paid leave, and travel funding to attend a research conference.[4] A file of research articles could be developed for each of the problems. New information about the problem could be disseminated on unit bulletin boards, flyers, during small unit conferences, journal clubs, inservice education programs, or nursing grand rounds.[4] Consultants might be used to assist the nurses in synthesizing the information, making recommendations for implementing the findings into practice, or developing a research investigation.

Priorities in Critical Care Research

When the intuitive feelings, conflicts, and hunches of many nurse experts from across the country are pooled, the "big picture" of current clinical questions emerges. In an attempt to best use personnel, time, and resources, the American Association of Critical-Care Nurses (AACN) did just that: They carried out a research study to identify and assign priorities to the most important problems affecting critical care nursing that could be answered by nursing research.[23] As part of this study, experts in critical care nursing were identified throughout the country. These nurses were asked to take part in a study using a Delphi technique to identify questions that were affecting patient welfare most significantly. The Delphi technique is a process of gaining consensus by soliciting, evaluating, and tabulating the opinions of experts in the field. Data were obtained through four rounds of questionnaires from a total of 206 expert panelists who ultimately identified 74 research questions concerning their potential impact on the welfare of critically ill patients. The top 15 questions are outlined in Table 7-1 and are listed in order of priority.[23]

An important question to be considered is whether the priorities reported in 1983 have, in fact, guided the efforts of researchers. To answer this question, the AACN's Research Committee examined 11 pertinent journals from 1983 through 1987 to identify research articles related to the top 15 questions.[9] The number of research studies conducted per question are presented in Table 7-1.

No studies were found in the areas of reducing burnout, interventions for patients with impaired communication, or incorporating research findings into practice. Conversely, many articles were found in the areas of reducing staff stress, effects of patient positioning on cardiovascular and pulmonary functioning, and nursing measures to prevent infections related to invasive lines or procedures. A reason cited for the lack of research in some areas is the difficulty inherent in researching some of the questions (e.g., question 14, which deals with developing effective methods to incorporate research findings into practice, is a difficult study to design). Another reason cited is that some of the questions require intervention studies that are more difficult to develop and carry out than simple descriptive studies (e.g., question 9 which deals with efforts to minimize anxiety, helplessness, and pain in patients with impaired verbal communication requires an intervention study).[9] This explanation is supported by a study in 1988 that analyzed nursing practice research from 1977 to 1986. Of the 720 research articles analyzed, almost two thirds were categorized as assessment-focused (descriptive) studies, whereas only one third were described as intervention studies.[25]

Currently, we must continue to focus research efforts on priority areas in which there is a paucity of research. Also, in the areas judged to have a sufficient number of studies, the

Table 7-1
Priority Research Questions Affecting the Welfare of Critically Ill Patients and Number of Reported Research Studies Per Question

RESEARCH QUESTION	NUMBER OF RESEARCH STUDIES REPORTED FROM 1983–1987
1. What are the most effective ways of promoting optimum sleep-rest patterns in the critically ill patient and preventing sleep deprivation?	1
2. In light of the critical care nursing shortage, what measures can be taken to prevent or lessen burnout among critical care nurses?	0
3. What type of orientation program for critical care nurses is most effective in terms of cost, safety, and long-term retention?	2
4. What effects do verbal and environmental stimuli have on increased intracranial pressure in the patient with a head injury?	3
5. What are the most effective, least anxiety-producing techniques for weaning various patients from ventilators?	2
6. What types of patient classification systems are the most valid, reliable, and sensitive in determining staffing ratios in critical care units?	1
7. What types of incentives (e.g., wage scales, recognition programs, "clinical ladder", etc.) will retain nurses in critical care units?	3
8. What are effective ways of reducing staff stress in critical care areas?	5
9. What are effective nursing interventions in patients with impaired communication (e.g., intubated patients, aphasic patients) to minimize anxiety, helplessness, and pain?	0
10. What are the effects of patient positioning on cardiovascular and pulmonary functioning of various types of critically ill patients?	7
11. What are the most effective staffing patterns (e.g., 12-hour shifts, rotating nurses to noncritical care areas) to reduce burnout and provide continuity of patient care?	1
12. What nursing measures (e.g., frequency of intravenous tubing or dressing changes, use of antibiotic ointment) are most effective in preventing infections in patients with invasive lines or those undergoing invasive procedures?	8
13. What is the maximum time a patient on a mechanical ventilator with positive end-expiratory pressure can be off the ventilator during suctioning without significantly lowering the PaO_2?	2
14. What are the effective methods of encouraging the incorporation of research findings into critical care nursing practice?	0
15. What nursing measures singly or in combination are most effective in assessing and relieving pain in various types of critically ill patients (e.g., infants, children, burn patients, patients with neurologic impairment, etc.)?	3

Data obtained from Funk, M. Research priorities in critical care nursing. *Focus Crit. Care* 16:135, 1989, and Lewandowski, L. A., and Kositsky, A. M. Research priorities in critical care nursing: A study by the American Association of Critical Care Nurses. *Heart Lung* 12:35, 1983.

research must be critiqued carefully and the results synthesized to judge if the findings should be applied to practice.[9] Moreover, it must be determined whether the priority areas cited in 1983 need to be expanded and updated as critical care nursing practice continues to change.

The last section in each of the clinical chapters in this book (Chaps. 20 to 47) contains a list of potential research questions, conflicts, and ideas that may be suitable topics for future research. Some of these questions fall within the realm of the AACN's priority areas, whereas others are the product of our conflicts with patient care situations in clinical practice. They are presented in each chapter to stimulate thinking and encourage future research.

QUANTITATIVE AND QUALITATIVE RESEARCH METHODS

Regardless of whether one is evaluating the results of a completed research study or just beginning one, the inherent advantages and constraints of the research methodologies used must be considered carefully. The following paragraphs discuss two important research methodologies that may be used in nursing—the qualitative and quantitative approaches.

Much of medical and nursing research as we know it today has been influenced greatly by the 17th-century teachings of Descartes. Descartes taught the concept of reductionism in research or the idea of breaking down every question into its smallest possible part as a way of systematically studying a problem. The concept of reductionism has been enormously beneficial in advancing medical science. For example, the person is broken down into a physiologic part and then further subdivided into organs, cells, biochemical substances, molecules, atoms, and subatoms. In this way, scientists can study and identify the etiology of disease (e.g., identifying that *Staphylococcus aureus* is one cause of bacterial endocarditis). The findings from such investigations then offer direction for isolating the cure (e.g., sterilizing the bacterial vegetations of

Staphylococcus endocarditis with antibiotics).[13] Thus, biomedical research continues to abound throughout the world as demonstrated by the enormous numbers of personnel, resources, and money that are allocated toward finding cures, at the molecular level, for such problems as the common cold, coronary artery disease, acquired immunodeficiency syndrome (AIDS), cancer, essential hypertension, thyroid disease, and many others.[13]

The reductionistic approach has evolved over the centuries, resulting in the scientific or *quantitative method* used today. This method is used to predict and control the outcomes of illness and its treatment. This approach enables scientists to formulate hypotheses, by reducing the area of interest to its smallest possible part, formulate and test the hypotheses, and reject or accept the hypotheses using statistical analyses. Based on the findings, scientists are then able to replicate similar studies and generalize the findings to other similar patient populations.

The success of biomedical research in isolating the cause and finding a cure for many illnesses has been important in legitimizing medicine as a scientific discipline. This success has greatly influenced the direction of research in nursing. Within the past few decades, however, nurse researchers have begun to realize that the reductionistic approach does not account for the whole person as an integrated unit. We also have begun to understand that the fit between quantitative research methods and holistic nursing practice is not always an ideal one.[13] The central tenet underlying the holistic framework is that the whole is greater than the sum of its parts.[8] Because quantitative methods seek only to find answers to parts of the whole, nurse researchers have looked to alternate philosophies of science and sought additional research methods that are compatible with investigating humanistic and holistic phenomena.[29,35] Such methods are called *qualitative research*. Qualitative research is used to study the context and meaning of observed patterns. Its scope is holistic, and its method incorporates interactions of variables.[26]

A holistic approach to research, for example, might explore descriptively all possible variables in the life of an individual with a specific problem (*e.g.*, coronary artery disease).[24] The data might be analyzed to determine the impact of such variables on the person's illness, what combination of variables affect this problem in the individual, and how these variables represent patterns that characterize the person's pathway to coronary artery disease. When the results are understood, other individuals with coronary artery disease could be evaluated to identify similarities and differences. The results can lead to theory development regarding the interactive nature of such variables on the development of the illness. Intervention studies can then be designed and tested to repattern the patients' pathways toward wellness.

In contrast, the quantitative method is used to identify an isolated cause that is producing an undesirable effect. Cause and effect are validated by using control or comparison groups and statistical analysis. The quantitative method, however, does not consider the phenomenologic nature of a particular problem or the unique patterns manifested by one individual.[3] More importantly, it does not explain why one individual becomes ill and why another does not given a similar set of circumstances. This issue has never been relegated any importance in medicine because it is not a concern of the biomedical paradigm.[5]

The roots of the scientific paradigm have been challenged over the past few decades, however, by the astounding research findings supporting the interactive nature of psychophysiologic variables. The research done in the field of psychoneuroimmunology has provided conclusive evidence that thoughts, emotions, attitudes, and feelings affect the immune, autonomic, endocrine, and neuropeptide system at the cellular and subcellular levels, establishing proof of bodymind connectedness. From this research, it is clear that any attempts to explain health and illness must take into consideration the central role of human consciousness.

It has taken centuries to progress beyond Cartesian dualism and generate convincing data that refute the idea that the mind and body are separate. Thus, we are currently taking part in a revolutionary change in thinking regarding health and illness. Many individuals remain tied to the biomedical model, however, and view holistic principles and its corresponding research as unscientific. Such individuals criticize the psychophysiologic link between health and illness because evidence to support the link traditionally has been provided in the form of anecdotes or personal testimonials. "Hard-core" researchers who embrace the quantitative method also have not placed much value on the "softer data" obtained from qualitative studies. Even when quantitative methods have been employed to support the link, such studies have been criticized because of their methodologic problems, such as the use of data collection instruments lacking psychometric properties.[11]

Although the evidence to support the bodymind link is convincing, it is clear that additional scientifically sound research must be generated before the link is accepted universally. Nurses, by virtue of their day-to-day care of the patient, are in the unique position to observe, document, analyze, and quantify the interactive relationship of the psychophysiologic variables affecting various illness states. In the past, however, qualitative methods have not been taught in nursing and medical schools, thereby significantly reducing their worth in the minds of individual nurses and physicians who simply do not understand the importance and benefits of these methods. The value of qualitative research will undoubtedly be realized in the future as nursing and medical professors begin to introduce these methods into their curricula. The respectability of qualitative methods will make rapid gains as important bodymind variables continue to be discovered in future studies, research journal editors begin to accept more qualitative studies for publication, and authors of nursing research texts dedicate more time to this content area.[3]

It is important to point out that the decision to use qualitative versus quantitative methods should not be viewed as an either/or issue. A strong case has been argued for use of both methods in nursing research.[4,33] Qualitative research is needed to explore patterns and variables about which little is known. It is also used to investigate variables whose meanings cannot be understood when they are broken down into isolated parts. The results from qualitative studies also supply researchers with a plethora of potential research hypotheses for quantitative investigation. Quantitative research, on the other hand, is needed to validate new knowledge, identify etiologies, and predict outcomes of nursing interventions.

Within a particular research design, both qualitative and quantitative methods may be considered. In a recent study that investigated the effects of relaxation and music therapy on the psychophysiologic stress levels of patients with acute myocardial infarction, for example, both approaches were built into the design.[14] The quantitative method analyzed the effects of the interventions on psychophysiologic variables and compared them with those of a control group, and the qualitative method analyzed the subjects' evaluation of the interventions. The qualitative findings proved to be a rich source of data on the effects of these therapies on the subjects' own estimation of their behavior and outcomes. The findings from both data sources offered a better reflection of the whole than either method alone.[14,27] Both approaches are needed in nursing research in the 1990s.[3]

TAKING RESEARCH FINDINGS BACK TO THE BEDSIDE

When a problem area has been investigated sufficiently by research, the scientific basis for changing practice becomes possible. The challenge to professional nursing is how to bring such findings back to the bedside. Because there tends to be a long delay from the time research is conducted, written into a report, and then published in the journals, a thorough search of the literature for answers to a clinical problem is recommended. Nurses can run a library computer search on the subject and search the *Cumulative Index to Nursing, Index Medicus,* and the *Social Science Citation Index* for related articles.

After the pertinent literature has been found, the credibility of the research studies and their findings must be evaluated. Not all research published is scientifically sound; therefore, it must be critiqued to determine violations in "research rules." To help develop the necessary evaluation skills, books and articles dealing with criteria by which to critique investigations can be made available and discussed with staff nurses by educators or inservice instructors.[7,18,32,39]

It is critical to remember that the results from one study alone are not enough to prove a point; *i.e.,* one study, regardless of its quality, generally does not provide enough data to change current nursing practice.[16] Changes in practice must be directed by the combined results of several supportive studies that have been repeated or replicated. It is not unusual, however, for the results of several studies to conflict or at least differ. Thus, after the studies have been read critically, the results must be synthesized and consolidated.[19]

Several nursing and medical journals have recognized this need and have begun publishing review and synthesis articles on a particular topic. Within these articles, studies related to a specific problem are critiqued, results are synthesized, and implications for practice are offered. Good examples of such articles are back massage after acute myocardial infarction,[6] use of heparinized intra-arterial lines to obtain coagulation samples,[15] atypical manifestations of acute myocardial infarction,[28] effects of relaxation training on clinical symptoms,[17] minimizing hypoxemia due to endotracheal suctioning,[1] needs and concerns of families of critically ill adults,[36] and prevention of intensive care unit psychosis.[21] Nurses can use the methodology in these articles to consolidate findings on a topic so that recommendations for incorporating the findings into practice can be made.

After the problem has been defined and the relevant research critiqued and synthesized, the next step is to determine whether it is appropriate to change practice by implementing the research results at the bedside. It may be decided, after the critique of the literature, however, that insufficient or conflicting data are found that do not support a change in practice. On the other hand, one might determine that the benefits of the change are not warranted but that the findings from various studies might be cognitively applied to enhance the understanding of a particular problem. Conversely, one might conclude that the research findings justify a change in practice and that direct application is favored. In this case, a written plan should be developed to serve as a road map for implementation.[19]

The plan should describe the specific problem, the need or desirability for a change, and its effectiveness, safety, and benefits. For example, if the results of a quality-assurance study have uncovered a high incidence of catheter-related infections and a new method to prevent these infections has been identified and supported through research, then the advantages, disadvantages, and constraints of that new procedure should be outlined carefully. The advantages might be a lowered incidence of infection, reduced length of stay in intensive care, or other improved patient outcomes. The disadvantages or constraints also are appraised. The cost of the new procedure or equipment necessary to carry it out might be prohibitive. The cost in terms of training personnel to use the new equipment or learn a new procedure must also be considered.[19]

A timetable for implementing the change also is recommended. The timetable includes how the current unit procedure will be modified in order to implement the change, the steps of the new procedure, the plans for inservicing the nurses who will implement the change, and the method of evaluating the change.[19] The length of the evaluation phase is specified, and the method for evaluating the short- and long-term effects on patient outcomes is identified carefully.

To evaluate the outcomes, consider the objectives of the change, the results of the change, and whether the results observed are the ones that were expected.[19] If the objective of a new procedure was to reduce catheter-related infections, then the results might be evaluated by identifying the number of current infections and comparing this figure with the infection rate before the new procedure was implemented. An evaluation data sheet might be developed that includes nursing notes, results of patient records, physical assessment data, and results of laboratory cultures. Interviews with staff nurses also might be conducted to determine their responses to the new procedure and personal observations. After the evaluation phase, a decision is made to determine whether the outcomes of the change favor retaining, modifying, or discarding the new procedure.[19]

ADVANCING YOUR RESEARCH ROLE

Nursing will never develop a scientific basis for its practice until the practitioners themselves become more involved in research. Practitioners need to assess their current research skills and determine the best way to advance their role as researchers. The most obvious role is one of an independent researcher. In such a role, the nurse identifies a problem, designs a research study to help find answers to it, collects and analyzes the data, and interprets and writes up the findings. The role of an independent researcher usually involves additional education and training.

Nurses who have not had this additional education may wish to begin their involvement by becoming an interdependent researcher. This can be accomplished by several approaches. Nurses who identify a clinical problem or conflict can take their ideas and questions to resource nurses (*e.g.,* clinical nurse specialists, staff development nurses, or faculty at schools of nursing). Such resource individuals can join forces with bedside clinical nurses, who are intimately aware of the clinical patient care problems, and share in designing the research study and carrying out the investigation.

Becoming a member of the quality-assurance team or the hospital research or ethics committee also can provide valuable experience. In addition, nurses can become involved in an ongoing research project at their institution. They also can collaborate with nurses in different settings who have established a collaborative research study and are in need of additional sites for data collection. They can become involved with physician-directed research or a project developed by non-nurses to resolve a problem that necessitates a multidisciplinary approach. In each of these examples, nurses can help primary researchers design realistic studies, identify potential subjects for a study, obtain informed consent, collect data, assist in analyzing data, write up and publish the findings, and discuss ways to implement the findings into clinical practice. Finally, nurses can become participants in research projects when appropriate.

Becoming involved in clinical research can take place at a number of levels. We challenge all nurses to cultivate their intuitive thinking and curiosity-seeking behaviors. We encourage nurses to assess their research skills and experience and seek creative opportunities to advance their roles as nurse researchers.

SUMMARY

Research is a critical mandate for advancing nursing practice. The results of research provide the scientific principles to guide assessment, diagnoses, patient outcomes, and nursing interventions. Nurses face the challenge of exploring creative ways to implement research findings into practice and advance their role as researchers.

REFERENCES

1. Barnes, C. A., and Kirchhoff, K. T. Minimizing hypoxemia due to endotracheal suctioning: A review of the literature. *Heart Lung* 15:164, 1986.
2. Berlyn, D. E. *Conflict, Arousal, and Curiosity.* New York: McGraw-Hill, 1960.
3. Bockmon, D. F., and Riemen, D. J. Qualitative versus quantitative nursing research. *Holistic Nurs. Pract.* 2:71, 1987.
4. Briones, T., and Bruya, M. A. The professional imperative: Research utilization in the search for scientifically based nursing practice. *Focus Crit. Care* 17:78, 1990.
5. Clark, C. C. *Wellness Nursing: Concepts, Theory, Research, and Practice.* New York: Spring Publishing Co., 1986.
6. Dunbar, S., and Redlick, E. Should patients with acute myocardial infarctions receive back massage? *Focus Crit. Care* 13:42, 1986.
7. Fleming, J. W., and Hayter, J. Reading research reports critically. *Nurs. Outlook* 22:172, 1974.
8. Flynn, P. *Holistic Health: The Art and Science of Care.* Bowie, MD: Brady Co., 1980.
9. Funk, M. Research priorities in critical care nursing. *Focus Crit. Care* 16:135, 1989.
10. Garrity, P. L. Perception in nursing: The value of intuition. *Holistic Nurs. Pract.* 1:63, 1987.
11. Guzzetta, C. E. The human factor and the ailing heart: Folklore or fact [editorial]? *J. Intensive Care Med.* 2:3, 1987.
12. Guzzetta, C. E. Nursing Process and Standards of Care. In B. M. Dossey, L. Keegan, C. E. Guzzetta, *et al. Holistic Nursing: A Handbook for Practice.* Rockville, MD: Aspen, 1988.
13. Guzzetta, C. E. Research and Holistic Implications. In B. M. Dossey, L. Keegan, C. E. Guzzetta, *et al. Holistic Nursing: A Handbook for Practice.* Rockville, MD: Aspen, 1988.
14. Guzzetta, C. E. Effects of relaxation and music therapy on patients in a coronary care unit with presumptive acute myocardial infarction. *Heart Lung* 18:609, 1989.
15. Harper, J. Use of heparinized intra-arterial lines to obtain coagulation samples. *Focus Crit. Care* 15:51, 1988.
16. Haughey, B. P. Consideration in applying research findings to practice. *Dimens. Crit. Care Nurs.* 3:288, 1984.
17. Hyman, R. B., Feldman, H. R., Harris, R. B., *et al.* The effects of relaxation training on clinical symptoms: A meta-analysis. *Nurs. Res.* 38:216, 1989.
18. Jacox, A., and Prescott, P. Determining a study's relevance for clinical practice. *Am. J. Nurs.* 78:1882, 1978.
19. Jennings, B. M., and Rogers, S. Using research to change nursing practice. *Crit. Care Nurs.* 9:76, 1989.
20. Jung, C. *Psychological Types.* New York: Harcourt, Brace, 1959.
21. Kloosterman, N. D. Prevention of ICU psychosis. *Focus Crit. Care* 10:59, 1983.
22. Lewandowski, L. A. Research: It doesn't pertain to me—or does it? *Focus Crit. Care* 8:27, 1981.
23. Lewandowski, L. A., and Kositsky, A. M. Research priorities for critical care nursing: A study by the American Association of Critical-Care Nurses. *Heart Lung* 12:35, 1983.
24. Mehl, L. *Mind and Matter: Foundations for Holistic Health.* Berkeley, CA: Mindbody Press, 1981.
25. Moody, L. E., Wilson, M. E., Smyth, K., *et al.* Analysis of a decade of nursing practice research: 1977–1986. *Nurs. Res.* 37:374, 1988.
26. Mullen, P., and Iverson, D. Qualitative methods for evaluative research in health education programs. *Health Ed.* May-June:11, 1982.
27. Myers, S. T., and Haase, J. E. Guidelines for integration of quantitative and qualitative approaches. *Nurs. Res.* 38:299, 1989.
28. Neill, K. M. A review of atypical clinical manifestations of acute myocardial infarction. *J. Intensive Care Med.* 2:25, 1987.
29. Newman, M. A. *Health as Expanding Consciousness.* St. Louis: C. V. Mosby, 1986.
30. Polanyi, M. *Personal Knowledge.* New York: Harper & Row, 1958.
31. Polanyi, M. *The Tacit Dimension.* New York: Anchor Press, 1966.
32. Polit, D., and Hungler, B. *Nursing Research: Principles and Methods* (4th ed.). Philadelphia: J. B. Lippincott, 1991.
33. Porter, E. J. The qualitative-quantitative dualism. *Image* 21:98, 1989.
34. Schraeder, B. D., and Fisher, D. K. Using intuitive knowledge in the neonatal intensive care nursery. *Holistic Nurs. Pract.* 1:47, 1987.
35. Silva, M. C., and Rothbart, D. An analysis of changing trends in philosophies of science on nursing theory development and testing. *Adv. Nurs. Sci.* 6:1, 1984.
36. Simpson, T. Needs and concerns of families of critically ill adults. *Focus Crit. Care* 16:388, 1989.
37. Van Bree Sneed, N. Curiosity and the yen to discover. *Nurs. Outlook* 38:36, 1990.
38. *Webster's New Universal Unabridged Dictionary* (2nd ed.). New York: Simon and Schuster, 1979.
39. Wilson, H. S. *Research in Nursing.* Menlo Park, CA: Addison-Wesley, 1985.
40. Young, C. E. Intuition and nursing process. *Holistic Nurs. Pract.* 1:52, 1987.

8

Psychosocial Assessment and Intervention for the Critically Ill Adult

Marilyn B. Chassie
Dora Headrick Bradley

REAL LISTENING

In order to listen to your patients, colleagues, family, and friends tell the meaning surrounding their life and circumstances, you must listen actively. Being quiet while someone else is talking is not equivalent to real listening. The key to real listening is *intention,* which helps facilitate the healing process. Intention occurs when you focus with someone in order to move with purpose in your responses and interventions. This can lead others or yourself toward effective action steps or forward in personal growth. Real listening occurs when you have the intention to understand someone, help someone, enjoy someone, or learn something.

Good listening is achieved by quieting your inner dialogue. Good listening has an enormous quality of *nowness.* Nowness involves throwing away your intellectualization when a person goes off in an unexpected direction. How often, when listening to a person who is intent on telling their story, do you stop the flow of the story and bring the person back to a certain point that then blocks the person's insight? Perhaps you get intent on a personal view of what you think should be happening in an exchange of ideas because you start your inner dialogue of analysis and intellectualization.

Developing skills of intention and nowness is an ongoing process. It also allows the person to move to a state of nowness that allows inner wisdom to emerge. Questioning and listening that do not structure the answers, except minimally, is a great art.

One may lapse into pseudolistening when trying to meet the needs of others. The following list identifies examples of pseudolistening and times when you are trying to meet your own needs and not actively listening:

* Silence as you buy time preparing for your next remark
* Listening to others so that they will listen to you
* Acting interested when you are not
* Listening in order not to be rejected
* Searching for a person's weaknesses in order to take advantage of them
* Searching for a person's weak points so that you can be stronger in your response
* Listening only to specific information while deleting the rest
* Partially listening because you do not want to disappoint the other person

Active listening requires that you first focus on what is going on with another person. Secondly, you must try to live in what is, not avoid it, and to let it be.

Active listening helps clarify the message. As you receive the message, you can verify nonverbal messages communicated through body language or by what is not said by the other person. Real listening creates healing moments because you have a greater acceptance of the person's thoughts and emotions; thus, you can facilitate the choosing of the most effective behaviors that will lead the person toward health and wholeness.

LEARNING OBJECTIVES

After reading this chapter, the nurse should be able to do the following:

1. Describe alternative responses of the patient and the patient's family to critical illness and the critical care setting.
2. Evaluate responses of the caregiver to the critically ill patient, the family, and the critical care environment.
3. Formulate specific psychosocial nursing diagnoses and associated nursing orders for critically ill patients.
4. Delineate nursing interventions to support the critically ill patient and the patient's family.
5. Evaluate physiologic and psychosocial outcomes of nursing interventions.
6. Identify common stress-related behaviors in critical care nurses.

PSYCHOSOCIAL ASPECTS

In recent years, increasing attention has been directed toward investigating, describing, interpreting, and understanding psychosocial aspects of critical care, namely, factors of the environment that influence onset, development, or exacerbation of critical illnesses; factors that affect search for medical attention; and factors that affect responses of patients, families, and staff to illness, treatment, the critical care environment, and recovery or death.[1-3,6,7,9,12,13,16-20,22,30,31,34,38,47,53,65,69,70,76,90] Awareness of these factors, acceptance of their importance in critical care, and planning and implementation of psychosocial nursing interventions for the critically ill will greatly enhance the potential for positive outcomes of care.

This chapter focuses on potential patient responses to critical illness, factors that affect patient responses, psychosocial nursing diagnoses applicable to critically ill patients, nursing interventions associated with those diagnoses, and evaluation of patient responses to nursing interventions. The psychosocial impact of illness on the family and the nursing staff is also discussed.

PSYCHOSOCIAL RESPONSES TO ILLNESS

Although patients differ in terms of their preparation for critical illness, rapidity of illness onset, number of presenting problems, personal responses, and nature of illness, they share the experience of being acutely ill. Critical illness alters sense of well-being, physical integrity, and ability to be independent and self-sufficient in the most basic of self-care measures. Because they are attached to equipment, invaded by tubes, covered with dressings, experiencing nausea, pain, or alterations in sensation, or having difficulty in breathing, swallowing, or moving, critically ill patients are dependent on others to meet their most intimate needs. Altered self-concept frequently leads to loss of self-esteem and accompanying grief over what is lost or changed. Feelings of anxiety arise over uncertainty of the future. Critically ill patients face coping with feelings arising from their illness or accident. Fears about living and dying predominate.

Admission to a critical care unit constitutes a significant life disruption. Critically ill patients are controlled by other people, procedures, schedules, and unit policies. They are in pain and bombarded by unfamiliar sights, sounds, and odors. Interactions with family, friends, and employers are interrupted or suspended. They do not know whether, when, how, or if they will want to resume former activities and relationships.

It is no wonder that patients in critical care settings feel sad, anxious, angry, frightened, dependent, frustrated, helpless, and possibly hopeless. Although some patients express these feelings directly, many others communicate only indirectly through words or behaviors. The important point is that most patients use coping mechanisms, either consciously or unconsciously, to deal with the critical situation and to allay anxiety.[63] The most common patient coping mechanisms in the critical care settings are listed in Table 8–1.

ASSESSMENT OF PATIENT RESPONSES

One tool to help the nurse identify patient responses to critical illness is the mental status evaluation. This evaluation consists

---

Coping Mechanisms Used by Patients

NAME	MECHANISM	EXAMPLE
Displacement	Unconscious transfer of feelings from an object, situation, or idea to one more acceptable	"You don't know how to change burn dressings; all of you are so darned incompetent, you make me sick."
Projection	Unconscious attribution of one's own ideas or impulses, usually unacceptable, to another person	"The doctors don't think I'm going to pull through; in fact, none of you do."
Suppression	Conscious and deliberate refusal to consider mind anxiety-producing thoughts	"I don't want to talk about the accident right now. I would get too upset."
Repression	Involuntary blocking of painful thoughts or memories from consciousness	"I don't remember being in the accident."
Rationalization	Justification of behavior or decisions that are not necessarily rational or logical	The patient with severe burns who says "I pulled off the dressings because they were not put on straight."
Regression	Returning to an earlier level of emotional development or adaptation	The previously independent patient who becomes childlike, clinging, dependent, and helpless following a tracheostomy. "I am just not able to do that. Will you do it for me?"
Denial	"Conscious or unconscious repudiation of all or a portion of the total available meaning of an illness in order to allay anxiety and to minimize emotional stress"[39]	"Who me? A heart attack? Ha, you've got the wrong man, Doc."

of systematic observation of patient behavior in order to determine and record observable aspects of psychologic functioning.[52] The following paragraphs discuss components of the mental status evaluation.

General Appearance and Attitude
In a critical care setting, the nurse cannot accurately assess the patient's grooming, dress, posture, and gait, but the nurse can observe the following:
- Facial expression (*e.g.*, wide-eyed, tense, sad, no expression)
- Unique mannerisms (*e.g.*, eye rolling, fist clenching, sighing, pulling hair)
- Motor behavior (*e.g.*, movements of entire body or parts of the body, fidgeting, turning, picking, thrashing)
- Attitude toward the nurse (*e.g.*, smiles, turns toward or away from the nurse, avoids eye contact, makes no response)
- Response to nursing care (*e.g.*, attempts to keep the nurse longer, is not satisfied, is grateful, tries to prevent or interfere with care)

Speech Activity
- Presence or absence of verbal communication
- Rate of speech (*e.g.*, rapid, slow, lack of pauses)
- Tone (*e.g.*, high-pitched, shrill, flat, barely audible, deep)
- Quality of response (*e.g.*, repetitive statements, monosyllabic answers, avoidance of certain subjects)
- Unique characteristics (*e.g.*, pressure of speech, loosening of associations, slurring and stuttering, peculiar use of words, irrelevance)

Affective Behavior
- Mood (*e.g.*, depressed, elated, apathetic, anxious, hostile, spontaneous, negativistic, cheerful, labile, irritable)
- Methods used to deal with or control emotions (*e.g.*, crying, throwing objects, complaining, swearing, shouting, remaining silent, talking, joking, rationalizing, displacing or projecting feelings, sexually acting out, denying concern, withdrawing, regressing)
- Manifest needs (*e.g.*, need for security, need to be cared for, need to be submissive)
- Patient's evaluation or description of mood or feelings

Distorted Thought Content
- Hallucinations (imaginary sense perceptions), such as hearing voices or seeing bugs
- Delusions (false, fixed beliefs that cannot be changed by logic), such as "You are putting poison into that IV."
- Ideas of reference (interpretation of incidents incorrectly as having direct reference to self), such as a patient who hears staff members talking about someone who is dying and assumes that they are referring to him or her
- Suicide ideation, such as when a patient states, "I'm not going to take this any longer; I'd rather be dead."
- Phobias, obsessions, grandiose ideas
- Psychotic ideation

Intellectual Functioning
- Orientation to person, place, time
- Memory for recent and remote past, as well as for immediate recall of what was just discussed
- Insight concerning current situation
- Judgment (tested by asking a question such as, "What would

you do if you found an addressed, stamped letter on the sidewalk?")
- Abstract thinking (tested by asking the patient to interpret proverbs)
- General information (tested by asking the patient to name the presidents of the United States)

A mental status evaluation done on admission serves as a baseline to which future mental status evaluations can be compared. Other tools to assess patients' feelings and reactions are the Holland-Sgroi Anxiety-Depression Scale for Medically Ill Patients,[35] the Hackett-Cassem Denial Scale,[36] and Murray's instrument to assess the psychologic status of the patient in surgical intensive care.[66]

Mattson[59] offers a theory to explain the general psychologic reaction of critically ill patients to severe physical injury. Patient response is categorized by six phases: the emergency reaction, the psychologic shock, the contrashock, the psychologic resistance, the psychologic convalescence, and the psychologic outcome. Each phase has its unique characteristics. The nurse familiar with these phases can formulate nursing diagnoses and draft nursing orders for appropriate nursing interventions to diminish anxiety and enhance psychologic support.

FACTORS AFFECTING PSYCHOSOCIAL RESPONSES

What determines the critically ill patient's response to illness and the coping mechanisms he employs? In the following paragraphs, four major factors are discussed: the "personhood" of the patient, the nature of the illness, the critical care environment, and the timing of the illness. In discussion of each factor, consideration is given to nursing assessment, diagnoses, intervention, and evaluation.

"Personhood" of the Patient

The term *personhood* refers to all that makes the patient a unique human being: strengths, weaknesses, life-style, goals, aspirations, character traits, previous experiences, and demographic characteristics. On arrival in the critical care unit, when a physiologic assessment is being carried out and appropriate life-saving and maintenance measures are introduced, the nurse can also begin to determine the following:

- Who is this patient? What is his or her age, sex, religion, ethnic background, life-style, marital and family status, education, employment? What are typical activities, life interests, plans, goals?
- What are characteristic personality traits? How does the patient describe himself or herself?[62] To what values might the nurse appeal to elicit cooperation? How is pain perceived, and what measures might increase comfort? What is the patient's intellect, sense of order, desire to comply? What are areas of vulnerability?
- What are previous experiences with hospitalization?
- How has the patient coped with illness or other stressors in the past? How effective were these coping mechanisms? What coping mechanisms are employed now, and how effective are they?
- What are the patient's life-style patterns? What evidence

exists that the patient successfully regulates diet, exercise, smoking, alcohol consumption, and drug usage.

- How does the patient express concerns? Are questions asked about this illness and its outcome?
- What is the predominant mood? What are current feelings? What needs are expressed?
- How does the patient perceive this illness will affect family roles and relationships?

If the patient is unable to supply information, family members may be a source of help. The information is collected neither to change the patient's personality nor to strip defenses. Rather, the nurse uses information to help the patient participate in care, to support effective coping mechanisms, and to select alternative support measures when those selected are ineffective.[67] Information gathered will be crucial in evaluation of responses to nursing interventions. Assessment reassures the patient that someone cares and recognizes the individuality of reactions to illness. The patient may experience relief from tension through talking about and sharing the illness experience.

In planning nursing care that supports the personhood of the patient, the nurse should do the following:

- Observe social amenities. It has been said that patients receive more courtesy and respect in an airline terminal than in a hospital. Although some patients prefer being called by their first names or nicknames, others may be offended. Ribbons in the hair of a 70-year-old woman may look "cute" to the staff but embarrass the patient. Determining patient preferences is essential to successful interventions and outcomes.[23]
- Foster independence. Although dependence is initially useful because it helps the patient tolerate care, dependence ultimately contributes to depression and interferes with rehabilitation. The nurse should look for ways, however small, to support patient self-care.
- Emphasize the patient's active participation in the care regimen, such as coughing, deep breathing, notifying the nurse when pain is experienced.
- Encourage patient decisions consistent with personal needs and state of health.[41] Likewise, the nurse should be alert to the danger of expecting or forcing the patient to make decisions beyond present capabilities.
- Recognize the importance of personal hygiene and personal items to self-image. An inability to care for oneself in the accustomed manner fosters feelings of powerlessness. Stripped of personal clothing, hairstyle, makeup, jewelry, teeth, personal care items, and money, the patient may feel naked, vulnerable, and exposed. Scrupulous attention to aspects of personal hygiene, coupled with flexibility in individualizing and personalizing care, fosters self-esteem.
- Consult with and refer to professional resources such as the chaplain, social worker, volunteer, psychiatric nurse, clinical nurse specialist, and psychiatrist.

By examining the patient's responses to an intervention or group of interventions, the nurse can determine the effectiveness of intervention. Based on this evaluation, the nurse can revise the plan of care to attain desired outcomes. In evaluating the effectiveness of interventions the nurse would:

- Compare the results of the intervention with the expected outcome. Is the patient closer to the goal attainment than before the intervention?
- Examine specific responses to the intervention. Has the patient's behavior changed? Does the patient talk more? Are more positive or negative feelings expressed? Is the patient less agitated, restless, or upset? Is there a change in appearance (less grimacing, posture change)? Is participation in self-care increased?
- Decide if the intervention was the basis for behavioral change. Record findings and conclusions regarding intervention effectiveness and subsequent plans.

Nature of the Illness

This is the second major category of factors contributing to patient responses to illness. It can be subdivided into two sections: the nature of the illness as perceived by the patient, and the objective nature of the illness.

The Illness as Perceived by the Patient

Patient perceptions of the illness include knowledge, understanding, fantasies, and misconceptions. The nurse is interested in the patient's perceptions of physical functioning, effects of the illness on the sense of general well-being, emotional or psychologic meaning of affected body parts, and how these contribute to the definition of total body image.

The patient with heart involvement perceives the heart as more than a pump, as do people with healthy hearts. Literature, folklore, poetry, and songs abound with images of the heart as the seat of love and affection. Male patients often associate the heart with virility. They view an insult to the heart, such as a myocardial infarction, as an attack on their masculinity.

The following suggestions help to determine patients' perceptions of illness and assist in developing interventions to reduce anxiety associated with these perceptions:

- Find out what the patient thinks is wrong. Be sure to include specific statements in the medical record; patient quotations are a good barometer of adjustment to illness when noted throughout a hospitalization.
- Encourage the patient to clarify or elaborate on words used in describing the problem. Consider the following dialogue:

Patient: I've had a heart attack.
Nurse: What do these words mean to you?
Patient: A heart attack means you die.
Nurse: Heart attack means death?
Patient: Sure, all my friends who had heart attacks died.

- Assess what immediate feelings, fears, or threats are present. The nurse might ask something such as, "What's it like to be so sick?" or "What do you find yourself thinking about?" or "What are some of your worries?"

Patient: I feel sad.
Nurse: What does this feel like? (or, Tell me what it's like to feel sad.)
Patient: Like being half a man.
Nurse: Half a man? What do you mean?

Patient: What the hell good am I? They might just as well dig a hole in the ground, put me in a box, and cover me up.

- Listen for the patient's ideas about cause of illness. Does the patient feel illness is punishment for past sins or misdeeds? Does the patient feel that some behavior directly led to the illness, such as driving too fast or taking drugs, or are others blamed? What feelings are expressed? If the patient expresses guilt, the nurse listens, without expressing an opinion as to whether the guilt feelings are justified.
- Determine the patient's perception of the recovery process. Does the patient believe recovery is progressing satisfactorily? Too slowly? Not at all? Are complications or problems in recovery anticipated by the patient? Is death the inevitable outcome? Are disabilities, loss of function, or disfigurement feared or envisioned?
- Listen for consistency in communication appropriateness. If the patient's responses have been appropriate and change to inappropriate, the nurse needs to assess alternative causative factors. Perceptions of his illness can be affected by physiologic and environmental factors such as hypoxia, electrolyte imbalance, sensory overload or deprivation, or sleep deprivation.[31]
- Clarify long-range concerns resulting from this illness. Clarification is appropriate when the nurse believes progress is hampered by concern over the future, such as job availability or resumption of sexual activity. The nurse might inquire, "What do you think your life will be like following this illness?" Concerns mentioned are addressed at the time they are identified. Some answers must wait until convalescence. The nurse cares for the patient by listening, focusing and clarifying concerns expressed, agreeing that the future is a source of worry, and assuring the patient that concerns are recorded and dealt with during hospitalization.
- Listen for patient omissions. If the patient never mentions the illness, diagnosis, medications, or procedures, the nurse may broach these subjects. For example, "We've talked about so many things this morning, but one thing we haven't talked about is your illness. What is it like for you to be a patient?" If resistance is met, the nurse does not push but encourages the patient to talk. "Patients often have questions or concerns about being sick and all the things being done for them. Asking questions and talking about concerns seem to help some people. If you would like to talk, be sure to let me know."
- Provide updated information. Health care personnel constantly obtain data to reassess the status of the patient's health, but the patient is rarely given this information as a basis for reinterpreting initial perceptions of health status. Lack of updated information can interfere with the patient's acceptance of progressive ambulation, increased responsibility for self-care, and transfer. It is extremely important for the patient involved in care to be knowledgeable about progress.
- Realize that the patient's perception of and response to this illness may be affected by folklore, literature, knowledge of others with the same illness, and responses of family, employer, community, or hospital personnel to the illness. It does little good to focus on return to a previous job if the employer prohibits persons with the patient's diagnosis from performing that job.

- Assess secondary gains associated with the illness, such as more attention or permission to be dependent. Does the patient suggest that transfer from the unit, assumption of new activities, or discharge from the hospital are impossible for the duration of the illness? Rewards stemming from illness include regressive and dependent postures with less responsibility.
- Provide accurate information when the patient is ready. Having clarified the patient's perceptions and understanding of the illness and determined needs for learning, the nurse plans and implements a teaching program to meet these needs. Pictures, brochures, anatomic models, samples of equipment, on-the-spot drawings, and other visual aids are helpful teaching aids. Ongoing records of specific topics discussed with the patient contribute to continuity in the teaching program.

The Illness as It Is in Reality

In addition to the patient's perception of personal illness, realistic aspects of the illness affect responses and mechanisms of coping. The following points must be considered:

- Did this illness or trauma occur suddenly, or did it develop over a period of time? Was the patient fully conscious during onset of illness?
- What is the present effect of the illness on total body systems? What are current vital signs, electrolyte levels, blood gas levels, metabolic status, and fluid balance?
- Is cerebral hypoxia present?
- Is the patient in pain, sedated, recovering from anesthesia, withdrawing from drugs or alcohol?
- What medications are being administered? Is the patient receiving atropine? Is lidocaine infusing at the proper rate? Is the patient receiving steroid therapy? If so, what kind and for how long? Is a drug reaction present?
- Is the patient septic?
- Are casts, traction, or splints constraining mobility or restricting normal functions? Is the patient covered with dressings or bandages or isolated from others?
- Are body orifices and vessels invaded by tubes, infusions, wires, leads, catheters? Is the patient dependent on tubes and machines to assist or totally support normal physiologic functioning?
- Does the patient require suctioning, chest physiotherapy, or injections? Must nurses assume responsibility for feeding, bathing, turning, positioning, and other aspects of care?
- Are any body parts missing or deformed? Do odors emanate from orifices, wounds, or the person in general?
- Is the sleep pattern normal? To what degree do treatments and procedures interfere with normal sleep patterns? Does the patient have nightmares?
- Does the patient require specific isolation precautions? Do individuals approaching the patient require gowns and masks?
- Is a malignancy present? Is the patient terminally ill? Is this the first stage or the end stage of the illness?
- Are required painful procedures repeated as part of the care regimen?

To lessen generalized anxiety generated by the illness and its treatment, the nurse should do the following:

- Continually evaluate the patient's feelings and concerns about staff activities and interventions. Initiation of routine intravenous infusion may not seem routine to a patient whose father arrested while an infusion was being started. Obtaining a blood pressure reading is a simple enough procedure, but the patient may view it as a means of torment used by night staff.
- Identify oneself by name and position and continue attempts to elicit verbal or nonverbal signs of patient recognition.
- Provide explanations about treatments and procedures before touching or uncovering the patient.
- Maintain the patient's dignity and modesty by closing curtains or doors and by limiting unnecessary exposure.
- Emphasize the temporary nature of aspects of treatment or the effects of illness that are transient. Give the patient goals that are realistic, and point out progress made, however minute.
- Continuously evaluate the need for specific procedures or treatments. Assessment of intervention necessity may result in discontinuance of unnecessary procedures or rearrangement of the care schedule to permit uninterrupted sleep.
- Assess degree of orientation and level of awareness. If patients are not completely oriented, identification of date and time and repeated simple explanations of who they are, where they are, and why they are in critical care are indicated.
- If the patient is having nightmares after an accident, burns, or surgery, provide reassurance that frightening dreams are common, temporary, and do not indicate loss of control or mental illness. Encouraging talk about nightmares and arranging for someone to remain at the bedside during sleeping hours may reduce anxiety and help the patient obtain restful sleep.[48]

Environmental Characteristics

The third major category of factors contributing to patient responses to illness is environmental characteristics. The following considerations come under this category:

- The physical characteristics of the hospital room. How many windows? Beds? Are there cubicles, or are patients separated by curtains? Are bright lights on constantly, or are they lowered at night? Are calendars and clocks within patient sight? Does the patient have control over bedside lighting? Where is the nurse's station in reference to the patient? How close is the patient to doors, hallways, utility areas?
- Equipment. Kind? Amount? Size? Sounds? How close is the equipment to the patient?
- Other patients in the room. How many? What sex? How close are they to the patient? How sick are they? What sounds do they, their relatives, or their equipment make?
- Are objects meaningful to the patient present? Does the patient have any personal possessions, such as pictures, clothes, Bible, or other books?
- Are there any symbols of affection from others, such as cards, letters, flowers, or fruit?
- What is the nature of conversations that occur within the patient's hearing?
- Who comes in contact with the patient (*e.g.*, patient care personnel, support staff, family, other visitors)?

- How much activity can the patient see and hear (*e.g.*, noise,[91] confusion, many people moving about, emergencies)?

The environment of a critical care unit can be highly traumatic for patients.[31,38,50,76] With appropriate nursing interventions, however, the environment can become less stressful for some patients and highly positive and supportive for others. The nurse should do the following:

- Assess the patient's response to the immediate environment. Look at the room from the patient's vantage point (Fig. 8–1). Is there anything in the patient's line of vision that is not in an ordinary hospital room? If there is, assume that the patient at least wonders about it and at most is frightened by it. Mention aspects of the immediate environment in conversation if the patient does not. For example, ask the patient, "Is there anything you see or hear that you wonder about?" The nurse can preface her questions with, "This may be a strange and unfamiliar place for you. Patients often have questions and concerns about being here." The words used are not as important as the feelings conveyed, namely, that the nurse cares about the patient's comfort and is open to hearing of fears and worries.
- Explain the equipment, its purpose, sounds (*e.g.*, hissing), side-effects (*e.g.*, alarms), and sights (*e.g.*, IV lines) in terms the patient understands. The nurse may demonstrate equip-

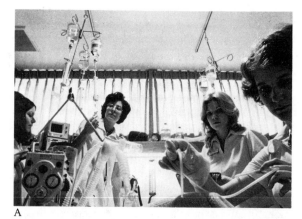

A

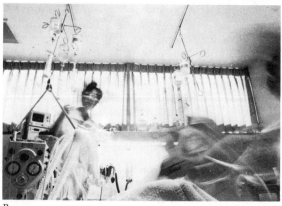

B

Figure 8–1

Look at the room from the patient's vantage point (*A*), and remember that movement may blur what the patient sees and perceives (*B*).

ment function, or the patient can be shown equipment in use on another patient. The nurse's aim is to help the patient tolerate the equipment rather than be made anxious by it. In fact, with the nurse's help, the patient may focus on positive aspects of the equipment and experience less anxiety after learning how specific equipment helps the nurse provide necessary care. If at all possible, equipment should be positioned in such a way that the patient's line of vision is not obscured.

- Control sounds. In one recovery room, nurses routinely discarded glass vials and other used supplies in a large metal trash can. Although they had become accustomed to the resultant din, the patients found the sound extremely disturbing. Some noises, such as the one just described, can be eliminated when the nursing staff becomes aware of deleterious effects on patients. Other sounds cannot be reduced. It is essential that the nurse explain unfamiliar sounds in simple terms. A special attempt should be made to control noise during the night. Conversations with the patient should be concrete to avoid distortion or confusion. It is important to remember that the patient's hearing may extend beyond the immediate bedside area. One patient who was recovering without incident heard a nurse outside his room say, "That old thing won't last much longer." He assumed that the nurse was talking about him. In reality, she was discussing a piece of equipment.
- Control lighting so that the patient can experience a day-night cycle as close to normal as possible.
- Control sights. The patient is often in close proximity to staff members and can observe facial expressions and gestures. Staff activities may be frightening. One patient in a surgical intensive care unit witnessed resuscitation attempts on a patient across the room. His impression was that a sexual orgy was taking place. Another patient who witnessed a tracheostomy being performed assumed that the patient was being murdered. Her suspicions seemed confirmed when she later saw the bed empty.

If a patient witnesses a cardiac arrest, resuscitation efforts, and death, it is important to discuss what he heard, saw, and felt. The patient may experience or express sorrow over the loss, anger over the inconvenience or noise, relief that it was the "other guy," or reassurance at the speed and competence of staff. The patient may feel, but not directly express, anxiety over a possible similar fate. Anxiety may be manifested in an elevated blood pressure or pulse, more frequent request for pain medication, or increased use of the call buzzer, especially in the 24-hour period after the incident. As the patient talks about the incident, the nurse should listen for indications that aspects of similarity between the patient and the deceased are being repressed. A focus on differences is healthy ("He was much older than me" or "He didn't follow the doctor's orders" or "His heart attack was worse than mine"). If the patient is unable to focus on differences, the nurse can point these out to the patient.

- If no outside window exists in the hospital cubicle or room, the patient has no visual contact with the outside world. The patient cannot see the sun, rain, or snow or differentiate day from night. Familiar, comforting objects in the external environment, such as trees, birds, or clouds cannot be seen. Even with an outside window, the patient may need a radio, newspaper, television, telephone, calendar, clock, family,

and the nurse to help maintain contact with and orientation to the world outside the critical care unit.

- Realize that a patient may be made anxious by close proximity to a patient of the opposite sex. Also, the patient may feel uncomfortable expelling flatus, talking about bowel movements and other body functions, or giving out information considered intimate.
- Make the environment as personal as possible. Try to include some objects that are meaningful to the patient. For example, if a pet dog is highly valued by the patient, perhaps someone can bring the patient a picture of that dog.
- Give the patient some control of the environment, if possible. For example, allow the patient to turn off a radio or adjust lighting. Even minimal control of the environment supports feelings of competence and effectiveness.
- Recognize the importance of a patient's space or territory. The patient who is not acutely ill has an opportunity, when admitted, to walk around new surroundings and to become familiar with sights, sounds, and activities. An ambulatory patient can unpack suitcases, arrange belongings, and, thus, in a sense, delineate personal space or territory. The patient in a critical care unit cannot. The nurse decides which belongings go where and which ones are sent home. The patient has no opportunity to explore, to define, or to identify personal territory. This situation can heighten feelings of helplessness and powerlessness. To diminish those feelings, the nurse can help the patient delineate personal territory through a brief verbal orientation to the nursing unit and a description of the space that "belongs" to the patient. Also, the nurse can ask advice about the placement of personal objects in the patient's unit.
- Realize that several kinds of sensory alterations can occur. The term *sensory deprivation* refers to the elimination, reduction, or stereotyping of sensation from vision, hearing, or touch. The term *sensory monotony* refers to continuous sensory input along with the elimination or reduction of other sensations (*e.g.*, the constant sound of the cardiac monitor, which blocks other sounds). The term *sensory overload* refers to a condition of highly intense stimulation that is not patterned, such as might be experienced in the recovery room.

The patient who is experiencing sensory alteration may show signs of decreased ability to solve problems and reason; loss of accuracy in tactual, spatial, and time orientation; deficiencies in visual and motor coordination; change in size, shape, and color perception; boredom; restlessness; fatigue; drowsiness; and feelings of being dazed, confused, or disoriented. Thus, the patient may fall out of bed because perception of the boundaries of the bed have been altered. The patient may turn to the left when the nurse says right because left-right discrimination is lost in fatigue and early sensory deprivation. The patient may be unable to make simple decisions or may forget directions, simple instructions, or other kinds of information.

The nurse must repeatedly assess the effects of sights, sounds, and smells on the patient. In addition, the nurse must determine what effect the illness and its treatment have on the patient's ability to receive and sort out sensory input. Answers are sought to the following questions: Does the patient usually wear dentures, glasses, or a hearing aid? Does the patient have dressings or patches over eyes or ears? Is the patient restrained from moving or touching anything?

Is the patient physically active within constraints of the medical condition? Can the patient understand English and expressions used by the health care team? Does the patient's position in bed prevent or obstruct observation of activities and people in the immediate environment? Are adequate uninterrupted rest periods provided? Was the patient taking any medications routinely? Does the patient have a fever or some other medical problem that interferes with perception and integration of stimuli? Knowing answers to these questions can help in planning care that diminishes the effects of sensory alteration.

- Realize that the presence of people valued by the patient is probably the single most important factor in making the environment a secure, caring one. The category includes significant persons in the patient's life and the members of the health care team on whom the patient relies. It is important to manage visiting hours in terms of length of visit and time of day, visitor numbers, and specific individual visitors.[16,57] Nurses have long known that some patients become more relaxed, less fretful, and less restless when someone they love is near; however, nurses often do little to encourage others to remain with the patient.

Although it is generally accepted that parents accompany ill children, hospital personnel are still uncomfortable when children visit ill parents. Values and attitudes of hospital personnel may prevent or delay the assessment and fulfillment of the needs of hospitalized critical care patients and their children. Short, frequent visits may be highly beneficial for both. If children cannot be brought into the unit, possibly the patient can be taken outside to visit for brief periods. Also, children can be encouraged to send in drawings and notes, and the patient can be helped to respond in some fashion. Exchanges of cassette tapes and telephone calls can help maintain family ties.

Nurses play a vital role by monitoring the environment and its effects on the patient and by sharing themselves. Through the use of touch,[21,61,74,80] presence, listening,[27,29] talking, observing, carrying out procedures and treatments, and monitoring vital signs, nurses share their personhood, their acceptance, their concern, and their health. Conversely, for a variety of reasons, including personal responses to working in a critical care unit, nurses can contribute to the patient's anxiety and diminish feelings of self-worth. Deleterious behaviors include the following:

- Offering superficial reassurance (e.g., "Don't worry. Everything will be all right.")
- Lacking sensitivity to expressed feelings (e.g., "There's really nothing to cry about.")
- Frightening the patient (e.g., "I've never seen this reaction before" or "I don't like the looks of that.")
- Disparaging or contradicting other personnel
- Checking equipment too frequently
- Ignoring the patient when coming to the bedside to carry out a procedure or to check equipment
- Delaying response when summoned by the patient
- Complaining to the patient about the workload and the number of patients assigned
- Belittling patient concerns
- Changing the subject when the patient asks questions that make the nurse feel uncomfortable
- Rushing in and out of the patient's room or cubicle
- Asking the patient a question and then either "tuning out"

the answer or exhibiting impatience because response isn't instantaneous
- Disregarding common courtesy
- Removing equipment without appropriate psychologic weaning and support
- Ignoring or minimizing learning needs of the patient
- Overprotecting the patient for a period of time, then suddenly expecting autonomy and independence in self-care
- Promising to visit after transfer and not following through
- Shouting or calling out to other staff members across the room
- Even actions viewed by personnel as benign or routine, such as taking a pulse, walking into the patient's room, or giving the patient a pill, can arouse both physiologic and psychologic responses.[57]
- Prepare the patient for transfer from the critical care environment. Because dependence on personnel, equipment, and the secure environment is likely to increase over time, early transfer from the unit is desirable. Encourage the patient to share feelings, reactions, and fears relating to transfer. Many patients speak about sadness and loss at leaving the critical care unit. They express feelings of anxiety over what the new unit will be like, whether personal needs will be met, whether the staff will know how to carry out specific care and handle emergencies that might arise, and whether the necessary equipment and medications will be available. The nurse can be helpful by accepting these feelings and pointing out gains the patient will make after transfer. The nurse should emphasize that staff members on the receiving unit have skills, equipment, and medications necessary to handle any emergency that might occur, although this particular patient is not expected to become emergent. If possible, the patient should be weaned from equipment, such as a monitor or respirator, at a time other than at transfer.

If possible, transfer should occur during the day, with familiar people accompanying the patient. The patient should be introduced to someone on the receiving unit and be told that individualized information regarding ongoing care has been shared with responsible team members, both in writing and verbally. Later, members of the critical care staff with whom the patient has established rapport might visit to provide additional continuity and reassurance.[60]

Timing of the Illness

The timing of the illness, the fourth major category of factors that affect response to illness, has, until recently, received relatively little attention. This category includes the role of stress and the "anniversary reaction."

Role of Stress

Although feelings of loss have long been recognized as a reaction to illness, only recently have illness and death been recognized as responses to loss and other stress producers.[72,73,79,81,84] Stress is a generalized physiologic response of the body to any demand made on it. Each stressor, a stimulus that upsets physiologic homeostasis, calls forth specific and nonspecific responses. A specific response to a stressor is localized, such as the skin's response to heat. A nonspecific response is generalized. All stressors have something in common: They increase demand for adjustment. It is immaterial whether the stressor is pleasant or unpleasant, desirable or undesirable. The intensity of the demand for readjustment or adaptation is of importance. The more stressful an event or happening, the more intense the demand on the organism to adapt, and the greater the physiologic response. Energy necessary to acquire and maintain adaptation, apart from caloric requirements, is called *adaptation energy*.[79] Selye[79] has coined the term *general adaptation syndrome* to describe the three-phased generalized physiologic response by which the autonomic nervous system and endocrine glands mobilize to resist stressors and regain equilibrium.

In recent years, researchers have attempted to develop tools to measure stress and the effects of stress on health status. Holmes and Rahe[46] compiled a list of life events that occur around the time of disease onset. Each event places an adjustment demand (stress) on the person involved. The Social Readjustment Rating Scale measures, in life-change units, the amount of readjustment required by each event on the list. Using this instrument to gather life-change data from 279 survivors of documented myocardial infarction and from 226 cases of abrupt coronary death, Rahe *et al.*[73] found significant elevation in life-change units during the 6 months before infarction or death. For victims of sudden death, elevation was particularly evident. On the basis of their research, Holmes and Rahe suggest that when total life-change units equal or exceed a score of 300 in any given year, a danger point has been reached. In one study of subjects who scored in excess of 300, 80% had heart attacks, became seriously depressed, or experienced other serious illnesses.[82]

Knowledge that stressors evoke both physiologic and psychologic responses has implications for the critical care setting. The patient who comes to the hospital in the process of dealing with social stressors, such as a new job or recent divorce, may need special help. The burden of coping with multiple stressors and resulting autonomic stimulation may exceed the patient's adaptation capacity. Without appropriate intervention, the patient may succumb to the illness or its complications. Whatever the nurse can do to identify recent stressful life events, assess the degree of unresolved conflicts, identify stressors in the present situation, and intervene with appropriate measures to reduce effects of these stressors[44,64,66,76,83,84] will enhance the patient's psychologic comfort and foster physical well-being.

Techniques used to reduce impact of stressors may be more widely applied in critical care areas in the future. Biofeedback, meditation, and relaxation, used individually or in combination, assist the patient in coping. The relaxation response counteracts the physiologic effects of stressors by lowering heart rate and metabolism and decreasing respiratory rate.[56,60,79] Lown *et al.*[56] discussed the effective use of meditation in a 39-year-old patient who twice experienced ventricular fibrillation and exhibited numerous ventricular premature beats. Biofeedback, a technique using instrumentation to give a person immediate and continuing information on specific automatic body function, has been used to teach patients greater awareness of mind-body correlates and conscious control of certain body functions. Lowering of blood pressure and pulse, reduction of tension headaches and lower back pain, and improvement in muscle function have been cited as results of these techniques (see Chap. 1).

Anniversary Reaction

Another factor to consider in the category of timing is that of the "anniversary reaction." This phenomenon occurs when others in the patient's family contracted or died of similar illnesses on the same date, at the same time, or at the same age. For example, a 50-year-old patient with a myocardial infarction whose father died from infarction at a similar age may feel that his death is inevitable. If evidence of an anniversary reaction exists, the patient may need help in grieving the loss of the relative, in expressing anxiety at having contracted the same illness, and in pinpointing how this case is different from that of the deceased relative.

Four determinants of patient responses to critical illness, *i.e.*, personhood of the patient, nature of the illness, environmental characteristics, and timing of the illness, have been discussed individually for purposes of description and clarity. These factors do not affect the patient separately but interact to affect how a patient responds to and copes with critical illness.

NURSING INTERVENTIONS FOR SPECIFIC NURSING DIAGNOSES

In addition to general nursing measures suggested to assist the patient in coping with critical illness and in expressing generalized fears and anxieties, specific nursing interventions are based on nursing diagnoses of particular responses to critical illness. Interventions discussed in this chapter are specific to denial, anxiety, ineffective individual or family coping, disturbance in self-concept, sensory/perceptual alteration, altered verbal communication, anticipatory grieving, potential for violence, and hopelessness.

NURSING DIAGNOSIS

1. *Ineffective denial, nonacceptance of critical diagnosis, related to inability to cope with fear and anxiety (choosing pattern)*

Patient Outcomes	*Nursing Orders*

1. The patient can discuss the critical diagnosis and ask questions.	1. Assess for the readiness to explore underlying reasons for denial, or leave the process intact because the denial is acting as a protective mechanism.
	  A. Offer feedback of expressed feelings.
	  B. Ask questions that encourage answers that reflect reality perception.
	  C. Explore how this patient has handled other threatening situations.
	  D. Explain that persons pace themselves in emotional adjustment to critical illness.

(continued)

NURSING DIAGNOSIS Continued

1. *Ineffective denial, nonacceptance of critical diagnosis, related to inability to cope with fear and anxiety (choosing pattern)*

Patient Outcomes	Nursing Orders
2. The patient cooperates with the care regimen.	2. Ask for cooperation with the medical regimen. Do not directly challenge denial.

Implementation and Evaluation

Denial is a protective mechanism that can take several forms:

- Verbal denial (*e.g.,* "I don't have cancer.")
- Minimizing severity (*e.g.,* "Yes, I had a heart attack yesterday, but it's all gone now.")
- Displacing symptoms on another organ system (*e.g.,* "It wasn't my heart; it was indigestion.")
- Behavior contrary to medical advice (*e.g.,* "Sure, I still smoke. Cigarettes aren't going to bother my lungs.")

Some of the manifestations of denial are excessive cheerfulness, joking, use of cliches in reference to death, conversation focused on issues other than illness, and use of dismissive gestures when referring to distressing events.[17,22,69]

If a patient is verbally denying seriousness of the illness but allows treatments and care to be carried out, denial may be serving a highly useful purpose. Denial is maladaptive when behavior interferes significantly with care (*e.g.,* patient pulls off monitor leads, refuses medication, or gets out of bed when contraindicated). In these instances, arguing with a patient makes the nurse and the patient angry and reinforces the patient's denial. Teaching is likewise generally ineffective. If a patient does not believe a particular illness has been contracted, why learn about that illness?

The nurse attempts to clarify the underlying threat without challenging denial directly. This is done by asking the patient to talk in general terms about the problem or illness, without having to personalize the problem. The nurse acknowledges the patient's comments or description and affirms that others have similar perspectives. The nurse can also ask for cooperation rather than intellectual assent (*e.g.,* "You tell me you don't believe you had a heart attack. Many people feel the same as you do; they don't believe it either. In fact, at this point, we're not expecting you to believe it. We're just asking you to go along with us and keep these leads on.")

Evaluation of the patient's use of denial is based on the degree, intensity, and appropriateness of the denial demonstrated.[5] The effectiveness of an intervention is determined by change in the patient's behavior or verbalization. Progress might be measured by observing the increase of patient participation in self-care. Significant progress has occurred when the patient begins to talk about the illness in personal terms.

CASE STUDY

A 54-year-old man was admitted to a four-bed coronary care unit with the diagnosis of massive myocardial infarction. The day after his admission, he pulled off the leads and began walking in the hall. When told by the staff he could not do this, he threatened to sign out of the hospital.

Nurse: You've removed the monitor leads several times today and gotten out of bed. What makes it so hard to keep them on and stay in bed?

Patient: I'm an ex-con. Being strapped with those things and the side rails up reminds me of solitary confinement. I can't stand it; I'm getting out of the hospital.

Nurse: You're telling me you can't stay here with activities restricted so much. If there was one thing I could change to make the situation tolerable enough for you to stay, what would it be?

In such a way, the nurse communicates concern, recognition of the patient's need to control, and willingness to compromise. Modifications of what nursing personnel consider "ideal" are not always easy to make. Yet these modifications may induce the patient to remain in the hospital and receive care that is desperately needed.

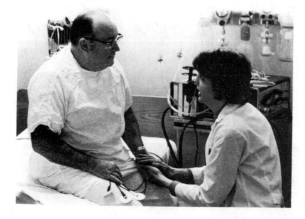

Figure 8–2

"I hear you say you can't stand being so restricted. If there was one thing I could change that would help, what would it be?"

NURSING DIAGNOSIS

2. *Anxiety related to acute illness, life-threatening illness, and unknown resolution of illness (feeling pattern)*

Patient Outcomes	Nursing Orders
1. The patient verbalizes anxious feelings.	1. Explain the typical course of illness, including sensations that might be expected.
2. The patient's agitation eases in response to specific therapeutic relaxation interventions.	2. Teach relaxation exercises for initiation at the onset of anxious feelings. At appropriate time, introduce imagery and music therapy.
3. The patient, family, or significant others exhibit a reduction in anxiety.	3. Inform the patient and family of progress toward recovery. Maintain all aspects of hope and the will to live.
4. The patient initiates measures to allay the onset of anxiety.	4. Explain the purpose of interventions and changes in the care regimen.

5. The patient should feel secure in the critical care unit, and the environmental stresses should be minimized.	5. Familiarize the patient with the environment and the protocols. Tell the patient about the following:
	A. Staff members
	B. Nurses' bell call
	C. Monitoring equipment
	D. Hospital routine
	E. Treatments and medications
	F. Visiting hours
	  (1) Provide care in an interested, knowledgeable manner.
	  (2) Assess the patient's pain, and use comfort measures as well as analgesics to alleviate any pain.
	  (3) Provide the patient with a clock and a calendar.
	  (4) Relieve the monotony. If possible, increase the patient's mobility.
	  (5) Plan nursing procedures to allow the patient uninterrupted periods of sleep.
	  (6) Use reality orientation principles.
	  (7) Have the patient's family bring in familiar objects from home.
	  (8) Assess the patient's knowledge and anxiety levels, and give the information necessary about the critical care unit.
	  (9) Keep noises to a minimum, and provide pleasing sounds, such as music and soft voices.

6. The patient will be treated as an individual.	6. Provide individualized nursing care.
	A. Assess the patient for psychologic as well as physical problems, using an assessment tool as an outline.
	B. Use the data collected to plan and evaluate care.
	C. Coordinate care and communicate information to the staff of the unit to which the patient is transferred.
	  (1) Be sensitive to the patient's feelings, and take time to assess his behavior.
	  (2) Help the nurses to get in touch with their own feelings.
	  (3) Have the same staff care for the patient as much as possible.
	  (4) Use eye-to-eye contact when talking with the patient.

7. The patient will maintain a sense of self.	7. Demonstrate respect for the patient by addressing the patient properly and by including the patient in conversations, particularly on rounds. A. Have respect for the patient's privacy, shielding the patient as necessary. B. If the patient's scheduled activities must be changed, ask the patient to confirm the changes. C. Provide uninterrupted periods for talking with the patient, and talk with the patient during care. D. Listen to what the patient says. E. Use good communication techniques with the patient. F. Encourage communication.
8. The patient should be included in personal care.	8. If the patient is not too ill, have the patient plan personal care with the nurse. A. Allow the patient to know when painful procedures may be carried out and include regular rest periods. B. Assist the patient in making menu selections as soon as the patient is able.
9. The patient will maintain a sense of control and involvement during hospitalization.	9. Let the patient have as many responsibilities as can be handled. Teach the patient the value of self-care.

Implementation and Evaluation

The acutely anxious patient may exhibit one or more of the following: rapid, high-pitched voice; incessant talking; fidgeting, twisting, or restless movements; rapid pulse; increased respirations; elevated blood pressure; increased perspiration; difficulty sleeping; tense expression; and wide, staring eyes.[36,66,69] One patient may say outright, "I'm scared" or "What's going to happen to me?" or "Am I going to die?" Another may call for the nurse frequently and cling verbally or physically once the nurse is at the bedside. In either instance, the nurse should encourage the patient to talk about anxious feelings and affirm fear as normal.

Nurse: You tell me you are feeling anxious. What does this feel like?
Patient: I don't know; I just don't feel right.
Nurse: Describe how you just don't feel right.
Patient: Well [pause], I feel restless, nervous. I want to get this over with.
Nurse: Get what over with?
Patient: They tell me I have to go back for another operation to change these dressings.
Nurse: Is something about this especially upsetting?
Patient: I don't know [pause]. I wonder if it will hurt. I know it will. Will I have anesthesia? I want to be asleep. I don't want any more pain.

The more the patient can identify the factors that contribute to feelings of anxiety, the more data the nurse has for planning. Each factor should be examined individually with the patient. Some problems can be solved with simple explanations. Others may require the help of resource people. Some problems cannot be fully resolved, but at least the nurse and the patient are aware of specifics and can deal with them directly.

The presence of a significant other, a family member, or someone else the patient trusts may diminish anxiety and help induce rest. Likewise, having the same nurses, with whom a relationship can evolve, is very helpful. Planned, frequent visits by the nurse reassures the patient; confidence and trust can be transferred to nursing colleagues. The patient should be informed of changes in caregivers and, if possible, introduced to individuals responsible for providing care. When responsibility for care is passed from one nurse to another, reviewing procedures or routines with which the patient feels comfortable, in the presence of the patient, is comforting and facilitates the transfer of patient trust from one nurse to another.

The severely anxious patient needs reassurance about routine aspects of treatments, progress being made, and preparation for what is to come. Anticipating reactions to surgery or procedures (e.g., pain or nausea), along with reassurance that medication is available to relieve these responses, diminishes anxiety. Explanations, directions, or information should be brief, simple, and repeated at frequent intervals. Some patients also seem calmed by knowledge that they are being treated in a specialized unit staffed with educated nurse experts. The effect of verbal assurance is strongly enhanced if nurses go about their work calmly, appear in control of the environment, and are flexible within a structured framework.

Finally, in the strange environment, the patient may need medication for reduction of anxiety or sleep. Some patients require reassurance that such medication is an important adjunct to treatment. The anxious patient should not be responsible for determining the need and requesting this medication. Assessment of patient need for medication to reduce anxiety or aid sleep and administration of medication are the nurse's responsibility.

Evaluation centers on interpretation of the patient's behaviors and verbalizations. Effective intervention results in verbal expression of anxious feelings. If the patient is unable to speak, the nurse evaluates effectiveness of intervention by observing the patient's behavior to include reduction in irritability or restlessness. Another significant evaluation finding for this diagnosis is patient initiation of strategies to reduce anxious feelings at onset.

NURSING DIAGNOSIS

3. *Ineffective individual or family coping related to feelings of a depressive nature (mild, moderate, severe) or acute illness (choosing pattern)*

Patient Outcomes	Nursing Orders
1. The patient will be able to express feelings of sadness and loss.	1. Maintain sensory function and stimulation through frequent contact, movement, touch, or speech. Express empathy, warmth, and friendliness.
2. The patient will be able to cry if appropriate.	2. Encourage awareness and expression of feelings from patient or significant others. Foster family interaction and support.
3. The patient will begin to verbalize feelings of hope and speak of transfer or discharge.	3. Direct attention to the future, reassuring the patient that the present situation will pass.
4. The family and friends will effectively cope with the patient's illness.	4. The following interventions are suggested to help family and friends cope effectively with the patient's critical illness and the critical care unit: A. Orient the family to the critical care unit, waiting room, protocol, visiting hours, and staff. B. Provide written information on the unit and visiting hours.

(continued)

NURSING DIAGNOSIS Continued

3. *Ineffective individual or family coping related to feelings of a depressive nature (mild, moderate, severe) or acute illness (choosing pattern)*

Patient Outcomes	*Nursing Orders*
	C. Allow for flexible visiting hours as needed; assess each family and its needs concerning length of stay and number of visits. Families view the nurse as communicator, gatekeeper, and caregiver.
	D. Encourage the family to turn to other family members and friends during the acute phase for additional support.
	E. Encourage the family to feel there is reason for hope when appropriate, answer questions honestly, and let the family have frequent progress reports on the patient.
	F. Encourage the family to write questions when they arise so that they can be answered by the health care staff.
	G. Interview family members to complete gaps in the patient data base. Assess responses to questions such as anxiety, fear, and guilt.
	H. Identify other resource people for the family, such as the chaplain, dietitian, social worker, or patient advocate.
	I. Assess family members' desires for involvement in the patient's care. Does the family encourage the patient's independence or dependency?
	J. Encourage the family to help the patient maintain involvement in life by bringing cards or small special, personal, or meaningful items. Encourage the family with storytelling and reflections on positive life events and the patient's strengths.
	K. Make provisions for family members to phone the nurse's station so that they can leave the hospital to go home or to the hotel for rest and relaxation.
	L. Help family members with problem solving and decision making.
	M. Introduce family members to support groups that relate to the patient's illness such as cardiac and cancer support groups. Families in crisis benefit from such groups.
	N. Identify the special needs of family members of dying patients. Provide specific resource people to help.

Implementation and Evaluation

Depression is a response to a narcissistic injury, a blow to the image of oneself as whole, intact, and independent. With increasing awareness of the reality of the situation, the patient may become withdrawn, listless, apathetic, and pessimistic; show retarded speech and motor activity; cry; have a decrease in appetite; express feelings of hopelessness; and look sad.[21] Some individuals may ruminate about what life will be like as a result of this illness.

Anticipate feelings of sadness and depression, and reassure the patient that these are normal. The nurse can encourage the patient to share these feelings. If focus on the illness persists to exclusion of all other topics, the nurse may need to direct attention to another more optimistic time in the patient's life. Patient tears about changes, losses, or fears are generally healthy; for some patients, tears may be accompanied by a sense of loss of control. Matter-of-fact acceptance rather than an overly sympathetic approach to patient crying is most supportive.

Nurses need not join the patient in feeling that the situation is hopeless; nor should they be overly optimistic. They can refer to the future in their conversations and promote future-oriented thinking. Taking an activity history and beginning a program of planned activity early in the hospitalization will lessen the incidence of depression and foster the patient's sense of well-being.[19]

It is helpful to look for ways to increase the patient's self-esteem. They can encourage the patient to focus on small gains rather than long-term goals. Patients need nurses' input to do this. For example, a nurse might say, "From now on, your blood pressure will be evaluated every hour instead of every 15 minutes because you are doing so well." The nurse can accentuate the positive, pointing to patient capabilities rather than to activities curtailed.

Recognize that the depressed patient does not appreciate an exuberant approach; it serves only to heighten feelings of sadness. Sometimes superficial attempts to be cheerful are seen as just that—superficial. It would be more helpful to say, "I notice that you look sad and have been crying [pause]. Tell me about it." Again, the words the nurse uses are not so important as the message of concern and caring transmitted to the patient. Sometimes, words are not necessary. Just being with the patient, touching an arm or hand, and sharing oneself are sources of great comfort.

The patient may begin to express anger as a means of diminishing feelings of helplessness. Anger is not a personal attack on the nurse. Rather than respond to the patient defensively, the nurse can encourage the patient to focus on the source of distress.

Patient: The food is always cold, the nurses sure don't know much about giving shots, and then there's that parking lot! Why, they charge my wife $3.50 every time she comes in!

Nurse: Seems like many things are really upsetting you today. Wonder if you are also upset about being sick and being here in the unit?

Patient: No, it's not that. It's the parking lot. I hate it with a purple passion.

This patient was not ready to confront the issue of his illness and all that it meant. The nurse listened as the patient expressed more anger. Two days later, during a similar conversation, she again raised the point of the patient's illness and related feelings. At that time, he was able to talk about his sadness and fear.

Evaluation of the patient's progress is often very difficult in these situations. What may initially seem like inappropriate behavior may actually be a significant step toward acceptance of the illness. Patient's interest in the surroundings is important. Progress toward desired outcomes is seen when the patient is able to verbalize feelings of sadness, anger, and fear.

NURSING DIAGNOSIS

4. *Self-esteem disturbance manifested by sexual aggressiveness that is related to maladaptation to psychological stress (perceiving pattern)*

Patient Outcomes	Nursing Orders
1. The patient will refrain from inappropriate sexual behavior.	1. Recognize sexual behavior or innuendos. Inform the patient that sexual behavior is inappropriate at this time, in this place, and with this individual.
2. The patient will verbally express anxiety related to sexual adequacy and future sexual functioning.	2. Reassure the patient that concerns about sexual functioning are normal and may be discussed legitimately. Answer questions about sexual identity and functioning.

Implementation and Evaluation

Sexual acting-out can occur verbally when the patient tells off-color jokes, makes seductive remarks, cites details of past sexual accomplishments, invites discussion of personal life, or suggests the nurse participate in sexual activities. Also, sexual aggression can occur behaviorally, with the patient pinching, poking, fondling, or kissing the nurse; exposing breasts or genitalia; or masturbating in the nurse's presence.

Sexual acting-out may be the result of anxiety over an altered self-image.[86] The patient fears loss of personhood as a whole man or woman and wonders whether others recognize him or her as a sexual being. The patient acts out this concern through comments and behavior. Nurses often feel anxious, angry, frightened, or embarrassed, and respond by disparaging the patient. The patient may then try harder through words or actions to communicate sexual competency. Nursing intervention can be considered effective if there is a decrease in exhibited behavior and verbalized feelings of self-worth.

NURSING DIAGNOSIS

5. *Sensory/perceptual alteration related to decreased level of conciousness (perceiving pattern)*

Patient Outcomes	Nursing Orders
1. The patient will be free from episodes of disorientation and fluctuating states of consciousness.	1. Assess the following physiologic parameters associated with altered levels of consciousness: A. Temperature B. Neurologic signs of increased intracranial pressure C. Drug infusion rates and levels D. Blood gas levels
2. The patient's physiologic status will return to equilibrium.	2. Protect the patient from self-injury.
3. The patient will have regular patterns of sleep and wakefulness.	3. Provide for periods of uninterrupted sleep. Reassure the patient that nightmares associated with critical illness are usually transient.
4. The patient will be oriented as appropriate.	4. Orient patient as appropriate. A. Talk to patients while caring for them. B. Record exactly the patient's reaction to touch, visual, and voice or other auditory stimuli.

(continued)

NURSING DIAGNOSIS Continued

5. *Sensory/perceptual alteration related to decreased level of conciousness (perceiving pattern)*

Patient Outcomes	*Nursing Orders*
	C. Ask the patient to perform certain activities every 4 hours.
	D. Encourage the patient's family to talk to the patient during visits. Ask them to bring in family pictures or tape recordings of family messages, and involve them in ways to stimulate the patient in their absence (*e.g.*, through poster boards or telephone conversations).
	E. See that the patient has a clock and a calendar.
	F. Keep a radio in the patient's room. Play music and change stations, even if the patient is unconscious.
	G. Be creative with music and sound.
	H. Employ reality therapy.
	I. If the patient has a speech impairment, consult with a neurologist, a clinical specialist, and a speech therapist.

Implementation and Evaluation

Delirium is a reversible psychotic state related to a variety of factors, including the nature and severity of the illness, the degree of cerebral hypoxia, metabolic disturbances, medications, procedures, treatments, environment, sadness, pain, and anxiety.[1,31,72,88] Symptoms may include restlessness, agitation, mild confusion, memory loss, disorientation, fluctuating states of consciousness, and perceptual distortions. Delirium occurs more frequently in surgical intensive care units than in medical intensive care units.

Many nursing measures discussed earlier are useful in minimizing the potential for delirium. These are measures to provide adequate sleep, to monitor and minimize harmful effects of the environment, to determine emotional responses to illness, to prevent sensory alterations, and to isolate and deal with factors that contribute to anxiety. Establishing rapport with a patient preoperatively, teaching about sensations that will be experienced, and introducing the possibility that bad dreams may occur after surgery should reduce the likelihood of delirium.

If delirium does develop, the nurse must assess what physiologic factors might have contributed to its onset (*e.g.*, a very high temperature, too rapid an infusion of lidocaine or atropine, a low PaO_2), and the impact of environmental and psychologic factors. The delirious patient may find it helpful to talk about what is being experienced. Presence of family members may calm the patient and diminish the need for restraints. Although the patient needs protection from self-injury, restraints may only increase agitation. Once the delirium has passed, the patient may wish to talk about the experience.

Level of consciousness is an evaluative indicator for this diagnosis. The nurse needs to evaluate the patient's status relative to expected effects of the disease process, medications administered, the environment, and psychologic factors that impact level of consciousness. Effectiveness of interventions is evaluated by change in the patient's level of consciousness and orientation.

NURSING DIAGNOSIS

6. *Impaired verbal communication patterns related to intubation, depressed cerebration, or loss of physical strength coupled with fear and anxiety (communicating pattern)*

Patient Outcomes	*Nursing Orders*
1. The patient will be able to communicate needs and wishes.	1. Ask simple, direct questions. Position the patient so that a signal for help can be communicated.
2. The patient will be able to express fears and anxieties associated with loss of speech.	2. Allow time for the patient to receive, interpret, and respond to verbal messages. Provide a pad and pencil for the patient's use.
3. The patient will be a participant in two-way communication.	3. Identify consistent, simple signals for yes and no responses from the patient. If patient is unable to communicate because of intubation, give him a pencil and paper or have him start to spell key words on the nurse's hand with his fingers. Spelling of the entire word is usually not necessary because the letter **P** will frequently prompt the nurse to ask if the patient requires pain medication, or the letter **C** may elicit a question concerning whether the patient needs to cough or is cold.

Implementation and Evaluation

The patient who cannot communicate verbally faces the task of coping with the loss of a capability available since birth. Speech loss may be unexpected, as in traumatic injury or anticipated as in intubation. Even patients who have been prepared for intubation find loss of speech a frightening and anxiety-provoking experience. Patients wonder whether they will ever be able to speak again.

Unable to communicate verbally, the patient writes or signals a response to questions, uses body language, signals a response by using cards with letters, words, or pictures, or takes specific actions. The nurse with sensitivity and empathy can help the patient communicate. While carrying on a monologue, the nurse observes patient reactions and uses these responses to determine the trend of the conversation. The nurse must stand or sit so that the nurse and patient are in eye contact. A hand on the patient can be reassuring as well as sensitive to the patient's responsive movements. The following is an example of communication with a nonverbal patient.

Example

"I'd like to spend a few minutes talking with you about what it's like for you to be a patient here [pause]. Most people tell us it's not easy to be a patient [pause]. They have many questions, concerns, or worries about being ill [pause]. Talking about these concerns and getting answers to questions help them feel more comfortable [pause]. I wonder what some of your thoughts might be or what some of your questions are [pause]. Let's work together to look at these."

After such a beginning, the nurse can become more specific. The more such an approach is used and the broader an understanding of the common areas of concern, the easier and more helpful the approach becomes. Whatever assumptions the nurse makes should be confirmed by the patient. The nurse should accept whatever feelings are expressed, assure the patient that these feelings are shared by others, and plan for appropriate supportive measures. When a patient's anxiety is lessened, concentration and relaxation during potentially stressful procedures, such as being taken off the respirator, are enhanced.

Initially, patient progress toward desired outcomes is evident when the verbally impaired patient is able to communicate "yes" and "no." Further progress is evident when the patient succeeds in communicating additional information. An intervention that results in patient expression of frustration and anxiety without verbalization is significant evidence of intervention effectiveness.

NURSING DIAGNOSIS

7. *Anticipatory grieving related to the terminal nature of the patient's critical illness (feeling pattern)*

Patient Outcomes	*Nursing Orders*
1. The patient, family, and significant others will express fears and other feelings associated with dying and death.	1. Assist the patient and family to focus on what has been accomplished in life. Provide as much privacy as possible.
2. The patient will experience closure on matters of daily living.	2. Provide the opportunity to complete "unfinished business." Fulfill the patient's requests to see a member of the family, lawyer, member of the clergy, or a physician.
3. The patient will be comfortable and participative until death occurs.	3. Evaluate the procedures and treatments that can be discontinued to make the patient more comfortable. Make provisions for someone to remain with the patient all the time if so desired by the patient.

Implementation and Evaluation

Most patients hospitalized in critical care units consider the possibility of dying at one point or another. Those who survive critical illness find that thoughts of death diminish and finally disappear as they progress toward health. The others, the dying patients, face the awesome task of preparing for and adjusting to their impending death. Much has been written about the needs of the dying patient, the stages of the dying process, and predominant feelings during these stages.[16,51] The empathetic nurse recognizes professional responsibility in guiding and supporting the dying patient.

Sensitive, empathetic communication is essential to caring for the dying. Without it, the patient may be isolated, alone, and without solace and comfort. How can communication with the dying patient be initiated and enhanced? First, the nurse must be available, respect needs of the patient relative to pain relief, use touch appropriately, and provide physical care. Caring for repugnant wounds or malodorous drainage can be very difficult. The nurse should anticipate needs for fresh air, mouth care, frequent turning and positioning, light, rest, water, and comfort.

If the patient gives verbal or nonverbal cues that thoughts of death and dying exist, the nurse provides an opportunity for the patient to discuss these thoughts. For some patients, an appropriate answer to the question "Am I going to die?" might be "I don't know, but I wonder what you feel" or "That's a question I don't know how to answer, but what do you think? It must be on your mind."

As in other issues, the words the nurse uses are not as important as the message communicated, namely, that the nurse has heard the patient's words, is willing to hear more, and wonders what thoughts or fears prompted the question or the statement. Whatever the patient answers, the nurse invites elaboration and explanation but accepts patient refusal to share further at any point in the discussion. The nurse clarifies the questions asked and refrains from answering questions immediately or superficially. Honesty, appropriateness, and maintaining hope for the future and trust in the present are considered. If the patient has misinterpreted some information, the nurse may be able to clarify or correct misinterpretations. The nurse also encourages the patient to raise questions and discuss concerns with the physician and significant others.

As the patient talks more about approaching death, the nurse may learn of specific concerns, needs, or fears. Careful listening helps to identify areas for intervention and support.

Patient: I'm dying, you know.
Nurse: Yes, I know. (Gets closer to the patient.) What's it like for you?
Patient: Oh, it's not so bad, I guess, once you get over the shock of it. I mean, there's nothing I can do to stop it; that's the worst of it. It's like looking up and seeing this avalanche of rocks and dirt coming down toward you and knowing you can't get out of the way, no matter what. (Note the denial, then the expression of loss of control, helplessness, and fear of a catastrophic ending.)
Nurse: That seems pretty frightening.
Patient: It is. (Begins to sob.)
Nurse: (Reaching out to patient and putting a hand on his arm, the nurse remains silent while patient cries.)

After this exchange, the nurse might look for ways, however small, to increase the patient's feelings of control over personal care. Measures may be instituted to help the patient view dying as less catastrophic or as less lonely. These measures include reassuring the patient that someone will be available to provide comfort; asking the patient for help in identifying what might make death less frightening and then incorporating these suggestions into the care plan; ensuring effective pain control; administering medication for anxiety or sleep as indicated; allowing the patient either to talk of important matters or to keep silent; helping the patient meet needs for closeness, security, affection from family, friends, or members of the health care team; and accepting the patient's expressions of feelings.

Even though the goal of patient acceptance of impending death is "ideal," it may not be realistic.[77] Progress toward acceptance can be estimated by the degree of comfort and extent of well-being the patient is experiencing. This comfort and well-being may be the consequence of the nurse supporting the patient's coping strategies or the nurse providing the patient opportunities to make decisions regarding personal care.

In the course of listening to a dying patient, the nurse may be struck by the patient's enumeration of and preoccupation with failures, poor decisions, and missed opportunities in life. While refraining from denying nor attempting to argue the patient's statements away, the nurse focuses on what has been accomplished, created, or contributed, such as children, a garden of fresh vegetables, getting to work on time, tolerance of the illness, humor with colleagues at work, a good bowling score. Death may be easier to accept if the patient feels a mark has been left in this world and that others will remember him with fondness and pride.

The nurse cannot take away a patient's death. Through sharing presence, caring, and being, the nurse can provide support so that the patient can participate in defining circumstances of life during the dying process.

NURSING DIAGNOSIS

8. *High risk for violence (self-directed) related to act of sucidial ideation or aggressive suicidal behaviors (feeling pattern)*

Patient Outcomes	*Nursing Orders*
1. The patient will be protected from further self-inflicted injury.	1. Remove harmful objects from the immediate environment. A. Refer the patient to the psychiatric liaison nurse. B. Provide ongoing physical support. C. Permit the patient to talk about the suicide attempt. D. Evaluate the patient's mental status periodically, and report changes promptly. E. Participate in assessing the patient's current suicide risk. F. Observe the patient's reactions to telephone calls, mail, and visitors, as well as the visitors' responses to the patient. G. Be aware of the patient's mood and content of conversation. H. Use resources to help family members deal with feelings about the patient, as well as to gain vital information about the circumstances surrounding the event. I. Chart observations about the patient's behavior or appearance, as well as comments made by the patient.
2. The patient will identify alternatives to suicide for dealing with life problems.	2. After an acute suicide attempt, refer the patient for individual or group therapy. Reassess the patient's ability to deal with life stressors.

Implementation and Evaluation

The patient admitted to a critical care unit after a suicide attempt presents a special challenge to nursing personnel.[32,45,69] Nurses may experience conflicting feelings while caring for such a patient: loathing and contempt, compassion and concern, annoyance and anger, anxiety and fear. Although committed to doing all possible to save the patient, the nurse may also question why time, energy, and effort are spent to save someone who wanted to die. Feelings may be heightened if previous suicide attempts were made, especially if the same nurses cared for the patient in the previous recovery process; if the suicide attempt seems manipulative; if the patient had no "good" reason (in staff judgment) to attempt suicide; or if the patient expresses hostility toward the rescuers. If the patient acknowledges foolishness, expresses remorse, vows not to attempt suicide again, accepts psychiatric intervention, or has a "good" reason for the suicide attempt, staff may respond more positively. Feelings may intensify as the nurse observes reactions of and interacts with family members.

Example

A 31-year-old married mother of two daughters was admitted to the respiratory critical care unit following an overdose of glutethimide. As she regained consciousness, she attempted to remove herself from the respirator and pull out her intravenous infusion. Given a pad of paper and pencil, she scribbled on the pad, "Let me die." Her husband remained in the waiting room, alternately wringing his hands in despair and asking angrily, "Why did she do this to me? What's wrong with her?" The patient's mother shouted to the husband through her tears, "It's all your fault. You drove her to it!" Two small girls were huddled together on the waiting room couch crying quietly for their mother. Their father and grandmother appeared unaware of their presence.

It is important for the nurse to acknowledge personal feelings and responses to the patient who has attempted suicide, so that nursing care is not hindered. It is not necessary for the nurse to accept or agree with the patient's desire to die in order to accept the patient as someone who needs care.

Use of psychiatric resource personnel after admission may help with interviewing the patient, assessment of mental status and suicide risk, suggestions for management and treatment, and provision of ongoing support or therapy. The patient may require constant observation and protection from further self-injury. Unnecessary and potentially dangerous supplies and equipment should be removed from the patient's immediate environment. The nurse should note when and if the patient talks of further suicide attempts and be sensitive to changes in mood.

NURSING DIAGNOSIS

9. *Hopelessness related to perceived change in quality of life and impending death (perceiving pattern)*

Patient Outcomes	*Nursing Orders*

1. The patient participates in identifies short-range goals or activities for self-care and personal management.
2. The patient expresses feelings regarding loss of valued friends, activities, and future-oriented dreams.
	1. Be physically available to the patient at frequent intervals.
	   A. Involve patient in decisions regarding personal care.
	   B. Develop a plan for each shift with the patient.
	2. Provide truthful information to the patient and family.
	   A. Focus conversations on current patient capabilities.
	   B. Involve significant others in the patient's care.
	   C. Use role rehearsal with the patient to practice responses to life-event changes.

Implementation and Evaluation

Manifestations of hopelessness include apathy and inability to perceive acceptable resolution of problems. Expressions of hopelessness may be as follows: I just have no reason to live; I know I will never achieve what I had wanted; I have no future. Nursing observations of hopelessness include passivity, decreased verbalization, lack of interest, and decreased problem solving ability.[11,14,15,71,77] The hopeless patient is unable to identify personal coping resources.

Hope is often contagious.[77] If people around the patient are hopeful, this encourages patient hopefulness. The nurse is in a key position to assist the patient in re-evaluating goals and identifying ways to participate in self-care and decision mak-ing. Nursing interventions for the patient experiencing hopelessness include involvement of significant others in patient care. The nurse may need to assist the family and friends in providing an environment that provides warmth, genuineness, and truthfulness.

Sometimes persons hospitalized with illnesses secondary to human immunosuppressive viruses have lost social support that was available in the past because fear and social stigma surround the disease.[34,54,69] False optimism and benign reassurance do not provide hope for these patients. Hope must evolve from the belief that better times are ahead, perhaps a moment with less pain or easier breathing. Interventions are derived using the patient's current status as a baseline.

As in other situations, patients experiencing hopelessness

use coping mechanisms for self-protection. The nurse can be truthful while assisting the patient to focus on goals for the present. The nurse needs to help the patient deal with current reality and exercise choices available at each point during hospitalization.

The nurse evaluates effectiveness of interventions based on change in patient's behavior. Does the patient turn toward visitors? Is there less sighing?[11,15] Effectiveness of interventions is also reflected in a patient's reference to the future or a spontaneous expression that the patient is "feeling better." If the patient begins to make plans for discharge and realistic life changes, the nurse's plan of care has been successful.

FAMILY RESPONSES TO CRITICAL ILLNESS

Just as the patient experiences a variety of feelings in response to illness, so do the relatives experience anger, sadness, guilt, frustration, fear, anxiety, and hope. They cope with these feelings in many ways, including being overprotective, crying, holding a "living wake" at the bedside, complaining about care, blaming the patient, seeking reassurance, expressing anger, and using denial. The family may even abandon the patient. The nurse may need to shield the patient from the wrath of the family. Nurses are appropriately concerned about how relatives express their needs, how those needs are met, and how they affect the patient.[12,13,22,28,34,37,42,68,70,85,92]

As soon as possible, the nurse should orient the family to the unit. The nurse should give them a tour, introduce them to staff, and acquaint them with protocol. Family members should be encouraged to write down questions to facilitate asking for answers during patient visits. Relatives can be given written information about the unit to read at a less anxious moment. A comfortable and convenient visitor's lounge with a rest area and hot plate, where visitors can relax, rest, wait, cry, eat, and talk informally with members of other families, reduces the discomfort and distress of families of patients in intensive care. Volunteer personnel assigned to the visitors' lounge may be useful in supporting family members, answering simple questions, and explaining hospital routine.

The patient's relatives or significant others should be interviewed by the nurse to complete gaps in information about the patient and to assess the relatives' response to illness and need for support. A supportive comment and question such as "Your husband is stable today. How have you been holding up through all of this?" gives the wife an opportunity to share reactions to the patient's illness. The nurse may learn that the wife or some other relative feels guilty about having contributed to the patient's trauma or illness (e.g., driving the car in which the patient was injured or carelessly disposing of cigarettes that started the fire in which the patient was burned). Relatives may express anger that the patient became ill or that the patient is not cooperating in getting better. Some people may have ambivalent feelings toward the patient and feel frightened or guilty about their wish to see the patient dead. In addition to meeting the initial needs expressed by relatives, the nurse can introduce family members to one or more resource people available for support: a social worker, psychiatric nurse clinician, psychiatrist, dietitian, chaplain, ombudsman, patient advocate, or volunteer.

Many relatives are reluctant to approach the critically ill patient. Initially, the nurse accompanies visitors to the bedside and encourages them to touch and talk with the patient. If possible, equipment that precludes close contact with the patient should be removed. Specific procedures for visitors of the critically ill patient (e.g., gowning and gloving) or patient restrictions (e.g., oral intake) must be explained. Evaluation of relatives' attitudes and behaviors assists in planning appropriate patient care interventions and family teaching. Do the patient's relatives want to be involved or uninvolved? Do they have a need to keep the patient ill? Are they pushing the patient to be independent too soon or keeping the patient dependent too long? Do their values support the patient's wishes for care and possible intervention limitations?

Relatives may want to be supportive of the patient, but they need help in doing so. They need preparation for questions patients may ask of them, such as questions about dying, or behavior the patient may exhibit, such as attempting to get out of bed. Those who show a willingness to become involved in the patient's care can be given tasks such as helping to bathe the patient, reading to the patient, or bringing some special food from home. Through observation and interaction with the family, the nurse can determine which relative is most supportive. A significant family member may be willing to be "on call" if the patient requires a visit, especially during the night. A family contact person can be kept informed of changes in the patient's condition and communicate the news to other family members.

Relatives might also help the patient maintain an interest in life. Perhaps they will contact employers, friends, or an organization that would wish to remember the patient with cards or notes. Being remembered by family and friends is especially important when illness extends over several weeks.

Some nursing units permit the relative closest to the patient to call at any time. Relatives find this option highly supportive, and staff members say relatives rarely abuse it. Other units have a calling hour in which one phone call per family is encouraged. Still others have a policy by which the nurse caring for the patient telephones the family daily and gives a report on patient progress or condition. A provision for relatives to talk with knowledgeable nurses by telephone enables family members to ask questions about the patient, relay messages, and alleviate anxiety without having to travel to the hospital.

The group setting can be an effective means of providing support to family members. For example, when a patient is admitted to the critical care unit, relatives may be informed that group discussions for relatives are held routinely at specific times, locations, and days. When family members participate in such meetings, the nurse leader introduces participants and explains that discussions are held to provide an opportunity to share reactions and feelings related to the experience of having a critically ill relative. Information about the condition of specific patients need not be given in the meeting, but issues of general concern can be discussed and questions answered. Group meetings can be both informative for the staff and supportive to the family members. Relatives who attend may become more comfortable at the patient's bedside, develop rapport with and trust in staff members, and meet needs for information and support. Techniques of group intervention have been used with relatives of patients who have myocardial infarctions,[13] relatives of burned patients,[12] and relatives of renal transplant patients. Regardless of the support method (telephone, individual contact, or group contact), caring for relatives and their reactions diminishes feelings of neglect or jealousy about the care and attention the patient is receiving.

Relatives of dying patients may have additional needs and heightened emotional reactions.[43,80] Some may need help in dealing with feelings so that they can be available and supportive to their loved one. Most need affirmation in discussing the illness and death and in showing emotion, such as crying or hugging the patient. They also need to know that laughter and joking, a sense of humor, have a place in relating to the patient. Those who say they do not want the patient to know that death is near may need to hear that the patient already "knows" the diagnosis, even though he was not specifically "told."[16] Fears of "falling apart" might concern the relatives rather than the patient. Some relatives may ask for information about autopsy or donating organs for transplantation. Referring to autopsy as an "examination after death" may make it more acceptable to family members.

When the patient dies, relatives need to hear from the physician what occurred and why. Although people are never totally prepared for the death of a loved one, relatives of a patient who dies suddenly have had no time to anticipate and to prepare for their loss; they may be in severe shock. The family requires privacy, support, and an opportunity to talk about and react to the loss. Family members may withdraw, cry, or get angry. An unaccompanied relative should not leave the hospital alone, especially after an unexpected death. A member of the staff or a sensitive volunteer might wait with the relative until transportation has been arranged.

After relatives have begun adjustment, they may wish to learn and talk more about the circumstances surrounding the loved one's death. The need for information and closure may not occur for several days or even weeks. After the funeral, family members may return to the hospital one more time to bring closure to the relationship developed with the patient's caregivers.

One hospital has attempted to meet relatives' needs for support not only while the patient is hospitalized but also after death. During the patient's hospital stay, a chaplain visits frequently with family members and establishes a relationship. Periodic phone calls are made to the family. After the patient dies, the chaplain is available to participate in whatever rituals are observed or burial services held. Once a month, a religious memorial service is held at the hospital to remember all patients who died in the previous month. Relatives of deceased patients, and staff who cared for them, are invited to attend. At that time, many relatives finish their "unfinished business." They approach staff members who cared for their loved one and ask, "How was it?" or "What did he or she say?" Staff members find in the service an opportunity to say good-bye to the patient and the family. This ritual, a formalization of the grieving process, is healthy; it permits discharge of pain and restores equilibrium.[26]

THE NURSE'S RESPONSE

Highly motivated, highly dedicated, highly skilled—these adjectives only partially describe nurses working in critical care. Critical care nursing requires technical competence, knowledge of physiologic and psychologic responses to injury or illness, ability to make perceptive observations and critical judgments, and, above all, compassion for and commitment to patients. At its best, critical care nursing can be rewarding, challenging,

satisfying, and fulfilling. At its worst, it can be depressing, demoralizing, frustrating, infuriating, exhausting, and heart rending.

A wide range of feelings are evoked in the critical care setting: joy, fulfillment, satisfaction, sadness, anger, guilt, fear, and anxiety. These feelings can be uncomfortable, threatening, and even frightening to nurses who experience them and to nurses who perceive them in colleagues. Nurses deal with these feelings in a variety of ways. If ways of coping increase anxiety, diminish self-esteem, decrease patient care quality, or foster job dissatisfaction, they are maladaptive. Some examples of maladaptive behaviors are as follows:

- Forming close bonds with critical care staff and disassociating with others
- Withdrawing from or avoiding patients
- Experiencing exhaustion
- Having nightmares about work
- Displacing feelings on others
- Denying or repressing feelings
- Criticizing involvement, commitment or performance of others
- Fostering overdependent behavior in the patient
- "Acting-out" feelings by calling in ill, coming to work late, drinking excessively, leaving work before completing assigned responsibilities
- Focusing on technical aspects of care
- Exercising excessive control, such as by enforcing rigid visiting hours
- Manifesting hyperkinetic behavior
- Regressing
- Rationalizing actions or behavior

Nurses in critical care settings have consistently identified the following as sources of stress in their work that generate uncomfortable feelings:[7,18,34,39,40,42,50,80] the patient and patient care; nurse-nurse relationships, including relationships with peers, head nurse, supervisor, and nurses on other units; nurse-doctor relationships; families; and the work environment. In addition, there are some sources of stress peculiar to individual units, such as required gowns and masks, too few ancillary or clerical staff, and lack of supportive resources.

In each critical care unit, nurses need to assess continually their responses to work as a whole as well as to particularly stressful aspects of the job. Sometimes assessment is done in an informal way, such as over coffee or after the change-of-shift report. Some critical care units have regularly scheduled weekly meetings with resource persons or facilitators and informal "as-needed" meetings to identify, acknowledge, and share feelings; clarify and review the realistic aspects of the work situation; and receive feedback and support. Nurses often feel relieved, replenished, and supported by such meetings and are able to integrate what they have learned and experienced into their care of patients. When continuing sources of stress for the group are identified, the nurses plan how to eliminate or reduce them. Likewise, through group processes, nurses collectively identify satisfying aspects of work and share ways to enhance or increase these aspects.

The nurse who accepts and expresses feelings appropriately and copes effectively with stressors experienced feels happier and more satisfied, and can be more open and giving to patients, families, and colleagues.[33]

SUMMARY

Patients' responses to acute illness, the assessment of those responses, and the factors affecting those responses have been discussed. Suggestions have been offered for nursing intervention in general and specific situations. The responses of families and nurses have been discussed briefly.

The objectives of the critical care nurse are the reduction of patient anxiety and the promotion of patient comfort. Intervention, therefore, includes learning and fostering that which is essential, desirable, or supportive to the patient. The critical care nurse also learns about and attempts to minimize anything that is demeaning, frightening, anxiety provoking, or nonsupportive to the patient. The burden is not carried in isolation; there are numerous resources within the community and hospital setting to help nurses identify and meet emotional needs of patients. Nurses in critical care settings play unique and meaningful roles in assessing reactions, identifying needs, and initiating the interventions responsive to those needs. Thus, critical care nurses contribute to patients' immediate comfort and well-being and to long-range adjustment to critical illness.[48]

DIRECTIONS FOR FUTURE RESEARCH

Researchable questions concerning psychosocial aspects of critical care nursing have been ranked in high priority in a study conducted by the American Association of Critical-Care Nurses. For example, the question receiving the highest priority was "What are the most effective ways of promoting optimum sleep-rest patterns in the critically ill patient and preventing sleep deprivation?"

Other possible questions include identification of specific interventions to involve families in stress reduction; the timing of relaxation techniques relative to physiologic indices of stress; effects of positioning, touch, and social support on recovery time; and development of modalities to increase tenure of nursing personnel in critical care settings. Research is vital to the development of nursing practice and science. The practitioner needs only to look at those aspects of the critical care environment that stimulate the question, "Why?"

REFERENCES

1. Adams, M., Hanson, R., Norkool, D., *et al.* Psychological responses in critical care units. *Am. J. Nurs.* 78:1504, 1978.
2. Adler, M. L. Kidney transplantation and coping mechanisms. *Psychosomatics* 13:337, 1972.
3. Andreasen, N. J. C., Noyes, R., Hartford, C. C., *et al.* Management of emotional problems in seriously burned adults. *N. Engl. J. Med.* 286:65, 1972.
4. Barry, P. D. *Psychosocial Nursing Assessment and Intervention.* Philadelphia: J. B. Lippincott, 1984.
5. Beck, C. K., Rawlins, R. P., and Williams, S. R. *Mental Health Nursing—A Holistic Life-Cycle Approach* (2nd ed.). St. Louis: C. V. Mosby, 1988.
6. Benoliel, J. O., and VanDeVelde, S. As the patient views the intensive-care unit and the coronary-care unit. *Heart Lung* 4:260, 1975.
7. Bilodeau, C. B. The nurse and her reactions to critical-care nursing. *Heart Lung* 2:358, 1973.
8. Bohachick, P. Progressive relaxation training in cardiac rehabilitation: Effect on psychological variables. *Nurs. Res.* 33:283–287, 1984.
9. Bolin, R. H. Sensory deprivation: An overview. *Nurs. Forum* 13: 240, 1974.
10. Breu, C., Dracup, K., and Walden, J. Integration of nursing diagnoses in the critical care nursing literature. *Heart Lung* 16:(6): 605–616, 1987.
11. Brockopp, D. Y., Hayko, D., Davenport, W., *et al.* Personal control and the needs for hope and information among adults diagnosed with cancer. *Cancer Nurs.* 12:112–116, 1989.
12. Brodland, G. A., and Adreasen, N. J. C. Adjustment Problems of the Family of the Burn Patient. In R. H. Moos (ed.), *Coping with Physical Illness.* New York: Plenum, 1977.
13. Brown, A. J. Effect of family visits on the blood pressure and heart rate of patients in the coronary-care unit. *Heart Lung* 5:291, 1976.
14. Bruss, C. R. Nursing diagnosis of hopelessness. *J. Psychosoc. Nurs.* 26(3):28–31, 1988.
15. Carpenito, L. J. *Handbook of Nursing Diagnosis 1989–90.* Philadelphia: J. B. Lippincott, 1989.
16. Cassem, N. H. What you can do for dying patients. *Med. Dimens.* 2:29, 1973.
17. Cassem, N. H., and Hackett, T. P. Psychiatric consultation in a coronary-care unit. *Ann. Intern. Med.* 75:9, 1971.
18. Cassem, N. H., and Hackett, T. P. Sources of tension for the CCU nurse. *Am. J. Nurs.* 72:1426, 1972.
19. Cassem, N. H., and Hackett, T. P. Psychological rehabilitation of myocardial infarction patients in the acute phase. *Heart Lung* 2: 382, 1973.
20. Cassem, N. H., and Hackett, T. P. Stress on the nurse and therapist in the intensive-care unit and coronary-care unit. *Heart Lung* 4: 252, 1975.
21. Clark, P. E., and Clar, M. J. The therapeutic touch: Is there a scientific basis for the practice? *Nurs. Res.* 33(1):37, 1973.
22. Clark, S. Nursing diagnosis: Ineffective coping. II. Planning care. *Heart Lung* 16:677–683, 1987.
23. Cosgrove, S. The nurses' contribution to the humanisation of health services in the presence of increasing technology. *NZ Nurs. J.* November: 12, 1982.
24. Cronin, S. N., and Harrison, B. Importance of nursing caring behaviors as perceived by patients after myocardial infarction. *Heart Lung* 17:374–380, 1988.
25. Davidson, S. P. Nursing management of emotional reactions of severely burned patients during the acute phase. *Heart Lung* 2: 370, 1973.
26. Deliman, T., and Smolowe, J. S. *Holistic Medicine: Harmony of Body-Mind-Spirit.* Reston, VA: Reston Publishing Co., 1982.
27. Dossey, L. Care giving and natural systems theory. *Top. Clin. Nurs.* 3(4):21, 1982.
28. Dracup, K., and Breau, C. Helping the spouses of critically ill patients. *Am. J. Nurs.* 78:51, 1978.
29. Drew, N. Exclusion and confirmation: A phenomenology of patients' experiences with caregivers. *IMAGE: J. Nurs. Scholarship* 18(2):39–43, 1986.
30. Dunnington, C. S., Johnson, N. J., Finkelmeier, B. A., *et al.* Patients with heart rhythm disturbances: Variables associated with increased psychologic distress. *Heart Lung* 17:381–389, 1988.
31. Easton, C., and MacKenzie, F. Sensory-perceptual alterations: Delirium in the intensive care unit. *Heart Lung* 17:229–235, 1988.
32. Farberow, H. Suicide prevention in the hospital. *Hosp. Community Psychiatry* 32:99, 1981.
33. Ferrucci, P. *What We May Be.* Los Angeles: J. P. Tarcher, 1982.
34. Flaskerud, J. H. AIDS: Psychosocial aspects. *J. Psychosoc. Nurs.* 25(12):9–16, 1987.
35. Froese, A., Hackett, T. P., Cassem, N. H., *et al.* Trajectories of anxiety and depression in denying and nondenying acute myocardial infarction patients during hospitalization. *J. Psychosom. Res.* 18:137, 1974.
36. Froese, A., Vasques, E., Cassem, N. H., *et al.* Validation of anxiety, depression and denial scales in a coronary care unit. *J. Psychosom. Res.* 18:137, 1974.

37. Gilliss, C. L. Reducing family stress during and after coronary artery bypass surgery. *Nurs. Clin. North Am.* 19(2):103, 1984.

38. Hackett, T. P., Cassem, N. H., and Wishnie, H. A. The coronary care unit: An appraisal of its psychologic hazards. *N. Engl. J. Med.* 279:1365–1370, 1968.

39. Hackett, T. P., and Cassem, N. H. Development of a quantitative rating scale to assess denial. *J. Psychosom. Res.* 18:93, 1974.

40. Hau, S., and Wray, L. Codependency: Nurses who give too much. *Am. J. Nurs.* 89:1456, 1989.

41. Hanlon, R. Contracting for care. *Am. J. Nurs.* 84:335, 1984.

42. Hickey, M., and Lewandowski, L. Critical care nurses' role with families: A descriptive study. *Heart Lung* 17:670–676, 1988.

43. Hine, V. H. Holistic dying: The role of the nurse clinician. *Top. Clin. Nurs.* 3(4):45, 1982.

44. Hoffman, M., Donckers, S., and Hauser, M. The effect of nursing intervention on stress factors perceived by patients in a coronary care unit. *Heart Lung* 7:804, 1978.

45. Holland, J., and Plumb, M. Management of the serious suicide attempt: A special ICU nursing problem. *Heart Lung* 2:376, 1973.

46. Holmes, T. H., and Rahe, R. H. The social readjustment rating scale. *J. Psychosom. Res.* 11:213, 1967.

47. Johnson, J. E., and Lauver, D. R. Alternative explanations of coping with stressful experiences associated with physical illness. *Adv. Nurs. Sci.* 11:39–52, 1989.

48. Johnston, R. L. The holistic experience of stress: Opportunity for growth or illness. *Occup. Health Nurs.* 28(12):15, 1980.

49. Klein, R. F., Kliner, V. A., Zipes, D. P., et al. Transfer from a coronary care unit: Some adverse responses. *Arch. Intern. Med.* 122:104, 1968.

50. Kornfeld, D. S. The Hospital Environment: Its Impact on the Patient. In R. H. Moos (ed.), *Coping with Physical Illness.* New York: Plenum, 1977.

51. Kubler-Ross, E. *On Death and Dying.* New York: Macmillan, 1969.

52. Langsley, D. G. The Mental Status Examination. In G. Usdin and J. M. Lewis (eds.), *Psychiatry and General Medical Practice.* New York: McGraw-Hill, 1979.

53. Lanuza, D. M., and Marotta, S. F. Endocrine and psychologic responses of patients to cardiac pacemaker implantation. *Heart Lung* 16:496–505, 1987.

54. Lasher, A. T., and Ragsdale, D. The significant other's role in improving quality of life in persons with AIDS dementia complex. *J. Neurosci. Nurs.* 21:250–255, 1989.

55. Lewandowski, L. A., and Kositsky, A. M. Research priorities for critical care nursing: A study by the American Associate of Critical-Care Nurses. *Heart Lung* 12:35, 1983.

56. Lown, B., Temte, J. V., Reich, P., et al. Recurring ventricular fibrillation in the absence of coronary heart disease. *N. Engl. J. Med.* 294:623, 1976.

57. Lynch, J. J., Thomas, S. A., Paskewitz, D. A., et al. Human contact and cardiac arrhythmia in a coronary care unit. *Psychosom. Med.* 39:188, 1977.

58. Maron, L., Bryan-Brown, C. W., and Shoemaker, W. C. Toward a unified approach to psychological factors in the ICU. *Crit. Care Med.* 1:81, 1973.

59. Mattsson, E. I. Psychological aspects of severe physical injury and its treatment. *J. Trauma* 15:217, 1975.

60. McClure, D. L. Wellness: A holistic concept. *Health Values* 6(5): 23, 1982.

61. McCorkle, R. Effects of touch on seriously ill patients. *Nurs. Res.* 23:125, 1974.

62. McGlashan, R. Strategies for rebuilding self-esteem for the cardiac patient. *Dimens. Crit. Care Nurs.* 7(1):28–38, 1988.

63. McKay, S. Wholistic health care challenge to health care providers. *J. Allied Health* 9(3):194, 1980.

64. Minckley, B. B., Burrows, D., Ehrat, K., et al. Myocardial infarct stress-of-transfer inventory: Development of a research tool. *Nurs. Res.* 28:4, 1979.

65. Mumford, E., Schlesinger, H. J., and Glass, G. V. The effects of psychological intervention on recovery from surgery and heart attacks: An analysis of the literature. *Am. J. Publ. Health* 72(2): 141–151, 1982.

66. Murray, R. L. E. Assessment of psychologic status in the surgical ICU patient. *Nurs. Clin. North Am.* 10:69, 1975.

67. Nelms, B. C., and Mullins, R. G. Evolution of holistic practice in nurse practitioners. *Pediatr. Nurs.* 6(5):27, 1980.

68. Nyamathi, A. D. The coping responses of female spouses of patients with myocardial infarction. *Heart Lung* 16:86–92, 1987.

69. Nyamathi, A., and van Servellen, G. Maladaptive coping in the critically ill population with acquired immunodeficiency syndrome: Nursing assessment and treatment. *Heart Lung* 18:113–120, 1989.

70. O'Keeffe, B., and Gilliss, C. L. Family care in the coronary care unit: An analysis of clinical nurse specialist intervention. *Heart Lung* 17:191–198, 1988.

71. O'Malley, P. A., and Menke, E. Relationship of hope and stress after myocardial infarction. *Heart Lung* 17:184–190, 1988.

72. Rahe, R. H., McKean, J. D., and Arthur, R. J. A longitudinal study of life change and illness patterns. *J. Psychosom. Res.* 10:355, 1967.

73. Rahe, R. H., Romo, M., Bennett, L., et al. Recent life changes, myocardial infarction, and abrupt coronary death. *Arch. Intern. Med.* 133:221, 1974.

74. Randolph, G. L. Therapeutic and physical touch: Physiological response to stressful stimuli. *Nurs. Res.* 33(1):33, 1984.

75. Richards, K. C., and Bairnsfather, L. A description of night sleep patterns in the critical care unit. *Heart Lung* 17:35–42, 1988.

76. Rowe, M. A., and Weinert, C. The CCU experience: Stressful or reassuring? *Dimens. Crit. Care Nurs.* 6:341–348, 1987.

77. Scanlon, C. Creating a vision of hope: The challenge of palliative care. *Oncol. Nurs. Forum* 16:491–496, 1989.

78. Schoenhofer, S. O. Affectional touch in critical care nursing: A descriptive study. *Heart Lung* 18:146–154, 1989.

79. Selye, H. *Stress of Life* (2nd ed.). New York: McGraw-Hill, 1976.

80. Simon, L. The therapist-patient relationship: A holistic view. *Am. J. Psychoanal.* 41(3):213, 1981.

81. Slaby, A. E., and Glicksman, A. S. *Adapting to Life-Threatening Illness.* New York: Praeger Publishers, 1985.

82. Slay, C. L. Myocardial infarction and stress. *Nurs. Clin. North Am.* 11:329, 1976.

83. Solack, S. O. Assessment of psychogenic stresses in the coronary patient. *Cardiovasc. Nurs.* 15:116, 1979.

84. Stephenson, C. A. Stress in critically ill patients. *Am. J. Nurs.* 77: 1806, 1977.

85. Thornton, J., Berry, J., and Dal Santo, J. Neonatal intensive care: The nurses's role in supporting the family. *Nurs. Clin. North Am.* 19(1):125, 1984.

86. Van Bree, N. S. Sexuality, nursing practice, and the person with cardiac disease. *Nurs. Forum* 14:397, 1975.

87. Van der Poel, C. J. Suffering and healing: the process of growth. *Hosp. Prog.* 62(2):42, 1981.

88. Wall, T. Creating a healthy psychic environment. *Dimens. Health Serv.* 57(9):38, 1980.

89. Welch-McCaffrey, D. Cancer, anxiety, and quality of life. *Cancer Nurse* 8:151–158, 1985.

90. Wilson, V. S. Identification of stressors related to patients' psychologic responses to the surgical intensive care unit. *Heart Lung* 16:267–273, 1987.

91. Woods, N. F., and Falk, S. A. Noise stimuli in the acute care area. *Nurs. Res.* 23:144, 1974.

92. Zbilut, J. P. Holistic nursing: The transcendental factor. *Nurs. Forum* 19(1):45, 1980.

9

Legal Aspects of the Care and Treatment of the Critically Ill Patient

R. Jack Ayres, Jr.

HEALING AND WHOLENESS

Healing can be related to spiritual experiences, because it is also a state that requires its own kind of oneness. Healing is that process of bringing all the parts of yourself (the physical, mental, emotional, social, and spiritual) together at deep levels of inner knowing. When healing or wholeness is experienced, a sense of living in peace results that can be similar to the universal expression of oneness and unity. The result is a higher degree of integration, balance, and happiness in your life as you become aware of the importance and relationship of all parts of life. To be healed, then, is to become whole, and in the highest forms of healing, it is to know and feel the wholeness, the unity, that has occurred. This experience is extraordinarily spiritual in its essence.

Higher health, spirituality, and wholeness necessitate a world view different from that of ordinary day-to-day experience. You become more aware of the patterns and processes that evolve as you open yourself to life's journey. This journey also involves being with others as they explore their spirituality. Higher health and wholeness do not require health insurance, for they cannot fail. Spirituality is timeless and infinite; thus, you can neither attain it nor escape it. It is here now, and it belongs, at this very moment, to everyone. It is in you, now.

LEARNING OBJECTIVES

After reading this chapter, the nurse should be able to do the following:

1. State three levels of patient consent.
2. Compare and contrast consent protocol for the adult and the child.
3. Act according to the law when faced with special problems in consent protocol.
4. Identify common theories of liability and responsibility for patient care.
5. Differentiate individual responsibilities in claims prevention, counseling, and personal conduct.

PATIENT CONSENT AND THE LAW

Obtaining and maintaining patient consent for treatment should be one of the first considerations in every encounter between the practitioner and the patient. In the past, the legal concept of consent has, to a regrettable degree, been bound up in rumor, myth, half-truth, and outright gossip. Accordingly, it is necessary to discuss the concept of patient consent in some detail, particularly as it applies to the emergent or critically ill patient.

The word *consent*, in a medicolegal context, describes a situation in which the patient has given permission to a health care provider to enable the practitioner to treat or care for the patient. Generally speaking, consent may be either "expressed," in the sense that it is affirmatively communicated by words or actions, or "implied" by legal presumption. It is imperative that the patient's consent be obtained before treatment is instituted because (1) the rational and conscious patient has a substantial constitutional right to refuse or accept treatment that must be scrupulously observed and respected, (2) treatment of a patient without consent may give rise to potential civil and criminal liability, and (3) the practitioner's knowledge of the law of patient consent may reduce or avoid entirely critical delay in initiating required patient care.

Several years ago, the author, at Parkland Memorial Hospital in Dallas, TX, developed a medicolegal system for determining patient consent that has been in use for some years with considerable apparent success. The Parkland system involves recognition of consent at three levels (Table 9–1).

The first level of consent, which is the highest and most desirable level, is referred to as *voluntary consent*, or what may be described as "expressed" consent. The essence of this level of consent is a voluntary and informed agreement between the practitioner and the patient about the scope and course of the patient's treatment.

The second level of consent is referred to as *involuntary consent*, in which the patient's consent is supplied by the process of the law itself, regardless of the patient's wishes. Examples are treatment that is ordered by a court because the patient is mentally ill, under arrest, or unable to consent for some other exceptional reason. In cases of involuntary consent, treatment may be rendered only in strict compliance with the order of the court and the directions of the judge issuing the order.

The third level of consent, and consent of last resort, is referred to as *implied consent*. Implied consent is said to exist when the patient is unconscious or unable to communicate and is suffering from what reasonably appears to be a life-threatening disease or illness. In such cases, the law presumes that the patient would desire treatment to be instituted and, thus, would deem the patient to have consented implicitly to the indicated care or treatment. (Each of these levels of consent

should be considered in connection with the following section on special problems in consent as well.)

Having considered the levels of consent necessary to obtain the required permission to treat the patient, the practitioner should next adopt a systematic approach to analysis of consent. The practitioner must first consider and exhaust all possibilities of consent at the first level before proceeding to the second and all alternatives at the second level before proceeding to the third. By using this systematic approach to patient consent, the chance of error in determining the presence or absence of consent may be reduced significantly, if not eliminated.

The first step in systematic consent is determining whether the patient is an adult or a minor under the laws of the state in question. Generally, an adult is any person over the age of 18 years, any person who is or has been validly married, or any person who has had the disabilities of minority removed by court order. All other persons may be legally considered to be minors.

Having determined that the patient is either an adult or a child, the practitioner proceeds to an analysis under each category.

THE ADULT

The first level of the systematic approach is to seek the adult's voluntary and informed consent to treatment. In this case, the practitioner simply asks for or responds to the patient's request for treatment. The patient's response should be charted and thoroughly documented in the patient's record. If there are any factors that may influence or affect the patient's ability to make a knowledgeable and informed choice, such as the administration of medications, intoxication, or other conditions, these likewise should be charted. Generally speaking, the requirement for obtaining a so-called informed consent in most jurisdictions at present rests on the treating physician or consulting physician rendering the treatment. However, given the rapid rise of technology, the accompanying sophistication of the nursing profession, and the advent of the nurse practitioner, it is not unreasonable to assume that at some point in the future courts will require professional nurses to likewise obtain informed consent before initiating patient treatment. If any question of informed consent arises, the nurse or practitioner involved should seek competent legal advice before proceeding.

If the practitioner is unable to obtain voluntary consent for patient treatment, the second level—involuntary consent—is reached. The circumstances in which involuntary consent arises clinically are limited and are strictly and narrowly defined by the court order in question. In general, involuntary consent does not authorize the rendering of general or palliative care or, indeed, any care that is not necessary to treat a life-threatening disease or illness without advance and specific permission of the court.

If the practitioner is unable to obtain either voluntary or involuntary consent, there is one final recourse, which is consent of last resort: implied consent. Implied consent requires that the patient must be unconscious or unable to communicate and suffering from what reasonably appears to be a life-threatening disease, illness, or injury. Several of the features of implied consent should be discussed. First, the truly unconscious patient is unable to maintain protective reflexes, including a patent airway, and may therefore be considered

Table 9-1
Schematic Diagram of the Parkland Model of Consent

PATIENT	
Adult	**Child**
Voluntary Consent	
By patients themselves	Special circumstances
	Pregnancy
	Armed Forces
	VD
	Drug abuse
	Child abuse
	Emancipated
	Surrogate or substitute
	Parent or guardian
	Grandparent
	Adult aunt or uncle
	Adult sibling
	Written consent
Involuntary Consent	
By court order	By court order
From peace officer in some circumstances	From peace officer in some ciurcumstances
	From child welfare worker in case of abuse or delinquency
Implied Consent	
Unconscious patient	No parental refusal
Life-threatening illness or disease	Life-threatening illness or disease

to have a life-threatening disease or illness by definition. Second, the ability of the patient to communicate should not be confused with his or her competence or inability to communicate medically relevant information. As will be noted in the section on special problems of consent, if patient competence is an issue, different rules apply. Finally, the determination of the life-threatening character of the disease, illness, or injury should be weighted heavily in favor of the patient's longevity. Stated differently, only in cases in which a clear threat to life can be ruled out affirmatively should treatment be withheld in the implied-consent case.

THE CHILD

The systematic approach to obtaining consent applies with equal facility to the treatment of minors or children, with some modification. Generally, children may not legally consent to their own treatment. Therefore, in order to obtain the first level of voluntary consent, the practitioner must identify one of two subcategories: so-called special circumstances or surrogate consent (*i.e.*, consent by another on the child's behalf). If special circumstances are absent, the practitioner should proceed to the determination of surrogate consent, in that order.

Generally, special circumstances enable the practitioner to treat the child with the child's own cognitive consent if the child is capable of such consent. Examples are a child who is on active duty with the armed services of the United States, a pregnant child, a child suffering from a venereal disease, or such other serious contagious disease that would be reported to public health officials under applicable state law, a victim of child abuse due to physical or emotional mistreatment, and the so-called emancipated minor.

Several observations should be made concerning certain of these categories of special circumstances. First, in acting on special circumstances, the practitioner may reasonably rely on the assumed truthfulness of information given by the child in instituting or withholding care. For example, a nurse would be justified in treating a 16-year-old female with a chief complaint referrable to possible spontaneous abortion if the patient informs the nurse that she is or may be pregnant, whether the patient should be ultimately medically determined to be pregnant. Stated differently, the practitioner will have consent to treat the patient under special circumstances if the information related by the patient had been true. Consent does not depend on the future determination of whether such information was in fact true. Also of note is the fact that in most states it is a criminal offense to fail to report circumstances that justify the reasonable belief that a child has been physically, emotionally, or mentally abused. Finally, the so-called emancipated minor is essentially the common-law equivalent of a minor whose disabilities have been removed by a formal court order. The emancipated minor ordinarily is a child who is at least 16 or 17 years of age and lives away from home without being substantially dependent on the parents for financial support.

If the practitioner cannot determine and confirm the existence of special circumstances, it is necessary to obtain substitute or surrogate consent. The purpose of the law in requiring surrogate consent is to be certain that only a person standing in a special relationship to the child may authorize or control the child's medical treatment. Thus, generally, a natural parent or court-appointed guardian is the primary, if not exclusive, source of surrogate consent. Neither step-parents nor foster parents have parental rights to consent or refuse to consent to treatment for the child except by court order.

In attempting to obtain surrogate consent, first every reasonable effort should be made to locate the natural parent to obtain voluntary consent for treatment of the child. In most states, if a parent cannot be readily located, consent may be given by other "surrogates," including a natural grandparent, natural adult aunts or uncles, or an adult sibling. Moreover, in most states, the natural parent may authorize treatment by signing a particular written instrument in the form and manner required by state law. Finally, in almost every state, the emergently ill or critically ill child may be treated, as will be illustrated, by the doctrine of implied consent or by other considerably more liberal rules than would obtain for an adult.

Assuming that the practitioner has attempted but failed to obtain voluntary consent for treatment of the child by either special circumstance or surrogate consent, the next level of consent is involuntary consent. Involuntary consent for the child is similar to that for an adult, with one important addition. In most states, the abused child may be treated by order of the child welfare worker who has the child in custody under an order of the court. As with the adult, involuntary consent for the treatment of children is ordinarily permitted only to the limited emergency conditions specified by state law.

The final consent and consent of last resort for treatment of the child is implied consent. Implied consent for treatment of children is significantly different from implied consent for treatment of adults. To obtain implied consent for treatment of a child, the child must have what appears to be a life-threatening disease or illness, and there must be no parental refusal of treatment. There is no requirement that the child be unconscious or unable to communicate, because obtaining permission from a child in such circumstances would be ineffective. As will be noted in the next section, it is important to remember that implied consent to treat a child does not, as a rule, override a parental refusal to give consent.

SPECIAL PROBLEMS IN CONSENT

Occasionally, the health care practitioner will encounter a patient or members of the patient's family who, for whatever reason, resist or oppose treatment. This situation occurs rarely, but it is essential that the practitioner be able to recognize the problem immediately and know how to deal with it effectively and appropriately.

Before proceeding to medicolegal analysis of special problems in consent, two preliminary matters must be discussed and resolved. First, the health care practitioner should recognize that the ultimate determination of the presence or absence of patient consent will be judged by a legal standard, not by a medical or ethical one. Accordingly, when faced with a problem in obtaining consent, practitioners should disregard everything they have learned from the "grapevine" about the law that pertains to such cases or how such cases may necessarily have been handled in the past. Only a handful of medical or nursing schools in the United States provide their students with any meaningful amount of legal training. As a result, in a critical or emergency case, many decisions that should be made on the basis of the law are made instead on the basis of happenstance, or misunderstood "policy," to the resulting detriment of the patient and, ultimately, the practitioner as well.

Second, in order to deal effectively with the "problem" patient or the family, the health care practitioner must integrate fundamental principles of behavior assessment and modification into the treatment process. Almost without exception, the patient or family member who resists or opposes treatment has mental or emotional difficulties that are at least as incapacitating as the medical problem. Unless the practitioner can assess and deal effectively with the mental and psychologic as well as the physical aspects of the patient's treatment, frequently it will be impossible to obtain consent or treatment may be rendered fragmented and ineffective.

We proceed now to an analysis of several special problems in consent that are being confronted presently in critical and emergency care of patients.

The Patient Who Needs but Refuses Treatment

One of the most perplexing problems in medicine and nursing today is that of the conscious, rational adult patient who has an actually or potentially life-threatening disease or illness but who, for whatever reason, refuses treatment entirely or rejects given modalities of therapy, thereby fragmenting treatment. In dealing with this patient, the first priority is to exercise professional judgment to determine if in fact the patient has a truly life-threatening disease or illness. If so, every reasonable and lawful effort should be made to convince the patient, the patient's family, or anyone who has any influence with the patient to urge the patient to accept the treatment required. As previously noted, if an adult patient who is conscious and rational refuses consent, the patient cannot be treated without risk of civil and criminal liability.

If despite all reasonable efforts the patient persists in refusing consent, the refusal should be documented carefully in the chart, signed by the patient, and preferably witnessed by an impartial observer. Generally, patient care advocates, members of the clergy, or family members who desire the patient to be treated make excellent witnesses in such cases. The chart should contain a complete description of the patient's condition, the time and number of efforts made by the health care team to obtain consent, and, as nearly as possible, the patient's verbatim responses thereto.

The law recently has undergone a revolutionary change in the rights of patients, particularly institutionalized mental patients, to refuse consent to treatment that may otherwise be appropriate and even medically required. The health care practitioner should recognize that, under the law, it is extremely hazardous to attempt to force a patient to submit to treatment, and to do so may subject the practitioner to civil and criminal liability, as well as ethical or professional reprimand. In a case of sufficient gravity, many hospitals and medical staffs have recognized the need to seek court-ordered treatment if the competence of the patient is in any way at issue. A patient need not be literally insane or wholly mentally deranged to be unable to make appropriate decisions regarding a specific course of medical treatment.

When confronted with a patient refusal by an adult with a viable prognosis if treated, coupled with substantial risk of

mortality or morbidity without treatment, the health care professional is placed in what may be considered an untenable position. If the patient is treated against his or her will, the practitioner will be subject to claims of liability on that account, but if the practitioner honors a refusal that is not in fact competent or informed, this may likewise form a basis for subsequent complaint in a legal context. To remedy such situations, all critical care hospitals or health care practitioners who treat critically or emergently ill patients should have developed in advance a program whereby such a case can be communicated to competent legal counsel selected in advance for familiarity with medicolegal problems, the staff, and with litigation and court procedures. If appropriate in such a case, counsel for the hospital or practitioner should not hesitate to seek court authority by order, if required, to stabilize the patient's condition until the issue of competence can be determined fully and finally.

The Parent Who Refuses Permission to Treat a Child with a Life-Threatening Illness

Very rarely, a health care practitioner will encounter a parent who refuses consent, usually on moral, ethical, or religious grounds, to treat a seriously ill child. In some cases, the child may have a viable prognosis with treatment, and in others, particularly infants with congenital defects or with other profound or terminal disease processes, the prognosis is hopeless. Understandably, these situations may evoke intensely bitter conflict within the health care professions with regard to an appropriate course of action. The case of a child who suffers from a life-threatening disease or illness is, under the law, a very different situation from that of an adult. Generally, the courts will intervene immediately to require emergency treatment for a child who has a viable prognosis regardless of the moral, ethical, or religious views of the parent. However, the treatment of a child without a viable prognosis and therefore suffering from a terminal illness is considerably more complicated. Recently, the Department of Health and Human Services, through the Department of Justice, has instituted suits to attempt to review the necessity for treatment on behalf of neonates or infants with profound congenital defects and mental retardation. Again, faced with such a situation in which there cannot be an agreed resolution between the parents or responsible individuals, the reasonable health care practitioner and the hospital should promptly resort to the courts for the protection of all concerned. The risk of legal and ethical liability for failing to act appropriately in such cases cannot be overstated.

Should a parent refuse requested and desired permission to treat a child, every effort should again be made to convince the parent of the seriousness of the problem and the necessity for treatment. If agreement is not possible, again, competent legal counsel should be consulted.

The Mentally Ill Patient

Under the law, individuals who by reason of mental defect or disease are unable to handle their own business or personal affairs and thus require supervision by the court or a qualified person (usually called a guardian) are referred to as *non compos mentis* ("not of sound mind"). The determination of whether a patient is sufficiently mentally incompetent or irrational as to require court-ordered supervision is one of the most difficult and complex of all legal proceedings. Although every state has a procedure for both voluntary and involuntary commitment of a patient who is truly mentally ill, there is no reliable way of determining ultimate mental competence quickly in a crisis or emergency situation. In most states at present, only a qualified physician may determine that a patient is mentally incompetent according to required legal standards so as to obtain an order for medical treatment over the patient's objections, and physicians themselves may disagree in given cases. For this reason, mental illness proceedings themselves are generally an undesirable alternative in obtaining the required consent necessary for treatment of the emergently or critically ill patient.

Nonetheless, on confronting a patient who health care practitioners suspect is mentally ill, routine rules of professional conduct, compassion, sincerity, and caring will aid immeasurably. Practitioners without "pressure" should in the normal case encourage patients, if at all possible, to seek treatment for all their problems by committing themselves voluntarily to the hospital. If patients cannot be convinced to commit themselves voluntarily, involuntary commitment procedures may be required. Almost all such procedures require formal written application to a county or local law enforcement authority, coupled with a court order of commitment for protective custody or a warrant of confinement or arrest. Generally, there are stringent limitations on the length of time an individual may be confined under such order, and the procedures involved are complicated and cumbersome. Only on a court order or with the permission of the guardian is the health care practitioner justified in instituting treatment against the will of a mentally ill patient.

The Inappropriate, Intoxicated, or Belligerent Patient

Many patients present initially or at varying stages of the treatment process with metabolic, neurologic, or psychologic overlays that impair judgment. The effects and characteristics of acute drug or alcohol intoxication are a medical and social phenomenon that is well understood by most health care providers. Not so well understood, however, are the serious legal consequences that flow from dealing with these patients. If a critically ill patient refuses care while intoxicated, the practitioner should follow the protocol previously advised for dealing with patient refusals. Every effort should be made to persuade the patient to consent to treatment voluntarily, and, if consent is refused, the refusal should be documented carefully and witnessed. If the patient's condition is sufficiently grave, legal consultation may be indicated.

If, however, the intoxicated patient consents to treatment, care should be taken in assessment, diagnosis, and therapy. Alcohol, drugs, and the underlying metabolic derangement may mask vital symptoms, so a seriously compromised patient with these conditions has a higher than average risk of death or disability. The principal barrier to appropriate care of such patients is that the practitioner will become "turned off" by the patient's demeanor or conduct and may overlook signs and symptoms that would otherwise be recognized as vital.

The Patient Who Gives and Then Withdraws Consent for Treatment

Occasionally, the practitioner will encounter a patient who originally agrees to treatment but later withdraws consent during the treatment process. These patients may feel that the therapy has become too invasive or painful. Under the law, the practitioner may treat the patient only as long as the practitioner has the patient's effective consent.

In most cases, treatment must be discontinued when the patient withdraws consent. There are, however, certain instances in which it is medically inappropriate to discontinue treatment once it is instituted. For example, a patient who has a chest tube placed in a surgical intensive care unit simply cannot be permitted to leave the hospital with the chest tube inside the chest with or without medical advice. Likewise, the patient with narcotic overdose who has received drug therapy that is ephemeral in effect cannot be permitted to leave the hospital without risk to the patient's life. In such cases, if the patient's consent cannot be obtained, immediate resort should be made to legal counsel for assistance in compelling treatment as may be required.

The Decision to Resuscitate and "No Code" Orders

Ordinarily, a patient who suffers a cardiac or respiratory arrest in the hospital should receive vigorous advanced life support to restore vital functions. However, when a patient has a terminal illness, has no viable prognosis, or has executed a so-called living will or directive to physicians, the stage is set for a medicolegal decision of momentous importance: the right to life and the duty to preserve life versus the right to die and the duty to alleviate pain and suffering.

Although the complex problems regarding resuscitation decisions are beyond the scope of this chapter, substantial legal difficulties arise in selecting or refusing patients for resuscitation based on arbitrary criteria such as age, economic status, or living arrangements. Some physicians have advocated openly that certain classes of patients, particularly patients over a certain age, should not be resuscitated at all. In one case, a municipal nursing home had a standing instruction that cardiopulmonary resuscitation was *not* to be performed routinely on any resident, regardless of prognosis. A patient aspirated a bolus of food that was dislodged using the Heimlich maneuver, but the patient was not ventilated and subsequently died. Suit was filed for alleged violation of the patient's civil rights and for the wrongful death of the patient. Practitioners should beware of such arbitrary selection of patients for resuscitation on any basis of age, economic status, or living circumstances. Such an undertaking is fraught with legal peril.

The Living Will

Many states have enacted statutes that permit an individual who has been diagnosed as having a terminal disease or illness to execute a document that directs that physicians and other health care practitioners shall not prolong or extend the patient's life in the hospital or otherwise by extraordinary or heroic means. The living will is ordinarily binding on the physician and the health care practitioner as fully and to the same extent as would be the patient's expressed conscious desire even if the patient should be rendered unconscious subsequently or should be unable to communicate. Many authorities argue that when a state has enacted so-called living will legislation, the living will becomes the exclusive method by which patients can express in advance the desire that they not be resuscitated in the event of clinical death. Accordingly, these authorities would argue that unless the patient has executed a living will in the form and manner prescribed by statute, the hospital and health care practitioners within the hospital cannot withhold life-sustaining or life-prolonging treatment regardless of prognosis. Further, they would argue that without a living will, all patients who undergo clinical death should be resuscitated aggressively until resuscitation has been demonstrated to be futile, at which time the patient may be pronounced dead.

The Terminal Patient Who has Not Executed a Directive to Physicians

The majority of patients in the hospital with a terminal illness have not executed a directive to physicians or a living will in accordance with state law. Many times the patient's failure to execute a directive may be explained by virtue of a sudden and rapid onset of the disease process, coma, physical or mental inability, or reluctance to face one's own mortality. With alarming frequency, physicians confronted with the terminal patient have customarily, after consultation with the patient or family, entered "no code" or "do not resuscitate" orders, which direct the nursing staff or other physicians not to resuscitate the patient in the event of a cardiopulmonary arrest. This situation has produced conflicting legal results and widely divergent views among medical and legal commentators.

One school of thought holds that the patient and not the family or physician should determine what treatment will be given or withheld because of the patient's terminal condition. This school would argue that if the patient desires to live and receive maximal therapy, neither the doctor nor the hospital should have the power or ability to override the patient's wishes. Accordingly, these authorities would contend that unless the patient has executed a living will in compliance with the statute governing such matters, neither the hospital nor the physician has any discretion in treating the patient but must treat the patient in accordance with an objective standard of care, including vigorous resuscitation where indicated. This school of thought would advocate further that the practitioner or institution is authorized to approve withholding treatment for patients in comatose or vegetative states under the law only after hearing before a court and, if necessary, a jury. Some members of this school of thought would argue that the voluntary withholding of life support from any patient without legal authority should give rise to criminal charges of homicide or to civil liability.

The other school of thought basically recognizes that the living will is a preferable method of expressing the patient's wishes but is not necessarily exclusive, particularly in cases in which the patient was deprived of the opportunity to consider the necessity for a living will. Accordingly, these groups believe that the decision to give or withhold medical treatment should be made in consultation between the patient and family and the physician and is primarily a medical as opposed to a legal choice. This school of thought would permit the use of "no code" orders under policy or guidelines approved by the hospital without court authority.

Faced with these divergent views and the obvious legal issue, some hospitals and health care practitioners have adopted the extremely dangerous policy of a "code gray" or "slow code" protocol in dealing with terminally ill patients. In these situations, rather than accept the responsibility for writing a "no code" or "do not resuscitate" order, physicians and hospital personnel have an informal understanding or agreement that such patients will not in fact be treated or resuscitated vigorously, but merely that the cardiac arrest team will "go through the motions." This approach is legally and factually dishonest, compromises the integrity of the providers, and increases the risk of liability. It is mentioned only to be condemned. If life support should be withheld from the patient, the decision should be made openly and honestly and, wherever possible, with due regard and respect for the wishes of the patient and the patient's family.

It should also be remembered that assumed reliance on the wishes of the patient as articulated by the "family" may be misplaced. The phrase "blood is thicker than water" frequently is coined by undeserving relatives. The law historically has been jealous of its prerogatives in such cases by reason of the historical unreliability of assumed familial loyalty and the potential for abuse of undisclosed financial or personal interest in connection with the treatment process. It is not difficult to understand why the sole heir of a viable 78-year-old person would suggest that the patient had lived a full life and should be permitted to die with dignity.

Many problems could be avoided if health care practitioners, consistent with the medical needs of the patient, would promptly and honestly discuss prospects for treatment or withholding life support under extraordinary circumstances. If the terminal patient expresses the desire that extraordinary measures be withheld, the patient should be encouraged and the physician should insist that the patient obtain competent legal advice to embody those wishes in a living will or a directive to physicians in compliance with state law. If this is not practical, hospitals and physicians should adopt comprehensive policies respecting the rights of terminally ill patients. In no case should an individual physician be permitted to determine the issue by inserting a "do not resuscitate" order in the absence of compliance with objective criteria set out by the hospital and the medical and nursing staff in advance. Finally, if there is any question of patient competence or any indication of improper motivation on the part of attending family members, resort to the court should be made for decision-making authority.

THEORIES OF LIABILITY

Under the laws of the United States, any person has a constitutional right to institute a legal proceeding against a health care provider or anyone else thought to be legally responsible for improper conduct in regard to patient treatment.

One type of legal proceeding is referred to as a *civil action.* A civil suit is instituted by one private individual against another private individual and usually seeks the recovery of money damages as the result of a judgment or favorable determination by the court in favor of the plaintiff, the person who institutes the suit, against the defendant, the party who is sued. The statutes in various jurisdictions often will require that certain forms of notice be given to the health care practitioner before suit can be instituted. Such notice, along with formal requests for medical records, is often a prelude to the institution of either a personal injury or wrongful death suit. Any health care practitioner receiving notice of this type should immediately contact independent counsel capable of evaluating the claim and responding to it.

Occasionally, a provider's conduct may give rise to a *criminal proceeding*. In a criminal proceeding, the party seeking relief is the United States or a state in which the professional has practiced. In such a case, if a criminal complaint is filed with the law enforcement agency, it is ordinarily referred to a grand jury. If the grand jury determines that there is reasonable basis to believe that a crime has been committed, the defendant is indicted, at which time the defendant is required to appear and post bond to ensure his or her appearance. In a criminal case, the government has the burden to prove guilt of the accused beyond a reasonable doubt. A defendant found guilty of a felony can, at the discretion of the court or the jury, be punished by fine, imprisonment, or both.

By comparison, in a civil case, because the plaintiff, the moving party, usually seeks only monetary damages, he or she is required to prove his or her claim only by a preponderance of the evidence, which is the greater weight and degree of the testimony believed or accepted by the trier of fact. The burden and the result are considerably different in civil and criminal proceedings.

With these principles in mind, we proceed to explore theories of liabilities that may be urged against health care providers.

Assault and Battery

An *assault* occurs when the defendant, without privilege or excuse, *threatens* an unlawful invasion of the plaintiff's right to bodily security, whether or not that threat was actually carried out. *Battery*, however, is committed when the defendant, without privilege or excuse, actually *touches* or *has contact* with the plaintiff's body or items closely related thereto, such as clothing or articles the plaintiff may be carrying. Both assault and battery are civil wrongs referred to as *torts*, but the same conduct may give rise to criminal responsibility as well. Virtually any act of medical treatment could be considered an assault or battery if it is undertaken without consent. Assault and battery, therefore, are prime examples of the absolute necessity for patient consent before treatment is begun.

False Imprisonment

False imprisonment occurs when the defendant, without privilege or excuse, restrains the right of the plaintiff to freedom of movement. In the field of medicine, charges of false imprisonment may be brought if the practitioner restrains the patient illegally or refuses to permit the patient to leave if the patient has the right to do so. Again, obtaining adequate patient consent, whether voluntary, involuntary, or implied, provides the privilege necessary to provide care and treatment and avoid liability.

Invasion of Privacy and Defamation

The law recognizes that a citizen has the right to be free of invasion of privacy or from unwarranted or defamatory disclosures. *Defamation* consists of making an untrue statement about a person's character or reputation without privilege or consent. If a defamation is made orally, it is called *slander*. If it is made in writing or by the use of mass media, it is called *libel*.

The courts have also recognized the existence of a tort called *invasion of privacy*. An invasion of privacy occurs when the defendant ascertains private or personal information about the plaintiff and in some fashion reveals this information or allows someone else to reveal it to cast the plaintiff in a false or ridiculous light to the public or by disclosing some natural defect or condition about the plaintiff.

In order for defamation to be actionable, the disclosure must be false. With invasion of privacy, the statement that is made may be true but conveys a false impression or subjects a person to ridicule without justification or excuse. The relevance of these torts to critical care nursing should be obvious. Health care practitioners are privy on a daily basis to a wealth of information that is highly confidential and would be extremely embarrassing to the patient or patient's family should it be revealed publicly.

One of the most recent examples of claims made in the area of privacy and defamation are claims resulting from disclosure that a patient has the acquired immunodeficiency syndrome (AIDS) virus or has been tested or treated for the AIDS virus. One physician was sued for disclosing that a patient did *not* have AIDS based on the theory that even to suggest that the patient had AIDS is a defamation of character. Extreme attention should be given to the privacy rights of patients and their families in the area of highly communicable diseases to avoid possible legal problems.

The practitioner should be extremely cautious about communicating medical information about a patient to anyone who does not have a medical need to know the information without the advance knowledge or consent of the patient or family. Likewise, the practitioner should exercise extreme professional judgment in writing information concerning the patient's care or condition in the chart or medical records. The best policy is not to discuss the medical condition of a patient or information ascertained as a result of a confidential relationship with anyone other than an individual who has a medical need to know and then to communicate medical information only.

Civil Rights Violations

The United States and several states have comprehensive laws that prohibit discrimination in granting or denying health care services to a patient by reason of the patient's race, color, sex, national origin, age, or, in some cases, the patient's ability to pay for the services rendered. It is imperative that all health care professionals understand that a patient's right to critically needed emergency treatment may not be abridged or denied because of any of these factors.

Negligence

By far the most common theory of recovery against health care providers is a claim of professional negligence, which is sometimes referred to as *malpractice*. The circumstances under which a patient may bring a civil action for professional negligence vary from state to state. In general, however, the plaintiff must plead, prove, and obtain favorable findings by the court or jury of the following:

- The defendant had a legally recognized duty to provide health care to the plaintiff.
- The care the defendant provided to the plaintiff was substandard and was thus a breach of duty.
- The defendant's breach of duty was a proximate cause of damage to the plaintiff.
- The nature and extent of the damages suffered by the plaintiff.

Each of these factors will be discussed in detail.

Duty

In the claim of professional negligence, the concept of *duty* is simple and straightforward. There must be a relationship between the plaintiff and defendant that obligates the defendant to act toward the plaintiff in a certain way. Generally, a defendant has no affirmative obligation or legal duty to undertake a person's medical care if there is no antecedent or present relationship between the defendant and the plaintiff based on professional function or the medical needs of the patient. In some jurisdictions, however, the concept of duty presently is undergoing changes such that a health care practitioner's duty to the patient may be determined in the future not so much by voluntary undertaking by the practitioner but by the health care practitioner's relationship to the state in general. For these reasons, health care practitioners should be cautious in refusing to care for or treat a patient who is in need of treatment regardless of the legal duty owed. Moreover, courts generally recognize a heightened standard of care for specialists in any given medical activity. Thus, critical care nurses typically will be held to the standard of other persons of similar background, experience, and training.

Breach of Duty

Generally, a *breach of duty* arises from an act of commission or an act of omission. An *act of commission* is the affirmative doing of an act or practice that a reasonably prudent health care practitioner would not have done under the same or similar circumstances. An *act of omission* is the failure to do that which a reasonably prudent health care practitioner would have done under the same or similar circumstances. Proof of breach of duty involves producing evidence of the standard of care owed to the patient. The standard of care owed is not a guarantee that the plaintiff will receive the best care available, but only that the defendant will perform in a reasonably prudent fashion consistent with his or her training under the circumstances. In almost all cases of health care liability, expert testimony is required to establish both the standard of care and whether or not the duty of care has been breached.

Proximate Cause

The third requirement of a successful claim for professional negligence is that the plaintiff establish that the defendant's breach of duty was a proximate cause of damages sustained by the plaintiff. *Proximate cause* is a term that embodies at least two concepts in regard to medical care: cause in fact, and foreseeability.

The concept of *cause in fact* embodies the law's requirement that the defendant be responsible only for the effect of the defendant's conduct that actually results in injury or damage to the plaintiff. Cause in fact may become an issue in medical liability cases in which the plaintiff claims the defendant gave improper treatment for a pre-existing illness or injury or failed to make a correct diagnosis that resulted in delay in treatment. In such cases, a dispute may develop in the evidence as to whether the undesirable result was caused in fact by the alleged breach of duty. If the undesired result would have occurred regardless of the defendant's conduct, the plaintiff's case fails, even though the defendant may have admittedly acted inappropriately.

The other component of proximate cause is *foreseeability*. Foreseeability requires that the defendant should reasonably have known or anticipated that the plaintiff would sustain injury or damage as a result of the defendant's conduct. The defendant will not be held liable for an injury sustained by the plaintiff, even if the injury was caused in fact by the defendant's conduct, if the injury or complication was so bizarre that no reasonable person situated as the defendant would have foreseen that it would occur ultimately. It is not necessary that the defendant foresee the specific injury that the plaintiff suffered, but rather only that he or she should reasonably foresee the general type or category of injury that actually occurred.

Damages

Finally, the successful plaintiff in the professional negligence action must prove *damages*. In most health care liability claims, the plaintiff commonly seeks compensation for physical pain and suffering, mental anguish, hospital and medical expenses, sometimes loss of earnings and earning capacity, and other items of pecuniary loss. An unfortunately high number of claims against health care professionals involve brain or spinal cord injury or death. It is not unusual in such claims for the amount of damages sought to exceed several million dollars. The amount of money to be awarded the plaintiff in damages is ordinarily determined by the jury or judge in a civil case. Such a determination generally is not set aside on appeal unless the award is grossly excessive or inadequate by objective standards.

Further, most states allow the plaintiff to plead and prove a right to punitive or exemplary damages in cases in which the defendant has been guilty of gross negligence or willful or malicious misconduct. Punitive or exemplary damages are not imposed to compensate the plaintiff, but to punish the defendant and to deter others from committing similar acts by making the case example. Gross negligence in most jurisdictions differs only in degree from ordinary negligence. The same facts that give rise to a claim for negligence may also give rise to a claim for gross negligence if the defendant's action was sufficiently reckless and improper under the circumstances. Willful and wanton conduct, however, requires an element of actual or intentional desire to injure or carelessness with some element of conscious disregard of another's rights.

INDIVIDUAL RESPONSIBILITY AND CLAIM PREVENTION

Health care practitioners have not only ethical and moral obligations to their professions but a duty to the public as well. Therefore, it is important that all health care practitioners understand the dimensions of their personal responsibility for patient care under the law.

Government Immunity

Hundreds of years ago it was thought that the sovereign ruler derived authority directly from God and, accordingly, that such rulers and, by extension, their governments, were answerable only to God for their actions. This principle was originally referred to as the *doctrine of sovereign immunity* and arrived in the United States at the time of the formation of the original constitution and its government. Over the years, however, and in modern times the courts have shown decreasing sympathy for such doctrine.

Most states and the United States government have enacted what are called *tort claims*—laws that allow an individual to sue the government under limited circumstances. Health care practitioners who practice in government institutions should be aware that there are dramatic differences in liability that may be imposed on government employees and government institutions as opposed to private employees of private institutions. These differences will be determined by the applicable so-called tort claims statutes. These statutes vary dramatically from state to state and from the state government to the federal government. It is important that a health care practitioner bear in mind the crucial distinction between individual and governmental liability in such cases.

Good Samaritan Legislation

Some time in the early 1960s, a number of states began enacting statutes that were originally designed to provide freedom from liability to individuals who stopped and aided others at the scene of an emergency. Although the intention behind the so called good samaritan statute may have been laudable, the results have been mixed in effect. The original good samaritan concept was designed to promote broad-based community involvement by the well-intentioned nonprofessional bystander. Thus, most states denied good samaritan immunity to individuals who received compensation for their services or to health care practitioners. Several cases have held good samaritan legislation to be inapplicable to health care providers who are providing services that are in the ordinary and expected course of their practice (emergency room or critical care). In addition, good samaritan statutes are subject to serious constitutional question, and, finally, these statutes protect health care providers only if they are alleged to have acted in good faith and without gross negligence or willful misconduct. Accordingly, the allegation that the practitioner was guilty of gross negligence or malicious misconduct will avoid the effect of the statute almost entirely. The most serious effect of the existence of good samaritan legislation is to create a false sense of security in the minds of some health care professionals. Accordingly, good samaritan legislation is no substitute for personal competence and personal liability insurance.

Liability Insurance

Liability insurance is a contract between a health care provider and an insurance company that in consideration of the payment of a premium the company will provide the insured, subject to the terms and conditions of the policy, with a defense for the claims made by the plaintiff, and further that the company will pay any judgment against the professional up to and including the maximum limits of coverage provided by the policy.

A health care professional should keep in mind when obtaining liability insurance that it is important to understand the terms and conditions of coverage, particularly the exclusions and limitations. One should be aware that liability insurance not only protects against a money judgment but provides payment for legal fees, court costs, costs of investigation and discovery expenses, and costs of litigation generally. Knowledgeable observers have estimated that defending the average health care liability claim may result in expenses and legal fees in excess of $30,000 to $40,000, depending on the nature of the case and jurisdiction in which it is tried.

Some health care professionals, notably physicians, have advocated "going bare," a situation in which they have no professional liability insurance at all. These naive individuals argue that liability insurance is merely an incentive for claims-minded lawyers to sue. There is no statistical support for this belief, and on the contrary, in almost every instance in which a physician without insurance has been successfully sued, the physician has faced serious financial deprivation or potential bankruptcy. In our contemporary society, there is no effective alternative to having adequate liability insurance. Again, the advice of a competent attorney should be obtained with regard to the requirements of insurance for a given profession.

Claims Prevention

Claims of liability may be avoided in several statistically validated ways. Each will be discussed in brief detail.

Providing Competent Treatment

Clearly, the best defense to a claim of liability is that the health care practitioner provided competent and favorable treatment.

Good Medical Records

Much has been written about the necessity for a complete and well-documented patient record. An accurate and thorough record aids in the evaluation, management, and improvement of the patient's condition and is integral to the treatment process. Thus, the medical record is designed primarily for the benefit of the patient. The record also serves a valid legal purpose by documenting the care and treatment given the patient. For this reason, medical records should be complete, accurate, legible, and free of extraneous information. In addition, the patient chart should be protected scrupulously from intrusion and maintained to safeguard confidentiality. Careful documentation and charting provide perhaps the most economical and accessible means of claims prevention. By taking sufficient time to record data as treatment is rendered, the health care practitioner avoids substantial difficulties later.

Continuing Education

Another excellent way to prevent claims is by maintaining one's professional competence. Assuming that a practitioner was educated adequately and received adequate clinical training, such training and academic knowledge must be maintained throughout the length of practice. Accordingly, all health care practitioners should attend continuing educational programs regularly that emphasize intellectual information and clinical and technical skills so as to maintain overall competence. Keeping abreast of developments by regular professional reading will likewise ensure that the provider has the most current information to provide ongoing competent care.

Demeanor

The term *demeanor* emcompasses the physical and personal appearance of the health care practitioner as well as the overall impression of personal well-being and credibility conveyed to the public or the patient. Numerous statistical studies have shown that if the health care practitioner is neat and well-groomed, whether uniformed or not, a belief is created in the patient's mind that the practitioner is well organized, competent, and professional. High health care standards depend rightfully on cleanliness and sanitation. Accordingly, the practitioner should take considerable care to see that she or he presents an appearance consistent with the required respect for the profession and patient confidence.

Attitude

The health care professional's attitude is perhaps the greatest single determining factor in claims prevention. If the practitioner is hostile, belligerent, or sarcastic toward the patient or the family, almost without exception the patient and family will return hostility, belligerence, and sarcasm. Such a negative interchange affects the quality of care given the patient and greatly increases the likelihood of punitive legal action to correct the practitioner's perceived attitude. It is undoubtedly true that thousands of health care liability claims were precipitated because the patient or family viewed the health care provider or the institution as a whole as being indifferent or hostile to the patient's needs. A positive and professional approach may have avoided some of these cases.

Counseling and Therapy

Physically, psychologically, and emotionally, the delivery of health care to the emergent or critically ill patient is one of the most demanding of all professions. Critical care practitioners work at odd hours, under intense stress, under adverse conditions and sometimes in unstable social and personal environments. To add to these difficulties, the critical care practitioner sees all stages and degrees of human suffering and degradation and deals frequently with death and human tragedy. It is important for the health care practitioner to remember that the healing professions enjoy no immunity from grief, anger, frustration, or dangerous depression. The health care practitioner should remain alert constantly to personal signs of psychologic or emotional imbalance and promptly seek referral for counseling as may be indicated.

SUMMARY

The nurse practicing at the bedside of the critically ill patient must be cognizant of the legal aspects of nursing practice. Fundamental to care is the concept of consent. A systematic approach in obtaining consent is part of the initial care of the patient. Nurses need to be aware of the common theories of liability and be able to outline their individual responsibilities in claims prevention. Many times critically ill patients have completely entrusted their being to the nurse, and the nurse must act in a professional, ethical, moral, and legal manner.

SUGGESTED READINGS
Journal Articles

Bennett, H. M. Personal liability insurance coverage. *Crit. Care Nurse* 3(2):79–80, 1983.

Cushing, M. A matter of judgment. *Am. J. Nurs.* 82(6):990–992, 1982.

DiFabio, S. Nurse's reactions to restraining a patient. *Am. J. Nurs.* 18(5):972–975, 1981.

Fry, S. T. Accountability in research: The relationship of scientific and humanistic values. *Adv. Nurs. Sci.* 4(1):1–13, 1981.

Greenlaw, J. Documentation of patient care: An often underestimated responsibility. *Law Med. Health Care* 10(5):172–174, 1982.

Greenlaw, J. Failure to use siderails: When is it negligence? *Law Med. Health Care* 10(3):125–128, 1982.

Greenlaw, J. Communication failure: Some case examples. *Law Med. Health Care* 10(2):77–79, 1982.

Guarriello, D. L. Nursing malpractice litigation: Toward better patient care. *Trial* 18(10):78–90, 1982.

Haynes, B. E., and Niemann, J. J. Letting go: *DNR* orders in hospital care. *JAMA* 254(4):532–533, 1985.

Katz, B. F. Reporting and review of patient care: The nurse's responsibility. *Law Med. Health Care* 11(2):76–79, 1983.

Penticuff, J. H. Resolving ethical dilemmas in critical care. *Dimens. Crit. Care Nurs.* 1(1):22–27, 1982.

Rawnsley, M. M. The concept of privacy. *Adv. Nurs. Sci.* 2(2):25–31, 1980.

Regan, W. A. Transplants: Confidentiality of transplant records. *Regan Rep. Hosp. Law* 24(2):4, 1983.

Regan, W. A. Hospitals and life-support systems: Regulations. *Regan Rep. Hosp. Law* 23(12):1, 1983.

Rizzo, R. F. The living will: Does it protect the rights of the terminally ill? *New York State* 1(2):72–79, 1989.

Robb, S. S. Nurse involvement in institutional review boards: The service setting perspectives. *Nurs. Res.* 30(1):27–29, 1981.

Walker, D. Nursing 1980: New responsibility, new liability. *Trial* 16(12):42, 1980.

Watson, A. B. Informed consent of special subjects. *Nurs. Res.* 31(1):43–47, 1982.

Books

Annas, G. J., Glantz, L. H., and Katz, B. F. *The Rights of Doctors, Nurses, and Allied Health Professionals.* Cambridge, MA: Ballinger, 1981.

Benesch, K., Abramson, N., Grenvik, A, Meisel, A. (eds.). *Medicolegal Aspects of Critical Care.* Rockville, MD: Aspen Publishers, 1986.

Curtain, L., and Flaherty, M. *Nursing Ethics: Theories and Pragmatics.* Bowie, MD: Robert J. Brady, 1982.

Davis, A. J., and Krueger, J. C. (eds.). *Patients, Nurses, Ethics.* New York: American Journal of Nursing Company, 1980.

Doudera, A. E., and Peters, J. D. (eds.). *Legal and Ethical Aspects of Treating Critically and Terminally Ill Patients.* Washington: AUPHA Press, 1982.

Fenner, K. M. *Ethics and Law in Nursing.* New York: Van Nostrand Reinhold, 1980.

Gadow, S., and Spicker, S. (eds.). *Nurses: Images and Ideals.* New York: Springer, 1979.

Hemelt, M. D., and Mackert, M. E. *Dynamics of Law in Nursing and Health Care.* Reston, VA: Reston Publishing Co., 1982.

Humber, J. M., and Almeder, R. F. (eds.). *Biomedical Ethics and the Law.* New York: Plenum, 1979.

Levine, R. J. *Ethics and Regulation of Clinical Research.* Baltimore: Urban and Schwarzenberg, 1981.

Meyers, D. *Medico–legal implications of death and dying.* San Francisco: Bancroft Whitney, 1990.

Murchison, I. *Legal Accountability in the Nursing Process.* St. Louis: C. V. Mosby, 1981.

President's Commission for the Study of Ethical Problems in Medicine and Biomedical Research. *Deciding to Forego Life-Sustaining Treatment.* Washington, D.C.: U.S. Government Printing Office, 1983.

Reiser, S. J., (ed.). *Ethics in Medicine.* Cambridge, MA: MIT Press, 1977.

Robertson, J. A. *The Rights of the Critically Ill.* New York: Bantam Books, 1983.

Rocereto, L. R., and Maleski, C. M. *The Legal Dimensions of Nursing Practice.* New York: Springer, 1982.

Rozovsky, F., and Rozovsky, L. *Consent to Treatment: A Practical Guide* (2nd ed.). Boston: Little, Brown, 1990.

Sadoff, R. L. *Legal Issues in the Care of Psychiatric Patients.* New York: Springer, 1982.

Shannon, T. A., and Manfra, J. A. (eds). *Law and Bioethics: Major U.S. Court Decisions.* New York: Paulist Press, 1981.

Shaw, M. W., and Doudera, A. E. (eds.). *Defining Human Life: Medical, Legal, and Ethical Implications.* Washington: AUPHA Press, 1983.

Ziegenfuss, J. T. *Patient's Rights and Professional Practice.* New York: Van Nostrand Reinhold, 1983.

10

Living Your Ethics

Sarah E. Shannon

THE POWER OF MEANING

Meaning is the particular significance or importance we attach to events in our lives. Sometimes meaning enters the body with profound effects.

One woman, on being told that her husband was suing her for a divorce, experienced immediate emotional shock, suffered a cardiac arrest, and died abruptly. Another woman with severe heart disease and incapacitating angina pectoris was told precisely the same thing—that her husband was suing her for a divorce. She was delighted, having endured a miserable marriage for decades. She experienced an amazing clinical improvement. Her angina disappeared, her physician was able to stop her heart medications, and she took up a jogging program.

These life events were the same, but the meaning they held for each of the women differed. The difference in meaning was a difference in life and death.

Nurses must be sensitive to the potent effects of meaning. Even innocent words may carry powerful meanings for a patient and can trigger surprising effects. This requires a "sixth sense" on the nurse's part that involves being sensitive to the needs of our patients and intuiting their emotional requirements. This is not as difficult as it might seem, if we remember always to give undivided attention, to be fully present, and to care genuinely for those we serve.

LEARNING OBJECTIVES

After reading this chapter, the nurse should be able to do the following:

1. Describe three models of patient advocacy.
2. Discuss four arguments against the role of the nurse as the patient advocate.
3. Describe the four areas common to all clinical ethics cases.
4. Discuss five strategies for acting on an ethical choice.

ETHICS IN CRITICAL CARE

Current advances in health care have been accompanied by a dramatic increase in the frequency and complexity of ethical challenges faced by health care practitioners. In critical care units, ethicists debate issues such as patient autonomy, medical futility, and resource consumption while professionals and lay people struggle to make the "right" choices. This chapter offers the critical care nurse practical advice about how to make ethical decisions at the patient's bedside and how to act on those choices in the challenging professional environment in which nurses practice. You will not find a prescription for what is the "right" thing to do or a philosophical discussion of ethics. Rather, this chapter is a hands-on discussion of how to reason through patient care issues and then act effectively on your convictions.

ETHICAL THEORIES

When clinicians find themselves confused about the right thing to do in a patient care situation, they may sign up for an ethics course or attend a lecture on ethics. These good intentions turn to frustration as they are taught about theories of ethics that seem far removed from their patient's bedside. Similarly, lectures on specific issues such as abortion or organ transplantation may have little application to their own clinical area. What these clinicians are seeking is help in making the difficult decisions that they face daily at the bedside. What they may get at ethics offerings often seems decontextualized and overly specific. The clinicians may leave asking, "Yes, but what do I *do* in these situations?"

Ethical theorists attempt to identify the key principles that ought to guide moral action. Utilitarianism, by Jeremy Bentham and John Stuart Mill, Kant's categorical imperative, or Rawl's theory of justice represent a division of ethics called *normative ethics,* or ethics that are concerned with standards for moral behavior and how these standards apply to real-life behavior.[2] Becoming familiar with theories of ethics is a good way to begin thinking about major principles in ethics, such as justice or beneficence. However, theories of ethics may not tell the clinician what is the ''right'' action in a specific patient situation. In a similar way, discussions of controversial areas such as organ transplantation can be helpful in getting an overview of the main concerns around the issue, but these discussions will not always tell the nurse what to do when faced with an actual patient who has a transplant. *The decisions that critical care nurses face at the bedside require careful analysis and creative intervention.*

ETHICS IN NURSING

What is nursing ethics and how does it relate to bioethics? Tristan Engelhardt defined *bioethics* as the ''disciplined puzzling of people attempting to understand the significance of birth, copulation, illness, and death especially as these are touched on by health care and the biomedical sciences.''[1] The issues facing health care practitioners do center around these areas. Ethical issues are the ones that keep nurses up at night asking, ''Did I do the right thing?'' These are the cases that are pondered in a quiet moment at the nursing station. They are the situations that are among the most difficult to handle as a professional and as an individual.

Nurses, physicians, social workers, respiratory therapists, and other professionals who practice in critical care units have unique interests but also share a large area of overlapping concerns. For example, all health care professionals identify decisions about whether the care a patient is receiving is futile as problematic ethically. For nurses, however, the issue may be deciding when it is ethically permissible to use restraints, chemical or mechanical, on a patient. For physicians, the concern may be deciding when diagnostic tests no longer offer any benefit to a patient.

Health care workers also have ethical concerns that are not in the area of bioethics. For instance, professional ethics are examined when one must confront a co-worker who is believed to be taking drugs on the job. This ethical problem could be faced by any health care professional. Similarly, macro-level bioethics are concerned with resource allocation and rationing (*i.e.,* deciding how to spend the shrinking American health care dollar).

In contrast to macro-level bioethics or professional ethics, this chapter focuses on clinical or bedside ethics, which involve interactions between health care providers and patients. In nursing, *clinical ethics* most often is associated with the role of the nurse as the patient advocate. Nurses adopted the legal metaphor of the nurse as patient advocate after rejecting the historical view of the nurse as the physician's handmaiden, a metaphor that reflected nursing's military roots.[10]

Sara Fry critiqued the multiple views of the role of the nurse as the patient's advocate, and identified three main schools of thought concerning patient advocacy: the rights protection model, the values-based decision model, and the respect-for-persons model.[3] The rights protection model came out of the consumer rights movement and reflected the concern that patients, like other consumers, were not adequately protected by the law. In this model, nurses should defend the rights of their patients in a highly technologic health care environment.

The values-based decision model emphasizes that the role of the nurse is not only to provide information to patients but to assist them actively to discover their own preferences regarding health care. Finally, the respect-for-persons model includes situations in which patients are unable to make their own preferences known because of their illness. This model asserts that unconscious and otherwise nonautonomous patients deserve respect for their human dignity. The nurse may need to speak for the patient to promote what the nurse believes would be in the best interests of the patient. These beliefs are usually based on any knowledge the nurse may have about the patient's wishes and on the nurse's own preferences.

Common to all three models of patient advocacy is the nurse's accountability to the patient. *Accountability* is the fundamental value of nursing; that is, accountability to patients is the most basic and underlying value of nursing. Therefore, nurses are morally obligated to protect their patient's right to autonomy in health care decision making, to support and respect their patient's values, and to preserve their patient's human dignity even when the patient may no longer be able to act autonomously.

The role of the patient's advocate has been beneficial to nursing as a profession and to nurses as professionals. Patient advocacy has helped nurses to prioritize, at least theoretically, their responsibilities and accountabilities. Because nurses are held accountable to multiple sources (such as physicians, hospitals, patients, families, and themselves), deciding which source takes precedence can be difficult. Furthermore, thinking in terms of advocating for the patient assists nurses to clarify their judgments about what is right or wrong in specific situations.

Arguments Against Patient Advocacy

It may be time for nurses to move beyond the role of patient advocate. This is not to suggest that nurses should no longer act as advocates for their patients. Rather, nurses may be ready to move beyond this role of patient advocacy by finding a new model to help guide their actions. There are four main arguments against the metaphor of the nurse as the patient advocate: the best advocate argument, the physician-as-adversary argument, the coercive nurse argument, and the powerless nurse argument.

The Best Advocate Argument

Some authors in nursing suggest that nurses may be the best advocates for patients because of their special relationship with their patients. After all, nurses spend more time with patients than other health care professionals, and they have more intimate knowledge of their patients' values and wishes. Furthermore, nurses are naturally better at being advocates because they do not define their own success based on whether the patient survives at all costs, as physicians appear to do sometimes. These statements about why nurses are the best advocates for patients deny the relationships patients do have with other health care professionals: the family doctor who the patient has known for years, the dialysis nurse or technician who has cared for the patient throughout the progression of the disease, the social worker who helped the family cope in the initial crisis period, or the emergency room physician who spoke briefly (but compassionately) with the patient during his or her immediate fear of dying. *Patients need all their health care professionals to be advocates for them.* Adhering rigidly to the view that the nurse is the best advocate may deny the meaningful connections patients have made with other caregivers.

The Physician-as-Adversary Argument

In the legal sense, the term *advocate* implies that a person needs support and protection from a potential threat. Therefore, the language of patient advocacy suggests that some *adversary* exists. The rationale for needing a patient advocate often begins with a description of today's highly technologic and impersonal health care environment. The rationalization then undergoes a transformation to the need to protect the patient from the technology-driven, impersonal *physician*. Somehow the environmental threat has been changed into an individual threat in the form of a physician concerned only with curing the patient at all costs. Perhaps by using language that requires an adversary to play the "bad guy" (to the "good guy" advocate), actual individuals are miscast in these roles! This is not to suggest that impersonal physicians do not exist, because they do; however, by starting with a dichotomous position, advocate against adversary, the patient's needs may not be met.

Based on recent research findings, authors in both medicine and nursing are pleading for a more collaborative relationship. For example, mortality rates have been found to be significantly better (*i.e.*, lower than predicted by the APACHE instrument) in hospitals in which physicians and nurses verbally coordinated the care of critical care patients.[5] Decreasing the perception that nurses are patient advocates and physicians are patient adversaries may improve collaboration between these two groups and improve the care patients receive.

The Coercive Nurse Argument

When nurses focus on their role as the patient's advocate, they may overlook the potentially coercive aspects of the nurse-patient relationship. A great deal has been written about *paternalism* in health care (*i.e.*, deciding what is best for the patient without obtaining the patient's opinion). Less attention has been focused on *maternalism*. Susan Taylor suggested that the difference between maternalism and paternalism is that with maternalism one person not only decides what is best for others, but then makes them think they agree with the decision.[9] When nurses act maternalistically (parentally), they elicit cooperation from their patients by confronting them with the consequences of their behavior, not with alternatives. An example is when the nurse says, "I'm sorry, Mr. Jones, but if you can't cough I'm going to have to put that little tube down your nose again." Sometimes we clothe our parentalism with the subterfuge of participation and even fool ourselves along with our patients.

The Powerless Nurse Argument

Can a group, nurses, that lacks power itself advocate successfully for a more vulnerable group such as patients? This might be called the pessimistic pragmatist view: If you don't have it, how can you give it away? Perhaps when nurses struggle to protect their patients, they end up expending more energy trying to elevate their own status as a group instead of actually helping achieve the patient's goals. Could there be a better way to accomplish the overall goal of supporting the rights of patients to participate in the decision-making process regarding their health care?

What lies beyond the role of patient advocacy for nursing ethics? Perhaps the answer to that question is *a common ground where health care professionals, patients, and their families work together to make the difficult choices that are a part of critical care.* To accomplish that goal, health care professionals will need a shared framework for ethical decision making at the bedside.

ETHICAL DECISION MAKING

As critical care nurses, we become comfortable making complex assessments of a patient's physiologic and psychologic state, weighing the treatment options appropriate to the problem, and then making a choice about which action to take. In cases of hemodynamic compromise, this reasoning might include continuing to monitor the problem, hanging a medication drip that is ordered on an as-needed basis, or calling the physician to discuss other options. We learn to trust our clinical judgment and to act appropriately.

Edmund Pellegrino analyzed the process of clinical judgment and concluded that it could be captured in three questions: What is wrong with this patient? What can be done for this patient? What should be done for this patient?[7] Most critical care nurses become competent at answering the first two questions. They use their clinical judgment based on "book" knowledge, experience, and intuition to assess and choose appropriate, individualized treatment. However, the final question (What should be done for this patient?) does not use the same set of information or the same clinical reasoning. This last step in the process of clinical judgment is clinical ethics. Clinical ethical decision making, like the other parts of clinical judgment, requires specific information and analysis to arrive at a good decision.

Albert Jonsen, a philosopher and theologian, Mark Seigler, a physician, and William Winslade, a lawyer and psychoanalyst, have developed a practical framework for making clinical ethical decisions.[4] This model helps clinicians analyze a patient's case effectively. It provides a systematic way to ask what should be done for this patient in this situation. The framework will not help in the analysis of professional ethics issues or in resource allocation problems, but it will offer the nurse clinician a model to review a patient's case critically, organize a care conference, or identify the most important issues before discussing these concerns with the patient's family or other health care professionals in order to decide what should be done.

A Model for Clinical Ethical Decision Making

In analyzing a clinical ethics case, four areas are considered: medical indications, preferences of patients, quality of life, and external issues.

Step One: Medical Indications

When you pause for a moment during your care of a critical care patient and say to yourself, "Wait a minute . . . what is it we are really doing here," you are beginning your analysis of an ethics case. The first task in analyzing a patient's case is to step back and consider the overall pathophysiologic aspects of the case. Sometimes you will discover you do not have an ethical issue at all, because although a situation may be tragic, you may have no treatment to offer the patient except supportive care.

The underlying ethical principle in considering the medical indications is beneficence: Be of benefit and do no harm. When we make treatment decisions regarding the care of a patient, we are acting on the principle of beneficence. For example, when we cajole a postoperative patient to cough and breathe deeply, we are acting primarily to be of benefit to the patient, not to support their individual autonomy or promote fairness.

Medical indications can be thought of as encompassing the first two considerations in Pellegrino's clinical judgment model: what is wrong with this patient, and what can be done for the patient. Health problems are not merely "facts" but are problems that imply an action. Therefore, the presence of Down's syndrome may be a fact in a case, but it does not by itself imply a specific treatment. In a similar way, the fact that a patient lives in a nursing home does not imply only certain treatment options. These facts, plus the mental status or living situation of the patient, are important pieces of information in the decision-making process. However, they are considered separately in this model.

After you have decided what the health problem is, you can ask, "What ought to be the next step?" For the patient who has returned from coronary artery bypass graft surgery and now is bleeding profusely from the chest tube, the answer to this question is usually obvious: The patient has a leak from one or more of the vessels and is in need of surgical repair. However, in a case in which the health problem is end-stage cardiac disease, it may be difficult to decide what the next treatment ought to be. The appropriate treatment might depend on the stage of the disease (e.g., aggressive treatment for an exacerbation of a chronic disease versus supportive care during the dying process). Therefore, the next questions to consider regarding the medical indications of the case are "What is the overall goal in this case?" and "What should be the goal in cases such as this one?" For the case of the patient bleeding after bypass surgery, the goal is to support the patient through the postsurgical period with the expectation that the patient will recover at least to his or her previous state of health. However, for the patient who is in end-stage disease, the goal is not as defined or predictable. In this type of case, there may be disagreement about whether further treatment would be of meaningful benefit to the patient (i.e., is further treatment futile?).

Who defines futility? Is it the patient or the family, the surgeon or the oncologist? Futility is a central concept in considering treatment options. Clearly, treatments such as dialysis for end-stage lung disease would not be expected to have any positive effect and would not be offered to a patient. What about offering cardiopulmonary resuscitation (CPR) in a situation in which the patient is already being maximally supported—that is, when there is nothing left to offer the patient except CPR? In cases like this, CPR may be futile because the patient is already receiving all the treatment options that are appropriate. It might be helpful to consider what more could be done in this case? As clinicians, we tend to remember the

miracle "saves" most vividly. These unusual cases may alter our judgment about whether a treatment is futile and whether it could be expected to have the desired effect?

In considering the medical indications in a case, you will probably arrive at several conclusions. Usually one outcome of this process is the identification of incomplete information regarding the case. Possible sources for further information might be the primary physician or a specialist, a text on the disease, or a recent article on the disease prognosis given various treatments. It is important for effective care conferences to make sure you have the necessary resources (either human or written) available to discuss the medical indications issues of the patient's case. For example, it may be useful to do more diagnostic tests to get a clearer picture of the patient's prognosis.

The most important conclusion to reach about medical indications, however, is a sense of where this case falls on a continuum. Is this a case in which we have a treatment to offer that has a clear benefit and few risks? For example, antibiotics can cure a life-threatening illness with few side effects. At the opposite end of the continuum may be a case in which the treatment we have to offer is unsure and may even carry significant burdens. An example of this situation might be a bone marrow transplantation for radiation sickness. Where a case is situated on the continuum—from clear, beneficial treatment options to unsure, burdensome treatments—affects the urgency with which you seek out the patient's wishes.

Step Two: Preferences of Patients

Autonomy, the individual's right to be self-determining, is the underlying ethical principle guiding this need to determine the patient's preferences. The patient's wishes are considered *after* examining the medical indications in the case in order to be clear about what options are available to the patient.

What are the patient's preferences? A surprising number of competent patients are not consulted about their wishes regarding treatment. The reasons for this are numerous. There may be a perception that the discussion will "upset" the patient, or the treatment may not be perceived as optional or subject to veto by the patient.

For patients who are not able to speak for themselves at the time of decision making, an effort can be made to find out if they have ever expressed their preferences. For example, did they sign a living will, or do they have a durable power of attorney? Have they talked with family members, a primary physician, or a close friend about health care situations? Have they experienced the illness of a parent or other relatives and perhaps expressed how they would have wanted the situation handled if it had been them? In many cases, it is possible to get a good idea about what a person might say in a situation through a bit of detective work with friends and family.

Once you have a picture of what the patient's preferences are, whether that is from the individual or other sources, the major issue to be resolved is, "Can we trust this patient (or family)?" It is easy to feel supportive of the patient who agrees with the recommendations made to them, but what about the patient who listens carefully, but then chooses to take an alternate path. These patients often get labeled as noncompliant owing to a strong bias in health care against noncooperators. Health care professionals in general tend to prefer "active" treatment versus withdrawal of care.

Step Three: Quality of Life

After evaluating what is wrong, what options are available, and what the patient's preferences are regarding the treatment, it may be necessary to consider the quality-of-life issues embedded in the case. What is quality of life? Is it being able to think clearly, to laugh, to walk, to love, or some combination of all these? If a dozen people are asked what makes life worth living, a dozen answers will emerge. So, how can quality of life be considered in a systematic way when analyzing the ethical aspects of a patient's case? *Separate the discussion about quality-of-life issues from statements about medical indications or the patient's preferences.* By doing so, the subjective nature of quality-of-life evaluations can be acknowledged and debated openly.

The central question to ask in considering quality of life in a patient situation is this: By whose standards do we judge quality of life? If patients are able to speak for themselves, we should use their standards, but what if we do not believe the patient? For example, consider the situation of a patient who appears to be depressed by the diagnosis of a chronic and potentially life-threatening illness. Do we support this patient's "right" to discouragement in the face of adversity, or do we work with such a patient to help him or her see options that might be available to cope with his illness? When are we intervening appropriately, and when are we imposing our view of the situation on the patient?

To make this question even more difficult, what if the patient's judgment of his or her quality of life cannot be known? For example, in cases of a persistent vegetative state or coma, it may be impossible to obtain the patient's judgment of what quality of life is. If the patient is not able to judge quality of life, then whose evaluation do we accept—the physician's, the critical care nurse's, the rehabilitation nurse's, or the family's? There are no easy answers to whose standards are most accurate, or when we can trust the judgment of patients regarding their quality of life. However, by separating these issues out from the discussions about medical indications and patient preferences, this subjectivity and ambiguity can be acknowledged openly. The advantage of open discussion is that the inevitable biases regarding quality of life that each person has can be discussed. We make better decisions when we are able to see our prejudices and attempt to set them aside.

In the section on medical indications, it was noted that Down's syndrome or living in a nursing home is not an indication for treatment but rather the facts of the case. This type of information regarding a patient's mental status or living situation may actually be a judgment of the health care professional about the quality of the patient's life. The statement, "The patient lives in a nursing home," actually could be stated as, "The patient lives in a nursing home and, therefore, his or her quality of life would not be acceptable to me." Sorting these issues out can facilitate clarification of the case.

Step Four: External Issues

The last step in clinical ethical decision making is to consider whether any extraneous issues are relevant to the case being discussed. These may be varied but center around two general principles: justice or fairness, and utilitarianism, or the greatest good for the greatest number.

When considering justice or fairness, it may be useful in a particular case to consider who will be the primary beneficiary of this treatment. Is it the researcher who wants to keep the patient in the study? Is it the students in a teaching hospital environment? Perhaps the person benefiting most from the treatment is the spouse of the patient who is coping with feelings of guilt or remorse. Or, maybe the primary beneficiary is the neonatal intensive care nurse who has bonded to the patient. In any case, a frank discussion of who is benefiting from the treatment the patient is receiving can be helpful.

A second issue to consider is whether the resources being consumed by this patient could be of more benefit to others. A related issue concerns whether the costs of care are unduly burdensome to the patient. The main purpose in discussing the use of resources and cost of care is to bring these issues to the foreground and allow open discussion of sensitive areas. Issues such as use of resources and cost of care might be expressed as a vague concern or recurrent theme in the discussion of a patient's case. In reality, these issues rarely "decide" the case. How to spend the health care dollar should be a decision debated at the policy level for a group of patients, not a bedside decision made for one individual.

Putting the Steps Together

The four steps described—medical indications, preferences of patients, quality of life, and external issues—represent the four areas that are common to all clinical ethical cases. Using a systematic model for clinical ethical decisions allows health care professionals, patients, and families to work together in making the difficult decisions that are a part of critical care today. The process for decision making described will not produce the "right" answer, but it will encourage the asking of the right questions. In turn, asking good questions assists one in making good, thoughtful, and caring choices.

ACTING ON YOUR DECISION

Sometimes it feels like the hard part is over when one has thought through a patient case and arrived at a choice that one believes is the best possible given in the situation. Inevitably, however, the real work begins when one acts on that decision. Clinical ethics cases almost always involve many players: the patient, family members, friends, critical care nurses, physicians, specialists, social workers, nutritionists, and physical therapists. Acting on the decision involves articulation with the other people invested in the case.

The American Association of Critical-Care Nurses Demonstration Project found mortality rates in the critical care units of a community hospital in the northwest were 50% of the predicted rate based on the physiologic instability of the patients.[6] The critical care nursing staff was more experienced, older, and had been employed at the institution longer than national averages for those variables. To answer the question of what was different about this group of nurses that characterized a "sample of excellence," a qualitative research study was completed.[8] Twenty-one critical care nurses were interviewed using an open-ended question format to understand how the clinical practice of this group might be unusual. Of the 21 nurses, 19 recounted patient care situations that were examples of clinical ethics. In the stories the nurses shared, the role of being the patient advocate was overshadowed by an emphasis on negotiating and collaborating with others. The nurses talked of more than just protecting their patient's autonomy, although supporting the right of the patient to be self-determining was a foundational value on which they based their care. However, these nurses also talked of doing what was "best" and doing what was "right" for their patients.

Their stories included five strategies for acting on ethical decisions: recognizing the accountability of others; arguing the case, not personal issues; seeking to know the patient; challenging yourself to see beyond what you would want; and never accepting a dead end.

Recognizing the Accountability of Others

In the complex environment of critical care, a team of health care professionals must work together with patients and families to achieve the best outcomes. It is not surprising that the team may not share the same vision. The experienced nurses in the qualitative clinical judgment study spoke of getting involved when their patients needed them but also of allowing the other team members to do the same.

Sometimes it is the family who is "most" accountable to the patient. Consider, for example, the case in which a nurse encourages a family member to begin thinking about the issue of a do-not-resuscitate order for a critically ill patient. One nurse in the research study spoke of gently preparing and supporting the legal surrogate of a patient, the wife, to anticipate the difficult decision regarding code status. The nurse began with teaching about what was happening to the patient. She provided information and supported conversations with the physician. The nurse supported the wife; she held her while she cried. She allowed the wife to deal with not wanting to have to make this difficult decision. A week later, when the patient had deteriorated further, the wife spoke with confidence and conviction that it was time to let her husband go.

Physicians have accountabilities to patients that may seem to be in conflict with those of nurses. One nurse shared a story of a patient with pneumocystic pneumonia who had asked his physician to "do everything." A month and a half later, the physician felt obligated to continue mechanical ventilation even though there was no hope for recovery. The primary nurse initiated a discussion with the physician each day, asking questions like, "What is our goal now?" After 3 days, the physician was able to talk about the situation with the family and recognized that he had fulfilled his promise to the patient to "do everything."

Recognizing the accountability of others requires understanding their ethical analysis of a patient's case and respecting their choices. It does not mean "giving in" or "giving up." In contrast, by communicating about how another person has considered a case, you may have the opportunity to reach a consensus through mutual understanding of the patient's case.

Arguing the Case, Not Personal Issues

Conflicts are inevitable when dealing with sensitive issues such as withdrawal of care. These conflicts may be mistaken for personality disagreements and, thus, result in a discussion of "who's right" instead of a systematic analysis of the patient's case. Conversely, the fear of challenging another person on

their views may discourage some professionals from discussing an ethics case with colleagues.

Disagreement about what should be done for the patient can be expected. The key to managing this disagreement effectively is return the focus of the discussion to the patient's case when necessary. In addition, it can be helpful to reflect another's personal preference back to them in a nonjudgmental manner. For example, a colleague might assert that no one would want to be "kept alive after a C 3-4 fracture." A response might be, "So, you would not want to be kept alive given the quality of life we can expect for this patient. Has the patient expressed a view about how he or she feels about his or her expected quality of life?"

Talking openly and honestly about the issues of the case is the best way to ensure that a good choice is made. Sometimes this will take on the form of arguing or debating the case. Keeping the discussion focused on the questions described earlier for ethical decision making may help to discourage arguments about personal issues with colleagues, patients, or families.

Seeking to Know the Patient

Clinical ethics is concerned with decision making for a particular patient in a particular situation. In contrast, general rules of ethics are intended for groups of people. The goal of general rules or principles is fairness, whereas the goal in clinical ethics cases is to ensure that the best choice is made for the individual. When we decide to withdraw a ventilator, we want to be right, not just fair!

The nurses in the qualitative clinical judgment study worked to get to know their patients as individuals. They interacted with the patient's family and friends to gain a more complete picture of the patient's previous choices and preferences. These nurses reported that in order to analyze the patient's case, they needed to know the patient as an individual and as a person connected to others. This information allowed the nurses to consider the unique aspects of the patient's case in evaluating what should be done.

Challenging Yourself to See Beyond What You Would Want

When our patient's values and life-styles are congruent with our own, it may be easier to understand and accept the choices they make. The challenge to each health care professional is to see beyond these personal preferences to understand the patient's view.

A situation that challenged a nurse in the clinical judgment study was the case of a 30-year-old man who worked in the computer industry. This man lived at home with his mother and chose not to get a driver's license. He accepted a high degree of dependency on his mother, particularly around health care decision making. The nurse acknowledged that she could not understand the patient's choices because they were so divergent from her own. However, she talked with the patient to verify that he was comfortable with his mother's influence over decision making and then supported the patient's choice. Sometimes a decision about what should be done for a patient seems obvious or simple for the health care professional but is in conflict with what the patient wants. This disagreement may be an indication of different values and goals. The challenge to all health care professionals is to acknowledge their own values but to strive to see the situation from the patient's perspective.

Never Accepting a Dead End

The last strategy for acting effectively on your ethical decision is never to accept a dead end! A correlate to this strategy is to keep discussions flowing by discouraging premature closure. Adopting a stance of exploring the issue instead of becoming mired in vigorously defending opinions can encourage reflective discussion about a patient's case.

Sometimes, even with the best efforts, discussion can be blocked by others involved in the decision-making process. At these times, the nurse may need to enlist the assistance of nursing or medical colleagues, supervisors, or others. In some hospitals, a multidisciplinary ethics committee or an ethics consultation team provides another resource.

SUMMARY

What lies beyond the role of patient advocate for nurses? Perhaps a collaborative role in ethical decision making is possible with health care professionals, patients, and families in order to sort through the challenges that critical care offers. By using a shared framework for ethical decision making, the common ground between each person may be nurtured.

Sometimes, because there is little opportunity to act on ethical decisions, it can be discouraging for nurses to become involved in the ethical dimensions of their patients' care. Trying new strategies aimed at collaboration and negotiation, rather than protection and conflict, may decrease this frustration and encourage open communication and involvement in clinical ethics. For the critical care nurse, it is the opportunity to live your ethics.

DIRECTIONS FOR FUTURE RESEARCH

Research in the area of ethics has focused on the role of individual differences (such as age, religion, stage of moral de-velopment) to explain differences in ethical action. The results of these studies have been mixed and inconclusive.

There does not appear to be a set of individual characteristics that account for differences in ethical reasoning or action. The environment in which the nurse practices may be the key to understanding why different choices are made. Rather than focusing on the individual's ethical decision-making process, it may be more useful for future investigations to examine the environmental characteristics that support or constrain ethical reasoning and action.

REFERENCES

1. Engelhardt, H. T. *The Foundations of Bioethics*. New York: Oxford University Press, 1986, p. 9.
2. Fowler, M. D. M. Introduction to ethics and ethical theory: A road map to the discipline. In M. D. M. Fowler & J. Levine-Ariff, *Ethics at the Bedside: A Source Book for the Critical Care Nurse*. Philadelphia, PA: J. B. Lippincott Co., (pp. 24–38), 1987.
3. Fry, S. T. Autonomy, advocacy, and accountability: Ethics at the bedside. In M. D. M. Fowler & J. Levine-Ariff, (eds.), *Ethics at the Bedside: A Source Book for the Critical Care Nurse*. Philadelphia, PA: J. B. Lippincott Co., (pp. 39–49), 1987.
4. Jonsen, A. R., Siegler, M., & Winslade, W. J. *Clinical Ethics* (2nd ed.). New York: Macmillan, 1986.
5. Knaus, W. A., Draper, E. A., Wagner, D. P., & Zimmerman, J. E. An evaluation of outcome from intensive care in major medical centers. *Annals of Internal Medicine*, 194:410, 1986.
6. Mitchell, P. H., Armstrong, S. & Simpson, T. F. American Association of Critical-Care Nurses Demonstration Project: Profile of excellence in critical care nursing. *Heart & Lung* 18:219, 1989.
7. Pellegrino, E. The anatomy of clinical judgments. In H. T. Englelhardt, Jr., S. F. Spicker & B. Towers (eds.), *Clinical Judgment: A Critical Appraisal* (pp. 169–194), 1979.
8. Shannon, S. E. Living your ethics: Strategies of experienced nurses. Paper presented at the American Association of Critical-Care Nurses National Teaching Institute, San Francisco, CA, May, 1990.
9. Taylor, S. Rights and responsibilities: Nurse-patient relationships. *Image* 18:9, 1985.
10. Winslow, G. From loyalty to advocacy: A new metaphor for nursing. *The Hastings Center Report* June:32, 1984.

11

Patient and Family Teaching in Critical Care

Donald A. Bille

GETTING READY FOR SURGERY: BEING IN CONTROL

I met Mr. D while he was awaiting open heart surgery. He was scheduled for coronary artery bypass surgery the next day, and my role that day as Cardiac Surgical Nurse Teacher was to provide preoperative teaching and support. It was obvious after introductions were made that Mr. D was anxious and would not benefit from any teaching at this time. He was easily distracted, avoided eye contact, fidgeted with objects on his table, and seemed to have difficulty concentrating on any conversation.

I proceeded to talk with Mr. D about his recent change in life-style and hospitalization. As the conversation continued, Mr. D relaxed in his chair, stopped fidgeting, made eye contact, and began to breathe more deeply. We then discussed methods he had used successfully in the past to reduce anxiety and stress. He stated that he focused on his breathing and would slow it and consequently feel more relaxed. However, this method had not been successful since he was hospitalized. He was amenable to learning new methods to reduce stress and anxiety, so we explored other methods of focused breathing.

I wanted to use a technique that was quick to learn and could be used by Mr. D himself when a coach might not be available and to promote his need for control. I taught him to think or say "I am" on inspiration and "relaxed" on expiration. Mr. D practiced this with me and felt it would be helpful when he awoke from surgery. He was concerned he would be anxious after surgery and "out of control."

At this time, I was able to discuss his open heart surgery and explore perceptions and concerns to reduce anxiety further. By the time I left Mr. D, he stated he was "ready" for surgery.

The following day, I visited Mr. D 4 hours after surgery. His nurse stated he was waking from anesthesia calmly and was hemodynamically stable. While I visited, he opened his eyes, smiled, and proceeded to "mouth" words around his endotrachial tube. I came closer, trying to understand what he was trying to communicate. The ventilator was cycled, and he took a deep breath in, assisting the ventilator. As he exhaled, the word he mouthed was *Relaxed.*

Pam Davis, RN, BSN, RNC, CCRN
Special Care Unit
Maine Medical Center
Portland, Maine

LEARNING OBJECTIVES

After reading this chapter, the nurse should be able to do the following:

1. State a philosophy of patient teaching.
2. List four assumptions of adult education, and explain their implications for patient teaching.
3. Explain the phases of the teaching-learning process and the importance of each phase.
4. Describe a conceptual framework for arriving at nursing diagnoses in patient teaching.

PHILOSOPHY OF PATIENT TEACHING

The overall objective of teaching carried out by professional nurses is to make changes in health-relevant behavior; ultimately, it aims at adjustment to life-altering behavioral changes with compliance to the medical regimen. Increasingly, nurses have come to realize that a philosophy for patient teaching cannot be separated from the practice of nursing.

Some of the more common beliefs about patient education include the following:

- Patient education is an integral part of comprehensive patient care.
- Patients, as health care consumers, have a right to know what is being done to, for, and about them and their illnesses.
- The patient and family have a need for health care information in order to prevent disease and to improve and maintain health.
- Optimal health is the right of everyone. Inherent in such a right is the person's responsibility to attain or maintain optimal health through his or her own actions.
- Health care knowledge may be instrumental in decreasing the length of the patient's hospitalization or the number of readmissions for the same condition.
- At times, patients may not "learn" at all, making it essential that at least one family member be taught what the patient needs to learn.

ASSUMPTIONS OF ADULT EDUCATION

In the past few years, a distinctive theory about how adults learn has begun to evolve. Educators have known for a long time that they cannot teach adults in the same way that they teach children. Adults are nearly always voluntary participants in a learning experience, and they simply do not continue to participate in learning experiences that do not satisfy them. Even though adults who are "captive audiences" (such as hospitalized patients) may be physically present in a learning environment, they will most likely tune out any instructions that they do not wish to learn. Instructions given while patients are tuned out will be a waste of time for both nurse and patient.

The theory of education that deals with the adult learner is known as *andragogy,* which derives from the Greek stem *andr-,* meaning "man." Andragogy is the art and science of helping adults learn. Adult educators have identified at least four ways in which adult learners differ from child learners:[10] the adult's self-concept has changed from that of a dependent person to that of a person who is capable of self-direction; adults have a large resource for learning based on their life experiences; the adult's motivation to learn is more frequently oriented to problem solving than to learning for the sake of learning; and the adult's time perspective has changed in that the adult desires immediate applicability of knowledge gained. In the following paragraphs, each of these differences is described briefly, and the implications for the nurse who is doing patient teaching are pointed out.

Self-Concept

The adult's self-concept may rule out certain teaching approaches, especially when a disease or injury presents an added burden. Adults see themselves as producers or doers—the breadwinners. They learn their adult role through conscious choice. They do not, however, choose to become sick; therefore, they do not choose the sick role.

The adult who has suffered an illness or injury that is serious enough to warrant admission to a critical care unit may also be suffering from a threat to self-concept. Questions such as "Am I ever going to be the same?" or "Am I ever going to be able to work again?" come from the patient, whereas questions such as "What will my loved one (family member) be like after this?" may be of concern to the family. Patients and family members may not be totally aware of these feelings of threat to self-concept; therefore, it is important for the critical care nurse to listen carefully to what patients and family members are saying.

Experience

Every adult has had a variety of experiences—good and bad—as a part of growing up. Adults become what they have done, and they therefore have a great investment in their accomplishments. For the most part, serious illness is not part of becoming an adult. Thus, coping with illness is not something that an adult can readily call up from past experiences.

Sometimes a patient or a family member may have had some prior experience with a critical care unit or critical illness. If the patient (or a family member) has been hospitalized before, teaching outcomes might need to be aimed more at stress reduction than at knowledge levels.

Patients need a great deal of information about their environment and what is going to happen to them. Even though the information might not stay with the patient permanently (sometimes it is forgotten within 5 to 10 minutes), the time that elapses between teaching and forgetting will be less anxious, thus promoting greater comfort for the time being.

Readiness to Learn

Adults pass through various phases of growth as they respond to the developmental tasks before them. The socially acceptable roles for adults include those of worker, mate, parent, homemaker, son or daughter of aging parents, citizen, friend, organization member, religious affiliate, and user of leisure time.[11] The sick role is not one of the "normal" developmental roles, and the adult who is ill needs time to adapt. Adults are ready to learn (the teachable moment occurs) only when they are able to recognize that a need to learn exists.

Orientation to Learning

Adults need to be able to apply learned material immediately. They participate in the learning process more willingly when the learning activities respond to needs arising from pressures in their current life situation.

Not all the learning needs of critical care patients or their family members relate to the diagnosis or self-care needs after discharge. Thus, patient/family teaching in the critical care setting must be done with a "process" orientation, not a "product" orientation. In the process orientation, the nurse is much more concerned with relieving patient/family anxieties, relieving stressors, and promoting comfort than with a concern for knowledge. Many times, critical care patients and their family members do not remember a word the nurse has said 5 minutes after an interaction with the nurse, but the result may be lowered blood pressure, less nausea, or other physiologic outcomes.[4]

Adults have a problem-centered focus to their learning activities. It will be extremely important for the critical care nurse to determine what problems the patient and family are having as a result of the hospitalization and to deal with these problems before any other teaching-learning content is attempted.

THE TEACHING-LEARNING PROCESS

Efforts at patient/family teaching that are not well organized may take too much of the practitioner's valuable time and may not always produce optimum learning. Organizing patient/family teaching-learning into a particular framework, although it may take some time, may actually save time for the practitioner, and may ultimately achieve a higher degree of success in getting the patient and family to learn what they need to learn, as well as what they want to learn. The patient/family teaching-learning process is a set of seven activities organized and structured to maximize the results for the patient and family (in terms of new knowledge, skills, or attitudes) and to minimize the time and effort of the practitioner. These seven steps include: assessment, nursing diagnosis, planning, implementation, evaluation, documentation, and referral.

Assessment

In patient/family teaching, assessment is the activity of gathering facts and information that assist the practitioner in identifying the patient's or family's needs for learning. Assessment is a vital component in an organized patient/family education program, because it will serve many purposes for both the teacher and the learner. It identifies what the patient/family wants to learn, allows therapeutic seeding, establishes a point of reference in learning, identifies incorrect knowledge, identifies limitations to learning in the patient's home environment, establishes a baseline for evaluation, builds trust and rapport, provides for family involvement, and begins the discharge planning process.

Purposes of Teaching-Learning Assessment

Identify What the Patient and Family Want to Learn. An adult learns best those things that are related to identified problems. If the adult does not yet recognize a problem (*e.g.*, denial is still in effect), it is unlikely that a significant amount of learning will occur. It is impossible to make the adult learn. The practitioner can teach, but unless the patient or family member identifies the need to learn, efforts to teach may fail.

Assessing what the patient and family want to learn is often no more difficult than asking "What concerns you?" or "As a result of your hospitalization, what questions do you have?" Once the patient expresses a concern or question, the need to learn is clearly identified, and learning can take place efficiently and effectively.

Allow Therapeutic Seeding. Anyone who has ever tried to teach patients or their families probably realizes that they often will not express questions or concerns, thus making the teaching-learning process more difficult. At such times, the practitioner cannot make the adult learn. A technique called *therapeutic seeding*, however, can be used to plant ideas in the learner's mind. After the patient and family member have had a chance to think about the idea, needs for learning may be more easily identified and satisfied. Consider the following example.

Mrs. George is a 40-year-old woman who is recovering from a lateral wall myocardial infarction. Conversations with the nurse have already indicated that Mrs. George has not identified any learning needs. The practitioner's therapeutic seeding would consist of statements such as "Mrs. George, many women who have had a heart attack express concerns about how this may affect their diet. What concerns do you have about your diet?" (Note that the practitioner has provided some direction for the assessment—diet—but leaves the decision making up to the patient.)

The practitioner thus inserts externally generated objectives (those thought of by the practitioner and not the patient) into the teaching program by making them part of the therapeutic seeding approach. The patient or family member hears the fact that other patients have problems and can feel comfortable with the fact that he or she too can have problems.

Three different types of responses are likely to be elicited from the patient or family through this technique. First of all, the patient may state, "Oh, I'm not concerned about that." He or she may really be saying "I'm not ready to learn about that yet." The teacher should not become discouraged if the patient is not ready to identify concerns the first time a subject is approached.

A second type of response to "What concerns do you have about your diet?" may be the identification of a specific need to learn. For instance, Mrs. George might say, "You know, I have been wondering about the foods I can eat when I go to someone else's house to play bridge. . . ." She has identified a specific need to learn and, as a result, will learn quickly and efficiently.

The final type of response might be "You know, I don't know enough about diets to even ask. You tell me what I will need to learn about it!" The patient (or family member) has just given the practitioner permission to teach the necessary information.

When used with patience and persistence, therapeutic seeding is a successful technique because it lets adult learners make some decisions about their own teaching program.

Establish a Point of Reference for Learning. It is much easier to learn something when the new information can be related to pre-existing knowledge. Some time and effort will be required during the assessment phase to identify the patient's (or family's) knowledge level. The knowledge may or may not be in a subject directly related to what the patient wants to learn.

Identify Incorrect Knowledge. Gibson[6] has stated that the patient's knowledge "is a hodgepodge of folklore, handed-down family experience, hearsay, bits of advertising, much misinformation, [and] many misconceptions."

The mass media (television, newspapers, magazines, and so forth) convey a great deal of health-related information every day. Information gained from the media or even from friends may be factual but irrelevant to the patient's current illness. It is often difficult for patients to make this differentiation, however, and they may be inclined to believe something because they heard it on television or from a relative. During the teaching-learning process, the practitioner must identify and dispel any incorrect information (including superstitions and folklore) before the process of teaching the correct information begins.

Identify Limitations to Learning in the Patient's Home Environment. During the assessment phase, the patient's environment must be assessed and examined. Patients who do not own a stove or refrigerator will have difficulty complying with their dietary instructions if it is assumed that these appliances are present.

When the home environment cannot be assessed adequately through the interview, it may become necessary to arrange a home visit.

Establish Baseline Data for Evaluation. Evaluation may be conducted for many reasons. Two of the most common reasons for evaluation, however, are to prove that the patient has learned (by measuring the individual patient's knowledge) and to justify the existence of the overall patient/family teaching program (by examining the results of measurements of all patients who have been taught).

The patient and the family should be asked specific questions before one begins teaching each objective. This technique is called *pretesting*. The same questions may be asked again after the teaching has been done (posttesting), and the answers are then compared to determine the change in the patient's knowledge level.

The administration of a pretest is another means of performing therapeutic seeding, because patients are able to see the types and amount of information they do not know. Once the pretest results are shown to the patient, a greater degree of motivation to learn may appear, because the patient is now more aware of the need to learn. An example of a pre- and posttest is presented in Figure 11–1.

When the pretests of all patients are compared with their posttests, the overall success of the patient education program can be seen. If many patients are showing little or no increase in knowledge between the pretest and posttest, the patient/family teaching program should be re-evaluated carefully.

Build Trust and Rapport. One of the most important factors in achieving successful teaching-learning outcomes is establishing trust and rapport, or a situation of mutual respect between the patient and the teacher.[1,3] The teacher's approach to the patient will not only determine the amount of information the patient receives but may affect the accuracy of this information. When the patient senses an attitude of sincerity, integrity, and warmth in the caregiver, the freedom to discuss all matters relating to health is more likely to exist, regardless of how personal those matters may be.[14] Patients will reveal their inner feelings only when they perceive that the teacher accepts them unconditionally. This does not mean that the teacher has to agree with the patient but that the teacher refrains from making moral judgments about the patient's actions or beliefs. "The establishment of rapport or lack of it explains why one examiner may elicit a significant history from a patient when another fails to obtain clear-cut information from the same person."[14]

Provide for Family Involvement. The learning needs of the family, like those of the patient, are essential in achieving optimum health care outcomes.[2] It is essential that the family be involved in the assessment phase as well as in the remainder of the teaching-learning process.

The effective patient/family teacher will determine the family's needs for learning as well as the family's perceptions

of the patient's needs. The family also can provide information about the home environment and the resources they can provide to ease the patient's transition from hospital to home. These resources may be personal (assisting the patient with procedures, cooking, dressing), material (providing finances or equipment), or architectural (moving the patient's bedroom to the first floor).

Begin the Discharge Planning Process. The Joint Commission on Accreditation of Healthcare Organizations (JCAHO) states that "patients who are discharged from the hospital requiring nursing care should receive instructions and individualized counselling prior to discharge, and evidence of the instructions and the patient's or family's understanding of these instructions should be noted in the medical record."[7] Thus, discharge planning must be accomplished for every patient in order to fulfill accreditation criteria.

Although assessment is required to identify nursing diagnoses, teaching needs, and discharge teaching needs, one assessment, if done properly and completely, can be used to evaluate each of these areas. To some extent, the remaining steps of the teaching-learning process are similar to the steps of the nursing and discharge planning processes. Thus, it is useful to think of one overall, organized process, the nursing-teaching/learning-discharge planning process, which encompasses all those activities that the practitioner does with and for the patient and family members. The work done for one activity (*e.g.*, providing care) serves well for all of the other activities (*e.g.*, teaching-learning and discharge planning) (Fig. 11–2).

Assessment of the teaching-learning process takes place throughout the entire program. Information is obtained during each teacher-learner contact. Even the most ideal situation will not yield a complete picture of the patient's learning needs during one encounter, especially the initial contact. As additional information is gained, the patient's teaching/care plan should be revised accordingly.

Conducting the Teaching-Learning Assessment

Assessing the patient's and family's needs for teaching-learning is done through a good interview, which is conducted in much the same way as history taking.[14] The components of a thorough interview have been discussed in Chapter 5.

Analysis (Nursing Diagnosis)

Information about the concerns and needs of the patient and the family as well as the limitations of their knowledge that was gathered during the assessment phase of the teaching-learning process is analyzed by the practitioner. The data gathered during the assessment form the basis for all other activities occurring throughout the remainder of the teaching-learning process (as well as the nursing process and the discharge planning process).

Conceptual Framework for Analysis

The activities of the analysis, or nursing diagnosis, phase of the teaching-learning process are intellectual. It is easier to carry out this intellectual function (and therefore establish a nursing diagnosis) if the practitioner uses a conceptual frame-

Pre- and Post-diabetic Test

Name: _____ Identification Number: _____

Part A: 50 Points

Please check the correct answers to the following questions:

1. Diabetes will "go away" when the blood sugar and urine are kept normal.
   True _____ False _____
2. The pancreas plays an important role in diabetes.
   True _____ False _____
3. Diabetes only occurs in the 30- to 60-year age group.
   True _____ False _____
4. Calories are made up of carbohydrate, protein, and fat.
   True _____ False _____
5. All diabetic persons must take insulin.
   True _____ False _____
6. Routine exercise and foot care are important to the diabetic patient.
   True _____ False _____
7. A diabetic patient must always eat at home—never in restaurants or at parties.
   True _____ False _____
8. Margarine has fewer calories than butter.
   True _____ False _____
9. Regular canned fruit may be used by washing with cold water.
   True _____ False _____
10. Black coffee, tea, and broth are "free foods."
    True _____ False _____

Part B: 50 points

Answer the following questions. Use the back of this page if necessary.

11. What is diabetes?

_____
_____
_____

12. How is diabetes controlled?

_____
_____
_____

13. Describe how you might feel if your blood sugar is too <u>low</u>?

   a. _____   d. _____
   b. _____   e. _____
   c. _____   f. _____

14. Describe how you might feel if your blood sugar is too <u>high</u>?

   a. _____   d. _____
   b. _____   e. _____
   c. _____   f. _____

15. Name two complications of diabetes. Write the symptoms and the causes.

   a. _____
      _____
   b. _____
      _____

Figure 11–1

Pre- and post-diabetic test. This test, which was developed from and based on the objectives for the diabetes education classes, is used before teaching as a "needs assessment" (as well as an external motivator for learning) and as a "summative evaluation" at the end of the teaching program.

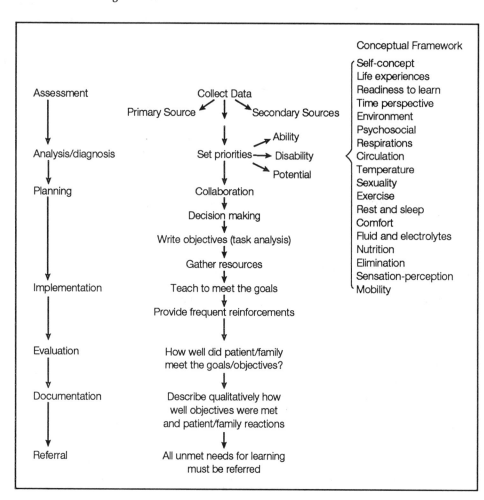

Figure 11–2

The patient's and family's teaching-learning process. The seven steps of the process are seen as flowing from each other, continuous, and often simultaneous. The conceptual framework (seen at the upper right of the figure) is used to organize one's thinking as well as each of the activities in the process.

work (*i.e.,* a "package" of ideas by which to organize one's thinking).

A practical conceptual framework for patient and family teaching is one that combines the activities and demands of daily living[13] with the assumptions about adults as learners.[10] An activity of daily living (ADL) is something that someone needs to do on a regular, if not daily, basis (*e.g.,* eating, or nutrition). Patients and their families often are placed into situations in which one or more ADL needs to be changed because of disease or injury. Each ADL places certain demands on the individual. With the ADL of nutrition, for instance, someone will have to shop for groceries, carry the food home, store it, cook it, serve it, wash dishes later, and then finally carry out the garbage. Each of these demands of daily living (DDL) must be carried out to meet one ADL.

Mitchell and Loustau[13] proposed that chronic illness might affect 13 different ADLs. Knowles[10,11] proposed that four assumptions (self-concept, life experiences, readiness to learn, and orientation to learning) are unique to each individual adult learner. By using the list of ADLs along with the assumptions about the adult learner, the practitioner can quickly determine what learning needs the patient and family may have (Table 11–1). During the assessment phase, if the list of ADLs and assumptions also are used as a framework for data collection, the practitioner can arrive more easily and quickly at a complete list of teaching-learning needs for both the patient and the family. For the patient or family who needs information on nutrition, the nursing diagnosis would read "knowledge

deficit about nutrition related to newly prescribed diet (low sodium)."

Set Priorities for Learning

Although it is the learner (patient or family member) who really decides what is to be learned (whether consciously or not), the practitioner can assist the patient and family member in the determination of what their strengths are, what the most urgent needs seem to be (related to the patient's condition), and what learning needs can be left for sometime in the future. Setting priorities for learning is the final part of the analysis phase of the teaching-learning process.[16]

In analyzing the collected data, three distinct categories of data, including abilities, disabilities, and potential disabilities, are established. Each of these categories is then used to determine the priority of needs for teaching-learning. *Abilities* are those aspects of self-care (such as the ADLs and DDLs) that the patient or family is managing well. These abilities also are called strengths. It is helpful to begin teaching-learning interactions with a review of the patient's strengths (*e.g.,* "Mr. Jones, you are already doing a fine job of managing your diet and your medications.") and, in this way, reward the patient and family member for skills they have already mastered. In addition, this prevents the practitioner from reteaching items the patient already knows.

Disabilities are those self-care abilities that the patient or family member is not able to do because he or she lacks the

Table 11-1
Activities of Daily Living

ACTIVITY	SAMPLE DESCRIPTION
Environment	What is the atmosphere surrounding the patient and family at home, at work, in the community?
Psychosocial	What stage of adaptation are the patient and family in?
	What types of social activities are important to the patient and family?
Respiratory	Are there any breathing difficulties or potential for respiratory complications?
Circulatory	Are there any circulatory complications, such as edema or arteriosclerotic changes?
Temperature	Is there any exposure to extremely hot or cold temperatures?
Sexuality	Does the patient and significant other have a comfortable sexual relationship?
Rest and sleep	Are the patient and family able to sleep soundly, without interruption?
Comfort	Does the patient have any pain or other feeling that is discomforting?
Fluid and electrolytes	Is intake and output adequate?
	Is there a need to restrict either the amount of fluids or the type of fluids?
Nutrition	Is body weight adequate, or is some adjustment necessary?
Elimination	Is there any problem with either bowel movements or urinary output?
Sensation and perception	Does tactile, visual, or hearing loss exist?
Mobility	Are the patient and family able to move around freely, without pain or limitation?

Modified from Mitchell, P. H. and Loustau, A. *Concepts Basic to Nursing* (3rd ed.). New York: McGraw-Hill, 1981:118; with permission.

knowledge, skill, or will to do so. Also called weaknesses or self-care deficits, the disabilities are viewed as short-term needs for learning. They involve the immediate need to learn activities in order to "survive" on discharge from the hospital; they represent the "need to know" category of learning objectives. Examples of survival skills might be medication administration, dressing changes, intake and output measurement, and vital signs.

Potential disabilities are those long-term learning needs that are "nice to know" aspects of one's self-care. The learning needs represent self-care knowledge, skills, and attitudes that may not be essential today but might be essential sometime in the future. For instance, if someone is a few pounds overweight, this may not be a priority problem today, but if the weight gain continues, it could be a problem a year from now. This patient might be referred to a community-based agency for help with this problem.

Planning

The next step of the teaching-learning process begins as soon as a learning need has been identified. A teaching-learning plan is focused on the patient's or family member's need to learn and contains objectives for the patient's or family's learning. The learning objectives are goals, ends, or outcomes desired from the teaching-learning interactions and are written in terms of those things the patient and family should be able to do after such interactions have occurred.

Purposes of Learning Objectives

Writing learning objectives is probably one of the most difficult aspects of the teaching-learning process, especially for the beginning teacher. It is also one of the most time-consuming aspects. With experience, however, writing objectives becomes easier and more meaningful.

The usefulness of learning objectives far outweighs the effort needed to write them, because the objectives clarify what is to be taught and learned as well as clarify what (and how) to evaluate, what to document, and what may need to be referred on the discharge plan.

Objectives Clarify What Is to Be Taught. Many different practitioners interact with each patient or family member every day. A written teaching care plan containing objectives for the patient's or family's learning, aims to achieve continuity of all teaching efforts toward specific goals.

Objectives Clarify What Is to Be Learned. Objectives for the patient's and family's teaching-learning process should be established together with the patient and the family. Once learning needs are identified, these needs are discussed and the planning of objectives (and the learning experiences that follow) becomes a mutual undertaking between the learner(s) and the teacher.

Mutual teacher-learner planning fits into the philosophy of adult education. The mutual planning of objectives is sometimes called a *learning contract*.[11,16] Contracting is a vital component of a successful patient/family education program because "the learner develops a sense of ownership of (and commitment to) the plan."[11]

A simplified way to view the learning contract can be illustrated as follows: After the list of abilities, disabilities, and potential disabilities has been translated into learning needs, the practitioner shows the complete list (with the three categories) to the patient or family member. The conversation might sound something like this: "Mr. Smith, as a result of the things you have told me about yourself and your lifestyle, I have written a list of items that we need to discuss to help you adjust to your heart disease. Take a look at this list. You can see that there are quite a few things that you are doing very well already; therefore, we don't need to go over these things again unless you would like to. I also see a few things on this list that you may want to consider learning or changing. Is there anything on this list that you disagree with? Is there anything that you think might be important that is not on this list?" Finally, "Which of the items on this list is most important to you? Would you like to start by learning more about this item?"

Once the patient or family member has had the opportunity to critique the list, make additions or deletions, and choose where on the list to begin, the level of commitment and readiness to learn will have increased to a point where the patient is more likely to be motivated to learn.

Objectives Clarify What (and How) to Evaluate.   At the time an educational plan is written out, the patient and teacher agree on what is to be learned. Evaluation involves determining whether the patient and family have learned adequately to satisfy the objective. A well-written objective specifies what the patient will be able to do and the particular behavior that will demonstrate that learning has occurred. For instance, one typical objective for learning for a patient with ulcerative colitis is the following: "List stress factors in your own life-style that aggravate ulcerative colitis." Evaluation of this objective would be accomplished by having the patient write or verbalize a list of the various life stressors that increase the symptoms of ulcerative colitis.

Objectives Clarify What to Document.   Documentation of the patient's learning outcomes is problematic for many practitioners. As a result, few medical records have adequate documentation of teaching-learning outcomes.[5] A well-written objective, however, assists the practitioner in documentation as well as evaluation. To document the objectives for the patient with ulcerative colitis, for instance, one might simply ask the patient to accurately list those stress factors in his or her own life-style that aggravate ulcerative colitis.

Objectives Clarify What Is to Be Referred.   Once objectives have been written, the entire learning package for the patient and the family has been determined. Any portion of that package that has not yet been satisfactorily learned before hospital discharge will need to be referred to the community health agency.

The Components of an Objective

Each objective for patient teaching must contain two important components: an observable verb (*i.e.*, a verb that denotes an observable behavior) and the content.

The first part of each learning objective contains a verb, or action word, that states what the learner is to do to demonstrate achievement of the objective. Verbs such as *know, understand,* or *comprehend* are poor terms because they are neither observable nor easily interpreted. On the other hand, terms such as *identify, list, state, plan, give, define,* and *read* relate to more easily observed actions, have fewer interpretations, and thus are more useful to the patient's learning program.

The second part of each objective is the content (in terms of knowledge, attitudes, or skills) that the patient will learn. The content is the substance of the objective that meets the assessed learning need. Examples of the content part of objectives include life-style factors in heart disease, signs and symptoms of postoperative infection, reasons for a low-residue diet, and high-protein diet for 24 hours. By combining the two components (the verb and the content), complete, observable objectives, such as the following, are written:

Identify life-style factors in heart disease.
List signs and symptoms of postoperative infection.
State reasons for a low-residue diet.
Plan a high-protein diet for 24 hours.

The Usefulness of an Objective

Once an objective has been written, it must be examined for four qualities in order to be useful. Objectives must be specific, inclusive, measurable, and realistic.

An objective is *specific* if it contains a singular idea. Although combining similar ideas into one objective (*i.e.*, list signs and symptoms of postoperative infection and necessary wound care) may shorten the list of objectives, it encumbers the teaching and evaluation stages, making more work for the teacher later on.

The amount of information contained in an objective may also make it more *inclusive.* For instance, if all persons involved in teaching the patient and the family about the signs and symptoms of postoperative infection know and agree on what those signs and symptoms are, there is no need to list them in the objective. If one or more persons disagree, however, then the content portion of the objective should be expanded to include the information the patient and family should learn. The more inclusive objective now reads as follows: List signs and symptoms of postoperative infection, including heat, redness, swelling . . . (etc.).

An objective becomes more easily *measurable* if the number of items in the content portion is mentioned. For instance, one may ask the patient to list the four Es that may precipitate angina. (*Note*: The four Es are emotion, eating, exercise, and exposure to cold.)

An objective is *realistic* only if it can be attained by the patient and family member(s). This quality can be ascertained by assessing with the patient and the family the ability to achieve the objective. At times, an objective that is not realistic for the patient may need to be taught to a family member (*e.g.*, instructing the patient to give himself or herself 40 units of NPH insulin daily may not be realistic for the patient who has crippling rheumatoid arthritis, but it might be managed by a family member). When a specific objective, such as grocery shopping, is the usual responsibility of one family member, it may not be realistic to teach other family members about it. In this situation, the objective would become "Mrs. Jones will demonstrate what to look for on food container labels."

Implementation

Once a teaching-learning need has been identified and an objective agreed on by the teacher and learner, the most difficult parts of the teaching-learning process have been accomplished. Implementation is accomplished by communicating information about specific objectives to the patient and family.

This author firmly believes that skill in the art of teaching is not the result of an advanced college education but the result of actual practice. Thus, the lack of a college diploma should not be an excuse for not teaching. Knowledge of what is to be taught, the ability to communicate that knowledge to others, and the sensitive observation of the patient's or family's reactions likely will promote successful outcomes of most teaching-learning interactions.

Determine Content to Be Taught

Ideas are more easily understood if they are organized in a logical sequence, from simple to more complex. The practitioner must analyze all the material to be presented before beginning. Does the patient or family need background information before teaching a specific objective? Is there a logical progression inherent in the material itself?

One of the greatest fears expressed by most practitioners is that the patient or a family member will ask questions for which they may not know the answer. Undoubtedly, this situation does occur, but it can be handled best by saying something like, "That's a very good question, and I don't know the answer, but I'll find out for you." Thus, the patient, family members, and nurse have learned new information.

Determine Method of Presentation

In the past, teacher-learner interactions have been based on the false belief that exposure to material assures learning. "Yet each generation rediscovers the fact that in the end it is the learner who must do the learning, and no amount of communication by lecture, by book, by film, by radio, or by television will make the slightest difference unless he or she does something with what he or she receives."[15]

Several factors have an influence on whether the learner does anything with what is received, including the teaching methods used. Various methods for conveying information exist, and each one has its own strengths and weaknesses. Regardless of the method used, the practitioner must pay attention to one important characteristic that makes the adult learner unique—the need for immediate, present-tense application.

Lecture.   The lecture traditionally has been the most widely used, and therefore abused, method of presenting material to the adult learner. A large amount of content can be presented easily, either to an individual or a group, through the lecture, but the amount of material actually learned or implemented may not be in proportion to the amount of material presented.

Many barriers exist in the patient or family member that interfere with the receipt of information from a lecture delivered without any other aids. It has been estimated that a human being hears only about 24% of the material that is being delivered through a lecture.[8,15] Listening is the body's most passive activity. Listeners can also daydream, become confused, or even refer to inappropriate experiences for help in understanding something new, "hoping to draw conclusions which may then apply to the new problem."[15]

A lecture will be more effective if it is combined with one or more of the body's senses. For each sense that is added, in addition to hearing, the learning process becomes not only more active but also more efficient.

The practitioner can involve the patient's senses by teaching while performing a procedure. For instance, while giving foot care to a diabetic, the practitioner can explain the procedure to the patient or family member; the procedure can then be seen and felt by the patient. If an infection is present, the sense of smell may enter into the teaching-learning process. All five senses can be involved by teaching about a therapeutic diet while the patient is eating. The patient will be able to hear the explanation, see, smell, and taste the food, and may even learn useful information by touching the food.

When material is presented by lecture, the practitioner strives immediately to apply the material just taught. This can be done by designing a case study or some other teaching method. Once the adult has had a chance to practice what has been taught, learning and retention will be greater.

Demonstration.   When any skill is being taught, the demonstration method (often combined with a lecture) is an effective teaching method. Once the theory or rationale for a particular skill has been presented, the actual skill can be demonstrated to the patient or family member, and they can then be provided with an immediate chance to return-demonstrate the skill (the return demonstration is the chance for immediate application necessary for learning).

Audiovisuals.   During the past decade, the field of audiovisual education has proliferated. This proliferation has spilled over into the field of patient and family teaching, and many educators now rely heavily on mediated presentations. The rationale behind mediated instruction is accurate; humans do learn better when more than one of their body's senses is involved in the teaching learning process.

Color slides, particularly 35 mm, can be made cheaply and easily. Although the practitioner should check copyright laws carefully, many times slides can be taken of textbook illustrations and used to explain concepts. Statistical, numerical, and other factual data (such as definitions) also can be used as teaching slides.

Overhead transparencies may be handwritten or drawn. Many photocopy machines also reproduce typed, graphic, or other illustrative materials on specially prepared transparencies. These special transparencies often come in various colors, providing variety for the viewer and organization of material by the presenter.

Films, such as 16 mm or super 8 movies, can be used to teach or to supplement teaching by other methods. This type of medium, however, tends to be more expensive than some others, and it can be less flexible and harder to keep current. Many practitioners function under the misconception that the entire movie must be shown during a teaching-learning session. If a film has only 1 minute of worthwhile material essential to the understanding of a concept, the movie can be turned on for that 1 minute, and then stopped. As the film is being introduced, the practitioner should inform the viewers what to look for, what to remember, and what points will be discussed after viewing.

Television is an easily portable method for teaching. Videocassettes are a relatively inexpensive item and can easily be played for the viewer at any time without changing the lighting or other conditions of the classroom. Many times, universities, associations, and organizations have materials on videotape that can be procured without charge simply by sending them a blank cassette. Videotapes already in possession of the health care organization also can be easily duplicated to provide the patient or family with a copy for viewing at home.

Audiotapes are another cheap means of conveying information. As in a lecture, the length and amount of information conveyed by this medium are limited. Audiotapes have the additional limitation that the listener cannot see the speaker and his or her body language. Ideally, audiotapes should be accompanied by illustrative materials that the listener can refer to while listening to the tape.

To organize audiovisuals into an effective presentation takes time and effort (plus money) on the part of the educator. As Prior and Silberstein state, "The time and effort involved, however, are well spent; for, when used with skill and zeal, each type of media can help to make an instructor a more effective communicator."[14]

Many different methods of presentation can be used successfully within the same teaching-learning interaction, but they must be viewed as supplements to the human teacher. Whereas audiovisual materials may be able to convey all of the information needed in a high school or college course, patient and family teaching will always require human interactions because of the psychosocial adjustments the patient and family undergo.

Computer-Assisted Instruction.   Computers are now being used to a wide extent to facilitate teaching-learning. Computers can be used in many different ways and can facilitate both cognitive and psychomotor learning. Demonstrations of skills can be provided by interactive computer software just as effectively as a live instructor. The computer cannot observe the patient and family members while they give a return demonstration, however.

Computers are still very expensive, and software (the actual materials used to teach) is limited at this time for patient and family teaching. In addition, many adults may never have had hands-on experience with a computer and therefore may not feel comfortable learning on the computer.

Simulation.   The simulation of an experience is one more method the practitioner can use to promote effective learning through immediate application. Once the content has been presented, a situation can be set up to provide an opportunity for practice and application. This method is probably best used when some skill has been taught during the program, but it also allows the practitioner to measure knowledge effectively.

Simulations have been used effectively in such content areas as grocery shopping, cooking, managing home-based intravenous infusion and hemodialysis, and recognizing a wound infection during dressing changes. Thus, the practitioner can use the simulation method for almost any situation in which skills are involved.

Provide Frequent Reinforcements of Teaching and Learning

Learning that is reinforced will become stronger and is more likely to have an influence on health-related behaviors. A principle learned early in almost any psychology course is that behavior that is rewarded tends to be repeated. Therefore, whenever the patient and family responds to a teaching-learning interaction by giving the expected (correct) response (knowledge, attitude, or skill), the practitioner provides a reward, such as praise for a job well done, to reinforce that learning.

Reinforcements can be provided verbally or in writing. Written reinforcements provide immediate rewards for learning and continuing reinforcement each time the patient or family looks at the written material. Written reinforcements can be individualized (*i.e.,* information is written at the time a reinforcement is given). For instance, after teaching a patient or family member about a prescription drug, the pharmacist can review and reinforce what has been learned by writing the information on a sheet of paper.

Preprinted information can also be used to reinforce teaching-learning interactions. When content to be learned is always identical, with little or no room for individualization (*i.e.,* certain prescription drugs), forms can be developed and then handed out after a teaching-learning interaction has been completed successfully.

Evaluation

The process of evaluation, or determining whether the patient and the family has achieved the learning objectives, is easy once the objectives have been written. The objectives tell what the patient will be able to do and specify the particular behavior that demonstrates that learning has occurred.

For instance, the objective "Identify risk factors that contribute to coronary heart disease" can be evaluated by asking the learner to talk about the various factors that probably contribute to this condition. The objective "List signs and symptoms of postoperative infection" can be evaluated by saying, "Tell me what things you should look for around your incision?" or "What would you notice if your incision was becoming infected?" The objective "State reasons for low-residue diet" can be evaluated by asking, "Why has your doctor placed you on a special diet?" or "Why are you supposed to avoid foods with high residue?"

Once the practitioner is sure the patient knows the correct answer or can perform a skill properly, this provides an opportunity to re-evaluate the patient's learning and to raise the patient's self-esteem when the patient successfully explains, defines terms, or demonstrates skills to a family member. During this brief period, the patient is "promoted" or steps out of the sick role, and assumes the role of teacher.

Documentation

The outcome of the teaching-learning interaction is recorded in the medical record. According to the JCAHO, "nursing documentation should address the patient's needs, problems, capabilities, and limitations. Nursing intervention and patient response must be noted."[7] Documentation has at least three purposes: It provides valuable communication to all other members of the health-care team, it serves as a legal record of what happened to the patient during hospitalization, and it helps to satisfy accreditation standards of the JCAHO. Documentation, however, is often not sufficient by itself to meet any of these purposes,[5] and it must still be accompanied by verbal communication to other practitioners.

Documentation of the patient's learning outcomes can be simplified to a point where it becomes less difficult for the busy practitioner to remember what to chart. According to the JCAHO, "the nursing department or service is encouraged to standardize documentation of routine elements of care and repeated monitoring of, for example, personal hygiene, administration of medication, and physiologic parameters."[7]

Documentation of the patient's learning program must contain two components. First, documentation contains notations on how well the patient and family achieved the learning objectives. This component is met adequately by using a standardized form such as the one presented in Figure 11–3. The practitioner also makes notations on the patient's and family's reactions to the teaching-learning situation and the content of this instruction. This can only be done in narrative form,

---

Patient Education Guide for Hypertension

Directions: Enter date of teaching session at column head. If you supply or review information suggested by objective, enter "R." If patient gives satisfactory response, enter "S," if unsatisfactory, enter "U."

Objective: Date: _____   Comments:

1. Defines blood pressure (B/P)   _____

2. Defines hypertension   _____

3. Defines systolic blood pressure   _____

4. Defines diastolic blood pressure   _____

5. States that the cause of hypertension is unknown   _____

6. States that hypertension is a lifetime condition that can be
    controlled but not cured.   _____

7. States that hypertension is often asymptomatic.   _____

8. Lists the complications of hypertension   _____

9. Defines the following:
    a. Stroke or cerebrovascular accident (CVA)   _____

    b. Heart attack or myocardial infarction (MI)   _____

    c. Kidney failure   _____

10. States common symptoms of:
    a. CVA   _____

Figure 11–3

Patient education guide for hypertension. This preprinted form (first page only is shown here) is used for documentation of teaching-learning interactions with the patient and family. Blank spaces are added at the end of the guide for individualized patient and family teaching objectives. This form can be printed on pressure-sensitive, multiple-copy forms, such that the original stays on the medical record, a copy is sent to the community or home health agency as a referral, a copy goes home with the patient, and one goes to the physician's office. A separate form can be developed for each diagnosis, saving a great deal of time and effort for the busy practitioner.

but the narrative can be included either in a "comments" section of the preprinted form or as a separate entry in the "progress notes" of the patient's medical record.

Note Patient and Family Achievement

Each time a teaching-learning interaction occurs, especially when an objective is achieved, a notation should be made in the patient's medical record. The information includes a qualitative description of how well the patient achieved the objective. For instance, the documentation might read as follows: "Accurately identified life-style factors contributing to heart disease; listed four signs and symptoms of postoperative infection; will reteach swelling and heat; planned high-protein diet for 24 hours; needs to pay more attention to a variety of foods in the three meals."

Note Patient Reactions

The teaching-learning process also requires the teacher to make particular observations throughout each interaction. The teacher needs to be alert to subtle cues that the patient or family does not understand information being taught or does not accept the information or the condition itself. This observation is sometimes helpful in predicting how closely the patient will follow posthospitalization prescriptions as well as in deciding how much or what kind of follow-up is needed by other health care agencies when the patient leaves the hospital.

Observations should be recorded as they are seen or heard, without subjective information or opinions. For example, if the patient has expressed doubts as to why life-style factors

in heart disease need to be changed, documentation might reads as follows: "Accurately identified life-style factors that contribute to heart disease, but stated 'I don't see what this has to do with me! There's nothing wrong with my life-style!'"

Referral

Any teaching-learning need that has not been met must be referred to another organization (such as a home health agency or the community health nursing department) or another individual (such as the physician or the office nurse).[9] The process of referral, or discharge planning, is easier because of the objectives that were written during an earlier phase of the teaching-learning process. When these objectives have been preprinted on a form, such as that seen in Figure 11–3, a copy of that form can be sent to the referral agency; in this way, the agency is able to see which learning objectives have already been met and which objectives remain to be taught.

SUMMARY

Patient and family teaching is a responsibility of the professional nurse. Many nurses have philosophies of nursing care that include teaching as a direct or indirect function within patient care.

The steps of the teaching-learning process help to organize teaching and learning and provide for the assessment of knowledge, nursing diagnosis of learning needs, planning of teaching-learning, implementation of teaching, evaluation and documentation of learning outcomes, and referral of learning needs after discharge from hospital.

REFERENCES

1. Bille, D. A. Patients' knowledge and compliance with posthospitalization prescriptions as related to body image and teaching format. Ph.D. dissertation. Madison: University of Wisconsin, 1975.

2. Bille, D. A. The role of body image in patient compliance and education. *Heart Lung* 6:143, 1977.

3. Bille, D. A. *Practical Approaches to Patient Teaching.* Boston: Little, Brown, 1981.

4. Bille, D. A. Process-oriented patient education. *Dimens. Crit. Care Nurs.* 2:108, 1983.

5. Bille, D. A. Personal conversations with Joint Commission on Accreditation of Healthcare Organizations Nurse Surveyors, June 4, 1987.

6. Gibson, W. B. But who teaches the patient? *Arch. Dermatol.* 88: 1935, 1963.

7. Joint Commission on Accreditation of Hospitals. *Accreditation Manual for Hospitals.* Chicago: Joint Commission on Accreditation of Hospitals, 1985.

8. Klevins, C. *Materials and Methods in Adult Education.* New York: Klevins, 1972.

9. Klis, M. A. Discharge Planning and Patient Teaching. In Bille, D. A. (ed.), *Practical Approaches to Patient Teaching.* Boston: Little, Brown, 1981:113–130.

10. Knowles, M. S. *The Modern Practice of Adult Education.* New York: Association Press, 1970.

11. Knowles, M. S. *The Adult Learner: A Neglected Species* (2nd ed.). Houston: Gulf Publishing, 1973.

12. Miller, G. E. The continuing education of physicians. *N. Engl. J. Med.* 269:298, 1963.

13. Mitchell, P. H., and Loustau, A. *Concepts Basic to Nursing.* New York: McGraw-Hill, 1981.

14. Prior, J. A., and Silberstein, J. S. *Physical Diagnosis: The History and Examination of the Patient* (4th ed.). St. Louis: C. V. Mosby, 1973.

15. Whittich, V. A., and Schuler, C. F. *Audiovisual Materials: Their Nature and Use* (4th ed.). New York: Harper & Row, 1967.

16. Ziemann, K. M., and Dracup, K. How well do CCU patient-nurse contracts work? *Am. J. Nurs.* 5:691–693, 1989.

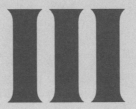

III

Technology in Critical Care Nursing

RECOGNIZING THE DIFFERENCE BETWEEN PHYSICAL HEALTH AND SPIRITUAL HEALTH
There are many flaws in contemporary thinking about the relationship between physical and spiritual health. One of these is equating spiritual health with bodily health. On the surface, it would appear, because healing and spirituality seem so closely related, that those who are highly evolved spiritually would be supremely healthy. It is not that simple. When we explore the lives of people who are ''spiritual giants''—those who are indeed highly evolved spiritually—we discover the complexity of the relationship between spiritual and bodily health. For example, the beloved saint of modern India, Sri Ramana Maharshi, died of cancer in 1950. Although he demonstrated unquestioned transcendent spiritual attainment, he died with much physical pain and suffering. When his devotees asked him to explain the great contradiction between his pain and suffering and his enlightened state, he offered a large, compassionate, loving smile and responded, ''You take my body for Bhagavan and attribute the suffering to him. [But] I am not identified with the body. I am the Self. If [my] hand . . . were cut with a knife, there would be pain, but because [I am] not identified with the body, [I would remain] in bliss despite the pain.''*

   If you search the mystical literature of both the East and the West, bodily health and spiritual attainment do not always correlate. Sometimes an inverse correlation seems to occur, for with physical illness many persons experience a sense of wholeness. Yet it is true that physical illness may disappear as one moves forward on a spiritual path, but when this happens, it seems to be almost a grace or an aside. What is most important in all the great spiritual traditions is the inner life of the spirit, not the outer health of the body.

* Osborne, A. *Ramana Maharshi and the Path of Self-Knowledge.* New York: Samuel Weiser, 1973: 186.

12

Cardiac Monitoring and Dysrhythmias

Linda C. Gary   *Cathie E. Guzzetta*

SCIENTIFIC LOGIC AND INTUITION

Some people have a love-hate attitude toward science and the rationality and logic it stands for. They see the scientific mind as hostile toward intuition, that inner kind of knowing that so often is impossible to describe and with which they feel most comfortable. Some believe they have to make a choice between being either "right-brained intuitives" or "left-brained rationalists."

A look at the lives of the greatest scientists shows that this choice is artificial. They combined high degrees of intuition with analysis, logic, and reason. Einstein is a case in point. He thought in images and "dressed them up" in mathematical formulas as a last step.* Michael Faraday, who preceded Einstein, was also an interesting example. Faraday was poorly schooled in mathematics. Like Einstein he arrived at his scientific theories through rich visual and mental images and could even see invisible "lines of force" between physical bodies.†

All of us are rich tapestries of *both* modes of mental function—the intuitive and the rational. When we elevate one mode over the other, we cut off an essential part of our psyche. Being a nurse requires *all* we are, not just a part.

LEARNING OBJECTIVES

After reading this chapter, the nurse should be able to do the following:

1. Discuss the electrostatic and chemical events for each of the five phases of the action potential.
2. Identify the normal placement and configuration of the standard 12 electrocardiogram leads and MCL₁ lead.
3. Calculate and interpret the electrical axis from a 12-lead electrocardiogram.
4. Calculate heart rate from a 6-second rhythm strip.
5. Outline a systematic approach for assessing cardiac rhythm strips.
6. Discuss the significance, pathology, electrocardiographic criteria, treatment, and nursing responsibilities for patients with cardiac dysrhythmias and cardiac conduction disturbances.

* Koestler, A. *The Act of Creation.* New York: Dell, 1964: 171.
† Kendall, J. *Michael Faraday.* London: Faber, 1955: 138.

PROPERTIES OF CARDIAC MUSCLES

Cardiac muscle (the atrial and ventricular muscle and the specialized conduction muscle fibers) has characteristics that determine its function, such as automaticity, excitability, conductivity, and contractility.

Automaticity refers to the ability of the heart to initiate its own impulse. *Excitability* is the heart's ability to respond to an impulse. The ability of the heart to transmit electrical impulses to other areas of the heart is referred to as *conductivity.* *Contractility* may be defined as the heart's ability to achieve tension and muscle fiber shortening.

AUTONOMIC NERVOUS SYSTEM CONTROL

The heart is influenced by the two divisions of the autonomic nervous system—the sympathetic system and parasympathetic system, which maintain a balance by their opposing forces.

The origin of the sympathetic nerves supplying the heart is at the level of the first thoracic through the second lumbar vertebrae of the spinal column. Sympathetic nerve endings are located in the atria and the ventricles. Stimulation of those nerve endings releases norepinephrine, which produces an increase in the overall activity of the heart by increasing the rate of discharge from the sinoatrial (SA) node, increasing conduction through the atrioventricular (AV) node, augmenting the force of atrial and ventricular contraction, and increasing the excitability of the heart. The sympathetic system is referred to as the *adrenergic system*.

Parasympathetic nerve endings, on the other hand, are found primarily in the atria, and they leave the central nervous system through the cranial and sacral spinal nerves. The vagi are the parasympathetic nerves of the heart. When stimulated, acetylcholine is released at the vagal nerve endings, producing a reduction in the rate of discharge from the SA node, a decrease in the excitability of the AV junctional fibers, a slowing of AV node conduction, and a slight reduction in ventricular contractility. The parasympathetic system is generally referred to as the *cholinergic system*.

ELECTROCHEMICAL PHYSIOLOGY

The electrical activity of the heart consists of depolarization (stimulation) and repolarization (relaxation). These two events are the results of electrochemical changes in the membrane potential of cardiac cells. In these cells, there is a larger concentration of potassium inside the cell in contrast to a larger concentration of sodium and calcium outside the cell. In the resting cell, there is also an intracellular negativity that establishes a membrane potential between the inside and outside of the cell (Fig. 12–1).

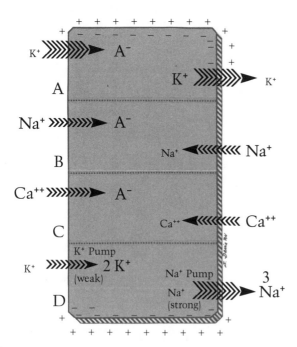

Figure 12–1

Factors responsible for the resting membrane potential. Left side of (A), (B), and (C) illustrate the electrostatic forces that balance the chemical forces on the right side of (A), (B), and (C). The size of the *arrows* represents the relative importance of the forces acting on the resting membrane potential. The size of the *ions* represents their concentration inside and outside the cell. (D) illustrates the effects of the sodium-potassium pump on the resting membrane potential.

Membrane Potential

An electrical potential gradient exists across the cell membrane. The interior of the cell is negative with respect to the outside of the cell. This resting membrane potential (Vm) is −80 to −90 mV in all areas of the heart except the SA and AV nodes. This resting membrane potential is determined primarily by two mechanisms: active transport of ions across the membrane (sodium-potassium pump), and concentration gradient for potassium.[5,10]

When the cell is at rest, ions are actively transported by the sodium-potassium pump, which pumps sodium out of the cell and potassium into the cell. Because the sodium pump is stronger than the potassium pump, three sodium ions are pumped out of the cell for every two potassium ions pumped into the cell, contributing approximately 10 mV to the negative intracellular potential. Because the sodium-potassium pump results in an excess of negative charges inside the cell, the pump has been termed the *electrogenic pump*.

The membrane potential is also maintained because of the concentration gradient for potassium. The resting membrane is much more permeable to potassium than to either sodium or calcium. Because there is a higher concentration of potassium inside than outside the cell ($K_i^+ > K_0^+$), intracellular potassium readily diffuses to the outside of the cell in the direction of its concentration gradient.[5] Potassium leaving the cell causes a net deficit of positive ions on the inside of the cell and accounts for the remainder of the −90 mV transmembrane potential.

When considering the movement of sodium across the cell, diffusional factors play only a small role in the development of the resting Vm. This is because the membrane is only slightly permeable to sodium ions. Because of the electronegativity inside the cell, electrostatic forces are present to pull sodium from the outside to the inside of the cell. Although the chemical and electrostatic forces are pulling extracellular sodium into the cell, the net influx of sodium is small because of the low membrane permeability to sodium. In addition, the sodium pump is pumping sodium against its electrostatic and chemical gradients, removing sodium from the cell, and further creating an electronegativity inside the cell.[5]

In summary, the negative resting Vm develops in cardiac cells because the high permeability of the membrane to potassium allows potassium to diffuse easily out of the cell; the low permeability of the membrane to sodium limits the influx of sodium that will not offset the negative electrical gradient; and the sodium-potassium pump removes more sodium from the cell than it pumps potassium into the cell.

Action Potentials

A current flows when there is a reversal in the polarity of the cell. In the normal resting cell, the ions of opposite polarity are lined up on either side of the semipermeable membrane, negative on the inside and positive on the outside. There is no current flow, and the cell is said to be *polarized*. As long as the membrane remains undisturbed, the cell remains in its resting state (see Fig. 12–1).

Any factor that suddenly alters the membrane permeability produces rapid changes in the transmembrane potential. The sequence of changes in which the intracellular potential briefly becomes positive and then returns to its original negative level is termed the *action potential*. Factors that can elicit an action potential are electrical or chemical stimulation, heat, cold, ischemia, injury, or any other phenomenon that disturbs the normal resting state of the cell temporarily.

The action potential includes two separate stages of the cardiac cycle, depolarization and repolarization, which are divided into five phases (Fig. 12–2).[5] The first phase of the action potential is called phase 0, or the rapid phase of depolarization. Phase 0 is characterized by a rapid upstroke of the action potential as a result of reaching threshold, which causes the cell to depolarize (be stimulated) and reverses the electrical membrane potential. The interior of the cell becomes 20 mV more positive than the outside of the cell (overshoot). Phase 1 is characterized by a brief period of early repolarization. Phase 2 is a plateau period that is 0.1 seconds to 0.2 seconds in duration and is maintained by the influx of calcium. Phase 3 is a period of rapid repolarization that occurs as increased potassium leaves the cell. Phase 4 is the period of polarization (or rest) that extends from completion of repolarization to the next action potential. During phase 4, nonpacemaker cells maintain this potential until the SA node drives them to threshold. Slow diastolic depolarization (the reduction of the resting membrane potential to a less negative value) occurs in pacemaker cells. This results from an increased entrance of sodium into the cell. When the voltage in the cell is reduced to −30 to −40 mV, it reaches *threshold* and can be activated.

In the normal heart, electrical activity precedes mechanical contraction. These electrical and chemical events (the action potential), occurring at the cellular level, initiate cardiac contraction.

There are two types of action potentials in the heart (Fig. 12–3). The *fast response* is found in the atria, ventricles, and Purkinje system and consists of the five phases described previously (Fig. 12–3A).[5,9,11,15] The resting Vm of fast-response cells is −85 mV (−80 mV to −90 mV), with a depolarization (stimulation) threshold of −65 mV. The heart also has *slow-response* action potentials in the SA node, the natural pacemaker of the heart, and around the AV node (Fig. 12–3B). In these cells, phase 0 is characterized by a slow upstroke, reduced rate of conduction, a minimal overshoot, no period of early repolarization, and no plateau phase. Phase 3 (repolarization) and phase 4 (slow diastolic depolarization) are present in slow-response action potentials. Such cells have a resting Vm of −60 mV and a depolarization threshold of −40 mV (−35 mV to −45 mV).

Electrochemical Changes That Cause the Fast Response

Changes in the membrane permeability that result in the action potential occur because of the opening and closing of special membrane channels controlled by gates. The gates are said to be voltage-dependent, which means that they open and close according to the level of the membrane potential.

During phase 4 of the action potential, the *m* gates are closed and the *h* gates are open. Although the electrostatic and chemical forces are drawing sodium into the cell during phase 4, the *m* gates obstruct the fast sodium channels, thereby making the membrane relatively impermeable to sodium (low P_{Na}) (Fig. 12–4A). When fast-response cells are stimulated, the Vm becomes less negative and the *m* gates (activation gates) begin to open, unblocking some of the fast sodium channels and allowing sodium to enter the cell. As sodium enters the cell, the membrane potential becomes even less negative, which in turn causes more fast sodium channels to open. This process, called the *regenerative process for sodium*, continues until the membrane potential reaches threshold (−65 mV). At threshold, all *m* gates swing open and there is a sudden rapid influx of sodium, causing the Vm to increase abruptly and produce phase 0 of the action potential (Fig. 12–4B).

Likewise, the *h* gates (inactivation gates) begin to close as the Vm becomes less negative. The *h* gates, however, are slow, taking about 1 m/second to close, in contrast to the *m* gates, which are fast, taking 0.1 to 0.2 m/second to open. Thus, when the Vm becomes less negative, the *m* gates are opening at a rapid rate, whereas the *h* gates are starting to close slowly (see Fig. 12–4B). When the *h* gates are completely closed, the fast sodium channels are blocked and the permeability to sodium is once again low (Fig. 12–4C). When the *h* gates close, they terminate phase 0 and remain closed until the middle of phase 3. Until the *h* gates open partially, the cell remains refractory to stimulation.[5]

Phase 1 is seen as a brief period of early repolarization, in which the cell becomes less positive, which is probably caused by the flux of chloride into the cell.

Phase 2, or the plateau of the action potential, is a specialized process characterized only by fibers in the fast-response cell of the heart. It is produced by the opening of the slow sodium and calcium channels, which are activated and inactivated by gates similar to but at a slower rate than the gates in the fast sodium channels. The slow channels are activated at a Vm of −35 mV to −45 mV. The influx of sodium and calcium through the slow channels can be increased by catecholamines and reduced by verapamil.

The fast-response cardiac cells are characterized by a decreased P_K, whereby the permeability of potassium outward decreases during phase 2. Reducing the permeability of potassium during phase 2, called anomalous rectification, is responsible for prolonging the plateau and maintaining the Vm at 0 mV. Thus only a small amount of potassium actually

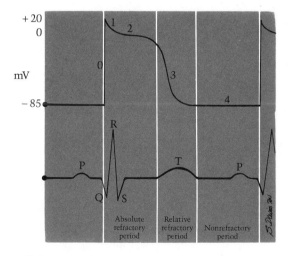

Figure 12–2
Cardiac action potential and ECG tracing of refractory periods. (Lauer, J. M. Electrical Activity of the Heart and Dysrhythmias. In C. E. Guzzetta and B. M. Dossey, *Cardiovascular Nursing: Bodymind Tapestry*. St. Louis: Mosby, 1984; with permission.)

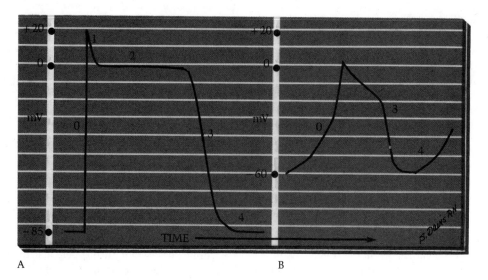

Figure 12–3

(*A*) Fast-response action potential, characteristic of atrial, ventricular, and Purkinje's fibers. The resting membrane potential is −85 mV. The threshold for stimulation is −65 mV. When the membrane potential reaches the threshold, there is a rapid rise in the upstroke of the action potential (phase 0) due to a sudden influx of extracellular sodium through the fast channels and an overshoot of the membrane potential (to +20 mV), a short period of early repolarization (phase 1), a plateau phase (phase 2) due to the influx of extracellular calcium through slow channels, a repolarization phase (phase 3), and a diastolic depolarization phase (phase 4). Fast-response cells can be converted to slow-response cells under abnormal conditions, such as myocardial ischemia and hypoxemia. (*B*) Slow-response action potential, characteristic of the pacemaker cells of the sinoatrial (SA) and atrioventricular (AV) nodes. The resting membrane potential is only −60 mV (a level at which the fast sodium channels are inactivated). The threshold for stimulation is −40 mV. When the membrane potential reaches the threshold, depolarization (phase 0) is characterized by a slow upstroke and reduced rate of conduction because of the influx of extracellular calcium through the slow channels and a minimal overshoot, no period of early repolarization, no plateau phase, a repolarization phase (phase 3), and a slow diastolic depolarization phase (pacemaker potential or phase 4), which may be due to the influx of sodium or calcium or a decreased efflux of potassium. (Guzzetta, C. E. The Person Requiring Cardiovascular Drugs. In C. E. Guzzetta and B. M. Dossey, *Cardiovascular Nursing: Bodymind Tapestry*. St. Louis: C. V. Mosby, 1984, with permission.)

leaves the cell, which is balanced by the slow influx of sodium and calcium to maintain the plateau.

Phase 3 of the action potential occurs because of a sudden increase in the P_K and by inactivation of the slow channels to obstruct the influx of sodium and calcium. The increase in P_K is responsible for restoring the Vm to its resting state.

Phase 4 of the action potential represents the period of rest, in which the sodium-potassium pump is actively working. The sodium pump works to pump out the excess sodium that entered the cell during phase 0 and phase 2, whereas the potassium pump works to pump in the potassium that left the cell during phases 2 and 3.[5]

Electrochemical Changes That Cause the Slow Response

Slow-response cells in the SA node and around the AV node are depolarized by an inward current of sodium and calcium through slow channels. This process is similar to the events that occur during phase 2 of the fast-response action potential. Slow-response action potentials contrast sharply with fast-response action potentials because they do not possess the fast sodium channels discussed previously. Slow-response action potentials are characterized by the following:

- Less negative resting Vm
- Less negative threshold for stimulation
- A reduced upstroke or slope of phase 0
- Reduced overshoot
- A slower impulse conduction velocity
- A greater potential for blocked impulses

Fast-response cells can be converted to slow-response cells by causing the resting Vm to become less negative during such conditions as myocardial ischemia.

IMPULSE CONDUCTION

An action potential produced at any point on a cell membrane can excite adjacent membranes, resulting in propagation (spread) of the action potential (cardiac impulse). A local circuit of current flows between the depolarized and resting membrane sections until all parts of the membrane and adjacent interconnecting fibers have been stimulated. The current flows quickly between cells because of the low resistance through the intercalated discs.

When the threshold is reached in the fast-response cells, all the fast sodium channels are activated, producing a wave of depolarization. The conduction velocity of the impulse is

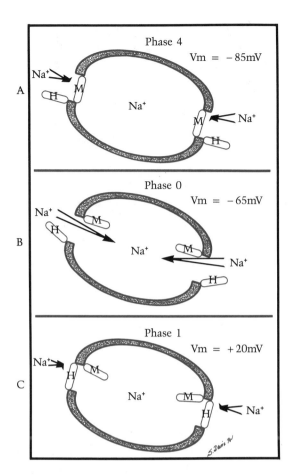

Figure 12-4

Fast-response action potential. (A) During phase 4, *m* gates are closed, obstructing fast-response sodium channels and reducing P_{Na}. (B) During phase 0, the *m* gates swing open to activate the fast sodium channels and increase the P_{Na}. (The *h* gates are slowly starting to close.) (C) During phase 1, the *h* gates are completely closed, inactivating the fast sodium channels and reducing the P_{Na}. Vm: membrane potential.

dependent on three factors: the rate of change in the membrane potential; the amplitude of the action potential (*i.e.*, the difference in potential between the polarized and maximally depolarized zone); and the level of the resting Vm. The greater the rate of change in the membrane potential, the greater the amplitude of the action potential; also, the more negative the resting Vm, the faster the depolarization wave is transmitted down the fiber.

Fast-response action potentials can be converted to slow-response action potentials by raising the resting Vm when the potassium outside the cell is abnormally elevated. When the potassium is normal, for example, fast-response cells, when stimulated, will demonstrate the five phases of the fast-response action potential, as described previously. Should the serum potassium become elevated, however, the resting Vm will become less negative than normal (*e.g.*, from −85 mV to −60 mV). Under such circumstances, the amplitude and duration of the action potential will be reduced, the slope of phase 0 will be less, and the conduction velocity will be diminished. This occurs because, as the *m* gates swing open during phase 0, the *h* gates will be partially closed (due to the

elevated resting Vm) and will partially block the fast sodium channels.

It is estimated that half of the fast sodium channels are activated at −70 mV and all the fast sodium channels are inactivated at −55 mV.[5] Should the serum potassium become excessively elevated, such that the resting Vm is elevated to −50 mV, the *h* gates will be closed and all fast sodium channels will be inactivated. The fast-response action potential will then be converted to a slow-response action potential, in which depolarization occurs because of the influx of calcium and sodium through the slow channels.

REFRACTORY PERIODS

Once the membrane is depolarized from the preceding action potential, a second action potential cannot occur because the sodium channels have become inactivated and will not respond to any amount of excitation. This period is called the *absolute (effective) refractory period*. In fast-response cells, the cell is not excitable from the beginning of phase 0 until phase 3, at which point repolarization has reached about −50 mV.[5] In slow-response cells, the absolute refractory period extends well beyond phase 3 and into phase 4.

After the absolute refractory period, a stronger than normal stimulus can excite the cell.[10] This is the *relative refractory period*. This period results from an increasing number of available sodium channels.[16] When a fast-response cell is activated during the relative refractory period, the shape of the action potential will depend on the membrane potential at the time of stimulation. As the cell is stimulated progressively later and later during the relative refractory period, the greater will be the amplitude and upstroke of the action potential and the greater the conduction velocity of the impulse. At the beginning of phase 4, the *m* and *h* gates are reset and the cell is said to be nonrefractable or fully excitable, responding easily to another stimulus (see Fig. 12-2).

In slow-response cells, impulses occurring earlier in the relative refractory period are conducted slower than if they occurred later during this period. The long refractory periods and reduced impulse conduction observed with slow-response cells are associated with a greater tendency for conduction blocks than in fast-response cells.[5]

EXCITATION

Pacemaker cells in the heart exhibit the unique property of self-excitation. The SA node, called the natural pacemaker of the heart, has the highest order of rhythmicity. In comparison with other pacemaker cells, the SA node has also the highest (least negative) resting Vm. Its impulse therefore, is conducted slowly, and its action potential exhibits an absent plateau and a gradual phase 3 repolarization. The most important characteristic of the SA node (and other pacemaker cells) is its slow diastolic depolarization during phase 4, called the *pacemaker potential*. In nonpacemaker cells, the Vm during phase 4 remains constant, whereas in pacemaker cells, the cell slowly becomes less negative during phase 4, until threshold is reached and the action potential begins. The slow diastolic depolarization that occurs during phase 4 in most pacemaker cells may be the result of a reduction in the P_K (thus, less potassium progressively leaves the cell, making the Vm less negative) or an increase in P_{Na} (thus, more sodium enters the

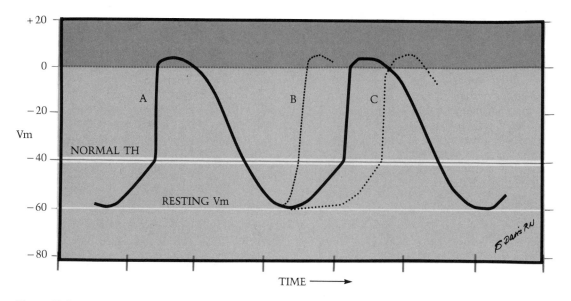

Figure 12–5

(A) Normal frequency of discharge from the sinoatrial (SA) node. (B) Effects of increasing (raising) the slope of phase 4. (C) Effects of reducing the slope of phase 4. Vm: membrane potential; TH: threshold.

cell, making the Vm less negative). In SA node pacemaker cells, however, it is believed that the slow diastolic depolarization may actually be due to a slow influx of extracellular calcium in through the slow calcium channels.

In comparison with other pacemaker cells, the SA node has the greatest slope of phase 4. Because the slope is steeper than other pacemaker cells, the threshold is reached earlier and the frequency of discharge of the SA node is faster (Fig. 12–5A). Thus, the SA node overrides other potential pacemaker cells and is normally the dominant pacemaker. Three mechanisms can change the frequency of pacemaker firing: changing the slope of phase 4, changing the threshold, and changing the resting Vm.[5,6]

Changing the slope of phase 4 can be accomplished by autonomic nervous stimulation. Sympathetic nervous system stimulation increases the slope of phase 4, allowing the membrane potential to reach threshold earlier and increasing the heart rate (Fig. 12–5B). The slope of phase 4 also can be increased with myocardial ischemia, and this increased automaticity can result in dysrhythmias. Conversely, parasympathetic nervous system stimulation reduces the slope of phase 4, which prolongs the slow diastolic depolarization phase and the time necessary for the membrane potential to reach threshold (Fig. 12–5C). Because the onset of phase 0 is delayed, the heart rate decreases.

Increasing the threshold (making it less negative) (Fig. 12–

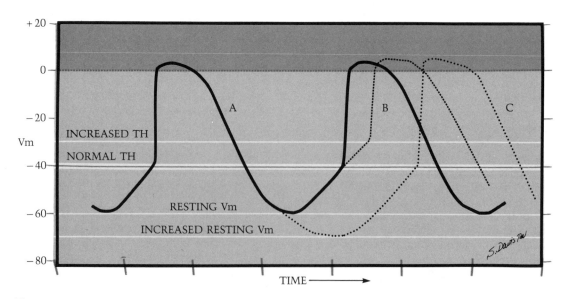

Figure 12–6

(A) Normal frequency of discharge from the sinoatrial (SA) node. (B) Effects of increasing the threshold (TH) for stimulation. (C) Effects of increasing the resting membrane potential (Vm).

6A,B) with such drugs as bretylium tosylate will prolong the slow diastolic depolarization phase, delay the onset of phase 0, and, consequently, decrease the rate. The threshold can be lowered (made more negative) by myocardial ischemia to shorten the slow diastolic depolarization phase, increase the rate, and produce dysrhythmias.

Increasing the resting membrane potential (making it more negative) (Fig. 12–6C) will prolong the time necessary to reach the threshold and will reduce automaticity. Conversely, when the resting Vm becomes less negative as a result of myocardial ischemia, dysrhythmias can develop because the time necessary for the Vm to reach the threshold is shortened.[5]

CONDUCTION SYSTEM

The conduction system of the heart comprises the SA node, the AV node, the bundle of His, the left and right bundle branches, and the Purkinje network (Fig. 12–7). These specialized areas initiate and conduct the impulse that results in electrical activation of the myocardium, which then results in systole (or contraction).

The dominant pacemaker of the heart, the SA node, which normally fires 60 to 100 times/minute, is located in the right atrium near the superior vena cava. The characteristic of automaticity is found within the SA node, allowing it to initiate its own impulse. Because the SA node fires faster than other areas of the electrical conduction system, it overrides the lower slower pacemakers (overdrive suppression) and is the primary pacemaker of the heart. The rate of firing of the SA node is influenced by both divisions of the autonomic nervous system, being increased with sympathetic stimulation and decreased with vagal activity. If the SA node should fail as the primary pacemaker, one of the other components of the conduction system can act as a secondary pacemaker. If that occurs, the farther the secondary pacemaker is from the SA node, the slower the rate will be.

Once the impulse is fired from the SA node, it spreads through both atria in a wavelike manner to the AV node located in the inferior wall of the right atrium near the tricuspid valve. The conduction tissue that connects the atria and the ventricles is referred to as AV junction. It is composed of the A-N region (between the atrium and remainder of the node), the N region (mid-portion of the node), and the N-H region (AV node merges with the bundle of His).[5] It is in the A-N region that the principal delay in impulse conduction occurs, thereby allowing the atria to contract to augment ventricular filling before the onset of ventricular contraction. An intact, healthy pathway across the AV junction is needed for normal ventricular activation. Under abnormal circumstances, the AV junction can take over as a secondary pacemaker, firing at its inherent rate of 40 to 60 beats/minute. Such a rhythm is called an AV junctional rhythm.

Once it enters the bundle of His, the impulse moves rapidly into the right and left bundle branches. The right bundle branch is located on the right side of the interventricular septum and extends almost to the apex of the right ventricle, where it branches to all areas of the right ventricle through the Purkinje system. The left bundle crosses to the left side of the interventricular septum and divides immediately into the anterior and posterior branches. The left anterior branch (anterior fascicle) spreads superiorly, and the left posterior branch (posterior fascicle) spreads inferiorly to the diaphrag-

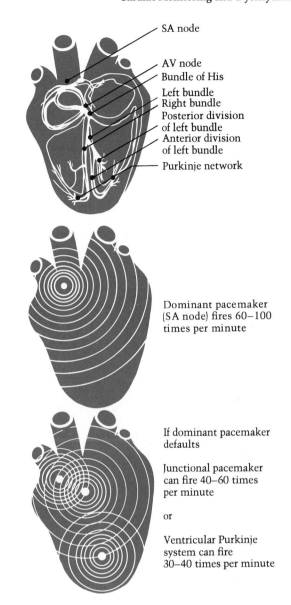

SA node

AV node
Bundle of His
Left bundle
Right bundle
Posterior division
of left bundle
Anterior division
of left bundle
Purkinje network

Dominant pacemaker
(SA node) fires 60–100
times per minute

If dominant pacemaker
defaults

Junctional pacemaker
can fire 40–60 times
per minute

or

Ventricular Purkinje
system can fire
30–40 times per minute

Figure 12–7
Conduction system of the heart. AV: atrioventricular; SA: sinoatrial.

matic wall of the left ventricle. Once the impulse has passed through the bundle branches, it spreads quickly through the Purkinje network found within the ventricular myocardium. Being the largest cells in the heart, the Purkinje fibers have the fastest conduction velocity, which permits rapid activation of the entire endocardial surface of the ventricles. If the SA node or AV junction defaults, the ventricular Purkinje system can fire at 30 to 40 beats/minute and become the pacemaker of the heart.

THE ELECTROCARDIOGRAM

As the normal impulse travels through the conduction system, the electrocardiogram (ECG) or oscilloscope records the electrical forces. Because the body acts as a conductor of electrical currents, any two points on the body can be connected to record the heart rhythm. A series of waves and intervals that are recorded during each cardiac cycle have been labeled ar-

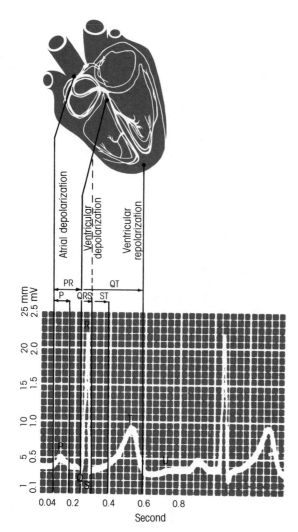

Figure 12–8
Electrical impulse recording.

a downward deflection after the R wave. Not every QRS complex, however, will show a Q or an R or an S wave. A QRS complex, for example, may consist only of an R wave, or only of an RS wave. Nevertheless, it is still referred to as the QRS complex. The duration of a normal QRS complex is 0.04 second to 0.10 second.

The *T wave* represents ventricular recovery or repolarization and results from currents generated during phase 3 of the action potential. The T wave generally is upright and of the same polarity as the QRS, although it may be abnormal as a result of ischemic changes, electrolyte abnormalities, medications (*e.g.*, digitalis, quinidine), or other conditions that alter repolarization as well as the depolarization process. The absolute refractory period occurs during the ST segment and the beginning of the T wave and ends approximately at the peak of the T wave. The relative refractory or vulnerable period is from the peak to the end of the T wave. Should a stimulus occur during the relative refractory period, serious ventricular dysrhythmias may be precipitated.

The *ST segment* is the time interval from the end of the QRS complex to the onset of the T wave. It represents phase 2 of the action potential, the early phase of ventricular repolarization. The point at which the ST segment takes off from the ventricular complex is the *J point*. The ST segment is usually flat, producing an *isoelectric line* that curves slightly into the T wave and represents a period of electrical quiet. Sometimes, however, the ST segment is abnormally elevated or depressed (above or below the isoelectric line) because of cardiac disease or drugs (*e.g.*, digitalis).

The *QT interval* represents electrical systole and lasts from the beginning of the QRS complex to the end of the T wave. It varies particularly with the heart rate. Serial measurements of the QT interval may be important to determine the effects of certain medications, particularly quinidine.

The significance of the *U wave* is still not understood. When present, the U wave is smaller than the P wave, follows the T wave and is of the same polarity, and appears with a variety of phenomena, such as electrolyte shifts, digitalis, and premature ventricular contractions. It may be inverted with ischemia and is more prominent in women than in men.

bitrarily on the ECG as the P, QRS, T, and U waves, the PR and QT intervals, and the ST segment (Fig. 12–8).

Waves and Intervals

The *P wave* represents depolarization of the atria. The P wave generally is upright and rounded in leads 1, 2, aV_F, and V_4, V_5, and V_6. The P wave may be found to be upright, diphasic, flat, or inverted in leads 3, aV_L, V_1, V_2, and V_3, depending on the position of the heart. Because atrial depolarization travels away from the positive electrode, the P wave in aV_R normally is inverted. Because the atria are thin-walled structures, P waves are small (not more than 3 mm in height) and not more than 0.11 second in duration. If P waves are taller or wider, atrial enlargement is suspected. The *PR interval* lasts from the beginning of the P wave to the beginning of the QRS complex; it represents the time period from atrial depolarization to the beginning of ventricular depolarization (see Fig. 12–8). The PR interval, normally 0.12 second to 0.20 second, includes the normal conduction delay in the AV node.

The *QRS complex* represents ventricular depolarization. An initial downward deflection is the Q wave. The first upward deflection of the QRS complex is the R wave. The S wave is

Isoelectric Line

A baseline, known as the isoelectric line, may be seen to run through the length of the ECG tracing. It represents complete cardiac rest or electrical inactivity, and it is present whenever there is no flow of electrical current. The isoelectric line is determined by running an imaginary line across the ECG tracing from its origin at the TP interval (end of the T wave to the beginning of the next P wave).

The ECG Paper

Each small square on the ECG paper is 1 mm square. *Time* is measured on the horizontal axis. Each small square represents 0.04 second in time. The larger square (or five small squares) represents 5 mm in length and 0.20 second in time (see Fig. 12–8). The interval between the two vertical lines above the ECG grid represents 3 seconds.

Amplitude or *voltage* is measured on the vertical axis. The height or depth of a wave is measured from the isoelectric

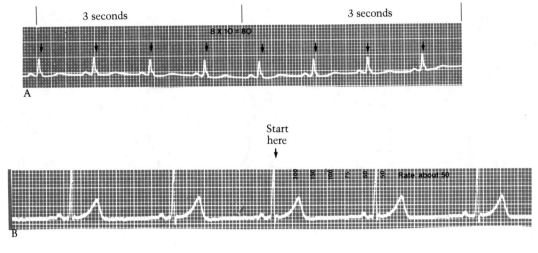

Figure 12-9

Two methods of calculation of heart rate. (*A*) Count the number of QRS complexes within a 6-second strip and multiply by 10. (*B*) Identify a QRS complex that falls on a heavy line. Count off the numbers 300, 150, 100, 75, 60, and 50 for each heavy line that follows.

line. Twelve-lead ECGs are usually standardized so that 1 mV is equal to 10 mm, or two large vertical squares.

Calculation of Heart Rate

The single ECG tracing can be used to calculate the heart rate by several different methods. The first method involves finding a QRS complex that lands on and within the vertical line above the ECG grid. The number of complexes within 6 seconds (two 3-second intervals) multiplied by 10 gives the approximate number of beats per minute (Fig. 12–9A). This method can be used when the rhythm is regular or irregular.

A second method of determining the rate when the rhythm is regular is to find a QRS complex that falls on a heavy line and then count off the numbers 300, 150, 100, 75, 60, and 50 for each heavy line that follows. The next QRS complex determines the rate (Fig. 12–9B). The rationale for the counting system is that the distance between heavy lines is 1/300 minute. Therefore, the method seen on Figure 12–9B shows that from a QRS complex on a heavy line to the next QRS complex (R to R interval) are six large squares. The rate is determined by dividing 6 into 300.

Leads

A normal ECG is composed of 12 leads: three standard leads and three augmented leads in the frontal plane, which give information about current flow that is right, left, inferior, or superior; and six precordial leads in the horizontal plane, which give information about current flow that is anterior or posterior (Fig. 12–10). The ECG records the same electrical activity in each lead, but the morphology of the waves is different because the activity is viewed from different positions. The 12 leads represent depolarization and repolarization of the heart from 12 different perspectives.

Standard Limb Leads

The standard limb leads (*i.e.*, 1, 2, and 3) are bipolar leads with a positive and negative electrode on the body, all about

equally distant from the heart, to record the difference in electrical potentials between two connected limbs.

The axis of lead 1 (an imaginary line between the two electrodes) extends from shoulder to shoulder, with the negative electrode on the right arm and the positive electrode on the left arm. The axis of lead 2 extends from the right shoulder to the left leg, with the negative electrode on the right arm and the positive electrode on the left leg. Lead 3 extends from the left shoulder to the left leg, with the negative electrode on the left arm and the positive electrode on the left leg (Fig. 12–11A). Remembering that placement, one can see that the axes of the three bipolar limb leads form a triangle around the area of the heart known as Einthoven's triangle (Fig. 12–11B). The triaxial reference system is formed by the sides of Einthoven's triangle as the centers bisect one another (Fig. 12–11C). The sum of the potentials of those leads is zero. (The P waves in lead 2 should be the tallest, and the QRS complex in lead 2 should equal the sum of the corresponding complexes in leads 1 and 3.)[14]

Augmented Leads

The augmented unipolar extremity leads are leads aV_R, aV_L, and aV_F (Fig. 12–11D). The letter *a* means augmented. A lead may be augmented by disconnecting the central terminal at-

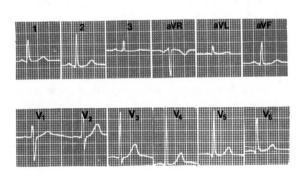

Figure 12-10

The 12 leads in a normal electrocardiogram.

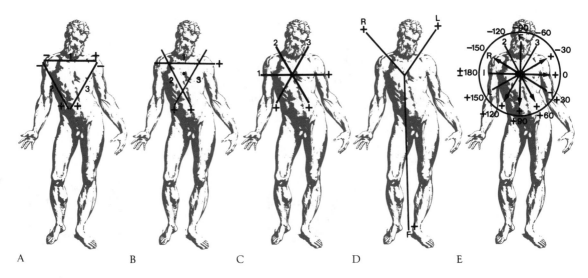

A   B   C   D   E

Figure 12-11

Intersection of standard limb leads and augmented leads. (*A*) The three limb leads create Einthoven's triangle. (*B*) The three limb leads come together to form a zero potential point. (*C*) The triaxial reference system is formed by the sides of Einthoven's triangle as they bisect. (*D*) The unipolar leads come toward the zero potential point. (*E*) The hexaxial reference system consists of six limb leads as they bisect each other.

tached to the explored limb, thereby causing the amplitude of the deflection to be increased by 50% without changing the shape of the waveform. The *V* stands for vector, and the letters *R*, *L*, and *F* indicate the placement of the positive electrode (*e.g.*, right arm, left arm, left leg [foot]). The other two electrodes are used as a common ground.

Those leads intersect at a 60° angle, and when they are superimposed on the standard limb leads, they intersect at 30° angles to form the frontal plane, which is referred to as the hexaxial reference system (Fig. 12–11E). Progressing clockwise from lead 1 (0 degree), the 30° increments are positive, whereas progressing counterclockwise from lead 1, the 30° increments are negative.

Precordial Leads

The precordial (or chest) leads are unipolar, with each lead consisting of one positive electrode and a zero potential reference point. The axis of those leads is an imaginary line drawn from the positive electrode toward the center of the heart, and it identifies the horizontal plane. The precordial leads are placed at the following positions (Fig. 12–12):

V_1—fourth intercostal space, at the right sternal border
V_2—fourth intercostal space, at the left sternal border
V_3—midway between positions V_2 and V_4
V_4—fifth intercostal space, at the left midclavicular line
V_5—fifth intercostal space, in the left anterior axillary line
V_6—fifth intercostal space, in the left midaxillary line
V_3R—not shown, not used unless right ventricular infarction is suspected; midway between V_2R, the fourth intercostal space at the right sternal border, and V_4R, the fifth intercostal space at the right midclavicular line

Electrocardiographic Vectors

The term *vector* can be defined as an electrical force characterized by magnitude and direction. The wave of depolariza-

tion produces many small electrical forces. Each small electrical force, called an *instantaneous vector*, varies in magnitude and direction. The average of all the small electrical forces is termed the *mean vector*, which represents the general direction of the wave of depolarization.[15] The mean vector can be inferred from the morphology of the QRS complexes.

The ECG can inscribe on paper QRS complexes that are biphasic, equiphasic, or isoelectric. The magnitude and direction of the mean vector determining the shape of the QRS complex inscribed will depend on the placement of the positive and negative electrodes. The following three principles are given to illustrate this concept:[1]

• The more the mean vector moves toward the positive electrode of a given lead, the larger will be the *positive* QRS deflection (Fig. 12–13A).

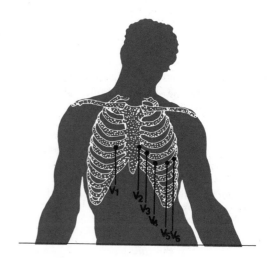

Figure 12-12
Precordial leads (unipolar leads).

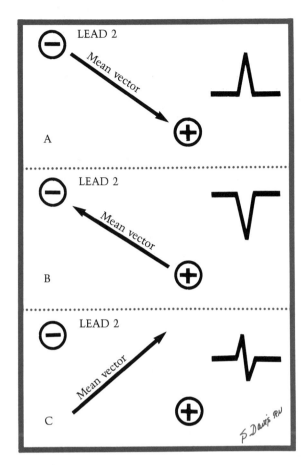

Figure 12–13

Orientation of the mean vector with respect to lead 2 and the resultant QRS complex. (*A*) Mean vector directed toward the positive lead, producing a maximally upright QRS complex. (*B*) Mean vector directed toward the negative lead, producing a maximally inverted QRS complex. (*C*) Mean vector directed perpendicular to lead 2, producing an equiphasic QRS complex.

- The more the mean vector moves toward the negative electrode of a given lead, the larger will be the *negative* QRS deflection (Fig. 12–13B).
- The more the mean vector moves perpendicular to the positive and negative electrodes of a given lead, the more isoelectric, or equiphasic, the QRS deflection (Fig. 12–13C).

To determine the general direction and magnitude of the mean QRS vector, the net QRS deflection must be assessed.[1] The *net QRS deflection* is calculated by subtracting the height (in millimeters) of the positive portion of the QRS deflection from the height of the negative portion of the QRS deflection. Figure 12–14A illustrates a net positive deflection of 2 mm, and Figure 12–14B illustrates a net negative deflection of 5 mm. An *equiphasic deflection* has an equally positive and negative deflection, producing a net deflection of zero (Fig. 12–14C). An *isoelectric deflection* has such an extremely small positive and negative deflection that the net QRS deflection is also zero (Fig. 12–14D).

The mean QRS vector can travel in five different directions to any given lead. In relation to lead 1, for example, the mean QRS vector can travel in the following directions:[1]

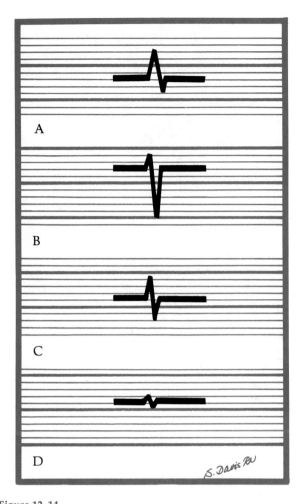

Figure 12–14

Calculation of net QRS deflection. (*A*) QRS deflection is 4 mm positive and 2 mm negative, producing a 2-mm positive net QRS deflection. (*B*) QRS deflection is 2 mm positive and 7 mm negative, producing a 5-mm negative net QRS deflection. (*C*) QRS deflection is 3 mm positive and 3 mm negative, producing a 0 net QRS deflection. (*D*) QRS deflection is so small that net QRS deflection cannot be calculated.

- Parallel toward the positive electrode of lead 1, producing a maximally positive QRS deflection (Fig. 12–15A)
- Obliquely toward the positive electrode of lead 1, producing a smaller positive QRS deflection (Fig. 12–15B)
- Parallel toward the negative electrode of lead 1, producing a maximally negative QRS deflection (Fig. 12–15C)
- Obliquely toward the negative deflection of lead 1, producing a smaller negative QRS deflection (Fig. 12–15D)
- Perpendicular to lead 1, producing an equiphasic or isoelectric QRS deflection (Fig. 12–15E)

Electrical Axis

The *electrical axis* refers to the direction of the depolarization wave. It identifies the intensity and direction of the electrical impulses, providing information about the mean QRS vector. The mean QRS vector is the average of the smaller vectors that all contribute to the sum of the electrical forces occurring during ventricular depolarization. The mean QRS vector can be located in one of four quadrants in the heart: down (inferior)

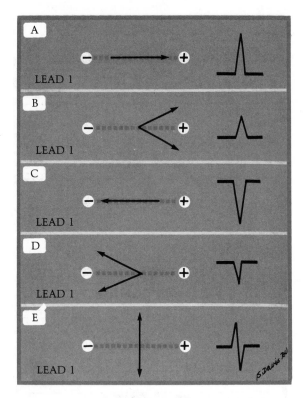

Figure 12–15

Five different directions in which the mean QRS vector can travel in relation to lead 1: (*A*) parallel to positive; (*B*) obliquely toward positive; (*C*) parallel to negative; (*D*) obliquely toward negative; and (*E*) perpendicular to lead 1.

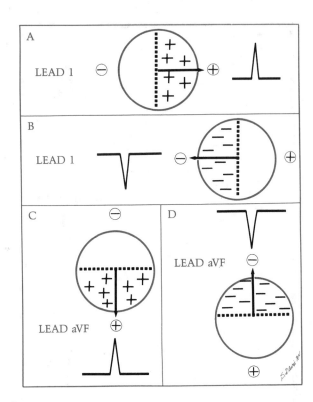

Figure 12–16

Direction of mean vectors and resultant QRS complexes in relation to lead 1 (*A* and *B*) and lead aV_F (*C* and *D*).

and to the left, down and to the right, up (superior) and to the left, and up and to the right.

In persons with normal hearts, the mean QRS vector is down and to the left. Thus, when the mean QRS vector lies between 0° and +90°, the patient is said to have a *normal axis*. The normal mean QRS axis is located in this area, because the left ventricle has the greatest muscle mass and, therefore, produces most of the electrical forces. Should the mean QRS vector lie between 0° and −90° (up and to the left), the patient is said to have *left-axis deviation*. If the mean QRS vector is located between +90° and ±180° (down and to the right), the patient is said to have *right-axis deviation*. Should the mean QRS vector lie between −90° and ±180° (up and to the right), the patient is said to have *indeterminate axis*. The axis could be either an extreme right or extreme left axis. This quadrant is also known as *no-man's land*. When the axis is beyond 0°, it is left, but it is not abnormally left until it is beyond −30°. Similarly, when the axis is beyond +90°, it is right, but it is not abnormally right until it is beyond +120°. Thus, normal axis generally is considered between −30° and +120°.

Two-Lead Method for Determining Axis (Quadrant Method)

Frequently, the electrical axis can be determined by examining two of the six leads in the frontal plane (leads 1, 2, 3, aV_R, aV_F, aV_L). For the purpose of this discussion, leads 1 and aV_F will be examined. When assessing lead 1 from Figure 12–16A, it can be observed that one half of the heart is considered to

be positive and the other half of the heart is considered to be negative. Thus, if the mean QRS vector is moving toward the positive electrode of lead 1, the QRS deflection will be positive on the ECG, indicating that the mean QRS vector is moving toward the left. Conversely, if the mean QRS vector is moving toward the negative electrode of lead 1, the QRS deflection will be negative on the ECG, indicating that the mean QRS vector is moving toward the right (Fig. 12–16B).

After determining whether the mean QRS vector is directed right or left, it must then be determined whether it is directed up or down. This information can be obtained by assessing lead aV_F. From Figure 12–16C, it can be seen that the bottom half of the heart is considered to be positive, whereas the top half is considered to be negative. If the mean QRS vector is moving toward the positive electrode of lead aV_F, the QRS deflection will be positive, indicating that the vector is directed downward. Conversely, if the mean QRS vector is moving toward the negative electrode of aV_F, the QRS deflection will be negative, indicating the vector is directed upward (Fig. 12–16D). Thus, the information obtained from the QRS complexes in leads 1 and aV_F will provide an orientation concerning whether the mean QRS vector is traveling left or right and up or down. The direction of the electrical axis can, therefore, be estimated.

The following examples are given to illustrate the two-lead method for calculating axis. Look at leads 1 and aV_F on an ECG. If the QRS complex is positive in lead 1 (vector moving left) and positive in lead aV_F (vector moving downward), the mean QRS vector is estimated to lie between 0° and +90°, and the patient is said to have a normal axis (Fig. 12–17A). If the QRS complex is positive in lead 1 (left) and negative in

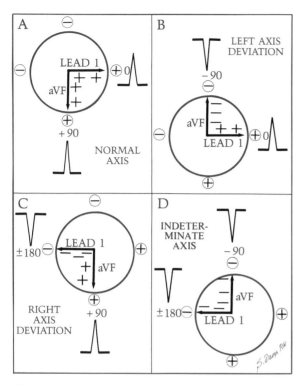

Figure 12-17

Calculation of electrical axis, using leads 1 and a V_F.

traveling toward the positive or negative electrode by assessing whether that lead is positive or negative on the ECG. If positive, it is traveling toward the positive electrode. If negative, it is traveling toward the negative electrode.

4. Identify the electrical axis (degree designation) of the QRS complex in step 3 by using the hexaxial reference system.

To illustrate this method, evaluate the six-limb leads in Figure 12–10 using the following four steps:

1. Smallest (most equiphasic) QRS complex is aV_L.
2. Lead perpendicular to aV_L is lead 2. (The axis lies parallel with lead 2.)
3. Lead 2 is positive on the ECG. Therefore, current is traveling toward the positive electrode of lead 2.
4. The positive end of lead 2 is at +60° on the hexaxial system.

Interpretation: Normal axis.

Left-axis deviation can be illustrated from Figure 12–18A using the following four steps:

1. Smallest (most equiphasic) QRS complex is aV_R.
2. Lead perpendicular to lead aV_R is lead 3. (The axis is paralleled to lead 3.)
3. Lead 3 is negative. Therefore, current is traveling toward the negative electrode of lead 3.
4. The negative end of lead 3 is at −60° on the hexaxial system.

Interpretation: Left-axis deviation.

Right-axis deviation (Fig. 12–18B) and indeterminate axis also can be determined using these four steps.

ELECTROCARDIOGRAPHIC MONITORING

Patients are monitored in order to recognize dysrhythmias. The 12 leads can be adapted to monitoring by placing the right and left arm electrodes on the upper right and left chest and the right and left leg electrodes on the lower right and

aV_F (upward), the mean QRS vector is estimated to lie between 0° and −90°, indicating left-axis deviation (Fig. 12–17B). Should the QRS complex in lead 1 be negative (right) and positive in aV_F (downward), then the mean QRS vector is estimated to lie between +90° and ±180°, indicating right-axis deviation (Fig. 12–17C). If the QRS complex is negative in lead 1 (right) and negative in aV_F (upward), then the mean QRS vector is estimated to lie between −90° and ±180°, indicating indeterminate axis (Fig. 12–17D).

Six-Lead Method for Determining Axis (Hexaxial Figure)

When the nurse desires a more precise estimate of the electrical axis (e.g., to determine if left-axis deviation is > −30° and, therefore, abnormal, or when the QRS complexes in leads 1 and aV_F are equiphasic or biphasic), the six-limb leads of the frontal plane are used to extimate axis in degrees.[1] From the 12-lead ECG, only leads 1, 2, 3, aV_R, aV_L, and aV_F need to be assessed. From those leads, identify which leads from the three standard limb leads lie perpendicular to the three augmented leads. From Figure 12–11E, it can be observed that lead 1 lies perpendicular to lead aV_F, whereas lead 2 lies perpendicular to aV_L, and lead 3 lies perpendicular to aV_R.

The six-lead method involves the following four steps:

1. Identify the smallest (or most equiphasic) QRS complex from leads 1, 2, 3, aV_R, aV_L, or aV_F.
2. Determine the lead lying perpendicular to the lead with the smallest (or most equiphasic) QRS complex. (The QRS vector lies parallel with this perpendicular lead.)
3. Determine whether the mean QRS vector from step 2 is

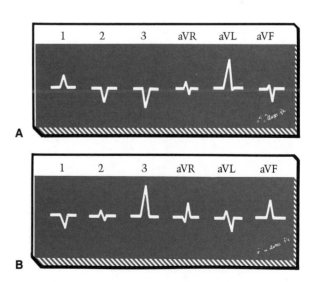

Figure 12-18

(A) Left-axis deviation. (B) Right-axis deviation.

left chest. The electrode site should be clean, dry, and smooth. Shave excessive hair and mildly abrade skin to break down the high-impedance epidermal layer. Some electrode companies recommend a rub with gauze to be sure the site is dry and to help prevent skin irritation and poor electrode adhesion. Excessive moisture or skin oils can be removed with alcohol or acetone. If these solvents are used, be sure the site is completely dry before electrode application.

In positioning the electrodes, avoid placing them over muscles in order to reduce motion artifact. To optimize signal amplitude, have adequate distance between the positive and negative electrodes. This will ensure that the amplitude of the QRS complex is sufficient to trigger the cardiac monitor rate meter properly. When possible, the patient's chest should be left loosely covered and electrode pads should be positioned carefully so that defibrillation paddles may be easily placed, if necessary, and the usual areas for auscultation are accessible.

When monitoring the patient's rhythm, the nurse must be constantly alert for changes. Alarms are kept on at all times. Extreme vigilance is required to detect subtle changes, especially if the change is not rate-dependent. It has been shown that detection of serious dysrhythmias by conventional monitoring averages 60%, whereas computerized systems detect 98% to 100%. The following conditions are recommended for nurses or technicians who are assigned to watch cardiac monitors.[7] The monitoring person does best when he or she does the following:

- Has normal or usual sleep patterns before the monitoring period
- Uses auditory and visual signals for dysrhythmia detection
- Has supervision
- Supervisoring person gives correct dysrhythmia detection information to the monitoring person as soon as possible
- Performs monitoring for periods limited to 60 minutes

MCL$_1$ Lead

A monitoring lead that frequently is preferred is the modified CL (chest) lead, or MCL$_1$ (Fig. 12–19). A bipolar lead, it is

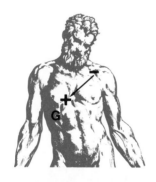

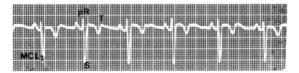

Figure 12–19
MCL$_1$ monitoring (bipolar lead), where G represents the ground lead.

similar to the unipolar precordial lead V$_1$. The positive electrode is placed in the fourth intercostal space at the right sternal border, and the negative electrode is placed just below the left midclavicle. The MCL$_1$ lead has diagnostic value as a monitoring lead because it is extremely useful for differentiating supraventricular beats with aberrancy from ventricular tachycardia, for recognizing and recording atrial activity, for distinguishing right from left bundle branch block, and right from left ventricular ectopic beats.

Artifact

Frequently, artifacts are observed on the cardiac monitor. An artifact is any movement on the ECG that is not due to currents generated during the cardiac cycle.[19] For example, when patients are tensing their muscles, electrical potentials are picked up by electrodes and recorded on the ECG as irregular jerks or a grossly uneven baseline (Fig. 12–20A). A wandering baseline reveals easily identified complexes, but the baseline is undulating (Fig. 12–20B). Alternating current interference that produces regular deflections at 60 cycles/second (Fig. 12–20C) is usually due to a leakage of electrical power during the recording of the ECG. A standardization artifact is introduced deliberately by the person recording the ECG. The artifact is generally a 10-mm deflection (two large squares) that is used to standardize the machine and to compare the size of the recorded cardiac complexes (Fig. 12–20D). Complexes produced during external cardiac massage can easily be identified (Fig. 12–20E) and resemble regular, wide ventricular beats. Some artifacts may mimic dysrhythmias (*e.g.*, a patient scratching or brushing the teeth may suggest ventricular tachycardia on the cardiac monitor). However, careful assessment will reveal regular QRS complexes in the midst of the "apparent" ventricular tachycardia (Fig. 12–20F). Similarly, the oscilloscope may show a straight line if one of the electrodes has lost contact with the skin. Regardless of the presumptive observation, the findings must always be correlated with the nurse's observation of the patient.

SYSTEMATIC ASSESSMENT OF CARDIAC RHYTHM

When assessing the patient's cardiac rhythm, the critical care nurse combines findings of the patient's clinical status with a systematic assessment of the rhythm strip. The following is carefully assessed on each strip:

1. P waves (atrial activity)
   A. Are there P waves present?
   B. Are they normal in configuration?
   C. If abnormal, are they peaked, notched, diphasic, flat, inverted, or missing?
   D. Are they regular?
   E. Is each P wave followed by a QRS?
   F. Is there more than one P wave for each QRS?
   G. What is the atrial rate?
2. QRS complex (ventricular activity)
   A. What is the contour of the complex?
   B. Are the QRS complexes of normal duration (0.04 second–0.10 second)?
   C. Are they occurring regularly?
   D. What is the ventricular rate?

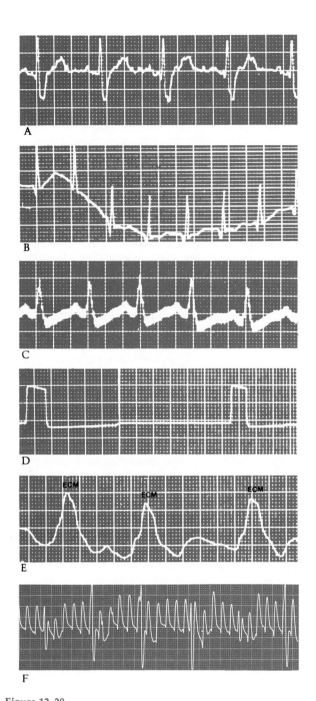

Figure 12-20

(*A*) Muscle tremor. (*B*) Wandering baseline. (*C*) Alternating current interference. (*D*) Standardization mark. (*E*) Complexes during external cardiac massage (ECM). (*F*) Patient scratching.

3. PR interval
   A. Is it normal (0.12 second–0.20 second)?
   B. Is it constant for each QRS complex (relationship between atrial and ventricular activity)?
4. QT interval
   A. Is it normal (0.3–0.4 second)?
5. ST segment
   A. Is it normal? (isoelectric)
   B. Is it elevated?
   C. Is it depressed?

6. T wave
   A. Is it normal?
   B. Is it peaked or inverted?
7. Extra beats
   A. Are there any atrial, junctional, or ventricular premature beats?
   B. Are there any escape beats?
   C. Are there any aberrantly conducted beats?
8. General
   A. What is the underlying rhythm?
   B. Considering the clinical status of the patient, how should the rhythm be treated?

Success in recognizing and interpreting dysrhythmias depends largely on developing and using a consistent, systematic method of assessment.

CAUSES OF DYSRHYTHMIAS AND CONDUCTION DISTURBANCES

The term *dysrhythmias* is used throughout this text to refer to a dysfunction of the cardiac rhythm.[17] Dysrhythmias can be caused by several cellular mechanisms, such as altered automaticity, afterdepolarizations, and re-entry or the circus movement.[5,6,9,15] Dysrhythmias occurring because of *altered automaticity* may occur in the His-Purkinje fibers or in the cells of the working atrial or ventricular myocardium. Because of a declining membrane potential during phase 4 (diastole), the membrane can reach threshold earlier and result in a spontaneous action potential (spontaneous diastolic, or phase 4, depolarization).[16] Altered automaticity can be due to the enhancement of the normal automaticity in the His-Purkinje fibers as a result of an increase in catecholamines or due to abnormal automaticity as a result of an increased influx of sodium. Abnormal automaticity is seen with such conditions as ischemia, infarction, hypokalemia, hypocalcemia, and cardiomyopathy.

Afterdepolarizations are responsible for producing dysrhythmias due to triggered activity. The afterdepolarization is always coupled to a preceding beat and causes the membrane potential to become less negative; this may or may not cause it to reach threshold. Afterdepolarizations may occur during phase 3 (early afterdepolarizations) or during phase 4 (late afterdepolarizations).[5,9] If the upstroke of the afterdepolarization does not reach threshold, no action potential is elicited. If the upstroke of the afterdepolarization reaches threshold, it can initiate a depolarization or action potential (extrasystole) that itself may be followed by an afterdepolarization that may or may not reach threshold. Thus, afterdepolarizations can lead to repetitive beats, resulting in a paroxysmal tachycardia. The afterdepolarizations occur as a result of elevated intracellular calcium that occurs with excess extracellular calcium and toxic levels of digitalis. The calcium activates channels that allow a transient influx of sodium and potassium.[5]

Dysrhythmias also can be caused by a re-entry mechanism. *Re-entry* occurs when a cardiac impulse restimulates a portion of the heart that it has already stimulated. Three conditions, which all must be present, are necessary for re-entry to take place:[5,6,9]

• An appropriate autonomic pathway consisting of an initial common pathway, a dual pathway, and a final common pathway

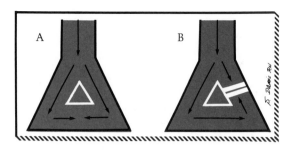

Figure 12-21

Impulse conduction in a loop of cardiac tissue, consisting of an initial common pathway, a right and left branch (dual pathway), and a final common pathway. (*A*) Impulse is conducted down the initial common pathway, right and left branches, and collides in the final common pathway, where it is extinguished. (*B*) Impulse is conducted down the initial common pathway, blocked in the left branch, conducted rapidly down the right branch, and final common pathway, and is extinguished at the site of the block because the tissue is still refractory to stimulation.

• A region of slow conduction
• A region providing a unidirectional conduction block

Under normal conditions, an impulse can enter the initial common pathway of the loop, traveling down both sides of the dual pathways, and become extinguished at the point of collision in the final common pathway (Fig. 12-21A).

A unidirectional block can be established in a dual pathway, such as in the AV node, because the branches have unequal conduction velocities and refractory periods. Should a premature beat occur, the impulse may find one pathway refractory or blocked.[15] Thus, for example, if a unidirectional block is present in the left branch of the dual pathway, an impulse will enter the initial common pathway and will be blocked in the left branch while traveling down the right branch. If the impulse from the right branch is conducted rapidly around the loop, the impulse will find the blocked site still refractory and the impulse will be extinguished (Fig. 12-21B).

If, however, a unidirectional block and slow conduction are both present, an impulse will enter the initial common loop and will be blocked in the left branch (Fig. 12-22A), but it will travel down the right side. If this impulse is conducted slowly enough through the common pathway and back up to the blocked site, the fibers in the left branch may have been able to recover sufficient excitability. The impulse may then be able to pass the point of the one-way block and re-enter the initial common pathway and the right branch thereby

developing a re-entrant pathway (Fig. 12-22B,C). The re-entrant mechanism for dysrhythmias may occur in the Purkinje fibers, the bundle branches, or the AV node.[5,9,15]

DYSRHYTHMIAS

All nurses working in critical care must be able to recognize the major dysrhythmias. Although dysrhythmias can be classified as minor, major, or lethal, critical care patients must always be assessed carefully and re-evaluated frequently when they are having dysrhythmias, regardless of how the dysrhythmia is classified.

When a dysrhythmia is identified, the nurse should assess the patient's color, mentation, apical-radial heart rate (noting any deficits), blood pressure, respiration, and urinary output. Depending on the situation, a 12-lead ECG may be indicated. The nurse should also know whether the patient had experienced such a dysrhythmia previously and how it was treated. The nurse should continue to re-evaluate the patient's vital signs and, when appropriate for the situation, contact the physician or initiate therapy, or both, based on the critical care unit's medical protocols for patients with dysrhythmias (*e.g.*, cardiopulmonary resuscitation, defibrillation, oxygen, antidysrhythmic drugs, parasympatholytic drugs, sympathomimetic drugs, etc.).

Normal Sinus Rhythm

Because the sinus node normally maintains the fastest rate of impulse formation over other pacer sites, it is the dominant pacemaker of the heart. Normal sinus rhythm (Fig. 12-23) occurs at a rate of 60 to 100 beats/minute. The P waves are normal and uniform in appearance. Each P wave will be followed by a QRS complex. The PR interval is 0.12 second to 0.20 second and constant. The QRS complexes are uniform in configuration and are essentially regular. If the cardiac cycle varies from these defined parameters, a dysrhythmia or conduction disturbance is present.

Dysrhythmias From the Sinoatrial Node
Sinus Tachycardia

Sinus tachycardia is caused by an increase in automaticity due to sympathetic nervous system activity and the release of catecholamines due to fear, anxiety, tension, exercise, fever, myocardial disease, anemia, anoxia, hyperthyroidism, or medications, such as atropine sulfate, isoproterenol, and epinephrine.

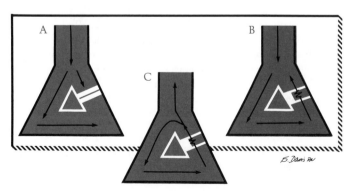

Figure 12-22

Impulse conduction in a loop of cardiac tissue when a unidirectional block and slow conduction are present. (*A*) Impulse is conducted down the initial common pathway, blocked in the left bundle, and conducted slowly down the right bundle and final common pathway. (*B*) Impulse continues slowly around the loop and up the left bundle. Conduction has been slow enough that the tissues around the block have regained excitability and the impulse is permitted to penetrate the blocked region. (C) Impulse re-enters the common initial pathway and the right branch of the loop to establish a re-entrant circuit.

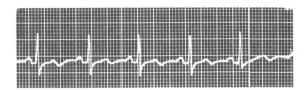

Figure 12-23
Normal sinus rhythm.

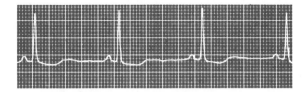

Figure 12-25
Sinus bradycardia.

A sinus tachycardia is present when the rate of normally conducted beats that originate from the SA node exceeds 100 beats/minute. The atrial and ventricular response is generally 100 to 160/minute (Fig. 12–24). The rhythm is regular, with a P wave preceding each QRS complex. The PR interval is normal. With very rapid rates, the TP interval is shortened, causing the P wave to be superimposed on the preceding T wave. Sinus tachycardia reduces diastolic ventricular filling and coronary artery filling and, consequently, may produce angina pectoris. The rapid rate also may decrease cardiac output and precipitate congestive heart failure in the patient with myocardial disease or injury. The treatment depends on the underlying cause of the dysrhythmia.

Sinus Bradycardia

A sinus rhythm of less than 60 beats/minute is referred to as a *sinus bradycardia*. It is normally observed in physically fit individuals, and it can be produced by changes in automaticity due to excessive vagal tone, which is caused by a variety of circumstances. It is seen in patients with severe pain, myxedema, and atherosclerotic heart disease, and it may be produced by drugs, such as digitalis, reserpine, or propranolol. It is observed frequently after acute inferior myocardial infarction and commonly occurs with sleep, vomiting, and suctioning.

Sinus bradycardia is a regular rhythm that rarely falls below 45 beats/minute. A normal P wave precedes each QRS complex. The PR interval is normal (Fig. 12–25). The slow rhythm may predispose the person to premature ectopic beats. If ventricular filling or stroke volume is reduced significantly, the slow rate may decrease cardiac output and play a major role in the development of congestive heart failure, dizziness, or syncope.

Bradycardias are observed during the first few hours after an acute myocardial infarction. Bradycardias that can produce a ventricular rate below 60 beats/minute include sinus bradycardia, junctional escape rhythms, and AV block (at the AV node level). The treatment for such dysrhythmias is outlined in Box 12–1.[2]

In the asymptomatic patient, sinus bradycardia requires no intervention except for continued assessment. If the sinus

bradycardia is associated with symptoms (such as chest pain or dyspnea) or hypotension, or predisposes the person to premature ventricular contractions, intravenous atropine sulfate may be given.

Sinus Exit Block and Sinus Arrest

Sinus exit block (SA block) and sinus arrest (pause) may be caused by vagal stimulation, atherosclerotic disease involving the SA node, occlusion of the SA nodal artery, acute infections, and medications, such as digitalis, quinidine sulfate, and procainamide. *Sinoatrial block* implies that the SA node fires but the conduction pathway from the SA node to the atria is blocked. Sinoatrial block is recognized by the absence of an expected P wave from the SA node. Because the sinus node is not able to release a rhythmic discharge, the entire cardiac cycle of P-QRS-T waves is missing. If a sinus beat is blocked, the resulting pause is exactly equal to some multiple of the sinus cycle (*i.e.*, the pause is equal to two sinus cycles or 2:1 SA block). That occurs because the timing cycle of the SA node has not been reset and the SA node continues to fire at the same rate, whether or not the impulse is released or its exit is blocked (Fig. 12–26A).

A *sinus arrest* or a *sinus pause*, on the other hand, exists when there is an abrupt failure of the SA node to send out a pacemaking stimulus. The resulting pause, however, is not equal to a multiple of the sinus cycle (Fig. 12–26B). After the pause produced by SA block or arrest, there may be a resumption of the sinus rhythm or a junctional or ventricular escape beat may occur, thereby replacing the sinus cycle. Sinus or atrial standstill is observed when there is a total absence of all P waves, indicating complete SA block or sinus arrest.

The most common clinical symptoms associated with these dysrhythmias result from the pause in rhythm and cardiac activity. Patients may be completely asymptomatic, or they may complain of angina pectoris, dizziness, or syncope. The treatment depends primarily on the cause of the SA block or arrest and on the clinical manifestations. Therapy may include the use of such medications as atropine sulfate, epinephrine, and isoproterenol. When pharmacologic measures are not effective, artificial cardiac pacing is indicated.

Sinus Arrhythmia

When all impulses originate from the SA node but the rate of discharge increases and decreases, a sinus arrhythmia is present. The dysrhythmia is generally a physiologic variation of normal sinus rhythm, and it is not believed to indicate underlying heart disease. It is prominent from childhood through adolescence and it may also be found in old age.

Sinus arrhythmia most commonly corresponds with respiration because of the variations in venous return, ventilation,

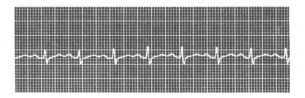

Figure 12-24
Sinus tachycardia.

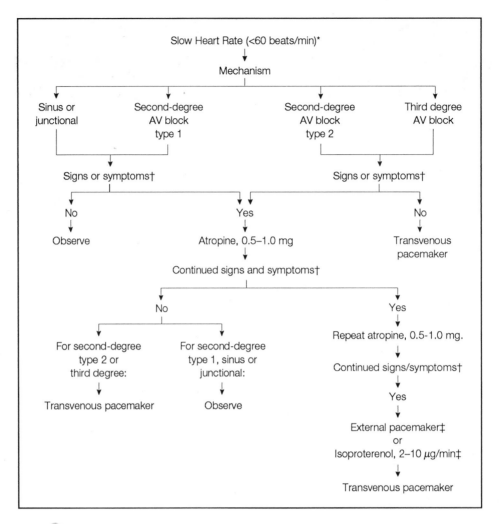

Box 12-1

Bradycardia. This sequence was developed to assist in teaching how to treat a broad range of patients with bradycardia. Some patients may require care not specified herein. This algorithm should not be construed to prohibit such flexibility. AV: atrioventricular. (McIntyre, K. M., and Lewis, A. J. Standards and guidelines for cardiopulmonary resuscitation and emergency cardiac care. *J. Am. Med. Assoc.* 255: 2841, 1986; with permission.)

 * A solitary chest thump or cough may stimulate cardiac electrical activity and result in improved cardiac output and may be used at this point.

 † Hypotension (blood pressure < 90 mm Hg), premature ventricular contractions, altered mental status or symptoms (e.g., chest pain or dyspnea), ischemia, or infarction.

 ‡ Temporizing therapy.

and vagal tone. The rhythm is irregular as it speeds up slightly during inspiration as the right heart distends with an increased venous return, and it slows slightly during expiration. A sinus arrhythmia is present when the difference in time between the two fastest continuous beats and the two slowest continuous beats exceeds 0.12 second (Fig. 12–27). To verify the rhythm, it is important to run a rhythm strip that includes the entire respiratory cycle. The patient is generally asymptomatic, and treatment is not necessary.

Sick Sinus Syndrome

The term *sick sinus syndrome* has been used to describe a variety of dysrhythmias and associated clinical manifestations produced by some pathologic dysfunction of the SA node. The

signs and symptoms result from failure of adequate escape pacemakers rather than sinus node dysfunction per se.

Damage to the SA node may be caused by ischemia, rheumatic, inflammatory, sclerotic, or hypertensive disease.[12] Sick sinus syndrome appears in about 5% of patients who have acute myocardial infarction. Many patients with inferior wall infarctions develop SA node dysfunction because the SA nodal artery usually branches off of the right coronary artery. The term *sick sinus syndrome* is used to describe syncope or other manifestations of cerebral dysfunction associated with one or more of the following:[9]

* Severe sinus bradycardia
* Sinus arrest with or without replacement by atrial or junctional escape rhythms

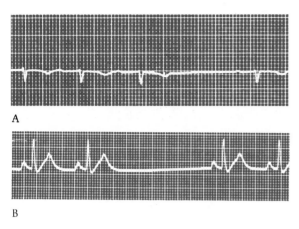

A

B

Figure 12–26

(A) Sinus exit block. The pause is equal to a multiple of the sinus cycle. The sinus node rhythm is not reset. (B) Sinus arrest. The pause is not equal to some multiple of the previous sinus rhythm.

- Sinus node exit block
- Bradycardia-tachycardia syndrome
- Carotid hypersensitivity
- Inability of the heart to resume a sinus rhythm after electrocardioversion

Symptomatic sick sinus syndrome is generally refractory to pharmacologic therapy and usually requires the insertion of a permanent cardiac pacemaker.

Dysrhythmias from the Atria

Premature Atrial Contractions

Premature atrial contractions (PACs) occur during the cardiac cycle when an impulse or ectopic focus, located in either the right or left atrium, discharges earlier than the next expected sinus impulse. Premature contractions can be caused by an increase in automaticity, afterpotentials, or re-entry. Premature atrial contractions are common among all age groups, and they may result from the use of tobacco, caffeine, or alcohol, or from stress or heart disease. Although isolated PACs are common in the normal person, frequent PACs may indicate organic heart disease and may predispose the person to congestive heart failure or to other supraventricular dysrhythmias, such as atrial flutter, atrial fibrillation, and atrial tachycardias.

The ventricular rate will depend on the number of PACs, and the rhythm is essentially irregular because of the premature beats. The P wave of the PAC has a different contour and configuration than the P wave that originates from the SA node, or it may be buried in the preceding T wave (Fig. 12–28A). The PR interval may be normal or prolonged, or the P wave may occur with no QRS complex. The QRS complex that follows the P wave is usually normal in contour, but it may appear distorted as a result of aberrant conduction (Fig. 12–28B), which may occur when the conduction pathway is still partially refractory. If the P wave occurs during the absolute refractory period, it will not conduct and the PAC is said to be blocked or nonconducted (Fig. 12–28C).

The patient may experience a pause in the cardiac rhythm or a feeling of palpitation. The palpitation is not due directly to the PAC but to the beat after the ectopic one. Generally,

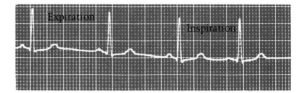

Figure 12–27

Sinus arrhythmia. The rhythm slows with expiration and speeds up with inspiration. The time difference between the two fastest beats and the two slowest beats is 0.20 second.

there is an incomplete compensatory pause associated with the PAC that allows greater ventricular filling time and stroke volume to be associated with the impulse after the PAC and thus produces a sensation of jumping or skipping.

An *incomplete compensatory pause* is determined by measuring the distance between three consecutive normal P waves (or 2×; see Fig. 12–28A) preceding the PAC. That distance is then compared with the distance between the P waves immediately preceding and immediately following the PAC. If the distance between the P waves preceding and following the PAC is less than the distance between the three consecutive normal P waves (<2×), an incomplete compensatory pause is present (see Fig. 12–28A). If both distances are equal, a *complete compensatory pause* exists.

Treatment is rarely necessary. If the PACs are frequent, one should omit alcohol or stimulants, such as tobacco and caffeine. Relaxation techniques or sedation may lower a patient's stress level and thus may reduce the number of PACs. In rare situations, digitalis, propranolol, verapamil, quinidine sulfate, or procainamide may be used.

Atrial Flutter

Atrial flutter may be defined as an abnormally fast but regular atrial rhythm that originates from an accelerated atrial focus. It occurs most commonly in patients who have ischemic myocardial disease. It is observed in 2% to 5% of patients with acute myocardial infarction,[3,6] and it may be precipitated by many kinds of acute illness (*e.g.*, hypoxia and pericarditis).

The physiologic mechanism involved in atrial flutter is probably the result of a re-entry pathway, although enhanced automaticity also may be involved.

Electrocardiographically, atrial flutter is identified by flutter or F waves and an atrial rate of 220 to 350 beats/minute. The common flutter waves are regular and sawtooth in configuration, especially in leads 2, 3, and aV_F. Other leads in the same ECG may not, however, reveal typical flutter waves. The PR interval is not measurable. The QRS complex is normal in configuration except when bundle branch block or aberrant conduction is present. Because the ventricles cannot respond to the rapid atrial rate, a QRS complex usually does not follow every flutter wave. The ventricular rate is generally a whole number fraction of the atrial rate (*e.g.*, 3:1, 4:1, or 5:1), and usually results in a regular ventricular response (Fig. 12–29A). The ventricular response may, however, disclose an irregular rhythm because of an alternating variation in AV conduction (*e.g.*, both 2:1 and 4:1 conduction). This is called variable atrial flutter (Fig. 12–29B).

On physical examination, flutter *a* waves may be observed

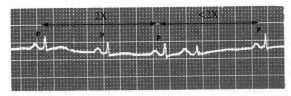

A

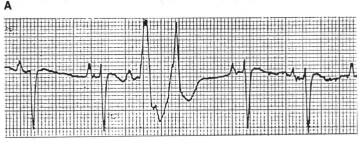

B

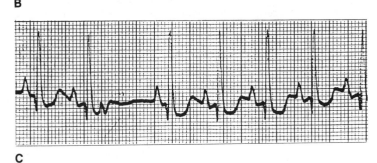

C

Figure 12–28

(*A*) Normal sinus rhythm with premature atrial contraction (PAC). The fourth beat is premature, and the QRS complex is preceded by a P wave. An incomplete compensatory pause associated with the PAC is present (the interval between the P wave before and the P wave after the PAC is less than two normal P-P intervals). (*B*) Normal sinus rhythm with PAC's with aberrancy. The third and fourth beats are premature, preceded by P waves with distorted QRS complexes. (*C*) Normal sinus rhythm with nonconducted PAC. After the second beat is an early P wave with no QRS complex.

in the jugular venous pulse. Although atrial flutter may be suspected, it may be difficult to differentiate 2:1 flutter from paroxysmal atrial tachycardia. Carotid sinus pressure is helpful diagnostically because it will increase the degree of AV block temporarily, thereby slowing the ventricular response and uncovering additional flutter waves (*e.g.,* from a 2:1 atrial flutter with a ventricular response of 150 before carotid sinus pressure to a 4:1 atrial flutter with a ventricular response of 75 during massage). After the carotid stimulation has ceased, the 2:1 atrial flutter will reappear.

Patients may be totally unaware of the dysrhythmia, or they may complain of symptoms that are primarily dependent on the rate of the ventricular response. If the ventricular response is rapid, as in 2:1 atrial flutter, the patient may complain

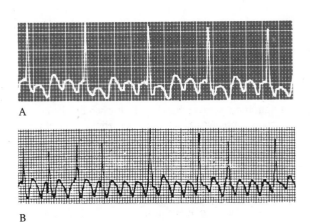

A

B

Figure 12–29

(*A*) 4: 1 atrial flutter with a regular ventricular response. (*B*) Atrial flutter with a variable ventricular response.

of palpitations, angina pectoris, dyspnea, or symptoms of pulmonary edema and cerebrovascular insufficiency.

Treatment of atrial flutter consists of treating the underlying cause and converting the rhythm to normal or controlling the ventricular response. Elective cardioversion or countershock, usually using low voltage levels, is very effective in converting the dysrhythmia and is generally the treatment of choice. If the patient's condition permits, atrial overdrive pacing may successfully convert the dysrhythmia. Cardioversion and overdrive pacing are effective because they evoke a depolarizing stimulus, causing a portion of the myocardium to become refractory, thus interrupting the circus movement that perpetuates the dysrhythmia. Digitalis, verapamil, or propranolol is used in some situations, however, to slow the ventricular rate. Quinidine sulfate, procainamide, or disopyramide is then frequently used to restore the rhythm to normal.

Atrial Fibrillation

Atrial fibrillation results from a rapid and uncoordinated atrial movement in which all of the atrial cells are depolarizing and repolarizing at different times and in different directions. The chaotic atrial flow may be triggered by a PAC or by atrial tachycardia. Generally, atrial fibrillation is a more stable dysrhythmia than is atrial flutter, and it is associated with such disease states as rheumatic mitral valve disease, hypertension, ischemic heart disease, or thyrotoxicosis. It may also be seen in patients with acute myocardial infarction, atrial septal defects, chronic obstructive lung disease, pericarditis, congestive heart failure, and cocaine overdose. In addition, it may be seen in apparently normal individuals.

The ECG characteristically reveals two important features with atrial fibrillation: the absence of P waves, and "irregularly irregular" ventricular response. There are fibrillatory or *f* waves

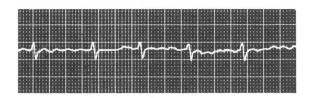

Figure 12-30

Atrial fibrillation with a normal ventricular response. Note the absence of P waves and the irregularly irregular ventricular response. Coarse *f* waves are seen between the QRS complexes.

that reflect the chaotic atrial activity. These may vary in amplitude, spacing, and contour. The *f* waves may be coarse and irregular, resembling flutter waves, or they may be fine fibrillatory waves that look much like a wavy baseline or, occasionally, like a straight line in some leads. Because there are no P waves, the PR interval is not measurable (Fig. 12-30). The QRS complex is generally of normal configuration as a result of normal ventricular conduction.

Because of the rapid number of atrial impulses, the atrium does not depolarize or contract as a unit. The ventricles, therefore, do not receive the benefit of the atrial "kick," or atrial contraction, which may augment ventricular filling by as much as 20% to 30%. As a result, the cardiac output can diminish. Furthermore, because of the uncoordinated, passive, and dilated state of the atrium, thrombi can develop on the atrial walls to produce systemic or pulmonary embolism.

Patients in atrial fibrillation frequently complain of palpitations or symptoms consistent with heart failure or embolism. Atrial fibrillation is suspected immediately when an irregularly irregular pulse is discovered. With rapid ventricular rates, many of the audible apical impulses fail to produce peripheral arterial pulsations, causing an apical-radial deficit to occur. The jugular neck veins may reveal a rippling from the fibrillatory waves, but more frequently it is found on inspection that *a* waves are missing from the jugular venous pulse. On auscultation, the first heart sound varies in intensity from one beat to the next and is louder at the end of shorter cycles.

Treatment is aimed at controlling the ventricular response or attempting to convert the dysrhythmia to a normal sinus rhythm. The approach to treatment depends on the degree of symptoms. Should the patient be hemodynamically unstable, immediate synchronized cardioversion is indicated. Synchronized cardioversion is successful in converting most acute cases of the dysrhythmia.

When countershock is not successful and when the ventricular response is rapid, intravenous propranolol, calcium channel-blocking drugs, or digitalis may be used to slow the ventricular rate. Quinidine sulfate or procainamide may then be added to convert the rhythm back to normal. If the dysrhythmia has had a recent onset, treatment should also be directed toward correction of the underlying disturbance (*e.g.,* heart failure, hyperthyroidism, or hypertension).

Synchronized cardioversion generally is ineffective for patients with long-term atrial fibrillation. The treatment for the patient with chronic atrial fibrillation usually consists of controlling the ventricular response rather than converting the rhythm to normal.

Atrial Tachycardia

Atrial tachycardia is a rapid, regular supraventricular rhythm from an ectopic atrial focus. Atrial tachycardia can be caused by the rapid firing of an ectopic pacemaker due to altered automaticity, triggered activity due to afterdepolarizations, or re-entry.[5] The normal response of the AV node to this rapid rate is to block; thus, atrial tachycardia occurs frequently with 2:1 (or 3:1, 4:1) conduction. As the rate increases, the P wave that is not conducted may be buried in the preceding T wave. The atrial rate may be slightly irregular, with the P-P interval without the QRS greater than the P-P interval with the QRS (ventriculophasic). Most commonly, this dysrhythmia is associated with digitalis toxicity (Fig. 12-31).

Wandering Atrial Pacemaker

A wandering atrial pacemaker results when at least three supraventricular foci are initiating impulses. The pacemaker of the heart "wanders" between the SA node, the AV node, and the atrial muscle. Consequently, the P waves vary in size and configuration, and the PR intervals may vary depending on the proximity of the pacemaker to the AV node. Conduction from the AV node through the ventricles is usually normal, producing a normal QRS. Treatment is generally not indicated (Fig. 12-32).

Multifocal Atrial Tachycardia (Chaotic Atrial Rhythm)

Multifocal atrial tachycardia is actually a fast wandering atrial pacemaker. Multiple ectopic atrial foci are reflected on the ECG as at least three different P waves. Multifocal atrial tachycardia is seen commonly in patients with chronic pulmonary problems. Treatment, if required, is directed at controlling the rate (Fig. 12-33).

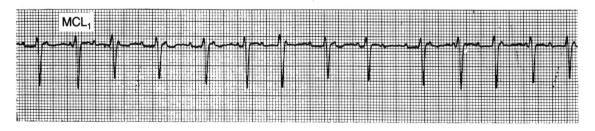

Figure 12-31

Atrial tachycardia with block. (Jacobson, C. Basic arrhythmias and conduction disturbances. In S. L. Underhill, S. L. Woods, E. S. Silvarajan Froelicher, et al., *Cardiac Nursing,* 2nd ed., Philadelphia, J. B. Lippincott, 1989 with permission)

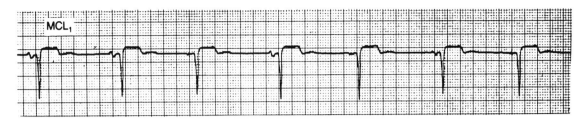

Figure 12–32

Wandering atrial pacemaker. (Jacobson, C. Basic arrhythmias and conduction disturbances. In S. L. Underhill, S. L. Woods, E. S. Silvarajan Froelicher, et al., *Cardiac Nursing*, 2nd ed., Philadelphia, J. B. Lippincott, 1989 with permission)

Dysrhythmias From the Atrioventricular Junction

AV Junctional Rhythms

If the SA node fails to fire or if atrial impulses are not transmitted through the AV node, the AV junction may take over as the primary pacemaker to produce a *junctional rhythm*. Any problem that suppresses SA node activity, such as sinus bradycardia, SA block, and digitalis-induced vagal stimulation, can result in a junctional rhythm. The rhythm may also be a result of any problem that enhances AV junctional automaticity, such as digitalis intoxication, acute inferior myocardial infarction, or rheumatic fever.

Impulses arising from the AV junction spread simultaneously upward to the atria and downward to the ventricles. The ECG displays a normally conducted QRS complex. The atria are usually, but not always, activated by retrograde conduction from the AV junction. The resulting P waves will be inverted in leads 2, 3, and aV$_F$, and they may occur before, during, or after the QRS complex depending on the speed of retrograde conduction compared with anterograde conduction. When present, the PR interval is generally less than 0.12 second. The premature junctional beat may or may not be associated with a complete compensatory pause.

When the sinus pacemaker has been suppressed, junctional pacemaker sites can assume the role of primary impulse formation, usually at a rate of 40 to 60 beats/minute, producing a *junctional rhythm* (Fig. 12–34A). When the junctional rhythm is a result of enhanced AV junctional activity, with a rate of 60 to 100 beats/minute, an *accelerated AV junctional rhythm* is present. An *AV junctional tachycardia* exists when the rate exceeds 100 beats/minute (Fig. 12–34B). If there is blocked retrograde conduction to the atria, there will be AV dissocia-

tion, and the rhythm is called *accelerated idiojunctional*. Impulses arising prematurely from the AV junction are known as *premature junctional contractions* (Fig. 12–34C).

The clinical signs and symptoms depend on the ventricular response. The physical examination may be normal, or it may reveal cannon *a* waves in the jugular venous pulse together with a loud S$_1$. The treatment involves increasing the discharge rate of higher pacemakers, improving the AV conduction, or using artificial cardiac pacing (see Box 12–1). Premature junctional contractions generally require no treatment. Escape rhythms and beats are protective and are not treated.

Paroxsymal Supraventricular Tachycardia

Paroxysmal supraventricular tachycardia can be caused by AV nodal re-entry or a re-entry pathway involving an accessory pathway in Wolff-Parkinson-White syndrome. Atrioventricular nodal re-entry, the most common form, is usually initiated by a PAC with a prolonged PR interval (from traveling down the slower pathway). It returns up the recovered fast pathway, resulting in a P wave lost in the QRS or just at the end of the QRS (Fig. 12–35). Often the P wave looks like an r wave in V$_1$ or an S wave inferiorly. Paroxysmal supraventricular tachycardia is characterized by an abrupt onset and abrupt cessation, has a rate greater than 150 to 160 beats/minute, and generally has a narrow QRS.

When paroxysmal supraventricular tachycardia involves an accessory pathway, there are retrograde P waves following the QRS (closer to the preceding R wave, resulting in an RP interval that is less than the PR interval). The initiating PR interval is normal.

Treatment of paroxysmal supraventricular tachycardia is directed toward elimination of the cause and slowing the ven-

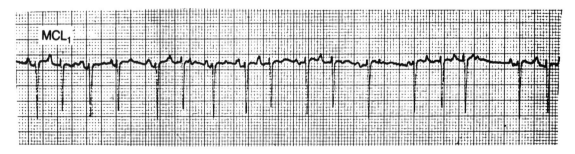

Figure 12–33

Multifocal atrial tachycardia. (Jacobson, C. Basic arrhythmias and conduction disturbances. In S. L. Underhill, S. L. Woods, E. S. Silvarajan Froelicher, et al., *Cardiac Nursing*, 2nd ed., Philadelphia, J. B. Lippincott, 1989 with permission)

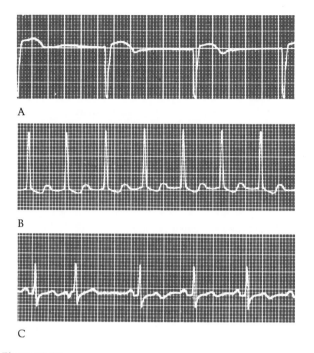

Figure 12–34

(A) Junctional rhythm. The ventricular rate is 55. No P waves are present. (B) Junctional tachycardia. The ventricular rate is 125. (C) Normal sinus rhythm with premature junctional contraction (PJC). The second beat is a PJC with an inverted P wave.

tricular rate. Sedation and vagal stimulation, including vasopressors, may be used to slow or terminate the rhythm. Digitalis, propranolol, or verapamil may be given to slow the ventricular rate, or to prevent recurrences of the rhythm. If the patient is symptomatic with the rapid rate, cardioversion may be used. (See the treatment algorithm for paroxysmal supraventricular tachycardia in Chap. 14).

Heart Blocks

The electrical connection between the atria and ventricles is through the AV junction. When an impulse has difficulty getting through the AV junction, some degree of heart block results.

First-Degree Atrioventricular Block

In first-degree AV block, which is actually a delay in conduction rather than a block, all of the sinus beats conduct. First-degree AV block can result from ischemia of the AV node or the effects of drugs (primarily digitalis).

First-degree AV block exists when the PR interval (in adults) exceeds 0.20 second (Fig. 12–36A). The patient usually has no symptoms. When first-degree AV block is noted in a patient who is receiving digitalis, digitalis intoxication should be suspected, and the physician should be consulted before the drug is given again. Usually the PR interval will revert to normal and not progress to a higher degree of AV block, although the patient must be observed closely. If the patient has a slow heart rate and is symptomatic, atropine sulfate, 0.5 mg to 1 mg, may be administered intravenously to correct the problem.

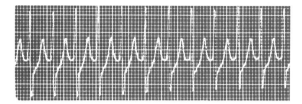

Figure 12–35

Paroxysmal supraventricular tachycardia.

Second-Degree Atrioventricular Block

In second-degree AV block, some of the sinus beats are not conducted to the ventricles. It may be due to ischemia or injury of the AV node, drug intoxication, coronary artery disease, rheumatic fever, or various viral infections. Second-degree AV block is divided into two major types: Mobitz type 1 (Wenckebach phenomenon) and Mobitz type 2.

Type 1 block characteristically has a progressive lengthening of the PR interval (and a progressive shortening of the R-R interval) for several successive beats until a P wave occurs that is not followed by a ventricular response. The QRS complexes are narrow, because the block occurs in the AV node above the bundle of His. The PR interval after the dropped beat is prolonged (Fig. 12–36B). Occasionally, the conduction ratio will be 2:1. In such cases, there will not be PR lengthening. However, the QRS complexes will be narrow, and the PR intervals will usually be prolonged.

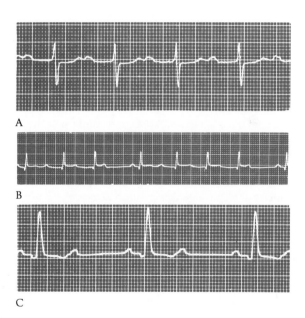

Figure 12–36

(A) First-degree atriaventricular (AV) block. The PR interval is 0.36 second. (B) 5 : 4 Wenckebach phenomenon (Mobitz type 1 AV block). The fourth beat begins the cycle. Note the progressive lengthening of the PR interval in the fourth, fifth, sixth, and seventh beats, but by decreasing increments, such that the ventricular cycle (R-R interval) shortens (particularly between the fourth and fifth beats, and the fifth and sixth beats). Note the blocked P wave resulting in no QRS complex (dropped beat) following the seventh beat. (C) 2 : 1 Mobitz type 2 second-degree AV block. There are two P waves for each QRS complex—hence 2 : 1 AV block (every other sinus beat is blocked). Note that the atrial rate is 90, whereas the ventricular rate is 45; the PR interval is normal, and the QRS complex is greater than 0.12 second.

Type 1 block is associated with acute inferior wall myocardial infarction, digitalis toxicity, and myocarditis, and may occur after open heart surgery. The patient is usually asymptomatic. Type 1 heart block is a transient form of heart block and usually does not advance to a higher degree of block. Generally, it is not treated, but the patient should be observed closely (see Box 12–1).

Mobitz type 2 second-degree AV block is a more serious form of heart block. Characteristically, a sudden drop in AV conduction occurs in which only every second, third, or fourth impulse reaches the ventricles. That drop results in a ventricular rate that is one half, one third, or one fourth of the atrial rate (*i.e.,* the ratio is 2:1, 3:1, or 4:1) (Fig. 12–36C).

Type 2 block is commonly associated with anterior myocardial infarction. The patient may or may not be symptomatic. When the ventricular rate becomes excessively slow, cardiac output falls and the patient may complain of dizziness or syncope. The QRS complexes are usually wide, because the block develops in the His-Purkinje system or below the bundle of His. The PR intervals are normal.

Because Mobitz type 2 block may progress to complete AV block with a ventricular escape rhythm in the presence of acute myocardial infarction, a temporary demand cardiac pacemaker is always indicated (see Box 12–1).

Third-Degree Atrioventricular Block

In third-degree AV block, none of the sinus impulses conduct. Third-degree AV block can be caused by ischemia or injury to the AV node, bundle of His, or bundle branches; drug intoxication; trauma; or congenital abnormalities. Classically, in third-degree AV block, there are two active pacemakers within the heart, one in the atria and one in the ventricle, causing the atria and ventricles to depolarize and contract independently (Fig. 12–37). P waves and QRS complexes appear at regular intervals, but they are completely independent of each other. P waves that have plenty of opportunity to conduct do not conduct; consequently, AV dissociation is present. Typically, the ventricular rate is slower than the atrial rate. If the ventricular pacemaker is higher in the region of the AV junction, the QRS complexes will be narrow and will range from 40 to 60 beats/minute. When the pacemaker is lower in the ventricles, the QRS complexes will be wide (greater than 0.12 second) and will range from 20 to 40 beats/minute.

If the rate becomes excessively slow and thus produces a reduction in cardiac output (most likely with a lower ventricular pacemaker), the patient may complain of dizziness and syncope (Stokes-Adams syndrome). Congestive heart failure may be precipitated or aggravated. In symptomatic patients, an emergency situation exists that requires the use of atropine

or isoproterenol and the insertion of a temporary demand cardiac pacemaker (see Box 12–1). If third-degree heart block persists, implantation of a permanent pacemaker is considered.

Atrioventricular Dissociation

In AV dissociation, the atria and ventricles are controlled by separate pacemakers and are beating independently. Atrioventricular dissociation is a result of some other basic disorder, not a primary rhythm itself. The usual causes of AV dissociation include the following:

Sinus bradycardia (escape rhythm takes over)
Accelerated idiojunctional rhythm
Accelerated idioventricular rhythm
Complete AV block (causes AV dissociation, but AV dissociation is not necessarily complete heart block)

Bundle Branch Block

Bundle branch blocks are caused frequently by ischemia, rheumatic heart disease, aortic valvular disease, hypertension, and congenital abnormalities (specifically septal defects).[16] Normally, both the right and left bundles receive the excitatory impulse about the same time, depolarizing the entire ventricular muscle. An obstruction or delay in impulse conduction from the bundle of His to the right or left bundle branch can cause one of the ventricles to depolarize and contract before the other. When impulse conduction is blocked on one side, a bundle branch block pattern is produced on the ECG.

Right Bundle Branch Block. When the right bundle branch is blocked, the impulse goes down the left side first and the right ventricle is activated late. The delay in conduction results in a QRS interval that is greater than 0.12 second. In addition, an rSR′ pattern is seen in V_1, and a small Q wave and broad prominent S wave are seen in leads 1 and V_6 (Fig. 12–38). The R′ in lead V_1 and the terminal S wave in leads 1 and V_6 result from the delayed right ventricular activation. There may be secondary T wave changes in the right ventricular leads

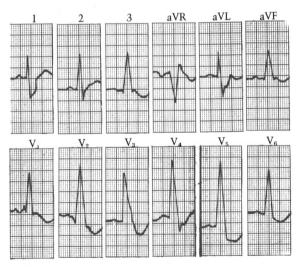

Figure 12–38
Right bundle branch block.

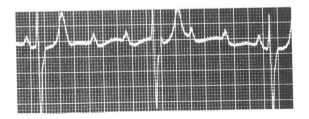

Figure 12–37
Third-degree (complete) atrioventricular block

(V_1–V_3) and a delayed intrinsicoid deflection in V_1 (time from the beginning of the QRS to the peak R wave).

Left Bundle Branch Block. When the left bundle branch is blocked, the right ventricle is depolarized first and then the left ventricle. The septum is abnormally activated from right to left. The QRS complex is wide (>0.12 second). There is a positive QRS in leads 1, aV_L, and V_6, usually slurred or with a notched R wave. Because of the abnormal septal activation, there is no Q wave in lead 1, aV_L, or V_6. The right ventricular leads V_1 to V_3 reflect the delayed left ventricular activation with a mainly negative complex (QS or rS). There are altered ST interval and T-wave changes over the lateral leads and a delayed intrinsicoid deflection over the left ventricle (Fig. 12–39).

Hemiblocks. The left bundle branch divides into an anterior and posterior fascicle (see Fig. 12–7). When a block is observed on the ECG in only half of the left bundle, it is termed a *hemiblock.* The term *bifascicular block* describes an existing right bundle branch block in combination with a left anterior or left posterior hemiblock. The term *trifascicular block* describes a block in the right bundle branch and in both the anterior and posterior branches of the left bundle or main left bundle (resulting in complete heart block). Patients with bundle branch blocks and hemiblocks must be observed closely for the development of second- and third-degree AV blocks.

Left Anterior Hemiblock. Left anterior hemiblock occurs more frequently than does left posterior hemiblock because the anterior fascicle is a more vulnerable structure. It is particularly vulnerable because it is long and thin and is not a highly diffuse structure; it receives its blood supply from only one source (the septal branch of the left anterior descending coronary artery), and it lies in the left ventricular outflow tract.[15] Because its blood supply is from the left anterior descending coronary artery, left anterior hemiblock is usually seen with anteroseptal or anterolateral myocardial infarctions.

Because the left anterior fascicle is blocked, the impulse spreads through the left ventricle by way of the posterior fas-

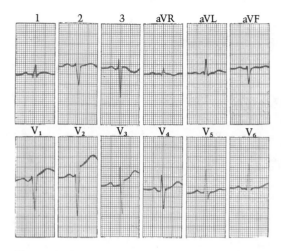

Figure 12–40
Left anterior hemiblock.

cicle located inferiorly and then travels superiorly upward and to the left. This abnormal depolarization results in a left-axis deviation, which is the main criterion for diagnosing left anterior hemiblock. The ECG diagnosis includes left-axis deviation (at least −45°), a small Q in lead 1 and a small r in lead 3. The QRS duration is usually normal (Fig. 12–40).

Left Posterior Hemiblock. Left posterior hemiblock is seen with more extensive myocardial damage, usually with two areas of infarction, and is almost always associated with right bundle branch block. Left posterior hemiblock is less common than left anterior hemiblock because the posterior division of the left bundle branch has a dual blood supply—from both the right and left circumflex coronary arteries.

The impulse spreads through the left ventricle by way of the anterior fascicle superiorly and then travels inferiorly, down and to the right. This results in a right-axis deviation, the primary ECG abnormality in left posterior hemiblock. The ECG diagnosis includes right-axis deviation (+120 or greater), a small r wave in lead 1, and a small Q wave in lead 3. The QRS is normal duration if left posterior hemiblock occurs alone. However, it most commonly is seen in combination with right bundle branch block (Fig. 12–41).

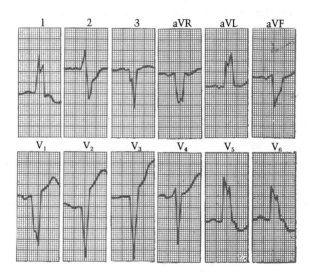

Figure 12–39
Left bundle branch block.

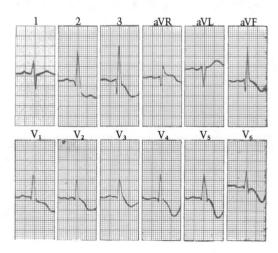

Figure 12–41
Left posterior hemiblock.

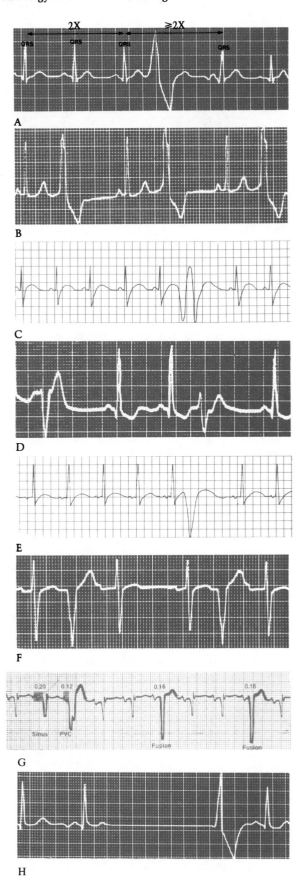

A

B

C

D

E

F

G

H

Dysrhythmias from the Ventricles

Premature Ventricular Contractions

A premature ventricular contraction (PVC) originates from an ectopic focus in the wall of the ventricle and may develop because of enhanced automaticity, afterpotentials, or re-entry. Although they can occur in healthy individuals, they are caused most frequently by ischemia, hypoxia, heart failure, acute myocardial infarction, digitalis intoxication, or electrolyte imbalances.

There are generally no P waves preceding the QRS complex. Because the impulse originates in an ectopic center in one of the ventricles and spreads anomalously, the QRS complex is distorted, bizarre, and prolonged. The PVC occurs prematurely in the cycle, and it is usually followed by a complete compensatory pause (Fig. 12–42A).

Premature ventricular contractions may have characteristic patterns. When every other beat is a PVC, the phenomenon is termed *bigeminy* (Fig. 12–42B); if every third beat is a PVC, the phenomenon is termed *trigeminy;* and if every fourth beat is a PVC, the phenomenon is termed *quadrigeminy.* If two or more PVCs are consecutive, they are referred to as *coupled* or paired PVCs (Fig. 12–42C). When the PVCs have different configurations, they are termed *multifocal* PVCs. The term indicates that the vector is different to the axis of the lead with each ectopic beat (*i.e.,* the PVCs originate from different foci within the ventricle), and the phenomenon generally reflects a very sick and irritable heart (Fig. 12–42D).

The R-on-T phenomenon exists when a PVC occurs during the vulnerable phase of recovery. Actually, the PVC (R wave) occurs during the relative refractory period (T wave) of the previous impulse. During that period of time, a dangerous ventricular dysrhythmia can occur, because the heart is not yet ready to respond to the ectopic stimulus in a normal, organized manner (Fig. 12–42E).

One type of PVC that does not interrupt the regular basic rhythm is the *interpolated PVC,* which falls between two normal sinus beats. The interpolated PVC does not have a compensatory pause. It can occur only when the normal rate is slow enough to find the myocardium physiologically nonrefractory for a period sufficient to complete the response to an ectopic stimulus and then return to a nonrefractory state before the next normal sinus impulse (Fig. 12–42F).

A *fusion beat* is one PVC that will be preceded by a P wave. The sinus node discharges at its regular rate and initiates the P wave. Before the sinus beat captures the ventricles, a PVC occurs and activates the ventricles. The two impulses merge

Figure 12–42

(*A*) Normal sinus rhythm with premature ventricular contraction (PVC). The fourth QRS complex is wide, bizarre, and premature. A complete compensatory pause associated with the PVC is present (the distance between the QRS complex before and the QRS complex after the PVC is equal to the distance between two normal R-R intervals). (*B*) Bigeminy of PVCs. (*C*) Paired PVCs. (*D*) Multifocal PVCs. (*E*) R-on-T phenomenon. (*F*) Interpolated PVCs. (*G*) Fusion beat. (*H*) Ventricular escape beat.

(or fuse) in the ventricles, and the resultant beat is a combination of a sinus beat and a PVC (Fig. 12–42G). Fusion beats, often called *end-diastolic* or *late* PVCs, are seen frequently at the beginning and end of accelerated idioventricular rhythm.

Premature ventricular contractions are considered dangerous, and they must be treated aggressively in patients with ischemic heart disease in the following situations:

- When they occur frequently (more than six PVCs per minute)
- When they are coupled, paired, or in short runs
- When they are multifocal
- When the R-on-T phenomenon is present

The drug therapy of choice is a bolus of lidocaine followed by a continuous lidocaine infusion (see the treatment algorithm in Box 12–2). Some PVCs may be innocuous, but often, especially in the presence of acute myocardial infarction, they can be forerunners of ventricular tachycardia or ventricular fibrillation.

Ventricular Escape Beat

When the sinus node fails to conduct impulses to the ventricle, a ventricular escape beat may occur. Escape beats occur late, after a pause in the rhythm. The ECG reveals a broad ventricular beat because the impulse originates below the bifurcation of the bundle of His (Fig. 12–42H). This is one situation in which lidocaine is not the drug of choice to treat ventricular beats. If the patient is symptomatic, with a ventricular rate below 60 beats/minute, and has frequent ventricular escape beats, the drug of choice is intravenous atropine sulfate.

Ventricular Tachycardia

Ventricular tachycardia is a dangerous dysrhythmia resulting from irritability of the ventricles. It may be caused by ischemia, hypoxemia, acidosis, acute myocardial infarction, or drug toxicity. The ECG reveals wide, bizarre ventricular complexes at a rate of 100 to 250 beats/minute. Three or more PVCs that occur sequentially are called *ventricular tachycardia.* The rhythm is usually regular, but it may be slightly irregular. The P waves are often lost in the QRS complexes or may appear with AV dissociation, and the QRS interval is greater than 0.12 second (Fig. 12–43A).

Ventricular tachycardia is extremely dangerous in the setting of acute myocardial infarction, because it will cause mild-to-severe hemodynamic changes that can precipitate heart failure or shock and that may also be a precursor to ventricular fibrillation.

Treatment is aimed at quick recognition. The drug of choice is an intravenous bolus of lidocaine and then a lidocaine infusion (see Appendix II). When ventricular tachycardia does not respond to such treatment, electrical cardioversion may be indicated. In patients who are hemodynamically unstable, electrical cardioversion is the initial treatment followed by lidocaine, as described previously. Patients who are pulseless with ventricular tachycardia are treated as if they are in ventricular fibrillation. (See treatment algorithm for ventricular tachycardia in Chap. 14.)

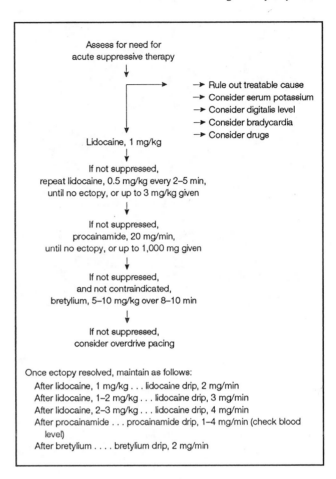

Box 12–2

Ventricular ectopy: acute suppressive therapy. This sequence was developed to assist in teaching how to treat a broad range of patients with ventricular ectopy. Some patients may require therapy not specified herein. This algorithm should not be construed as prohibiting such flexibility. (McIntyre, K. M., and Lewis, A. J. Standards and guidelines for cardiopulmonary resuscitation and emergency cardiac care. *J. Am. Med. Assoc.* 255:2841, 1986; with permission.)

Accelerated Idioventricular Rhythm

Accelerated idioventricular rhythm is a ventricular rhythm between 40 to 100 beats/minute. Formerly called *slow ventricular tachycardia,* this rhythm has the same ECG characteristics as ventricular tachycardia (except rate). Accelerated idioventricular rhythm is seen when an automatic focus in the ventricles exceeds the rate of the sinus node or when the sinus node slows down. It commonly begins and ends with a fusion beat. Accelerated idioventricular rhythm frequently is seen with acute myocardial infarction, is generally benign, and is not treated.

Ventricular Fibrillation

Ventricular fibrillation occurs when myocardial function is severely compromised by ischemia, drug toxicity, high-voltage

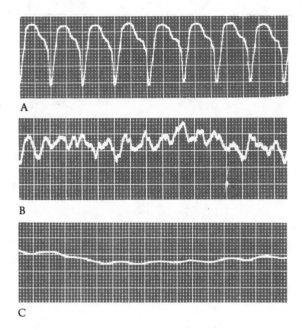

Figure 12–43

(*A*) Ventricular tachycardia. (*B*) Ventricular fibrillation. (*C*) Cardiac standstill.

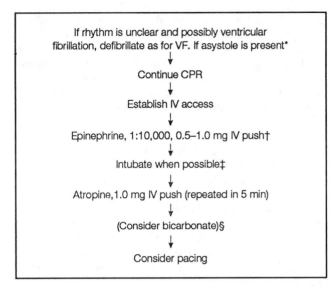

Box 12–3

Asystole (cardiac standstill). This sequence was developed to assist in teaching how to treat a broad range of patients with asystole. Some patients may require care not specified herein. This algorithm should not be construed to prohibit such flexibility. Flow of algorithm presumes asystole is continuing. VF: ventricular fibrillation; IV: intravenous. (McIntyre, K. M., and Lewis, A. J. Standards and guidelines for cardiopulmonary resuscitation and emergency cardiac care. *J. Am. Med. Assoc.* 255:2841, 1986; with permission.)

  * Asystole should be confirmed in two leads.

  † Epinephrine should be repeated every 5 minutes.

  ‡ Intubation is preferable; if it can be accomplished simultaneously with other techniques, then the earlier the better. However, cardiopulmonary resuscitation (CPR) and use of epinephrine are more important initially if patient can be ventilated without intubation. (Endotracheal epinephrine may be used.)

  § Value of sodium bicarbonate is questionable during cardiac arrest, and it is not recommended for the routine cardiac arrest sequence. Consideration of its use in a dose of 1 mEq/kg is appropriate at this point. Half of original dose may be repeated every 10 minutes if it is used.

electrical shock, or trauma. There are no P waves or definite QRS complexes (Fig. 12–43B). Because there is no uniform ventricular depolarization, there is no ventricular contraction, and there is an abrupt cessation in cardiac output. The patient becomes unconscious and is considered clinically dead. Basic life support should be instituted, and, in the hope of converting the dysrhythmia to a normal sinus rhythm, a precordial thump may be delivered immediately in a witnessed situation.[2]

The immediate treatment of choice is direct-current countershock. It is known that successful defibrillation is related to the time that elapses before the countershock is administered. If unsuccessful, epinephrine, lidocaine, or bretylium may be given.[2] After successful defibrillation, lidocaine is given intravenously. (See treatment algorithm for ventricular fibrillation in Chap. 14.)

Cardiac Standstill

Cardiac standstill is the total absence of electrical activity and contraction of the heart. The ECG reveals a straight line, and the patient loses consciousness, pulse, and blood pressure (Fig. 12–43C). Death results unless treatment is immediate. Cardiopulmonary resuscitation is the treatment of choice. Epinephrine, atropine, and oxygen may also be used.

Insertion of a transvenous pacemaker may be indicated (see treatment algorithm in Box 12–3).

Aberrant Ventricular Conduction

Aberrant ventricular conduction is a term that applies to transient abnormal conduction of a supraventricular impulse. It results most commonly from stimulation of the bundle branches while one of the bundle branches is still refractory

(phase 3 aberration).[8] Because the right bundle branch repolarizes slightly later than the left, most aberrancy has the configuration of right bundle branch block.

Aberrant ventricular conduction can easily be mistaken for—and inappropriately treated as—PVCs or ventricular tachycardia (Fig. 12–44). Thus, the ability to differentiate aberrancy is of great clinical significance. Several studies have identified ECG features that help distinguish supraventricular tachycardia with aberrancy from ventricular tachycardia.[8,13,21] The following are most significant and favor ventricular tachycardia:

* Atrioventricular dissociation
* QRS duration greater than 0.14 second (fascicular ventricular tachycardia may be less)
* QRS axis greater than −30° (abnormal left) or indeterminate
* QRS morphology. When V_1 has a positive QRS, the following favor ventricular tachycardia:
  * Bi- or monophasic QRS
  * In V_6, S wave > R wave

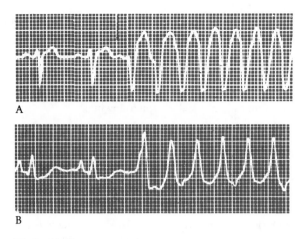

Figure 12-44

(*A*) Aberrant ventricular conduction. (*B*) Ventricular tachycardia.

- When V_1 has a negative QRS, the following favor ventricular tachycardia:
  - r wave is >0.03 second
  - Slurred downstroke of S wave
  - Delayed nadir in V_1 (>0.06 second)
  - Q wave in V_6
- Precordial concordance (QRS in V leads are all positive or all negative) favors ventricular tachycardia when negative

The QRS morphology, width, and axis are particularly important in atrial fibrillation when there is no preceding P wave to aid in diagnosis. Vera and colleagues[20] found that the rSR' in V_1 favored aberrant ventricular conduction in atrial fibrillation 24:1. A qR or monophasic R of right bundle branch block or QS or RS of left bundle branch block in V_1 favored ventricular ectopy, as did bizarre axis, concordance, and malignant PVCs. Ashman's phenomenon (which states that the refractory period for a beat varies with the length of the previous cycle) is considered unreliable in the differentiation of aberrancy and ectopy in atrial fibrillation.[18]

Electromechanical Dissociation

In patients who have electromechanical dissociation, the ECG reveals organized electrical activity, but clinically, ventricular contractions are inadequate to support life. Electromechanical dissociation is a serious problem that can be caused by hypoxemia, severe acidosis, pericardial tamponade, tension pneumothorax, hypovolemia, vagotonia, and pulmonary embolus. Treatment includes cardiopulmonary resuscitation, epinephrine, and treatment of the underlying cause (see treatment algorithm in Box 12–4).

Wolff-Parkinson-White Syndrome

The Wolff-Parkinson-White syndrome, a pre-excitation syndrome, is produced when accelerated conduction through an accessory pathway between the atria and ventricles results in abnormal early excitation of the ventricles. The ECG reveals a PR interval of less than 0.12 second due to accelerated conduction across an accessory pathway rather than the normal

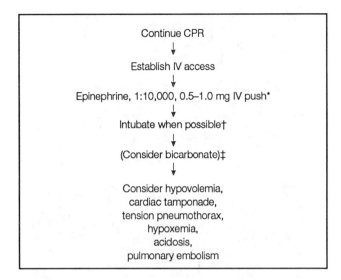

Box 12-4

Electromechanical dissociation. This sequence was developed to assist in teaching how to treat a broad range of patients with electromechanical dissociation. Some patients may require care not specified herein. This algorithm should not be construed to prohibit such flexibility. Flow of algorithm presumes that electromechanical dissociation is continuing. CPR: cardiopulmonary resuscitation; IV: intravenous. (McIntyre, K. M., and Lewis, A. J. Standards and guidelines for cardiopulmonary resuscitation and emergency cardiac care. *J. Am. Med. Assoc.* 255:2841, 1986; with permission.)

* Epinephrine should be repeated every 5 minutes.

† Intubation is preferable. If it can be accomplished simultaneously with other techniques, then the earlier the better. However, epinephrine is more important initially if the patient can be ventilated without intubation.

‡ Value of sodium bicarbonate is questionable during cardiac arrest, and it is not recommended for routine cardiac arrest sequence. Consideration of its use in a dose of 1 mEq/kg is appropriate at this point. Half of original dose may be repeated every 10 minutes if it is used.

conduction pathway through the AV node. The QRS complex is 0.12 second or more. This results from the *delta wave*, an initial slurring of the QRS complex as the impulse begins early depolarization of the ventricles. In addition, there may be secondary T-wave changes from abnormal ventricular repolarization.

In the past, Wolff-Parkinson-White syndrome was classified according to specific ECG patterns as type A or type B. This classification is felt to be an oversimplification and Wolff-Parkinson-White syndrome is now classified according to the location of the accessory pathway determined by the initial force of the QRS complex (Fig. 12–45A,B).[16]

Patients with Wolff-Parkinson-White syndrome are usually asymptomatic while in sinus rhythm. However, they are prone to develop paroxysmal supraventricular tachycardia due to circus movement tachycardia or atrial fibrillation with rapid ventricular rates. Circus movement tachycardia (seen with Wolff-Parkinson-White syndrome) differs from AV nodal reentry tachycardia in the following ways:

- The PR interval that initiates the circus movement tachycardia is not prolonged.

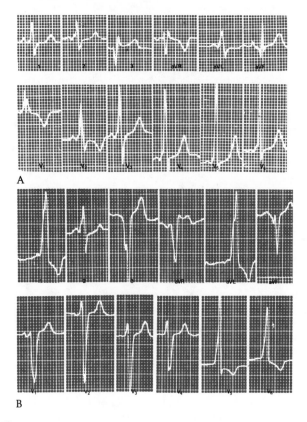

Figure 12–45

(*A*) Wolff-Parkinson-White syndrome with left-sided accessory pathway. Note the negative delta wave in leads 3 and aV$_F$ and the positive delta wave in the precordial leads. (*B*) Wolff-Parkinson-White syndrome with right-sided accessory pathway. Delta wave is positive in leads 1, 2, and aV$_L$.

• The R-P interval is less than the PR interval. (In AV nodal re-entry, the P wave is hidden or is at the end of the QRS.)
• Approximately one third of patients with circus movement tachycardia have electrical alternans.

Also, with circus movement tachycardia, there will be no AV dissociation, no AV block, and no absence of visible P waves.[18]

Atrial fibrillation in Wolff-Parkinson-White syndrome is described as fast, broad, and irregular. It is fast because of the shorter refractory period in the accessory pathway; the QRS complexes are broad because of starting outside the normal conduction system; and the rhythm is irregular because of concealed conduction in the accessory pathway from the rapid stimulation from the atria.

It is important to recognize circus movement tachycardia and atrial fibrillation in Wolff-Parkinson-White syndrome in order to ensure proper treatment. Because of the involvement of the accessory pathway, several of the usual medications used to treat atrial fibrillation are contraindicated because they alter or do not affect conduction through the accessory pathway. For example, digitalis is contraindicated for patients with Wolff-Parkinson-White syndrome in atrial fibrillation because it speeds conduction through the accessory pathway and will, consequently, increase a rapid response to an even faster, and

potentially lethal, rate. The treatment of choice for symptomatic patients is surgical ablation of the accessory pathway.

NURSING DIAGNOSES

Common cardiovascular nursing diagnoses for patients with dysrhythmias might include the following:

• Altered cardiac output related to electrical factors (rate, rhythm, or conduction)
• Anxiety related to
  • Acute illness
  • Fear of death
  • Critical care unit environment and monitoring equipment
• High risk for noncompliance related to inadequate knowledge about acute illness and discharge regimen for health maintenance.

Details of patient outcomes, nursing plans, interventions, and evaluation related to cardiovascular dysfunctions are found in Unit V.

SUMMARY

Caring for patients with dysrhythmias or the potential for the development of dysrhythmias is both challenging and exciting. Critical care nurses must continue to increase their knowledge and skill in this specialized area to provide quality care to acutely ill patients.

REFERENCES

1. Alspach, J. G. Electrical axis: How to recognize deviations on the ECG and how to interpret them. *Am. J. Nurs.* 79:1976, 1979.
2. American Heart Association. *Textbook of Advanced Cardiac Life Support* (2nd ed.). Dallas: American Heart Association, 1987.
3. Andreoli, K., Fowkes, V., Zipes, D. D., *et al. Comprehensive Cardiac Care* (5th ed.). St. Louis: C.V. Mosby, 1983.
4. Belic, N., and Talano, J. Current concepts in sick sinus syndrome. *Arch. Intern. Med.* 145:722, 1985.
5. Berne, R. M., and Levy, M. N. *Cardiovascular Physiology* (5th ed.). St. Louis: C.V. Mosby, 1986.
6. Braunwald, E. *Heart Disease.* Philadelphia: W.B. Saunders, 1988.
7. Daly, B. The effect of fatigue on the vigilance of nurses monitoring electrocardiograms. *Heart Lung* 12:384, 1983.
8. Dancy, M., *et al.* Misdiagnosis of chronic recurrent ventricular tachycardia. *Lancet* 2:320, 1985.
9. Goldberger, E. *Textbook of Clinical Physiology.* St. Louis: C.V. Mosby, 1983.
10. Guyton, A. *Textbook of Medical Physiology.* Philadelphia: W.B. Saunders, 1986.
11. Guzzetta, C. E. The Person Requiring Cardiovascular Drugs. In C. E. Guzzetta and B. M. Dossey, (eds.), *Cardiovascular Nursing: Bodymind Tapestry.* St. Louis: C.V. Mosby, 1984.
12. Hurst, J. W., Logue, R. F., Rackley, C., *et al. The Heart* (5th ed.). New York: McGraw-Hill, 1986.
13. Kindwall, K., *et al.* Electrocardiographic criteria for ventricular tachycardia in wide complex left bundle branch block morphology tachycardias. *Am. J. Cardiol.* 61:1279, 1988.
14. Krasover, T. A conceptual approach to the electrocardiogram. *Crit. Care Nurs.* 1:27, 1981.
15. Lauer, J. M. Electrical Activity of the Heart. In C. E. Guzzetta and B. M. Dossey, (eds.), *Cardiovascular Nursing: Bodymind Tapestry.* St. Louis: C.V. Mosby, 1984.

16. Mandel, W. J. *Cardiac Arrhythmias: Their Mechanisms, Diagnosis, and Management.* Philadelphia: J.B. Lippincott, 1987.

17. Marriott, H. J. L. Arrhythmia versus dysrhythmia. *Am. J. Cardiol.* 53:626, 1984.

18. Marriott, H. J. L., and Conover, M. B. *Advanced Concepts in Arrhythmias* (2nd ed.). St. Louis: C.V. Mosby, 1989.

19. Smith, M. Rx for ECG monitoring artifact. *Crit. Care Nurs.* 4:64, 1984.

20. Vera, Z., *et al.* His bundle electrography for evaluation of criteria in differentiating ventricular ectopy from aberrancy in atrial fibrillation. *Circulation* (suppl. II) 46:90, 1972.

21. Wellens, H. J. J., *et al.* The value of the electrocardiogram in the differential diagnosis of a tachycardia with a widened QRS complex. *Am. J. Med.* 64:27, 1978.

13

Pacemakers and Automatic Implantable Cardioverter-Defibrillator

Doris McGirt   *Linette Klevan*

PEACEFUL BEING

Throughout this book, we discuss research that demonstrates the intimate connections between body, mind, and spirit. Indeed developments in many areas of science tell us we cannot understand our world without taking into account the connectedness and relatedness of what we once called separate parts. To experience peaceful being is to experience and know this oneness between all human beings, between man and nature, and between man and God. This has been hailed as the eternal task of the mystic: to participate in the oneness of all things. It would seem, then, that we face a paradox in our culture: if we scientifically know so much about this oneness, relatedness, and connectedness, why does "loss of meaning" become such a common complaint? Why are so many people searching for ways to create new perceptions for their life in order to enhance healing, wholeness, and spirituality?

Do you ever feel like your life has lost meaning? If so, answer or begin a process of answering the following questions:

- How do I define spirituality?
- What is my life purpose?
- What gives my life meaning?
- When I use the words *Guiding Force, Higher Power, God,* or *Absolute*, what kind of link with a universal wholeness do I experience?

LEARNING OBJECTIVES

After reading this chapter, the nurse should be able to do the following:

1. Identify the chamber paced, chamber sensed, and mode of response as classified by the NASPE/BPEG pacemaker code.
2. Define the terms *capture, inhibited mode, sensitivity,* and *threshold.*
3. Differentiate the terms *failure to capture, failure to fire,* and *failure to sense.*
4. Explain the appropriate troubleshooting pacemaker interventions to correct failure to capture, failure to fire, and failure to sense.

5. Describe the purpose of the automatic implantable cardioverter-defibrillator.

ADVANCES IN CARDIAC PACING

The technologic advances in cardiac pacing over the past 10 to 15 years have not only enhanced our ability to treat life-threatening dysrhythmias but also have improved the quality of life for all patients with pacemakers. This chapter presents critical pacemaker concepts as they apply to both temporary and permanent pacing. Owing to the potential hazards and emergencies faced in the critical care environment, however, emphasis is placed on temporary cardiac pacing. The automatic implantable cardioverter-defibrillator also is presented in this chapter because many of the concepts, patient experiences, and teaching associated with this modality are similar to those associated with a cardiac pacemaker.

Pacemaker Identification Code

The pacemaker identification code was first developed in 1974 by the Intersociety Commission for Heart Disease (ICHD) Resources and expanded upon in 1983. The basic code consists of three letters that designate, in order, the chamber paced, the chamber sensed, and the mode of response to a sensed event. Two other letters, for the fourth and fifth positions, were proposed to designate the level of programmability and the capability for tachycardia termination. In 1987, the North American Society for Pacing and Electrophysiology (NASPE) and the British Pacing and Electrophysiology Group (BPEG) revised and updated the system to include the fourth and fifth letters.[1] The code serves to identify the basic functions and programmability of a pulse generator (Table 13–1).

The basic description of pacemakers can thus be explained by using the first three letters of the identification code found in Table 13–2. However, with the recent increase in the use of rate-responsive and antitachycardic pacemakers, we will be seeing more use of the fourth and fifth letters.

Pacemaker Terminology

Understanding pacemakers is dependent on knowledge of cardiac anatomy and physiology, pathophysiology, and electricity. The following terms are provided to facilitate your understanding of this section on pacemakers. Some pacing terms are common to both temporary and permanent pacing, and others are more specific to either temporary or permanent pacing. To aid in the interpretation of these terms, the following key will be used: T/P (term used in both temporary and permanent pacing); T (term used in temporary pacing); P (term used in permanent pacing).

Ampere (T/P): Unit of electrical current; the amount of electrical current being delivered to the myocardium. The unit usually is expressed in milliamperes (ma).
Anode (T/P): The positive pole of the pacemaker circuit.

Asynchronous (Fixed-rate) mode (T/P): Pacemaker fires independently of the intrinsic rhythm.
Atrial tracking (P): In DDD pacing, (see Table 13-1) ventricular paced event after a sensed atrial event. DDD pacing permits pacing and sensing of both chambers; and inhibiting and triggering of the pacemaker. The ventricular pacemaker is triggered to respond to a sensed atrial event at the end of the programmed atrioventricular (AV) interval, allows for AV syncrony and, in the presence of normal atrial response to exercise and stress, provides a dynamic rate response.
Atrioventricular interval (T/P): Amount of time in a dual-chamber pacemaker between an atrial event (sensed or paced) and the paced ventricular event; corresponds to our intrinsic PR interval
Capture (T/P): Successful depolarization of the chamber being paced due to electrical stimulation from the pacemaker
Cathode (T/P): The negative pole of the pacing circuit
Current (T/P): Rate of transfer or flow of electricity; measured as amperes
Escape interval (T/P): The time between a consecutive sensed (intrinsic) event and a paced event; usually the same as the pacing interval or rate
Fusion beats (T/P): Depolarization of the atria or ventricles resulting from combined depolarization from intrinsic and paced impulses; has characteristics of both intrinsic and paced beats
Hysteresis (P): Characteristic of some ventricular pacemakers that allows the escape interval to be significantly longer than the pacing interval; permits the intrinsic rhythm to control the heart rate, even when the rate is lower than the programmed pacing rate
Impedance (T/P): Often used interchangeably with the term *resistance*; a more comprehensive description of opposition to current flow
Inhibited mode (P): Represented by an *I* in the third letter of the classification code. Pacemaker responds to the sensed intrinsic activity by being inhibited
Magnet rate (P): Rate of a pulse generator elicited by placing a magnet over the pulse generator
Milliamperes (T): The amount of current being delivered to the myocardium
Ohm's Law (T/P): Voltage = current × resistance

Table 13–1
The NASPE/BPEG Generic (NBG) Pacemaker Code

POSITION	I*	II	III	IV	V
Category	Chamber(s) paced	Chamber(s) sensed	Response to sensing	Programmability, rate modulation	Antitachydysrhythmia function(s)
	0 = None	**0** = None	**0** = None	**0** = None	**0** = None
	A = Atrium	**A** = Atrium	**T** = Triggered	**P** = Simple programmable	**P** = Pacing (antitachydysrhythmia)
	V = Ventricle	**V** = Ventricle	**I** = Inhibited	**M** = Multiprogrammable	**S** = Shock
	D = Dual (A + V)	**D** = Dual (A + V)	**D** = Dual (T + I)	**C** = Communicating	**D** = Dual (P + S)
				R = Rate modulation	
Manufacturers' designation only	**S** = single (A or V)	**S** = single (A or V)			

* Positions I through III are used exclusively for antibradydysrhythmia function.

(Bernstein, A. D., Camm, A. J., Fletcher, R. D., *et al.* The NASPE/BPEG generic pacemaker code for antibradyarrhythmia and adaptive-rate pacing and antitachyarrhythmia devices. *PACE* 10:794–799, 1987; with permission.)

Table 13–2
Descriptions of Pacemakers

CHAMBERS PACED	CHAMBERS SENSED	MODE OF RESPONSE	DESCRIPTION (COMMON NAMES)
V	O	O	Ventricular pacing, no sensing function (fixed rate)
A	O	O	Atrial pacing, no sensing function (fixed rate)
D	O	O	Atrial and ventricular pacing, no sensing function (fixed rate)
V	V	I	Ventricular pacing and sensing, inhibited response to sensing (ventricular demand)
V	V	T	Ventricular pacing and sensing, triggered response to sensing (ventricular demand)
A	A	I	Atrial pacing and sensing, inhibited response to sensing (atrial demand)
A	A	T	Atrial pacing and sensing, triggered response to sensing (atrial demand)
V	A	T	Ventricular pacing, atrial sensing, triggered response to sensing (A-V synchronous)
D	V	I	Atrial and ventricular pacing, ventricular sensing, inhibited response to sensing (AV sequential)
V	D	D	Ventricular pacing, atrial and ventricular sensing, triggered response in the atrium and inhibited in the ventricle (ASVIP)
D	D	D	Atrial and ventricular pacing and sensing, triggered response in the atrium and inhibited in the ventricle (universal)

(Sager, D. The person requiring cardiac pacing. In C. E. Guzzetta and B. M. Dossey, (eds.), *Cardiovascular Nursing: Bodymind Tapestry.* St. Louis: C. V. Mosby, 1984; modified from Parsonnet, V., Furman, S., and Smyth, N. *Circulation* (Suppl.) 50:A21, 1974; with permission.)

Oversensing (T/P): Inappropriate or inaccurate sensing of signals by the cardiac pacemaker

Pacemaker syndrome (T/P): Episodes of weakness and dizziness during a paced ventricular rhythm due to loss of atrial kick or loss of AV synchrony

Pacing interval (P/T): The period of time between two consecutive pacing spikes; also known as the automatic interval; measured in milliseconds

Pacing rate (T/P): The rate at which the pacemaker is programmed to discharge

Pulse amplitude (P/T): The amount of current being delivered to the myocardium; measured in milliamperes

Pulse width or pulse duration (P/T): The width of the pacemaker spike in time; the amount of time programmed for the pacemaker to deliver the electrical energy (not a programmable feature of most temporary pacemakers)

Resistance (T/P): Opposition to the flow of electric current through a material due to its physical characteristics; expressed in Ohms

Sensitivity (T/P): Refers to the pacemaker's ability to sense intrinsic cardiac activity

Synchronous (demand) mode (T): Pacemaker senses intrinsic rhythm and fires with it as needed to prevent heart rate from falling below pacing rate; another term for triggered

Threshold (T/P): Minimum amount of electrical energy required to produce consistent cardiac depolarization

Triggered mode (P): Represented by a *T* in the third letter of the classification code. Pacemaker responds to sensed intrinsic activity by firing an impulse simultaneously with the sensed beat

Undersensing (T/P): Ineffective sensing of signals by the cardiac pacemaker

Voltage (T/P): Difference in potential energy between two points; causes current to flow from negative to positive in a circuit

Temporary Cardiac Pacing in Emergency Cardiac Care

Temporary cardiac pacing can be an important mode of therapy in a cardiac emergency. The indications for its use in an emergency are related to the development of life-threatening dysrhythmias. Drug therapy used to treat these acute problems, particularly complete AV block, is less reliable and successful than is artificial cardiac pacing. Cardiac pacing involves delivering an artificial stimulus to the heart to cause electrical depolarization and myocardial contraction.

Indications

The primary indications for temporary cardiac pacing are AV block, certain AV conduction deficits, and symptomatic bradydysrhythmias or tachydysrhythmias.[4] These rhythm disturbances may precede, follow, or occur during a cardiac arrest. As a result, temporary pacemakers are used prophylactically as well as therapeutically.

The most common indication for insertion of a temporary pacemaker is complete AV block. Heart block results from congenital defects, or it can be surgically induced as a result of edema or inflammation around the AV node or bundle of His. It may also be caused by aortic or mitral valvular disease, and it can be linked to myocardial ischemia. Drugs such as digitalis, potassium, quinidine, and procainamide are known to produce AV block. Infections such as scarlet fever, influenza, measles, pneumonia, and tuberculosis also have been found to be causative factors. In the majority of cases, complete AV block is due to sclerodegenerative disease that causes fibrosis of the peripheral bundle branches and their divisions.

Bilateral bundle branch block is commonly observed to occur before the development of complete heart block. A common bilateral bundle branch block is right bundle branch block, in association with left anterior hemiblock. This bifascicular block maintains intraventricular conduction by means of the remaining left posterior fascicle of the left bundle. The posterior fascicle, however, can become blocked intermittently, producing a Mobitz type 2 second-degree AV block or spontaneous complete AV block (other types of bilateral bundle branch block are described in Chap. 12). Depending on the situation, temporary cardiac pacing may be needed in the management of any of these conduction disturbances.

Bradydysrhythmias, which frequently are severe enough to produce a drastic reduction in cardiac output secondary to depressed cardiac rates, may require cardiac pacing. Reduced cardiac output can result in dizziness, syncope, ventricular irritability, and cerebral or tissue hypoxia. The bradydysrhythmias associated with sick sinus syndrome (Chap. 12) frequently produce rates below 60 beats/minute. These dysrhythmias respond poorly to treatment with atropine or isoproterenol. In some cases of sinus arrest, sinus exit block, or sinus bradycardia, the dysrhythmia is transient and can be demonstrated only intermittently by continuous cardiac monitoring. Sinus bradycardias are commonly seen in patients with acute myocardial infarction, particularly an infarction involving the inferior or posterior wall.

Temporary cardiac pacing is occasionally indicated to overdrive, or suppress, atrial or ventricular tachydysrhythmias. Overdrive pacing is used to stimulate the myocardium at a rate above the patient's own intrinsic cardiac rhythm and thus suppress impulse formation.[2] *Atrial overdrive pacing* may be used to convert atrial flutter, supraventricular tachycardia, and tachycardias associated with Wolff-Parkinson-White syndrome to normal sinus rhythm.

Ventricular overdrive pacing may be useful in treating patients with refractory ventricular dysrhythmias. It is used, for example, to suppress an irritable ventricular focus, such as one that produces ventricular tachycardia or frequent premature ventricular contractions (PVCs). The overdrive pacing rate, however, does not need to be faster than the ectopic rate, and it may need to be only slightly faster than the normal sinus pacemaker.

Methods

Temporary cardiac pacing is accomplished by one of four methods: external pacing, transthoracic pacing, epicardial pacing, or transvenous endocardial pacing.

External Pacing.   External cardiac pacing was developed to manage temporary and permanent heart blocks that arose as complications of open heart surgery. It is accomplished by placing skin electrodes on the patient's precordium and administering repeated shocks.

New technology has allowed this method to become the most frequently used form of pacing in emergencies. Anterior and posterior electrode patches are placed, and rate, sensing, and output are established.

Transthoracic Cardiac Pacing.   Transthoracic cardiac pacing is a rapid procedure that is generally used only in emergencies. A large-bore needle is inserted in the fourth to fifth intercostal space at the left sternal border to provide an entry into the right ventricle. A pacing wire is inserted through the needle and embedded in the ventricle. The needle is removed, and

the pacing wire is connected to a pulse generator (a temporary pacemaker). The procedure may be associated with severe complications, such as cardiac tamponade, coronary artery laceration, and pneumothorax.

Epicardial Pacing.   Cardiovascular surgeons insert temporary epicardial pacing wires during open and closed heart surgery prophylactically to treat dysrhythmias or conduction disturbances. Wires are sewn loosely to the epicardium of the atrium and ventricle. If postoperative dysrhythmias occur, the epicardial wires are connected to the pacemaker and the patient is paced as indicated. The wires are easily removed by pulling them through the skin.

Transvenous Endocardial Pacing.   Transvenous endocardial pacing is the method of cardiac pacing used most commonly.[3] The pacing wire is passed into the brachial, femoral, subclavian, or jugular vein by a percutaneous stick or by cutdown. The catheter wire is advanced through the vein, into the right atrium, and generally on through the tricuspid valve and embedded in the trabeculae of the right ventricle.

The transvenous endocardial pacing electrode is inserted with the guidance of fluoroscopic or electrocardiographic (ECG) monitoring. Fluoroscopy is not recommended in the emergency situation because it usually involves moving the patient from the critical care area to a radiology department or cardiac catheterization laboratory.[6] If portable fluoroscopy is not available, electrode placement under ECG control (blind pacemaker insertion) is a relatively rapid procedure that can be carried out at the patient's bedside.

The first step in the blind insertion of a pacemaker involves attaching the patient to the limb leads of the ECG. An intravenous line must be in place, and a defibrillator and emergency cardiac drugs should be at the patient's bedside. A balloon-tipped catheter is inserted aseptically into the patient's vein (the balloon on the catheter must be checked before it is inserted). When the balloon is inflated, it causes the catheter to float with the venous blood into the right ventricle. After the catheter is inserted into the vein, the external end of the catheter is attached to lead V on the ECG with a wire that has two insulated alligator clamps. One clamp is attached to lead V. The other clamp is attached to the electrode on the external catheter that corresponds to the tip electrode (the distal end of the catheter inside the heart); it serves as the exploring electrode within the heart. The lead V selector switch on the ECG is turned on to provide an intracardiac ECG.

As the tip electrode approaches the right atrium, large negative P waves and small QRS complexes are recorded on the ECG. At this point, the balloon on the catheter is inflated to the recommended volume (usually 1.5 cc). As the tip electrode approaches the low right atrium, the P waves become positive and smaller than the QRS complexes. The catheter is passed through the tricuspid valve and the balloon is deflated. When the catheter is in the right ventricle, a large rS deflection is observed on the ECG, with ST-segment elevation as the tip electrode touches the endocardium, indicating good endocardial placement of the catheter. The patient is disconnected from lead V, and the external catheter is connected to the pacemaker.

After the pacemaker settings have been chosen (see Pacemaker Settings), the catheter is sutured in place and the insertion site is covered with an antibiotic ointment and a sterile dressing. A posteroanterior chest radiograph is taken to check for the presence of pneumothorax or other possible complications of the catheter insertion. A lateral chest radiograph is also taken to check the positioning of the catheter. If the catheter tip is in the right ventricular apex, it points anteriorly on the lateral chest radiograph, but if the catheter is in the coronary sinus or has perforated the right ventricle, it points posteriorly and it must be repositioned.

Right ventricular pacing is also assessed electrocardiographically by observing a wide QRS complex and left-axis deviation with deep S waves in leads 2, 3, and aV$_F$ and a left bundle branch block pattern in the right precordial leads. Although ventricular pacing is used most commonly, atrial or AV pacing may be indicated occasionally.

Classification of Temporary Pacemakers

The temporary pulse generators available currently are limited in their programmability. The *single-chamber pulse generators* have four programmable functions: rate, output (milliamperes), sensitivity, and mode (VVI, VVO). The rate establishes the rate or frequency of discharge of the pacemaker, the output, or milliamperes, sets the amount of current to be delivered to the myocardium, and the sensitivity programs the pacemaker to the synchronous (*i.e.*, inhibited demand) or asynchronous mode. Thus, a pacemaker connected to a ventricular lead and programmed at a rate of 72, 1.5 ma, and in the synchronous mode will discharge 1.5 ma of current at a rate of 72 if the patient's heart rate drops below 72. The result is a temporary pacemaker functioning in the VVI mode (pace-ventricle; sense-ventricle; inhibited when intrinsic ventricular activity sensed) (Fig. 13–1). The pacemaker spikes preceding the wide, bizarre QRSs complexes represent discharge of electrical current by the pulse generator.

The opposite of this VVI mode would be a temporary pacemaker programmed to the asynchronous or VOO mode (Fig. 13–2). Using the same pacing rate and milliamperes, this pacemaker would deliver 1.5 ma of current to the myocardium at a rate of 72 without sensing the heart's natural rhythm. This VOO pacing could result in a competitive rhythm if the patient's heart rate is the same or higher than the pacing rate (Fig. 13–3).

The problems associated with a competitive rhythm are related to the vulnerable period that occurs during the T wave,

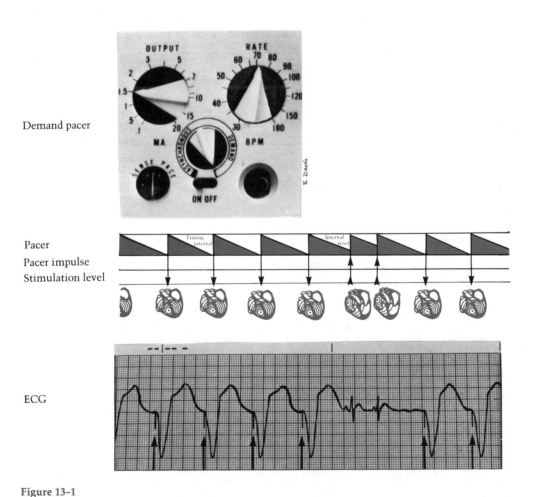

Demand pacer

Pacer
Pacer impulse
Stimulation level

ECG

Figure 13–1

A demand pacemaker. The rate is 72 beats/minute; the output is 1.5 ma. The first four beats illustrate the release of pacemaker impulses at 72 beats/minute. The fifth and sixth beats reveal the temporary return of inherent cardiac functioning. The timing interval is reset on the demand pacemaker when it senses the return of the inherent rhythm; thus, the pacemaker impulse (output) is inhibited. The seventh and eighth beats occur when the heart rate falls below the preselected interval (72 beats/minute) and the pacemaker impulse is released to stimulate the ventricle.

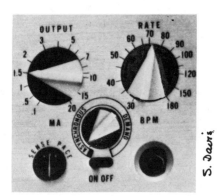

A　Fixed-rate pacer

B　Pacer
　　Pacer impulse

C　Stimulation level

D

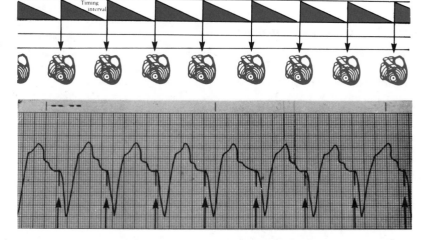

E　ECG

Figure 13–2

(*A*) Fixed-rate pacemaker: The rate is 72 beats/minute; the output is 1.5 ma. (*B*) The pacemaker has a circuit that measures off the timing interval to release 72 impulses/minute. (*C, D*) The pacemaker impulse is released at a high enough stimulation (capture) level (*C*) that the ventricle is depolarized (*D*). (*E*) The pacemaker impulse is represented on the electrocardiogram (ECG) as a spike (artifact) followed by ventricular capture (a wide QRS complex).

the period when the myocardium is partially but not completely recovered. If the pacemaker spike strikes during this period, ventricular fibrillation may develop (see section on pacemaker malfunctions). Fortunately, there is a wide safety margin between the amount of energy needed to produce ventricular fibrillation. The presence of myocardial ischemia, anoxia, infarction, electrolyte disturbances, or metabolic disturbances can reduce the ventricular fibrillatory threshold, extend the vulnerable period, and narrow the margin of safety. As a result, less energy is needed to produce ventricular fibrillation. Because of these problems, fixed-rate pacemakers have limited clinical use.

Dual-chamber temporary pacemakers have five programmable features: pacing rate, atrial output (milliamperes), ventricular output (milliamperes), sensitivity, and AV interval/delay. These programmable functions, in addition to establishing rate and sensitivity, permit different amounts of current to be delivered to the atria and ventricles and set the AV interval. (As defined in the section on pacemaker terminology, the *AV interval* is the amount of time after intrinsic or paced P wave and the following paced QRS complexes).

Power Supply

Most artificial temporary cardiac pacemaker batteries have a life span of 2 to 4 months (keeping the batteries in a cool

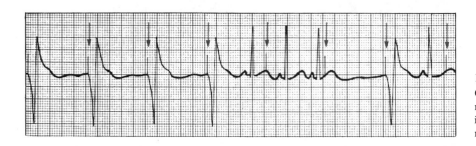

Figure 13–3

Competitive rhythm. The cardiac pacemaker does not sense inherent activity, owing to fixed rate/asynchronous programming, releases pacemaker impulses (*arrows*).

place, such as a refrigerator, helps them stay charged). Each time a temporary pacemaker is inserted, new batteries should be installed and tested for proper functioning. The time and date that the battery was inserted should be written on a piece of adhesive tape attached to the back of the pacemaker. The nurse should routinely check the pulse generator's battery-life indicator every 8 hours. The batteries should be replaced at the first sign of failure. It is advisable, however, to change them prophylactically every 2 or 3 days when the pacemaker is in continuous use (see section on electrical hazards).

Types of Pacing Leads

Artificial pacing is accomplished by means of a unipolar or a bipolar pacing lead. The impulse generated from the pacemaker must flow between two poles or electrodes to create an electric circuit.

Unipolar Electrode.   In the unipolar electrode, one wire is in the catheter that is positioned in the heart. It is known as the *intracardiac electrode,* and it senses and stimulates electrical heart activity. It is connected to the negative terminal on the pacemaker. The other electrode needed to complete the circuit is known as the *indifferent,* or *ground electrode.* It consists of an electrode skin plate placed on the extremity nearest the lead insertion. To ensure good contact with the skin, conductive paste is placed under the plate, which is then secured with tape. A wire with two alligator clamps is then attached to the electrode plate, and the other end is attached to the positive terminal on the pacemaker. The advantage of the unipolar electrode is that it needs a lower threshold of stimulation. The ground electrode must be used with caution; it should be insulated and protected from electrical interference.

Bipolar Electrode.   The bipolar electrode contains both the sensing (or stimulating) electrode and the ground electrode. It is useful because it provides better contact with endocardial tissue. The electrode at the far end of the lead is the *distal electrode* and is in direct contact with the endocardium. Above the distal electrode is a *proximal* (or ring or *indifferent*) *electrode.*

When the distal electrode is connected to the negative terminal on the pulse generator and the proximal electrode is connected to the positive terminal, current will flow. Such current will flow from the negative electrode to the endocardium and then back to the positive electrode. Ventricular, atrial, and AV sequential bipolar endocardial leads are available for temporary cardiac pacing.

If one of the bipolar wires malfunctions, it can be converted to a unipolar electrode by the addition of a skin electrode. To convert a bipolar electrode to a unipolar electrode, one electrode, usually the distal electrode, if intact, is connected to the negative terminal, the proximal electrode is disconnected, and the positive pole is grounded to the patient's subcutaneous tissue, as described for the unipolar electrode. Converting the electrode from a bipolar to a unipolar mode is particularly helpful when a pacemaker fails to sense the patient's intrinsic QRS complex because the complex is generating an inadequate intracardiac voltage. Unipolar electrodes act like antennas because of the large interelectrode distance, and they can therefore pick up a greater voltage for a given QRS signal as compared with the bipolar electrode.

Pacemaker Settings

Before artificial pacing is begun, one must consider the pacemaker settings. Selecting the appropriate *pacemaker rate* depends on the patient's need for pacing. The lowest rate that controls the dysrhythmia and produces a maximum cardiac output at rest is chosen. Rates above those that are hemodynamically necessary can cause a rise in myocardial oxygen consumption and, perhaps, a decline in cardiac output.

The stimulation threshold is the minimum amount of energy necessary to stimulate the heart.[6] The *energy output* control, calibrated in milliamperes, is raised slowly until a QRS complex is seen to occur after every pacemaker artifact. This point is called the *stimulation threshold.* It is the amount of current needed to produce a 1:1 *capture* (one QRS complex for every pacemaker artifact (Fig. 13–4). The capture level helps to indicate whether the electrode is positioned properly in the endocardium. If less than 1.5 ma is needed to capture the heart,

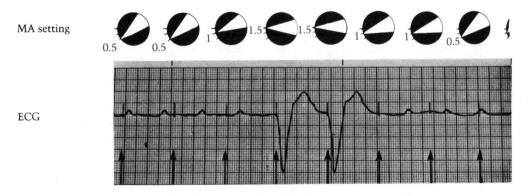

Figure 13–4

Threshold (capture) level. The first and second pacemaker impulses are released at an energy output of 0.5 ma, and the third impulse is released at 1 ma. The energy output is insufficient to stimulate (capture) the ventricle. The electrocardiogram (ECG) reveals a pacer artifact (*arrows*) followed by no QRS complex. The fourth and fifth impulses are released at an energy output of 1.5 ma. That level of energy is sufficient to stimulate the ventricle, and it is known as the threshold (capture) level. The ECG shows a pacer artifact followed by a QRS complex. The output on the pacer is again turned down to 1 and 0.5 ma in the sixth, seventh, and eighth impulses. Once again, the ventricle is no longer stimulated, and the ECG reveals loss of capture.

the electrode is in good position. The threshold level rarely stays constant after insertion; it often changes in time. Factors that increase the threshold include eating, sleeping, anesthetics, mineralocorticoids, and fibrosis around the tip of the catheter. When one or more of these factors are present, the heart demands a greater amount of energy (a higher milliamperes) for stimulation. The threshold is lowered by such factors as exercise, a low blood sugar level, glucocorticoids, and sympathomimetics, resulting in the need for less current—or a lower milliamperes—to capture. Because the threshold level is unpredictable and resistance generally rises several days after the catheter has been inserted, the energy output (maintenance level) is set two or three times above the stimulation threshold needed for capture to ensure consistent pacing. The energy output should not be set too high, however, because the fibrillation threshold ranges from 10 to 30 times that of the capture level.

The *sensitivity control* of pacemakers frequently is numbered from 1 mV to 20 mV. Such numbers represent the amplitude or the millivolt size of an R or P wave that is sensed by the pacemaker. The lower number represents the most sensitive setting for the pacemaker, whereas the higher number represents the least sensitive setting. After 20 mV, the pacemaker may read "asynchronous," indicating that the pacer will function at a fixed rate without sensing.

Securing the Pacemaker

To prevent catheter dislodgement, most pacemaker electrodes are sutured to the skin. If the catheter is placed in the arm, to prevent displacement of the wire, the arm should be rendered immobile using armboards, Kling or Ace bandages, and pillows. The reasons for limiting the movement of the arm are explained to the patient. Analgesics can help to relieve the pain and stiffness associated with immobility. After removal of the pacemaker, range-of-motion exercises are begun.

Securing the pacemaker unit to the patient avoids accidental breakage and permits the patient to turn in bed. Pacemaker or colostomy belts or Kling or Ace bandages are wrapped around the patient's arm or leg and are tied to the pacemaker.

Care of the Insertion Site

The area around the insertion site is checked daily for signs and symptoms of infection or inflammation. The dressing is changed daily. The nurse, using sterile gloves, cleanses the area with iodine and applies antibiotic or bacteriostatic ointment and a sterile dressing. The date and time of the dressing change are recorded on the dressing. This information and information about the general appearance of the insertion site are recorded in the nursing notes. Extreme caution is used to prevent catheter dislodgment during the dressing change, especially if the catheter is placed in the arm.

Patient Teaching

When inserting a temporary pacemaker in an emergency, generally there is not enough time to teach the patient completely about the procedure. Although explanations may need to be brief, one must not forget to reassure the patient. In the elective and stable situation, patients are told why they need the pacemaker and are taught how it works. A picture can be used to explain the location of the catheter in the heart. Patients should know that the procedure will take about an hour and that they will be awake. They should understand that they will be connected to a continuous cardiac monitor, have an intravenous line in place, and have their face covered if the site of insertion is the subclavian or the jugular vein. The discomforts associated with the procedure, such as stiffness and pain at the insertion site, should be discussed. Patients should be assured that they will receive analgesics and a local anesthetic to relieve any discomfort associated with the procedure. If possible, the nurse should explain briefly what the patient can expect with regard to care and management in the postoperative period.

Troubleshooting Temporary Pacemakers

Nurses must thoroughly understand the principles of cardiac pacing, and the equipment, leads, and pulse generators used in their institution. They must know why a pacemaker was inserted in their patient, and they should know their responsibilities. The rate, energy output, and sensitivity controls; mode of pacing; and time, date, and site of insertion should be written in the patient's care plan. The settings may change frequently, and the records must be updated as needed.

When a problem arises with a temporary pacemaker, the nurse must first assess the patient's color, pulse, blood pressure, and respiration. Signs and symptoms of confusion, restlessness, or unresponsiveness are evaluated. Also, the nurse should observe the patient for rhythmic hiccoughing or diaphragmatic twitching, which indicates that the electrode has perforated the right ventricle.

Troubleshooting must be systematic. After a rapid assessment of the patient, determine whether the pacemaker is turned on. Most temporary pacemakers have a sense/pace dial. If the pacemaker is turned on and the batteries are working, the needle on the dial indicates whether the pacemaker is sensing or pacing the cardiac rhythm. The battery-life indicator, rate of pacing, mode of pacing, and the energy output and sensitivity control levels are checked for proper settings. Most pacemaker units have a plastic cover to prevent the patient or hospital personnel from inadvertently changing the settings. Nevertheless, the settings should be checked. The connection between the pacemaker generator and leads is checked. Finally, the insertion site is checked to be sure that the pacing wire has not been pulled out accidentally.

If pacing problems occur, repositioning the patient to the left lateral recumbent position is sometimes helpful in restoring contact with the endocardium if a transvenous lead has been displaced. Atropine or isoproterenol often is given in an attempt to accelerate the cardiac rhythm until pacing is restored. Basic and advanced cardiac life support should be initiated as appropriate.

Pacemaker Malfunctions

A pacemaker malfunction is generally one of three types: failure to fire, failure to capture, or failure to sense.

Figure 13–5A illustrates a *failure to fire* because the pacemaker artifact is absent. The pacemaker output is not entering the electrode to stimulate the heart. The problem may be a result of pulse generator malfunction, broken or loose connections, battery exhaustion, circuitry failure, or inhibition of

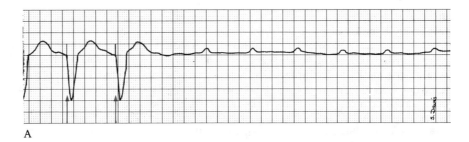

A

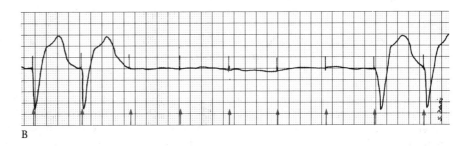

B

Figure 13-5

(*A*) Failure to fire. No pacer artifact is observed on the electrocardiogram (ECG) after the second beat. (*B*) Failure to capture. The pacer artifact is present but is not capturing the ventricle. The ECG reveals several pacer artifacts followed by no QRS complex. (*C*) A runaway pacemaker. The pacemaker impulses are firing faster than the preset rate. Fortunately, each artifact is not followed by ventricular capture. The *large arrow* indicates a pacer artifact hitting the T wave.

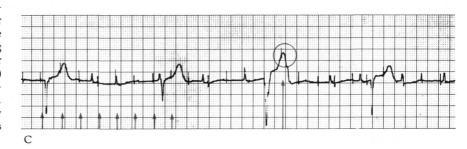

C

the pacemaker stimulus. Correction of the problem involves assessing the patient, checking the on-off switch, the output setting and other pacemaker settings, checking the connection between the pacemaker terminals and electrode, increasing the milliamperes to the highest level, and changing the batteries or the pacemaker unit.

Inhibition of the pacemaker output can be caused by electromagnetic interference and oversensing. Oversensing can produce pauses in the output and can be remedied easily by lowering the sensitivity setting until normal sensing is seen. Sources of electrical interference, which can cause pacemaker inhibition and produce failure to fire, also should be identified and removed (see the section on electrical interference).

Figure 13-5B illustrates *failure to capture;* the pacemaker artifact is not followed by a QRS complex. This problem may be a result of catheter dislodgment, electrode perforation of the ventricle, electrode fracture, or an increase in the threshold needed for capture. Occasionally, the amplitude of the pacemaker artifact is large enough to be interpreted by the cardiac monitor as a QRS complex. Because the cardiac monitor "sees" the pacemaker spike as a stimulated ventricular complex, the rate meter will continue to function normally and fail to trigger the cardiac monitor alarm system, unless an ECG lead has been used to monitor the QRS alone. In this potentially lethal situation, the pacemaker spikes will continue to trigger the cardiac monitor even though the patient has a serious brady-

cardia or is in standstill. When failure to capture is discovered, a quick assessment of the patient and the pacing system is performed. While supporting the patient with cardiopulmonary resuscitation (CPR) if necessary, quickly increase the energy output and check and tighten all connections. The patient can be repositioned onto the left side or to a sitting position while leaning forward if hypotension is not present. These maneuvers are helpful if the electrode catheter is displaced minimally.

If a *lead fracture* is suspected, the pacing catheter can be evaluated by connecting first one and then the other electrode terminal of the catheter to lead V on the ECG. The wires in the catheter are intact if the ECG can be recorded through both electrodes. If a wire is fractured, a straight line is recorded on the ECG; a partial break will reveal small QRS complexes. If a fracture is found but only one wire within the lead is broken, the electrodes can be reversed on the pacemaker terminal or the system can be converted to a unipolar lead to bypass the break by connecting the remaining intact lead to the negative terminal on the pacemaker.

Another serious but less frequently encountered malfunction is the runaway pacemaker. In this situation, the pacemaker rate control is not operating correctly, allowing the repeated firing of pacemaker output beyond the pacemaker's upper rate limit (see Fig. 13-5C). Each of the pacemaker artifacts may capture the myocardium, resulting in a life-threatening rapid heart rate. When this occurs, the pacemaker must be disconnected immediately and changed. To prevent reuse of this defective unit, it must be labeled and sent for repair.

Problems associated with *failure to sense* are evidenced electrocardiographically by an intrinsic QRS complex that is preceded or followed by an inappropriately timed pacemaker artifact. This malfunction is also known as *competitive rhythm* (see Fig. 13–3). Figure 13–6 shows a pacemaker artifact falling within the vulnerable period of the ventricle on the T wave in a patient with an ischemic myocardium. Ventricular fibrillation results. In this case, the pacemaker is turned off and basic cardiac life support initiated until defibrillation can be performed (see the section on cardiac arrest and cardiac pacing).

The first action to take when failure to sense is identified is to check the sensitivity setting and increase it until capture is seen. If the mode setting has been set on VOO, change it to VVI. Next, because the electrode may be malpositioned, repositioning the patient may be useful. Other methods of intervention might be turning the pacemaker off, changing the batteries or the pacemaker unit, converting the bipolar electrode to a unipolar one, or increasing the pacing rate to override the intrinsic rate. The pacemaker will not sense an intrinsic cardiac impulse if the complex is small and less than the sensitivity setting on the pacemaker. If the sensitivity control is set at 4 mV, for example, and the intrinsic beat is 3 mV, the pacemaker will not sense until the sensitivity setting is adjusted to 3 mV or less. Thus, some sensing problems can be corrected by increasing the sensitivity (decreasing the millivolt control).

Electrical Hazards

The person who does not have an artificial pacemaker is generally protected by the high resistance of the skin and other body tissue against small amounts of electric current arising from improperly grounded, line-powered equipment. Electric current seeks the path of least resistance (see Chap. 15). An electrode that is placed directly in the heart bypasses the protective resistance of the skin and provides a low-resistance pathway to electric current. Ventricular fibrillation can be produced by low-voltage current if the current is applied directly to the heart.

The use of two-pronged plug equipment, extensions, adapters, or cheater cords near the patient with an artificial pacemaker is strictly forbidden because such devices are potential sources of "hot" or stray current. Hot current seeks a ground by using the path of least resistance (the patient). Most patients who have temporary artificial pacemakers are also connected to a well-grounded cardiac monitor. If an ungrounded piece of equipment (one with a two-pronged plug), such as line-powered radio, is placed at a patient's bedside, it

is a potential source of hot current. Should the patient touch the radio, stray current may pass through the patient's body to seek the ground of the cardiac monitor. Because of the low resistance provided by the electrode that is placed directly into the patient's heart, the stray current may cause ventricular fibrillation. This danger also can arise if the nurse (or anyone else) touches the radio and the patient simultaneously, causing the current to pass through his or her and into the patient. Nurses must be careful to avoid contact with the patient while they are operating such electrical equipment. The problem is avoided by ensuring that all electrical equipment is grounded properly and checked periodically (see Chap. 15).

The exterior end of the pacer catheter must be insulated carefully to prevent contact with stray current. Most of the newer models have well-insulated pacemaker terminals. Many of the older pacemakers, however, have exposed electrode tips sticking through the terminal poles of the unit. If the tips are exposed, they must be insulated by placing the temporary pacemaker and electrode connections in a dry surgical rubber glove so that they do not come in contact with liquids or other conductive substances. When handling the electrode terminals, the nurse should wear rubber gloves. If alligator clamps are used, the connections between the electrode terminals and the clamps must be insulated.

Batteries should not be replaced while the pacemaker is in use on the patient. Contact with the battery terminals may be as dangerous to the patient as contact with the electrode terminals. The catheter should be disconnected from the pacemaker (contact with the electrode terminals should be avoided) and the battery replaced. If the patient cannot be disconnected from the pacemaker, rubber gloves should be worn to change the batteries; extreme caution should be used to avoid touching the pacemaker battery terminals. Also, prophylactic pacing wires, which are placed in a patient after open heart surgery, should be insulated with a dry rubber glove. Patients with temporary pacemakers should not use electric razors, electrical bed controls, or other electrical equipment. A sign should be placed over the patient's bed that reads, "Temporary Pacemaker—Electrical Safety Precautions."

Environmental Interference

Demand pacemakers are able to respond to environmental electrical signals, causing the inhibition of their demand function. Many newer pacemakers have developed better shielding and filtering devices, but the danger of external interference still exists. Environmental interference may suppress demand pacemaker functioning, leaving the patient unprotected. Pacemakers may be disrupted by radar, diathermy, or electrocautery equipment. Because patients with temporary pacemakers are generally restricted to the critical care area, such

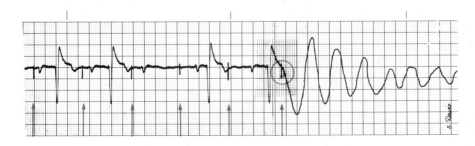

Figure 13–6

Failure to sense. Competitive rhythm with a pacemaker artifact hitting on the T wave to produce ventricular fibrillation.

disruptions are rare. They occur more frequently in the patient with a permanent pacemaker. Should a problem arise, however, the treatment is to move the patient away from the environmental interference or to remove the source. The demand pacemaker will then resume normal functioning. Anytime pacemaker inhibition is suspected, such as when electrocautery equipment must be used, the pulse generator can be set in the asynchronous (fixed-rate) mode to avoid sensing electrical interference.

Complications of Temporary Pacemakers

The problems of failure to sense, failure to fire, failure to capture, local infection at the lead insertion site, catheter dislodgment, electrode fracture, electrical hazards, battery failure, and myocardial perforation have been discussed. The nurse must also assess the patient for signs and symptoms of other complications of cardiac pacing. They include pneumothorax, hemothorax, dysrhythmias, infection, bleeding from the insertion site, pulmonary embolism, venous thrombosis, and potential hazards of immobility related to restricted activities.

Cardiac Arrest and Cardiac Pacing

If the patient has a cardiac arrest after the insertion of a temporary pacemaker, CPR must be initiated. Also, the pacemaker unit should be checked to be sure that it is turned on. The energy output level should be raised to 20 ma, if necessary, to obtain capture. The rate should be set above 60. The functioning of the pacemaker is assessed by observing the ECG and the sense/pace dial while palpating the carotid pulse simultaneously. A new pacemaker may be needed. If the patient is in ventricular fibrillation, the pacemaker is turned off and disconnected from the patient before defibrillation is attempted, to prevent pacemaker damage and to be sure that the electric current is not diverted from the cardiac pathway. After defibrillation, the rhythm is checked again and, if necessary, the pacemaker is reconnected and turned on.

Permanent Pacemakers

Some patients suffer from continuous or intermittent rhythm disturbances. These patients are observed to determine whether they need permanent pacemakers. Permanent pacemakers are indicated for patients with complete, intermittent, or incomplete AV block with Stokes-Adams syncope or congestive failure, sinus bradycardia, sinus arrest or symptomatic sinoatrial block, permanent postoperative surgical heart block, or uncontrollable tachydysrhythmias.

Permanent pacemakers usually are inserted while the patient is under local anesthesia. An incision is made over the right or left external jugular or subclavian vein. The pacing catheter is passed into the heart. A subcutaneous pocket is made in the upper chest to implant the pacemaker. A tunnel is formed under the skin between the two incisions. The distal end of the pacing catheter is pulled under the skin from the insertion site to the subcutaneous incision. The catheter is attached to the pacemaker and is placed in the subcutaneous pocket and sutured.

Attachment of pacing wires to the epicardial surface of the myocardium is the second method of inserting a permanent pacemaker. The pacing wires are sutured or screwed into the myocardium and then tunneled to the pacemaker generator pocket in a similar method to transvenous insertion. This more invasive technique is used less often than the transvenous method, but it is indicated in infants and children with small vessels and adults who are simultaneously undergoing cardiac surgery.

The general principles for the preoperative preparation of the temporary pacemaker patient apply also to the permanent pacemaker patient. Postoperatively, the nurse must assess pacemaker functioning by checking the patient's apical and radial pulses, blood pressure, and cardiac rhythm. The nurse must help patients to become independent with regard to their care and to realize their ability to return home to an active and productive life. After postoperative instruction, patients should be able to demonstrate to the nurse how to take their pulse; identify the activities that should be restricted; discuss the environmental and electrical hazards and how to prevent them and what to do if they occur; describe their diet, medications, and the signs and symptoms of incisional infection; and explain signs and symptoms of pacemaker malfunction and what to do if they occur.

Hospital nurses are generally less familiar with permanent pacemakers than temporary generators. Permanent pacemakers require special programmers to reset the rate, milliamperes, and so forth, and rarely are these adjustments made during hospitalization. However, hospital nurses must be familiar with particular aspects of permanent pacemakers.

In order to interpret permanent pacemaker ECG rhythm strips, nurses need to know how the pacemaker mode is programmed (i.e., VVI, VVT, DDD, and so on), pacing rate(s), and whether hysteris is on or off (VVI only). This information is available in the progress or procedure notes of patients with new implants, and it should be noted in the history and physical examination of those with older implants. If the patient's current or old hospital records do not contain this information, ask the attending physician and document the information on the cardiac monitor or care plan. In the event that the attending physician does not have this information, call the physician who follows this patient for pacemaker checks to obtain the most recent programed data. Remember, a pacemaker ECG rhythm strip is difficult to interpret as normal or abnormal if the programmed data are not known.

AUTOMATIC IMPLANTABLE CARDIOVERTER-DEFIBRILLATOR

At least half of the deaths from coronary artery disease occur suddenly, with little or no warning. Many times there is no accompanying myocardial infarction. In the majority of patients with sudden cardiac deaths, ventricular fibrillation is presumed to be the primary mechanism. Despite the use of prophylactic antidysrhythmic drugs and public awareness of CPR, health care providers recognize their inability to prevent lethal ventricular dysrhythmias and, consequently, recurrent episodes place the individual at high risk for sudden cardiac death. This has prompted the exploration and development of several new medications, procedures, and devices.

One of these innovations is the automatic implantable cardioverter-defibrillator. The development and implementation of the automatic implantable cardioverter-defibrillator (AID), more recently referred to as AICD, has been pioneered by Dr. Michael Mirowski. On recognition of ventricular tachycardia or fibrillation, the device delivers an internal electrical discharge to terminate the dysrhythmia. With a 98.8% survival at 1 year,[7] the AICD has been called the "gold standard"[5] of device therapy designed to reduce mortality from sudden cardiac death.

Description

The AICD is composed of a pulse generator and lead system. The pulse generator is similar in size to earlier pacemaker models, weighing approximately 10 ounces. It consists of sensing circuitry, lithium batteries, and energy storage capacitors. Today's devices have the potential of delivering over 300 impulses or a monitoring life of 5 to 6 years. The system also includes two epicardial leads for sensing rate and rhythm and synchronizing the discharge to the QRS complex, and two epicardial patch leads placed over the left and right ventricles for monitoring QRS durations and delivering the discharge.

The AICD continuously analyzes the patient's rhythm. It can sense dysrhythmias and deliver converting shocks. Once a preprogrammed rate cutoff limit is met, the unit can charge and deliver between 0.1 joules to 30 joules for the first shock energy. If the dysrhythmia persists, the second shock will occur within seconds and deliver a 12-joule to 30-joule shock. The third, fourth, and fifth shock energies are 30 joules if the dysrhythmia persists. If after the fifth shock the dysrhythmia does not terminate, no more shocks will be delivered. The storage and retrieval of shock information is now available with a programmer, similar to that of a pacemaker. By interrogating the AICD with the hand-held programmer, the operator has a clear picture of how many shocks and what type of shocks have been delivered to the patient.

Patients may or may not experience symptoms in association with their dysrhythmia. Awareness and recall of the episodes depend on the level of consciousness at the time the unit fires. Those who are aware describe the shock as being unpleasant but less noxious than external cardioversion-defibrillation. Some equate it to a "blow to the chest." The newer devices have the ability to deliver lower energy for the first shock. At 0.1 joules, most patients may not feel the shock. Some patients equate this to a "hiccough."

Indications

Patients who are survivors of sudden cardiac death that is not associated with an acute myocardial infarction are candidates for placement of an AICD. They may or may not have their dysrhythmia reproduced in the cardiac electrophysiology laboratory. Also, patients who have had sustained ventricular tachycardia who have failed serial electrophysiologic testing or had a recurrence on antiarrhythmic medications are also candidates.

Procedure

The AICD is inserted under general anesthesia. The approach used most widely today is through median sternotomy or lateral thoracotomy. The epicardial patch leads, which are the defibrillating electrodes, are sutured directly to the ventricular wall. Two unipolar leads are also attached to the epicardium and serve as the rate-sensing leads.

To create a pocket for the pulse generator, a subcutaneous incision is made in the abdomen. The leads are then tunneled under the skin and connected to the generator. The operation of the device is tested before closure.

The unit remains operational unless it has been deactivated using the hand-held programmer. Patients with a deactivated AICD need continuous cardiac monitoring.

Postoperative Care

Postoperative nursing care depends, in part, on the surgical approach. The care is similar to other cardiac procedures; thus, infection, cardiac tamponade, and thromboemboli are possible complications regardless of the approach. Initially, the nurse assesses hemodynamic stability, cardiac rhythm, and respiratory status.

Should dysrhythmias recur during the hospital recuperation, the nurse must record each event to document the response of the device. Additional intervention may be unnecessary; however, advanced cardiac life support (ACLS) should be instituted if the dysrhythmia persists. Cardioversion or defibrillation can be performed without damage to the device.

The unit itself may fail to respond appropriately as a result of dislodgment or fracture of a lead wire, isolated component failure, or battery depletion. Environmental interference such as diathermy or electrocautery may also affect sensing capabilities of the AICD, causing inadvertent delivery of an impulse.

Patient outcomes may be influenced by any number of factors, such as the underlying cardiac condition, frequency of the dysrhythmia, prior life experiences, coping skills, and social support. Consequently, these factors should be included in the nurse's assessment. Further research will guide future nursing interventions. Issues to discuss with the patient in preparation for hospital discharge include what to expect should dysrhythmias recur, the appropriateness of CPR training for family members or significant others, recognition of signs and symptoms of infection, instructions pertaining to environmental interference, activity limitations, medications, and plans for follow-up care.

SUMMARY

This chapter has presented the fundamental pacemaker concepts as they apply to both temporary and permanent pacing. This information will assist the nurse in administering appropriate nursing care, interpreting pacemaker data, and troubleshooting malfunctions.

This chapter also has presented the role of the automatic implantable cardioverter-defibrillator (AICD) in reducing mortality from sudden cardiac death. Nursing care of the patient with an AICD was developed with guidelines for specific discharge teaching.

REFERENCES

1. Bernstein, A. D., Camm, A. J., Fletcher, R. D., et al. The NASPE/BPEG generic pacemaker code for antibradyarrhythmia and adaptive-rate pacing and antitachyarrhythmia devices. PACE 10:794–799, 1987.
2. Frye, R. L., Collins, J. J., DeShanetis, R. W., et al. Guidelines for permanent cardiac pacemaker implantation. J. Am. Coll. Cardiol. 4:2, 1984.

3. Gillette, P. C. Transvenous Implantation Technique. In P. C. Gillette and J. C. Griffin (eds.), *Practical Cardiac Pacing.* Baltimore: Williams & Wilkins, 1986.

4. Horowitz, L. N. Temporary Cardiac Pacing: Indications, Techniques, and Management. In A. H. Hakki (ed.), *Ideal Cardiac Pacing.* Philadelphia: W. B. Saunders, 1984.

5. Lehmann, M. H., Steinman, R. T., Schuger, C. D., *et al.* The automatic implantable cardioverter-defibrillator as antiarrhythmic treatment modality of choice for survivors of sudden cardiac arrest unrelated to myocardial infarction. *Am. J. Cardiol.* 62:803–805, 1988.

6. Moses, H. W., Taylor, G. J., Schneider, J. A., *et al.* Clinical Electrophysiology of Pacing. In H. W. Moses, Taylor, G. J., Schneider, J. A., *et al. A Practical Guide to Cardiac Pacing.* Boston: Little, Brown, 1987.

7. Winkle, R. A., Mead, R. H., Ruder, M. A., *et al.* Long-term outcome with the automatic implantable cardioverter-defibrillator. *J. Am. Coll. Cardiol.* 13:1353–1361, 1989.

14

Defibrillation and Cardioversion

Linda A. Prinkey

EXPERIENCING TIME

In the West, emphasis is placed on an outmoded concept of time. The common-sense approach to time, or the classical Newtonian model of time, states that time is the same for everybody—that real time flows and is divisible into past, present, and future. The notion is that life is lived in a linear sequence, a series of episodic events from birth, health, illness, and death. This view of the world has been discarded by modern physics because no experiment has ever been done that proves this sense of moving time.

When we think of these events in a linear fashion, we are dependent on an external reality that is determined by what is outside of us. The only way we can experience birth, health, illness, and death is by our senses, by our own internal experience. Thus, if we are to be consistent with modern concepts of time, we must think about birth, health, illness, and death in a way in which we turn inward to personal experiences. It is our meaning in life that determines our sense of time.

In reflecting on death, what words come to your mind? For most people, the words are *desperate, panic, final, always, ending,* or *forever.* These words create a constricted sense of time, and fear and urgency are inflicted on our experiences. If we revise our idea of time to be consistent with the modern physical world views, we realize our experience of time is bound to our senses; it is part of us, not "out there."

An outmoded sense of time is what creates the fears surrounding death—avoidance, denial, and a tragic, final event. The dualism that characterizes the Western world view of living and dying must be altered if one is to die in peace. Modern physics can help us in that it can reshape our view of time by proving that time does not flow, that time is now. The self-regulation strategies developed in Chapter 3 enable us to become familiar with states of awareness of being in the moment. You can learn to expand time, not constrict it with fear and worries.

LEARNING OBJECTIVES

After reading this chapter, the nurse should be able to do the following:

1. State the difference between defibrillation and cardioversion.
2. Describe the principles of effective defibrillation and cardioversion.
3. List the indications for defibrillation.
4. Describe appropriate nursing care for patients undergoing defibrillation.
5. List the indications for cardioversion.
6. Describe appropriate nursing care for patients undergoing cardioversion.

ELECTRICAL THERAPY

The notion that electricity could affect life-sustaining bodily functions was first explored by Abilgaard in 1775.[8] Early researchers used electricity to induce pulselessness and fibrillation. It was not until 1900 that Prevost and Batelli discovered that stronger shocks could cause the heart beat and pulse to return.[7] The first successful human defibrillation was accomplished much later, in 1947, using specially designed internal paddles.[2]

Today, defibrillation and cardioversion are commonly used forms of cardiovascular electrical therapy. In theory, these interventions cause the simultaneous depolarization of myocardial cells, which then allows normal impulse formation and conduction to resume. *Cardioversion* is the delivery of an electrical shock timed to occur approximately 10 msec after the peak of the R wave. In contrast, *defibrillation* is the application of asynchronous or untimed shocks. The indications and nursing care related to these interventions are discussed later in this chapter.

PRINCIPLES OF ELECTRICAL THERAPY

Equipment

The devices used to defibrillate and cardiovert are referred to collectively as *defibrillators*. In general, these devices possess the ability to deliver both synchronous and asynchronous shocks depending on user selection. Similarly, the amount of energy delivered is also controlled by the operator. Portable defibrillators use batteries as their primary power source. Other defibrillators contain AC to DC converters that change the electrical power obtained from standard wall sockets to direct current. All defibrillators possess capacitors that store the selected amount of energy until it is discharged through the electrodes or paddles. Most defibrillators also offer electrocardiographic (ECG) monitoring capabilities. Some models provide "quick-look" ECG monitoring when the defibrillator paddles are applied to the chest. Other devices offer transcutaneous pacing capabilities in addition to defibrillation and cardioversion.

To ensure the proper functioning of defibrillators, the actual energy delivered through a 50-ohm resistance load (which simulates body resistance) should be measured by biomedical engineering personnel for each setting of stored energy. Critical care personnel should charge the defibrillator to the highest energy level and discharge it into a test load once a week. They should also perform a visual inspection and a charge/discharge test at 50 joules into a 50-ohm test load daily.[4] Visual inspection includes examining the paddles for pitting and oxide-film build-up. Biomedical engineering personnel and critical care staff should also check the batteries of battery-powered defibrillators according to service manual recommendations.[1] Logs recording these maintenance activities should be kept near the defibrillator.

Defibrillators deliver energy that is quantified as joules (J) or watt-seconds:

Energy (Joules) = power (watts) × duration (seconds)

However, it is the current flow that actually defibrillates.[12] The amount of current flow depends on the strength of the shock and the impedence between the defibrillator electrodes.[13] Because *transthoracic impedence* is mainly resistive, the greater the resistance, the less current is delivered.[1]

$$\text{Current (amperes)} = \frac{\text{Potential (volts)}}{\text{Resistance (ohms)}}$$

Therefore, successful defibrillation, in part, depends on effective resistance reduction efforts.

Electrical Resistance

The main resistance to be overcome during cardioversion and defibrillation is transthoracic impedance. Factors affecting transthoracic impedance include the following:[1]

Energy delivered
Electrode size and composition
Interface between the electrode and the skin
Number of shocks delivered and the time interval between them
Patient's phase of ventilation
Distance between electrodes

Resistance related to energy level cannot be controlled by the defibrillator operator.[9]

The optimal size for electrodes varies. Much depends on the type of electrode used. For instance, research indicates that the optimal external paddle for adults is between 10 cm and 13 cm in diameter.[10,15] The optimal size for self-adhesive defibrillator electrodes is thought to be 11 cm, although 8-cm apical electrodes used in combination with 12-cm parasternal pads have also been effective.[6,14] Paddles for infants and children should be 4.5 cm and 8 cm, respectively.[1]

The interface between defibrillator paddles and the skin is very important. This is the factor most easily affected by technique of critical care personnel. First, transthoracic resistance can be reduced by applying conductive cream or gel to the paddles. Care must be taken to spread the gel or cream evenly across the paddle surface and to prevent any excess from being smeared across the chest between the paddles. Saline-soaked gauze pads may also be used. However, electrode cream is more effective.[13] Alcohol pads should never be used because they can cause serious skin burns.

Because electricity follows the path of least resistance, any connection between paddles created by conductive material will cause the current to flow along this connection and not through the chest. The passage of current through the chest is necessary to depolarize the critical mass of myocardium required for successful defibrillation.[18] Excess cream or gel can also create a shock hazard for the defibrillator operator and other rescuers if allowed to come in contact with their bodies. Conductive gel pads and self-adhesive electrodes can reduce this risk.

The pressure used to apply hand-held paddles to the chest also affects the electrode to skin interface and, therefore, the transthoracic resistance. Firm pressure of approximately 25 lb/paddle is recommended.[1] Interestingly, self-adhesive pads used without the added benefit of firm pressure have been demonstrated to have comparable defibrillation success rates.[14]

Other factors that affect impedance include the number of shocks delivered, the distance between paddles, and the phase of ventilation. Transthoracic resistance is lowered by previous shocks and during full expiration. Decreasing the distance between paddles or electrodes also reduces resistance.[1]

Electrode Placement

Standard paddle or self-adhesive electrode placement consists of one electrode placed to the right of the sternum just below the right clavicle and one electrode placed just left of the left nipple with the center of the electrode in the midaxillary line (Fig. 14–1). Anteroposterior positioning consists of placing one electrode anteriorly over the left precordium and the other electrode posteriorly, behind the heart. When patients have permanent pacemakers, electrodes should be positioned a minimum of 5 in from the pacemaker generator.[1]

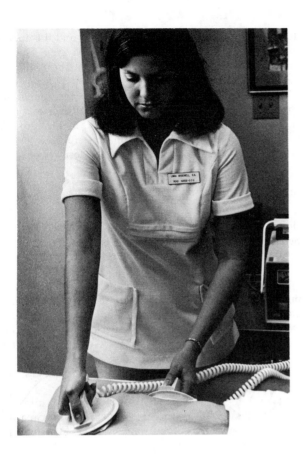

Figure 14-1
Electrode placement for defibrillation (anterior placement of electrode paddles).

TECHNIQUE BOX 14-1. Precordial Thump*

Mechanism of Action

Mechanical energy from a blow to the chest creates an electrical stimulus that can potentially depolarize the heart.

Technique

Raise a closed fist no more than 12 in above the center of the patient's chest.
Deliver a single sharp blow to the mid-sternal area using the fleshy portion of the fist.

Guidelines for Use

Deliver only a single blow. Do not delay defibrillation to deliver. Use only in the following situations:

- A witnessed cardiac arrest while awaiting arrival of the defibrillator
- Monitored patients with ventricular fibrillation
- Monitored patients with asystole or marked bradycardia *and* hemodynamic instability
- Monitored patients with ventricular tachycardia *and* a palpable pulse *only* when a defibrillator is immediately available (precordial thump may induce ventricular fibrillation in these patients)

(* The precordial thump is an ACLS technique only)

(Modified from Standards and guidelines for cardiopulmonary resuscitation [CPR] and emergency cardiac care [ECC]. *JAMA* 255(21):2915, 1986; with permission.)

DEFIBRILLATION

Procedure

Defibrillation, the delivery of unsynchronized shocks, is indicated for ventricular fibrillation and for pulseless ventricular tachycardia. Ventricular tachycardia associated with hypotension, unconsciousness, or pulmonary edema also requires defibrillation.[13] If the development of these conditions is witnessed, the nurse should check for a pulse. If a pulse is not found, the nurse may administer a *precordial thump* (see Technique Box 14-1). After rechecking for a pulse, the nurse initiates cardiopulmonary resuscitation (CPR) for pulselessness (see Appendix I). When the arrest is unwitnessed, the nurse confirms pulselessness and starts CPR without first delivering a precordial thump while awaiting the arrival of a defibrillator.

Once a defibrillator arrives, the nurse should check the rhythm with "quick-look" paddles or by placing ECG electrodes on the patient. Paddle monitoring has the advantage of being faster; however, fine ventricular fibrillation can mimic asystole. Because confirmation of asystole requires observation of a "flat line" pattern in at least two leads,[1] ECG electrodes will need to be applied. Therefore, when an unmonitored patient arrests, it is recommended that one nurse use the "quick-look" paddles while another applies ECG electrodes.

If the rhythm is confirmed to be ventricular fibrillation or pulseless ventricular tachycardia, conductive material is applied to the paddles or to the chest (saline-soaked gauze or gel pads). The defibrillator is set to charge the capacitor to 200 J. While the capacitor is charging, the paddles are positioned on the chest and 25 lb of pressure are applied. Before discharging the defibrillator, the paddle operator should ensure that all personnel have no direct or indirect contact with the patient. The paddle operator then delivers the countershock. Usually, this is accomplished by depressing the buttons located on each paddle simultaneously. In certain instances, the defibrillator is discharged by other personnel positioned at the defibrillator's controls.

If the electrical energy is delivered to the patient, the patient's chest wall muscles will contract. If the muscles do not contract, the nurse should check to assure that the synchronizer mode is off and that the defibrillator is plugged in or has adequate battery charge levels.

Once the shock has been delivered, the nurse should assess the patient's pulse and rhythm. If the patient continues to remain pulseless and in ventricular tachycardia or fibrillation, the defibrillator is set to charge to either 200 J or 300 J. The defibrillation procedure is then repeated. If pulseless ventricular tachycardia or fibrillation persists, a third shock of 360 J is delivered.

If no pulse is present after the third shock, CPR is resumed and an intravenous line established. Epinephrine is then given. The patient also is intubated if possible. After these interventions have been completed, the patient is defibrillated with 360 J. If no pulse is established, drug therapy alternating with shocks of 360 J is initiated (Fig. 14-2). The patient's pulse and rhythm are checked after each defibrillation attempt.

Energy Levels

Because up to 90% of adult patients weighing up to 90 kg who are in ventricular fibrillation can be successfully defibrillated using 200 J,[11] this energy level is recommended for the first shock. The energy required for the second shock is more controversial. Considering the changes in impedance and the predictability of delivered energy, the second shock can be 200 J to 300 J.[1] Higher energy levels can cause dysrhythmias and myocardial damage.[17] The maximum recommended energy level is 360 J.[1]

Open-chest defibrillation requires far less energy than does transcutaneous defibrillation. When specially designed sterile

electrodes are placed over the right atrium and the apex of the heart, shocks starting at 5 J can be delivered. The recommended maximum energy level for open-chest interventions is 50 J.[13]

The recommended defibrillation energy for infants and children is 2 J/kg, initially. If this level is insufficient to convert the patient's rhythm, two additional shocks of 4 J/kg may be given. If the second 4 J/kg shock is unsuccessful, interventions should be initiated to correct existing acidosis, hypoxemia, and hypothermia.[1]

Other Defibrillation Techniques

Automatic external defibrillators (AEDs) can be used by both medical personnel and nonmedical rescuers. Automatic external defibrillators have defibrillator pads that must be applied after pulselessness has been determined. Once the pads are applied, the device uses preprogrammed algorithms to determine the rhythm and energy level for the shocks to be delivered. AEDs also provide messages informing the user of poor lead contact, charging activity, and when to check pulses. Once the device is charged, the only way to prevent firing is to turn the machine off. Semiautomatic models inform the user of ventricular fibrillation or ventricular tachycardia and advise the user to press the defibrillation button.

It takes 6 to 12 seconds for AEDs to commit to firing. An additional 8 to 15 seconds is required to charge the capacitor. Therefore, there will be approximately 15 to 30 seconds between shocks delivered by an AED if the patient remains in ventricular tachycardia or fibrillation. The unit should be turned off during CPR and when the patient is moving or having a seizure.[3]

The effectiveness and feasibility of using AEDs in the homes of high-risk patients are being studied. Initial results are disappointing. Skill retention and the emotional impact of family

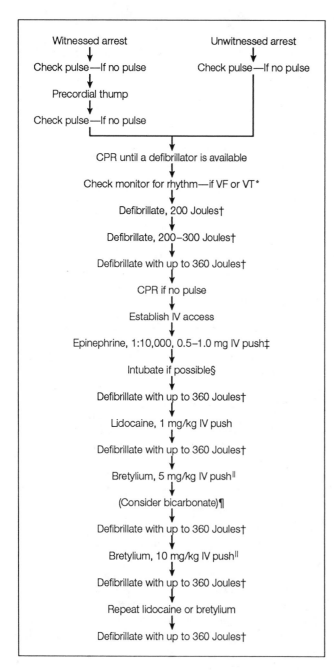

Figure 14-2

Ventricular fibrillation (and pulseless ventricular tachycardia). This sequence was developed to assist in teaching how to treat a broad range of patients with ventricular fibrillation (VF) or pulseless ventricular tachycardia (VT). Some patients may require care not specified herein. This algorithm should not be construed as prohibiting such flexibility. Flow of algorithm presumes that VF is continuing. CPR: cardiopulmonary resuscitation. (McIntyre, K. M., and Lewis, A. J. Standards and guidelines for cardiopulmonary resuscitation and emergency cardiac care. *J. Am. Med. Assoc.* 255:2841, 1986; with permission.)

* Pulseless VT should be treated identically to VF.

† Check pulse and rhythm after each shock. If VF recurs after transiently converting (rather than persists without ever converting), use whatever energy level has previously been successful for defibrillation.

‡ Epinephrine should be repeated every 5 minutes.

§ Intubation is preferable. If it can be accompanied simultaneously with other techniques, then the earlier the better. However, defibrillation and epinephrine are more important initially if the patient can be ventilated without intubation.

‖ Some may prefer repeated doses of lidocaine, which may be given in 0.5-mg/kg boluses every 8 minutes to a total dose of 3 mg/kg.

¶ Value of sodium bicarbonate is questionable during cardiac arrest, and it is not recommended for routine cardiac arrest sequence. Consideration of its use in a dose of 1 mEq/kg is appropriate at this point. Half of original dose may be repeated every 10 minutes if it is used.

members with life-threatening dysrhythmias are two factors affecting home-use success rates.[5]

Automatic implantable cardioverter-defibrillators (AICDs) can be surgically placed in patients at high risk of sudden death. Unlike AEDs, AICDs do not depend on human operators to activate them. Once implanted and activated, AICDs continuously monitor the patient's rhythm. Automatic implantable cardioverter-defibrillators use QRS morphology and heart rate to determine when to discharge. They can deliver up to five shocks per dysrhythmia occurrence. However, they require at least 35 seconds of a rhythm other than ventricular tachycardia or fibrillation in order to reactivate the defibrillation cycle.[16] If an unconscious AICD patient has muscle contractions indicating internal defibrillation but does not have a pulse when muscle contractions cease, the patient should receive external shocks according to the previously outlined defibrillation procedure. Automatic implantable cardioverter-defibrillators are protected against external defibrillator shocks.[1]

Transtelephonic defibrillation is another new intervention for high-risk patients. A trained family member or other individual applies self-adhesive monitor defibrillator pads to the patient. The pads are then attached to the cables of a device that transmits the rhythm by telephone to a remote base station. Emergency personnel at the base station control the charging and discharging of the home device. These devices also offer two-way voice communication.[5]

Factors Affecting Defibrillation Outcomes

In addition to techniques and protocols, other factors affect the success of defibrillation attempts. The duration of the ventricular fibrillation or pulseless ventricular tachycardia influences outcomes. Long periods of these rhythms decrease the chances of successful countershock.[1] Early, effective CPR improves the chance for positive outcomes. Conditions such as acidosis, hypoxemia, hypothermia, drug toxicity, and electrolyte imbalance can make the heart more refractory to defibrillation.[1]

CARDIOVERSION

Procedure

Cardioversion, or synchronized shock, is indicated for unstable ventricular tachycardia (except for patients who are pulseless, hypotensive, or in pulmonary edema) and rapid supraventricular tachycardias (Figs. 14–3 and 14–4). The principles of electrical therapy discussed earlier apply to cardioversion as well as defibrillation. Cardioversion, however, requires the application of ECG electrodes and the selection of a monitoring lead that best facilitates recognition of the QRS complex. Additionally the synchronization switch must be activated.

Patients requiring cardioversion are conscious. Because cardioversion is potentially uncomfortable, anesthesia or analgesia is necessary. If the cardioversion is emergent, sedation should be considered.[1] A physician skilled in airway management, preferably an anesthetist, should be present. In addition, a patent intravenous line should be established. Emergency drugs and equipment also should be available. The procedure is explained to the patient as conditions permit. Informed consent is obtained from patients undergoing elective cardioversion.

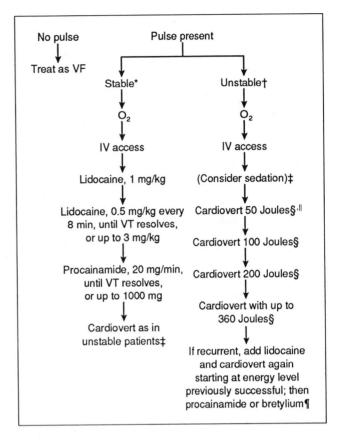

Figure 14–3

Sustained ventricular tachycardia (VT). This sequence was developed to assist in teaching how to treat a broad range of patients with sustained VT. Some patients may require care not specified herein. This algorithm should not be construed as prohibiting such flexibility. Flow of algorithm presumes that VT is continuing. VF: ventricular fibrillation. (McIntyre, K. M., and Lewis, A. J. Standards and guidelines for cardiopulmonary resuscitation and emergency cardiac care. *J. Am. Med. Assoc.* 255:2841, 1986; with permission.)

* If patient becomes unstable (see footnote † for definition) at any time, move to "unstable" arm of algorithm.

† Unstable indicates symptoms (*e.g.*, chest pain or dyspnea), hypotension (systolic blood pressure < 90 mmHg), congestive heart failure, ischemia, or infarction.

‡ Sedation should be considered for all patients, including those defined in footnote † as unstable, except those who are hemodynamically unstable (*e.g.*, hypotensive, in pulmonary edema, or unconscious).

§ If hypotension, pulmonary edema, or unconsciousness is present, unsynchronized cardioversion should be done to avoid delay associated with synchronization.

‖ In the absence of hypotension, pulmonary edema, or unconsciousness, a precordial thump may be employed prior to cardioversion.

¶ Once VT has resolved, begin intravenous (IV) infusion of antiarrhythmic agent that has aided resolution of VT. If hypotension, pulmonary edema, or unconsciousness is present, use lidocaine if cardioversion alone is unsuccessful, followed by bretylium. In all other patients, recommended order of therapy is lidocaine, procainamide, and then bretylium.

Once all the preparations have been completed, the paddles or self-adhesive electrodes are placed on the patient's chest as described previously. The synchronizer switch is activated, the energy level is selected, and the defibrillator is charged. When the operator depresses the buttons to deliver the shock,

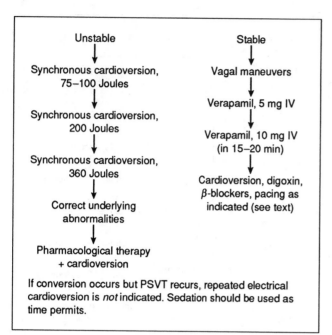

Unstable	Stable
↓	↓
Synchronous cardioversion, 75–100 Joules	Vagal maneuvers
↓	↓
Synchronous cardioversion, 200 Joules	Verapamil, 5 mg IV
↓	↓
Synchronous cardioversion, 360 Joules	Verapamil, 10 mg IV (in 15–20 min)
↓	↓
Correct underlying abnormalities	Cardioversion, digoxin, β-blockers, pacing as indicated (see text)
↓	
Pharmacological therapy + cardioversion	

If conversion occurs but PSVT recurs, repeated electrical cardioversion is *not* indicated. Sedation should be used as time permits.

Figure 14–4

Paroxysmal supraventricular tachycardia (PSVT). This sequence was developed to assist in teaching how to treat a broad range of patients with sustained PSVT. Some patients may require care not specified herein. This algorithm should not be construed as prohibiting such flexibility. Flow of algorithm presumes PSVT is continuing. (McIntyre, K. M., and Lewis, A. J. Standards and guidelines for cardiopulmonary resuscitation and emergency cardiac care. *J. Am. Med. Assoc.* 255:2841, 1986; with permission.)

the paddles must be held in place until the synchronizer discharges the energy. This is necessary because the energy is not released until the machine senses the appropriate portion of the QRS complex. This avoids delivering the shock during the vulnerable period of the T wave and reduces the probability of inducing ventricular fibrillation. Should the patient's rhythm be cardioverted to ventricular fibrillation, the synchronizer switch should be turned off and the unit charged to 200 J. The patient is then defibrillated immediately. If necessary, the rest of the ventricular fibrillation treatment algorithm should be implemented.

Energy Levels

The energy required for cardioversion depends on the type of dysrhythmia being treated. For cardioversion of atrial fibrillation, the recommended energy level is 100 J for the first shock, 200 J for the second, and 360 J for the third. For paroxysmal supraventricular tachycardia, the recommended initial energy level is 75 to 100 J. The second and third shocks should be 200 J and 360 J, respectively. The initial energy used to cardiovert atrial flutter should be 25 J. For urgent or emergent treatment of unstable ventricular tachycardia, the initial shock should be 50 J followed by subsequent shocks of 100 J, 200 J, and 360 J, if necessary.[1]

SUMMARY

Tachydysrhythmias and ventricular fibrillation can be treated successfully with direct-current electrical shock. The appropriate use of cardioversion and defibrillation theoretically depolarizes a critical mass of myocardium and allows normal impulse formation and conduction to be restored. Knowledge of the principles of electrical therapy and the procedures appropriate for the treatment of the patient's dysrhythmia can lead to positive patient outcomes from potentially life-threatening situations.

REFERENCES

1. American Heart Association. *Textbook of Advanced Cardiac Life Support.* Dallas: American Heart Association, 1987.
2. Beck, C. S., Pritchard, W. H., Feil, S. A. Ventricular fibrillation of long duration abolished by electric shock. *J.A.M.A.* 135:985, 1947.
3. Bocka, J. J. Automatic external defibrillators. *Ann. Emerg. Med.* 18:1264, 1989.
4. Creed, J. D., Packard, J. M., Lambrew, C. T., et al. Defibrillation and Synchronized Cardioversion. In K. M. McIntyre and A. J. Lewis (eds.), *Textbook of Advanced Cardiac Life Support.* Dallas: American Heart Association, 1981.
5. Cummins, R. O. From concept to standard-of-care? Review of the clinical experience with automated external defibrillators. *Ann. Emerg. Med.* 18:1269, 1989.
6. Dalzell, G. W., Cunningham, S. R., Anderson, J., et al. Electrode pad size, transthoracic impedance and success of external ventricular defibrillation. *Am. J. Cardiol.* 64:741, 1989.
7. DeSilva, R. A., Graboys, T. B., Podrid, P. J., et al. Cardioversion and defibrillation. *Am. Heart J.* 100:881, 1980.
8. Driscol, T. E., Ratnoff, O. D., Nygaard, O. F. The remarkable Doctor Abildgaard and countershock. *Ann. Intern. Med.* 83:878, 1975.
9. Ewy, G. A., Ewy, M. D., Nuttall, A. J., et al. Canine transthoracic resistance. *J. Appl. Physiol.* 32:91, 1972.
10. Kerber, R. E., Grayzel, J., Hoyt, R., et al. Transthoracic resistance of human defibrillation: Influence of body weight, chest size, serial shocks, paddle size and paddle contact pressure. *Circulation* 63: 676, 1981.
11. Myerburg, R. J., Castellanos, A. Cardiac arrest and sudden cardiac death. In E. Braunwald (ed.), *Heart Disease: A Textbook of Cardiovascular Medicine* (3rd ed.). Philadelphia: W.B. Saunders, 1988.
12. Patton, J. N., Pantridge, J. F. Current required for ventricular fibrillation. *Br. Med. J.* 1:513, 1979.
13. Standards and guidelines for cardiopulmonary resuscitation (CPR) and emergency cardiac care (ECC). *J.A.M.A.* 255(21):2915, 1986.
14. Stults, K. R., Brown, D. D., Cooley, F., et al. Self-adhesive monitor/ defibrillator pads improve prehospital defibrillation success. *Ann. Emerg. Med.* 16(8):872, 1987.
15. Thomas, E. D., Ewy, G. A., Dahl, C. F., et al. Effectiveness of direct current defibrillation: Role of paddle electrode size. *Am. Heart. J.* 93:463, 1977.
16. Verseth-Rogers, J. A practical approach to teaching the automatic implantable cardioverter-defibrillator patient. *J. Cardiovasc. Nurs.* 4(2):7, 1990.
17. Warner, E. D., Dahl, C., Ewy, G. A. Myocardial injury from transthoracic defibrillator countershock. *Arch. Pathol.* 99:55, 1975.
18. Zipes, D. P., Fischer, J., King, R. M., et al. Termination of ventricular fibrillation in dogs by depolarizing a critical amount of myocardium. *Am. J. Cardiol.* 36:37, 1975.

15

Electrical Precautions and Safety

Doris A. McGirt   Cornelia Vanderstaay Kenner

SELF-TALK
Have you ever thought about the fact that the person you talk to the most in a day is yourself? Learning to recognize your constant inner dialogue is helpful, particularly when that dialogue is negative. The reason for this is that your body's physiology responds to images that are created from your senses and the words of your inner dialogue. Your reactions and patterns of behavior are based on your self-talk. Self-regulation accompanied by self-reflection skills help you recognize your bodymind connections. Here are two acronyms with definitions to help you increase both your self-regulation and self-reflection skills—**STOP** and **FOCUS.** Use these techniques when your dialogue is negative or destructive:

STOP	*FOCUS*
S—Self	F—Focus
T—Talk	O—On
O—Organizes	C—Communicating
P—Patterns	U—Understanding
	S—Self

As discussed in Chapter 3, images create either positive or negative physiologic effects. Your inner dialogue represents different levels of self-knowledge and may be thought of as your subpersonalities, or your truthful self, your critical self, your loving self, your perfectionist self, your wise mentors, and so forth. The purpose of developing self-reflection skills is to help you become more aware of your self-talk, your powerful healing voice, and to recognize when it is working against you.

LEARNING OBJECTIVES

After reading this chapter, the nurse should be able to do the following:

1. Identify the electrical hazards present in a critical care unit.
2. Differentiate between macroshock and microshock.
3. Identify appropriate nursing measures for the provision of electrical safety.

ELECTRICAL PRECAUTIONS

Patients in a critical care unit are in a hazardous position. They are connected to or located near any of a number of electric devices: pacemakers, cardiac and blood pressure monitors, volume infusion pumps, hypothermia blankets, electric beds, suction machines, or lamps. If the particular piece of equipment is not properly grounded, current can flow through any pathway with a low resistance.[1,2] Normal skin resistance (50,000 to 100,000 ohms) is reduced whenever the skin is wet or underlying moist tissue or mucous membranes are exposed—a frequent occurrence in the critical care unit.

Electric current is a flow of electrons that moves from areas of higher potential (*i.e.,* greater numbers of electrons) to areas of lower potential (*i.e.,* fewer electrons). Earth, usually referred to as *ground*, has the lowest possible potential to which current may flow, and current will flow to ground whenever possible. In order to get to the area of lowest potential, however, current must have a pathway, and current seeks the pathway that provides the least resistance. If a nurse provides the pathway of least resistance, the current will flow through the nurse. If a patient provides the path of least resistance the current will flow through the patient.

Electric current that flows from an electrical outlet is usually delivered to an appliance through a two-pronged plug. One prong is the "hot" side that sends electricity to the appliance; the other prong is the "neutral" side that is tied directly to an earth ground. If there is a third prong, it also provides a ground, an alternate pathway in case of current leakage of a short circuit, and it is essential in ensuring an electrically safe patient environment.

Most electrical appliances, and especially those used in critical care units, leak a minute amount of the current into the cabinet/chassis of the appliance. This leaked current, like any other kind of current, searches for a convenient pathway through which it can return to ground. If a two-pronged plug is used, connections that make a good pathway for this current to reach ground include the nurse touching the cabinet of the appliance or touching the patient and simultaneously touching the appliance so that the patient is part of the path of least resistance to the ground.

Small amounts of current leaked from electrical equipment are usually unimportant because of the high protective resistance of skin. However, an intracardiac electrode catheter circumvents the protective resistance of the skin and provides an excellent path of least resistance directly to the myocardium. A current as low as 20 MA can produce ventricular fibrillation if applied directly to the myocardium through the intracardiac catheter.

Because current leaking into the cabinets of equipment in critical care units can be hazardous, the best way to keep the amount of current leakage to a minimum is to provide the leaked current its own pathway to ground. Thus, three-pronged plugs should be placed on the electrical cords of all equipment used in critical care areas—one prong to carry the "hot" current, one prong to return the current, and the third prong to return the current leaked into the cabinet back to ground.

PHYSIOLOGIC EFFECTS OF ELECTRICITY

In order for electricity to have any effect on the body, the body must become part of the electric circuit itself. At least two connections must exist between the body and an external source of voltage to effect a current flow. The magnitude of the current flow is a function of both the voltage between the body connections and the resistance of the body:

Voltage = current × resistance

The electric current can affect tissue in two different ways. First, the current flow can induce an action potential, causing the transmission of impulses through sensory and motor nerves. Stimulation of motor nerves in such a manner can cause contraction of the muscle groups involved. A greater intensity of motor nerve or muscle stimulation can cause tetanus of the muscle. Stimulation of sensory nerves by small amounts of current flow can cause a tingling sensation, and greater amounts of current flow can cause extreme pain. Second, electric energy dissipated in the tissue resistance can cause a temperature increase, resulting in an electrical burn. This very principle is used in electrosurgery, in which concentrated electric current from an electrical surgery unit (a radiofrequency generator with a frequency of 2.5 to 4 MHz) is used to cut tissue or coagulate small blood vessels.

Figure 15–1 shows the approximate current range for and the resulting effects of a 1-second exposure to various levels of 60-cycle current applied externally to the body. The organ most susceptible to electric current is the heart. An electric current of sufficient magnitude can tetanize the myocardium, resulting in the cessation of circulation for the duration of the applied current. If a tetanizing current is applied for a long period of time, death can result from lack of systemic circulation.

A current of lower intensity that stimulates only a localized section of the heart can be considerably more dangerous than one sufficient to tetanize the entire heart. Local excitation of the myocardium can desynchronize the heart, causing random, ineffectual muscle activity known as *fibrillation*. Fibrillation in the ventricles can be fatal, and reversion to a normal rhythm usually does not occur when the electric current is removed. To restore synchronous activity to the heart, the myocardium must be tetanized by a sufficiently strong current pulse from an external defibrillator.

The magnitude of electric current required to produce a certain physiologic effect in a person is influenced by many factors. The voltage level required to effect a current flow is dependent on the resistance offered by the body. The skin offers the most body resistance. The skin provides a natural protection against electrical danger, but when it is permeated by a conductive fluid or when conductive objects such as temporary

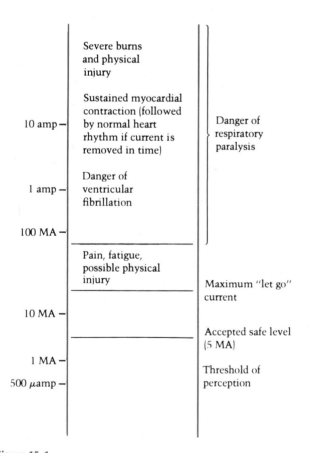

Figure 15–1

Physiologic effects of electric current from a 1 second external contact with the body (60 Hz AC).

pacemakers are introduced, the resistance of the skin is bypassed effectively.

Once the skin resistance is bypassed, the resistance between the contacts is determined only by the resistance of the tissue in the current path, which in most cases is extremely low. Many medical procedures involve the introduction of conductive objects into the body, such as catheters and needles, or the use of electrode paste to measure bioelectric potentials, such as an electroencephalogram (EEG) or electrocardiogram (ECG). In such procedures, the patient is deprived of the natural protection against electrical hazards that the skin normally provides. With such a resulting low resistance, voltages of even small magnitude can result in a fatal electric current flow.

MACROSHOCK VERSUS MICROSHOCK

In certain procedures (*e.g.*, cardiac catherization and cardiac pacing), electrically conductive catheters are introduced directly into the heart. These procedures pose unique problems. Introduction of an electrically conductive catheter into the heart can establish one of the two electrical contacts that can connect the heart directly to an external electrical source. In this situation, all the current introduced by the external electrical source flows directly through the heart itself. The current density in the heart can be several orders of magnitude higher than when the same current is applied to a contact more remote from the heart. As a result, patients with any type of indwelling or cardiac catheter are much more sensitive to electric current than they would otherwise be. Such patients are said to be "electrically susceptible." The effect of an electric current applied directly to the heart is known as *microshock*. In contrast, the effect of an electric current applied when no direct connection to the heart exists is referred to as *macroshock*.

How much electric current is required to induce ventricular fibrillation in humans has not been firmly established because of the obvious experimental difficulties. In a few measurements on humans whose hearts were intentionally fibrillated during open-heart surgery, currents of at least 180 A were required. In similar experiments on dogs, fibrillation could be achieved with as little as 20 A. For this reason, contemporary standards and specifications for medical equipment have set much lower limits than the 180 A found to cause fibrillation. For equipment to be used with electrically susceptible patients, a maximum leakage current of 10 A has been accepted by the majority of medical equipment manufacturers. Such a limit provides protection should the electric current accidentally flow into the patient.

IMPORTANCE OF THE EQUIPMENT GROUND

To understand any hazard presented by a piece of electrical equipment in the hospital environment, an understanding of the hospital's electric power distribution system is necessary. In Figure 15–2 the power distribution to the appliance is by a simple two-wire connection. In such a system, one of the wall receptacle contacts is connected to the "hot" wire, and the other "neutral" wire is tied directly to an earth ground. *Earth ground* (or ground) is a term used to denote any electrical conductor intimately in contact with the earth. Items typically connected to ground include water pipes, metallic room fixtures, or metallic building structures.

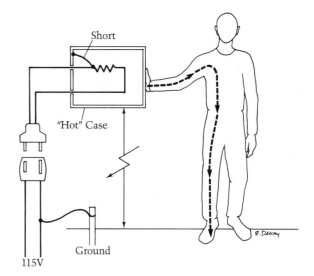

Figure 15–2

Electrical power distribution with a simple two-wire system. The person touching the equipment while in contact with the ground is exposed to a shock hazard.

To be exposed to an electrical macroshock hazard, a person must come in contact with both the hot and the neutral conductors, because two connections are required to afford a path for electrical flow. However, because the neutral wire is connected to an earth ground, a shock hazard exists between the hot wire and any conductive object in any way in contact with ground. Great care is taken with the use of insulating materials and in the design of electrical equipment to prevent accidental contact with the hot wire. However, through routine use, mechanical damage, or insulation breakdown, accidental contact between the equipment case and the hot wire can occur. In this simple "ungrounded" two-wire system, any person touching the equipment would be exposed to a severe shock hazard.

GROUNDED ELECTRICAL CONNECTIONS

The purpose of the equipment ground contact on the wall receptacle and the third conductor in a power cord is to provide an alternate path for electric current flow should current leakage or a short circuit occur. A short circuit, an accidental electrical connection (as illustrated in Fig. 15–3), can occur between a hot wire within an instrument and the equipment case. If a short circuit should occur, the current can return to ground through the equipment ground connection, minimizing the shock hazard. If the resultant current flow in this alternate circuit is sufficiently large, it will trip the circuit breaker for the hot conductor, thus interrupting the current flow.

The benefits of the three-wire system can be realized only if the continuity of the equipment ground connection is always guaranteed. Any interruption of the circuit because of the use of a three-to-two prong adapter ("cheater" plug) or broken ground pin completely negates the system's protective value. Even if the ground connection is not completely interrupted but exhibits a resistance in excess of about 1 ohm, the resulting voltage developed across the resistance due to the flow of the fault current can be dangerous. If there is any contact with

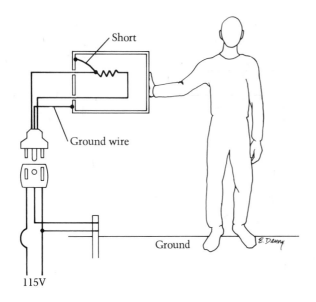

Figure 15-3
Third conductor in the electrical connection, an alternate pathway for electrical current flow. Should a short circuit occur, the current can return to the ground through the equipment ground connection and thereby minimize the shock hazard.

an instrument case exhibiting an elevated voltage, a macroshock hazard exists. For this reason, many hospitals have instituted a rigorous preventive maintenance schedule, checking various parameters of hospital equipment, including ground integrity, on a periodic basis.

NURSING MEASURES FOR ELECTRICAL SAFETY

Microshock is a great concern in the modern hospital environment, because a microshock hazard can be created by equipment with perfectly intact insulation.[1] This current leakage, which is frequently more than the 10 A present-day manufacturers use as a guideline, can result from a phenomenon known as *capacitive coupling*. Much of the patient monitoring and therapeutic equipment found in the hospital, in household appliances, and in lamps have capacitive leakages in excess of 10 A. Although such leakages are of no particular concern for normal operation in places other than a hospital, they can present a true microshock hazard to the electrically susceptible patient.

One way such a microshock hazard can occur is when a patient has an indwelling catheter to measure pressures. The catheter is part of an electronic line-powered monitoring system. The system establishes a path for current flow through the conductive fluid within the catheter, the pressure transducer, and the equipment ground lead in the line cord of the monitoring device. Such an arrangement establishes a ground connection directly to the patient's heart and, more importantly, a direct path for current flow. As a result, a microshock hazard is created by any conductive connection between the patient and an ungrounded electrical device having an excessive current leakage. If this were to occur, the path of current leakage would include the heart of the patient, because it is at that point that the patient is grounded.

Figure 15-4 shows a patient touching a hazardous piece of equipment directly. However, a similar conductive connection can be established by another person touching the device and the patient simultaneously. This is only one of the many ways a microshock accident can occur. What is important to note is that in every case a direct connection to the heart from outside the body is required. Therefore, special care must be taken with a patient with such a connection.

Numerous measures have been taken by equipment manufacturers to reduce the possibility of a microshock accident as a result of patient monitoring. Ultimately, the critical care personnel are responsible for preventing accidental electrocution.

Caution must always be taken with patients who are electrically susceptible. Catheters used to measure pressure and bioelectric potentials should be connected only to monitors that are specially designed to limit current leakage.

Patients with temporary or temporary-permanent pacing wires present a direct electrical connection to the heart. Care should be taken to ensure that no conductive portion of the pacing wire is exposed. No conductive portion of the wire should be touched by any person in contact with any piece of electrical equipment.

Specific measures for the provision of electrical safety are as follows:

1. Do not ignore interference on the ECG monitor.
   A. Check leads.
   B. Check electrodes and cables.
   C. Check the monitor.
   D. Disconnect the patient from the monitor.
   E. Call the maintenance department.
2. Report any problems with the electrocardiograph.
   A. Poor-quality tracing
   B. Alarm malfunction
   C. Automatic copies that fail to trigger
3. Report any unusual electrical interference on ECG that cannot be corrected by electrode adjustment.
4. Only use a battery-operated monitor or one with known

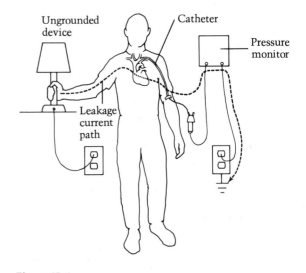

Figure 15-4
Patient touching hazardous object.

leakage current of less than 10 μa to assess position of pericardiocentesis needle or pacing catheter.

5. Use pacemakers that are battery-operated.
   A. Use a new, working battery every time pacemaker is used.
   B. Use nonconductive material to cover pacemaker terminals and tips of pacing catheter.
   C. Maintain a record of battery use (*i.e.,* manufacturer's date and hours of use) if used with pacemaker on demand or continuous mode.

6. Wear rubber gloves when connecting or disconnecting external pacemakers.

7. Maintain patient and personnel safety during defibrillation.
   A. Report any equipment malfunction (*i.e.,* long charging time, bent paddles, defibrillator not holding charge, slow response time).
   B. During defibrillation, all personnel should be clear of the patient, bed, and defibrillator.

8. Cover exposed electrodes or uninsulated pacemaker leads connected to patient with rubber gloves or other insulating material.

9. Always remove patient connections first, before unplugging the equipment.

10. If static electricity is a problem, touch the bed frame before touching the patient.

11. If electric tingle is felt when touching a piece of equipment, stop its use and call the maintenance department.

12. Check the grounding plugs of all electric appliances, especially the electric bed, frequently. The bed should be checked for leakage of current by the maintenance department. Leakage should be under 100 μa.

13. Do not touch patient while in contact with metal surface of an item that is plugged into an electrical outlet.

14. Inspect the cord and plug before using any piece of electrical equipment. Do not use equipment with frayed or damaged cords or plugs that are bent or have a ground prong missing. *Never* use ungrounded or "cheater" plugs.

15. Do not allow *any* patient-owned electrical equipment (*e.g.,* shavers, radios, fans, or heaters) until they are evaluated by the maintenance department.

16. When inserting or removing a plug from the wall, hold the plug cap. Do not pull on the cord. Protect the grounding prong.

17. Remember that moisture decreases resistance and increases the electrical conductivity of the skin.

18. Remember that a path for current can be provided to the patient without the nurse first feeling the shock.

SUMMARY

Critical care units promote unique electrical hazards owing to the presence of various indwelling lines and catheters and the presence of electrical equipment. A basic standard of critical care nursing involves understanding the effects of electricity, recognizing and preventing electrical hazards, and providing electrical safety measures.

REFERENCES

1. Meth, I. M. Electrical safety in the hospital. *Am. J. Nurs.* 7:1344, 1980.
2. Sundberg, M. C. *Fundamentals of Nursing with Clinical Procedures.* Boston: Jones and Barlett, 1989.

16

Airway and Ventilatory Management

Marianne Chulay

RELAXING WITH THE VENTILATOR

Mr. S. was a long-term patient in the Special Care Unit after having open heart surgery. His course was complicated by respiratory problems, and he became dependent on a ventilator. He progressed slowly but steadily with physical therapy and encouragement to the point of mobilizing him to the chair with assistance. We again tried to wean him from the ventilator. He managed to do quite well, and each day, he was weaned from one less ventilator-assisted breath. His most difficult time, however, was at night. He just could not relax and would end up losing all ground. We would then have to increase his rate on the ventilator again.

As I spoke with his wife on the phone one evening, she mentioned how much he had enjoyed golfing. I realized that I might be able to use this imagery to help him relax. I approached him with the plan, and he agreed. I turned the lights down and pulled the door closed. I suctioned his tracheotomy, made sure he was lying in a comfortable position, and began coaching him to slow his breathing down by counting ". . . in 2, 3 . . . out 2, 3. . . ." His respirations at that time were 36, he was slightly diaphoretic, and his blood pressure was elevated. Holding his hand and gently wiping his brow, I began a guided imagery of what I knew about golfing.

I continued to coach him with his breathing and told him to imagine his favorite golf course on a beautiful warm day, with a light breeze blowing. Not knowing too much about golf, I reminded him to just take note of things around him, what he saw and what he could feel and hear. Again I coached him to relax his body and use slow breathing.

As I let him image, I noticed that his blood pressure had come down considerably and his respirations had decreased. I stayed with him a few minutes longer, reminding him to continue this image. Then I slowly withdrew my hand and slipped out of the room, telling him I would check back soon. I found him sleeping a few minutes later. We did not have to increase the ventilator rate that night. We had broken the cycle. He continued to be weaned successfully.

Kim Tierney, RN, CCRN
Special Care Unit
Maine Medical Center
Portland, Maine

LEARNING OBJECTIVES

After reading this chapter, the nurse should be able to do the following:

1. List methods for oxygen delivery, the FiO_2 ranges of each, and their advantages and disadvantages.
2. Discuss the nursing management of patients with artificial airways.
3. Compare and contrast the modes of mechanical ventilation.
4. Discuss advantages and disadvantages of weaning from mechanical ventilation.
5. Identify areas for future research in airway and ventilator management.

OXYGEN THERAPY

Supplemental oxygen is administered for a variety of clinical disorders. The primary goal of oxygen therapy is to correct or prevent hypoxemia. Oxygen therapy should be used along with a therapeutic approach to the basic pathophysiology. An arterial oxygen tension (PaO_2) greater than 60 mm Hg is generally adequate if hemoglobin levels are normal.

An assortment of methods is available for oxygen delivery and can be divided into two main categories: low-flow oxygen systems, which achieve partial inspiratory requirements, and high-flow oxygen systems, which achieve complete inspiratory volumes. Selection of the appropriate oxygen delivery mode is based on the fraction of inspired oxygen (FiO_2) delivery required, patient tolerance and compliance, and cost.[8,20,29] Common methods for supplemental oxygen therapy are detailed in Table 16–1.

Nasal Cannula

Low concentrations of FiO_2 can be delivered by administering 1 to 6 L/minute of oxygen into a patient's nostrils with a nasal cannula or prongs (Fig. 16–1A). FiO_2 delivery with this device ranges from 0.24 to 0.38.[20] As long as the nares are not completely obstructed, FiO_2 delivery is accomplished whether mouth or nasal breathing is present. These devices are inexpensive and usually well tolerated by patients. Humidification of nasal oxygen at 1 to 6 L/minute, although not required, is commonly employed to prevent drying of the mucous membranes.

One disadvantage of nasal cannulas is the variability of FiO_2 delivery with changes in tidal volume and ventilatory rates. Low tidal volumes and rates result in higher FiO_2 delivery, and high tidal volumes and rates, such as occur with dyspnea, result in lower FiO_2 deliveries.

Masks

Several different types of masks that cover the nose and mouth are available for oxygen delivery. All require humidification of the oxygen during use. Although the design of each type is different, the masks differ primarily in their FiO_2 delivery capabilities and their consistency in oxygen delivery. The simple face mask (Fig. 16–1D) delivers an FiO_2 of 0.30 to 0.60 with 5 to 8 L/minute of oxygen inflow, but it does not allow

for controlled oxygen administration. Changes in tidal volume and rate will lead to alterations in FiO_2 delivery. The Venturi mask (Fig. 16–1C) overcomes these problems, delivering controlled levels of oxygen at specific oxygen concentrations from 0.24 to 0.50.[8]

In order to achieve an FiO_2 greater than 0.60 with a face mask, a reservoir bag must be attached to the face mask (Fig. 16–1B). An FiO_2 of 1.0 can only be achieved when a one-way valve is placed between the reservoir bag and the mask. The valve prevents exhaled gas from re-entering the reservoir bag and lowering the FiO_2. This type of device is called a *nonrebreathing mask*. When the one-way valve is not present, the mask is a partial rebreathing mask with an FiO_2 delivery range of 0.35 to 0.80.[8,20,29]

Manual Resuscitation Bags

Another method for oxygen delivery, is a manual resuscitation bag, sometimes referred to as an *ambu-bag* or *bag-valve device*. This device provides ventilation and oxygen by manually compressing the bag, which is attached to an artificial airway (endotracheal or tracheostomy tube) or to a mask fitted over the patient's nose and mouth. The oxygen delivery range of these devices is variable, dependent on the design, oxygen inflow, presence of an oxygen reservoir, tidal volume, and rate of delivery. In general, when used at adult tidal volumes and rates with 15 L/minute of oxygen inflow, manual resuscitation bags without oxygen reservoirs deliver FiO_2 levels of 0.30 to 0.40, compared with 0.60 to 1.0 for those with an oxygen reservoir.[3,9,14]

Hazards of Oxygen Therapy

Despite the benefits of oxygen therapy, several adverse effects can occur during or after use, including hypoventilation, absorptive atelectasis, and pulmonary oxygen toxicity. Most sequelae are observed when oxygen therapy has been prolonged and at high FiO_2 levels (*i.e.*, >0.50).

Hypoventilation may occur during oxygen therapy in individuals with hypoxic ventilatory drives, such as in some

Table 16–1
Types of Oxygen Delivery Systems and FiO_2 Ranges*

METHODS	FiO_2 RANGE	ADVANTAGES AND DISADVANTAGES
Nasal cannula, 1–6 L/min†	0.24–0.38	Well tolerated by patient Inconsistent FiO_2 delivery
Venturi masks	0.24–0.50	Consistent FiO_2 delivery
Simple masks	0.30–0.60	Inconsistent FiO_2 delivery
Partial rebreathing masks, 7–10 L/min	0.35–0.80	
Nonrebreathing masks, 4–10 L/min	0.40–1.0	Consistent FiO_2 delivery
Manual resuscitation bags— no oxygen reservoir, 15 L/min	0.30–0.40	
Manual resuscitation bags— with oxygen reservoir, 15 L/min	0.60–1.0	Large variations in model types

* Approximate ranges
† Oxygen inflow into the device

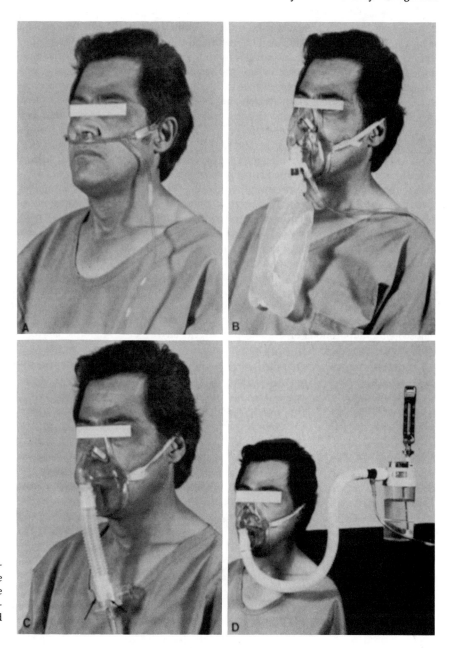

Figure 16-1
Different methods for delivery of oxygen therapy: (A) nasal cannula, (B) nonrebreather face mask, (C) Venturi facemask, (D) simple face mask. (Burton, G. G., and Hodgkin, J. E. *Respiratory Care: A Guide to Clinical Practice* (2nd ed.). Philadelphia: J.B. Lippincott, 1984)

forms of chronic obstructive pulmonary diseases. As the PaO_2 is raised with supplemental oxygen administration, the stimulus for the ventilatory drive is removed, leading to decreased ventilation or respiratory arrest. Oxygen must be administered with caution and at low levels for these individuals.

Absorptive atelectasis may occur with high FiO_2 administration because of a lack of nitrogen gas in the alveoli. Nitrogen normally is present in high concentrations in the alveoli and assists in keeping the alveoli open. As alveolar oxygen moves across the alveolar capillary membrane and is "absorbed" into the blood, the alveoli will collapse if minimal nitrogen gas is present in the alveoli.

The presence of a higher than normal amount of oxygen in the lower airways may lead to ciliary dysfunction, impaired removal of mucous, and respiratory distress syndrome. These sequelae of oxygen therapy are referred to as *pulmonary oxygen toxicity.*

AIRWAY ADJUNCTS

Prevention or treatment of transient, partial upper airway obstruction can be accomplished with a variety of different techniques. The use of oropharygeal, nasopharyngeal, and esophageal obturator airways facilitate patency of the upper airway.

Oropharyngeal Airway

The oropharyngeal airway is used to prevent upper airway obstruction from relaxation of the patient's tongue into the posterior wall of the pharynx. The oropharyngeal airway is semicircular and made of plastic, rubber, or metal materials (Fig. 16-2A). It is inserted upside down into the patient's oral cavity and then rotated to its proper position at the base of the tongue near the posterior pharyngeal wall. A tongue blade may also be used to move the tongue out of the way in order to place the airway. Care is taken to make sure that the patient's lips are not caught between the teeth and the airway. Improper placement or size of the airway traps the patient's tongue against the posterior pharynx and results in airway obstruction. Placement of the airway in an alert patient is not recommended because it may stimulate the gag reflex, causing retching and vomiting.

Nasopharyngeal Airway

A nasopharyngeal airway is used to maintain a patent airway in a semiconscious patient. It is inserted along the floor of the patient's nostril into the posterior pharynx behind the tongue (Fig. 16–2B). It is inserted gently with a water-soluble lubricant, preferably one containing a local anesthetic, to prevent trauma to the mucous membranes. The patency of the tube is checked after insertion. In patients with an intact gag reflex, the nasopharyngeal airway may be better tolerated than the oral airway. The nasopharyngeal airway also facilitates entering the trachea during nasotracheal suctioning and provides a less traumatic passageway for suctioning and fiberoptic bronchoscopy. Complications of the nasopharyngeal airway include sinusitis and erosion of the mucous membrane.[20]

ARTIFICIAL AIRWAYS

In many cases, the use of adjunct airways will be inadequate to facilitate ventilation and oxygenation. The insertion of a tube, or artificial airway, directly into the trachea is indicated for more severe upper airway obstruction, achievement of high levels of FiO_2, and when assisted ventilation is required. Criteria for intubation and ventilation are listed in Table 16–2.

Artificial airways may also be used to isolate or protect the lower airway from aspiration of secretions (oral, gastric) or foreign objects and to facilitate tracheal suctioning. A variety of artificial airways are available and include oral endotracheal tubes, nasal endotracheal tubes, and tracheostomy tubes.

Endotracheal Tubes

The endotracheal tube contains a standard universal adaptor for attachment to a manual resuscitation bag or mechanical ventilator tubing (Fig. 16–3). The end of the tube has an inflatable cuff that is used to seal off the airway after insertion, protecting the lungs from aspiration (Fig. 16–4). Tubes with high-volume, low-pressure inflatable cuffs should be used to avoid tracheal damage.

Endotracheal tubes may be inserted through either the nose or mouth. The oral endotracheal tube is passed directly into the trachea by means of laryngoscopic visualization of the glottis, larynx, and trachea (Technique Box 16–1). After insertion, the cuff is inflated with just enough air to create an airtight seal during ventilation with a manual resuscitation bag.[8,20,29] The position of the tube is determined by observing bilateral symmetric chest excursions and auscultating bilateral breath sounds. A chest radiograph is performed immediately after intubation, and periodically until extubation, to reveal any misposition of the tube in the trachea. After verification of proper placement, the centimeter marking on the endotra-

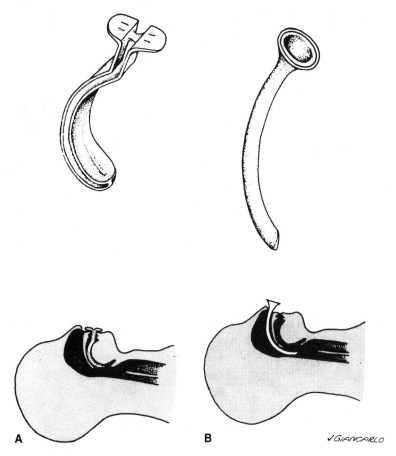

Figure 16–2

The oropharyngeal (*A*) and nasopharyngeal (*B*) airways. (Shapiro, B. A., Harrison, R. A., and Trout, C. A. *Clinical Application of Respiratory Care* (2nd ed.). Chicago: Yearbook Medical Publishers, 1979; with permission.)

Table 16–2
Assessment Parameters for Intubation and Ventilatory Assistance

	NORMAL	INTUBATION	VENTILATORY ASSISTANCE	PEEP	WEAN
Mechanics of ventilation:					
RR/min	12–16/min	>30/min	>35		<30
TV (ml/kg)	6–8 ml/kg	<5 ml/kg	<3.5		>5
VC (ml/kg)	50–60 ml/kg	<10 ml/kg	<10–15		>10–15
MIF cm H_2O	>−25 cm H_2O	<−20	<−25		>−20 cm H_2O
MV resting Lpm	<10 Lpm				<10 Lpm
Oxygenation:					
PaO_2 (mm Hg) 21%	80–90	Face mask < 70 mm Hg on 40%	<50	Ventilator < 65	>60
PaO_2 (mm Hg) 100%	550–630		<200		
P(A-a)O_2 21%	5–20	20–50	>50		
P(A-a)O_2 100%	20–60	>60	>350	>400	<350
Qs/Qt 5% CO	3%–8%	>15%	>40%	<20%	<15%
FRC					>50% of that predicted
pH	7.35–7.45	<7.25			
Ventilatory capability:					
$PaCO_2$ (mm Hg)	30–40	>50	>55		<40 or equal to preopertive level
VD/VT ratio	0.3–0.4	>0.6	>0.6		<0.6
Chest radiograph	Clear		Diffuse infiltrates		

CO: cardiac output; FRC: functional residual capacity; Lpm: liters per minute; MIF: maximum inspiratory force; MV: minute volume; P(A-a)O_2: alveolar-arterial oxygen difference; PEEP: positive end-expiratory pressure; pH: pH of the arterial blood; Qs/Qt: shunt fraction; RR/min: respirations per minute; TV: tidal volume; VC: vital capacity; VD/VT: dead space volume/tidal volume ratio.

cheal tube at the nasal or lip area should be marked and noted in the nursing record.

Nasal endotracheal tubes are often better tolerated by the conscious, nonsedated patient than are oral endotracheal tubes. Oral tubes are susceptible to occlusion from biting and cause increased salivation and stimulation of the gag reflex. Nasal endotracheal tubes permit the patient to close the mouth, are more easily anchored in place, and are less likely to move.

The disadvantages of nasal tubes are: that a smaller tube size is usually required, increasing the resistance to air flow; the tube is more difficult to keep patent and is more likely to kink owing to acute angulation in the nasal passage; the tube may obstruct drainage of the cranial sinuses; and the tube may cause nasal necrosis or epistaxis.[8] Nasal endotracheal intubation may be more technically difficult to perform than oral intubation. Endotracheal tubes are commonly left in place for extended periods of time, up to 6 weeks in some institutions. If an artificial airway is required for more than 6 weeks, a tracheostomy is usually performed.

Complications that may occur during endotracheal intubation include trauma to the nasal and oral mucosa, teeth, larynx, and trachea, and intubation of the esophagus or right main-stem bronchus. Intubation complications from endotracheal tubes include tracheal ischemia, necrosis, malacia, or stenosis; sinusitis (nasal tubes); occlusion of the airway by dried secretions or herniation of the cuff; and accidental extubation.

Tracheostomy Tubes

Tracheostomy tubes sometimes are used as the artificial airway when prolonged intubation is necessary (Fig. 16–5). A tracheostomy is performed rarely in an emergency situation but rather as an elective, operative procedure after successful endotracheal intubation. The tracheostomy tube (Fig. 16–5B) is a short, angulated tube that is inserted directly into the trachea while avoiding the upper airway and glottis. This allows for a larger-diameter tube, which decreases problems of airway resistance and occlusion. A standard connector and cuff are similar to those of an endotracheal tube. In addition, some types of tracheostomy tubes have an inner cannula (Fig. 16–5A) that is periodically removed for cleansing.

Many complications may develop after tracheostomy (Table 16–3). A rare but often dramatic and fatal complication of tracheostomy is innominate artery erosion. Although it occurs in less than 1% of tracheostomies, the peak incidence of innominate artery erosion occurs within 1 to 2 weeks after tracheostomy.[8] Patients at high risk for erosion include those with high- or low-placed tracheostomy stomas; overinflated cuffs; low-volume, high-pressure tracheostomy cuffs; and pulsation of the tracheostomy tube. If bleeding occurs, cuff inflation should be used to control bleeding until emergency surgery is performed.

Early dislodgement of the tracheostomy can often be avoided if the tube is secured at the flange with sutures as well as ties around the neck (Fig. 16–5D). The sutures may be left in place for 4 to 5 days until a tract is well formed to facilitate reinsertion.

NURSING MANAGEMENT OF PATIENTS WITH ARTIFICIAL AIRWAYS

The introduction of an artificial airway bypasses the upper airway, causing a loss of the filtering and humidification of inhaled gases, cough, and vocal functions. The majority of nursing interventions are designed to compensate for this loss

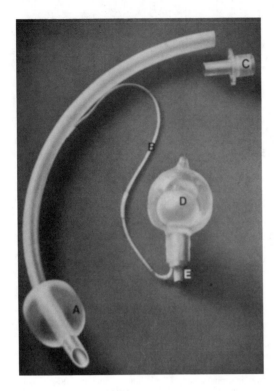

Figure 16–3
Lanz endotracheal tube: (*A*) tracheal cuff, (*B*) pilot line, (*C*) 15-mm adaptor, (*D*) pilot balloon reservoir, (*E*) pressure-regulating valve. (Burton, G. G., and Hodgkin, J. E. *Respiratory Care: A Guide to Clinical Practice* (2nd ed.). Philadelphia: J.B. Lippincott, 1984)

of upper airway function or to prevent complications associated with artificial airways.

Nursing Diagnosis: Ineffective Airway Clearance

The inability to generate a productive cough, humidify, and filter inspired gas can lead to secretion retention, inspissated

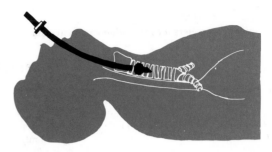

Figure 16–4
Placement of endotracheal tube in the trachea.

mucus, mucus plugging, and pneumonia. Nursing interventions to prevent these complications include encouragement of coughing, airway suctioning and humidification, and chest physiotherapy.

Suctioning

The removal of retained secretions through the endotracheal or tracheostomy tube should be performed whenever clinically indicated rather than on a fixed schedule.[8,20,29] Indications for suctioning include presence of coughing, auscultation of coarse crackles over the large airways, and higher-than-normal airway pressures during mechanical ventilation. Complications associated with suctioning include decreases in PaO_2,[2] increases in arterial carbon dioxide tension ($PaCO_2$),[2] increases in mean arterial pressure,[10,25] cardiac dysrhythmias,[22,30,35] and sudden death.[1] Trauma to the tracheal mucosa also occurs and includes bleeding and denuding of the tracheal cilia.[19]

Suctioning is always a sterile procedure (Technique Box 16–2) for critically ill patients, because they are at high risk for nosocomial pneumonias. Administration of hyperinflation and hyperoxygenation breaths before and after each pass of the suction catheter has been recommended to avoid some of the complications previously described.[11,12,27] A manual resuscitation bag or the mechanical ventilator may be used for this purpose. Depending on the model, use of the ventilator for

---

TECHNIQUE BOX 16–1.   Assisting With Insertion of an Endotracheal Tube

1. A stylet may be used to ease insertion of the tube. The stylet is a malleable wire that has a blunt end. It is placed in the endotracheal tube before insertion to make it stiffer. The stylet must be kept at least 1 inch back from the end of the tube. If it is not, the end of the stylet may perforate the trachea or bronchus during insertion.
2. Use a tube of the proper size (usually 7.5-mm and 8.5-mm tubes are used for female and male adults, respectively). All tubes have the standard adaptor.
3. Before insertion, check the tube to make sure it will inflate easily, hold air, expand evenly, and deflate completely.
4. If desired, lubricate the tip of the tube with a water-soluble or 5% lidocaine jelly.
5. Before intubation, position the patient with the head and neck in the sniffing position.
6. Ascertain that suction equipment, including a Yanhaeur suction tip, is available.

7. Administer 100% oxygen for 3 to 5 minutes to increase alveolar oxygen concentration. A manual resuscitation bag and mask must be available to administer ventilation in case of respiratory insufficiency.
8. Provide assistance while the physician performs the intubation.
9. When the tube has been placed in the trachea, inflate the cuff and ventilate with the manual resuscitation bag.
10. Immediately assess for correct placement of the tube by noting the adequacy of chest expansion and presence of bilateral breath sounds. If the tube is in the right main-stem bronchus, breath sounds may be decreased or absent on the left side.
11. Mark the endotracheal tube at the level of the patient's lip (nares for nasal endotracheal tube).
12. Secure the tube with an endotracheal tube fixation device or tape.
13. Obtain a stat portable chest radiograph to verify proper positioning of the tube in the trachea.

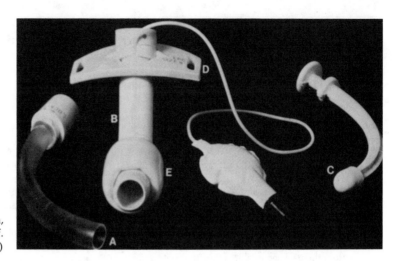

Figure 16-5

A standard tracheostomy tube showing (*A*) inner cannula, (*B*) outer cannula, (*C*) obturator, (*D*) flange, and (*E*) cuff. (Reproduced with permission of Shiley Laboratories, Inc.)

hyperinflation and hyperoxygenation may present hazards such as delays in achievement of high FiO$_2$ levels (up to 2 minutes for some models)[4] or the staff inadvertently forgetting to return to the presuction FiO$_2$ level.

Other measures that should be included in the suctioning interventions to prevent complications include the following: limit the length of time for each suction catheter pass to less than 10 to 15 seconds,[31] use small-diameter suction catheters (less than half the diameter of the artificial airway inner diameter),[6] and use coude (curve-tipped) catheters to improve intubation of the left main-stem bronchus.[18,24] The use of universal barrier precautions (*i.e.*, goggle, mask, gloves) is recommended during suctioning for the protection of the health care personnel.

Positioning the head to the right or left side does not improve suction catheter intubation of the left bronchus,[24] and the application of intermittent suction, rather than continuous suction, does not decrease damage to the tracheal mucosa.[23] The common practice of instilling sterile normal saline into the artificial airway before suctioning has not been shown to improve removal of secretions;[5,15] in fact, it may predispose the patient to bronchospasm[5] and increased risk of nosocomial pneumonia.[28]

Table 16-3

Complications Associated With Placement of a Tracheostomy Tube

Acute hemorrhage at operative site
Air embolism
Aspiration
Delayed tracheal stenosis
Dislodged tube
Erosion into the innominate artery with sudden exsanguination
Failure of the tracheostomy cuff
Left recurrent laryngeal nerve damage
Obstruction of tracheostomy tube
Placement in the right main-stem bronchus
Pneumothorax
Subcutaneous and mediastinal emphysema
Swallowing dysfunction
Tracheoesophageal fistula
Wound infection

The recent introduction of a closed-system in-line suction catheter system, although seemingly very practical, has several theoretical disadvantages. Suctioning in a closed airway space may remove large amounts of intrapulmonary gas and produce excessive intrapulmonary negative pressure, resulting in atelectasis. The impact of this technique on rates of nosocomial pneumonia is unknown. Until more data are available on the safety of the closed suctioning system, caution should be exercised in its clinical implementation.

Continuous assessment during suctioning is important to identify changes in cardiac rhythm, arterial pressure, development of hypoxemia, or other signs and symptoms of cardiovascular or pulmonary compromise. Suctioning should be discontinued if complications develop during suctioning.

Humidification

Humidification of gases inspired into the lungs is important to prevent damage (*i.e.*, bleeding, reduced mucociliary transport, bacterial invasion) to the tracheal and bronchial mucosa. The use of an artificial airway bypasses the humidification function of the nose and pharynx. Exogenous humidification of inspired gases is thus required to avoid excessive mucosal drying and retention of thickened secretions. A variety of devices can be used during spontaneous breathing or mechanical ventilation to provide humidification. Most function by passing the inspired gases through a container of heated sterile water before delivery to the artificial airway.

Chest Physiotherapy

Another method to improve removal of secretions from the large airways is chest physiotherapy. Chest physiotherapy consists of four different processes: the positioning of a specific lung area to maximize gravity (postural) drainage; gentle clapping with a cupped hand over the chest wall (percussion); mechanical or manual vibration of the chest wall (vibration); and removal of secretions from the large airways by coughing or suctioning. This intervention has been shown to increase secretion removal in a variety of acute and chronic pulmonary conditions, such as lobar atelectasis, chronic bronchitis, cystic fibrosis, and other conditions with large mucus production.[16,17] The "prophylactic" use of chest physiotherapy to prevent ac-

TECHNIQUE BOX 16–2. Procedure for Suctioning an Artificial Airway (Endotracheal or Tracheostomy)

Before beginning the suctioning, the nurse should explain the suctioning procedure to the patient, procure all the materials needed for suctioning, and make sure the equipment is functional.

1. Auscultate the chest for adventitious sounds before suctioning.
2. Gather necessary equipment (suction apparatus, sterile suction catheter kit, sterile H_2O, manual resuscitation bag (MRB) connected to oxygen, universal barriers).
3. Wash hands.
4. Adjust the suction control gauge to 80 to 160 mm Hg.
5. Adjust the oxygen inflow to the MRB.
6. Open the sterile catheter kit.
7. Don the universal barrier equipment, and connect the catheter to the suction tubing. The catheter should not be removed from the package until it is time to use it.
8. Put on sterile gloves.
9. Remove the ventilator tubing or humidification tubing from the artificial airway, protecting it from contamination.
10. Ventilate the patient with five to eight hyperinflation and hyperoxygenation breaths with the MRB or ventilator. *Caution:* If the setting on the ventilator is increased to an FiO_2 of 1.0, be sure to return it to the prescribed setting immediately after suctioning.
11. Insert the sterile catheter with the thumbhole open until resistance is met.
12. Apply suction as the catheter is withdrawn with a twirling motion.
13. Limit the suctioning and withdrawal time to 10 to 15 seconds.
14. Ventilate the patient with the MRB between each catheter insertion.
15. Repeat steps 10 to 14 for one or two more passes of the suction catheter if secretions are present.
16. Observe the cardiac monitor during suctioning for any dysrhythmias. Suctioning should be stopped and ventilation with the MRB provided if dysrhythmias develop.
17. Suction the posterior pharynx.
18. Reconnect the ventilator or humidification tubing to the artificial airway, checking the entire system for appropriate connections and settings.
19. Assess the patient for bilateral chest excursions, rate of respiration, and heart rate and rhythm, and auscultate the chest to see if the suctioning has decreased the adventitious sounds.

cumulation of secretions has not been supported by clinical research.[17]

Contraindications to chest physiotherapy include pulmonary hemorrhage, bronchospasm, rib fractures, thrombocytopenia, or tendancy to bleed. Chest physiotherapy should be administered with caution in individuals with low PaO_2 levels or hemodynamic instability.[20]

Nursing Diagnosis: Impaired Verbal Communication

The introduction of an artificial airway eliminates the patient's ability to communicate verbally, requiring the use of other communication methods. Alternative forms for communication include writing (*e.g.*, paper and pen, "magic" slates, chalk boards), pointing at drawings or letters on an alphabet and picture board; mouthing words; and using call lights, buzzers, or bells to gain staff's attention. Several of these forms should be readily available to facilitate communication, depending on the skills of the patient and nurses. One should consider deficits in manual dexterity or visual acuity that are often present in critically ill patients and make written communication difficult.

It is important to appreciate the frustration that can be associated with the inability to communicate one's thoughts, concerns, and desires rapidly and easily to others. The anticipation of patients' needs or questions is an important method to decrease frustration, as is the use of yes/no types of questions. (See also Nursing Diagnosis: Impaired Verbal Communication, Chap. 8.)

Nursing Diagnosis: High Risk for Complications Related to Artificial Airways

The introduction of an artificial airway predisposes the patient to a variety of complications, the most common of which are tracheal damage, pulmonary infection, and airway dislodgement. Nursing interventions to decrease or avoid these complications include stabilization of the artificial airway, maintenance of low cuff pressures, and stringent infection-control practices.

Airway Stabilization

Movement of artificial airways leads to oral, nasal, and epiglottic tissue trauma, tracheal mucosal damage, or unplanned extubation. Stabilization of the airway with tape or a commercially available fixation device (Fig. 16–6) is required to prevent in-and-out movement and excessive pressure on the oral or nasal cavities. In patients who require long-term airway management or in those with altered skin integrity, the use of a fixation device may be preferred.[32] In addition, most of these devices have a built-in bite block to prevent occlusion of the airway during biting.

Maintenance of Low Cuff Pressure

When the pressure of the airway cuff exceeds the capillary perfusion pressure, tracheal ischemia and necrosis can occur. The use of high-volume, low-pressure cuffs has greatly decreased the incidence of tracheal pressure damage. The pressure and volume within the cuff should be monitored periodically by connecting a three- or four-way stopcock to the cuff port, a syringe, and an aneroid or mercury manometer (Fig. 16–7). After cuff deflation, the volume of air required to prevent air leaks around the airway is noted, as well as the intracuff pressure. Pressures should be maintained below 20 mm Hg.[20]

Infection-Control Practices

Aseptic techniques for handling the patient's artificial airway, performing tracheal suctioning, and obtaining cultures of tra-

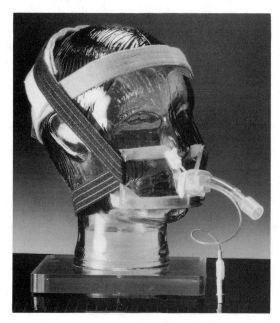

Figure 16-6

Endotracheal tube fixation device. (Reproduced with permission of Respironics, Inc., Murrysville, PA)

cheal secretions are important. Ventilator tubing and humidifiers should be changed every 24 hours and whenever contaminated.[8,20,29] Condensation that collects in the ventilator tubing should never be emptied into the humidifier. Manual resuscitation bags should be changed periodically.

VENTILATORS

The application of mechanical ventilation is indicated for a variety of clinical conditions that lead to inadequate ventilation or oxygenation. A variety of positive- and negative-pressure ventilators are available to provide assistance to the patient's ventilation. Negative-pressure ventilators, such as the iron lung or cuirass chest ventilator, are rarely used today in the acute management of respiratory failure. This section focuses on positive-pressure ventilators.

Classification of Ventilators

Positive-pressure ventilators force gas into the lungs during inspiration, generating positive alveolar pressure. Expiration occurs passively when the mechanical inspiratory gas flow ceases. Several types of positive-pressure ventilators exist and are classified according to how they terminate the inspiratory flow cycle: pressure-limited, volume-limited, and time-limited.

Pressure cycled ventilators deliver inspiratory gas until the pressure in the pulmonary airways reaches a predetermined level. Changes in airway resistance and pulmonary or chest wall compliance will alter the amount of gas delivered during inspiration (tidal volume). This variable tidal volume delivery, which is characteristic of pressure-limited ventilators, limits their use in acute ventilatory management because of frequent changes in airway resistance and compliance. An example of a pressure-limited ventilator is the Byrd Mark 6.

Volume-limited ventilators deliver inspiratory gas until a preset tidal volume is achieved, even if very high airway pres-

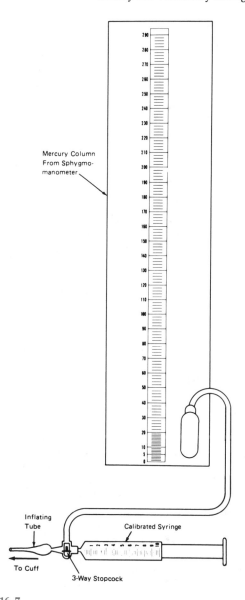

Figure 16-7

Measurement of artificial airway cuff pressures by connecting a three- or four-way stopcock to the inflating tube of the cuff, a 10-ml syringe, and a mercury manometer. (Burton, G. G., and Hodgkin, J. E. *Respiratory Care: A Guide to Clinical Practice* (2nd ed.). Philadelphia: J.B. Lippincott, 1984)

sures are required. These ventilators provide greater control over ventilation and oxygenation and are commonly employed in acute ventilatory management. Examples of volume-limited ventilators are the Puritan Bennett MA-1, MA-2, and 7200A, and the Bourns Bear I to V.

Time-limited ventilators deliver inspiratory gas for a predetermined interval of time. Changes in pulmonary airway resistance and compliance will lead to variability in tidal volume delivery. Examples of time-limited ventilators include the Siemens Servo 900, 900B, and 900C, and the Monaghan 225.

Many of the newer, microprocessor-type ventilators (*e.g.*, Servo 900C) are capable of functioning in more than one type of inspiratory flow cycle.

The majority of ventilators on the market today have built-in safety features to prevent excessively high pressure, volume, or flow delivery rates despite their classification type. The incorporation of these alarms prevents, for example, the delivery of dangerously high airway pressures during inspiration with a volume-limited ventilator. In addition, continuous monitoring exists to alert the practitioner to excessively high or low tidal volumes (TV), inspiratory/expiratory ratios, and respiratory rates.

Modes of Ventilation

Positive-pressure ventilators are capable of providing a range of ventilatory support, from total support to no support. There are four basic modes, or patterns, of ventilatory support: controlled mechanical ventilation, assist/control ventilation, intermittent mechanical ventilation, and spontaneous ventilation (Table 16–4). A new ventilation mode available on some ventilators is pressure support ventilation.[26,34]

During controlled mechanical ventilation, the ventilator delivers a set number of breaths per minute at a set tidal volume with no patient-initiated breaths. The total work of ventilation is accomplished by the mechanical ventilator.[21] The airway pressures, tidal volume, and pattern of ventilation during controlled mechanical ventilation are depicted in Figure 16–8A.

During assist/control ventilation, a preset minimum number of breaths per minute are delivered at a preset tidal volume by the ventilator ("controlled"), but the patient may initiate additional breaths ("assist"). These additional requested breaths are delivered at the same tidal volume as the "controlled" breaths. Virtually all the work of breathing is accomplished by the ventilator in the assist/control mode. Ventilatory patterns, airway pressures, and tidal volumes are shown in Figure 16–8B.

During intermittent mandatory ventilation, the ventilator delivers a set number of breaths per minute, at a set tidal volume, but allows the patient to breath spontaneously in-between "mandated" ventilator breaths. The spontaneous breaths are at whatever tidal volume the patient is able to achieve or generate on his or her own without ventilator sup-port. The FiO_2 level for these spontaneous breaths is the same as for the mandated breaths. The work of breathing with intermittent mandatory ventilation is shared by the ventilator (mandated breaths) and the patient (spontaneous breaths). Ventilatory patterns, airway pressures, and tidal volume delivery are shown in Figure 16–8C.

During spontaneous ventilation, the patient determines the respiratory rate, and tidal volume delivery is dependent on the patient's respiratory muscle capabilities. No assistance to breathing is provided by the ventilator. Delivery of FiO_2 during spontaneous ventilation is controlled at the preset level. Use of the ventilator during spontaneous ventilation is primarily to "monitor" the spontaneous tidal volume, respiratory rate, and a variety of other parameters. Use of the spontaneous ventilation mode on most ventilators causes a small increase in the work of breathing because of increased resistance to inspiration from the ventilator demand valve. The ventilatory patterns, airway pressures, and tidal volume delivery are shown in Figure 16–8D.

Pressure support ventilation is a mode of ventilation available on some of the new microprocessor ventilators (Servo 900C, Bennett 7200A). A high rate of gas flow is delivered by the ventilator at a preset level of positive pressure during spontaneous inspiration, augmenting the spontaneous tidal volume of the patient. The amount of tidal volume assistance contributed by the ventilator is a function of the level of airway pressure support level selected. Pressure support ventilation was designed initially to provide a small level of ventilatory assistance during spontaneous ventilation to overcome the resistance to inspiration caused by the ventilator circuit.[13] Recent application of high airway pressure levels during pressure support ventilation has expanded its use as a more complete ventilatory support[34] and as a weaning modality.[7] Figure 16–8E depicts the tidal volume, pressure, and ventilatory pattern seen during pressure support ventilation.

Positive End-Expiratory Pressure

Normally during expiration, airway pressures return to zero. The application of positive pressure to the airways at the end of expiration is termed *PEEP*, or positive end-expiratory pressure. Positive end-expiratory pressure increases the end-ex-

Table 16–4
Common Modes of Mechanical Ventilation

VENTILATORY MODE	DESCRIPTION
Continuous mandatory ventilation (CMV)	This is controlled ventilation with the ventilator delivering a set number of breaths per minute to the patient, allowing for no patient initiation of breaths.
Assist/Control (A/C)	Similar to CMV, it assures a minimum number of breaths per minute, but allows the patient to initiate the breaths and to increase above the minimum level.
Intermittent mandatory ventilation (IMV)	Periodic controlled ventilation. The inspiratory pressure is positive, and the patient breathes spontaneously between controlled breaths.
Spontaneous ventilation (SV)	The airway pressure is slightly negative during inspiration and slightly positive during expiration to move tidal volume.
Pressure support ventilation (PSV)	It augments the patient's tidal volume by delivering gas flow to a preset pressure level during spontaneous ventilation.
Positive end-expiratory pressure (PEEP)	At the end of expiration, a residual pressure is greater than atmospheric.
Continuous (or constant) positive airway pressure (CPAP)	Throughout a spontaneous breathing cycle, the pressure at the airway opening is greater than atmospheric.
High-frequency ventilation (HFV)	Ventilatory frequency of 60 to 100/minute or greater with small tidal volumes. The transpulmonary pressure is continuously positive throughout ventilatory cycle.

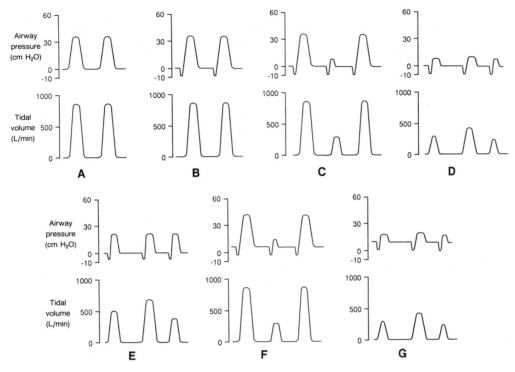

Figure 16–8

Examples of airway pressures and tidal volume delivery during mechanical ventilation modes: (*A*) controlled, (*B*) assist/control, (*C*) intermittent mandatory ventilation (IMV), (*D*) spontaneous ventilation, (*E*) pressure support ventilation, (*F*) positive end-expiratory pressure (PEEP) with IMV, (*G*) continuous positive-pressure ventilation (CPAP).

piratory lung volumes (functional residual capacity) and is employed to improve gas exchange, primarily oxygenation, in pulmonary conditions characterized by small airway collapse.[8,20,29] Positive end-expiratory pressure can be applied with the patient breathing spontaneously or while the patient is mechanically ventilated (Fig. 16–8F). Positive end-expiratory pressure generally is administered at pressures of 3 to 10 cm H_2O. High levels of PEEP (>15–20 cm H_2O) occasionally may be required in some patients with very low compliance and severe respiratory insufficiency.

Positive end-expiratory pressure increases intrathoracic pressure, which has a potentially negative effect on venous return to the right heart. Cardiac output and systemic arterial pressures may decrease with excessive levels of PEEP. Hypovolemia potentiates these hemodynamic changes. An optimal level of PEEP is characterized by a decrease in the percentage of shunt, an increase in the functional residual capacity, no significant increase in pulmonary capillary wedge pressure, maintenance of systemic blood pressure, an increase in the PaO_2, and minimal alteration in cardiac output.

The use of PEEP, especially high levels in lungs with low compliance, may cause an increase in the incidence of subcutaneous and mediastinal emphysema and tension pneumothorax. Therefore, PEEP should be maintained at the lowest level possible for optimal pulmonary function on a nontoxic concentration of oxygen.

Continuous Positive Airway Pressure

Continuous positive airway pressure (CPAP) is based essentially on the same principle as PEEP. The primary difference is that CPAP is positive expiratory airway pressure applied in patients breathing spontaneously without any ventilator support (Fig. 16–8G). Positive end-expiratory pressure is positive expiratory airway pressure applied during positive-pressure ventilation with a mechanical ventilator.

Continuous positive airway pressure can be applied through a mechanical ventilator circuit during spontaneous ventilation or, if an artificial airway is not present, by a special tight-fitting face mask. Continuous positive airway pressure delivered by face mask may be especially useful in alert, nonintubated patients who have inadequate PaO_2 levels despite delivery of maximal amounts of supplemental oxygen. Lethargic patients are not candidates for CPAP because they may not be able to remove the mask if vomiting should occur. Potential complications of CPAP therapy by face mask include aspiration, gastric dilatation, and facial pressure, which may cause discomfort and tissue necrosis.

High-Frequency Ventilation

During the past several years, three new techniques for high-frequency ventilation have evolved: high-frequency jet ventilation, high-frequency positive-pressure ventilation, and high-frequency oscillation.[26,34] Each system brings different physiologic effects and results. Many questions remain on how and whether any of these techniques are beneficial to ventilatory management.

Complications of Mechanical Ventilation

Many adverse sequelae are known to occur with mechanical ventilation (Table 16–5). The most significant complications

Table 16–5

Complications Associated With Mechanical Ventilation

ASSOCIATED WITH THE COMPLICATIONS TO OPERATION OF THE VENTILATOR

Failure of alarm or machine
Alarm "turned off"
Inadequate nebulization or humidification
Overheating of inspired air leading to mild hyperthermia
Fluid overloading compounded by humidified inspired air

ASSOCIATED WITH ALTERED PHYSIOLOGY DURING ASSISTED VENTILATION

Barotrauma
    Pneumothorax
    Pneumomediastinum
    Subcutaneous emphysema
Nosocomial pulmonary infections
Macroatelectasis secondary to obstruction of the left
    main-stem bronchus
Alveolar hyperventilation leading to hypocapnia and
    respiratory alkalosis
Alveolar hypoventilation leading to hypoxia, hypercarbia,
    and respiratory acidosis
Massive gastric distention
Microatelectasis after hypoventilation
Positive fluid balance
Depressed cardiac output and hypotension

are pulmonary barotrauma and cardiovascular compromise. Barotrauma includes several complications related to overdistention of the alveolar airways, including pneumothorax, pneumomediastinum, and subcutaneous emphysema. Increases in intrathoracic pressures cause decreased venous return and cardiac output, which lead to a compensatory fluid retention. Additional complications include acid-base disturbances, nosocomial infections, and mechanical ventilator failure.

NURSING MANAGEMENT OF PATIENTS ON MECHANICAL VENTILATION

The use of a mechanical ventilator to support ventilation and oxygenation places an enormous responsibility on the medical and nursing staff to ensure proper operation of the equipment. Nursing interventions associated with mechanical ventilation are directed at ensuring a safe and efficacious interface between this technology and the critically ill patient.

Nursing Diagnosis: High Risk for Inadequate Gas Exchange

Inadequate gas exchange may occur because of changes in the patient's condition or ventilator malfunction. Frequent assessment of the patient's response to mechanical ventilation is imperative to provide early detection of and intervention for changes in gas exchange. In addition to periodic arterial blood gas analysis, continuous monitoring (invasive and noninvasive) of cardiopulmonary response to ventilation may include electrocardiogram, arterial and pulmonary artery pressures, SaO_2, SvO_2, pulse oximetry, lung volumes and pressures, and exhaled gas tensions.

Another cause of inadequate gas exchange is dysynchrony between the patient and ventilator interface. "Fighting the ventilator" can be extremely detrimental to gas exchange and maintainence of low airway pressures. Causes of dysynchrony include inappropriate ventilator settings for the patient's current physiologic state, airway obstruction, ventilator malfunction, anxiety, or use of unusually high levels of ventilatory support (e.g., PEEP > 20 cm H_2O; respiratory rates > 40/minute).

Immediate intervention is indicated for "fighting the ventilator." The patient should be removed from the ventilator, and ventilation should be provided with a manual resuscitation bag while another person checks the ventilator for problems. A rapid assessment of the patient's cardiopulmonary status (i.e., blood pressure, heart rate, cardiac rhythm, color, breath sounds, chest wall movement, airway patency, arterial blood gas analysis) is performed while providing reassurance to the patient. Endotracheal suctioning may be appropriate to ensure a patent airway. Sedation or paralysis may then be required if agitation persists and gas exchange is affected negatively.

Nursing Diagnosis: High Risk for Complications Associated With Mechanical Ventilation

Frequent assessment for signs and symptoms of complications associated with mechanical ventilation (see Table 16–5) is essential to minimize the consequences to the patient. Of particular concern are complications associated with barotrauma, such as pneumothorax and subcutaneous emphysema, depressed cardiac output, and operational failures of the mechanical ventilator.

As the complexity of the ventilator design has increased to provide improved ventilatory support, so has the incidence of operational failures with the technology. Nurses must be knowledgeable and competent in the operation of each type of ventilator that is used in their institution in order to intervene appropriately when operational failures occur. The appropriate use of extensive alarm systems to monitor exhaled tidal volume, airway pressures, FiO_2 levels, and inhaled gas temperature continuously is essential to provide an early warning system for potential ventilator problems.

Weaning the Patient From Mechanical Ventilation

Immediately after placing a patient on mechanical ventilation, one must begin to determine when he or she can be removed from the ventilator. The three major complications of weaning are carbon dioxide retention, hypoxemia, and cardiovascular instability.

The criteria for weaning a patient from the ventilator are essentially the reverse of those for instituting ventilatory support (see Table 16–2). However, there are no simple determinations to indicate when mechanical ventilatory support should be terminated. Once oxygen and carbon dioxide tension levels in the arterial blood are within normal limits, there are few tests that accurately predict success or failure of weaning. Weaning should not be attempted in a patient who has too little strength to inspire (maximal inspiratory force is the amount of negative pressure the patient can generate when inhaling against a closed valve); a forced vital capacity of less than 10 ml/kg; hypovolemia; life-threatening dysrhythmias; a low cardiac index; an increased oxygen consumption; uncorrected acidosis or alkalosis; a V_D (dead space volume)/V_T (tidal volume) ratio of 60% or greater, or severe catabolism. When patients with chronic obstructive pulmonary disease are weaned from the ventilator, their PaO_2 and $PaCO_2$ levels should be as close as possible to their normal baseline levels.

Weaning the patient from mechanical ventilation generally is not begun until the level of FiO_2 is less than 0.50 and PEEP has been reduced to less than 10 cm H_2O. Before beginning the weaning process, the nurse must give the patient an adequate explanation of the purpose of the weaning procedure in order to avoid unnecessary anxiety. The patient should be reassured that someone will be in constant attendance, monitoring his or her response to the weaning process. The patient should be repositioned to facilitate diaphragmatic movement. A sitting or semirecumbent position is usually best tolerated. The airway should also be suctioned if secretions are present.

Baseline data should be obtained before weaning; these data include heart rate, cardiac rhythm and frequency of ectopy, blood pressure, respiratory rate, spontaneous minute volume, arterial blood gas values, and level of consciousness. Frequent assessment of these parameters should continue throughout the weaning process and guide decisions relative to the weaning success.

Weaning is accomplished with T-piece or CPAP trials of spontaneous breathing or intermittent mandatory ventilation. Recently, pressure support ventilation has also been advocated alone or in combination with CPAP or intermittent mandatory ventilation to facilitate the weaning process.

T-Piece and CPAP Trials

With T-piece weaning, the patient is removed from the ventilator and allowed to breath spontaneously for a period of time. Humidified oxygen is provided by way of a T-piece connection to the endotracheal or tracheostomy tube. There should be a continuous visible flow of humidified gas out of the exhalation port of the T-piece to avoid entrainment of room air into the delivered gas and a decrease in actual FiO_2 delivery.

Continuous positive airway pressure weaning is similar to T-piece weaning except that the patient remains on the mechanical ventilator during spontaneous breathing with a small amount of end-expiratory pressure. This method allows for more accurate FiO_2 delivery and monitoring of respiratory rate and tidal volume. Use of the mechanical ventilator during spontaneous breathing does slightly increase the work of breathing over the T-piece technique.

The length of time on the T-piece or CPAP trial is increased gradually as the patient's tolerance increases for spontaneous breathing. This continues until no ventilatory support is required to maintain cardiopulmonary stability.

Intermittent Mandatory Ventilation

Intermittent mandatory ventilation weaning is accomplished by a gradual decrease in the number of breaths per minute that the mechanical ventilator delivers, with the patient being allowed gradually to take over more of the work of breathing. Spontaneous ventilation by the patient progressively assumes a greater proportion of alveolar minute ventilation as mandatory breaths from the ventilator are decreased.

Pressure Support Ventilation

A relatively new method of weaning from mechanical ventilation is the use of pressure support ventilation. This technique can be accomplished only with the new microprocessor ventilators. With this technique, spontaneous breathing is augmented with gas flow from the ventilator to achieve a preset level of airway pressure. As the level of pressure support is decreased, the patient must assume a greater proportion of alveolar minute ventilation to maintain PaO_2 and $PaCO_2$ levels. As with CPAP, the use of the ventilator during the weaning process allows for greater control of FiO_2 delivery and monitoring of tidal volumes.

Failure to Wean

During weaning, if the spontaneous breathing effort is inadequate, the patient will develop acid-base or oxygenation disturbances that lead to respiratory distress. The development of any of the following signs and symptoms usually indicates respiratory distress, which requires the discontinuance of weaning: increases or decreases of greater than 10% in blood pressure, respiratory, or heart rates; tidal volumes of less than 300 ml; PaO_2 less than 60 mm Hg; $PaCO_2$ greater than 55 mm Hg; or pH less than 7.35.

Repeated failure to wean a patient from the ventilator is usually caused by one or more of the following basic problems:

- An increase in the alveolar ventilation requirement in the presence of an increase in V_D/V_T ratio or an increase in the $PaCO_2$ level
- A decrease in muscle strength secondary to metabolic wasting, inadequate nutrition, or respiratory discoordination
- An increase in the work of breathing after a decrease in lung compliance or an increase in airway resistance due to bronchospasm or mucous obstruction or narrowing of the air conduits with edema

Daily efforts should be made to strengthen the patient's respiratory muscles and ventilation ability by using a T-piece, CPAP, or pressure support ventilation for a few minutes and then returning the patient to mechanical ventilation. The period during which the patient is off the ventilator should be lengthened as the rest periods are shortened. The patient should be kept on the ventilator at night. Maximal nutritional efforts should be made to provide the energy needed for the work of spontaneous breathing.

Weaning From the Artificial Airway

If a patient tolerates spontaneous breathing without undue anxiety or inadequate cardiopulmonary function, extubation may be performed.

Before removal of the endotracheal tube, the patient should be suctioned adequately and placed in a sitting position. The cuff should be deflated and the tube removed quickly. Usually supplemental oxygen is delivered after extubation to ensure a PaO_2 level of 70 mm Hg.

After extubation, the patient may be hoarse and have some difficulty swallowing. Food and fluids by mouth are withheld for the first few hours. Bland liquids are given initially under supervision to determine the patient's ability to swallow. Upper airway obstruction secondary to edema of the vocal cords or larynx may occur. The patient should be observed for stridor and dyspnea. It may become necessary to re-establish an artificial airway.

A patient with a tracheostomy tube who has tolerated spontaneous breathing may have the cuffed tracheostomy tube replaced by a noncuffed fenestrated tracheostomy tube or have the tracheostomy tube removed and the stoma covered with a sterile, nonocclusive dressing. A fenestrated tube has a window that allows the patient to breathe through his or her own upper respiratory tract, to talk, and to cough if the external outlet is plugged. No inner cannula should be in place when the external outlet of a fenestrated tube is plugged.

Weaning from the inspired oxygen concentration may take several days. When supplemental oxygen therapy is discontinued, blood gas analyses should be made 30 minutes and 90 minutes after the discontinuation. If the patient seems hoarse, warm, humidified air may be administered through a face tent.

SUMMARY

Critically ill patients often require artificial airways and mechanical ventilation to support adequate respiratory function. A thorough understanding of these devices, their advantages and disadvantages, and the requirements for nursing management is imperative in order to provide quality care.

DIRECTIONS FOR FUTURE RESEARCH

Despite the large amount of nursing research on ventilatory support, many aspects of care, such as the following, need to be examined:

1. What are the most effective, least anxiety-producing techniques for weaning patients from mechanical ventilation?
2. What is the most effective method for decreasing the viscosity of pulmonary secretions?
3. What are the most effective methods for communicating with critically ill patients who are intubated?
4. What effect does closed-suction techniques have on cardiopulmonary function and rates of nosocomial infection?
5. What is the best method for artificial airway stabilization to prevent tracheal wall damage and accidental dislodgements?
6. In what conditions is chest physiotherapy beneficial for mechanically ventilated patients?
7. During chronic mechanical ventilation, does respiratory muscle "training" decrease the length of time for weaning?
8. What is the effect on cardiopulmonary function of a one-person suctioning technique?

REFERENCES

1. Anonymous. Cardiac arrest during therapeutic tracheal suction (case history). *Anesth. Analg.* 39:568–569, 1960.
2. Barnes, C., and Kirchoff, K. Minimizing hypoxemia due to endotracheal suctioning: A review of the literature. *Heart Lung* 15:164–176, 1986.
3. Barnes, T., and Watson, M. Oxygen delivery performance of four resuscitation bags. *Respiratory Care* 27:139–146, 1982.
4. Benson, M., and Pierson, D. Ventilator washout volumes: A consideration in endotracheal suction preoxygenation. *Resp Care* 24:832–835, 1979.
5. Bostick, J., and Wendelgass, S. Normal saline instillation as part of the suctioning procedure: Effects on PaO$_2$ and amount of secretions. *Heart Lung* 16:532–537, 1987.
6. Boutros, A. Arterial blood oxygenation during and after endotracheal suctioning in the apneic patient. *Anesthesiology* 32:114–118, 1970.
7. Brouchard, L., Harf, A., Lorino, H., et al. Inspiratory pressure support prevents diaphragmatic fatigue during weaning from mechanical ventilation. *Am. Rev. Respir. Dis.* 139:513–521, 1989.
8. Burton, G. G., and Hodgkin, J. E. *Respiratory Care: A Guide to Clinical Practice* (2nd ed.). Philadelphia: J.B. Lippincott, 1984.
9. Cardin, E., and Friedman, D. Further studies of manually operated self-inflating resuscitation bags. *Anesth. Analg.* 56:202–206, 1977.
10. Chase, D., Campbell, G., Byram, D., et al. Hemodynamic changes associated with endotracheal suctioning. *Heart Lung* 18:292–293, 1989.
11. Chulay, M. Hyperinflation/hyperoxygenation to prevent endotracheal suctioning complications. *Crit. Care Nurse* 7:100–104, 1987.
12. Chulay, M. Arterial blood gas changes with a hyperinflation and hyperoxygenation suctioning intervention in critically ill patients. *Heart Lung* 17:654–661, 1988.
13. Fiastro, J. F., Habib, M. P., and Quan, S. F. Pressure support compensation for inspiratory work due to endotracheal tubes and demand continuous positive airway pressure. *Chest* 93:499–505, 1988.
14. Fitzmaurice, M., and Barnes, T. Oxygen delivery of three adult resuscitation bags. *Respiratory Care* 25:928–932, 1980.
15. Hanley, M. Normal saline intratracheal instillation in intubated patients and dogs. Master's thesis. Seattle: University of Washington, 1977.
16. Holdy, B., and Goldberg, H. The effect of mechanical vibration physiotherapy on arterial oxygenation in acutely ill patients with atelectasis or pneumonia. *Am. Rev. Respir. Dis.* 124:373–375, 1981.
17. Kirilloff, L., Owens, G., Rogers, R., et al. Does chest physical therapy work? *Chest* 88:436–444, 1985.
18. Kirmili, B., King, J. E., and Phaeffle, H. H. Evaluation of tracheobronchial suction techniques. *J. Thorac. Cardiovasc. Surg.* 59:340–344, 1970.
19. Kleiber, C., Krutzfield, N., and Rose, E. Acute histologic changes in the tracheobronchial tree associated with different suction catheter insertion techniques. *Heart Lung* 17:10–14, 1988.
20. Luce, J. M., Tyler, M. L., and Pierson, D. J. *Intensive Respiratory Care.* Philadelphia: W. B. Saunders, 1984.
21. Marini, J. J., Capps, J. S., and Culver, B. H. The inspiratory work of breathing during assisted mechanical ventilation. *Chest* 87:612–618, 1985.
22. Marx, G. F., Steen, S. N., Arkins, R. E., et al. Endotracheal suction and death. *N.Y. State Med. J.* 68:565–566, 1968.
23. Ogburn-Russell, L. The effect of continuous and intermittent suctioning on the tracheal mucosa of dogs. *Heart Lung* 16:297, 1987.
24. Panacek, E. A., Albertson, T. E., Rutherford, W. F., et al. Selective left endobronchial suctioning in the intubated patient. *Chest* 95:885–887, 1989.
25. Preusser, B., Stone, K., Gonyon, D., et al. The effect of two methods of pre-oxygenation on mean arterial pressure, cardiac output, peak airway pressure and postsuctioning hypoxemia. *Heart Lung* 17:290–299, 1988.

26. Rasaneu, J., and Downes, J. B. New techniques of positive pressure ventilation. *Anesthesiol. Clin. North Am.* 5:893–900, 1987.

27. Riegel, B., and Forshee, T. A review and critique of the literature on preoxygenation for endotracheal suctioning. *Heart Lung* 14:507–518, 1985.

28. Rutula, W., Stiegel, M., and Sarubbi, F. A potential infection hazard associated with the use of disposable saline vials. *Infect. Control* 5:170–172, 1984.

29. Shapiro, B. A., Harrison, R. A., and Trout, C. A. *Clinical Application of Respiratory Care* (2nd ed.). Chicago: Year Book Medical Publishers, 1979.

30. Shim, C., Fine, N., Fernandez, R., *et al.* Cardiac arrhythmias resulting from tracheal suctioning. *Ann. Intern. Med.* 71:1149–1153, 1969.

31. Skelley, B., Deeren, S., and Powaser, M. The effectiveness of two preoxygenation methods to prevent endotracheal suctioning induced hypoxemia. *Heart Lung* 9:316–323, 1980.

32. Tasota, F., and Hoffman, L. Evaluation of two methods used to stabilize oral endotracheal tubes. *Heart Lung* 16:140–146, 1987.

33. Viale, J. P., Annat, G. J., Bouffard, Y. M., *et al.* Oxygen cost of breathing in postoperative patients. *Chest* 93:506–509, 1988.

34. Weilitz, P. B. New modes of mechanical ventilation. *Crit. Care Nurs. Clin. North Am.* 1:689–695, 1989.

35. Winston, S., Gavelyn, R., and Sitrin, S. Prevention of bradycardic responses to endotracheal suctioning by prior administration of nebulized atropine. *Crit. Care Med.* 15:1009–1011, 1987.

17

Hemodynamic Monitoring

Elaine Keiss Daily   *Cornelia Vanderstaay Kenner*

HEALING POWER OF TOUCH

Touch is a powerful way to share presence and love from our hearts when words are meaningless. Touch is keenly sensitive when people are ill or going through a crisis. Physical touch done lovingly, freely, and with joy conveys through our hands what our hearts are feeling. As a critical care nurse, you touch patients all the time. How often do you touch as routine, and how often do you think about the healing power of touch when done with intention?

Touch with intention can be a healing force that facilitates the patient knowing that you are a healer. When you touch with intention and an openness for the highest good, you are present with your patients in a healing way. Some of the special moments that critically ill patients remember that got them through the rough times are the fluffing of pillows or a straightening of sheets; a change of position, particularly to bony areas; or being given mouth care, a backrub, a foot massage, or light acupressure. They also remember being given a plastic urinal and smaller bedpans or metal or hard plastic equipment that had been warmed under warm water or a hot water bottle, or they remember when they were shivering and a nurse got a warm blanket from surgery.

How do you touch with intention? Start your touch by centering yourself with your breath or an image of healing light surrounding you and the person. Imagine that your hands are an extension of your heart. Warm your hands by rubbing them together or by using your hand-warming techniques. If you feel tense and cannot get them warm, place your hands in warm water for a few minutes. Slowly and gently uncover the person's body where you are touching, then place your hands gently on the person's body. Don't be afraid to ask the person how the touch feels and if it should be done with a lighter or firmer touch. You might find that if you are tense, your hands or upper body may cramp. If so, just back off, shake your hands, do a few shoulder rolls, and use your rhythmic breathing. Again, you will know when to stop the touch. Slowly and gently remove your hands, and once again cover the person so that they feel comfortable. Bring your touch to a close in whatever way seems right for you, such as shaking your hands or washing your hands in cool water to release the energy. You will be surprised at how calm and peaceful you feel.

Encourage family or friends to participate in touch, for it helps connect them with their loved ones and it humanizes the technologic environment. Remember that touch includes bathing, hair combing, feeding, changing the person's position, sheets, pillows, and sheepskins, and hugging and holding. These are powerful ways to break the illusion of separateness and loneliness and to alleviate the fears that build up in acute care. Touching with intention seems to shake loose fear, guilt, and loneliness and may evoke laughter, calmness, or tears. The emotions that come up with touch are the ones that need to be present.

As the nurse who cares for others, you must also care for yourself. Be sure and figure out a way to get your necessary hugs. Create times to give and get hugs with family, colleagues, and friends.

LEARNING OBJECTIVES

After reading this chapter, the nurse should be able to do the following

1. List the various types of patients in whom monitoring is used.
2. Describe the four factors that regulate the heart as a pump.
3. Define the correlating hemodynamic parameters used to assess the factors that affect heart function.
4. Discuss the normal and abnormal values obtained through hemodynamic monitoring.
5. Describe the physiologic and pathophysiologic factors that limit the interpretation of hemodynamic measurements.
6. List the complications of hemodynamic monitoring.
7. List the steps that should be used to assess problems with the monitoring equipment.

231

The word *monitoring* is derived from the Latin word *monere*, meaning "to warn, remind, or admonish." *Patient monitoring* consists of those protocols and devices that assess the patient's condition on a continuing basis. To expand patient assessment and obtain early warning of changes in a patient's condition, various monitoring devices are coupled with careful clinical surveillance. Unfortunately, many monitoring techniques are invasive and bring the inherent risks of invasive techniques to the bedside.

In the last 20 years, invasive monitoring techniques have progressed from complex cardiac cathether laboratory procedures to more simplified bedside assessment procedures. This has been primarily due to the development of the flow-directed, balloon-tipped catheter, which permits direct measurement of right-heart pressures in addition to indirect measurement of left-heart pressures. This assessment of cardiovascular function can provide general information regarding overall ventricular function and, more importantly, measure the cardiovascular response to specific therapeutic agents or maneuvers. In certain pathophysiologic states, hemodynamic data are useful in the differential diagnosis of the cause of shock.

When combined with careful clinical assessment of the patient, hemodynamic monitoring provides detailed information regarding the patient's cardiovascular status, and, thus, expands the scope of cardiovascular evaluation. It does not, of course, take the place of careful patient assessment and observation; rather, it serves as an adjunct to meticulous patient assessment.

INDICATIONS

Despite some recent controversy regarding the use (or abuse) of invasive hemodynamic monitoring,[2,17,36] as well as the lack of defined risk/benefit ratios, it remains a crucial tool in the management of critically ill patients.[3,27] In general, invasive hemodynamic monitoring is instituted in high-risk, hemodynamically compromised patients who are not responding well to therapy or whose care could be improved by more precise data. In this way, measured hemodynamic responses provide the basis for minute-by-minute titration of therapy. In addition, hemodynamic monitoring is indicated in patients with unexplained low-output syndromes to determine the underlying pathophysiology. Specific indications for use of invasive hemodynamic monitoring are listed in Table 17–1.

ANTECEDENT CONDITIONS

When evaluating the ill patient, a bedside assessment takes first priority. This assessment includes a thorough history and physical examination with heart rate, blood pressure, cardiac sounds, pulmonary sounds, electrocardiogram, chest x-ray data, and hemodynamic status (the reader should carefully review Chap. 5). Accurate monitoring by the primary care nurse to determine trends and assess the patient's changing status is vital. Whether the patient's condition is stable, unstable, or critical, data are needed.

Stable Patients

If the patient's condition is stable, vital signs are checked every 15 minutes at first and then at longer intervals. The most important indicators of the patient's condition are sensorium and hourly urinary output. Urinary output and renal blood flow are dependent on cardiac output. The presence and description of arterial pressure pulses provide a reliable parameter for assessing mechanical failure of the heart. The toe ambient temperature gradient is also reliable for assessing perfusion failure. When cardiac output is reduced, the blood flow to the skin (*e.g.*, of the big toe) is even more reduced. A reduction in skin temperature in relation to ambient temperature suffices to ascertain the reduction in blood flow to the skin. Careful evaluation of vital signs is a simple, noninvasive method that yields excellent data. The pulse can usually be palpated at the radial artery, and heart rate normally ranges from 60 to 100 beats per minute. Respirations should be carefully assessed; for example, one of the first indicators of clinical sepsis is an increased respiratory rate.

The sphygmomanometer can be used to make an adequate measurement of the patient's arterial pressure. The pulse pressure is related to stroke volume and the distensibility of the aorta, and many authorities consider a decrease in the pulse pressure an indicator of a decrease in stroke volume. The degree of vasoconstriction correlates with the increase in the diastolic pressure.

The amount and rate of blood flow are determined largely by mechanical properties. The difference in pressure between the proximal and distal ends of a vessel essentially determines the blood flow. The size of the lumen is particularly important to the rate of flow, in that the rate of flow in a vessel is directly proportional to the fourth power of its radius (Poiseuille's law). The amount of blood that flows through a vessel for a certain period of time is equal to the velocity of the flow multiplied by the area of the cross section. As the circulatory system proceeds from the aorta to the capillary beds, the area of the cross section increases and the rate of the flow decreases. The inverse proportion ranges from an area of 2 to 5 cm^2 and a rate of flow of 30 to 35 cm/second (in the aorta) to an area of 1500 to 2000 cm^2 and a rate of flow of about 0.5 cm/second (in the capillary beds). Other factors that affect flow are resistance, viscosity, the tone of the precapillary sphincter, and tissue oxygenation.

Table 17–1
Indications for Hemodynamic Monitoring

Complicated acute myocardial infarction
  Evidence of hypoperfusion
  Significant pulmonary congestion
  Unexplained dyspnea
  Refractory dysrhythmias
  Persistent myocardial ischemia
  Right ventricular infarction
Shock states
  Cardiogenic
  Hypovolemic
  Septic
Suspected anatomic lesions
  Ventricular septal rupture
  Papillary muscle rupture
  Pulmonary embolism
  Pericardial tamponade
High-risk patients undergoing surgery

Unstable Patients

If the patient's condition is not stable, monitoring of the electrocardiogram (ECG) and monitoring of the central venous pressure are added to the other types of monitoring. Monitoring of arterial oxygenation serially (blood gases) or continuously via pulse oximetry assumes an important role.

The use of serial central venous pressure readings has been endorsed, but then criticized by some authorities. However, readings taken from a catheter placed in the superior vena cava or in the right atrium yield critical data about the amount of blood coming into the right side of the heart and the ability of the right side of the heart to pump blood. Although right atrial pressures do not necessarily reflect the functioning of the left side of the heart, information about the status of right-sided heart functioning will suffice in many patients (*e.g.*, the hypovolemic patient with normal heart and lungs).[18]

One of the very best measures of perfusion failure is the arterial blood lactate level. Because the degree of lactic acidosis correlates with the severity of the oxygen deficit, the arterial blood lactate level essentially quantitates the oxygen deficit (and so, the degree of shock or perfusion failure).

Critically Unstable Patients

In a patient who is critically unstable, monitoring is expanded to make use of more sensitive and accurate devises to obtain more detailed assessment, to prevent complications, and to titrate therapy. Unfortunately, many of the devices used are invasive and thus bring risks as well as advantages to the patient. The best indication of the adequacy of tissue perfusion and, therefore, oxygenation is, of course, normal function of the body systems. Therefore, perfusion of the brain and kidneys remains a valuable indicator. Unless other conditions are present, restlessness, confusion, and disorientation indicate a critical stage of hypoperfusion, and perhaps shock.

The hourly urinary output should be kept within normal limits (about 50 ml/hour). In addition, osmolality, the sodium concentration, and the ratio of blood urea to urine urea must

be monitored. A decreased urine sodium concentration and an increased urine osmolality tend to be early indicators of shock, whereas decreased hourly urine volume is a later indicator of shock. For a detailed discussion of kidney perfusion, refer to Chapter 33.

VITAL SIGNS

Although monitoring vital signs is very important, the information obtained must be evaluated in terms of the individual patient. The body's mechanisms for maintaining temperature may be changed, and the patient's temperature may be very high or very low. For example, one common indicator of shock is a clinically subnormal temperature.

If palpation of the pulse at the radial artery is difficult, palpation at the carotid or femoral arteries is recommended. In selected instances (and combined with other measures), the carotid and femoral sites can be used to estimate the pulse volume and mean arterial pressure.

The arterial pressure measurement obtained with the sphygmomanometer is not necessarily accurate. As the stroke volume falls, the Korotkoff sounds become increasingly difficult to hear, and a wide variation in blood pressure readings occurs. Although Korotkoff sounds are quiet in the great majority of patients with low pressure, this is not necessarily the case. A Doppler ultrasonic flowmeter may be used to hear the arterial flow. If the Doppler measurement is not satisfactory, an intra-arterial catheter is used to identify trends and assess changes, because the mean arterial pressure is related more to blood flow than to sound. Usually, the measurement is made with an electronic transducer and monitor, but an anaroid manometer may also be used. The arterial line is generally used also to obtain samples to measure the arterial blood gases.

Hemodynamic monitoring with the pulmonary artery pressure catheter is used frequently in unstable patients. Table 17–2 shows several patient examples with potential therapies based on an assessment of their hemodynamic status.

Table 17–2
Assessment and Possible Therapies Based on Hemodynamic Parameters

PATIENT	BLOOD PRESSURE (mm Hg)	PULMONARY ARTERY WEDGE PRESSURE (mm Hg)	CARDIAC INDEX (L/min/m^2)	ASSESSMENT	THERAPIES
Ms. T.	120/80	25	2.5	Congestive heart failure, moderate	Diuretics, venovasodilators, and oxygen
Mr. S.	118/78	30	2.0	Congestive heart failure, severe	Diuretics, venovasodilators, inotropic agents, oxygen
Mr. B	94/76	3	1.8	Hypovolemic shock	Volume, inotropic agents
Mr. X.	84/58	10	3.8	Septic shock	Volume, dopamine, norepinephrine
Ms. G.	84/58	20	2.0	Cardiogenic shock	Norepinephrine, dopamine, oxygen, intra-aortic balloon pumping

RESPIRATORY MONITORING

Respiratory monitoring should focus on changes in the respiratory rate and especially changes in depth, in the alveolar ventilation, and in the arterial $PaCO_2$. The minute ventilation increases remarkably with tachypnea and respiratory alkalosis, a nonspecific response that occurs in early shock. If shock continues, metabolic acidosis becomes the primary derangement, and the body attempts to compensate with hyperventilation.

The serial assessment of the arterial blood gases must consider the inspired oxygen concentration, the alterations in oxygenation, the pH, the $PaCO_2$, and calculation of base excess. It must be emphasized that raising the hemoglobin from 10 to 12 mg/dl does much more for total oxygenation than does raising the percentage of inspired oxygen. (Assessment of the patient's respiratory status is discussed further in Chaps. 5 and 19.)

PHYSIOLOGY

The physiology of the circulatory system is dependent on a series of complex interactions between the heart as a pump, the vascular system as both a reservoir and conduit, and the kidneys as a regulator of blood volume and blood pressure. The nervous system mediates the interaction of the principal components and their adjustment to various physiologic demands.

The heart is a muscular organ that consists of two separate pumps. It is important to understand that the right and left sides of the heart function both together and, to some extent, independently of each other. The function of each is determined by its own pressures and any pathophysiologic mechanisms present.[1,6,26]

The system is pressure driven, with flow moving from an area of higher pressure to an area of lower pressure (Table 17–3). The system is dependent on electrical conduction causing rhythmic pumping and filling (i.e., systole and diastole). The efficiency of this pump is determined principally by four major factors: heart rate, contractility, preload, and afterload.

Diastole

Filling of the ventricles occurs during the diastolic phase of the cardiac cycle. Diastole is divided into three phases: early, middle, and late. These phases are also referred to as rapid filling and slow-filling phases.

Early diastole follows the opening of the atrioventricular valves, resulting in passive, rapid filling of the ventricle, and lasts for one quarter to one third of the total diastolic period. The pressure in the vena cava and pulmonary veins is slightly greater than the atrial pressure, and the atrial pressure is slightly greater than the ventricular pressure, causing rapid blood flow. By middle diastole, the ventricles are almost completely filled; however, the atria have not yet contracted. It is a period of slow filling.

In late diastole, electrical activity (atrial depolarization) produces atrial contraction, forcing a small volume to be ejected into the ventricles. Actually, atrial contraction contributes only a small amount to ventricular filling at normal heart rates. The contribution increases at faster heart rates.

Table 17–3

Normal Pressure Measurements in the Heart and Major Surrounding Vessels

SITE	MEAN VALUE (mm Hg)	RANGE (mm Hg)
Vena cava		
Maximum	7	2 to 4
Minimum	5	0 to 8
Mean	6	1 to 11
Right atrium		
Maximum	7	2 to 14
Minimum	2	−2 to +6
Mean	4	−1 to +8
Right ventricle		
Systolic	24	15 to 28
End-diastolic	4	0 to 8
Pulmonary artery		
Systolic	24	15 to 28
Diastolic	10	5 to 16
Mean	14	10 to 22
Pulmonary capillary wedge	7	4 to 12
Left atrium		
Maximum	13	6 to 20
Minimum	4	−2 to +9
Mean	7	4 to 12
Left ventricle		
Systolic	130	90 to 140
End-diastolic	7	4 to 12
Aorta		
Systolic	120	90 to 140
Diastolic	70	60 to 90
Mean	85	70 to 105

Systole

Following the spread of electrical activity to the ventricles (ventricular depolarization), ventricular contraction occurs. Myocardial fiber shortening causes the ventricular pressure to rise quickly and exceed atrial pressure. The increased pressure closes the atrioventricular valves, and the first heart sound in the cardiac cycle is heard. Because the ventricles are closed (and both valves are closed), the internal pressure rapidly increases. When the ventricular pressure exceeds the aortic and pulmonary artery pressures, the aortic and pulmonic valves are forced open and blood is ejected from the ventricles (Fig. 17–1).

Early in the ejection phase, the maximum ejection rate is achieved. The blood vessels expand and essentially "store" blood while the pressure continues to rise. The ejection rate then declines slowly at first and then more rapidly. Once the ventricular pressure falls below the pressure in the aorta and pulmonary artery, the semilunar valves close. This produces the second heart sound.

During contraction, the ventricles eject approximately 60% to 80% of their blood volume. The volume of blood still in the ventricles is considered a reserve, i.e., blood that can be ejected if and when increased demands are placed on the heart. The amount of blood ejected is termed the stroke volume and represents the difference between the end-diastolic vol-

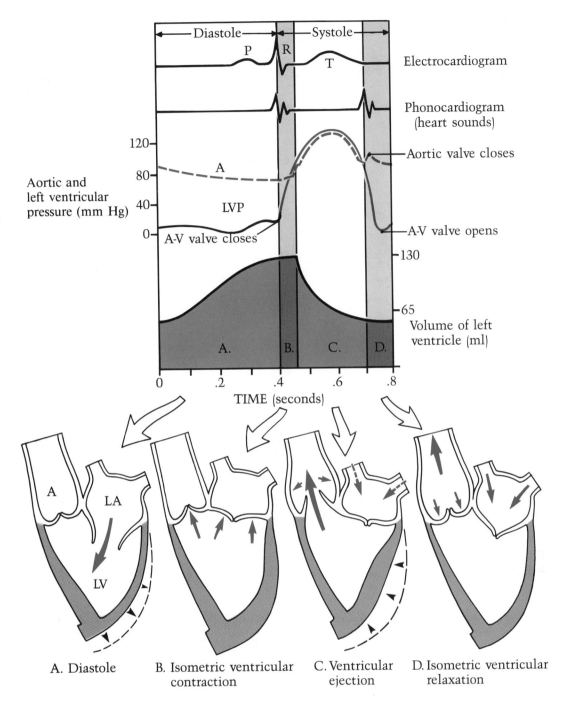

Figure 17-1

Mechanical and electrical events in the left ventricle during a single cardiac cycle.

ume and the end-systolic volume, *i.e.*, the difference between the ventricular volumes at the start and end of each contraction. The *ejection fraction* is the fraction of the end-diastolic volume ejected during systole and is normally greater than 0.5 (50%).

$$\text{Ejection fraction} = \frac{\text{stroke volume}}{\text{end-diastolic volume}}$$

Left ventricular ejection produces a pressure wave that travels through the arterial system and can be palpated as the peripheral pulse. The pulse strength is related to the stroke volume and pulse pressure. If the stroke volume is low, the pulse feels weak. If the stroke volume is high, the pulse feels strong.

Heart Rate

Heart rate is the major determinant of cardiac output, coronary blood flow, and myocardial oxygen utilization. Increasing the

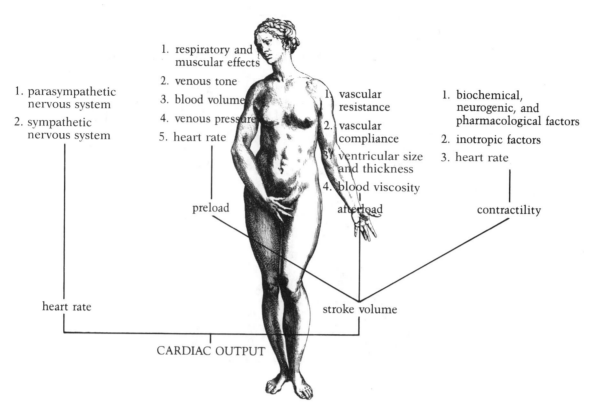

1. parasympathetic nervous system
2. sympathetic nervous system

1. respiratory and muscular effects
2. venous tone
3. blood volume
4. venous pressure
5. heart rate

1. vascular resistance
2. vascular compliance
3. ventricular size and thickness
4. blood viscosity

1. biochemical, neurogenic, and pharmacological factors
2. inotropic factors
3. heart rate

preload

afterload

contractility

heart rate

stroke volume

CARDIAC OUTPUT

Figure 17–2
Determinants of cardiac function.

heart rate is the primary means of increasing cardiac output (cardiac output = heart rate × stroke volume). The majority (approximately 75%) of coronary blood flow to the myocardium occurs during diastole. Rapid heart rates shorten the diastolic period and reduce the duration of coronary blood flow and may, in certain instances, result in myocardial ischemia. Rapid heart rates also dramatically increase myocardial oxygen consumption.

The heart has its own intrinsic regulatory mechanism in the sinoatrial node, but it also is regulated by the autonomic nervous system. During rest, vagal control predominates, and the sinus rate is kept slow (by the release of acetylcholine in the sinus node). During stress, sympathetic activity predominates, with increased norepinephrine concentration around the sinus node. Heart rate can range from 50 to 200 beats/minute. Factors such as pH, blood temperature, ionic composition, stretch of sinus node tissues, and hormone concentrations also affect the heart rate.

Stroke Volume

The volume of blood ejected with each heart beat is termed the *stroke volume*. It represents the difference between the volume of blood in the ventricle at the end of diastole (the end of filling) and the volume remaining at the end of systole (the end of ejection). Actual measurements of ventricular volume are difficult; however, a mean stroke volume can be calculated by dividing the cardiac output by the ventricular rate during that period. The normal range of stroke volume is 60 to 130 ml.

The stroke volume is determined by three factors: ventricular end-diastolic volume (preload), ventricular afterload, and contractility. Although these three factors operate simultaneously to determine the stroke volume, they are discussed separately.

Cardiac Output

The cardiac output is the volume of blood that the heart pumps per minute (Fig. 17–2), and it is equal to the venous return (the volume of blood that enters the heart on the venous side):

Cardiac output (L/min)

= heart rate (beats/min) × stroke volume (L/beat)

The average person's heart beats 72 beats/minute, and each ventricle ejects approximately 70 ml of blood per beat. Thus, the cardiac output is calculated as 72 beats × 70 ml, or approximately 5000 ml (5 L/minute).

The cardiac output can also be calculated as the cardiac index. The cardiac index is the cardiac output corrected for the person's physical size. In the normal adult, the cardiac index is approximately 3.5 L/minute/m^2, with a normal range of from 2.5 to 4.5 L/minute/m^2. A cardiac index less than 1.2 L/minute/m^2 is considered incompatible with life, and a cardiac index of 1.8 to 2.2 L/minute/m^2 is considered deleterious to the functioning of the vital organs (Table 17–4).

Table 17–4
Changes in Cardiac Index Indicative of Low-Output Failure

CARDIAC INDEX (L/min/m²)	PERFUSION
2.7–4.5	Normal
2.2–2.7	Subclinical
1.8–2.2	Clinical, low perfusion
<1.8	Shock

Preload

Preload refers to the volume of blood in the ventricles at the end of diastole, just before contraction, and is dependent on the capacity of the venous system and the distribution of blood volume. For example, venoconstriction causes a marked increase in blood return to the right side of the heart, whereas venodilation decreases blood return.

Preload is a determination of the length of muscle fiber stretch before the beginning of contraction and is measured indirectly in terms of the ventricular end-diastolic volume or end-diastolic pressure. The length or stretch of the myocardial muscle fiber is proportional to the force of the following contraction until a critical length is reached. Once the critical length is exceeded, the resultant force of contraction decreases. This relationship between the length of muscle fibers and the force of contraction is known as the *Frank-Starling Law of the heart*. The strength of contraction of a heart muscle varies with its length, *i.e.*, increasing the volume filling the heart increases the muscle fiber length and leads to increased output (within limits). Essentially, this mechanism is one of autoregulation, because the more the muscle is stretched, the greater is the following contraction. The relationship between cardiac output and preload can be expressed as a cardiac function curve. As shown in Figure 17–3, as preload increases, cardiac output increases up to a point. Increases in preload beyond this point cause the heart to fail.[5] The cardiac function curve is a series of plots of systolic work or cardiac output as a function of preload. Increases in preload represent an important compensatory mechanism invoked to maintain adequate cardiac output.

The preload of the right side of the heart refers to the filling pressure of the right ventricle. Although filling occurs during all of diastole, the end-diastolic pressure in the right ventricle represents the maximum filling pressure, or preload, of the right heart. Clinically, this is measured as the mean right atrial or central venous pressure. Figure 17–4 illustrates the close correlation between the mean right atrial pressure and the right ventricular end-diastolic filling pressure. Thus, the central venous pressure or mean right atrial pressure reflects the preload of the right heart.

Likewise, the left ventricular preload is synonymous with left ventricular end-diastolic volume (LVEDV), which is reflected by left ventricular end-diastolic pressure (LVEDP).

Clinically, left atrial volume and its corresponding pressure may be used as an indicator of LVEDP. If left atrial pressure is measured at end-diastole, the mitral valve is open and the left atrium and left ventricle are as one chamber. An indirect means of measuring left atrial pressure is to measure the pulmonary artery wedge pressure (PAWP).[22,24]

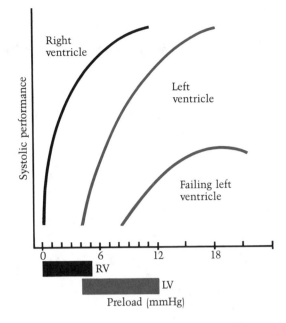

Figure 17–3
The effect of preload on cardiac output. For the right side of the heart, central venous pressure as preload is graphed versus cardiac output. For the left side of the heart, pulmonary artery wedge pressure as preload is graphed versus cardiac output. To a point, increasing the preload on the volume of blood in the heart leads to a greater cardiac output. Once this point is reached, a larger preload no longer produces an increase in cardiac output.

The PAWP is the pressure measured via a catheter located within a small branch of the pulmonary artery. Forward blood flow is occluded by inflation of the balloon of the catheter (see Fig. 7–15). The pressure measured is the retrograde transmission of the left atrium through the pulmonary venous system. The PAWP is thus used as an indicator of left atrial and ventricular end-diastolic pressure, and is therefore a reflection of preload of the left heart. The factors that determine the PAWP are blood volume, atrial and ventricular contractile force and compliance, ventricular and venous capacity, and the duration of diastole.

Afterload

Afterload is the tension developed by the ventricles during contraction. It is the force opposing ventricular ejection or the resistance that the heart must overcome in order to pump blood around the body. Afterload is inversely related to cardiac output, *i.e.*, the higher the afterload or force opposing ejection, the lower the stroke volume, and vice versa. Afterload is determined by ventricular size and thickness, blood viscosity, and arterial and arteriolar resistance.[37] Clinically, the determinant that changes most acutely, and most commonly, is the arterial/arteriolar resistance. For this reason, vascular resistance is used as the clinical measurement of afterload. Afterload of the left heart is usually estimated by calculating the systemic vascular resistance (normal range from 900 to 1400 dyne-seconds–cm⁻⁵) as follows:

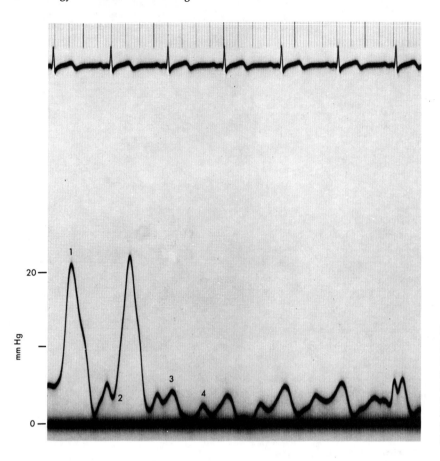

Figure 17–4

Normal right ventricular (RV) and right atrial (RA) waveforms. Note the similarity between RA a wave and the RV end-diastolic pressure (1 = RV systole; 2 = RV end-diastole; 3 = RA a wave; 4 = RA v wave). (Daily, E.K., and Schroeder, J.S. *Hemodynamic Waveforms: Exercises in Interpretation and Analysis* [2nd ed.]. St. Louis: C.V. Mosby, 1990; with permission.)

Systemic vascular resistance

$$= \frac{\text{mean arterial pressure} - \text{central venous pressure}}{\text{cardiac output}} \times 80$$

Afterload of the right heart is calculated as pulmonary vascular resistance (normal range from 20 to 130 dyne-seconds–cm^{-5}) as follows:

Pulmonary vascular resistance

$$= \frac{\begin{array}{c}\text{mean pulmonary artery pressure}\\ - \text{ pulmonary artery wedge pressure}\end{array}}{\text{cardiac output}} \times 80$$

Contractility

Contractility refers to the inotropic state of the myocardium or the velocity of fiber shortening during systole. The heart is influenced by a variety of biochemical, neurogenic, and pharmacologic factors. Some factors, such as circulating epinephrine, digitalis, or tachycardia, increase contractility, whereas other factors, such as hypoxia or acidosis, have a negative effect. Positive inotropic agents increase contractility, and negative inotropic agents decrease contractility.

Although contractility cannot be directly measured or even approximated in the clinical setting, an index of ventricular work (stroke work index) is used to assess changes in contractility. The stroke work indices of either ventricle can be calculated according to the formulae listed in Table 17–5. Studies by Shoemaker and colleagues have shown that maintenance of a left ventricular stroke work index greater than 55 g/m/beat is associated with improved survival in shock patients.[40]

PRESSURE MONITORING TECHNIQUES

Monitoring of central venous pressures, pulmonary artery pressures, and cardiac output is important in evaluating a person's pump effectiveness, blood volume, tissue perfusion, and vascular capacity.

Central Venous Pressure

Central venous pressure (CVP) is a direct measurement of the right atrial pressure via the superior vena cava or right atrium. Central venous pressure reflects venous return as well as right ventricular filling pressure (preload) (Fig. 17–5).

Clinically, the CVP is most valuable in monitoring blood volume or venous return, and right ventricular function. In postoperative patients with normal cardiopulmonary function, the CVP has been found to be an accurate and reliable estimate of left atrial pressure.[33] Although the CVP will eventually reflect left-sided heart failure, the timing and sequence of the pressure changes in the superior vena cava are less predictable.

Catheter Placement

The CVP catheter is placed percutaneously or via venous cutdown in the medial basilic, internal or external jugular, or subclavian veins. Introducer needles range from 24 gauge (small) to 14 gauge (large) in size. A smaller intracatheter comes

Table 17-5

Calculation of Common Parameters Used for Monitoring Critically Ill Patients

Central venous pressure (CVP) in mm Hg = CVP (cm H_2O) ÷ 1.36

Mean arterial pressure = arterial diastolic pressure + ⅓ (arterial systolic pressure − arterial diastolic pressure)

Mean pulmonary arterial pressure = pulmonary arterial diastolic pressure + ⅓ (pulmonary arterial systolic pressure − pulmonary arterial diastolic pressure)

Cardiac index (in L/min/m²) = cardiac output (CO) in L/min ÷ body surface area (BSA) (in m², as calculated by height and weight)

Stroke volume (SV) = CO ÷ heart rate

Stroke index (ml/beat/m²) = SV ÷ BSA

Right ventricular stroke work (RVSW) = SV × (mean pulmonary arterial pressure − CVP) × .0136

Left ventricular stroke work (LVSW) = SV × (mean arterial pressure − wedge pressure) × .0136

Stroke work ratio = RVSW ÷ LVSW

Systemic vascular resistance (SVR) = (mean arterial pressure − CVP ÷ CO) × 80

Pulmonary vascular resistance (PVR) = (mean pulmonary arterial pressure − wedge pressure ÷ CO) × 80

SVR index = SVR ÷ BSA

PVR index = PVR ÷ BSA

Filling ratio = CVP mm Hg ÷ wedge pressure

Arterial oxygen content = Hgb × arterial saturation × 1.34 + arterial P_{O_2} × 0.003

Venous oxygen content = Hgb × venous saturation × 1.34 + venous P_{O_2} × 0.003

Arteriovenous oxygen content difference = arterial oxygen content − venous oxygen content

Oxygen delivery = arterial oxygen content × 10 × CO

Oxygen consumption = arteriovenous oxygen content difference × CO × 10

Oxygen utilization = oxygen consumption ÷ oxygen delivery

Shunt = (capillary content − arterial content) ÷ (capillary content − venous content) × 100

with an introducer needle and remains in the vein after the needle is removed. The physician chooses the catheter based on the patient's body build, age, and clinical assessment.

Although arm vein cannulation for insertion of CVP catheters is associated with the lowest complication rate, the catastrophic complication of acute cardiac tamponade is more likely to occur when this insertion site is used.[10] Movement of the arm can cause forward migration of the CVP catheter tip, resulting in perforation of the wall of the right atrium with subsequent tamponade.

After selection of the site, the area is cleansed with an antibacterial solution such as povidone-iodine (Betadine solution). The needle and intracatheter are inserted until the tip of the intracatheter is in the superior vena cava near the right atrial junction. Antimicrobrial ointment and an occlusive dressing cover the site. A chest x-ray is obtained as soon as is practical

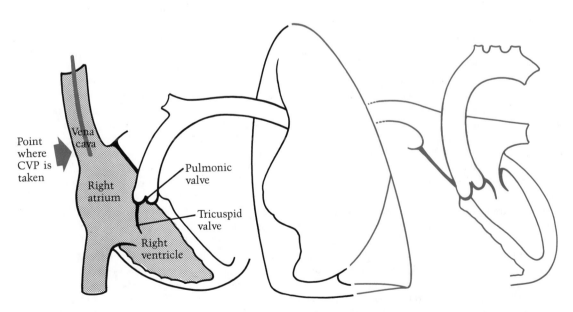

Figure 17-5

Measurement of central venous pressure. Central venous pressure (CVP) reflects the pressure in the right atrium. Right atrial pressure is usually low and offers little resistance to the systemic circulation. When the tricuspid valve is open, CVP is equal to right ventricular end-diastolic pressure.

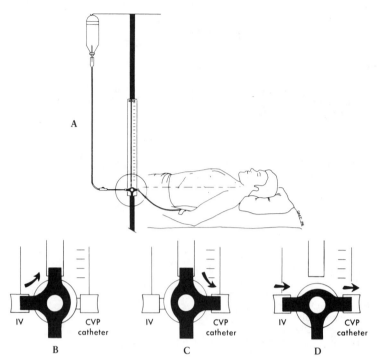

Figure 17–6

Procedure for measuring central venous pressure (CVP) with a water manometer. (*A*) Manometer and intravenous tubing in place. (*B*) Turn the stopcock so that the manometer fills with fluid above the level of the expected pressure. (*C*) Turn the stopcock so that the intravenous line is off and the manometer flows to the patient. Obtain a reading after the fluid level stabilizes. (*D*) Turn the stopcock to resume the intravenous flow to the patient. (Daily, E.K., and Schroeder, J.S. *Techniques in Bedside Hemodynamic Monitoring* [4th ed.]. St. Louis: C.V. Mosby, 1989; with permission.)

after insertion to be sure a pneumothorax has not been created and to determine the appropriate positioning of the catheter tip.

Measurement

The CVP can be measured with a water manometer (the original technique) or with a pressure transducer. When the CVP is measured with a water manometer, its measurement is in centimeters of water (cm H_2O). When measured with the use of a pressure transducer, its measurement is in millimeters of mercury (mm Hg). These differences in units of measurement may cause some confusion, which can be avoided if the manometrically measured CVP is converted to mm Hg. This can be done simply by dividing the cm H_2O value by 1.36. For example, 10 cm H_2O divided by 1.36 gives a value of 7.4 mm Hg. Perhaps an even easier method is to multiply the cm H_2O value by 0.74 to convert to mm Hg.

Regardless of which method is used, the CVP pressure should always be read at end-expiration. It is also essential to place the zero-reference port at the level of the right atrium. This level can be estimated by measuring the mid-chest at the fourth intercostal space to determine the patient's phlebostatic point.

Figure 17–6 illustrates the set-up and procedure for measurement of the CVP with a water manometer.[12] If the CVP is measured with a transducer, the fluid-filled set-up is the same as that outlined for pulmonary artery pressure measurement. The waveform obtained will have the appearance of right atrial waveform with somewhat exaggerated respiratory response (Fig. 17–7). The normal CVP or right atrial pressure is 1 to 7 mm Hg (0 to 10 cm H_2O), with a normal average of approximately 3 mm Hg (4 cm H_2O). The application of the catheter has evolved in a manner that has expanded its initial measurement applications. These applications include pressure measurement, flow measurement, blood sampling, angiography, and drug-infusion.[8]

Pulmonary Artery Catheterization

Pulmonary artery pressures are measured by a catheter placed in the pulmonary artery.[41] This method of measurement is advantagous because it permits the measurement of the pulmonary artery diastolic and wedge pressures, the continuous monitoring of the pulmonary arterial systolic and mean pressures, the sampling of mixed venous blood for the measurement of the arteriovenous oxygen differences, and an estimate to be made of the cardiac output by the thermodilution method. In addition, if a fiberoptic pulmonary artery catheter is used, continuous monitoring of the oxygen saturation of mixed venous blood in the pulmonary artery (SvO_2) is available. From these measurements, numerous cardiovascular parameters can be calculated by a digital calculator or bedside computer (Table 17–5). Myocardial function can thus be evaluated in terms of contractility, preload, and afterload, and provide important data used to guide and evaluate therapy.

The flow-directed catheter is designed to monitor pulmonary artery pressure and PAWP and for sampling of mixed venous blood. The three-lumen catheter is designed for the measurement of right arterial pressure in addition to the previous functions. The third lumen ends at the site of the right atrium, 20 to 30 cm proximal to the catheter tip. This proximal lumen can also be used as an intravenous infusion site. The four-lumen catheter has a thermistor near the catheter tip to sense temperature and determine temperature change for the measurement of cardiac output (Fig. 17–8). The five-lumen catheter has, in addition, two ventricular electrodes and three atrial electrodes for use when atrial or ventricular pacing or atrioventricular sequential pacing is needed. Intra-atrial and intraventricular ECGs also may be recorded.

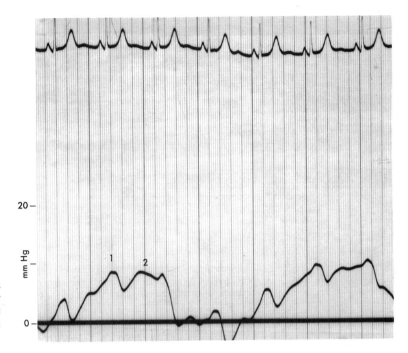

Figure 17–7

Normal central venous pressure (CVP) waveform showing *a* (1), and *v* (2) waves and normal respiratory variation. (Daily, E.K., and Schroeder, J.S. *Techniques in Bedside Hemodynamic Monitoring,* [4th ed.]. St. Louis: C.V. Mosby, 1989; with permission.)

All the catheters are flow-directed and balloon-tipped. The balloon sizes are 0.8 to 1.5 ml for the 5 F and 7 F catheters, respectively. Once inflated, the balloon directs the catheter through the right ventricle out into the pulmonary artery. The inflated balloon allows the catheter to be floated or pulled with the flow of blood through the heart and reduces the incidence of dysrhythmias, because direct endocardial contact with the catheter is prevented. The balloon lumen has a gate valve to protect against accidental locking in the inflated position. The catheter is radiopaque, so it can be seen on x-ray or under fluoroscopy.

Catheter Placement

Once the physician determines the need for catheter placement, it is the nurse's responsibility to obtain and prepare the equipment and the patient. The nurse should know if the percutaneous or cutdown approach is anticipated and if the brachial vein, internal jugular vein, subclavian vein, or femoral vein will be used. The physician is more likely to select per-

cutaneous venous cannulation than venous cutdown because it is a simpler, quicker, and less invasive procedure. It is also associated with a reduced rate of infection. A heparized flush solution (1 to 4 U of heparin/ml of saline) should be available, as well as a nonvented drip chamber, a sterile transducer, stopcocks, a flush connector, pressure tubing, and a monitor (Fig. 17–9). The monitor should be electronically calibrated, and the flush system should be connected to the transducer. All air bubbles should be expelled from the system.

The patient's and family's understanding of the procedure should be assessed. If the nurse has not been present during the physician's explanation, the patient's comprehension and desire for more information should be ascertained. Many people do not want details, and many are too sick to receive detailed information. Simple explanations are best. Most patients appreciate knowing what the experience of the procedure will be like, *i.e.,* what sensations will be experienced.

The catheter is placed under aseptic conditions; mask, cap, gown, and wide drapes are used. An antibacterial agent such as povidone-iodine is used to prepare the skin. Xylocaine hydrochloride or its equivalent is used as local anesthesia. Before actual catheter insertion, the integrity of the balloon of the pulmonary artery catheter is ensured by submerging the catheter under sterile water and inflating the balloon. All lumens are flushed to ensure patency. As in the introduction of all central catheters, the Trendelenburg position is generally used to facilitate location of the vein by engorgement of vessels and to prevent air embolism. After insertion of a 14-gauge needle, a guidewire is inserted 4 to 5 inches to allow removal of the needle. An introducer is then passed over the guidewire, and the guidewire is removed. The pulmonary artery catheter is then inserted through the sheath and advanced towards the heart.

Because the catheter tip may irritate the right ventricular wall and produce premature ventricular contractions, a lidocaine bolus and a defibrillator must be available during insertion, although manipulation of the catheter out of the right ventricle (into the right atrium or pulmonary artery) usually

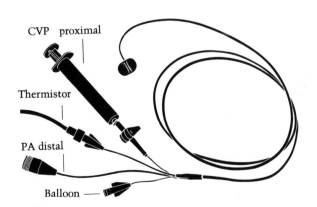

Figure 17–8

Four lumens of the flow-directed catheter. CVP: central venous pressure; PA: pulmonary artery.

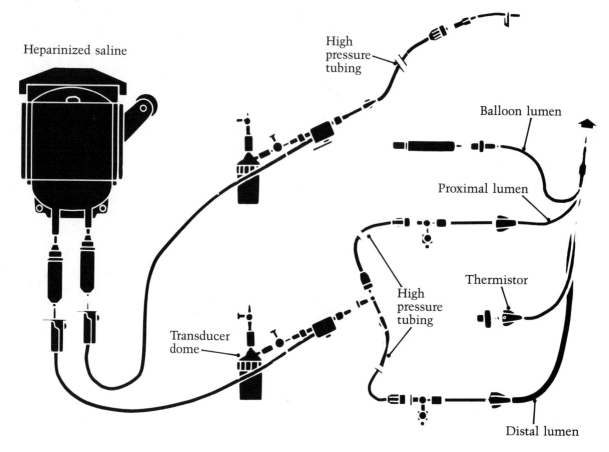

Figure 17–9
Fluid-filled system for hemodynamic monitoring of arterial and pulmonary artery pressures.

terminates any ventricular dysrhythmias. The location of the catheter is verified by the pressure tracings shown on the oscilloscope (Fig. 17–10). Once the right atrium is reached, the balloon is inflated and advanced slowly through the right ventricle into the pulmonary artery and then into the wedge position. Inflation of the balloon helps float the catheter through the chambers of the heart, and the inflated balloon covers the catheter tip so that the forces at the tip are distributed over a larger area (a phenomenon that minimizes the occurrence of premature ventricular contractions). Fluoroscopy, although not necessary, can facilitate rapid passage of the catheter. If the patient experiences a premature ventricular contraction, the physician inserting the catheter either retracts the catheter or orders the administration of an intravenous

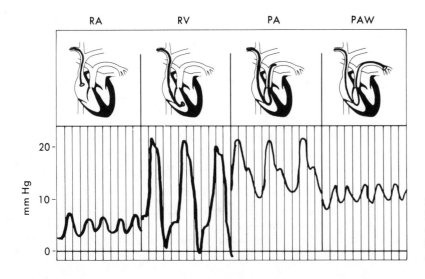

Figure 17–10
Flow-directed, balloon-tipped catheter locations with corresponding pressure tracings. (Daily, E.K., and Schroeder, J.S. *Techniques in Bedside Hemodynamic Monitoring* [4th ed.] St. Louis: C. V. Mosby, 1989)

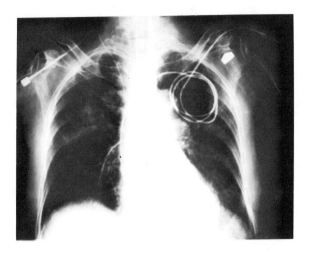

Figure 17–11
Chest radiograph verification of the position of the flow-directed catheter and the absence of pneumothorax. The tip of the catheter should not extend more than one half the distance to the chest wall.

bolus of lidocaine (50 to 100 mg). Besides the support and observation of the patient expected of the nurse in all such procedures, the nurse must also monitor the ECG and pressure tracings and notify the physician of any changes.

Once the wedge position is reached, PAWP tracing is seen on the oscilloscope. Deflation of the balloon produces a pulmonary artery tracing. If the PAWP tracing persists after deflation, the catheter may be wedged too far in the distal pulmonary artery and must be repositioned to the point at which a pulmonary artery wave form is visualized with a deflated balloon and a pulmonary artery wedge waveform is visualized when the balloon is inflated. Three criteria are used to ascertain

proper wedge position: characteristic pressure waveform, a PAW lower than the mean pulmonary artery pressure, and blood withdrawn from the wedge position that is nearly 100% saturated with oxygen. A follow-up chest x-ray verifies the position of the catheter (Fig. 17–11). The average catheter lengths from insertion site to wedge position are 30 to 35 cm from the subclavian vein, 30 to 40 cm from the internal jugular, and 50 to 60 cm from the antecubital site.

Pulmonary Artery Pressure

Advancement of the balloon floatation catheter out to either branch of the pulmonary artery provides measurement of the dynamic pressure changes within the pulmonary artery. During the systolic phase of the cardiac cycle, right ventricular ejection through the open pulmonic valve produces the pulmonary artery systolic pressure (Fig. 17–12). During the diastolic phase, the pulmonic valve is closed, isolating the pulmonary artery pressure from right-heart influence. The mitral valve, however, is open, permitting equilibration of pressures between the left ventricle, the left atrium, and the pulmonary veins and the pulmonary artery. Thus, the pulmonary artery diastolic pressure reflects LVEDP in the absence of pulmonary or mitral valve disease.

The pulmonary artery pressure is divided into two phases: systole and diastole (Fig. 17–13). Systole begins with the opening of the pulmonic valve with rapid ejection of blood into the pulmonary artery. On the pulmonary artery waveform, this is seen as a sharp rise in pressure, followed by a decline in pressure as the ejected volume decreases (Fig. 17–14). When the right ventricular pressure falls below the level of the pulmonary artery pressure, the pulmonic valve snaps shut, producing a notch (the dicrotic notch) on the downslope of the waveform. Diastole follows pulmonic valve closure with

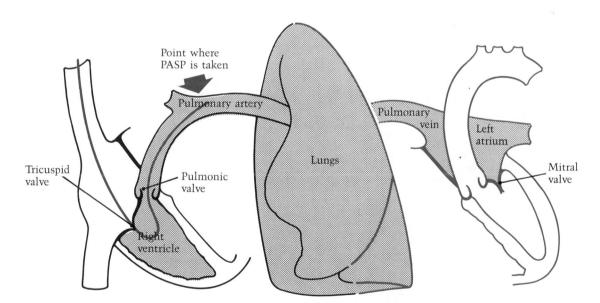

Figure 17–12
Measurement of pulmonary artery systolic pressure. Pulmonary artery systolic pressure (PASP) is the pressure in the pulmonary artery when the right ventricle is contracting and ejecting blood. Because the pulmonic valve is open, right ventricular and pulmonary artery systolic pressures are equal (unless the patient has pulmonary stenosis). Pulmonary artery systolic pressure, therefore, indicates right ventricular systolic function.

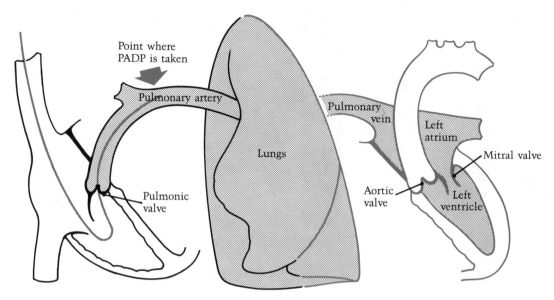

Figure 17–13

Measurement of pulmonary artery diastolic pressure. Pulmonary artery diastolic pressure (PADP) indicates left-sided heart pressures. In normal persons, it approximates the pulmonary artery wedge pressure (PAWP). However, in critically ill patients, especially in patients with pulmonary embolism or chronic obstructive lung disease, there may be differences, and PAWP must be measured directly.

runoff to the pulmonary artery, producing a further decline in pressure.

Normal peak systolic pulmonary artery pressure is 15 to 25 mm Hg, whereas the end-diastolic pressure ranges from 8 to 12 mm Hg. The systolic pressure measured in the pulmonary artery reflects the systolic right ventricular pressure (in the absence of pulmonic stenosis) and is, therefore, used clinically to assess right ventricular systolic function. The pulmonary artery end-diastolic pressure, on the other hand, reflects left

ventricular end-diastolic pressure (in the absence of pulmonary disease processes or mitral valve disease) and is used clinically to assess left ventricular diastolic function.

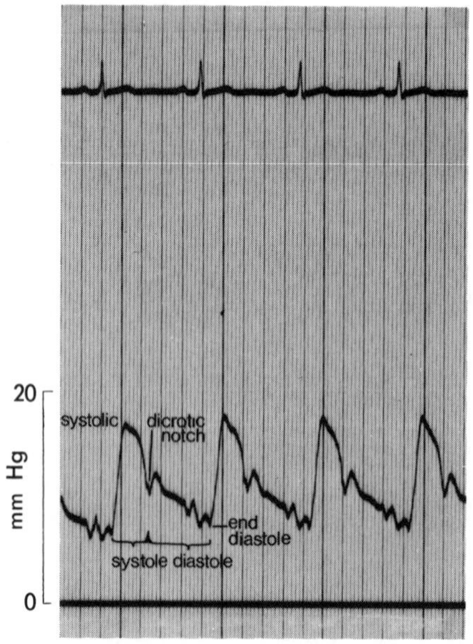

Abnormal elevation of the pulmonary artery pressure can occur secondary to increased pulmonary vascular resistance (PVR), increased pulmonary venous pressure, and increased pulmonary blood flow. Table 17–6 lists pathologic processes associated with each of these conditions.

Pulmonary Artery Wedge Pressure

The PAWP is obtained by inflating the balloon of the catheter to occlude a branch of the pulmonary artery (Fig. 17–15). This occlusion causes a cessation of forward blood flow in that branch of the pulmonary artery so that the catheter lumen at the tip senses only the pressure beyond it in the pulmonary venous system. Because there are no valves in the pulmonary venous system, this pressure is a direct reflection of the left atrial pressure. The pulmonary artery wedge waveform,

Figure 17–14

Normal pulmonary artery pressure. (Daily, E.K., and Schroeder, J.S. *Techniques in Bedside Hemodynamic Monitoring* (4th ed.) St. Louis: C.V. Mosby, 1989; with permission.)

Table 17–6
Causes of Pulmonary Hypertension

Increased pulmonary vascular resistance
   Pulmonary parenchymal disease
   Pulmonary embolus
   Essential pulmonary hypertension
   Hypoxia

Increased pulmonary venous pressure
   Mitral valve disease
   Left atrial myxoma
   Pulmonary venous obstruction
   Left ventricular failure

Increased pulmonary blood flow
   Left-to-right ventricular septal defect or atrial septal defect

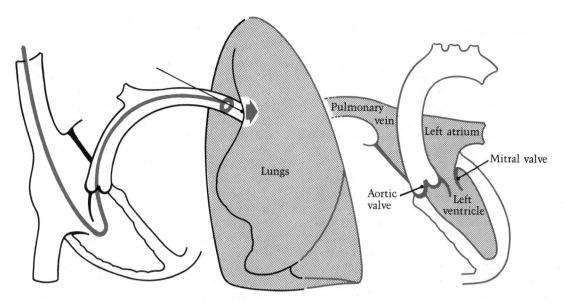

Figure 17-15

Measurement of pulmonary artery wedge pressure (PAWP). Pulmonary artery wedge pressure is obtained when the balloon of the pulmonary artery catheter is inflated and wedged into a branch of the pulmonary artery. Forward flow from the right side of the heart is blocked, and the wedge pressure reflects pressures from the left side of the heart.

therefore, reflects the left atrial pressure and is similar to the right atrial waveform in morphology, consisting of two or three positive waves (the *a*, *c*, and *v* waves) followed by negative waves (the *x*- and *y-descents*) (Fig. 17–16).[13] The a wave is a small rise in pressure produced by atrial contraction. It is followed by the *x-descent*, which represents a decline in pressure secondary to atrial relaxation. A small rise in pressure, the *c* wave, may occur during mitral valve closure, but it is

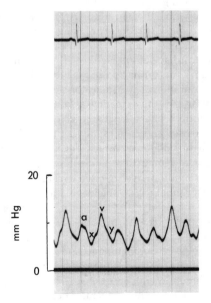

Figure 17-16

Normal pulmonary artery wedge pressure waveform showing *a* and *v* waves and *x*- and *y*-descents. (Daily, E.K., and Schroeder, J.S. *Techniques in Bedside Hemodynamic Monitoring* [4th ed.]. St. Louis: C.V. Mosby, 1989; with permission.)

not consistently transmitted to the pulmonary artery wedge waveform. The next positive wave is the *v* wave which represents an increase in pressure due to atrial filling. This is followed by opening of the mitral valve with rapid, passive filling of the LV. This rapid decline in atrial volume causes the pressure to fall, producing the *y-descent*.

Because both the *a* and *v* waves are of approximately the same magnitude (within a few mm Hg), a mean, or average of the components, is used to represent the average filling pressure of the left heart. Normally, this is between 4 to 12 mm Hg; however, if either one of the waves is more dominant than the other, the average height of each wave should be measured, and either the *a* wave or the *x* descent utilized as a reflection of left ventricular filling pressure. As with all hemodynamic pressure measurements, readings should be obtained at end-expiration when there is the least effect of pleural pressure changes.

The PAWP is clinically useful, not only as a reflection of LVEDP (LV preload) but as a direct measurement of pulmonary venous pressure, which is the primary determinant of pulmonary congestion.[7] Elevations in pulmonary venous pressure as measured by the PAWP are responsible for the movement of fluid out of the vascular space and into surrounding interstitial or intra-alveolar spaces and can be correlated with increasing evidence of pulmonary congestion both clinically (Table 17–7) and radiographically.[28]

Abnormal elevations in the PAWP can occur as a result of increases in left ventricular diastolic pressure (as in ventricular ischemia or infarction, or cardiomyopathy), increases in left atrial pressure (as in mitral stenosis or regurgitation), or increases in juxtacardiac pressure (cardiac tamponade, constrictive pericarditis, or high levels of positive end-expiratory pressure [PEEP] or continuous positive airway pressure [CPAP]. Elevations of the PAWP secondary to increased left atrial pressure, or increased pleural pressure are not reflective of changes in LVEDP. To assess LVEDP via the PAWP in

Table 17–7
**Changes in Pulmonary Artery Wedge Pressure (PAWP)
Associated With Pulmonary Congestion**

PAWP (mm Hg)	PULMONARY CONGESTION
18–20	Onset
20–25	Moderate
25–30	Severe
>30	Pulmonary edema

patients receiving PEEP greater than 10 cm H_2O, some clinicians approximate the transmural PAWP by subtracting one half of the PEEP level from the measured PAWP.[9] Removing PEEP for purposes of hemodynamic measurements is never recommended.

Patients with left ventricular dysfunction have decreased compliance with alterations in the pressure-volume relationship of the ventricle and, thus, require higher filling pressures to maintain adequate preload volume (Fig. 17–17). In these patients, efforts are made to maintain preload or PAWP between 15 to 20 mm Hg. These elevated pressures are not indicative of higher filling volumes, but rather the need for higher filling pressures for the same volume.

An elevated PAWP may also be obtained if the pulmonary artery catheter tip lies in zone 1 or 2 of the lung, in which the alveolar pressure exceeds pulmonary venous pressure. When the balloon of the catheter is inflated to obtain a PAWP reading in these locations, the higher alveolar pressure prevents accurate measurement of the pulmonary venous pressure. Accurate measurement requires that the catheter tip be located in a zone 3 location, in which pulmonary venous pressure always is greater than alveolar pressure, thus maintaining an open continuum between the catheter tip and the left atrium.[38] Fortunately, the pulmonary artery catheter, which is flow-directed, has a tendency to be carried to areas of greater flow, the zone 3 location.[3] Visual evidence of inaccurate PAWP measurement due to zone 1 or 2 conditions consists of the lack of normal waveform characteristics, a mean PAWP value greater than the pulmonary artery end-diastolic pressure, or

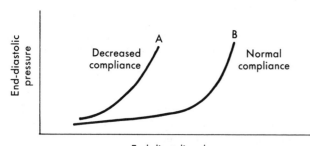

Figure 17–17

Relationship between ventricular end-diastolic volume and end-diastolic pressure. With normal ventricular compliance, relatively large increases in end-diastolic volume are accompanied by relatively small increases in end-diastolic pressure, up to a point (curve B). In the noncompliant ventricle, small increases in end-diastolic volume are associated with marked increases in end-diastolic pressure (curve A). (Daily, E.K., and Schroeder, J.S. *Techniques in Bedside Hemodynamic Monitoring* [4th ed.]. St. Louis: C.V. Mosby, 1989; with permission.)

an increase in the PAWP that exceeds more than half the increment in PEEP or CPAP.[29] Problems encountered with pulmonary artery catheters are discussed in Table 17–8.

Normally, the PAWP closely approximates the PAEDP (within 4 to 5 mm Hg). When such a close relationship has been established between the two pressures, the PAEDP should be monitored as a reflection of LVEDP. This eliminates the need to inflate the balloon of the catheter, with its potential risks of pulmonary infarction, pulmonary perforation, or hypoxemia.[21,24,52] However, in patients with increased pulmonary vascular resistance (PVR) due to pulmonary disease, pulmonary embolus or primary pulmonary hypertension, the PAWP must be obtained to assess the LVEDP accurately. A gradient greater than 5 mm Hg between the PAEDP and the PAWP is suggestive of pulmonary disease or hypoxia.[45] This observation is very useful in detecting underlying pulmonary disease.

Tachycardia (>130 beats/min) also invalidates the relationship between the PAEDP and the PAWP as the PAEDP becomes falsely elevated with the abbreviation of the diastolic period.

Cardiac Output

The development and refinement of the pulmonary artery catheter has produced an accepted and accurate method of determining cardiac output based on the principle of thermodilution. The cardiac output is calculated from changes in the blood temperature in the pulmonary artery.[25] A calibrated thermistor located approximately 4 cm from the catheter tip records changes in the temperature of the blood as a bolus that has been introduced into the right atrium circulates to the pulmonary artery. Because the quantity and temperature of the bolus are known, the difference in temperature between the bolus and the blood is the basis for the adjoining computer's calculation of the net blood flow during the time the temperature change was measured. (A constant number that stands for the gain of heat in addition to other minor variables are taken into consideration.) The change in pulmonary artery temperature creates a curve whose area is inversely proportional to the cardiac output (Fig. 17–18).[47] Patients with a low stroke volume and cardiac output exhibit a lower curve that is longer in duration as the indicator slowly circulates to the pulmonary artery, thus creating a larger area beneath the curve. In contrast, patients with a high cardiac output exhibit a curve that rises and falls rapidly as the indicator quickly circulates to the pulmonary artery. The injectate solution may be iced or room-temperature saline or dextrose in water.

Numerous studies have reported excellent correlation between cardiac output values obtained with either iced or room-temperature injectate.[11,30,39,50] However, the use of iced temperature is often necessary in patients who are significantly hypothermic, or whose fluid intake is very limited, necessitating the use of smaller (5 ml) injectate volumes. When using an iced solution, sufficient time should be allowed for the injectate solution to chill adequately. This time is reduced if the solution is kept in the refrigerator beforehand. The use of a closed injectate system with either room-temperature or iced injectate is preferred to reduce the risk of contamination and infection and improve accuracy.

The injectate solution can be injected manually or with the aid of an automatic injector. Whichever mode is used, the entire bolus must be injected smoothly and rapidly within 2 to 4 seconds. Faulty injection techniques are visually apparent on the upstroke of the cardiac output curve. A smooth, even upstroke represents a smooth, even injection, whereas an irregular upslope indicates an uneven or slow injection.

Normally, three cardiac output determinations are mathematically averaged as representative of the patient's average cardiac output. However, in patients with a wide range of cardiac output values, the number of determinations averaged may need to be increased to five or six.[11]

Alterations in stroke volume related to respiratory effects can result in widely varying cardiac output values. Timing all injections at the same point in the respiratory cycle may minimize some of this variation and increase the reproducibility of cardiac output determinations. However, such data represent the patient's flow rate at a specific time and are not reflective of the patient's average flow rate over time. Either random injections or injections made at varying times in the respiratory cycle are likely to represent more accurately the patient's average cardiac output per minute of time.

Fegler's initial description of the thermodilution technique recommended a 90-second interval between injections.[15] However, improved technology and thermistor sensitivity have shortened this time interval to approximately 1 minute.

It is important to remember that the thermodilution determination of cardiac output provides information over a very brief "window" of time, i.e., only several seconds of actual measurement. This number, then, is used as a reflection of the patient's flow rate per minute of time, and, depending on how frequently measurements are performed, it is assumed to reflect the patient's cardiac output over the ensuing hours. In addition to the patient's changing condition, the technique itself can introduce errors that further compound the problem.

Clinical Estimation

In the absence of more sophisticated techniques, many clinicians use a clinical estimate of the cardiac output. Stroke index is considered approximately equivalent to pulse pressure or to the volume of the radial pulse. In the pulse pressure estimate, the pulse pressure multiplied by the heart rate gives the estimated cardiac output (+20% to 35%). In the radial-pulse estimate, a full, strong pulse beat coupled with a rate within normal limits indicates a good cardiac output. However, preliminary studies indicate that the radial-pulse estimate varies from 30% to 200% of the anticipated levels, so the radial-pulse estimate must be used with this fact in mind. If the radial-pulse estimate is used, it should be used in combination with an evaluation of the patient's mental status, or degree of alertness, urinary output, and degree of blanching or skin color.

Ventricular Function Curves

With the measurement of cardiac output, data are available to calculate values that can be plotted on a series of ventricular function curves. A plotted curve is a representation of the Frank-Starling mechanism, with calculated or measured value representing systolic performance on the y-axis and a measured value representing preload on the x-axis. For example, cardiac output, stroke volume, or stroke work index can be placed on the y-axis and PAWP or PAEDP on the x-axis. The slope of the resulting curve signifies the response of the ventricle to an increase in preload.

Right ventricular stroke work index (RVSWI) and *left ventricular stroke work index* (LVSWI) reflect the amount of work performed by the heart. These parameters are used in accordance with PAWP as the basis for clinical decisions (Fig. 17–19). These values also can be used to plot a ventricular function curve for the patient and determine how the patient's functioning corresponds with normal contractility and the patient's own trends or past performance (see Fig. 17–19). In essence, the ventricular function curve reflects the overall performance of the heart. Therapy can be monitored and a visual picture formed for assessment purposes. For example, a therapy that is instituted may have more than one effect. These related effects can be determined by remeasuring the PAWP, recalculating the LVSWI, and determining if there is an overall improvement in cardiovascular function. In Figure 17–20, norepinephrine was administered, to a patient who had a subsequent rise in blood pressure (day 2). After measuring the hemodynamic parameters and calculating the LVSWI, however, the ventricular function curve indicates the patient's hemodynamic condition has deteriorated. Plotting ventricular function curves is very useful in assessing the patient's optimal preload level as well as visualizing changes in overall ventricular function.

INTRA-ARTERIAL MONITORING

Indwelling arterial catheters are common in critical care units. Because of the accuracy of direct pressure measurements, they are an ideal means to obtain continuous pressure readings. Serial samples for arterial blood gases and various hematologic samples can also be safely and easily obtained. Patients with multiple trauma, shock, dissecting aneurysms, extensive burns, and hyperthermia benefit from intra-arterial monitoring. It is also indicated in the patient who requires assisted ventilation for 3 to 5 days and needs frequent blood gas analysis.

Intra-arterial Pressure Measurements

Intra-arterial pressure can be measured directly by a small catheter placed in a peripheral artery. Directly measured arterial pressure is more accurate, and the ability to assess the arterial pulse waveform visually can often provide important diagnostic information.

The arterial system can be cannulated either percutaneously or by a cutdown at various sites, including the femoral, axillary, brachial, and radial arteries. Femoral and brachial arteries traditionally have been cannulated primarily in the cardiac catheterization laboratory on a short-term basis for pressure measurements and angiography, whereas the radial artery is commonly used for continuous intra-arterial monitoring at the bedside.

Catheter Placement

The physician selects the site for catheter placement from the radial, brachial, femoral, and dorsalis pedis arteries (Fig. 17–21). The radial artery is normally preferred because the hand usually receives collateral circulation from the ulnar artery.

Before cannulation of the radial artery, it is recommended to assess the adequacy of collateral blood flow to the hand.

Table 17–8
Problems Encountered With Pulmonary Artery Catheters

NURSING DIAGNOSIS	NURSING INTERVENTION(S)	RATIONALE
1. Decreased cardiac output		
Patient will demonstrate improvement in cardiac function	Measure SvO_2 and report reductions of 10% for 2–3 min or if <60%	Decrease in SvO_2 indicates inadequate tissue perfusion. SvO_2 < 60% associated with poor prognosis
	Reduce patient's activity and stress.	Reduced activity and stress will decrease O_2 demands
2. Altered peripheral tissue perfusion related to compromised circulation associated with invasive monitoring		
Patient will demonstrate optimal skin integrity, normal skin color and temperature, equal arterial pulses in all extremities	Assess catheter insertion site daily. Cleanse site, apply iodophor ointment and new sterile dressing.	Inflammation at catheter insertion site associated with infection or thrombophlebitis.
	Assess skin color, temperature and sensitivity in area around catheter insertion site. Report any significant changes.	Alteration in tissue perfusion may result in elevation in skin temperature below catheter site. An elevation in skin temperature with pain or tenderness is associated with thrombosis or thrombophlebitis.
	Palpate and compare pulses in each extremity. Report any changes.	A decrease or loss in arterial pulsations distal to catheter insertion site is associated with arterial insufficiency 2° thrombus formation.
	Assess catheterized extremity for evidence of edema by measuring like extremities at the same anatomic location.	Edema is characteristic manifestation when tissue perfusion is a result of venous interference.
3. High risk for infection related to invasive monitoring		
Patient will be free of infection as demonstrated by normal temperature, normal white blood cell count, negative cultures of blood or catheter tip	Check patient's temperature every 4 hr and as needed, and report any significant changes.	Increase in patient's temperature is associated with infectious process.
	Change catheter and catheter site every 4 days.	Risk of infection increases with duration of catheter placement > 5 days.
	Change IV fluid, tubing, stopcocks, and disposable transducer every 48–72 hr.	Static fluid is potential source for bacterial growth.
	Inspect and cleanse catheter insertion site every day, and apply iodophor ointment and clean sterile dressing.	Skin and old blood are potential sources for infection. Iodophor ointment reduces bacterial growth.
	Do not use IV solution containing glucose.	Glucose solutions promote growth of bacteria.
	Place sterile dead-ender caps on all stopcocks.	Open stopcock port allows bacteria to enter.
	Use aseptic technique when withdrawing from, or flushing the catheter.	Prevent contamination of open system.
	If reusable transducers are used, sterilize transducer before patient use.	Minute flaws in disposable transducer domes allow contact between infusing fluid and transducer, contaminating IV fluid.
	Carefully remove all traces of blood from stopcock ports after obtaining blood sample from catheter.	Old blood promotes growth of bacteria.
	Use sterile plastic sleeve over PA catheter.	Maintain external portion of catheter sterile to permit catheter advancement, if necessary.
4. High risk for injury related to hemorrhage, thromboembolism, venous air embolism, pulmonary infarction or hemorrhage, cardiac dysrhythmias or conduction disturbances		
A. Patient will remain without hemorrhage	Keep all catheter connecting sites visible, and observe frequently for possible hemorrhage.	Major blood loss can occur without notice from stopcocks or loose connections that are hidden beneath dressings or bed linens.
	Tighten all catheter connecting sites and stopcocks every 4 hr and as needed.	Plastic connections become loose over time and leakage can occur.

(continued)

Table 17-8   (*Continued*)

NURSING DIAGNOSIS	NURSING INTERVENTION(S)	RATIONALE
	Restrain patient, if necessary.	A restless or confused patient may pull catheter out, or connecting tubing apart.
	After removal of arterial catheter, apply firm pressure to insertion site for 10 min before checking and applying pressure dressing.	Allow clot to form at insertion site to seal vessel opening.
	Discontinue systemic heparinization several hours before catheter or sheath removal.	
B. Patient will remain without thrombus as evidenced by patent catheter, unimpeded infusion or flush, undamped waveform	Use heparinized IV solution with continuous-flush device to continuously infuse all catheter ports and sideport of sheath, if used.	Continuous forward flow and use of heparin is associated with decreased thrombus formation at catheter tip or around catheter in sheath.
	Always aspirate and discard before gently flushing any catheter. If unable to aspirate, do not flush catheter. Periodically aspirate and manually flush catheter or activate flush device (every 4–6 hr).	
	Do not fast flush arterial catheter longer than 2 sec; manually flush arterial catheter by gently tapping plunger of flush syringe with no more than 2–4 ml of fluid.	Vigorous flushing of arterial catheter with large amounts of fluid can result in cerebral embolization.
	Maintain 300 mm Hg pressure on IV cuff.	300 mm Hg ± required to maintain forward flow of heparinized solution via flush device.
	Remove all traces of blood from catheter, tubing, and stopcocks after withdrawing blood. Flush completely.	Residual blood in catheter, tubing, or stopcock can form small clots which can occlude catheter or be injected into patient.
C. Patient will remain without venous air embolism	Tighten all catheter connecting sites and stopcocks every 4 hr and as needed. Check frequently.	Plastic connections become loose over time permitting intake of air into system.
	Place dead-ender caps on all stopcock ports.	Open or vented ports permit intake of air.
	Keep all connections or possible openings into vascular system below level of heart.	Air intake more likely to occur through loose connection or open port when patient is in an upright position and takes a deep breath.
	Remove all air from IV solution bag.	Air in bag and solution enters tubing and catheter.
	Have patient hum or suspend respirations when vascular system is open and near or above heart level.	Air intake through open port occurs during inspiration.
	After removal of venous catheter that was in place for a long period of time, apply Vaseline and occlusive dressing to insertion site.	Air intake can occur through the open tract formed by long-dwelling catheter, especially in thin person with little subcutaneous tissue.
D. Patient will be free of pulmonary infarction or hemorrhage as evidenced by normal respirations, no hemoptysis, normal ABGs	Continuously monitor PA waveform at distal tip of PA catheter.	Forward migration of catheter into a wedged position will be evidenced by PAW waveform.
	Inflate balloon to wedge catheter briefly (<20 sec).	Minimize cessation in blood flow to reduce risk of pulmonary ischemia or infarction.
	Leave balloon of PA catheter deflated with stopcock open and syringe removed.	Open stopcock with syringe off permits passive deflation should any air remain in balloon.
	Monitor PAEDP instead of PAW (if close relationship).	Reduce risks caused by inflation of balloon and cessation of blood flow in branch of PA.
	Check location of catheter tip after insertion and as needed via PA chest film.	Catheter tip migrates forward along with blood flow into a wedge position (particularly during first 24 hr).
	Continuously observe waveform during *slow* balloon inflation; stop inflation at first appearance of PAW waveform. Do not inflate 7 F catheter with more than 1.5 cc air.	Overinflation of balloon can cause rupture of vessel.
	Do not inflate balloon with air if resistance is met.	Catheter may be in a small branch of the PA and already mechanically wedged, or balloon may already be inflated.
E. Patient will remain free of life-threatening dysrhythmias or conduction disturbances	Continuously monitor waveform from distal port of catheter.	Appearance of RV waveform indicates catheter tip has fallen into RV and could cause ventricular dysrhythmias.

(*continued*)

Table 17-8 (*Continued*)

NURSING DIAGNOSIS	NURSING INTERVENTION(S)	RATIONALE
	Monitor daily chest film.	Check for coiling of catheter in RV or RA, which could cause arrhythmias.
	If RV waveform appears, quickly inflate balloon of catheter.	Catheter tip in RV can produce ventricular dysrhythmias; with balloon inflation, catheter should float to PA.
	To remove catheter, deflate balloon actively and completely with syringe and quickly remove catheter.	Rapid removal of catheter with fully deflated balloon should result in few, if any, dysrhythmias.
	Follow emergency protocols for occurrence of life-threatening dysrhythmias.	

5. Anxiety related to fear of technologic equipment and procedures associated with hemodynamic monitoring.

Patient will verbalize feelings, demonstrate a relaxed manner, verbalize familiarity with hemodynamic monitoring procedures and equipment	Initiate interventions to reduce anxiety.	Readiness to learn facilitates meaningful learning and retention of knowledge.
	Assess ability and readiness to learn the following, when appropriate: 1. Reasons for hemodynamic monitoring 2. Function and purpose of hemodynamic monitoring equipment 3. Explanation of procedures related to hemodynamic monitoring	Knowing rationale and purpose of hemodynamic monitoring reduces anxiety.
	Instruct patient in relaxation techniques.	Use of energy release techniques helps reduce anxiety.
	Listen attentively, encourage verbalization, and provide a caring touch.	Reassurance to patient that he is not alone.

6. Sleep pattern disturbance related to invasive monitoring procedures

Patient will have undisturbed sleep	Do not awaken or reposition patient to obtain hemodynamic parameters.	Hemodynamic measurements may be obtained with patient in supine, right or left lateral positions, or 45° semi-fowler's position as long as air-reference stopcock is adjusted to mid-RA level and transducer is re-zeroed.
	Instruct in relaxation techniques.	Energy-release techniques help relax patient and aid in sleep
	Provide quiet, dimly lit environment.	Quiet, dark environment is more conducive to sleep.

ABG: arterial blood gas; PA: pulmonary artery; PAEDP: pulmonary artery end-diastolic pressure; PAW: pulmonary artery wedge; RA: right atrium; RV: right ventricle.

(Daily, E. K., and Schroeder, J. S. *Techniques in Bedside Hemodynamic Monitoring.* St. Louis: CV Mosby, 1989; with permission.)

This can be assessed by use of the ultrasonic Doppler test or the Allen test. In the ultrasonic Doppler test, the patency of the ulnar artery is ascertained by determining circulatory adequacy of an extension of the ulnar artery, the superficial palmar branch. The Doppler probe is positioned between the heads of the third and fourth metacarpals proximal to a line drawn along the medial edge of the outstretched thumb (Fig. 17–22). The probe is moved about until the pulse is located. Then the radial artery is manually compressed, and any circulation change to the superficial palmar arch is assessed by the Doppler probe. If there is no change, the radial artery can be used safely.

In the Allen test, the nurse visually inspects palmar circulation. Adequacy of ulnar circulation is assessed first by placing a finger or thumb over the patient's ulnar artery and the other thumb or finger over the patient's radial artery. The patient is asked to make a tight fist (squeezing blood from the palm and fingers) as the nurse increases pressure over the arterial site (Fig. 17–23). The nurse then asks the patient to open the fist and removes the pressure from the ulnar artery, leaving pressure over the radial artery. The nurse notes the time for return of color to the hand. If blood returns to the patient's palm and fingers within 5 seconds, the blood flow to the ulnar artery is adequate.

Before arterial catheter insertion, the nurse must evaluate the color, pulses, and warmth of the extremity. The condition of the extremity should be noted during the insertion, if possible, and immediately after insertion. Any changes should be reported to the physician immediately. The limb used for the arterial line insertion should remain uncovered or have easy access for observation. The pulses distal to the catheter should be checked every 2 hours for signs of thrombosis or total occlusion.

As with the venous cannulation technique, the area is scrubbed carefully with an iodine solution and a sterile drape is positioned around the site. A 1% solution of Xylocaine hydrochloride is used to anesthetize the area, and the percutaneous approach is used. The needle with catheter sheath is inserted into the artery. After the needle is withdrawn, the catheter is usually positioned 4 to 6 cm within the artery and a heparinized solution is attached under pressure to prevent clotting. The catheter is secured with sutures, and a sterile dressing is applied.

After the artery is cannulated, the nurse attaches the prepared arterial monitoring system, which comprises a flush bag of heparinized saline, nonvented pressurized tubing to the flush valve, a sterile disposible transducer with two stopcocks attached, and tubing from the transducer to the patient, with a stopcock placed near the insertion site for easy blood withdrawal. The transducer itself should be free of air bubbles and blood and should remain filled with heparinized sterile solution. The total assembly procedure is the same as that used with the pulmonary artery catheter. Any problems or potential problems should be investigated immediately and a solution identified (Table 17–9). In order to be sure no problems arise at the change of shifts as part of the caregiver-to-caregiver report, the nurse going off duty should accompany the oncoming nurse to the bedside and review all lines.

Arterial Pressure Pulse

The arterial pressure waveform resembles the pulmonary artery pressure waveform in contour and characteristics. Arterial systole begins with the opening of the aortic valve and rapid ejection of blood into the aorta associated with a rapid upstroke of the arterial pulse (Fig. 17–24). This is followed by runoff of blood from the proximal aorta to the peripheral arteries, which is associated with a decline in the arterial pressure. As the pressure falls, the aortic valve leaflets snap shut, causing a small rise or notch in the downslope of the pressure that is termed the *dicrotic notch*. Diastole follows closure of the aortic valve and continues until the next systolic ejection.

The peak systolic pressure, which reflects left ventricular systolic pressure, is normally 100 to 140 mm Hg in adults. Normal arterial end-diastolic pressure is 60 to 80 mm Hg.

The mean arterial pressure (MAP) represents the average pressure during the entire cardiac cycle and is dependent on the cardiac output and the elasticity or resistance of the vessels. Normal MAP is 70 to 90 mm Hg.

The pulse pressure is the difference between the systolic and diastolic pressure and is largely reflective of the stroke volume and arterial compliance. Wide pulse pressures are associated with large stroke volumes, whereas a narrow pulse pressure is seen in patients with low stroke volume.

The arterial pressure differs in both contour and value in various arterial locations. Arterial systolic pressures measured at sites distal from the aorta may be as much as 5 to 30 mm Hg higher owing to wave reflection and summation. Generally, the diastolic pressures become somewhat lower, whereas the mean values remain nearly the same.

BLOOD SAMPLES

The nurse will frequently need to obtain blood samples from the arterial line. The procedure is as follows:

1. Ascertain patency of the line by checking the pressure and waveform readings.
2. Turn the stopcock "off" to the patient and "open" to the

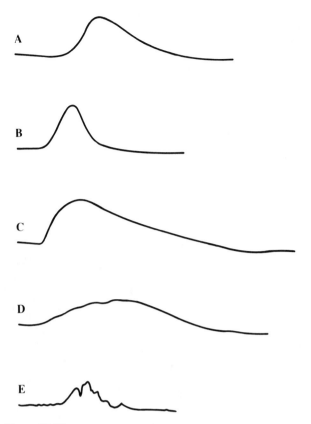

Figure 17–18

Schematic representation of various thermodilution cardiac output curves. (*A*) Normal cardiac output curve showing smooth, even upstroke. (*B*) Small area beneath the curve as seen in patients with high cardiac outputs. (*C*) Large area beneath the curve as seen in patients with low cardiac outputs. (*D*) Uneven injection indicated by uneven upstroke. (*E*) Artifact in both upstroke and decline of curve resulting in erroneous cardiac output measurement. (Tilkian, A., and Daily, E. K. *Cardiovascular Procedures: Diagnostic Techniques and Therapeutic Procedures.* St. Louis: C.V. Mosby, 1986; with permission.)

capped port site. Remove the cap and place a 10-ml sterile syringe to the port site.
3. Turn the stopcock "off" to the flush system and "open" to the port site syringe.
4. Draw 2 to 5 ml of blood from the line depending on the dead space of the catheter and tubing; turn the stopcock between ports "off" to all ports; discard the syringe.
5. Place a new sterile syringe in the port site.
6. Turn the stopcock "open" to the port site and the syringe; withdraw the amount of blood needed.
7. Turn the stopcock "off" to the port site and "open" between the flush system and the patient.
8. Remove the syringe, remove any air, place a cap on the tip and put in ice if necessary; fast-flush the line to the patient.
9. Turn the stopcock "off" to the patient and "open" between the flush system and port site. Fast-flush the open port site onto some sterile gauze without contaminating the port site.
10. Put a sterile cap on the port site. Turn the stopcock so that the system is on continual flush to the patient at 3 to 5 ml/hour.

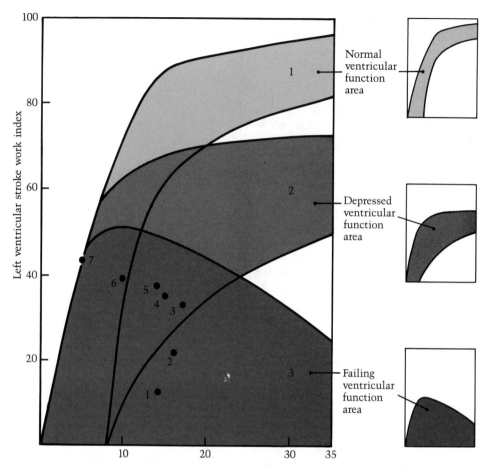

Figure 17–19

Ventricular function curve. A curve of cardiac function can be constructed for an individual patient. A measure of preload is plotted against a measure of systolic performance. Usually, pulmonary artery wedge pressure is used as the indicator for preload and left ventricular stroke work index as the indicator for systolic performance. The patient whose data are plotted here sustained significant multisystem trauma in a decelerating accident with subsequent hemodynamic instability. His ventricular performance improved significantly as treatment progressed (points 1 through 7).

MIXED VENOUS OXYGEN DETERMINATIONS

Measurement of the oxygen saturation in the venous blood is used clinically as a global reflection of tissue oxygenation.[45] When oxygen delivery to the tissues is normal (approximately 1000 ml/min) and the rate of oxygen extraction by the tissues is normal (approximately 25% at rest), the amount of oxygen remaining in the venous blood is about 75%. In fact, when mixed venous blood remains approximately 60% to 80% saturated with oxygen, it is generally assumed that oxygen delivery is adequate for the tissue's needs. On an even broader scale, a normal mixed venous oxygen saturation (SvO_2) usually reflects adequate cardiac output.

The saturation of oxygen in venous blood varies, depending on the organ system it serves. Venous blood returning from high flow areas such as the kidney or skin have higher concentrations of oxygen than venous blood from other areas (*e.g.*, from the heart). Complete mixing of these varying oxygen saturations occurs in the right ventricle, making the pulmonary artery blood reflective of the true mixed venous oxygen saturation. The oxygen saturation of pulmonary artery blood represents a flow-weighted average of all the different end-capillary oxygen saturations.

Measurement of the oxygen saturation of venous blood in the pulmonary artery can be done on an intermittent basis, with pulmonary artery blood samples sent to the laboratory for analysis, or on a continuous basis, with the use of a special SvO_2 catheter. This catheter is a modified 7.5 or 8 F thermodilution pulmonary artery catheter with one lumen containing optic fibers that transmit light to and from the blood stream. The light source consists of three diodes that emit alternating pulses of two or three wavelengths of red light through one of the optical fibers. This light is absorbed, refracted by the hemoglobin constituents of the blood, and reflected back through the second optical fiber to a light detector and data processor for analysis. The processed signal represents the percentage of total hemoglobin that has combined with oxygen

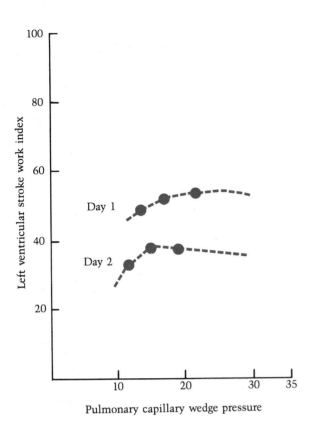

Figure 17–20
Ventricular function curve indicating hemodynamic deterioration. Although the patient's blood pressure increased after norepinephrine administration (day 2), the ventricular function curve indicates that the patient's overall hemodynamic condition has deteriorated.

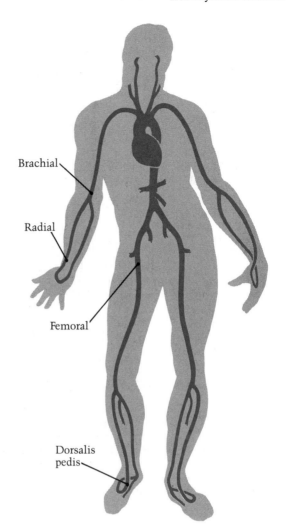

Figure 17–21
Arterial circulation. Arteries used for arterial cannulation are (1) radial, (2) brachial, (3) femoral, and (4) dorsalis pedis.

(oxyhemoglobin) and is continuously displayed digitally as well as visually on an attached monitor.

Continuous monitoring of SvO_2 with a fiberoptic catheter provides immediate "real-time" information on changes in the cardiopulmonary function and the balance between oxygen demand and supply. A decrease in any of the determinants of oxygen supply (cardiac output, hemoglobin, or arterial saturation) is usually associated with a decrease in SvO_2. In contrast, any change in oxygen demands, or oxygen consumption, is associated with an inverse change in the SvO_2.

Normal oxygen saturation of mixed venous blood ranges from 65% to 77%. SvO_2 levels below 60% occur because of increased oxygen extraction by the tissues and reflect an imbalance between the supply of and demand for oxygen. Most commonly, this is a result of cardiac decompensation, although sudden declines in SaO_2 or hemoglobin also can have the same effect. When SvO_2 falls to 50% or less, lactic acidosis can occur as a result of anaerobic metabolism.[16] The precise level at which anaerobic metabolism and lactic acidosis begin varies in each patient, but an SvO_2 of less than 40% likely represents the limits of compensation and impending lactic acidosis. Generally, an SvO_2 less than 30% (20 mm Hg) indicates insufficient oxygen availability to the tissues. Clinically, this degree of tissue hypoxia is usually accompanied by coma.

Table 17–10 lists the probably causes and clinical states associated with high and low SvO_2 readings. A fall in SvO_2 below 60% lasting for 5 minutes or longer indicates a compromise in at least one of the determinants of oxygen transport (cardiac output, hemoglobin, or arterial oxygen saturation) relative to oxygen demands. However, it is important to remember that a "normal" mixed venous oxygen saturation does not ensure adequate oxygen delivery to any one specific organ system but rather reflects an overall picture of tissue oxygenation.

Sustained reductions in SvO_2 of 10% or greater for 5 minutes or longer should prompt assessment of the determinations of oxygen delivery (Fig. 17–25) because this finding frequently warns of impending deterioration. Appropriate therapy directed towards correcting the decrease in oxygen supply controlling the oxygen demands can then be evaluated by assessing the subsequent response in the SvO_2.

Studies to assess the correlation between SvO_2 and any one of the individual determinants of oxygen delivery or of oxygen consumption have failed to show a consistent relationship.[4,49] However, correlation of SvO_2 and all the determinants is inversely high, suggesting that changes in SvO_2 occur not because of alterations in any one single determinant of the oxygen supply-demand balance but instead reflect an overall

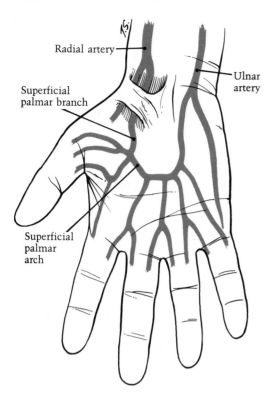

Figure 17–22

Palmar circulation. Before the placement of an arterial catheter, patency of the ulnar artery as it supplies the palm is evaluated with the ultrasonic Doppler test. The probe is placed over the superficial palmar arch and moved about until the pulse is heard. The radial artery is then compressed and the palmar circulation evaluated. If there is no change in the frequency of the signal heard, the radial artery can be used safely.

imbalance. Therefore, SvO_2 is used as a "barometer" to reflect overall tissue oxygenation.

RISKS AND COMPLICATIONS

Although valuable information can be obtained with hemodynamic monitoring, the invasiveness of the procedure places the patient at risk for the development of various complications ranging from minor, transient dysrhythmias to death. To date, there are no studies showing that the use of the pulmonary artery catheter has changed the outcome of the critically ill patient for most disease states,[35,42] and at least one study has suggested that pulmonary artery monitoring does *not* play a major role in influencing patient outcome after cardiac surgery.[48]

An awareness of potential complications that can occur in patients undergoing hemodynamic monitoring as well as steps to avoid such complications are key responsibilities of the critical care nurse. All efforts must be made continually to protect the patient from harm.

Cardiac Dysrhythmias

The occurrence of atrial or ventricular dysrhythmias during insertion of the pulmonary artery catheter is common and usually transient in nature. However, in patients with poor cardiac reserve, metabolic disorders, or underlying rhythm

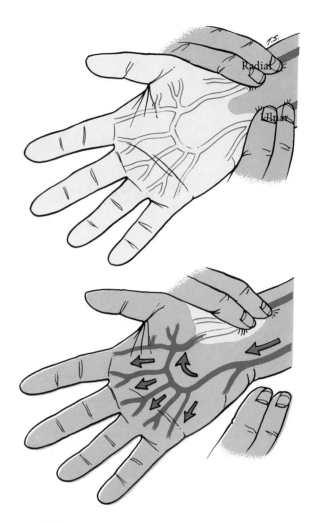

Figure 17–23

Allen test for palmar circulation. Prior to the placement of an arterial catheter, patency of the ulnar artery can be evaluated by the Allen test. The radial and ulnar arteries are compressed and the effect of the palmar circulation noted. The ulnar artery is then released. If return of circulation is seen within 5 seconds, ulnar circulation is ensured and the radial artery can be safely used for cannulation. If patency of the radial artery needs to be tested, the test can be repeated with release of the radial artery.

disorders, sustained ventricular tachycardia may develop, necessitating drug therapy or prompt cardioversion, or both. Ventricular fibrillation occurs rarely, necessitating immediate defibrillation. The occurrence of ventricular dysrhythmias correlates highly with shock, acute myocardial ischemia or infarction, hypokalemia, hypocalcemia, hypoxemia, acidosis, and prolonged catheter insertion times.

Prophylactic steps include the correction of electrolyte, oxygen, and metabolic disorders before catheter insertion in addition to a rapid placement of the pulmonary artery catheter. In general, the prophylactic use of lidocaine is not indicated, but in selected high-risk patients, it may be helpful.[43]

Bundle Branch Block

Right bundle branch block (RBBB) can easily occur during manipulation of the pulmonary artery catheter in the right

Table 17-9
Troubleshooting Problems Encountered With Intra-arterial Catheters

PROBLEMS	ASSESSMENT	NURSING ORDERS	PREVENTION
Bleeding related to arterial line disconnection	Separation of tubing with blood loss	Reattach connection. Estimate blood loss. Notify physician if over 50 ml.	Use Luer-Lock connections. Keep all connecting sites visible.
Infection related to local environmental characteristics, *e.g.,* no covering on stopcocks, blood back-up, encrusted blood surrounding stopcocks, prolonged catheter use	Increased temperature; redness, swelling at insertion site	Change occlusive dressing daily using aspectic techniques. Use antibacterial agent such as providone-iodine at site. Observe site carefully during daily dressing change. Notify physician when line has been in place 72 hr. Monitor extremity for distal ischemia, vasospasm, aneurysm, or hematoma, or signs of inflammation.	Maintain aseptic techniques. Use sterile caps to occlude all open parts. Carefully remove all traces of blood after blood sampling.
Damped pressure waveform related to partial occlusion by clot or catheter tip against vessel wall	Decreased amplitude of waveform	Observe waveform continuously. Reposition extremity while observing waveform. Observe catheter for any kinks. Check extremity for circulation Make sure stopcocks have been turned properly. Check for air bubbles. Aspirate clot with syringe; then flush system with sterile solution.	Use heparinized flush system with continuous drip. Fast flush after blood withdrawal.
Inaccurate pressure waveform and reading related to technical malfunction Decreased or absent distal pulse related to spasm or thrombosis of cannulated artery	Very high pressure, low to absent pressures Weak or absent pulses distal to catheter site; cool extremity distal to catheter site	Check transducer level and patient position. Re-zero and calibrate system. Check transducer calibration with mercury manometer. Check fast-flush dynamic response of system. Make sure transducer is open to catheter and that other settings on monitor are correct. Check connections. Notify physician if pulses are weak or absent. Prepare patient for catheter removal and Fogarty catheter procedure.	Understand workings of stopcocks and lines. Check for air bubbles within monitoring system each shift. Check fast-flush dynamic response of monitoring system each shift. Heparinize flush solution. Fast-flush monitoring line one to two times/shift. Occasionally use gentle manual flush with heparinized solution.

ventricle. This generally is not a problem, unless the patient has pre-existing left bundle branch block (LBBB), resulting in complete atrioventricular block and significant hypotension. In patients with LBBB, use of a pulmonary artery catheter with pacing electrodes or immediate availability of external pacing electrodes is recommended.[44]

The best prevention of this complication is rapid, gentle insertion of the pulmonary artery catheter, taking care to ensure that the balloon of the catheter is fully inflated before entering the right ventricle.

Pulmonary Infarction

Infarction of the lung can occur as a result of embolization of thrombus from the catheter or as a result of catheter migration and prolonged wedging that is preventing perfusion to an area of the lung. Forward migration of the catheter tip commonly occurs during the first 24 hours after insertion as the catheter loop in the right ventricle tightens with each contraction.

Steps to prevent this serious complication include continuous monitoring of the pressure from the distal lumen of the

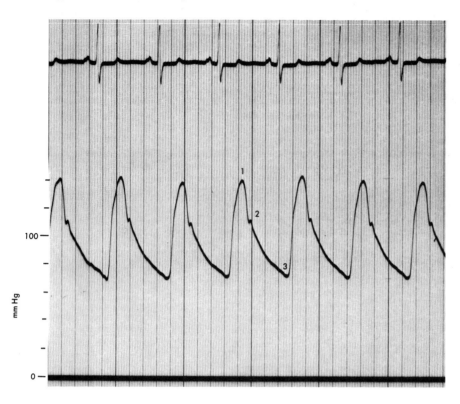

Figure 17–24
Normal arterial pressure waveform. 1: systole; 2: dicrotic notch; 3: diastole. (Daily, E.K., and Schroeder, J.S. *Hemodynamic Waveforms: Exercises in Interpretation and Analysis* [2nd ed.]. St. Louis: C.V. Mosby, 1990; with permission.)

catheter to detect any signs of self-wedging; monitoring the PAEDP rather than the PAWP (if there is good agreement); wedging the catheter, if necessary, for a very brief (<30 seconds) period of time; and carefully reviewing the chest x-ray in the first 12 to 24 hours. Chest x-rays should be repeated any time catheter migration is suspected.

Pulmonary Artery Rupture

Rupture of the pulmonary artery is a dramatic and usually fatal complication that occurs infrequently with the use of the pulmonary artery catheter. Patients with existing pulmonary hypertension, elderly patients (>60 years of age), patients re-

Table 17–10
Causes of Imbalance Between Oxygen Supply and Demand

	SvO_2 READING	PHYSIOLOGIC ALTERATION	CLINICAL CAUSES
High	80%–95%	Decreased O_2 consumption	Hypothermia Anesthesia Induced muscular paralysis Sepsis
		Increased O_2 delivery	Hyperoxia
		Mechanical interference	Catheter-wedged Left-to-right shunt
Normal	60%–80%	O_2 supply = O_2 demand	Adequate perfusion
Low	<60%	Increased O_2 consumption	Shivering Pain Seizures Activity/exercise Hyperthermia Anxiety
		Decreased O_2 delivery	Hypoperfusion (decreased cardiac output) Anemia Hypoxemia

(Daily, E. K., and Schroeder, J. S. *Techniques in Bedside Hemodynamic Monitoring*. St. Louis: CV Mosby, 1989; with permission.)

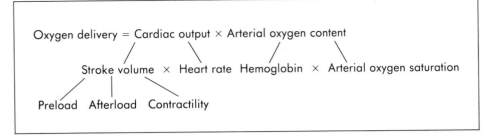

Figure 17-25

Oxygen delivery is a product of the cardiac output and the oxygen content of arterial blood. In turn, cardiac output is a product of stroke volume and heart rate. The stroke volume is subsequently determined by the preload, afterload, and contractility. The arterial oxygen content is a product of the patient's hemoglobin and oxygen saturation of arterial blood. Alterations in oxygen delivery can be achieved by manipulation of any of these parameters. (Daily, E.K., and Schroeder, J.S. *Techniques in Bedside Hemodynamic Monitoring* [4th ed.]. St. Louis: C.V. Mosby, 1989; with permission.)

ceiving anticoagulation therapy, and patients undergoing cardiac surgery with hypothermia are at increased risk for the development of this complication. For this reason, PAWP measurements in this subgroup should be avoided (if at all possible) or minimized. Pulmonary artery rupture may be caused by distal migration of the catheter tip, overinflation of the balloon, eccentric inflation of the balloon, and forceful manual flushing of a wedged catheter.

If pulmonary artery rupture is small, as indicated by a small amount of hemoptysis, the catheter should be immediately withdrawn to a proximal location, and the patient should be placed in a lateral recumbent position with the affected side down, with close observation and monitoring. If anticoagulation is being given, it should be stopped or reversed. Massive hemoptysis can be controlled with the insertion of a double-lumen endotracheal tube to prevent bleeding into the unaffected lung and improve ventilation. Prompt surgical repair may be necessary, along with pneumonectomy or lobectomy.

Prevention of this frequently fatal complication includes monitoring the distal lumen pressure continuously to ensure catheter tip location in the pulmonary artery; radiographically confirming a proximal location of the pulmonary artery catheter tip; monitoring the PAEDP rather than the PAWP (if close correlation); wedging the catheter, if necessary, for a very brief period of time (<30 seconds); slowly inflating the balloon while constantly monitoring the pressure and discontinuing balloon inflation *as soon as* the PAWP waveform appears; never using more than the recommended volume of air; making sure the waveform changes to pulmonary artery after balloon deflation; and always deflating the balloon before performing a gentle, manual flush of the catheter.

Cardiac Tamponade

Cardiac perforation resulting in cardiac tamponade can occur during movement of any catheter placed within the heart. This rare complication more commonly is associated with CVP catheters than pulmonary artery catheters, and can occur anytime from minutes to days after catheter insertion.[10]

Prevention of this complication includes radiographic documentation of appropriate location of the catheter tip; catheter insertion at a central site rather than in an arm vein, in which

movement of the extremity can promote catheter tip advancement; and careful suturing of the catheter at the insertion site.

Infection

Patients with pulmonary artery catheters may be more susceptible to nosocomial infections. Infection secondary to catheterization can range from contamination to colonization to sepsis. Although contamination or colonization reportedly occurs frequently (5% to 35% reported incidence), the development of sepsis related to pulmonary artery catheterization occurs in only 1% to 8% of patients with a pulmonary artery catheter.[19,31]

Prevention of infection includes meticulous technique during catheter insertion; daily care of the insertion site, including cleansing with a bactericidal agent and application of iodophor ointment and a sterile dressing; short duration of catheter placement (72 hours or less); use of a sterile sleeve in case catheter advancement is necessary; replacement of intravenous solution, tubing, stopcocks, and transducer every 48 hours; and use of nonglucose intravenous solution.

Thrombosis

All intracardiac and intravascular catheters are thrombogenic to some degree. Although thrombosis is frequently present along the pulmonary artery catheter or at the site of insertion, it infrequently represents a complication. Of concern, however, is the possibility of thrombus embolizing to the pulmonary artery. Overt signs of the presence of thrombus at the tip of the catheter are a damped appearance to the monitored waveform and difficulty in aspirating or flushing the lumen of the catheter. Preventative steps include the use of heparinized flush solution with a continuous flush system, occasional aspiration and gentle flushing of the catheter, short duration of catheter placement, and, possibly, the use of heparin-bonded catheters.

Arterial thrombosis occurs more commonly with the use of catheter sizes greater than 20 gauge and in catheters placed longer than 4 days.[14] Although arterial thrombosis can cause ischemia of the distal limb, it is reported to be asymptomatic in the majority of the patients.[8] Of concern is the potential for embolization to the systemic circulation. Prevention of arterial thrombosis is similar to that of venous thrombosis. However, particular care must be taken during manual flushing of arterial catheters, as even a small amount of flush solution (6 to 7 ml) has been shown to move retrograde into the cerebral circulation.[23] Flushing should be done very gently with tapping injections of a small amount of heparinized solution.

Air Embolism

The entry of air into the venous system can occur during catheter insertion, through an opening in the system after the catheter is in place, or after the catheter is removed and an open tract remains. The negative pressure generated during spontaneous inspiration can draw air into the venous system any time it is opened to ambient pressure. This complication reportedly occurs more commonly when either CVP or pulmonary artery catheters are inserted into the subclavian vein, rather than the internal jugular vein.[9] Treatment consists of placement of the patient in the left lateral position to promote movement of air to the right ventricular apex and away from the right ventricular outflow tract, where it would obstruct flow to the pulmonary artery. Administration of 100% oxyfjgen and aspiration of air through the catheter should also be carried out.[9]

Prevention of this complication includes placing patients in a Trendelenburg position during central catheterization, instructing the patient to stop breathing or to hum anytime the venous system is opened to air (during cannulation particularly), always making sure the fluid system is below the level of the heart when it is opened to air, using sheaths with self-sealing hemostatic valves, and placing vaseline and an occlusive dressing over the insertion site after catheter removal in patients who have had catheters in for extended periods of time.

SUMMARY

Patient monitoring is a rapidly expanding responsibility of the critical care nurse. The informed nurse plays a collaborative role with the physician in assessing changes in the patient's condition. The nurse is the constant caregiver at the bedside and is, therefore, the person who most readily identifies subtle changes in a patient's condition or initiates appropriate therapy according to specific protocols. When information from measurements with the flow-directed catheter is coupled with the calculations performed by a computer with a simple, programmable calculation, cardiovascular functioning can be assessed. Individual patient values can be evaluated with previous values and normal values and plotted on a curve to illustrate visually the patient's status.

The invasive nature of hemodynamic monitoring requires meticulous care and attention of the critical care nurse to prevent any possible harm to the patient. Equally important is the acquisition of accurate data on which subsequent therapies are based. This responsibility requires cognizance of the technical aspects affecting hemodynamic measurements. Standardization of associated technical procedures is necessary to ensure appropriate measurement. Hemodynamic data gathered in this way can positively impact care and management of the critically ill patient.

REFERENCES

1. Alpert, J. S. Hemodynamic monitoring: The basics. *Primary Cardiol.* 16:113, 1981.
2. Babb, J. D., and Leaman, D. M. Risks of cardiac catheterization today. *J. Cardiovasc. Med.* 5:941, 1980.
3. Benumof, J. L., Saidman, L. J., and Arkin, D. B. Where pulmonary arterial catheters go: Intrathoracic distribution. *Anesthesiology* 46:336, 1977.
4. Boutros, A. R., and Lee, C. Value of continuous monitoring mixed venous oxygen saturation in the management of critically ill patients. *Crit. Care Med.* 14:132, 1986.
5. Brantijan, C. O. Hemodynamic monitoring: Interpreting values. *Am. J. Nurs.* 82:86, 1982.
6. Branwald, E. Determinants and assessment of cardiac function. *N. Engl. J. Med.* 296:87, 1977.
7. Calvin, J. E., Driedser, A. A., and Sibbald, W. J. Does the pulmonary capillary wedge pressure predict left ventricular preload in critically ill patients? *Crit. Care Med.* 6:437, 1981.
8. Clark, C. A., and Harman, E. M. Hemodynamic Monitoring: Arterial Catheters. In J. M. Civetta, R. W. Taylor, and R. R. Kirby, (Eds.), *Critical Care.* Philadelphia: JB Lippincott, 1988.
9. Clark, C. A., and Harman, E. M. Hemodynamic Monitoring: Pulmonary Artery Catheters. In J. M. Civetta, R. W. Taylor, and R. R. Kirby, (Eds.), *Critical Care.* Philadelphia: JB Lippincott, 1988.
10. Collier, P. E., Ryan, J. J., and Diamond, D. L. Cardiac tamponade from central venous catheters. Reports of a case and review of the English literature. *Angiology* 35:595, 1984.
11. Daily, E. K., and Mersch, J. Comparison of Fick method of cardiac output with thermodilution method using two indicators. *Heart Lung* 16:294, 1987.
12. Daily, E. K., and Schroeder, J. S. *Techniques in Bedside Hemodynamic Monitoring* (4th ed.). St. Louis: CV Mosby, 1989.
13. Daily, E. K., and Schroeder, J. S. *Hemodynamic Waveforms: Exercise Waveforms: Exercises in Interpretation and Analysis* (2nd ed.). St. Louis: CV Mosby, 1990.
14. Downs, J. B., Chapman, R., and Hawkins, I. Prolonged radial artery catheterization. *Arch. Surg.* 108:671, 1974.
15. Fegler, G. Measurement of cardiac output in anesthetized animal by a thermodilution method. *Q. J. Exp. Physiol.* 39:153, 1954.
16. Gilbert, B. W., and Hew, E. M. Physiologic significance of hemodynamic measurements and their derived indices. *Can. Med. J.* 121:871, 1979.
17. Gore, J. M., Goldberg, R. J., Spodick, D. H., *et al.* A community-wide assessment of the use of pulmonary artery catheters in patients with acute myocardial infarction. *Chest* 92:721, 1987.
18. Hardaway, R. M. Pulmonary artery pressure versus pulmonary capillary wedge pressure and central venous pressure in shock. *Resuscitation* 10:47, 1982.
19. Hudson-Civetta, J. A., Civetta, J. M., Martinez, O. V., *et al.* Risk and deletion of pulmonary artery catheter-related infection in septic surgical patients. *Crit. Care Med.* 15:29, 1987.
20. Kahn, J. K., and Kirsh, M. M. The infusion delivery time of the flow directed pulmonary artery catheter: Clinical implications. *Heart Lung* 12:630, 1983.
21. Kainuma, M., and Shimada, Y. Decreased partial pressure of oxygen secondary to inflation of a pulmonary artery flow-directed catheter balloon. *Anesthesiology* 66:214, 1987.
22. Lamb, J. F., Ingram, C. G., Johnston, I. A., *et al. Essentials of Physiology.* New York: Blackwell, 1980.
23. Lowenstein, E., Little, J. W., and Lo, H. H. Prevention of cerebral embolization from flushing radial artery cannulas. *N. Engl. J. Med.* 285:1414, 1971.
24. McDaniel, D., Stone, J., Faltas, A., *et al.* Catheter-induced pulmonary artery hemorrhage. *J. Thorac. Cardiovasc. Surg.* 82:1, 1981.
25. Martin, C., Sanx, P., Auffray, J. P., *et al.* Thermodilution cardiac output measurements by injection in pulmonary artery vs CVP catheter. *Crit. Care Med.* 11(6):460, 1983.

26. Matthay, M. S. Invasive hemodynamic monitoring in critically ill patients. *Clin. Chest Med.* 2:233, 1983.

27. Mazzara, J. T., Parmley, W. W., and Russell, R. O. A close look at Swan-Ganz catheters. *Patient Care* 15(Feb):37, 1988.

28. Nemaans, E. J., and Woods, S. L. Normal fluctuations in pulmonary artery and pulmonary capillary wedge pressures in acutely ill patients. *Heart Lung* 11:393, 1982.

29. O'Quinn, R., and Marini, J. Pulmonary artery occlusion pressure: Clinical physiology, measurement and interpretation. *Am. Rev. Respir. Dis.* 128:319, 1983.

30. Pearl, R. G., Rosenthal, M. H., Nielson, L., et al. Effect of injectate volume and temperature on thermodilution cardiac output determination. *Anesthesiology* 64:798, 1986.

31. Pinilla, J., Ross, D., Martin, T., et al. Study of the incidence of intravascular catheter infection and associated septicemia in critically ill patients. *Crit. Care Med.* 11:21, 1983.

32. Quinn, K., and Quebbeman, E. J. Pulmonary artery pressure monitoring in the surgical intensive care unit. *Arch. Surg.* 116:872, 1981.

33. Rajacich, N., Burchard, K. W., Hasan, F. M., et al. Central venous pressure and pulmonary capillary wedge pressure as estimates of left atrial pressure: Effects of positive end-expiratory pressure and catheter tip malposition. *Crit. Care Med.* 17:7, 1989.

34. Riedinger, M. S., Shellock, F. G., and Swan, H. J. C. Reading pulmonary artery and pulmonary capillary wedge pressure waveforms with respiratory variations. *Heart Lung* 10:675, 1981.

35. Rinaldo, J. E. Risks and benefits of pulmonary artery catheters. *N.Y. State J. Med.* 84:484, 1984.

36. Robin, E. The cult of the Swan-Ganz catheter: Overuse and abuse of pulmonary flow catheters. *Ann. Intern. Med.* 103:445, 1985.

37. Ross, G. *Essentials of Human Physiology.* Chicago: Yearbook Medical Publishers, 1982.

38. Shasby, D., Dauber, I., Pfister, S., et al. Swan-Ganz location and left atrial pressure determine the accuracy of the wedge pressure when positive end-expiratory pressure is used. *Chest* 80:666, 1981.

39. Shellock, F. G., and Riedinger, M. S. Reproducibility and accuracy of using room temperature vs ice temperature injectate of thermodilution cardiac output determination. *Heart Lung* 12:174, 1983.

40. Shoemaker, W. C., et al. Clinical trial of survivors' cardiorespiratory patterns as therapeutic goals in critically ill postoperative patients. *Crit. Care Med.* 10:398, 1982.

41. Snow, N., Luces, A. E., and Richardson, J. D. Intra-aortic balloon counterpulsation for cardiogenic shock from cardiac contusion. *J. Trauma* 22(5):426, 1982.

42. Spodick, D. H. Physiologic and prognostic implications of invasive monitoring. Undetermined risk/benefit ratios in patients with heart disease. *Am. J. Cardiol.* 46:173, 1980.

43. Sprung, C. L., et al. Prophylactic use of lidocaine to prevent advanced ventricular arrhythmias during pulmonary artery catheterization. *Am. J. Med.* 75:906, 1983.

44. Sprung, C. L., Elser, B., Schein, R. M. H., et al. Risk of right bundle branch block and complete heart block during pulmonary artery catheterization. *Crit. Care Med.* 17:1, 1989.

45. Swan, H. J. C., Ganz, W., and Forrester, J. S. Catheterization of the heart in man with the use of a flow directed, balloon tipped catheter. *N. Engl. J. Med.* 283:447, 1970.

46. Swan, H. J., and Ganz, W. Hemodynamic measurements in clinical practice: A decade in review. *J. Am. Coll. Cardiol.* 1:103, 1983.

47. Tilkian, A., and Daily, E. K. *Cardiovascular Procedures.* St. Louis: CV Mosby, 1987.

48. Tuman, K. J., McCarthy, R. J., and Spiess, B. D. Effect of pulmonary artery catheterization on outcome in patients undergoing coronary artery surgery. *Anesthesiology* 70(2):199, 1989.

49. Vaughn, S., and Puri, V. K. Cardiac output changes and continuous mixed venous oxygen saturation measurement in the critically ill. *Crit. Care Med.* 16:495, 1988.

50. Vennix, C. V., Nelson, D. H., and Pierpont, G. L. Thermodilution cardiac output in critically ill patients: Comparison of room temperature and iced injectate. *Heart Lung* 13:574, 1984.

51. Vij, D., Babcock, R., and Magilligan, D. J. A simplified concept of complete physiological monitoring of the critically ill patient. *Heart Lung* 10:75, 1981.

52. Wiedemann, H., Matthay, M., and Matthay, R. Cardiovascular-pulmonary monitoring in the intensive care unit. *Chest* 85:537, 1984.

18

Mechanical Assistance for the Patient With a Failing Heart

Gayle Whitman

LOVE

True love makes you vulnerable. It allows you to accompany another person through crisis, change, pain, and dying. Love is the unconditional core that resides within you—the only thing that truly heals. When you acknowledge each day that you possess the qualities of unconditional love, then this experience is mirrored in much of what you do each day. This quality of unconditional love is that experience with another person when you feel connected. Your separateness is set aside, and you are present to serve and share with yourself and others.

From the center of love comes joy, because you can experience such profound joy about living life at this moment that nothing else matters. Being in this space allows for the true experience of time as being only the present moment. Unconditional love helps release you from fear because it helps you connect more with your source of joy and not focus on your weaknesses.

Part of human experience is being present for another and finding loving and compassionate ways to share and accompany others through all phases of life's journey. Caring and sharing with others is one of the important foundations of life. Your relationships with others—spouse, children, parents, friends, or companion—add to the richness and framework of your life tapestry.

In practicing the art and science of nursing, it is important to recognize your unconditional love. You move through many crises that can be healing or devastating. The outcomes depend on whether your journeys are unconscious or conscious. An unconscious journey means that you are not present in the moment and unaware of the qualities of the experience. A conscious healing journey means that you tell the truth to yourself whether it makes sense to anyone else or not. Your experiences through crises are real if you learn to share emotions with yourself and let others know when you are hurting and that you need help. Sharing with others your highs and lows leads to acknowledgment of your unconditional love and inner healing resources.

LEARNING OBJECTIVES

After reading this chapter, the nurse should be able to do the following:

1. Describe the major therapeutic goals of mechanical assist device therapy.
2. Discuss the major indications for the use of the various mechanical assist devices.
3. Compare and contrast the various mechanical assist device therapies.
4. Outline specific nursing care measures for patients receiving mechanical assist therapy.

INTRA-AORTIC BALLOON PUMP

First used successfully in 1967 by Kantrowitz,[48] the intra-aortic balloon pump (IABP) is currently the most commonly used assist device and consists of a polyurethane balloon attached to a catheter (Fig. 18–1). The catheter is generally a 10.5 or 12 French catheter onto which a 30-cc to 40-cc balloon is attached. The balloon catheter is placed in the descending thoracic aorta just distal to the left subclavian artery and generally exits by the femoral artery, where it attaches to the balloon console. Using the R wave of the electrocardiogram (ECG) as its trigger, the balloon is synchronously inflated and deflated, with deflation occurring just before systole and inflation occurring during diastole.

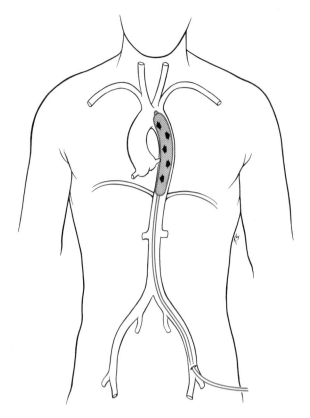

Figure 18-1

Placement of the intra-aortic balloon. The catheter is introduced through the femoral artery into the descending aorta with the balloon positioned above the renal arteries immediately distal to the left subclavian artery in order to prevent impairment of the cerebral circulation.

Mechanical Events and Physiologic Effects of Intra-aortic Balloon Pumping

Inflation of the intra-aortic balloon during diastole allows for displacement of blood cephalad into the aortic arch and cerebral vessels as well as downward toward the renal artery and peripheral areas (Fig. 18–2). With this action, aortic diastolic pressure has been demonstrated to increase as much as 10% to 40%.[16,25,58] This increase in aortic diastolic pressure augments coronary artery blood flow by 5% to 15%,[39] which is particularly important in ischemic myocardial states. Most studies demonstrate, however, that when coronary artery autoregulatory mechanisms are still functioning, an increase in aortic diastolic pressure does not increase coronary blood flow. This method of augmentation works only in the failing heart.

Deflation of the intra-aortic balloon occurs before the ejection phase of the next ventricular systole. This deflation decreases ventricular afterload. This decrease in resistance against the aortic valve allows left ventricular ejection pressures to be reduced by 10% to 15%. It also reduces the rate of left ventricular pressure rise (dP/dt) by 10% to 20%.[111] Both of these actions cause a significantly lesser amount of energy to be expensed in opening the aortic valve and commencing ejection. Because of enhanced ejection due to this ventricular unloading, ventricular stroke volumes can rise by 17%, and ventricular end-diastolic volumes and, hence, preload can diminish as much as 24%.[47,111] Clinically, cardiac output can increase by 10% to 40%,[47,111] and systolic arterial pressure can drop as

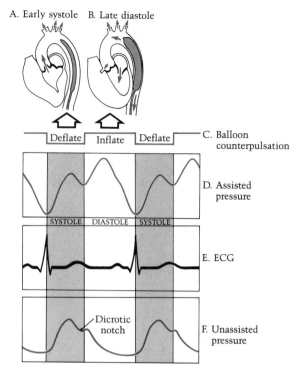

Figure 18-2

Cardiac cycle with the intra-aortic balloon. Timed and controlled augmentation of the diastolic blood pressure improves the hemodynamic functioning of the failing heart (*i.e.,* it increases myocardial perfusion, decreases preload, and decreases afterload). In systole, the balloon is deflated and blood is pumped into the systemic arterial circulation. In early diastole, balloon inflation is begun. In late diastole, the balloon is fully inflated. Inflation is synchronized using the R wave of the electrocardiogram (ECG). Incorrect inflation after a premature beat or after systole is prevented by the use of safety circuits. With counterpulsation, diastolic blood pressure is increased while systolic blood pressure and end-systolic blood pressure are decreased. The aortic pressure tracing is shown during counterpulsation. The augmented diastolic pressure in the tracing at the top is higher and more prolonged (almost until the next systole) than the normal aortic pressure tracing at the bottom. The ECG is shown for comparison in the cardiac cycle.

much as 10%.[47] Improved coronary artery blood flow facilitates returning the heart to a normal rate and diminishing or abolishing dysrhythmias.

Cerebral blood flow has been shown to increase by 56% during balloon pumping.[28] Renal blood flow is not increased, but urinary output generally increases as a result of the increase in cardiac output; thus, there is less of a need for diuretics.[7]

Clinical Indications for Intra-aortic Balloon Pumping

Indications for using the IABP are listed in Table 18–1. With many of these states, the patient's hemodynamic status may be anywhere on a spectrum from moderate stability to frank instability.

Generally, balloon pumping is instituted when the patient's hemodynamic profile demonstrates severe instability with a cardiac index (CI) less than 2.0 L/minute/m², a mean arterial pressure (MAP) of 60 mm Hg and falling, a pulmonary capillary wedge pressure (PCWP) greater than 20 mm Hg, and

Table 18-1
Clinical Indications for Intra-aortic Balloon Pumping

Angina
    Preinfarction
    Postinfarction
    Unstable
Malignant ventricular tachydysrhythmias
Acute myocardial infarction
Cardiogenic shock
    Acute myocardial infarction
    Cardiac contusion
Cardiac rupture
    Ventricular septal defect
    Mitral valve dysfunction
    Ventricular free-wall rupture
Postoperative low cardiac output states
Inability to wean from cardiopulmonary bypass
Prophylactic use in high-risk candidates undergoing
    Catheterization
    Percutaneous transluminal coronary angioplasty
    Cardiac surgery
Pulmonary artery pumping for right ventricular failure
Profound reversible myocardial depression due to
    Hypodynamic septic shock
    Anaphylaxis
Support during urgent noncardiac surgery in presence of
angina or recent myocardial infarction such as:
    Bleeding ulcer repair
    Resection of intracranial masses
    Small bowel obstruction

with the infusion of high dosage levels of inotropes.[25] In the settings of pre- or postinfarction angina, unstable angina, and malignant ventricular tachydysrhythmia, the effectiveness of balloon pumping is due largely to its ability to improve coronary blood flow, especially coronary collateral flow to the ischemic areas and their surrounding zones.[15,51] Relief of angina occurs in about 80% of patients with postinfarction angina.[69] During the early phases of acute myocardial infarction, balloon pumping can be used to limit the ultimate size of the infarction, prevent extension, support cardiac function, and decrease the incidence of postinfarction angina. Use in these situations is generally only a temporary therapy until definitive treatment such as revascularization or percutaneous transluminal coronary angioplasty can be performed.[2,16,54,55,72,108]

Use of IABP in cardiogenic shock is aimed at breaking the vicious cycle of poor perfusion to the organs, especially the myocardium, thus allowing the myocardium the chance to recover and assume its total function.[48,83,115] Ventricular septal defects, papillary muscle rupture, or ventricular free wall ruptures after acute infarction are also situations in which balloon pumping is efficacious. In these situations, the ventricular unloading capabilities of IABP are most important and assist in preventing the ventricle from becoming volume loaded. Definitive surgical therapy, however, is essential for survival in these patients. Surgical repair of a ventricular septal defect after an acute infarction generally can achieve an 80% survival rate.[4,17,27] Refractory cardiogenic shock from blunt cardiac injury also has been reported to be treated successfully with balloon pumping.[71]

Low cardiac output states or failure to wean from cardiopulmonary bypass after cardiac surgery is another indication for the use of IABP. The most common cause for these situations is inadequate myocardial preservation, preoperative left ventricular dysfunction, or intraoperative myocardial infarc-

tion.[9,18,56,80] Use of the IABP electively in patients who are high-risk candidates for cardiac catheterization, percutaneous transluminal coronary angioplasty, or cardiac surgery is another indication.[6,12,58,105,111] A high-risk patient generally is characterized as having an ejection fraction less than 30%, a CI less than 1.8 L/minute/m[2], left ventricular end-diastolic pressure greater than 22 mm Hg, or moderate left ventricular dysfunction accompanied by a recent myocardial infarction, unstable angina, or severe valve disease associated with coronary artery disease.[10]

In the setting of acute right ventricular failure due to an acute right ventricular infarction or pulmonary embolism, balloon pumping of the pulmonary artery has been performed successfully.[64,67] Intra-aortic balloon pumping has been shown to be effective in patients with profound reversible myocardial depression, which can occur in hypodynamic septic shock[1,94] or after anaphylaxis.[91] Finally, patients with a recent myocardial infarction or angina[11,22,34] who require urgent noncardiac surgical procedures such as repair of a bleeding ulcer or small bowel obstruction, or resection of an intracranial mass have been maintained successfully with balloon pumping.

In all of these situations, early insertion of the IABP is recommended in order to limit or prevent cardiac damage. Higher survival rates generally occur in those patients with normal left ventricular function. Survival in that group is reported to be 95%, whereas patients with moderately impaired left ventricles and poor left ventricular function survive at the respective rates of 82% and 42%.[1]

One study demonstrated that long-term (3 years or greater) survival of patients undergoing IABP for all reasons was 64%.[102] Sixty-three percent of patients in that study were still free of angina 3 years later, 52% were free of congestive heart failure, and only 43% reported mild heart failure. From a subjective perspective, 56% of patients reported returning to normal activity, 36% returned to moderate activity, and 7% reported that their activity was very limited. Balloon pumping is generally contraindicated in those patients with moderate to severe aortic insufficiency, because augmentation of these patients could increase ventricular loading.

Insertion Techniques for the Intra-aortic Balloon Pump

The most common insertion site for the balloon catheter is the left common femoral artery. A percutaneous or an arteriotomy approach can be used to place the catheter. With the arteriotomy approach, local anesthesia with 2% lidocaine is administered and an incision is made to expose the common femoral artery. After systemic and local heparization, an arteriotomy is performed on the vessel. A graft made of Dacron or a portion of saphenous vein or pericardium is attached to the arteriotomy site, and the balloon catheter is inserted through it and up into the aorta.[35,73,114] With a percutaneous insertion, the catheter is introduced by direct puncture or by a cutdown into the artery and is threaded up the aorta over a long guidewire.[3,113] Although the incidence of complications with these two techniques varies, the data conflict as to which approach is best.[7,25,49,111] There does seem to be agreement that fewer complications are associated with the use of smaller diameter catheters.[6,12]

If severe femoral artery disease exists, then an ascending

aorta or aortic arch approach can be performed.[47,61,62] This approach generally is reserved for surgical patients who have a thoracotomy or sternotomy incision. With this approach, an arteriotomy and a graft are attached to the aorta in a similar fashion to that described with the femoral technique. The balloon catheter is introduced through this graft and is situated in the descending thoracic aorta. A similar technique is used to place the pulmonary artery balloon catheter. In this technique, a portion of the balloon catheter resides in the pulmonary artery and the remainder of it resides in the Dacron graft, which serves as a reservoir.[64] Other sites not used commonly but applicable for use in patients with severe peripheral vascular disease are the right and left axillary artery, the subclavian artery, or the abdominal aorta.

Timing the Intra-aortic Balloon Pump

The trigger mechanism for the inflation and deflation of the intra-aortic balloon is the R wave of the ECG, which is generally the most reliable and clear signal. The upstroke of the arterial wave also can serve as a trigger source, and during cardiopulmonary bypass, when the heart is in standstill, an internal preset trigger logic can be used. All of these triggers will provide a single inflation and deflation for each cardiac beat (a 1:1 ratio). The bedside operator should fine tune the timing of inflation and deflation.[112] Inflation of the balloon should occur precisely on the dicrotic notch of the arterial wave. Figure 18–3F illustrates a nonassisted wave and can be contrasted with a properly timed arterial wave, which is shown in Figure 18–3A. Early inflation (Fig. 18–3B) is evidenced by an augmentation wave, which precedes the dicrotic notch. In this situation, the early inflation of the balloon will increase the pressure in the aorta, causing premature closure of the aortic valve. This will compromise cardiac output and increase myocardial oxygen consumption. Late inflation (Fig. 18–3C) occurs after the dicrotic notch and lessens the overall opportunity for augmentation.

Fine tuning of deflation is the responsibility of the bedside clinician. Ideal deflation occurs at the end of diastole synchronous with early ejection.[31] Ventricular unloading is not observed if deflation is completed before ejection. The largest reductions in systolic left ventricular pressures are associated with synchronized deflation with early ejection. Optimum unloading can be seen graphically when the balloon end-diastolic pressure wave is lower than the patient's own unassisted end-diastolic wave. In addition, a lower systolic pressure may be present on the unassisted wave. Assessment for these two criteria can be attained by switching the pumping frequency to a 1:2 mode so that assisted and unassisted waves can be compared with each other. When early deflation exists, a presystolic wave such as seen in Figure 18–3D will be present. With early deflation, aortic pressure rises as the root fills with blood, and the ventricle has to open against a higher pressure, thereby negating the effects of afterload reduction. When deflation is too late, the end-diastolic pressure wave will be blunted or rounded off and will produce a higher reading than an unassisted wave (Fig. 18–3E). In this situation, there will be impedance to ventricular ejection and a delay in aortic valve opening, resulting in an increase in myocardial workload and oxygen consumption.

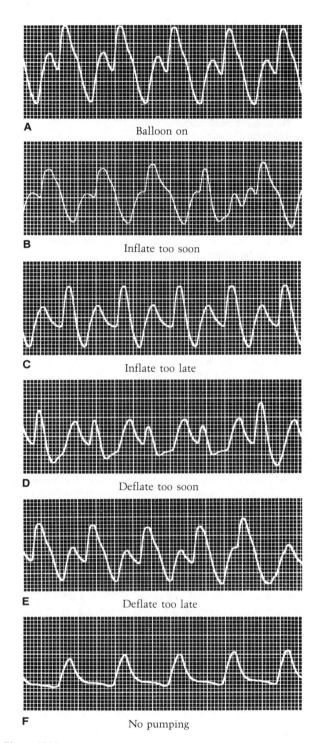

A   Balloon on

B   Inflate too soon

C   Inflate too late

D   Deflate too soon

E   Deflate too late

F   No pumping

Figure 18–3

Troubleshooting with the intra-aortic balloon. The most common problems are shown on the tracings: inflation too soon and too late, and deflation too soon and too late.

Complications Associated With Intra-aortic Balloon Pumping

The reported incidence of overall complications associated with IABP range from 10% to 45% (Table 18–2).[27,29,30,105] The most frequently occurring complications are those involving the

Table 18–2
Complications Associated With Intra-aortic Balloon Pumping

Vascular
    Embolization of arterial plaque with resultant
      ischemia or infarction
    Arterial dissection
    Arterial perforation
    Aortic dissection
    Aortic perforation
    Aneurysm formation
    Circulatory insufficiency of lower extremity
Infection
Balloon failure
Thrombocytopenia

vascular bed.[29,42,72,82] Limb ischemia is the most frequently occurring vascular complication[29,31,58,105] in patients with small vessels in which the diameter of the vessel is close to the diameter of the catheter, thereby impeding the distal flow. This situation also can enhance thrombus formation due to sluggish flow.[27,109] Use of smaller catheters when possible may lessen this complication.

Additional causes of ischemia include emboli. During insertion and removal of the balloon catheter, emboli can develop as plaque is dislodged. Difficult insertions, bed rest, and extended periods of balloon pumping are contributory factors to thrombus formation. In addition, removal of the balloon may lead to the release of platelets and fibrin as they are sheared off the catheter at the time of removal.[29] Preventive anticoagulation can be used to assist in thrombus reduction. Low molecular weight dextran can be infused in surgical patients, and subcutaneous heparin can be administered in medical patients to keep their prothrombin time 1½ to 2 times normal. If thrombus are on the catheter at the time of removal, proximal and distal thrombectomy are done.

Presenting signs and symptoms of peripheral ischemia consist of pain in the affected limb, pallor, cyanosis, decreased sensation, loss of motor function, and a decrease in toe temperature.[29,60] A loss of lower extremity pulses may develop. This occurs in 15% of patients who have catheters inserted whether they go on to develop significant ischemia.[21,29,72] This asymptomatic loss of pulses appears to be transient.

Compartment syndrome can develop as part of the lower extremity ischemic state. This syndrome occurs when there is an increase in pressure in the fascia, which is the tissue that holds together the nerves, muscles, bones, and blood in the lower leg. Because of thrombus formation, low flow, pre-existing vascular disease, or vasoconstricting drugs, an increase in pressure can develop. This further decreases blood flow and produces ischemic changes. Clinically, the lower extremity is swollen and tense to palpation, and the patient complains of continuous pressure, numbness, tingling, and excessive pain with passive movement. Sensory as well as motor loss can develop. As pressure continues to build, muscle and nerve damage can develop. In addition to these clinical signs, serum creatine phosphokinase increases to levels of 1000 to 5000 U and myoglobinuria develops; both are markers of muscle ischemia and damage. Needle pressure tests can be performed on the extremity. These will be elevated above their normal 0 to 12-mm Hg range, with readings sometimes as high as 30

mm Hg.[29] Treatment of compartment syndrome ideally consists of early prevention by removing the balloon catheter when initial signs and symptoms develop. Later therapy consists of performing fasciotomies. In some instances, owing to the patient's worsening cardiac status, removal of the catheter may be impossible and fasciotomies may be performed in the leg while pumping continues.

Ischemic complications are most likely to occur during the first 24 hours to 4 days after insertion of the catheter or after its removal. Depending on the patient's cardiac status, the catheter may be able to be withdrawn. With persistent severe cardiac compromise, it may become necessary to leave the catheter in place and risk continued vascular compromise. Although not a frequent consequence, gangrene can develop and amputation may become necessary. Even with early recognition of complications and removal of the catheter, corrective vascular repair may become necessary or there may be sustained neurologic impairment in the form of parasthenia or loss of motor function.

Other vascular complications that can develop include aortic dissection and pseudoaneurysm formation. These generally occur only 3% of the time, and many are not identified until after catheter removal.[21,58] Retrograde bleeding and hypovolemic shock can occur after catheter rupture of the aorta during insertion. These problems occur most frequently with the use of stiff introducers.[58] With perforation of the vessel and retroperitoneal bleeding, the first warning sign may be complaints of back pain by the patient during the insertion attempt. If this occurs, insertion should be halted. Paraplegia has developed when a percutaneously inserted catheter caused a critical occlusion of a spinal cord artery, a small dissection, or an arterial embolism to occur. The result was transient back pain and loss of motor function.[93,98,104] Another report detailed malposition of a percutaneously inserted catheter so that the flow to the internal mammary artery was obstructed.[96] In this situation, it was felt that the tip of the catheter entered the left subclavian artery. In this position, it attenuated forward flow, and because the internal mammary artery is generally the second major branch of the subclavian artery, flow to it was diminished.

Some studies support that there are predisposing factors to the development of vascular complications, suggesting that women are more prone to vascular complications owing to their smaller femoral artery lumen. This could potentiate intimal trauma[27,109] during catheter insertion. Additionally, diabetes is viewed as a risk factor, with one study reporting that only 14% of nondiabetic patients developed problems, whereas 22% of diabetic patients developed complications. Insulin-dependent patients were shown to have a 34% rate of complications.[7,34,110] However, despite this difference, overall survival did not vary. A history of smoking also has been associated with lower limb ischemic complications.[26] The length of counterpulsation correlates well with complications. Thirty-seven percent of patients who required pumping for more than 20 days developed complications, and only 15% of patients who required pumping for fewer than 20 days were affected. Again, overall survival did not differ.[24,78] Patients with pre-existing peripheral vascular disease are at a higher risk.[29,30] This group generally can be identified by their previous history of claudication, presence of femoral bruits, or absent pedal pulses. Long-term (greater than 3 years) vascular outcomes have been reported and demonstrate a 29% incidence of claudication after IABP.[102]

Bleeding from thrombocytopenia may develop owing to the trauma of the balloon against platelets. This generally does not require any therapy or removal of the catheter unless the platelets reach a level of less than 50,000 or there are clinical signs of bleeding.

The development of an infection can be a problem.[32] Infection at the insertion site is reported to occur at a rate as high as 22%.[49] Avoiding the use of graft material can minimize the risk of this complication.[105] Occlusion of the mesenteric artery by a balloon inserted through the ascending aorta has resulted in small bowel infarction.[13,44]

Balloon failure develops in about 1.3% of patients.[63,102] This includes balloon rupture or leakage of gas. In these instances, blood appears in the balloon catheter. The catheter then needs to be removed immediately in order to prevent further gas embolization. Rupture or fracture of the catheter can occur if the catheter comes in contact with certain chemicals such as acetone or ether. Overwrapping or instrument manipulation during insertion can provoke tears in the balloon membrane.[90] In addition, delayed abrasion of the balloon membrane due to repeated contact with calicified arterial plaque can cause balloon failure.[59] Helium embolisms can occur after rupture.

Their effects may range from unnoticeable deficits to global neurologic deficits that require hyperbaric oxygen treatments.[23]

Weaning and Removal of the Intra-aortic Balloon

Weaning generally is carried out by decreasing the frequency of balloon augmentation from every beat (1:1 ratio) to every other beat (1:2) to every third beat (1:3) and so on. In addition to decreasing the frequency of assistance, the amount of volume used to fill the balloon can be decreased. In this fashion, assistance to the myocardium is withdrawn slowly. While weaning, the patient continues to be monitored to ensure hemodynamic stability. After an appropriate period of stability, the catheter is removed. Distal pulses are monitored for 24 hours to assure early identification of vascular complications.

NURSING DIAGNOSES, PATIENT OUTCOMES, AND PLAN

The preceding knowledge base guides the nurse in establishing nursing diagnoses, patient outcomes, and the plan for the patient on the IABP.

NURSING CARE PLAN SUMMARY Patient on the Intra-aortic Balloon Pump

NURSING DIAGNOSIS

1. High risk for vascular injury related to intra-aortic balloon catheter trauma (exchanging pattern)

Patient Outcome	Nursing Orders

The patient will exhibit signs and symptoms of normal vascular integrity as evidenced by the presence of adequate peripheral pulses, normal color, warm extremities, normal chest radiograph, and normal organ and neurologic function.	1. Identify and describe mechanisms or factors that contribute to vascular complications during balloon pumping. Table 18-2 details specific vascular complications. Vascular complications result from catheter-induced dissection or perforation of the femoral artery or aorta or from embolization of arterial plaque or thrombosis. These complications develop most often during catheter insertion and removal.
	  A. Monitor, assess, and record the following signs and symptoms of vascular injury:
	  (1) Loss of peripheral pulses or uneven peripheral pulses. Most often pulses become diminished or are lost in the affected leg. An ankle-brachial index may be helpful as a quantitative measurement of peripheral flow. A *ankle-brachial index* is a ratio of a Doppler-recorded systolic dorsalis pedis or posterior tibial pressure compared with the brachial blood pressure. It is obtained by dividing the ankle systolic pressure by the brachial systolic pressure to determine the ankle-arm ratio. The normal value is 0.8 to 1.2. A ratio less than 0.8 is generally related to a diminished arterial flow.[29]
	  (2) Left radial artery pulses also should be carefully monitored for malposition of the tip of the catheter into the left subclavian vessel, which can cause a corresponding loss of left arm blood flow during balloon inflation. Baseline pulses are helpful for comparison.
	  (3) Cool, mottled, pale extremities
	  (4) Tender or painful extremities

(continued)

NURSING CARE PLAN SUMMARY *Patient on the Intra-aortic Balloon Pump* *Continued*

Patient Outcome	*Nursing Orders*
	(5) Loss of motor and sensory functioning peripherally
	(6) Complaints of back pain, particularly during insertion and removal
	(7) Pallor
	(8) Sudden hypotension
	(9) Unequal blood pressure in the right and left extremities
	(10) Distended, taut abdomen from aortic perforation
	(11) Falling hemoglobin and hematocrit
	(12) Sudden decrease in urine output, which could be related to a renal embolism or renal artery dissection
	(13) Absence of bowel sounds due to mesenteric ischemia or infarction
	B. Implement the following strategies to prevent, minimize, or alleviate vascular complications:
	(1) Obtain baseline peripheral pulses before balloon insertion.
	(2) Assess pulses every 15 minutes for an hour after insertion and removal, then every 30 minutes for 2 hours and then hourly.
	(3) Assure that catheter is securely sutured to insertion site to prevent upward movement.
	(4) Keep head of bed elevated no higher than 30° to prevent catheter from advancing upward and digging into the intima of the aortic arch.
	(5) Keep leg and hip straight at all times. Flexion could allow catheter movement. Use soft restraints on the affected leg with a sheet to prevent accidental movement by the patient.
	(6) Administer anticoagulation as ordered.
	(7) Monitor appropriate anticoagulation parameters.
	(8) Obtain chest film daily to check placement of balloon catheter.
	(9) Do not allow the balloon catheter to become noninflating for longer than 5 minutes. If this occurs, the catheter should be removed rather than reinflated, which brings with it a concomitant risk of embolization. The balloon should be discontinued if it remains in a 1:8 assist rate for longer than 4 hours.[90]
	(10) After percutaneous removal, apply sustained firm pressure for 15 to 20 minutes to prevent hematoma formation.[97]

NURSING DIAGNOSIS

2. *Actual or high risk for infection related to catheter insertion site, invasive lines, procedures, and possible debilitated state (exchanging pattern)*

Patient Outcome	*Nursing Orders*
The patient will remain infection-free as evidenced by lack of redness, drainage, or tenderness at the insertion site, absence of temperature elevation, normal white blood cell count, and negative cultures.	1. Identify and describe factors that contribute to the development of infection in a patient with an IABP. As an invasive procedure, the balloon insertion itself can result in an infection either locally or systemically. In addition, some patients are cachexic and nutritionally depleted before balloon-pump assistance. These states can alter their immunologic capabilities. Lymphorrhagia from injury to the lymph gland during insertion can develop. Although this generally resolves in a week or so, copious amounts of drainage are present. This drainage is an ideal medium for the development of infection.
	A. Monitor, assess, and record the following signs and symptoms of infection:
	(1) Fever
	(2) Chills
	(3) Diaphoresis
	(4) Warm peripheral skin temperature
	(5) Redness, induration, swelling, tenderness, and drainage from balloon insertion site

(continued)

NURSING CARE PLAN SUMMARY *Patient on the Intra-aortic Balloon Pump* Continued

Patient Outcome	*Nursing Orders*
	(6) Leukocytosis
	(7) Positive culture results
	B. Implement the following strategies to prevent, minimize, or alleviate infectious complications:
	(1) Provide meticulous care to catheter site.
	(2) Culture drainage.
	(3) Administer antibiotics per order.
	(4) Monitor temperature every 4 hours.
	(5) Monitor white blood cell count.

NURSING DIAGNOSIS

3. *Decreased cardiac output related to left ventricular failure (exchanging pattern)*

Patient Outcome

Nursing Orders

The patient will be free from left ventricular failure and need for balloon support as evidenced by adequate cardiac output (CO)/cardiac index (CI); normal systemic vascular resistance (SVR); adequate urine output; adequate or return to normal neurologic status; warm, dry skin; absence of chest pain; absence of hemodynamically unstable dysrhythmias; adequate oxygenation; absence of crackles; and absence of significant support from vasoactive drugs.

1. Identify and describe factors that contribute to the development of left ventricular failure (Table 18–1). Inappropriate balloon timing can also lead to impairment in left ventricular function. Additionally, during weaning of the intra-aortic balloon, signs and symptoms of failure may return. This may indicate that further temporary support is required. If multiple attempts at weaning are unsuccessful, the patient is considered to be dependent on the balloon pump. If no other definitive options, such as transplantation, are available, the decision to not add on any other supports (dialysis) or to withdraw the balloon pump is discussed with the family and the patient, if possible.
   A. Monitor, assess, and record the following signs and symptoms of ventricular failure or inability to be weaned from balloon pump:
      (1) Decreased CO/CI: CO less than 5 L/minute, or CI less than 2.7 L/minute/m^2
      (2) Hypotension: systolic pressure less than 90 mm Hg or mean arterial pressure less than 60 mm Hg
      (3) Elevated SVR or pulmonary vascular resistance (PVR): SVR greater than 1300 dyne-seconds/cm^5, and PVR greater than 240 dyne-seconds/cm^5
      (4) Elevated filling pressures
      (5) Urinary output less than 30 cc/hour or less than 0.5 cc/kg/hour
      (6) Presence of S_3 and S_4 heart sounds
      (7) Jugular venous distention
      (8) Bilateral crackles
      (9) Hypoxemia and acidosis
      (10) Tachycardia: heart rate greater than 110 beats/minute
      (11) Cyanosis
      (12) Rapid, shallow respirations
      (13) Cold, clammy, mottled skin
      (14) Decreased level of consciousness
   B. Implement the following strategies to minimize or avoid return to left ventricular failure:
      (1) Monitor hemodynamic parameters during weaning process.
      (2) Maintain optimum balloon timing. Significant changes in heart rate may require alterations in balloon inflation and deflation timing. Major criteria for a properly timed wave include inflation occurring just before the dicrotic notch, balloon-assisted end-diastolic pressure that is less than the patient's aortic end-diastolic pressure, and nonaugmented systole that is less than augmented systole.
      (3) Systematically decrease balloon support from a 1:1 ratio to 1:2, 1:3, and

(continued)

NURSING CARE PLAN SUMMARY   *Patient on the Intra-aortic Balloon Pump*   Continued

Patient Outcome	*Nursing Orders*
	so forth. Some researchers suggest that 4 hours of weaning for every 24 hours of pump support is required.[58]
	(4) Decrease volume in balloon in order to decrease augmentation support. This is generally done by decreasing the balloon volume 5 cc at a time until only 50% of the total volume remains. This assists in decreasing the patient's afterload and augmentation slowly.[58]
	(5) Continue weaning process only after the patient demonstrates hemodynamic stability at current weaning level.

NURSING DIAGNOSIS

4. *Sensory/perceptual alterations (auditory and visual) related to interrupted sleep/rest cycles and sensory deprivation (perceiving pattern)*

Patient Outcome	*Nursing Orders*
The patient will exhibit signs and symptoms of adequate sensory perception as evidenced by orientation to person, place, time, and situation; stable cognitive and emotional function; and verbalizing that they feel rested.	1. Identify and describe factors that contribute to the development of sensory/perceptual alterations. Inadequate periods of undisturbed sleep can evolve into episodes of irritability or delirium. Immobility, lack of privacy, and constant 24-hour attendance by nursing personnel can contribute to sensory deprivation and disorientation.

A. Monitor, assess, and record the following signs and symptoms of sensory/perceptual alterations:
  (1) Hypervigilance
  (2) Restlessness, confusion
  (3) Loss of orientation to person, place, time, and situation
B. Implement the following strategies to minimize or avoid impairment of psychologic functioning:
  (1) Maintain day/night cycles by dimming lights, and so forth.
  (2) Plan nursing care to provide for blocks of undisturbed rest.
  (3) Orient to time, place, person, and situation.
  (4) Explain function of balloon pump, tests, procedures, and so forth to patient and family in order to enhance their understanding and acquire their assistance in care as much as possible. A recent study demonstrated that families reported that the function of the IABP was explained to them 48% of the time by nurses and 37% of the time by physicians. When queried as to their understanding of the function of the IABP, 48% characterized it as "helping the heart" 22% stated that it helps the heart to rest, and 18% felt that it relieved the pressure in the heart.[28]
  (5) Involve patient and family in as much decision making as possible.
  (6) Provide methods of communication for intubated patients (see Impaired Verbal Communication, Chap. 8).
  (7) Provide diversional activities such as television, music, reading, and the like.
  (8) Assist patient with stress-reducing activities (*i.e.*, relaxation techniques, imagery, and so on). One study has reported that patients on IABPs rated many more situations stressful than did other patients in a coronary care unit.[79]

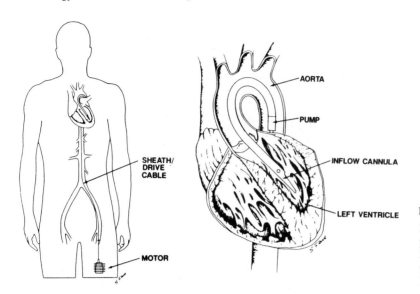

Figure 18–4

Placement of the Hemopump system cannula and pump through the femoral artery. (Rutan, P. M., Rountree, W. D., Myers, K. K., *et al.* Initial experience with the Hemopump. *Crit. Care Nurs. Clin. North Am.* 1:527, 1989; with permission.)

HEMOPUMP

Introduced in 1988 by Nimbus Medical, Inc., Rancho Cordova, CA, the Hemopump is an arterial pump used for closed chest temporary mechanical cardiac assistance.[46,53,100] Depicted in Figure 18–4, the Hemopump cannula is inserted through the femoral artery and is advanced upward into the aortic arch and past the aortic valve into the left ventricle. The cannula consists of very flexible silicone rubber. Blood is removed from the left ventricle through the tip of the inflow cannula. An axial flow pump is located on the distal portion of the cannula positioned in the descending thoracic aorta. The component parts of the cannula and axial flow pump are shown in Figure 18–5. A lifting of blood out of the ventricle develops when a portion of the pump begins to rotate rapidly. This rapid rotation in the tight cylinder of the cannula lifts blood out of the ventricle and ejects it into the descending thoracic aorta. The pump is capable of generating nonpulsatile continuous blood flow at rates ranging from 0.5 L to 3.5 L/minute/m^2. Because the pump rotates 25,000 revolutions/minute, the pump and the drive cable are lubricated with a dextrose solution.

The length of use of the Hemopump currently is limited to 7 days to prevent damage to the aortic valve. The Hemopump is not dependent on the cardiac cycle; therefore, unlike the IABP, it does not require synchronization. The Hemopump can be used on patients with the following hemodynamic criteria: CI less than 2 L/minute/m^2, systolic blood pressure less than 90 mm Hg, PCWP greater than 18 mm Hg, and insufficient response to maximal drug and volume therapy regardless of the cardiac etiology creating these parameters.[46]

Contraindications for the use of the Hemopump include patients with a femoral artery that cannot be dilated to accomodate the insertion of the cannula (21 French), patients with a prosthetic aortic valve, severe aortic wall disease, known or suspected dissecting aneurysm, or severe aortic stenosis or insufficiency. In patients who develop cardiogenic shock after an acute myocardial infarction, initial results have demonstrated a 50% survival rate, which is an improvement over the 80% mortality rate generally ascribed to this population.[46] In patients who developed postcardiotomy shock after myocardial revascularization, 33% were weaned successfully and discharged.[46] Nursing care of these patients is similar to the care of those receiving other types of ventricular assistance.

VENTRICULAR ASSIST DEVICES

Mechanical ventricular assist devices provide assistance to the failing myocardium by diverting blood flow from the myocardium to the systemic or pulmonary circulation. This is accomplished by inserting cannulas into the atriums or ventricles and diverting blood flow through these cannulas by way of an artificial pump into the aorta or pulmonary artery. Figure

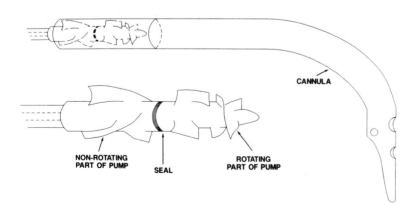

Figure 18–5

The cannula and axial flow pump components of the pump assembly. (Rutan, P. M., Rountree, W. D., Myers, K. K., *et al.* Initial experience with the Hemopump. *Crit. Care Nurs. Clin. North Am.* 1:527, 1989; with permission.)

18–6 depicts a left ventricular assist device in which a cannula inserted into the left atrium removes blood from the atrium and diverts it past the left ventricle and into the aorta. Although the ventricle can be used for placement of the outflow cannula, it has been found that in patients requiring temporary assistance, survival is enhanced when cannulation is performed through the atrium rather than through a direct ventricular entry, which would require the creation of a ventriculotomy incision that must heal later. Ventricular entry is used more commonly when the assist device is being used as a bridge to cardiac transplantation when the atrium needs to be left intact for the attachment of the donor heart. The disadvantage with atrial cannulation is that the left atrium is not always accessible owing to scarring and adhesions from previous surgery.

Figure 18–7 depicts a right ventricular assist device in which the outflow cannula is located in the right atrium and the inflow cannula is in the pulmonary artery. Both the left and right ventricular assist devices are used when there is isolated univentricular failure. In the case of biventricular failure, a biventricular assist device is used (Fig. 18–8). Ventricular assist devices can be pulsatile or nonpulsatile. Whereas the IABP is effective because of its ability to provide pressure assistance and therefore increase coronary artery perfusion and decrease

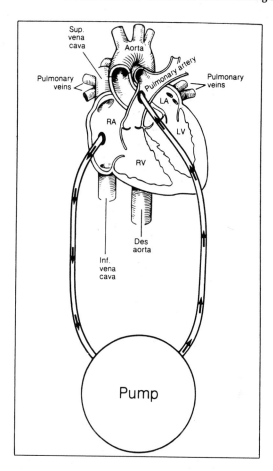

Figure 18–7
Right ventricular assist device (RVAD). LA: left atrium; LV: left ventricle; RA: right atrium; RV: right ventricle. (Barnes Brannon, P. H., and Batchelor Townes, S. Ventricular failure: New therapy using the mechanical assist device. *Crit. Care Nurse,* 6:70, 1986; with permission.)

left ventricular afterload, assist devices provide flow assistance and thus reduce ventricular ejection impedance, decrease volume loading, and provide for forward movement of blood. They do not require underlying ventricular function. The IABP is dependent on a certain level of ventricular function.

The current goal for assist device support is to provide temporary support until the myocardium recovers or can be replaced permanently with a transplant. In the future, a permanent implantable assist device for use in patients with severe and chronic left ventricular failure will be available. Currently in testing, these devices will be powered by transcutaneous energy transmission and will be totally implantable.[66]

Clinical Indications for Ventricular Assist Devices

Current clinical indications for use of mechanical ventricular assist devices include patients (Table 18–3) who are unable to be weaned from cardiopulmonary bypass despite adequate volume loading, pharmacologic support, or IABP support.[14,70,77] Other indications include patients awaiting cardiac transplantation[14,33,107] after acute cardiac graft rejection,[14,42] myocardial infarction shock,[14] or acute myocarditis,[14,106] or those requiring repair of traumatic tears of the aorta.[38] Re-

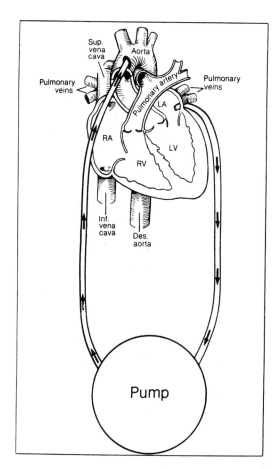

Figure 18–6
Left ventricular assist device (LVAD). LA: left atrium; LV: left ventricle; RA: right atrium; RV: right ventricle. (Barnes Brannon, P. H., and Batchelor Townes, S. Ventricular failure: New therapy using the mechanical assist device. *Crit. Care Nurse,* 6:70, 1986; with permission.)

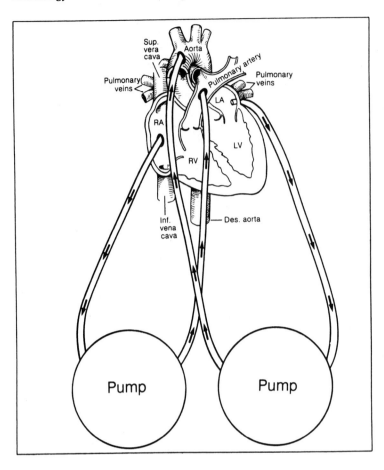

Figure 18–8

Right and left ventricular assist device (BiVAD). LA: left atrium; LV: left ventricle; RA: right atrium; RV: right ventricle. (Barnes Brannon, P. H., and Batchelor Townes, S. Ventricular failure: New therapy using the mechanical assist device. *Crit. Care Nurse,* 6:70, 1986; with permission.)

gardless of the etiology, patients generally considered as candidates for this therapy demonstrate the following:[84,85] a CI less than 1.8 L/minute/m², systolic blood pressure less than 90 mm Hg, MAP less than 60 mm Hg, systemic vascular resistance greater than 2100 dyne-seconds/cm⁵, right or left atrial filling pressures greater than 25 mm Hg, and a urine output less than 20 ml/hour in the presence of IABP support, maximum inotropic infusions, and adequate preload and cardiac pacing interventions. Maximal inotropic infusions can be characterized generally as doses of dopamine and dobutamine up to 25 µg/kg/minute, isoproterenol infusions up to 0.1 µg/kg/minute, and norepinephrine infusions up to 6 µg/kg/minute.[101]

Even with the aforementioned hemodynamic parameters, patients can be excluded from this intervention for a number of reasons. If the patient's body surface area is less than 1.0 m², the devices are too large to be implanted or cannula placement could be too difficult. Concurrent illnesses such as chronic renal failure; severe cerebrovascular, pulmonary, or hepatic disease; cancer with metastasis; or significant blood dyscrasia

place the patient in too high a risk category. If there is uncontrollable hemorrhage from the heart and great vessels, massive hemolysis, transfusion reaction, or massive air embolization, the patient is not considered a candidate. A technically unsatisfactory operative procedure or acute cerebral damage resulting in fixed pupils, a flat electroencephalogram, or both at 37°C would be other contraindications.[101]

Types of Ventricular Assist Devices

There are three basic types of assist devices (Table 18–4): roller pumps, centrifugal pumps, and pneumatic (air-driven) or heterotopic prosthetic ventricle systems. The roller-pump system (Fig. 18–9), devised by Litwak,[52] is a nonpulsatile system in which a roller pump is placed between the left atrium and aorta or the right atrium and pulmonary artery.[52,99] Blood is

Table 18–3
Clinical Indications for Use of Ventricular Assist Devices

Postcardiotomy failure to wean from bypass
Bridge to cardiac transplant
Cardiac graft failure
Myocardial infarction shock
Acute myocarditis

Table 18–4
Types of Ventricular Assist Devices

Roller-pump systems (Litwak)
Centrifugal pumps
    Bio-Medicus
    Centrimed
    Medtronic
Pneumatic (heterotopic prosthetic ventricles)
    Abromed
    Novacor
    Symbrion
    Thermedics
    Thoratec

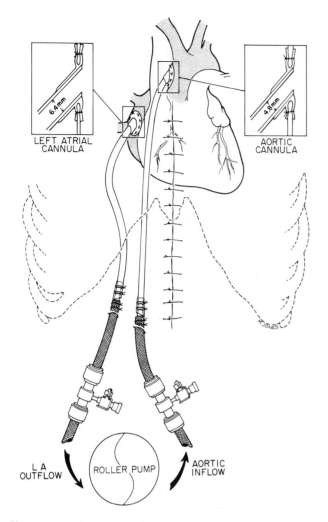

Figure 18–9

The roller pump assist device system. (Litwak, R. S., Koffsky, R. M., Jurado, R. A., *et al.* Use of left-heart assist device after intracardiac surgery: Technique and clinical experience. *Ann. Thorac. Surg.* 21:191, 1976; with permission.)

diverted constantly into the aorta, and maximal flow capacity is approximately 6 L/minute. Average flow is 2 to 4 L/minute, because flow rates that are too high can cause poor ventricle assist device filling and collapse of the atrium around the cannula. Generally, flow is not decreased to less than 1.5 L in order to prevent thrombus formation, and the left ventricle is allowed to eject minimally to prevent stasis and thrombus.[115] In addition to replacing ventricular forward flow, the roller-pump system allows preload to be decreased by emptying the left atrium.

One unique feature of this system is that discontinuation can be achieved without a sternal reoperation. Because the cannulas are tunneled out below the sternum through the abdomen, they can be obturated simply and the abdominal wound closed.[52] Potential problems with this system include tubing laceration due to wear and tear from the roller pump. Air emboli possibly can occur from leaks at the roller pump. Trauma to blood components is less likely to occur in systems in which both the roller heads and tubing are as large as practical.[52,99] When nonpulsatile systems are used, the IABP is

used to provide pulsatile flow. Having an IABP in place can serve as assistance when the patient is being weaned from the ventricular assist device.

Centrifugal pumps rely on kinetic energy to provide blood flow. In these systems, an impeller or rotary blade rotates at a high speed to provide an impulse in the direction of the flow.[8] This design allows large volumes of blood to be circulated at a low pressure. With this system, less turbulance is generated and, thus, there is reduction in air embolism formation. If air does enter the system, it remains within the vortex of the pumps and does not enter the arterial system. Examples of centrifugal pumps are illustrated in Figures 18–10 and 18–11.

Air-driven or pneumatic devices generally consist of a saclike chamber or bladder that has a diaphragm that can be compressed or expanded. When the diaphragm is expanded, the chamber fills with blood from the atria. Once the bladder is filled, the diaphragm is compressed and blood is ejected out of the chamber through a one-way valve into the aorta. Maximum flow rates from this device can be 6.5 L/minute/m^2.[42,65,81,85,115] The Thoratec Pierce-Donachy device (Thoratec Medical, Inc., Berkeley, CA) is an example of this type of system (Fig. 18–12).

The Novacor system (Novacor Medical Corp., Oakland, CA) (Fig. 18–13) is an implantable assist device. This left ventricular assist system is an electromechanically driven dual pusher-plate blood pump that derives its power from a percutaneous lead. It is capable of providing 10 L/minute of flow and can work synchronously at up to a heart rate of 240 beats/minute.[89,92] The Novacor cannulas are situated in the left ventricle and aorta. This device is not designed for right ventricular support, and it should be used only in a patient with isolated left ventricular failure. The pump is placed in the left upper quadrant of the abdomen either subcutaneously or preperitoneally. It is reported to cause only minimal trauma to red

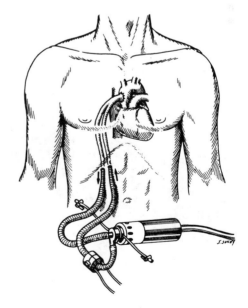

Figure 18–10

An example of a centrifugal pump system. (Golding, L. A. R., and Nose, Y. A simplified blood access method for a temporary left ventricular assist system in humans. *Artif. Organs* 2:317, 1978; with permission.)

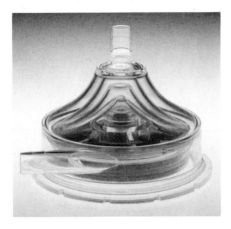

Figure 18–11

A Bio Medicus centrifugal pump. (Reproduced with permission of Bio Medicus Corporation, Eden Prairie, MN.)

blood cells and maintains a normal free plasma hemoglobin level,[107] two characteristics that would be required in permanent implantable assist devices.

Survival rates after use in cardiotomy and cardiogenic shock are generally 50%.[14,77,78,83,96] Causes of death most frequently include myocardial necrosis, hemorrhage, cerebrovascular accidents, and infections.[103] Long-term survival rates have been reported at 32%.[78] Higher survival rates of up to 66% to 71% have been reported in the bridge-to-transplant patient group.[11,20,47] Survival rates are generally highest in that group of patients in whom initiation of therapy occurred early, and in whom there was absence of biventricular failure, acute renal failure, and perioperative infarction.[14,42,77] In patients with acute myocardial infarctions, survival is only 25%, and if renal failure ensues, survival falls to 10%.[81] However, although perioperative infarction is a strong negative determinant of survival in postcardiotomy patients, it does not preclude that some patients may experience myocardial recovery.[82] Patients with preoperative histories of obstructive lung disease or he-

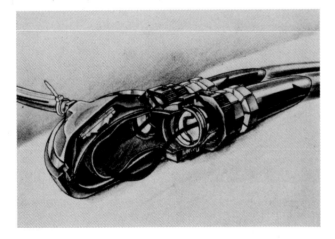

Figure 18–12

Internal design of the Pierce-Donachy Thoractec assist pump illustrating direction of blood flow through the pump. Bjork Shiley valves are used to direct flow. (Reedy, J., Ruzevich, S. A., Swartz, M. T., *et al.* Nursing care of a patient requiring prolonged mechanical circulatory support. *Prog. Cardiovasc. Nurs.* 4:1, 1989; with permission.)

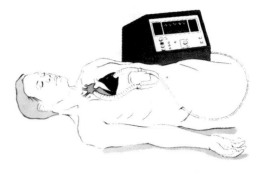

Figure 18–13

The Novacor ventricular assist system. The pump is implanted in the left upper abdominal quadrant and connected to a controller and power source by a cable, which is tunneled through the skin. (Reedy, J., Ruzevich, S. A., Swartz, M. T., *et al.* Nursing care of a patient requiring prolonged mechanical circulatory support. *Prog. Cardiovasc. Nurs.* 4:1, 1989; with permission.)

patic dysfunction, as evidenced by elevated liver enzymes and jaundice, and those undergoing emergency initiation of these devices do very poorly.[84] In addition, age plays a factor because regardless of the reason for ventricular support, patients over the age of 65 generally have only a 12% survival rate and those over 70 years of age have only a 6% survival rate.[83,84]

Complications Associated With Ventricular Assist Devices

The most frequent complication (Table 18–5) occurring in these patients is hemorrhage caused by surgical bleeding or coagulation derangements due to prolonged cardiopulmonary bypass times. This problem develops in approximately 30% to 50% of patients.[8,14,40,81,85,106] Surgical hemostasis is attempted first, and then neutralization with protamine sulfate is attempted. If the platelet count is less than 100,000 U/L, then transfusion of platelets is performed. Fresh frozen plasma is also administered, and fibrin glue is used on the operative sites. Decamino-D-arginine vasopressin (DDAVP) can also be given to improve platelet hemostatic plug formation because it includes Factor VIIIC and von Willebrand factor. However, it is only effective about once every 12 to 24 hours and lasts for only 30 to 90 minutes, so the timing of its administration is critical.[14]

Table 18–5

Complications Associated With Ventricular Assist Devices

Bleeding
    Coagulopathies
    Related to surgery
Thrombus formation and embolization
Infection
    Mediastinitis
    Septicemia
Acute renal failure
Adult respiratory distress syndrome
Neurologic deficits
    Transient ischemic attacks
    Cerebrovascular accidents
Multisystem organ failure
Device failure

Once the bleeding is halted, concern shifts to maintaining adequate anticoagulation. Anticoagulation is initiated once the chest tubes drain less than 100 cc/hour for a 2- to 3-hour period. At that time, a continuous intravenous infusion of heparin is begun to maintain the activated clotting times at 150 to 200 seconds or the activated partial thromboplastin time at 1.5 times its control. With pulsatile systems, low molecular weight dextran can be used to prevent thrombus. In patients who require long-term support, warfarin and dipyridamole can be administered in a dose that keeps the prothrombin time at 1.3 to 1.5 times the control.[92]

Serious infections develop in these patients 33% to 70% of the time.[8,81,85,106] These infections can be systemic or local. Local infections can affect cannula insertion sites or wounds. Owing to the patient's compromised state and the vascular nature of these sites, local infections can become systemic problems quickly. In cases in which the sternum cannot be closed, the risk of mediastinitis is large. Generally, attempts are made to close the sternum and broadly placed skin stitches are used to close the skin. Because re-entry into the chest is required for removal of the cannulas later, complete closure is not attempted. In some instances, closure is not possible because of lung and myocardial edema or ongoing bleeding. In these cases, the rib spreaders may be left in place, and the wound may be packed with gauze and then covered with a sterile drape to prevent entry of organisms.[40,50] Infections are treated aggressively with antibiotics. Evidence of infection can eliminate a patient from consideration for cardiac transplantation until the infection is treated effectively. Devices such as the Novacor generally have a lower incidence of infection, largely owing to their less invasive nature.[96]

Another major problem associated with assist devices is the development of acute renal failure which is associated with a higher mortality.[8,11,85,106] In addition to a low flow state to the renal beds, a contributing factor to acute renal failure is rhabdomyolysis, which occurs as a result of muscle ischemia in the leg in which the IABP is inserted. Many patients on ventricular assist devices have an IABP because it was the first therapy used but was unsuccessful, because pulsatile flow from the IABP is desired, or because the IABP will be used to assist with weaning. In any event, aggressive treatment of the renal failure is required to prevent volume overload and accumulation of nitrogenous waste products. Continuous arteriovenous hemofiltration and dialysis has been shown to be an effective method of assisting with volume and solute removal in hemodynamically unstable patients who require ventricular assistance.[74]

Other complications associated with ventricular assist devices include acute respiratory failure, cerebrovascular accidents, hemidiaphragm paralysis, multisystem organ failure, and device failure.[8,81,85,106] Respiratory failure develops for a number of reasons. Left ventricular failure can initiate hydrostatic pulmonary edema. With prolonged cardiopulmonary bypass times, multiple blood transfusions, and low flow to the lung parenchyma, a noncardiac or adult respiratory distress syndrome can develop. Together, this volume overload and lung tissue damage can result in severe and perhaps intractable respiratory problems. Injury to the phrenic nerve due to cannula placement can result in left hemidiaphragmatic paralysis, which generally is not identified until attempts are made at ventilatory weaning. In situations in which severe low flow is not resolved, multisystem organ failure develops. Cerebrovascular accidents can develop from either air or thrombus emboli. Rarely, irreversible neurologic ischemia also can occur. Lastly, device failure can become an issue. Fractured valves, split tubings, and drive-unit pump failures, although infrequent, are the most common complications.

Weaning of the Ventricular Assist Device

Weaning the patient of a ventricular assist device is carried out in the same systematic manner as for the IABP. In a patient who requires the ventricular assist device as a bridge to transplantation, there is no weaning. Once a donor heart is available, the patient goes to surgery. For other patients, the first assessment of a patient's readiness to wean is performed by turning the device off temporarily every day to evaluate ventricular function. This takes only a few minutes. If the patient can maintain a MAP of 60 mm Hg or greater, right-heart and left-heart filling pressures less than 20 mm Hg and a CI greater than 2.0 L/minute/m², then weaning is continued. At that point, the level of flow assistance is decreased gradually and the preceding parameters continue to be monitored. As the pump flow decreases, the cardiac output should remain the same, illustrating that the patient's myocardium is capable of resuming the workload. Cardiac output can be obtained by the thermodilution technique if a left ventricular assist device is used. In the presence of a right ventricular device, clinical assessment of cardiac output will be required. Observation of the arterial wave when the pump is momentarily off will illustrate the level of ventricular ejection. Weaning generally is not initiated until the patient has been on the ventricular assist device for at least 24 hours.[96] Studies suggest that weaning earlier, even if the patient is stabilized, is not as successful in the long term as allowing the patient at least a 24-hour run.

Weaning the patient to IABP support and mild vasoactive drug support is the goal of ventricular assist device weaning. If a biventricular assist device is used, weaning and removal of the device from each ventricle may occur at different times because their recovery may vary.

NURSING CARE PLAN SUMMARY Patient With Ventricular Assist Devices

NURSING DIAGNOSIS

1. High risk for injury related to excessive hemorrhage (exchanging pattern)

Patient Outcome

The patient will exhibit signs and symptoms of adequate coagulation as evidenced by normal parameters for activated clotting times (ACT), partial thromboplastin (PTT) and prothrombin times (PT), normal serum free hemoglobin levels, chest tube drainage less than 200 cc/hour, and absence of incisional or insertion site bleeding or oozing.

Nursing Orders

1. Identify and describe factors that can result in hemorrhage. The most common causes are prolonged cardiopulmonary bypass times, trauma to formed elements of the blood by the component parts of the assist system, and the need for anticoagulation.
   A. Monitor, assess, and record the following signs and symptoms associated with hemmorrhage:
      (1) Abnormal coagulation parameters (*i.e.*, ACT greater than 150 seconds, a PTT, and PT greater than two times the control)
      (2) Abnormal free plasma hemoglobin, which is indicative of hemolysis of red blood cells most likely associated with trauma from the pump head
      (3) Bloody or tarry stools
      (4) Hematuria
      (5) Bloody nasogastric tube drainage
      (6) Bloody endotracheal suctioning results
      (7) Oozing from incisions, ventricular assist device insertion sites, and invasive line sites
      (8) Chest tube drainage greater than 200 cc/hour
      (9) Development of petechiae
      (10) Development of hypovolemia
   B. Implement the following strategies aimed at eliminating or minimizing hemorrhagic complications:
      (1) Measure chest tube drainage frequently.
      (2) Measure nasogastric drainage and other drainages as accurately as possible. Observe amount and character.
      (3) Limit blood sampling and, thus, iatrogenic loss of blood volume.
      (4) Administer volume or blood component replacement agents as necessary. Fresh frozen plasma can be given for elevated PTT. Platelet units are given when the platelet count is less than 100,000/mm³. Cryoprecipitate and vitamin K are avoided owing to the risk of clot formation in the assist device.
      (5) Avoid bruising the patient.
      (6) Anticipate re-exploration for bleeding or cardiac tamponade. Keep equipment at bedside. Signs and symptoms of tamponade include an elevated right atrial pressure, widened mediastinum, falling blood pressure and cardiac output even with adequate volume loading, sudden cessation of chest tube drainage, and a pulsus paradoxus greater than 15 mm Hg.

NURSING DIAGNOSIS

2. Actual or high risk for infection related to ventricular assist device insertion, presence of multiple invasive lines, and debilitated state (exchanging pattern)

Patient Outcome

The patient will remain infection-free as evidenced by the absence of a temperature elevation as well as redness or drainage at any insertion sites, negative cultures, and normal white blood cell count.

Nursing Orders

1. Identify and describe factors that contribute to the development of infection in patients on ventricular assist devices. Prolonged operative times, debilitated states, multiple intravascular insertion sites, and open wounds provide ideal opportunities for infection. These patients also require prolonged ventilatory assistance, which can be associated with colonization.

(continued)

NURSING CARE PLAN SUMMARY *Patient With Ventricular Assist Devices* *Continued*

Patient Outcome	Nursing Orders

A. Monitor, assess, and record the following signs and symptoms of infection:
   (1) See Nursing Diagnosis: High Risk for Infection (IABP), page 267.
   (2) Abnormal sputum production
B. Implement the following strategies to prevent, minimize, or alleviate infectious complications:
   (1) See Nursing Diagnosis: High Risk for Infection (IABP), page 268.
   (2) Provide strict sterile technique when suctioning.
   (3) If chest remains open, place patient in either reverse or protective isolation.

NURSING DIAGNOSIS

3. *Decreased cardiac output related to ventricular failure (exchanging pattern)*

Patient Outcome	Nursing Orders

The patient will be free from ventricular failure and the need for ventricular assist support as evidenced by adequate cardiac output (CO)/cardiac index (CI); normal systemic vascular resistance (SVR); adequate urine output; adequate neurologic status; warm, dry skin; absence of hemodynamically unstable dysrhythmias; adequate oxygenation; absence of crackles; and absence of significant support from the assist device.

1. Identify and describe factors that contribute to the development of ventricular failure (see Table 18–3). Biventricular failure can develop in a patient who initially required only univentricular support. This usually occurs when there is an increase in atrial pressures in the unassisted ventricle with a concomitant decrease in CO in that ventricle. If right-sided failure results in a patient receiving left ventricular assistance, isoproterenol can be used to improve right ventricular contractility and decrease pulmonary vascular resistance. If left-sided failure develops in a patient with right-sided assistance, a biventricular assist device may be required.[57] Continued circulatory failure of the ventricle that is being assisted can be attributed to further myocardial deterioration or inadequate volume replacement. In addition, ventricular failure can reappear during the weaning process, indicating premature weaning.
   A. Monitor, assess, and record the following signs and symptoms of ventricular failure or inability to be weaned from assist devices:
      (1) See Nursing Diagnosis: Decreased Cardiac Output (IABP), page 268.
      (2) Decreased ventricular assist device flow. Flow is generally maintained at 2 to 4 L/minute.
      (3) Decreased CO/CI. Cardiac output is less than 5 L/minute, or CI is less than 2.7 L/minute/m². A thermodilution CO can be obtained when a left ventricular device is in place. Thermodilution CO is not a reliable parameter to use in the presence of right ventricular assist support because the injectate must travel from the right atrium through the pump before reaching the pulmonary artery. Because thermodilution is a measurement based on time and temperature change as blood moves from the right atrium to the pulmonary artery, this would be an inaccurate parameter.
      (4) Hypotension: systolic pressure less than 90 mm Hg or mean arterial pressure less than 60 mm Hg.
      (5) Elevated SVR or pulmonary vascular resistance (PVR): SVR greater than 1300 dyne-seconds/cm⁵, and PVR greater than 240 dyne-seconds/cm⁵.
      (6) Hemodynamically unstable dysrhythmias
      (7) Widened mediastinum
      (8) Increasing need for vasoactive drug support or volume loading
   B. Implement the following strategies to minimize or avoid return to ventricular failure:
      (1) Maintain optimum ventricular assist device flow.
      (2) Maintain optimum hemodynamic parameters.

(continued)

NURSING CARE PLAN SUMMARY *Patient With Ventricular Assist Devices* Continued

Patient Outcome	Nursing Orders

Nursing Orders

(3) Maintain optimum ECG rhythms. Ventricular dysrhythmias can be managed with routine antidysrhythmic agents. Conduction disturbances can be treated with a pacemaker.

(4) Maintain volume parameters.

(5) Administer vasoactive drugs as required.

(6) Observe skin color, temperature, and capillary refill time.

(7) Check quality and presence of peripheral pulses. If a nonpulsatile system is being used and the heart is contracting minimally, pulses may not be palpable.

(8) Record intake and output frequently.

NURSING DIAGNOSIS

4. *Impaired physical mobility (state level) related to ventricular assist device and severity of illness (moving pattern)*

Patient Outcome

The patient will be free from the consequences of immobility as evidenced by maintainance of skin integrity.

Nursing Orders

1. Identify and describe factors that contribute to the development of the loss of skin integrity. Low flow states, vasoconstriction from hypothermia and cardiopulmonary bypass, and lack of sufficient nutritional support and movement are etiologies for skin breakdown.

  A. Monitor, assess, and record the following signs and symptoms related to the complications:

    (1) Reddened areas on pressure points

    (2) Temperature elevations

  B. Implement the following strategies to prevent or minimize the complications of immobility:

    (1) Attempt to place an air mattress on the bed before the patient is moved from the operating table.

    (2) If patient can turn, gently turn patient from side to side to provide skin care.

    (3) Placing a pillow under the patient's shoulder or hip can tilt the patient slightly without altering functioning of ventricular assist device.

    (4) If patient is too unstable to be tilted, a five- to six-person lift can be performed to allow at least for placement of a clean bottom sheet.

    (5) Apply heel and elbow protectors.

    (6) Lubricate skin frequently with lotion.

    (7) Maintain proper body alignment to prevent contractures.

    (8) Provide nutritional support with a goal of 3000 calories a day.

    (9) Monitor as soon as possible weight and intake and output.

    (10) Monitor elimination patterns, and prevent impaction.

    (11) Perform passive range of motion at least twice daily.

    (12) With some of the implantable devices, getting out of bed, ambulation, and exercising on ergonomic bicycle apparatus can be performed. For patients awaiting transplantation, these activities are valuable in reversing the effects of immobility and permit patients to build themselves up from perhaps a previously cachexic state. The nurse needs to be in constant attendance for these activities.

(continued)

NURSING CARE PLAN SUMMARY Patient With Ventricular Assist Devices   Continued

NURSING DIAGNOSIS

5. *High risk for impaired gas exchange related to atelectasis, anesthesia, and ventilation/ perfusion mismatch (exchanging pattern)*

Patient Outcome	Nursing Orders
The patient will be free from impaired gas exchange as evidenced by adequate arterial blood gases, adequate lung sounds, and ability to be weaned from the ventilator.	1. Identify and describe factors that can contribute to impaired gas exchange. Anesthesia generally is not reversed after implantation of the assist device. This allows the patient to remain unresponsive and immobile for longer periods on arrival in the critical care unit. Although this facilitates the admission and assessment process, most importantly it saves the patient the energy of breathing and thus limits myocardial workload. As the anesthetic wears off, pain control with morphine or fentanyl is used as well as paralytic agents such as vecuronium or pancuronium. This sedation and paralysis will continue until the patient is hemodynamically stable. If the sternum was left open, the patient will remain sedated and paralyzed until it is closed.[5,19] Prolonged cardiopulmonary damage and interstitial edema and atelectasis all contribute to respiratory impairment. A. Monitor, assess, and record the following signs and symptoms of impaired gas exchange: (1) Inadequate rate, rhythm, depth of respiration, color, and level of consciousness (2) Inadequate arterial blood gases (3) Presence of abnormal breath sounds (4) Abnormal chest radiograph B. Implement the following strategies to eliminate or minimize impaired gas exchange: (1) Maintain adequate oxygenation by assuring optimum ventilator settings are maintained if the patient is intubated, and supplemental oxygen administration is maintained by way of face masks or cannulas in the extubated patient. (2) Suction the patient as necessary to minimize accumulation of secretions. (3) Assist the extubated patient with coughing and deep breathing exercises every 2 hours, or more often if necessary. (4) Administer bronchodilators as ordered. (5) If the patient can turn, gently turn patient from side to side to facilitate ventilation of poorly ventilated lung segments. (6) Place a pillow under the patient's shoulder or hip to tilt the patient slightly without altering functioning of ventricular assist device. (7) In patients awaiting transplantation, have patients sit out of bed in a chair or ambulate, which will also improve respiratory function.

NURSING DIAGNOSIS

6. *Ineffective patient/family coping related to unanticipated need for ventricular assist device (choosing pattern)*

Patient Outcome	Nursing Orders
The patient and family will be able to appraise the illness accurately, verbalize why the assist device and certain care are needed, express feelings appropriately, deal constructively with the crisis, and develop skills to reduce anxiety.	1. Identify and describe factors that can lead to ineffective family and patient coping. In some situations, such as in postcardiotomy cases, the family and patient may have had no warning that an assist device would be required. They may have anticipated an uneventful and usual recovery in which the patient would be discharged from the intensive care unit within a day and from the hospital within a week. They are most likely to be in a state of shock, denial, or

(continued)

NURSING CARE PLAN SUMMARY Patient With Ventricular Assist Devices *Continued*

Patient Outcome	Nursing Orders
	anger initially. In addition, although they may have prepared themselves for a small risk of death, they are now faced with a much larger one and the resultant loss and immediate role changes. For patients and families using assist devices as a bridge to transplant, the impact can generally be the same, even though they may have had years to deal with the patient's end-stage cardiac disease. Once a patient requires assist device support, the need to locate a donor heart accelerates. Potential transplant patients and their families know this is their last alternative.

A. Assess the family system.
B. Provide as much information as the patient and family need to deal with the situation in a supportive and empathetic fashion.
C. Supply constant reinforcement of this information and assure that all team members are providing the same information.
D. Answer all questions honestly about options and potential outcomes.
E. Encourage the family to verbalize their feelings.
F. Facilitate family strengths.
G. Assist family with problem solving, decision making, coping, and relaxation skills.
H. Allow as much visiting as is appropriate for both the patient and family.
I. Provide rest periods for both patient and family.
J. Encourage an attitude of realistic hope to deal with feelings of anxiety and hopelessness.

TOTAL ARTIFICIAL HEART

The first total artificial heart was used in the 1930s by a Russian who implanted it in an animal awaiting cardiac transplantation. In the 1960s, Dr. Kolff in the United States successfully accomplished the same task in a dog. Twenty-five years later, the Food and Drug Administration approved the permanent implantation of the Jarvik heart in patients who had end-stage cardiac disease but who were not considered candidates for cardiac transplantation. In 1982, Barney Clark became the first of a small group of patients who had the Jarvik heart permanently implanted. The longest surviving patient in this small group survived 660 days. The concept of permanent implantation of the Jarvik heart has ceased, at least for the time being, until further modifications can be produced to limit thromboembolism formation, hemorrhage, sepsis, and anticoagulation difficulties.

Although no longer used as a permanent replacement, the total artificial heart is now used successfully as a bridge to cardiac transplantation. As greater success has been achieved in the field of cardiac transplantation, more patients are being offered and are accepting this treatment modality. Unfortunately, the availability of donor organs has not increased to meet the demand, and the waiting period for cardiac transplantation has become longer. For those patients unable to maintain their physiologic stability with pharmacologic or balloon pump support while waiting transplantation, the temporary use of the total artificial heart is another option.

The total artificial heart consists of right and left hemi-spherical ventricles. A number are in use currently. Figure 18–14 depicts the Utah-100 and Jarvik-7 models. For implantation, the native heart is removed and the ventricles are connected to the remnant atria, pulmonary artery, and aorta. There are valves on the inflow and outflow tracts of the ventricles to assure unidirectional flow. Inside the ventricle, there is a dia-

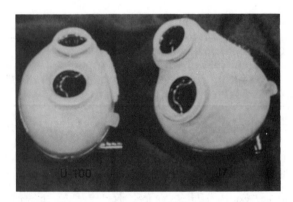

Figure 18-14

The Utah-100 and Jarvik-7 ventricles. (Robison, P. D., Pantalos, G. M., and Olsen, D. B. Pneumatically powered blood pumps used as a bridge to cardiac transplantation. *Crit. Care Nurs. Clin. North Am.*, 1:485, 1989; with permission.)

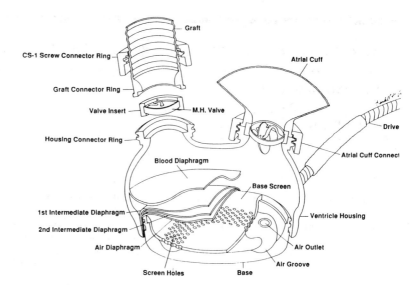

Figure 18–15

Cutaway view of the interior of the Utah-100 artificial heart. (Robison, P. D., Pantalos, G. M., and Olsen, D. B. Pneumatically powered blood pumps used as a bridge to cardiac transplantation. *Crit. Care Nurs. Clin. North Am.*, 1:485, 1989; with permission.)

phragm that, when collapsed by a vacuum, allows blood to enter and fill the ventricle (Fig. 18–15). When compressed air enters the diaphragm, it expands and fills the ventricular chamber, thereby causing blood to be ejected from the ventricle. The vacuum and pressure arrive through a drive line, which exits the body percutaneously and is attached to a drive console that controls the amounts and pressures delivered to the ventricles. The left and right ventricular pressures and rates may be varied independently of each other. This is useful in some patients in whom pulmonary edema can be avoided by turning down the cardiac output to the right ventricle and increasing cardiac output to the left. Maximum stroke volumes of 100 ml can be achieved for each side. The systems are sensitive to preload and afterload. Flow pressures of 5 to 7 mm Hg can generate a cardiac output of 4 to 5 L/minute. Increasing the inflow pressure to 10 to 15 mm Hg will create a 12- to 13-L cardiac output without any changes in heart rate.[45]

Clinical Indications for the Total Artificial Heart

The current use for the total artificial heart is to serve as a bridge to transplantation when pharmacologic, IABP, and mechanical ventricular assist devices are inadequate to support the patient. Generally, if a single ventricular assist device will provide enough hemodynamic stability, it is used rather than a total artificial heart. However, some authors believe that if a biventricular device is required, implantation of a total artificial heart would be better owing to the unknown length of time it may take to acquire a donor and the risk of infection associated with four cannulas exiting the body versus only one drive line used with the total artificial heart.[86]

The total artificial heart is generally indicated in patients with New York Heart Association (NYHA) class IV symptoms from idiopathic, viral, ischemic, or postpartum cardiomyopathies, or congenital heart disease. It is also indicated in patients with nonreparable surgical complications, inability to be weaned from cardiopulmonary bypass, or after acute transplant rejection.[95] Some studies report that up to 50% of these patients will survive long enough to receive a transplant.[86,95] Mortality is most often associated with infection, renal failure, and lack of donor availability. One study has reported supporting a patient for 379 days before he expired while awaiting a donor.[75]

Complications Associated With the Total Artificial Heart

As with all artificial devices, thrombus formation with resultant embolization is a major problem. Although the design of the total artificial heart chamber is as laminar as possible, there still remains areas in which turbulance can be created. Turbulance results in blood cell injury that activates platelets and thus initiates thrombus formation. Ideal media for turbulance are the crevices that exist in the valve rings and the connection sites of a total artificial heart. The converse of this complication is bleeding, which can occur from the anticoagulation these patients require. Careful monitoring and adjustments of heparin, dextran, and dipyridamole are essential. Infection is also a major complication because its occurrence can remove a patient as a potential transplant recipient. Likely sites for infection include the drive line, the total artificial heart itself, and the mediastinum. One predisposing factor that can lead to mediastinitis is the fact that, with the total artificial heart in place, there are still small open cavities in the chest that can serve as pockets for infection. Aggressive debridement and antibiotic coverage are required in this eventuality. Acute renal failure continues to play a major role in mortality and morbidity. It may result from hypoperfusion or from elevated free plasma hemoglobin levels, which are nephrotoxic. Finally, mechanical failure of the total artificial heart can develop that can be due to valve sticking, valve failure, drive failure, or air trapped in the diaphragm.[41]

NURSING CARE PLAN SUMMARY   *Patient With a Total Artificial Heart*

NURSING DIAGNOSIS

1. *High risk for decreased cardiac output related to mechanical dysfunction (exchanging pattern)*

Patient Outcome

The patient will maintain an adequate cardiac output as evidenced by adequate measurement of cardiac output; warm, dilated extremities; adequate blood pressure; normal sensorium; adequate urinary output; and optimum capillary refill.

Nursing Orders

1. Identify and describe factors that can contribute to an inadequate cardiac output. The diaphragm in the ventricle of the total artificial heart expands and causes systolic ejection as air is pumped through the drive line. This driving pressure must be set at a level high enough to overcome either the pulmonary artery pressure or the aortic pressure depending on whether right or left ventricular ejection is required. A drive pressure higher than the minimum required to exceed these pulmonary and systemic pressures is referred to as *overdriven*. Drive pressures higher than normal can impose stress on the valves and increase red blood cell destruction and platelet aggregation. *Underdrive* refers to a state in which inadequate pressure is applied and the ventricle is not completely emptied, thereby creating stagnation of blood. A major cause of inadequate cardiac output is suboptimal heart-driver settings. Alterations in venous return or in pulmonary and systemic vascular resistance can affect cardiac output, because these require changes in drive-pressure settings. (Other problems that can arise are mechanical failure of any internal and external components of the system.)
   A. Monitor, assess, and record the following signs and symptoms of alteration in cardiac output:
      (1) Alteration in drive console waveforms
      (2) Alteration in level of consciousness
      (3) Alteration in peripheral pulses
      (4) Pale, cool extremities
      (5) Hypotension
      (6) Urine output less than 0.5 cc/kg/hour
   B. Implement the following strategies to avoid or minimize alterations in cardiac output:
      (1) Ensure adequate drive pressures at all times.
      (2) Ensure that drive lines are unkinked and slack at all times.
      (3) Know troubleshooting techniques for equipment.
      (4) Be prepared to perform emergency procedures should equipment fail.
      (5) In the immediate postoperative period, keep head of bed elevated to 20°. Until adhesions form, the device can move in the chest, compressing the atria and thereby altering filling and emptying as resistances against chambers alter. Limiting motion is important to prevent these problems.
      (6) If hemodynamically stable, the patient can be turned from side to side as long as the cardiac output is monitored carefully and appropriate changes in drive pressure are performed.[36,37,41]
      (7) Early in the postoperative period, changes in intrathoracic pressure that develop with the use of positive end-expiratory pressure, coughing, or bagging can alter venous return and, consequently, cardiac output. Adjustment of drive pressures may also be required.[41]
      (8) Observe and record vital signs frequently.
      (9) Titrate vasoactive drugs as required.

NURSING DIAGNOSIS

2. *High risk for injury related to hemorrhage (exchanging pattern)*

Patient Outcome

The patient will remain free from hemorrhage as evidenced by absence of

Nursing Orders

1. Identify and describe factors that contribute to hemorrhage in patients undergoing implantation of a total artificial heart. Bleeding in the immediate

(continued)

NURSING CARE PLAN SUMMARY   *Patient With a Total Artificial Heart   Continued*

Patient Outcome	*Nursing Orders*
significant chest tube drainage; minimal need for replacement of blood products; normal hemoglobin, hematocrit, platelet counts, and coagulation parameters; absence of oozing and hematuria; and normal sensorium.	postoperative period is frequently surgical in nature as a result of the numerous suture lines and adhesions encountered by the surgeon. Coagulopathies can develop from prolonged cardiopulmonary bypass times and trauma to blood components from the total artificial heart. Lastly, as anticoagulation is started to prevent thrombus formation, bleeding can ensue. A. Monitor, assess, and record the following signs and symptoms related to hemorrhage: (1) Chest tube drainage greater than 200 cc/hour (2) Driver waveforms indicative of hypovolemia (3) Frank signs of bleeding (*i.e.,* oozing from incisions, chest tube sites, invasive line site, hematuria, and so on) (4) Occult signs of bleeding (*i.e.,* guaiac-positive nasogastric drainage, stools, and so forth) (5) Falling hemoglobin, hematocrit, and platelet levels (6) Elevated activated clotting time, prothrombin time, and partial thromboplastin times (7) Alteration in level of consciousness (8) Hypotension (9) Presence of petechiae or bruising (10) Decreased peripheral pulses (11) Increased systemic vascular resistance (12) Decreased central venous pressure B. Implement the following strategies to eliminate or minimize the risks of hemorrhage: (1) Monitor chest tube drainage closely, reporting levels greater than 200 cc/hour. (2) Monitor and report abnormal hematologic and coagulation parameters. (3) Administer volume replacement therapy as ordered. (4) Administer anticoagulation as ordered. (5) Protect patient from trauma. (6) Test urine, stool, and nasogastric drainage for presence of blood every 8 hours. (7) Limit iatrogenic loss of blood by using the least amount of blood required for each lab test. (8) Observe and record hemodynamic parameters.

NURSING DIAGNOSIS

3. *Actual or high risk for infection related to total artificial heart insertion, immobility, presence of multiple invasive lines, and debilitated state (exchanging pattern)*

Patient Outcome	*Nursing Orders*
The patient will remain infection-free as evidenced by the absence of an elevated temperature and elevated white blood cell count, absence of redness or drainage from incisions or insertion sites, negative cultures, normal sensorium, and continuation as a potential transplant recipient.	1. Identify and describe factors that contribute to the development of infection in patients who require a total artificial heart. Severe preimplantation cachexia, immobility, and invasive line catheterization predispose the patient to bacterial colonization before implantation of the total artificial heart. Additionally, preimplantation right-sided failure that results in abnormal liver function can alter the patient's immune capabilities. Prolonged periods for implantation of the device and numerous other invasive lines also add opportunities for infection. A. Monitor, assess, and record the following signs and symptoms of infection: (1) See Nursing Diagnosis: High Risk for Infection (IABP), page 267. B. Implement the following strategies to prevent or minimize the presence of infection:

(continued)

NURSING CARE PLAN SUMMARY *Patient With a Total Artificial Heart* Continued

---

Patient Outcome	*Nursing Orders*

(1) See Nursing Diagnosis: High Risk for Infection (IABP), page 268.
(2) Change dressings with strict aseptic technique.
(3) Limit visitor or personal contact with the patient.
(4) Remove all invasive lines as soon as possible.

NURSING DIAGNOSIS

4. *Impaired physical mobility related to total artificial heart device and severity of illness (moving pattern)*

Patient Outcome

Nursing Orders

The patient will remain free from the complications of immobility as evidenced by lack of contractures, skin breakdown, muscle atrophy, and atelectasis.

1. Identify and describe factors that contribute to immobility and its consequences. Initial restriction in movement is necessary until the patient becomes hemodynamically stable. Activities are then aimed at getting the patient out of bed and into a chair and gradually escalating the patient's activity to ambulation and riding of a stationary bicycle.
   A. Monitor, assess, and record the following signs and symptoms of the complications of immobility:
      (1) Reddened to broken skin
      (2) Elevated temperature
      (3) Atelectasis
      (4) Development of contractures
      (5) Deep vein thrombosis
   B. Implement the following strategies to prevent or minimize the complications of immobility:
      (1) Turn the patient frequently.
      (2) Perform passive then active range of motion.
      (3) Use low-pressure mattress, if possible.
      (4) Meticulously clean skin, wound, and insertion sites.
      (5) Maintain proper body alignment to prevent contractures.
      (6) Lift patient out of bed into a chair as soon as the patient is stable. Gradually increase activity to include ambulation and use of stationary bicycle.
      (7) Provide adequate nutrition.

NURSING DIAGNOSIS

5. *High risk for ineffective patient/family coping related to total artificial heart implantation (choosing pattern)*

Patient Outcome

Nursing Orders

The patient and family will exhibit signs of effective coping as evidenced by verbalizing an understanding of the situation and minimal levels of anxiety.

1. Identify and describe factors that can lead to ineffective coping. Major factors that contribute to ineffective coping consist of sleep pattern disturbances, depression, withdrawal, fear of death, loss of privacy and control, and alteration in self-concept.
   A. Implement the following strategies to diminish or alleviate these feelings:
      (1) Provide patient and family with as much information as possible.
      (2) Explain and re-explain procedures frequently.
      (3) Provide privacy.
      (4) Provide periods of undisturbed rest.

(continued)

NURSING CARE PLAN SUMMARY **Patient With a Total Artificial Heart** *Continued*

Patient Outcome	Nursing Orders
	(5) Remain calm and assuring yet realistic, in conversations with patient and family.
	(6) Assure that communication among all team members is consistent.
	(7) Allow as much decision making by the patient concerning care activities as possible.
	(8) Provide consistency with caregivers assigned to patient to allow relationships and trust to develop.
	(9) Provide divisional activities as much as possible.

SUMMARY

To provide quality care to the patient who requires mechanical cardiac assistance, the nurse needs to have an in-depth knowledge of the pathophysiologic changes of disease as well as the hemodynamic changes that occur after implantation of the various assist devices. Skill in clinically maintaining and managing the technologies associated with these therapies is also required. Lastly, it is important for the nurse to provide psychologic and emotional support to both patients and families caught in the crises associated with the use of these devices in order to help them achieve the best possible outcomes.

DIRECTIONS FOR FUTURE RESEARCH

1. What are the specific effects of positioning on the hemodynamic parameters in patients with mechanical assist device support?
2. What are the effects of various other nursing activities (*i.e.*, suctioning, range of motion, and so forth) on the hemodynamic parameters of patients requiring mechanical assist therapy?
3. What interventions would be most useful in decreasing stress and improving coping strategies in patients undergoing assist device support?
4. What are the best methods to provide information to patients and families during such high-stress situations as initiation of mechanical assist device support?

REFERENCES

1. Alcan, K. E., Stertzer, S. H., Wallsh, E., *et al.* Current status of intra-aortic balloon counterpulsation in critical care cardiology. *Crit. Care Med.* 12:489, 1984.
2. Alcan, K. E., Stertzer, S. H., Wallsh, E., *et al.* The role of intra-aortic balloon counterpulsation in patients undergoing percutaneous transluminal coronary angioplasty. *Am. Heart J.* 105:527, 1983.
3. Alderman, J. D., Gabliani, G. I., McCabe, C. H., *et al.* Incidence and management of limb ischemia with percutaneous wire-guided intra-aortic balloon catheters. *J.A.C.C.* 9:524, 1987.
4. Baillot, R., Pelletier, C., Trivino-Marin, J., *et al.* Postinfarction ventricular septal defect: Delayed closure with prolonged mechanical circulatory support. *Ann. Thorac. Surg.* 35:138, 1981.
5. Barnes-Brannon, P. H., and Towner, S. B. Ventricular failure: New therapy using the mechanical assist device. *Crit. Care Nurse* 6:70, 1986.
6. Beckman, C. B., Geha, A. S., Hammond, G. L., *et al.* Results and complications of intra-aortic balloon counterpulsation. *Ann. Thorac. Surg.* 24:550, 1977.
7. Bhayana, J. N., Scott, S. M., Sethi, G. K., *et al.* Effects of intra-aortic balloon pumping on organ perfusion in cardiogenic shock. *J. Surg. Res.* 26:108, 1979.
8. Bolman III, R. M., Cox, J. L., Marshall, W., *et al.* Circulatory support with a centrifugal pump as a bridge to cardiac transplantation. *Ann. Thorac. Surg.* 47:108, 1989.
9. Bolooki, H. (ed). *Clinical Application of Intra-aortic Balloon Pump* (2nd ed.). Mount Kisco, NY: Futura Publishing Co., 1984.
10. Bolooki, H., Williams, W., Thurer, R. J., *et al.* Clinical and hemodynamic criteria for intra-aortic balloon pump in patients requiring cardiac surgery. *J. Thorac. Cardiovasc. Surg.* 72:756, 1976.
11. Bonchek, L. I., and Olenger, G. N. Intra-aortic balloon counterpulsation for cardiac support during noncardiac operations. *J. Thorac. Cardiovasc. Surg.* 78:147, 1979.
12. Buckley, M. J., Craver, J. M., Gold, H. K., *et al.* Intra-aortic balloon pump assist for cardiogenic shock after CPB. *Circulation* (suppl II) 46:76, 1972.
13. Busch, H. M., Cogbill, T., and Gundersen, A. E. Splenic infarction: Complication of intra-aortic balloon counterpulsation. *Am. Heart J.* 109:383, 1985.
14. Copeland III, J. G., Harker, L. A., Joist, J. H., *et al.* Bleeding and anticoagulation. *Ann. Thorac. Surg.* 47:88, 1989.
15. Culliford, A. T., Madden, M. R., Isom, O. W., *et al.* Intra-aortic balloon counterpulsation: Refractory ventricular tachycardia. *J.A.M.A.* 239:431, 1978.
16. DeWood, M. A., Notske, R. N., Hensley, G. R., *et al.* Intra-aortic balloon counterpulsation with and without reperfusion for myocardial infarction shock. *Circulation* 61:1105, 1980.
17. Dougherty, J. E., Nino, A. F., and Rossi, M. A. Intra-aortic balloon counterpulsation: 1986 overview and perspective. *Emerg. Care Q.* 1:1, 1986.
18. Downing, T. P., Miller, D. C., Stofer, R., *et al.* Use of the intra-aortic balloon pump after valve replacement. *J. Thorac. Cardiovasc. Surg.* 92:210, 1986.
19. English, M. A. Preventing complications of ventricular assist devices. *D.C.C.N.* 8:330, 1989.

20. Farrar, D. J., Hill, D., Gray, L. A., *et al.* Heterotopic prosthetic ventricles as a bridge to cardiac transplantation. *N. Engl. J. Med.* 318:333, 1988.

21. Feola, M., Weiner, L., Walisky, P., *et al.* Improved survival after coronary bypass surgery in patients with poor left ventricular function: Role of intra-aortic balloon counterpulsation. *Am. J. Cardiol.* 39:1021, 1977.

22. Foster, E. D., Olsson, C. A., Rutenberg, A. H., *et al.* Mechanical circulatory assistance with intra-aortic counterpulsation for major abdominal surgery. *Ann. Surg.* 183:73, 1976.

23. Fredericksen, J. W., Smith, J., and Brown, P. Arterial helium embolism from a ruptured intra-aortic balloon. *Ann. Thorac. Surg.* 46:690, 1988.

24. Freed, P. S., Wasfie, T., Zado, B., *et al.* Intra-aortic balloon pumping for prolonged circulatory support. *Am. J. Cardiol.* 61:554, 1988.

25. Fuchs, R. M., Brin, K. P., Brinher, J. A., *et al.* Augmentation of regional coronary blood flow by intra-aortic balloon counterpulsation in patients with unstable angina. *Circulation* 68:117, 1983.

26. Funk, M., Gleason, J., and Foell, D. Lower limb ischemia related to use of the intra-aortic balloon pump. *Heart Lung* 18:542, 1989.

27. Goldberger, M., Labah, S. W., and Shah, P. K. Clinical experience with intra-aortic balloon counterpulsation in 112 consecutive patients. *Am. Heart J.* 111:497, 1986.

28. Goran, S. F. Family perceptions of the intra-aortic balloon pumping experience. *Crit. Care Nurs. Clin. North Am.* 1:475, 1989.

29. Goran, S. F. Vascular complications of the patient undergoing intra-aortic balloon pumping. *Crit. Care Nurs. Clin. North Am.* 1:459, 1989.

30. Gottlieb, S. D., Brinker, J. A., Boshom, A. M., *et al.* Identification of patients at high risk for complications of intra-aortic balloon counterpulsation: A multivariable risk factor analysis. *Am. J. Cardiol.* 53:1135, 1984.

31. Gould, K. A. Perspectives in intra-aortic balloon pump timing. *Crit. Care Nurs. Clin. North Am.* 1:469, 1989.

32. Grantham, R. N., Munnell, E. R., and Kanaly, P. J. Femoral artery infection complicating intra-aortic balloon pumping. *Am. J. Surg.* 146:811, 1983.

33. Gray Jr., L. A., Ganzel, B. L., Mavroudis, C., *et al.* The Pierce-Donachy ventricular assist device as a bridge to cardiac transplantation. *Ann. Thorac. Surg.* 48:222, 1989.

34. Grotz, R. L., and Yeston, N. S. Intra-aortic balloon counterpulsation in high-risk cardiac patients undergoing noncardiac surgery. *Surgery* 106:1, 1989.

35. Heberler, R. F. Simplified technique for organ placement and removal of intra-aortic balloon. *Ann. Thorac. Surg.* 48:134, 1989.

36. Henker, R., Smith, R. G., and Murdaugh, C. Effects of nursing interventions on cardiac output in the patient with a total artificial heart. *J. Cardiovasc. Nurs.* 2:56, 1988.

37. Henker, R., Shaffer, L., and Whittaker, A. Nursing care of a patient with a total artificial heart. *Heart Lung* 16:381, 1989.

38. Hess, P. J., Howe, H. R., Robicsek, F., *et al.* Traumatic tears of the thoracic aorta: Improved results using the Bio-Medicus Pump. *Ann. Thorac. Surg.* 48:6, 1989.

39. Hilberman, M., Derby, G. C., Spenser, R. J., *et al.* Effect of the intra-aortic balloon pump upon postoperative renal function in man. *Crit. Care Med.* 9:85, 1981.

40. Hill, J. D., Hardesty, R. L., Baumgartner, W. A., *et al.* Intra-operative management. *Ann. Thorac. Surg.* 47:82, 1989.

41. Hravnak, M., and George, E. Nursing considerations for the patient with a total artificial heart. *Crit. Care Nurs. Clin. North Am.* 1:495, 1989.

42. Icenogel, T. B., Williams, R. J., Smith, R. G., *et al.* Extracorporeal pulsatile biventricular support after cardiac transplantation. *Ann. Thorac. Surg.* 47:614, 1989.

43. Iverson, L. I., Herfindahl, G., Echer, R. R., *et al.* Vascular com-

plications of intra-aortic balloon counterpulsation. *Am. J. Surg.* 15:1, 1987.

44. Jarnolowski, C. R., and Poirier, R. L. Small bowel infarction complicating intra-aortic balloon counterpulsation via the ascending aorta. *J. Thorac. Cardiovasc. Surg.* 79:735, 1980.

45. Jarvik, R. K. The total artificial heart. *Sci. Am.* 224:66, 1981.

46. Johnson, D. Hemopump regulatory update. *Nimbus News* I, 1, 1989.

47. Kafrouni, G. Intra-aortic balloon counterpulsation. *Am. J. Surg.* 147:731, 1984.

48. Kantrowitz, A., Tjonneland, S., Freed, P. S., *et al.* Initial clinical experience with intra-aortic balloon pumping in cardiogenic shock. *J.A.M.A.* 203:113, 1968.

49. Kantrowitz, A., Wasfie, T., Freed, P. S., *et al.* Intra-aortic balloon pumping 1967 thru 1982: Analysis of complications in 733 patients. *Am. J. Cardiol.* 57:976, 1986.

50. Kron, I. L., Glover, W., and Tribble, C. G. A sterile, delayed-closure technique for placement of a left ventricular assist device. *Ann. Thorac. Surg.* 40:630, 1985.

51. Leinbach, R. C., Buckley, M. J., Austen, W. G., *et al.* Effects of intra-aortic balloon pumping on coronary flow and metabolism in man. *Circulation* (suppl) 43:I-77, 1971.

52. Litwak, R. S., Koffsky, R. M., Jurado, R. A., *et al.* Use of a left-heart assist device after intracardiac surgery: Technique and clinical experience. *Ann. Thorac. Surg.* 21:191, 1976.

53. Loisance, D. Left-ventricular support by intraventricular blood pumping during high-risk coronary angioplasty. *Lancet* (March): 561, 1989.

54. Lorente, P., Gourgon, R., Beaufils, P., *et al.* Multivariate statistical evaluation of intra-aortic counterpulsation in pump failure complicating myocardial infarction. *Am. J. Cardiol.* 46:124, 1980.

55. MacDonald, R. G., Hill, J. A., and Feldman, R. L. Failure of intra-aortic balloon counterpulsation to augment distal coronary perfusion pressure during percutaneous transluminal coronary angioplasty. *Am. J. Cardiol.* 59:359, 1987.

56. Maloney, J. V., and Nelson, R. L. Myocardial preservation during cardiopulmonary bypass. *J. Thorac. Cardiovasc. Surg.* 70:1040, 1975.

57. Marchetta, S., and Stennis, E. Ventricular assist devices: Applications for critical care. *J. Cardiovasc. Nurs.* 2:39, 1988.

58. Maurer, W. G., Kuntz, R. A., Dillard, R. E., *et al.* A proposed method for weaning from IABP assist following sequential hemodynamic assessment utilizing a micro computer. *J. Extracorporeal Tech.* 19:139, 1987.

59. Mayerhofer, K. E., Billhardt, R. A., and Codini, M. A. Delayed abrasion perforation of two intra-aortic balloons. *Am. Hosp. Assoc.* 108:1361, 1984.

60. McEnany, M. T., Kay, H. R., Buckley, M. J., *et al.* Clinical experience with intra-aortic balloon pump support in 728 patients. *Circulation* (suppl I) 58:124, 1978.

61. McGeehin, W., Sheikh, F., Donahoo, J. S., *et al.* Transthoracic intra-aortic balloon pump support in 39 patients. *Ann. Thorac. Surg.* 44:26, 1987.

62. Meldrum-Hanna, W. G., Deal, C. W., and Ross, D. E. Complications of ascending aortic intra-aortic balloon pump cannulation. *Ann. Thorac. Surg.* 40:241, 1985.

63. Milgalter, E., Mosseri, M., Uretzky, G., *et al.* Intra-aortic balloon entrapment: A complication of balloon perforation. *Ann. Thorac. Surg.* 42:697, 1986.

64. Miller, D. C., Moreno-Cabrol, R. J., Stinson, E. D., *et al.* Pulmonary artery counterpulsation for acute right ventricular failure. *J. Thorac. Cardiovasc. Surg.* 80:760, 1980.

65. Miller, K., and Pitz, K. Symbion acute ventricular assist device: Nursing challenge. *Crit. Care Nurse* 8:143, 1989.

66. Moise, J., Butler, K., Payne, J., *et al.* Experimental evaluation of complete electrically powered ventricular assist system. *Trans. Am. Soc. Artif. Intern. Organs* 31:202, 1985.

67. Moran, J., Opravil, M., and Gorman, A. J. Pulmonary artery balloon counterpulsation for right ventricular failure: II. Clinical experience. *Ann. Thorac. Surg.* 38:254, 1984.

68. Mulford, E. Nursing perspectives for the patient receiving postoperative ventricular assistance in the critical care unit. *Heart Lung* 16:246, 1987.

69. Mundth, E. D. Mechanical and surgical intervention for the reduction of myocardial ischemia. *Circulation* (suppl 1) 53:I-176, 1976.

70. O'Neill, M. J., Pierce, W. S., Wisman, C. B., *et al.* Successful management of right ventricular failure with the ventricular assist pump following aortic valve replacement and coronary bypass grafting. *J. Thorac. Cardiovasc. Surg.* 87:106, 1984.

71. Orlando, R., and Drezner, A. D. Intra-aortic balloon counterpulsation in blunt cardiac injury. *J. Trauma* 23:424, 1983.

72. O'Rourke, M. F., Norris, R. M., Campbell, T. J., *et al.* Randomized controlled trial of intra-aortic balloon counterpulsation in early myocardial infarction with acute heart failure. *Am. J. Cardiol.* 47:815, 1981.

73. Ortiz, A. F., Lukban, S. B., Jurado, R. A., *et al.* The use of vein allografts as sidearms for intra-aortic balloon insertion. *Ann. Thorac. Surg.* 19:574, 1975.

74. Paganini, E. P., Suhoza, K., Swann, S., *et al.* Continuous renal replacement therapy in patients with acute renal dysfunction undergoing intra-aortic balloon pump and/or left ventricular device support. *Trans. Am. Soc. Artif. Intern. Organs* 32:414, 1986.

75. Pae, W. E., Pierce, W. S., Myers, J. L. Staged cardiac transplantation: Total artificial heart or ventricular assist pump? *Circulation* (suppl III) 78:III-66, 1988.

76. Pappas, G. Intra-thoracic intra-aortic balloon insertion for pulsatile cardiopulmonary bypass. *Arch. Surg.* 109:842, 1974.

77. Parascandola, S. A., Pae, W. E., Davis, P. K. Determinants of survival in patients with ventricular assist devices. *Trans. Am. Soc. Artif. Intern. Organs* 34:222, 1988.

78. Park, S. B., Liebler, G. A., Burkholder, J. A., *et al.* Mechanical support of the failing heart. *Ann. Thorac. Surg.* 42:627, 1986.

79. Patacky, M. G., Garvin, B. J., and Schwirian, P. M. Intra-aortic balloon pumping and stress in the coronary care unit. *Heart Lung* 14:142, 1985.

80. Pennington, D. G., Swartz, M., Codd, J. E., *et al.* Intra-aortic balloon pumping in cardiac surgery patients: A nine-year experience. *Ann. Thorac. Surg.* 36:125, 1983.

81. Pennington, D. G. Seven years' experience with the Pierce-Donachy ventricular assist device. *J. Thorac. Cardiovasc. Surg.* 96:901, 1988.

82. Pennington, D. G., McBride, L. R., and Kanter, K. R. Effect of perioperative myocardial infarction on survival of postcardiotomy patients supported with ventricular-assist devices. *Circulation* (suppl III) 78:III-110, 1988.

83. Pennington, D. G. Emergency management of cardiogenic shock. *Circulation* (suppl I) 79:I-149, 1989.

84. Pennington, D. G., Lyle, J. D., Pae, W. E., *et al.* Patient selection. *Ann. Thorac. Surg.* 47:77, 1989.

85. Pennington, D. G., McBride, L. R., Swartz, M. T., *et al.* Use of the Pierce-Donachy ventricular assist device in patients with cardiogenic shock after cardiac operations. *Ann. Thorac. Surg.* 47:130, 1989.

86. Pennock, J. L., Pierce, W. S., Campbell, D. B., *et al.* Mechanical support of the circulation followed by cardiac transplantation. *J. Thorac. Cardiovasc. Surg.* 92:994, 1986.

87. Perler, B. A., McCabe, C. J., Abbott, W. M., *et al.* Vascular complications of intra-aortic balloon counterpulsation. *Arch. Surg.* 118:957, 1983.

88. Pierce, W. S., Gray, L. A., McBride, L. R., *et al.* Other postoperative complications. *Ann. Thorac. Surg.* 47:96, 1989.

89. Portner, P. M., Oyer, P. E., Pennington, D. G., *et al.* Implantable electrical left ventricular assist system: Bridge to transplantation and the future. *Ann. Thorac. Surg.* 47:142, 1989.

90. Purcell, J. A., Pippin, L., and Mitchell, M. Intra-aortic balloon pump therapy. *Am. J. Nurs.* 83:775, 1983.

91. Raper, R. F., and Fisher, M. M. Profound reversible myocardial depression after anaphylaxis. *Lancet* 1:386, 1988.

92. Reedy, J. E., Ruzevich, S. A., Swartz, M. T., *et al.* Nursing care of the patient requiring prolonged mechanical circulatory support. *Prog. Cardiovasc. Nurs.* 4:1, 1989.

93. Riggle, K. P., and Oddi, M. A. Spinal cord necrosis and paraplegia as complications of the intra-aortic balloon. *Crit. Care Med.* 17:475, 1989.

94. Roberts, A. J., Hoover, E., and Alonso, D. R. Prolonged intra-aortic balloon pumping in *Klebsiella*-induced hypodynamic shock: Cardiopulmonary, hematological, metabolic, and pathological observations. *Ann. Thorac. Surg.* 28:73, 1979.

95. Robison, P. D., Pantalos, G. M., and Olsen, D. B. Pneumatically powered blood pumps used as a bridge to cardiac transplantation. *Crit. Care Nursing Clin. North Am.* 1:485, 1989.

96. Rodigas, P. C., and Bridges, K. G. Occlusion of left internal mammary artery with intra-aortic balloon: Clinical implications. *J. Thorac. Cardiovasc. Surg.* 91:142, 1986.

97. Rodigas, P. C., and Finnegan, J. O. Technique for removal of percutaneously placed intra-aortic balloon. *Ann. Thorac. Surg.* 40:80, 1985.

98. Rose, D. M., Jacobowitz, I. J., Acinapura, A. J., *et al.* Paraplegia following percutaneous insertion of intra-aortic balloon. *J. Thorac. Cardiovasc. Surg.* 87:788, 1984.

99. Rose, D. M., Connolly, M., Cunningham, J. N., *et al.* Technique and results with a roller pump left and right heart assist device. *Ann. Thorac. Surg.* 47:124, 1989.

100. Rudan, P. M., Rountree, W. D., Myers, K. K., *et al.* Initial experience with the Hemopump. *Crit. Care Nursing Clin. North Am.* 1:527, 1989.

101. Ruzevich, S. A., Swartz, M. T., and Pennington, D. G. Nursing care of the patient with a pneumatic ventricular assist device. *Heart Lung* 17:399, 1988.

102. Sanfelippo, P. M., Baker, N. H., Ewy, H. G., *et al.* Experience with intra-aortic balloon counterpulsation. *Ann. Thorac. Surg.* 41:36, 1986.

103. Schoen, F. J., Palmer, D. C., Bernhard, W. F., *et al.* Clinical temporary ventricular assist: Pathologic findings and their implications in a multi-institutional study of 41 patients. *J. Thorac. Cardiovasc. Surg.* 92:1071, 1986.

104. Scott, I. R., and Goiti, J. J. Late paraplegia as a consequence of intra-aortic balloon pump support. *Ann. Thorac. Surg.* 40:300, 1985.

105. Shakian, D. M., Neptune, W. B., Ellis, F. H., *et al.* Intra-aortic balloon pump morbidity: A comparative analysis of risk factors between percutaneous and surgical techniques. *Ann. Thorac. Surg.* 36:644, 1983.

106. Starling, R. C., Galbraith, T. A., Baker, P. D., *et al.* Successful management of acute myocarditis with biventricular assist devices and cardiac transplantation. *Am. J. Cardiol.* 62:341, 1988.

107. Starnes, V. A., Oyer, P. E., Portner, P. M., *et al.* Isolated left ventricular assist as bridge to cardiac transplantation. *J. Thorac. Cardiovasc. Surg.* 96:62, 1988.

108. Verdouw, P. D., Hagemeiker, F., and VanDorp, W. G. Short-term survival after acute myocardial infarction predicted by hemodynamic parameters. *Circulation* 52:413, 1975.

109. Webber, K. T., and Janicki, J. S. Intra-aortic balloon counterpulsation: A review of physiologic principles, clinical results and device safety. A collective review. *Ann. Thorac. Surg.* 17:602, 1974.

110. Wasfie, T., Freed, P., Rubenfire, M., *et al.* Risks associated with intra-aortic balloon pumping in patients with and without diabetes mellitus. *Am. J. Cardiol.* 61:558, 1988.

111. Weiss, A. T., Engle, S., Gotsman, C. J., *et al.* Regional and global left ventricular function during intra-aortic balloon counterpulsation in patients with acute myocardial infarction shock. *Am. Heart J.* 108:249, 1984.

112. Whitman, G. R. Cardiac mechanics and intra-aortic balloon pumping. *Heart Lung* 7:1034, 1978.

113. Zada, F., McCabe, J. C., and Subramanian, V. A. Simplified technique for intra-aortic balloon insertion. *Ann. Thorac. Surg.* 29:573, 1980.

114. Zapolanski, A., Weisel, R. D., and Goldman, B. S. Pericardial graft for intraoperative balloon pump insertion. *Ann. Thorac. Surg.* 33:516, 1982.

115. Zumbro, G. L., Kitchens, W. R., Shearer, G., *et al.* Mechanical assistance for cardiogenic shock following cardiac surgery, myocardial infarction and cardiac transplantation. *Ann. Thorac. Surg.* 44:11, 1987.

IV

The Critically Ill Adult With Respiratory Problems

THE SOUL

The idea of the soul has long been thought to be only a religious concept with no scientific basis. Although there is no "soul meter" or device to measure it, there is nonetheless strong evidence that there is an aspect of the human psyche that is outside space and time that is omnipresent in space and infinite in time.

Studies done at Princeton University show that highly detailed mental images can be conveyed from one person to another by thought alone, when the two persons are separated by up to 6000 miles, and that the "receiver" gets the information up to 3 days before it is sent.* These studies, in addition to many others, strongly suggest that the mind is not confined to brains or bodies or to the present moment. It seems *nonlocal*, or not localized to the here and now.†

These data have profound implications for nursing. They suggest that death is impossible for this soul-like dimension of the psyche. This should come as comfort not only for the sick and dying patients that nurses care for but for everyone, including nurses themselves.

* Jahn, R. J., and Dunne, B. J. *Margins of Reality*. New York: Harcourt Brace Jovanovich, 1987: 149–190.

† Dossey, L. *Recovering the Soul*. New York: Bantam, 1989: 1–11.

19

Respiratory Assessment

Mary Elizabeth Egloff

REGULATING SELF

Working as a critical care nurse is challenging. To be as healthy as we can in this demanding environment requires that we take care of ourselves moment by moment. Self-regulation skills are important for health and effective coping with the daily demands. As discussed in Chapter 3, self-regulation is a process of learning to reverse the negative effects of stress and to select helpful bodymind responses to manage the numerous stressors with which you are faced each day. When you learn self-regulation skills, you will experience the following:

- An inward focus of attention
- Awareness of altered perception of linear time—past, present, and future
- Control of your state of awareness
- A relaxed inner calmness that may or may not be goal-directed

These experiences occur because you bring involuntary body responses (*i.e.,* heart rate, blood pressure, respirations, muscle tension) under voluntary control. The three steps in self-regulation are as follows:

1. Assess presence of negative bodymind responses to stress.
2. Evoke states of inner peace and calmness with healing rituals of relaxation and imagery skills.
3. Integrate relaxation and imagery in daily activities in order to make effective choices.

LEARNING OBJECTIVES

After reading this chapter, the nurse should be able to do the following:

1. Perform the techniques of inspection, palpation, percussion, and auscultation systematically and accurately.
2. Describe the characteristics associated with adventitious sounds.
3. Interpret arterial blood gas results correctly.
4. Describe how the following will augment a pulmonary assessment: chest radiograph, pulse oximetry, end tidal carbon dioxide monitoring, and pulmonary function tests.
5. Define compliance and discuss how a change in compliance may alter the care of the critically ill patient.
6. Explore the principles of ventilation and perfusion.
7. Analyze several factors that affect oxygenation.
8. Identify several nursing diagnoses pertaining to the care of the critically ill pulmonary patient.

OVERVIEW

The patients in critical care units collectively exhibit a gamut of respiratory problems. In some patients, the respiratory problem is the primary illness; in others, it is secondary to another illness.

It is important for the nurse to know that most patients in critical care units have some degree of respiratory difficulty. It is equally important (in the opinion of many authorities, more important) to know what respiratory problems are likely to occur while patients are in critical care units. Even if no other respiratory difficulty occurs, the supine position decreases the functional residual capacity of the patient's lungs and contributes to the development of atelectasis.

The major purpose of the respiratory system is to provide oxygen for the combustive process of metabolism and to remove carbon dioxide, the waste product of metabolism, from the body. The secondary functions of the respiratory system are acid-base balance, speech, the expression of emotion (laughing, crying, sighing), and, in a relatively minor way, maintenance of body water and heat balance.

The specific pulmonary problems exhibited by the critically ill patient are discussed elsewhere in the text. This chapter discusses a method of systematically assessing the respiratory system of the critically ill patient.

HISTORY

Years ago at the Johns Hopkins Hospital, Sir William Osler taught that if one listens to a patient long enough, the patient will tell one what's wrong. Unfortunately, this truth is easily forgotten in the hustle and bustle of the modern hospital.

The history clarifies why the patient has sought health care and how the problem has affected the patient and family. It paints a picture within whose framework therapy may be instituted.[3] The history need not be long. Relevant questions can pinpoint parts of the physical examination to be stressed.

Chief Complaint

The chief complaint is the reason the patient has sought medical attention, and, frequently, is obtained in the patient's own words. The complaint needs to be clarified further by the patient. For example, a constricting feeling in the chest may be dyspnea or pain. Open-ended questions are useful in starting the history. If patients give several complaints, ask them to identify first the one troubling them the most.

History of Present Illness

The history of the present illness dates from the time the patient noted a change. It is a chronologic review of the patient's immediate illness, including the initial symptoms and the development of the illness.

The cardinal symptoms of respiratory illness are carefully investigated, and information about onset and progression, frequency and duration, severity, precipitating factors, and aggravating and alleviating factors is recorded. The patient's past and present use of medications is reviewed.

Information about general constitutional symptoms, such as anorexia, weight loss, weakness, tiredness, sweating, chills, and fever, must be elicited.[8] Upper respiratory tract symptoms include nasal discharge (onset, character, precipitating factors, sneezing), obstruction of the nasal passages (pain or sinus tenderness), and hoarseness. Sputum is evaluated in regard to amount, consistency, color, odor, and presence of blood.

If patients complain of shortness of breath, they should be asked to describe any other changes in breathing. The subjective sensation of breathlessness may have various causes. Dyspnea needs to be differentiated from pressure sensations in the chest, weakness, and fatigability. For example, angina may be associated with a feeling of suffocation and may be mistaken for breathlessness. In addition, patients with hyperventilation often say that they are unable to take in enough air.[2]

The ongoing assessment in the critical care unit of subjective data considers the signs and symptoms the person has observed as well as any the medical team anticipates. For example, mental dullness or confusion may accompany hypoxemia, hyponatremia, or fluid volume depletion.

Past Health History

The past health history includes the patient's illnesses since birth. Frequency of illness and the treatment are noted, particularly with regard to pneumonia, pleurisy, fungal disease, tuberculosis, bronchiectasis, chronic obstructive lung disease, asthma, allergies, colds, sinus problems, and pneumothorax.[1] The patient's compliance with the various medical regimens, along with the dates of the last chest film, tuberculin skin test, and pulmonary function tests, is noted.

Family History

The family history includes information about the health status or causes of death of members of the patient's immediate family. If the patient has asthma or some other possible hereditary disease, the family history should include a review of similar problems in other family members.

Review of Systems

The review of systems is a rapid check to ensure that the patient has mentioned all signs and symptoms. Each body system is reviewed to obtain pertinent information. Any additional information uncovered may require further clarification.

Activities of Daily Living, Personal and Social History

A review of the patient's personal and social history not only gives information that describes the patient's life and helps to individualize care, but also gives clues to possible unidentified respiratory conditions.

The patient's job history may point to past or present factors conducive to the development of respiratory disease, as the following example shows. A 40-year-old man was admitted to a coronary care unit with severe chest pain. The early test results were negative for cardiac disease, but a detailed history revealed that years ago the man had been an asbestos pipe fitter. Further study established the diagnosis of asbestosis.

Geography may also be an important factor in the patient's background. The patient may have lived in a part of the country where certain fungal diseases are endemic.

PHYSICAL EXAMINATION

The next step in the assessment of the patient's respiratory functioning is the physical examination. Because most people in the critical care unit are in bed and have little physical stamina, the usual systematic approach after evaluation of the head and neck is examination of the anterior chest and then of the lateral and posterior chest.[4] The complete physical examination is described here, although nurses in the critical care unit would rarely do the entire examination. Rather, they would examine selected aspects determined by the patient's condition.

Inspection

The examination actually begins with observation of the patient by the nurse while eliciting historical data. General notations are made about the patient's overall condition. Then the nurse examines each area of the respiratory system and makes notes about normal and abnormal findings. Inspection and palpation are often done at the same time.

The nurse begins the inspection of the head and neck by noting any signs of respiratory distress: airway difficulty, gasping, cyanosis, open mouth, flared nostrils, or the use of accessory muscles. Bilateral jugular vein distention is indicative of elevated venous pressure. The examiner notes the sputum and the odor of the breath. The inspiratory–expiratory ratio is noted. The forced vital capacity may be estimated roughly by having the patient blow forcefully on the examiner's hand. (A Wright spirometer, which measures tidal volume and minute volume, can be used. Charts are available to determine normal volume values for different heights, weights, ages, and strengths.)

The patient's chest is inspected in regard to respiratory rate (normal = 16 to 18 respirations/minute), amplitude or depth of expansion, and rhythm. Abdominal breathing is more apparent in men, and thoracic breathing is more apparent in women. The breathing pattern is assessed (Fig. 19-1). Symmetry is ascertained, and any paradoxical movements are assessed immediately. Any other movements that denote labored inspirations, such as elevation of the clavicle and shoulder or retraction, are observed. Retraction on inspiration is indicative

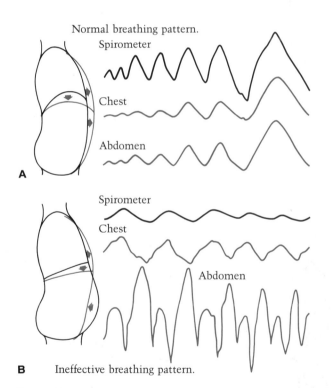

A Normal breathing pattern.

Spirometer

Chest

Abdomen

Spirometer

Chest

Abdomen

B Ineffective breathing pattern.

Figure 19–1
Normal contrasted with ineffective breathing pattern. All signals were recorded simultaneously. (*A*) Normal breathing pattern. Inspiration corresponds with downward movement of the diaphragm, outward movement of the chest and abdomen, and upward movement on spirometry. The reverse is true for expiration. (*B*) Ineffective breathing pattern. The chest and abdomen do not move in a synchronous pattern. During inspiration, the abdomen moves inward while the chest moves outward. During expiration, the abdomen moves outward.

of airway obstruction. Increased use of expiratory muscles may also be seen on forced expiration in a patient with a severe asthma attack or respiratory failure with chronic obstructive lung disease.[9] Observation is made of the contour and size of the chest, noting the anteroposterior diameter.

Examination of the extremities may reveal clubbing of the fingers or toes, suggesting the presence of a pulmonary disorder. The evidence may be difficult to evaluate. Normally, the angle at the nail bed is 160°, but early in pulmonary disease, hypertrophy of the nail bed is such that the angle increases to 180° or more.[4] Eventually the nail has a characteristic, bulbous, blunted appearance as the pulp under the nail enlarges further. In some instances, the changes in the nails are accompanied by a painful arthritis of the wrists and ankles termed *hypertrophic pulmonary osteoarthropathy.*

Palpation

The chest is palpated with the heel of the examiner's hand held flat against the person's chest or with the ulnar aspect of the hand. Palpation combined with inspection is particularly effective in assessing whether the movements of each side of the chest during deep inspiration and expiration are equal in amplitude and are symmetrical.

In an effective way of comparing chest excursions, the nurse first has the patient sit and then places his or her hands on the posterior aspects of the patient's chest, with the thumbs meeting in the midline. As the chest moves, the examiner's hands move, so the excursion of each side can be assessed simultaneously. Any unilateral asymmetry may be indicative of a disease process in that region. Evaluation also includes noting any tracheal deviation, crepitus, tenderness of the chest wall, muscle tone, swelling, and tactile (vocal) fremitus.

To assess tactile fremitus, the examiner palpates the patient's chest wall while the patient says phrases that produce relatively intense vibrations (*e.g.,* "99"). The vibrations are transmitted from the larynx through the airways and can be palpated at the chest wall. The intensity of vibrations on both sides is compared. Stronger vibrations are felt over areas where there is consolidation of the underlying lung. Decreased tactile fremitus is usually associated with abnormalities that move the lung further from the chest wall, such as pleural effusion and pneumothorax.

Percussion

If the chest is tapped with the finger, the vibrations of the tissues, lungs, and chest wall produce an audible sound wave. Just as with all musical tones, those vibrations are described in regard to their acoustic properties of frequency, intensity, duration, and quality. These four properties are then further evaluated and recorded as resonant, hyperresonant, dull, flat, or tympanic.

Frequency, or *pitch,* refers to the number of vibrations per second. *Intensity* refers to the amplitude of the sound wave. *Duration* is the length of time the sound is present. *Quality* is the characteristic most difficult to describe, comprising many subjective elements besides pitch, intensity, and harmonics.

Resonant sounds have a relatively low pitch (100 to 140 cycles/second), variable intensity, long duration, nonmusical quality, and are heard with percussion over normal lung tissue.

Hyperresonant sounds have an even lower pitch and overtones that are somewhat musical. An abnormal increase in the amount of air in the lungs or pleural spaces, such as with emphysema or pneumothorax, produces hyperresonant sounds. Dull sounds have a higher pitch (140 to 190 cycles/second), decreased intensity, short duration, and a nonmusical quality. Dullness is produced by percussion over tissue that is denser than lung tissue, for example, lung consolidation or tumor. Flat sounds have a higher pitch (190 cycles/second), even less intensity, a very short duration, and a nonmusical quality. Percussion over airless tissues results in a flat sound. This note can be simulated by percussing one's thigh. Tympanic sounds have an even higher pitch (200 to 350 cycles/second), a very loud intensity, a long duration, and a relatively rich (musical) quality. A large air-filled chamber or cavity such as a large tension pneumothorax results in a tympanic percussion note.

Percussion usually begins at the apices and proceeds to the bases, moving from the anterior areas to the lateral areas and then to the posterior areas. Ideally, the patient is seated, and percussion proceeds in an unhurried manner, with several points percussed in each intercostal space. If the patient is unable to sit up, he or she is examined first in one lateral decubitus position and then in the other. That procedure allows comparison of the two sides.

Auscultation

Auscultation, along with inspection, is the technique most frequently used in the critical care unit. By listening to the lungs with a stethoscope while the patient breathes with the mouth open, the nurse is able to assess three things: the character of the breath sounds, the character of the spoken and whispered voice, and the presence of adventitious sounds.[1] While listening, the nurse must keep in mind the segmental pulmonary anatomy (Fig. 19-2) in order to determine what segment of the lung is being listened to.

The breath sounds heard result from the transmission of vibrations produced by the movement of air in the respiratory passages from the larynx to the alveoli. The voice sounds heard result from the transmission of vibrations produced by sound waves from the larynx. The airways to the area examined must be open to have transmission of voice sounds. Adventitious sounds are extra sounds (crackles, rhonchi, wheezes, and pleural friction rub) superimposed on the breath sounds.

Breath Sounds

Breath sounds are termed *vesicular*, *bronchial*, and *bronchovesicular* (Table 19-1 and Fig. 19-3). Vesicular or normal breath

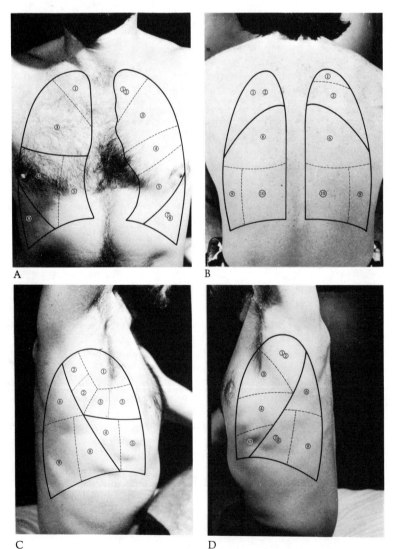

A   B

C   D

Figure 19-2

Location of the lung segments. (*A*) Front chest. (*B*) Dorsal chest. (*C*) Right lateral chest. (*D*) Left lateral chest. Right lung: *Upper lobe*—(*1*) Apical segment, (*2*) posterior segment and axillary subsegment, (*3*) anterior segment and axillary subsegment. *Middle lobe*—(*4*) Lateral segment, (*5*) medial segment. *Lower lobe*—(*6*) Superior segment, (*7*) medial basal segment, (*8*) anterior basal segment, (*9*) lateral basal segment, (*10*) posterior basal segment. Left lung: *Upper lobe*—Superior division: (*1, 2*) Apical-posterior segment, (*3*) anterior segment. Inferior division: (*4*) Superior lingular segment, (*5*) inferior lingular segment. *Lower lobe*—(*6*) Superior segment, (*7, 8*) antereomedial basal segment, (*9*) lateral basal segment, (*10*) posterior basal segment.

Table 19-1
Normal Breath Sounds

BREATH SOUND	NORMAL LOCATION	INSPIRATION/ EXPIRATION RATIO	PITCH	AMPLITUDE	QUALITY
Vesicular	Throughout the peripheral lung fields	3:1	Low	Moderate	Breezy
Bronchial	Over manubrium	2:3	High	High	Tubular
Bronchovesicular	Anteriorly over the central large airways	1:1	Moderate	Moderate to high	Breezy to tubular

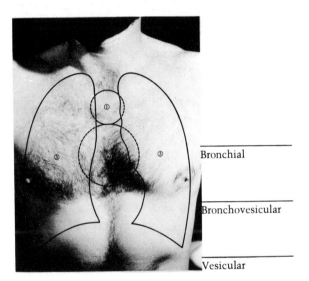

Figure 19-3

Sites of origin and graphic representations of various breath sounds: (1) bronchial, (2) bronchovesicular, and (3) vesicular breath sounds.

sounds are heard throughout the chest and best heard at the base of the lungs. During inspiration, the sound is heard longer and louder than during expiration. The sound during inspiration is produced by air moving into the terminal bronchioles and alveoli. Because airflow is greater during the earlier phase of expiration, more sound is heard early in expiration. In general, expiration is described as very quiet to silent. The inspiration–expiration ratio in vesicular breathing is normally 3:1. Decreased breath sounds are heard when there is fluid, air, or increased tissue in the pleural space that interferes with the transfer of vibrations to the chest wall. Absent or diminished breath sounds are heard also in bronchial obstruction, because there can be no airflow and thus no vibrations.

Bronchial breath sounds are produced by vibrations of air in larger airways. They are normally heard over the manubrium. No breath sounds are heard between inspiration and expiration, because there is no airflow. In the area between the trachea and the peripheral lung, a mixture of bronchial and vesicular sounds are heard. These sounds are called bronchovesicular sounds.

Voice Sounds

Auscultation also includes assessment of the spoken and whispered voice. Sounds produced by speaking are transmitted

from the larynx to the chest wall and may be heard with the stethoscope. In the normal lung, because most of the vibrations caused by the voice are absorbed by the lung tissue, the waves are not clear. A decrease in voice sounds can be caused by any factor that impairs the transmission of vibrations, such as airway obstruction. Voice sounds are also evaluated by having the patient whisper. With whispering, resonance and vibrations are less than with normal speech. Therefore, in the normal lung a weak sound is heard at the chest wall.

If consolidation develops, there is increased transmission of bronchial vibrations to the chest wall (since fluid is a better conductor of sound than is air). During the evaluation of bronchophony, vocal sounds are transmitted better and spoken words are clearer to the examiner. The patient's whisper is heard clearly and distinctly during the evaluation of whispered pectoriloquy. (Liquid in the airways caused by consolidation may also vibrate and cause rhonchi). Another valuable clinical test to assess consolidation is the evaluation of egophony. If consolidation is present in the patient's lung, the letter *E* spoken by the patient is not heard as *E* by the examiner. Rather, the examiner, listening with a stethoscope, hears the sound as *A*.

Adventitious Sounds

Adventitious sounds are extra sounds superimposed on breath sounds. They usually indicate disease. There is much discussion about the appropriate terminology in today's literature. The current American Thoracic Society and International Symposium on Lung Sounds nomenclature for adventitious sounds is used throughout this chapter.[6,7] Adventitious sounds are classified as crackles, wheezes, rhonchi, or pleural friction rubs.

Crackles. Sudden opening of a succession of small airways or the bubbling of air through secretions produces a crackle. Crackles have been referred to as *rales* in the past. The sound of a crackle can be reproduced by picking up a lock of hair with the thumb and forefinger and slowly rubbing the strands together close to the ear.

Crackles are classified as coarse or fine. Coarse crackles are discontinuous, interrupted explosive sounds. They are lower in pitch, louder, and longer in duration than fine crackles. Coarse crackles are found in patients with resolving pneumonia, pulmonary edema, and bronchitis.

Fine crackles are also discontinuous, interrupted explosive sounds but are softer, of shorter duration, and higher in pitch than coarse crackles. Conditions such as atelectasis, fibrosis, and pneumonia produce fine crackles.

Rhonchi. Rhonchi are continuous, low-pitched, snoring sounds. The passage of air through fluid-filled, narrowed air passages produces the sound. The term *gurgle* also has been used to describe this type of adventitious sound. Excess mucus or fluid production with such diseases as bronchitis, bronchiectasis, or pneumonia results in rhonchi.

Wheeze. A wheeze is another type of continuous lung sound but is higher-pitched and hissing. Narrowed airways cause the wheezes to have a musical or whistling quality. Wheezes are most commonly associated with asthma due to the presence of bronchoconstriction and edema, which narrow the airway. Foreign-body airway obstruction can also cause wheezing, so all wheezes are not necessarily from asthma.

Pleural Friction Rub. A pleural friction rub is produced from pleural inflammation. The cause may be pneumonia, pulmonary infarction, or pleurisy. The sound is described as rough, grating, and crackling, much like two pieces of leather being rubbed together. With inflammation, the pleural surfaces are roughened, and the normal lubrication between the visceral and parietal layers is lost. Usually these layers move noiselessly during inspiration and expiration. Because movement produces the sound, there is no sound when the person holds his or her breath. Timing of the sound in the respiratory cycle varies; it may be heard only during inspiration and expiration, or it may be heard in both phases. Usually increasing the pressure of the stethoscope on the chest wall increases the intensity of the sound. The rub is most commonly heard over the involved area.

Procedure

For the patient confined to bed, the physical assessment is done by using all four examination techniques for one body region and then repositioning the patient and using the techniques for another body region. The findings are recorded separately for each region (for example, left lower lobe: increased tactile fremitus, dull to percussion, breath sounds bronchial, crackles, bronchophony, and egophony) or the findings may be recorded according to techniques used (for example, inspection, percussion, palpation, and auscultation).

Anterior and Lateral Chest

Inspection (combined with palpation):

1. Skin: Color, lesions, edema, dilated veins, physical characteristics
2. Chest: Size and shape, symmetry and deformity, muscular size
3. Respirations: Rate and rhythm, inspiration-expiration ratio, depth, equality, symmetry, labored respirations, use of accessory muscles, retractions, abdominal or thoracic respirations

Palpation:

1. Tenderness in the skin, tissues, or bone
2. Tracheal deviation or crepitus
3. Muscle tone

4. Equal and synchronous movement
5. Tactile fremitus

Percussion:

1. Bilateral corresponding areas for resonance, hyperresonance, dullness, flatness, tympany
2. Note bases in particular.

Auscultation:

1. Bilateral corresponding areas for breath sounds, voice sounds, adventitious sounds

Posterior and Lateral Chest

(Patient may have to be turned and the examination repeated for opposite posterior chest.)

Inspection:

1. Skin: Color, lesions, edema
2. Chest: Symmetry, anteroposterior diameter, scapular position
3. Respirations: Symmetry

Palpation:

1. Tenderness
2. Muscle tone
3. Chest expansion

Percussion:

1. Corresponding bilateral intercostal spaces; note bases.
2. Diaphragmatic excursion after a deep inspiration and a deep expiration

Auscultation:

1. Bilateral corresponding areas for breath sounds, voice sounds, and adventitious sounds

DIAGNOSTIC STUDIES

Many parameters may be used to evaluate the patient's respiratory status. The choice depends on the patient's disorder. If the findings are abnormal, further examination is indicated. This section reviews several diagnostic studies that can augment one's respiratory assessment. The studies include chest radiograph, pulse oximetry, end tidal carbon dioxide monitoring, arterial blood gases, and pulmonary function tests.

Chest Radiograph

The best chest examination tool is the chest film, but alone it is not sufficient. The history and physical examination are essential accompaniments, because the chest film gives a picture of only one moment in time. Routine daily films are valuable in identifying abnormalities, even though most chest films in critical care units are taken with a portable machine and a suboptimal delivery system.[12]

The chest film is evaluated systematically in regard first to the normal areas and then to the abnormal areas. The bony structures and the diaphragm are examined, then the heart shadow, tracheobronchial tree, and lung parenchyma. On a normal chest film, the lung is black. The volume may be roughly estimated by the size of the lung fields. Atelectasis, the most common complication in the critically ill patient, is seen on the film as a density. The fine, white, wispy, thin structures that fan out from the hili are the shadows of blood vessels. These vascular markings are present over the entire lung field, and when they look enlarged and fuzzy, they are abnormal.

Pulse Oximetry

Pulse oximetry provides the clinician with a noninvasive measurement of arterial saturation. The current technology was developed over 50 years ago and today has become an integral part of the respiratory assessment. The principles of plethysmography and spectrophotometry are combined in the pulse oximeter. Light-emitting diodes transmit dual wavelengths—infrared and red light—through pulsating arterial blood to a photodetector. Oxyhemoglobin absorbs infrared light; reduced hemoglobin absorbs the red light. The photodetector transmits this information to a microprocessor which calculates the oxygen saturation. The oxygen saturation is the comparison of oxyhemoglobin, with the total functional hemoglobin present. Arterial saturations (SaO_2) have a close correlation with the saturations obtained from the pulse oximeter if the SaO_2 is 70% or greater.[11,14,15]

There are several advantages of use of the pulse oximeter. The monitors are easy to use and very portable. Pulse oximeters are used to monitor oxygen saturations during transportation and while weaning from mechanical ventilation. The latter use of the pulse oximeter may reduce the number of arterial blood gas tests needed.

Despite the advantages of pulse oximetry, physiologic, spectrophotometric, and instrumental limitations are present. Reduced arterial flow with hypotension, hypothermia, and vasoconstriction may cause signal loss and the inability of the oximeter to calculate a saturation. The oximeter cannot differentiate between oxyhemoglobin and carboxyhemoglobin and therefore might incorrectly interpret the hemoglobin as saturated. Extraneous digital motion may be interpreted as an arterial pulsatile motion and result in inaccurate readings. The following provides a quick guide to oxygen saturation:

O_2 saturation—PaO_2*
  50%—25 mm Hg
  75%—40 mm Hg
  90%—55 mm Hg
*PaO_2 values are approximate estimations taken from oxyhemoglobin curve.

End Tidal Carbon Dioxide Monitoring

End tidal carbon dioxide is a reflection of arterial carbon dioxide ($PaCO_2$). Carbon dioxide has a characteristic infrared absorption band and therefore can be measured. Capnometry is the measurement of the expired carbon dioxide or end tidal carbon dioxide ($etCO_2$). The tracing of the inhaled and exhaled carbon dioxide concentrations is referred to as *capnography*.

The recorded value refers to the amount of infrared light absorbed by the carbon dioxide molecules, with higher concentrations generating a higher value.[15]

The normal $PaCO_2$–$etCO_2$ gradient is 5 mm Hg in individuals with normal respiratory, cardiovascular, and metabolic function. Changes in any of these variables affect the $PaCO_2$–$etCO_2$ gradient. At this time, $etCO_2$ monitoring is limited to intubated patients, because capnography requires undiluted exhaled gas.

Clinical indications for $etCO_2$ monitoring include assessing the adequacy of ventilation, trending changes in deadspace ventilation, and, recently, assessing the adequacy of CPR.[14]

The clinician caring for a critically ill pulmonary patient would use the above assessment information to facilitate appropriate decision-making when planning care. For example, the physical examination reveals increased yellow sputum production with increased rhonchi in the left lower lobe. The chest radiograph reveals a new left lower lobe infiltrate. The oxygen saturations have dropped from 97% to 90% with an arterial blood gas PaO_2 of 55. Appropriate additions to the plan of care for this patient based on the above assessment would include frequent pulmonary assessments for suctioning and position changes. Consultation with the physician related to changes in oxygen therapy, antibiotic therapy, and intravenous hydration may be necessary.

Acid–Base Balance

Arterial blood gas measurements and pH are widely accepted physiologic parameters used to assess acid–base balance and cardiopulmonary functioning. In this section, the acid–base balance is discussed in terms of respiratory and metabolic abnormalities.

pH

Blood is either alkaline or acid as a result of a decrease or increase in free hydrogen ions (H^+). pH, the expression of the acid–base balance, is defined as the reciprocal logarithm of the hydrogen ion concentration expressed as the power of 10. In the following paragraphs, several principles are presented to help the learner understand acid–base balance.

Principles: H^+ can be thought of as an acid.

1. As the H^+ concentration increases, the blood becomes more acidic.
2. As the H^+ concentration decreases, the blood becomes more alkaline.

The normal serum pH is 7.4 (± 0.04) (the range is 7.36 to 7.44).

1. A pH below 7.36 is acidic (H^+ increase).
2. A pH above 7.44 is alkaline (H^+ decrease).

The acid–base balance is maintained by the special buffer systems found in the blood, lungs, and kidneys. An important blood buffer system is the bicarbonate–carbonic acid system, which prevents excessive changes in the hydrogen ion concentration. The system consists of 1 part carbonic acid (H_2CO_3) to 20 parts bicarbonate (HCO_3^-) in the extracellular fluid, and it may be expressed in a modified Henderson-Hasselbalch equation:

$$pH \propto \frac{base}{acid} = \frac{HCO_3^-}{H_2CO_3} = \frac{20}{1}$$

$$\uparrow \quad \downarrow$$
$$PaCO_2 \times 0.03$$

Carbon Dioxide

When the ratio of HCO_3^- to H_2CO_3 is altered, the acid–base balance (pH) will change. H_2CO_3 is formed at the cellular level by the production of carbon dioxide (CO_2) after the uptake of oxygen by the cell. H_2CO_3 then dissociates in the blood to form $CO_2 + H_2O$ ($H_2CO_3 \rightarrow CO_2 + H_2O$). Carbon dioxide is understood conceptually as the acid in the denominator of the Henderson-Hasselbalch equation. As carbon dioxide builds up, the blood becomes more acidic. The concentration of carbon dioxide is regulated primarily by the lungs.

Principles: CO_2 can be thought of as an acid.

1. As the carbon dioxide increases, the blood becomes more acidic and the pH decreases.
2. As the carbon dioxide decreases, the blood becomes more alkaline and the pH increases.

PaCO₂. The $PaCO_2$ is defined as the partial pressure exerted by the amount of carbon dioxide dissolved in the arterial blood. The tension that is produced by carbon dioxide is measured in torr units (1 torr = 1 mm Hg). The $PaCO_2$ is related directly to the rate and depth of respiration. It is a direct index of the effectiveness of ventilation. The normal value of the $PaCO_2$ is 40 (±4) torr (the range is 36 to 44 torr).

Principle: When the primary disturbance affects alterations in the $PaCO_2$, a *repiratory* derangement is present.

HCO₃⁻

Changes in the level of HCO_3^-, the numerator of the equation, also affect the acid–base balance. HCO_3^- is used to protect the blood against changes in pH because of its ability to take up and release H^+. The concentration of HCO_3^- is regulated mainly by the kidneys. The normal concentration of HCO_3^- in the blood is 22 to 28 mg.

Principles: HCO_3^- can be thought of as a base (alkaline).

1. As the HCO_3^- increases, the blood becomes more alkaline and the pH increases.
2. As the HCO_3^- decreases, the blood becomes more acidic and the pH decreases.

Principle: When the primary disturbance affects alterations in HCO_3^-, a *metabolic* derangement is present.

Acid–Base Abnormalities

The normal laboratory values for arterial blood gases are outlined in Table 19-2. Acid–base abnormalities may be produced by a respiratory derangement (expressed by a low or a high $PaCO_2$) or by a metabolic derangement (expressed by a low or a high HCO_3^-). Depending on the specific problem, the patient has acidosis (expressed by a low pH) or alkalosis (ex-

Table 19–2
Normal Laboratory Ranges for Arterial Blood Gases

TEST	READING
pH	7.36 to 7.44
$PaCO_2$	36 to 44 mm Hg
PaO_2	80 to 100 mm Hg
HCO_3^-	24 to 30 mEq/L
Base excess	+2 to −2 mEq/L
O_2 Saturation	Greater than 95%

pressed by a high pH). These abnormalities are discussed individually in the following paragraphs.

Respiratory Acidosis

Respiratory acidosis is defined as an abnormal physiologic process in which there is a primary reduction in the rate of alveolar ventilation relative to the rate of CO_2 production. Respiratory acidosis is caused by factors that produce hypoventilation. A pure respiratory acidosis is identified from arterial blood gas analyses in which the pH is shown to be low (acidosis) and the $PaCO_2$ (respiratory) is shown to be high (Table 19-3).

Respiratory Alkalosis

Respiratory alkalosis is an abnormal physiologic process in which there is a primary increase in the rate of alveolar ventilation relative to the rate of carbon dioxide production. It is caused by factors that produce hyperventilation. A pure respiratory alkalosis is identified when the pH is shown to be high (alkalosis) and the $PaCO_2$ (respiratory) to be low (Table 19-3).

Metabolic Acidosis

Metabolic acidosis is an abnormal physiologic process characterized by the primary loss of HCO_3^- from the extracellular fluid. It is identified from blood gas analyses when the pH is shown to be low (acidosis) and the HCO_3^- level (metabolic) to be reduced (Table 19-4).

Metabolic Alkalosis

Pure *metabolic alkalosis* is an abnormal physiologic process characterized by a primary gain in HCO_3^- in the extracellular fluid. Blood gas analyses reveal an elevated pH (alkalosis) and an increased HCO_3^- level (metabolic) (Table 19-4).

Compensation Versus Correction of Acid–Base Abnormalities

When acid–base abnormalities occur, one of two basic mechanisms may be used to return the pH to normal: compensation or correction.

In compensation, the pH is returned to normal by altering the system not primarily affected by the disturbance. If a primary respiratory disturbance is present, there is a change only in the $PaCO_2$. There is no immediate change in the overall base or bicarbonate system (the secondary system). Changes in $PaCO_2$ occur quite rapidly, because changes in respiration

Table 19-3

Respiratory Acidosis and Alkalosis

RESPIRATORY ACIDOSIS	RESPIRATORY ALKALOSIS
Causes	Causes
Hypoventilation	Hyperventilation
COPD	Pulmonary embolism
Sedation	Severe pain
Clinical manifestations	Anxiety
Dyspnea	Brain-stem disease
Headache	Chronic overventilation on
Mental confusion	controlled ventilator
Pallor	Clinical manifestations
Sweating	Dizziness
Apprehension, restlessness	Tingling, numbness
ABG measurements (example)	Restlessness, agitation
pH 7.24	Tetany
$PaCO_2$ 60	ABG measurements (example)
HCO_3^- 24	pH 7.48
Treatment	$PaCO_2$ 30
Determine and treat cause	HCO_3^- 22
Maintain adequate respiratory minute volume	Treatment
Increase tidal volume or increase respiratory rate	Identify and treat cause
Suctioning	Sedate patient
	Reduce respiratory minute volume
	Decrease tidal volume or decrease
	respiratory rate
	Reassure and support patient

ABG: arterial blood gas; COPD: chronic obstructive pulmonary disease.

cause carbon dioxide to be excreted or retained. In time, however, the kidneys attempt to compensate for the primary respiratory disturbance. In respiratory acidosis, for example, the kidneys help to compensate for the abnormally low pH by retaining HCO_3^- to return the base–acid ratio to 20:1. It should be noted that when the primary disturbance is respiratory, the secondary (compensatory) changes in the kidneys take

place only gradually to help return the pH to normal. Changes in HCO_3^- are primarily the result of the renal excretion of H^+ and retention of HCO_3^-. In contrast, if the primary disturbance is metabolic (as, for example, in metabolic acidosis), the lungs (the secondary system) immediately attempt to blow off excess acid as a compensatory mechanism to return the pH to physiologic neutrality.

The second mechanism to return the pH to normal is correction, in which the system primarily affected by the disturbance is treated. In the setting of respiratory acidosis, effective ventilation and suctioning may improve the $PaCO_2$ and return the pH to normal. In metabolic acidosis, a bolus of sodium bicarbonate is generally effective in combating the acidosis and correcting the abnormal pH. The general clinical approach used to deal with acid–base abnormalities usually is aimed at correcting the abnormality as quickly as possible rather than at helping the body to compensate (which may take a long and unpredictable period of time).

The critical care nurse has probably observed that acid–base abnormalities frequently are complicated. Assessing a pure respiratory or a pure metabolic disturbance is generally a simple procedure. More commonly, however, nurses observe both a primary metabolic and a primary respiratory disturbance (as, for example, in cardiac arrest), or they may observe acid–base abnormalities that are affected by the primary disturbance with compensated or uncompensated changes in the secondary system.

In evaluating complicated arterial blood gas measurements, the nurse must use a systematic approach. Blood gas analysis, like the physical examination and the analysis of a cardiac rhythm strip, demands patience and organization. One must first evaluate the patient's total clinical picture, the clinical signs and symptoms, the findings from the physical examination, and the presumptive diagnosis.

Table 19-4

Metabolic Acidosis and Alkalosis

METABOLIC ACIDOSIS	METABOLIC ALKALOSIS
Causes	Causes
Cardiac arrest	Vomiting
Diabetic ketoacidosis	Gastric suctioning
Poisoning (acetylsalicylic	Sodium bicarbonate overload
acid, methyl alcohol,	Diuretics
ethylene glycol,	Adrenal disease
paraldehyde)	Corticosteroids
Renal failure	Clinical manifestations
Diarrhea (loss of HCO_3^-)	Dullness
Clinical manifestations	Weakness
Lethargy	Dysrhythmias
Nausea, vomiting	Tetany
Dysrhythmias	Hypokalemia
Coma	ABG measurements (example)
ABG measurements (example)	pH 7.50
pH 7.30	$PaCO_2$ 40
$PaCO_2$ 40	HCO_3^- 40
HCO_3^- 15	Treatment
Treatment	Identify and treat cause
Identify and treat cause	Correct dehydration
Give sodium bicarbonate	Correct hypokalemia
	Acetazolamide (Diamox)
	Ammonium chloride
	Arginine monohydrochloride

ABG: arterial blood gas.

Systematic Approach to Arterial Blood Gas Analysis

The words "ABG interpretation" may cause panic and confusion. But once one develops a systematic approach, interpretation of arterial blood gases can become challenging and maybe even fun! Primary life-threatening physiologic abnormalities can be identified by using a systematic method of interpretation.

There are three basic steps as outlined by Sharpio[14]:

Step 1: Assessment of the ventilatory status
Step 2: Assessment of the hypoxemic state
Step 3: Assessment of the tissue oxygenation state

Step 1: Evaluation of the Ventilatory Status.   The first step is to evaluate the $PaCO_2$. The carbon dioxide tension is a direct reflection of the adequacy of alveolar ventilation. The $PaCO_2$ will fall into one of three categories: less than 30 mm Hg, alveolar hyperventilation (respiratory alkalosis); between 30 and 50 mm Hg, acceptable alveolar ventilation; or greater than 50 mm Hg, ventilatory failure or hypoventilation (respiratory acidosis).

Changes in the arterial pH in relation to the $PaCO_2$ indicate whether the problem is primarily ventilatory (respiratory acid–base) or primarily metabolic.

Step 2: Assessment of the Hypoxemic State.   Once the patient's ventilatory and acid–base status are known, the arterial oxygen tension can be evaluated. The arterial oxygen tension measurements—PaO_2 and oxygen saturation—indicate the existence or absence of arterial hypoxemia. Mild hypoxemia in a patient under 60 on room air is a PaO_2 less than 80 mm Hg; moderate hypoxemia is a PaO_2 less than 60 mm Hg; severe hypoxemia is a PaO_2 less than 40 mm Hg. It is important to remember that arterial hypoxemia may lead to ventilatory and acid–base disturbances.

Step 3: Assessment of the Tissue Oxygenation State.   Assessment of the tissue oxygenation state cannot be separated from the hypoxemic evaluation. During this step, cardiac status, peripheral perfusion status, and the blood oxygen transport mechanism are evaluated. Blood pressure, cardiac output, heart rate, skin color, capillary refill, mental status, electrolyte balance, and urine output are key factors in evaluating the cardiac and peripheral perfusion states. The arterial oxygen tension, blood oxygen content, and hemoglobin-oxygen affinity compose the blood oxygen transport mechanism. Proper interpretation of blood gases significantly enhances the clinical evaluation of the tissue oxygenation state.[14]

Arterial Blood Gas Problems

Using the information presented in this section, interpret the following blood gases:

	1	2	3	4
pH	7.2	7.2	7.4	7.6
$PaCO_2$ mm Hg	40	60	60	30
PaO_2 mm Hg	96	45	65	40
HCO_3^- mEq/L	15	25	40	25
Base excess mEq/L	−13	−4	+4	−2
O_2 Saturation	100%	79%	93%	77%

Answers:

1. Uncompensated metabolic acidosis
2. Acute respiratory acidosis with hypoxemia
3. Compensated metabolic alkalosis with hypoxemia
4. Acute respiratory alkalosis with hypoxemia

Pulmonary Function Tests

Pulmonary function tests frequently are used for clinical evaluation and research. In most respiratory care units, spirometric measurements are the nurse's responsibility. The cooperation of the patient is essential for an accurate spirogram.

Lung capacities are composed of two or more lung volumes and are useful measurements in the clinical situation. *Total lung capacity* (TLC), the maximum lung volume after full inspiration, is composed of four volumes (Fig. 19-4). At TLC, the force generated by a maximum contraction of the inspiratory muscles equals the recoil of the lung. Normal variations occur, depending on the person's age, sex, and height.[10] Because TLC is dependent on the strength of the respiratory muscles and the elastic resistance of the lung and the chest wall, abnormalities in these limit the volume obtained. For example, a person with a restrictive disease (*e.g.,* sarcoidosis) would have a decreased TLC.

The lung volumes that make up TLC are residual volume, tidal volume, expiratory reserve volume, and inspiratory reserve volume. *Residual volume* (RV) is the amount of air remaining in the lungs after a maximal voluntary expiration. Residual volume is approximately 20% of total lung capacity in younger adults, and it increases with age or any abnormal condition that involves high airway resistance. *Tidal volume* (TV) is the amount of gas expired during normal ventilation. The *expiratory reserve volume* (ERV) is the volume of gas between the residual volume and the tidal volume. The *inspiratory reserve volume* (IRV) is the volume of gas between the tidal volume and the upper limits of total lung capacity. The expiratory reserve volume and the inspiratory reserve volume are available to increase the tidal volume, but they are not used under conditions of normal resting ventilation.

Functional residual capacity (FRC) is the volume of gas remaining in the lungs at the end of a normal expiration. It

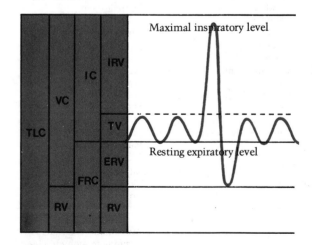

Figure 19–4

Lung volumes.

comprises the expiratory reserve volume and the residual volume. FRC is the volume at which the inward recoil of the lung is balanced by the outward recoil of the chest wall. Thus it is termed the *resting level* or the *midposition*. In addition to any existing pathophysiology, FRC is reduced in the supine patient, because the weight of the abdominal contents forces the diaphragm upward. FRC is also reduced by ascites or increased lung recoil, as in the patient with sarcoidosis.

Spirogram

Spirometry is the determination of lung volume that involves the forceful exhalation of air by the person being tested. The time volume indices used most frequently are the *forced vital capacity* (FVC), the *forced expiratory volume* (FEV_1), and the mean forced expiratory flow (forced midexpiratory flow, FEF25–75). Results on any of those tests may be reduced because of poor cooperation, poor muscular effort, fatigue, or airway obstruction.

The FVC is the total volume that can be expired after a maximal inspiration, and is the sum of the tidal volume plus the inspiratory-expiratory reserve volumes. The FVC is the maximum ventilatory volume or the maximum breathing ability of the patient. The patient makes the deepest possible inspiration and then expires as completely as possible. The exhalation is measured as the FVC. If the patient's FVC is less than 75% of the predicted normal vital capacity, the patient is said to have restrictive disease. In true restrictive disease, the FVC is small and the residual lung volume is unchanged, resulting in a decreased total lung capacity. The volume of gas in the lungs is also found to be small on posteroanterior and lateral chest films.

Example
Patient With Restrictive Disease From Pulmonary Fibrosis

FVC = 1.65 L
Estimated normal = 3.02 L
Percentage of normal = 55%

The FEV is the amount of gas exhaled over a given period (usually 1 second) during the performance of an FVC test. The volume is also expressed as a percentage of the FVC. The measurement is particularly indicative of obstruction of the larger airways and is one measurement that responds to bronchodilator therapy.

The FEF is the average rate of flow for a specified volume segment of the FVC. Usually a notation is made after the abbreviation to denote the volume segment in cubic centimeters or as a percentage. The middle segment of an FVC maneuver often is used as an index of disease of the small airways and as a means of evaluating the patient's response to bronchodilator therapy.[13] It is the FEF between 25% and 75% of the FVC (FEF25–75).

In obstructive disease, the results of pulmonary function tests show the following: The RV is increased, and the TLC is normal to increased. Chest film shows the volume of gas in the lungs to be increased.[10] The patient's FEV_1 is reduced because of the obstruction. If a person's FEV_1 is not 75% of the predicted normal value, the person is said to have obstructive lung disease. An FEV_1/FVC ratio of less than 75% also documents airway obstruction. An even more sensitive indicator is the FEF25–75 test. That test (flow rate) is so sensitive that in the presence of early airway obstruction, the FEF25–75 may be reduced even though other measurements are normal. After bronchodilator therapy, the two tests usually are repeated to assess the reversibility of the obstruction.

Example
Patient With Obstructive Disease From Asthma

	PREDICTED	OBSERVED	
	Normal	Before bronchodilator therapy	After bronchodilator therapy
FVC	4.66 L	4.16 L (89%)	4.54 L (97%)
FEV_1	3.92 L	1.42 L (36%)	2.32 L (59%)
FEF25-75	4.33 L/sec	0.81 L/sec (19%)	1.01 L/sec (23%)

In some patients, expiratory airway obstruction becomes so severe that they also develop what appears to be a restrictive ventilatory defect. The residual volume in their lungs is so large that their FVC is decreased even though their TLC is normal to increased. On chest film, a large volume of gas is seen in their lungs and their FEV is more severely impaired than is their FVC.

Example
Patient With Apparent Restrictive Lung Disease From Airway Obstruction

	PREDICTED	MEASURED	PERCENT
FVC	3.88 L	2.18 L	56
FEV_1	3.26 L	0.69 L	21
FEF25-75	3.57 L/sec	0.25 L/sec	7

The pulmonary function test changes associated with obstructive and restrictive diseases are outlined in Table 19-5.

Work of Breathing

Breathing is usually not associated with work in the same sense as the work of an Olympic swimmer because, for most people, breathing is effortless. But work must be thought of as anything that requires energy. The respiratory muscles—diaphragm, intercostal and abdominal muscles—contract, or work, to cause inspiration. This work of breathing is measured as pressure × volume.[16] The respiratory muscles work to overcome airway resistance and elastic forces (pressure) to create a flow rate and a tidal volume (volume). Pressure will change as airway resistance and elastic forces increase or decrease, resulting in changes in tidal volume and flow rates. Examples

Table 19-5
Pulmonary Function Test Changes With Disease

	OBSTRUCTIVE	RESTRICTIVE
FEV_1	Decreased	Decreased but not as much as with obstructive disease
FVC	Decreased	Decreased
FRC	Increased	Decreased
RV	Increased	Decreased
TLC	Increased	Decreased

of these changes in the work of breathing occur in patients with obstructive or restrictive lung disease. Obstructive disease increases airway resistance, so patients take slow, deep breaths in order to reduce work of the lung. Shallow, rapid breathing is present in patients with restrictive disease, because this helps to reduce the elastic work of the lung.

Compliance

Ventilation is determined ultimately by the interaction of volume, pressure, and resistance. Changes in airway resistance require that different pressures be exerted to maintain lung volumes and air flow.

What pressures must be exerted by the respiratory muscles is dependent on two factors: the resistance to the movement of gas through the airways, and the elasticity or stiffness of the lungs. Thus, while caring for critically ill patients, the nurse must remember that ventilation may be affected by changes in airway resistance or in the elasticity of the lungs.[16]

Compliance is the change in volume divided by the change in pressure necessary to produce that volume change. It is a gross reflection of the forces required to cause air to move into the lungs. A lung with low compliance (an inelastic lung) is one that requires a high distending pressure and is difficult to inflate.

A parameter that is useful in following the clinical course of critically ill patients undergoing mechanical ventilator therapy is effective compliance (dynamic effective compliance). *Effective compliance* is the ratio of tidal volume to peak airway pressure. Unless high airway resistance is present, it may be used as an indicator of the total compliance of the chest wall and lungs. Effective compliance is obtained by dividing the tidal volume (TV) by the peak airway inspiratory pressure (PAIP):

$$\text{Effective compliance} = \frac{TV}{PAIP}$$

Normal is 35 to 55 ml/cm H_2O.

It must be stressed that effective compliance is a measurement of both lung inelasticity and airway resistance. Patients with any change in effective compliance will, in all probability, be evaluated by a physician who specializes in pulmonary disorders. The physician will assess the patient's status by attempting to separate the effects of lung inelasticity from the effects of airway resistance. Because inspiratory airway pressure evolves during an inflow of air with turbulence, a more sensitive measurement would be that of compliance calculated when no airflow is occurring.

Static compliance measures pertain only to the inelasticity of the lung, because the measurements are made at the end of inspiration, when there is no airflow and therefore no airway resistance. With a patient using a ventilator, the lung is inflated, and the volume exhaled is noted during several inspirations. On a subsequent inspiration, the exhalation tube is occluded. Initially, the peak pressure on the manometer of the ventilator is noted, and the pressure decrease is noted when airflow stops at the end of inspiration (*plateau inspiratory pressure*, PIP), which is the static pressure. The plateau pressure will always be somewhat lower than the PAIP. If the patient is on end-expiratory pressure, the denominator used is the dif-

ference between airway pressure at the end of end-inspiratory pause (inflation hold) and end-expiratory pressure. To obtain static compliance, the static pressure is then divided into the average volume exhaled:

$$\text{Static compliance} = \frac{TV}{PIP}$$

Normal is 65 to 75 ml/cm H_2O.

In normal people, the values for static compliance and dynamic compliance are approximately the same. However, in patients with airway obstruction, dynamic compliance decreases, and it may be less than static compliance.

For example,

$$\text{Tidal volume} = 1000 \text{ ml}$$

$$\text{Dynamic pressure} = 50 \text{ cm } H_2O$$

$$\text{Static pressure} = 20 \text{ cm } H_2O$$

$$\text{Dynamic compliance} = \frac{1000}{50} = 20$$

$$\text{Static compliance} = \frac{1000}{20} = 50$$

HYPOXEMIA

Arterial hypoxemia is a decrease in the total arterial oxygen content of the blood. A lowered arterial oxygen results in tissue hypoxia. Because all four mechanisms of hypoxemia (hypoventilation, diffusion defects, ventilation-perfusion imbalance, and left-to-right shunting) involve a ventilation-perfusion imbalance, a discussion of alveolar ventilation and oxygenation must precede the discussion of the mechanisms.

Ventilation

The amount of inspired air that reaches perfused alveoli is referred to as the alveolar ventilation. The inspired volume that does not go to perfused alveoli is referred to as the dead space ventilation. In regard to only a single breath, the dead space volume (VD) is subtracted from the tidal volume to give the alveolar ventilation (VA).

$$V_A = TV - V_D$$

The minute ventilation is the total amount of gas exhaled by the patient per minute and is the sum of the dead space ventilation and the alveolar ventilation. Use of the minute volume and the alveolar ventilation is particularly helpful in determining the dead space ventilation for patients who are on ventilators. The following calculations are frequently done:

$$\text{Alveolar ventilation} = \left(\frac{\substack{\text{carbon dioxide tension} \\ \text{in venous blood to} \\ \text{determine carbon} \\ \text{dioxide production}}}{\substack{\text{carbon dioxide tension} \\ \text{in arterial blood}}} \right) 0.8$$

Dead space ventilation/min = minute ventilation

$$- \text{ alveolar ventilation/min}$$

$$\text{Dead space per breath} = \frac{\text{dead space ventilation}}{\text{respiratory rate}} \Big/ \min$$

When the air taken in during inspiration arrives in the alveoli, gas exchange takes place. Oxygen diffuses into the pulmonary capillary bed, and carbon dioxide diffuses into the alveolus. The exchange is effected by pressure differences. As carbon dioxide enters the alveolus, oxygen leaves the alveolus. Carbon dioxide is not present in the inspired air. Thus it does not exert any pressure and diffuses 20 times faster than oxygen. After gas exchange has taken place in the alveolus, the pressure of oxygen and of carbon dioxide is equal to the pressure that was exerted by the oxygen alone.

Alveolar oxygen pressure can be calculated by use of the alveolar air equation. Before considering the actual calculation, the components of the equation will be explained. The partial pressure of a gas is determined by multiplying the total pressure times the concentration of gas. For example, at sea level the barometric pressure is 760 mm Hg, and the concentration of oxygen in the air is 0.21. Thus the pressure of oxygen in the air is 160 mm Hg. Two important phenomena must be mentioned. First, air contains water vapor. The pressure exerted by water vapor is used as the standard measurement, 47 mm Hg. Second, because barometric pressure is different in different parts of the United States, the local standard pressure must be used. For example, if the barometric pressure is 747 mm Hg, then the pressure of oxygen in the air is (747 − 47) (0.21), or 147 mm Hg.

The respiratory quotient must also be understood. Because there is essentially no carbon dioxide in the inspired air, the amount of carbon dioxide leaving the body is usually less than the amount of oxygen consumed. The relationship of oxygen consumption divided by carbon dioxide production is commonly expressed as a decimal. The value varies: 0.8 is the average value. The alveolar air equation is as follows:

$$\text{Alveolar oxygen pressure} = \left(\begin{array}{c} \text{barometric} \\ \text{pressure} \\ - \text{ water vapor} \\ \text{pressure} \end{array} \right) \left(\begin{array}{c} \text{inspired} \\ \text{oxygen} \\ \text{concen-} \\ \text{tration} \end{array} \right) - \left(\begin{array}{c} \text{arterial plasma} \\ \text{pressure of} \\ \text{carbon dioxide} \\ \hline \text{respiratory} \\ \text{quotient} \end{array} \right)$$

Under normal circumstances, the mean alveolar oxygen pressure (P_AO_2) is higher than the peripheral arterial oxygen pressure (PaO_2). The reasons are that fully oxygenated blood from well-ventilated alveoli mixes with less well-oxygenated blood from poorly ventilated alveoli, and that a small amount of venous blood mixes with arterial blood from direct communications between the pulmonary artery and pulmonary vein and from the thebesian veins draining into the left heart. The difference between the mean alveolar oxygen pressure and the arterial oxygen pressure is referred to as the alveolar-arterial oxygen gradient (the A-a gradient, or difference). Approximately 3% to 6% of the normal cardiac output may bypass ventilated lung. Normally, the A-a gradient is 15 mm Hg or less on room air and 50 mm Hg or less on air that has high percentages of oxygen. To calculate the A-a gradient, the alveolar oxygen pressure is determined (using the alveolar air equation) and the arterial oxygen pressure is subtracted from the alveolar oxygen pressure.

Example

The patient is in Dallas, Texas, breathing room air (0.21). His arterial oxygen partial pressure is 90 mm Hg and arterial carbon dioxide pressure is 40 mm Hg.

$$\text{Alveolar oxygen pressure} = (747 - 47)(0.21) - \frac{40}{0.8}$$

$$= 147 - 50$$

$$= 97 \text{ mm Hg}$$

$$\text{A-a gradient} = \left(\begin{array}{c} \text{alveolar} \\ \text{oxygen} \\ \text{pressure} \end{array} \right) - \left(\begin{array}{c} \text{arterial} \\ \text{oxygen} \\ \text{pressure} \end{array} \right)$$

$$= 97 - 90$$

$$= 7 \text{ mm Hg}$$

Oxygenation

Determining the adequacy of tissue oxygenation is an important part of assessment. An intact circulatory system (Fig. 19-5) is fundamental for adequate oxygenation. The normal oxygen uptake and the normal carbon dioxide elimination are maintained by the ventilation-perfusion balance. The transportation of oxygen from the alveolus to the peripheral tissues depends on many factors: the oxygen concentration, the partial pressure of oxygen in the inspired air, the alveolar ventilation, the ventilation-perfusion relationship, the blood volume, the cardiac output, and the hemoglobin saturation.

Blood carries oxygen in two states: physically dissolved in plasma, and chemically combined with hemoglobin. The number of milliliters of oxygen/100 ml of blood can be calculated if the PaO_2, percent of saturation, and hemoglobin are known. Knowing the number of milliliters of oxygen/100 ml of blood allows a more accurate determination to be made of the adequacy of oxygenation than is afforded by the PaO_2 and percent of saturation alone. The number of milliliters of oxygen contributed by oxygen that is physically dissolved in the blood is a small portion of the total. The major part of the total oxygen content is combined with hemoglobin. The number of milliliters contributed by dissolved oxygen is calculated by multiplying the PaO_2 by 0.0031 ml/mm Hg. The number of milliliters contributed by oxygen that is combined with hemoglobin is calculated by multiplying the hemoglobin concentration by the percent of saturation by 1.39 ml/% saturation. The sum of the two is oxygen content. For example, assume that a patient has the following values: hemoglobin 15, PaO_2 90, percent saturation 96. The total content would be 20.30 ml/100 ml blood, with 0.28 ml/100 ml contributed by dissolved oxygen and 20.02 ml/100 ml blood contributed by oxygen that is bound to hemoglobin.

When the data are plotted on a graph, the relationship between the amount of oxygen combined with hemoglobin and the amount of oxygen dissolved in the arterial system is not shown to be a linear (or a straight-line) relationship. Rather, the relationship between arterial oxygen and percent saturation is depicted by an S-curve. (This curve, which is called the *oxyhemoglobin dissociation curve*, is shown in Fig. 19-6.) A change in the position of the curve to the right or left reflects

Pulmonary capillary bed

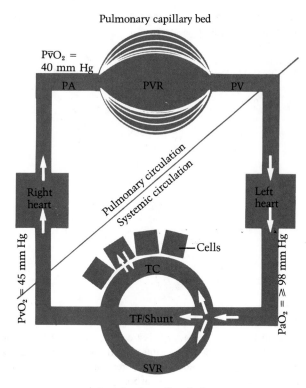

Peripheral capillary bed

Figure 19-5

The circulatory system. PA: pulmonary artery; PV: pulmonary veins; PVR: pulmonary vascular resistance; SVR: systemic vascular resistance; TF: thoroughfare channel, site of extrapulmonary arteriovenous shunting; TC: true capillary; $P\overline{v}O_2$: mixed venous oxygen tension; PvO_2: venous blood oxygen tension; PaO_2: arterial blood oxygen tension. The *single arrows* show the direction of blood flow. The *double arrow* indicates the nutrient and waste exchange between cells and blood perfusing the true capillaries.

the affinity of hemoglobin for oxygen and the transfer of oxygen from the hemoglobin to tissue cells.[16]

Study of the graph verifies several important points. It should be noted first that at an oxygenation of 100 mm Hg, hemoglobin is 97.5% saturated. Because the hemoglobin is almost saturated, it can accept little more oxygen. Even if the arterial oxygen pressure is raised above 100 mm Hg, the total oxygen content increases only slightly because oxygen may only be added to the blood in the dissolved form. Because the oxygen-carrying capacity of the blood is virtually dependent on the amount of hemoglobin present and on the percent saturation, maintenance of the hemoglobin levels is essential for adequate oxygenation.

Second, it should be noted that the curve is relatively flat between a PaO_2 of 70 and 100 mm Hg. At 70 mm Hg, the hemoglobin is 93% saturated, which means that even a severe drop in arterial oxygen pressure (*e.g.*, to 70 mm Hg) produces only a minimal change in the oxygen content of the blood because the hemoglobin saturation, the major determinant of the oxygen content, changes by only a small amount. However, below 60 to 70 mm Hg, the downward slope of the S-shaped curve is encountered. In this part of the curve, small changes in dissolved oxygen produce large changes in the percent saturation and total content. The curve is particularly steep between 10 and 40 mm Hg. Because small changes in

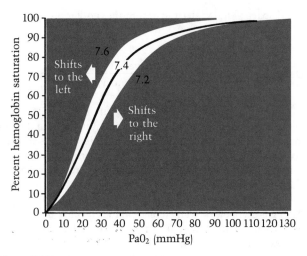

Figure 19-6

The oxyhemoglobin dissociation curve. The hemoglobin saturation is approximately 95% at a PaO_2 of 90 mm Hg. The slope of the curve is steep at a PaO_2 of less than 60 mm Hg. A shift of the curve to the right releases more oxygen at the peripheral tissue level. A shift to the left releases less oxygen.

arterial oxygen tension cause large changes in percent saturation in that part of the curve, one can produce large changes in total content simply by increasing the arterial oxygen level a small amount. In other words, because of the chemical characteristics of arterial oxygen and hemoglobin, values of arterial oxygen tension below 60 mm Hg produce a rapid decrease in the amount of hemoglobin saturated and the total oxygen content—and thus in the total tissue delivery.

The oxyhemoglobin dissociation curve is not a single curve but a series of curves. The shape of the curve changes with the hydrogen ion concentration, the partial pressure of arterial carbon dioxide, the temperature, 2,3-diphosphoglycerate (2,3-DPG), and electrolyte levels (Table 19-6). The effect the carbon dioxide tension and the hydrogen ion concentration have on the affinity of oxygen for hemoglobin is called the *Bohr effect.* An increase in any of the parameters just mentioned produces the release of oxygen by hemoglobin at a lower PaO_2. In other words, acidosis or an increased level of 2,3-DPG causes the dissociation curve to *shift to the right.* With a shift to the right, the hemoglobin binds oxygen less avidly, and the amount of oxygen given up to the tissues is increased.

The opposite is true for decreases in the hydrogen ion concentration, the arterial carbon dioxide tension, the 2,3-DPG level, the temperature, and the electrolyte levels. With decreases, the curve is *shifted to the left.* At a given level of arterial

Table 19-6

Factors That Increase Oxygen Release at the Systemic Cellular Level

Physical factors
    Large capillary-to-cell oxygen diffusion gradient
    Increase in body temperature
    Increase in $PaCO_2$
Chemical factors
    Increase in hydrogen ion (increase in acidity or decrease in pH)
    Increase in 2,3-diphosphoglycerate in red blood cells
    Increase in adenosine triphosphate

oxygen tension, the percentage of oxyhemoglobin is greater and less oxygen is given up to the tissues. Clinically, the patient's tissues may be oxygen deprived because the affinity of oxygen for hemoglobin is greater, and the amount of oxygen released is reduced.

As Figure 19-7 shows, the pressure of oxygen in the arteriolar sections of the capillary and the pressure of oxygen in the venular section of the capillary are greater than the oxygen tension in the interstitial fluid and the intracellular water. Because gases diffuse down a pressure gradient, oxygen diffuses toward the cell. Any increase in temperature or acidity gives more kinetic energy to a molecule. An elevation of body temperature or a decrease in pH consequently enhances the rates of oxyhemoglobin dissociation and of oxygen diffusion.

P_{50}

The P_{50} is the PaO_2 at which 50% of the available hemoglobin is saturated under the following standard laboratory conditions: T = 37°C, $PaCO_2$ = 40 mm Hg, and pH = 7.40. The

normal adult P_{50} is approximately 27 mm Hg. Under standard conditions, the P_{50} is a useful index of the position of the oxyhemoglobin curve.[5]

Oxygen Delivery

The amount of oxygen being delivered to the tissues is the important factor. It is up to the oxygen delivery system to make sure that the oxygen available equals the oxygen demand. If there is no equality, the body attempts to compensate by increasing cardiac output or by extracting more oxygen from the blood. Oxygen delivery is equal to the cardiac output multiplied by the oxygen content expressed in volumes per 100 ml. The A-V oxygen difference (the $C[a-v]O_2$) is the arterial oxygen content minus the venous oxygen content. Because the arteriovenous oxygen content difference increases in low cardiac output states, it can be used to assess changes in cardiac output at times when therapy is being titrated (*e.g.*, initiation or increase of respiratory support). A problem in oxygen delivery (or cardiac output) is determined by an increasing or widening difference. The actual oxygen extraction may be determined by multiplying the A-V oxygen difference by the cardiac output. Since the advent of the pulmonary artery catheter and the availability of mixed venous blood samples, this measurement can be determined accurately.

The oxygen extraction ratio or the utilization coefficient ($CaO_2 - C\bar{v}O_2/CaO_2$) defines the amount of delivered oxygen that is used (normal value approximates 0.25). If the ratio is high, the need for oxygen is greater than that available; thus the oxygen delivery is inadequate. If the ratio is low, the delivery is maldistributed (*e.g.*, suprahigh cardiac output or shunting).

Continuous monitoring of oxygen saturation in mixed venous blood is available in most critical care units. Because pulmonary and cardiac function are interrelated, a decrease in mixed venous oxygen saturation indicates an increase in peripheral oxygen consumption or a decrease in cardiopulmonary function (the principal exception is sepsis). The actual problem cannot be assessed, but the general trend in the overall clinical situation can be assessed. An improvement in cardiopulmonary function is indicated by a return toward normal values, indicating that the therapy is having a positive impact.

Mechanisms of Hypoxemia

The severity of hypoxemia is classically described in terms of arterial desaturation when the patient is breathing room air (0.21). In mild hypoxemia, the arterial oxygen is less than 75 mm Hg and more than 60 mm Hg. In moderate hypoxemia, the arterial oxygen is less than 60 mm Hg and more than 40 mm Hg. In severe hypoxemia, arterial oxygen is less than 40 mm Hg.

Four mechanisms of hypoxemia will be discussed in the following sections: hypoventilation, diffusion (or gas transfer) defects, ventilation-perfusion ($\dot{V}A/\dot{Q}$) inequality, and right-to-left shunt. All four involve a ventilation-perfusion inequality. The two mechanisms that produce hypercarbia are hypoventilation and $\dot{V}A/\dot{Q}$ inequality. In clinical practice, hypoventilation is the major cause of hypercarbia; however, $\dot{V}A/\dot{Q}$ inequality does add to the carbon dioxide retention seen in the later stages of diseases associated with low $\dot{V}A/\dot{Q}$ ratios. In addition to the four primary causes of a low PaO_2, a fifth

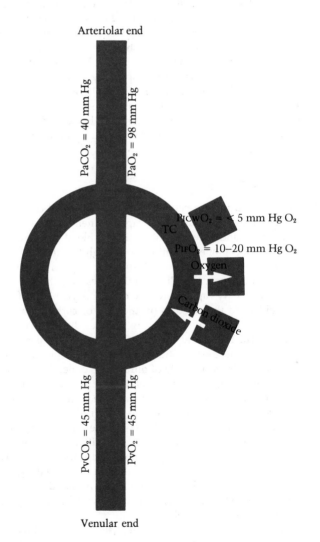

Arteriolar end

$PaCO_2$ = 40 mm Hg

PaO_2 = 98 mm Hg

$PICWO_2$ = < 5 mm Hg O_2

TC

$PIFO_2$ = 10–20 mm Hg O_2

Oxygen

Carbon dioxide

$PvCO_2$ = 45 mm Hg

PvO_2 = 45 mm Hg

Venular end

Figure 19–7

Gas diffusion gradients in the peripheral capillary bed. PaO_2: arterial oxygen tension; $PIFO_2$: interstitial fluid oxygen tension; $PICWO_2$: intracellular water oxygen tension; TC: true capillary. The *arrows* indicate the direction of passive gas diffusion down pressure gradients.

cause of hypoxemia is possible. At high altitudes, the inspired oxygen tension is reduced owing to the lower barometric pressure. The reduction results in a low alveolar oxygen tension which in turn lowers the PaO_2 and can ultimately result in hypoxemia. Inspired oxygen tension is also reduced when the person breathes mixtures with a low oxygen concentration. This circumstance occurs infrequently and is usually the result of an error in valving systems during the administration of anesthetic gases.

Hypoventilation

Impaired gas exchange related to hypoventilation means that the amount of new or fresh gas reaching the alveoli is reduced. The reduction causes both hypoxemia and hypercarbia. The degree of hypercarbia is an index of the degree of hypoventilation and is readily assessed by arterial blood gas analysis. The $PaCO_2$ reflects the balance between carbon dioxide production by the body cells and its elimination by the lung. Therefore, an increase in $PaCO_2$ (hypercarbia) indicates alveolar hypoventilation. Conversely, a decrease in $PaCO_2$ (hypocarbia) occurs during alveolar hyperventilation.

Examples of frequent causes of hypoventilation are brain and spinal cord injuries, respiratory center depression caused by narcotics, barbiturates, and tranquilizers; and neuromuscular disease such as Guillain-Barré syndrome, myasthenia gravis, or muscular dystrophy. In addition, some patients with increased work of breathing let their $PaCO_2$ drift up (hypoventilate) rather than do the work necessary to keep their $PaCO_2$ normal. Still other patients appear to have a primary lack of sensitivity to increased $PaCO_2$ or hypoxemia as stimuli to ventilation. Consequently, they fail to maintain normal arterial blood gas levels. Another less frequently recognized cause of hypoventilation is extreme obesity. The mechanisms of hypoventilation in the obese patient are not known for certain, but the increased work of breathing is probably contributory.

In hypoventilation, the arterial carbon dioxide levels are always elevated, because the lungs cannot maintain an alveolar ventilation that will eliminate the carbon dioxide produced by the body. The nitrogen equilibrium is not altered, and as the alveolar carbon dioxide level rises, the alveolar oxygen level falls.

Hypoxemia caused by hypoventilation alone is usually not severe. The reason for this is evident from the alveolar gas equation. The following example shows that when the $PaCO_2$ rises 20 mm Hg from a normal 40 mm Hg the PAO_2 falls to only 72 mm Hg:

$$PAO_2 = \text{Inspired oxygen tension} - \frac{PaCO_2}{RQ}$$

$$= 147 - \frac{60}{0.8}$$

$$= 147 - 75$$

$$= 72 \text{ mm Hg}$$

The PaO_2 is lower, of course, but it would not be severe unless, in addition to hypoventilation, one of the other causes of hypoxemia were present. Compared with the effect uncompensated respiratory acidosis ($PaCO_2$ of 60 mm Hg) will have on

the pH, it can be seen that the major concern in a patient with acute hypoventilation is likely to be a severe acid–base imbalance rather than severe hypoxemia.

If the patient does not have a respiratory disorder, the hypoventilation itself is corrected by breathing normal volumes of room air. For example, if the patient's tidal volume has decreased because of an overdose of analgesics, effective alveolar ventilation has decreased and produced the syndrome.

If the patient has a respiratory disorder and a defect in alveolar oxygenation from hypoventilation, a small increase in the oxygen concentration in the inspired gas will increase the oxygen pressure in the alveolus. If oxygen is administered through a nasal cannula at 3 L/minute, the oxygen is increased from about 21% (150 mm Hg) to 28% (200 mm Hg). Because of the corresponding increase, the alveolar oxygen tension increases by 50 mm Hg.

Patients with pure hypoventilation who require support with a mechanical ventilator can often be ventilated with room air. However, when hypoventilation is combined with another cause of hypoxemia, such as $\dot{V}A/\dot{Q}$ inequality or shunt, the hypoxemia will be much greater than would be anticipated with hypoventilation alone. In mixed causes of hypoxemia, the response to oxygen therapy depends primarily on whether the additional problem is one of shunt or $\dot{V}A/\dot{Q}$ inequality.

Frequently, the decision must be made about discontinuing oxygen when the patient has respiratory failure and when hypoventilation is the only mechanism of hypoxemia present. The anticipated alveolar oxygen pressure may be predicted by using the patient's values for arterial carbon dioxide tension and the concentration of oxygen for room air in the alveolar air equation.

Diffusion Defects

The overall diffusion capacity involves physical diffusion through the alveolar pulmonary capillary membrane and capillary plasma and diffusion within the red blood cell. The discussion here is limited to diffusion through the alveolar pulmonary capillary membrane. Diffusion is a passive process caused by the pressure gradient for the gases from the alveolus to the pulmonary capillary (in the case of oxygen) and from the capillary to the alveolus (in the case of carbon dioxide) (Fig. 19-8). The diffusion pathway includes the layer of pulmonary surfactant, the alveolar epithelium, the alveolar basement membrane, the interstitial fluid, and the pulmonary capillary endothelium. The rate of diffusion is dependent on the pressure gradient, the thickness of the membrane, the surface area available for diffusion, the membrane permeability characteristics, and the gas diffusion characteristics.

Loss of lung surface or thickening of the alveolar-capillary surface are the two processes associated with gas-transfer impairment. Diffusion is directly proportional to the surface area available and inversely proportional to the distance the gases have to travel. In addition, in the liquid phase, diffusion is proportional to the solubility of the gas divided by the square root of its molecular weight.

Impaired gas exchange related to diffusion impairment means that equilibration between the pulmonary capillary blood and the alveolar gas has not occurred. Under resting conditions, it takes only about one third (0.25 second) of the total time the blood is in the capillary (0.75 second) to equilibrate; therefore, there is time for equilibration in reserve. Even during

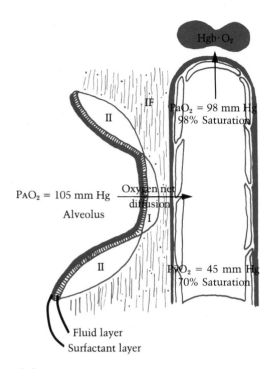

PAO$_2$ = 105 mm Hg

Oxygen net diffusion

Alveolus

PvO$_2$ = 45 mm Hg
70% Saturation

Hgb·O$_2$

PaO$_2$ = 98 mm Hg
98% Saturation

IF

II

I

II

Fluid layer
Surfactant layer

Figure 19–8

The alveolar capillary membrane (gas exchange unit). PAO$_2$: alveolar oxygen tension; PvO$_2$: mixed venous oxygen tension (dissolved oxygen); PaO$_2$: arterial oxygen tension (dissolved oxygen); Hgb·O$_2$: oxygen chemically combined with hemoglobin. The *arrows* indicate the direction of net diffusion of oxygen down the pressure gradient.

severe exercise, when contact time is reduced to about 0.33 second, gas equilibration is still assured. Thus diffusion abnormalities, although undoubtedly a factor in many diseases in which loss of surface area or thickening of the alveolar-capillary membrane is present, are almost never a physiologic cause of hypoxemia at rest.

People with such diseases as diffuse interstitial fibrosis, collagen diseases (such as scleroderma and lupus erythematosus), or severe emphysema (with loss of alveolar-capillary tissue) may have a decreased diffusion capacity during exercise. But these diseases are also associated with $\dot{V}A/\dot{Q}$ inequalities. Therefore, it is difficult to say how much hypoxemia should be attributed to $\dot{V}A/\dot{Q}$ inequality and how much to diffusion limitation.

The best measure of the diffusion process is the *diffusion capacity,* the total amount of gas transferred per minute across the alveolar membrane per millimeter difference in the pressure of the gas on the two sides of the membrane. In regard to the noncritically ill patient, a technician from the pulmonary function laboratory determines the diffusion capacity for carbon monoxide and, using that measurement, calculates the values for oxygen (normal is 20 to 30 ml carbon monoxide/minute/mm Hg). In the critically ill patient, determination would be made using the clinical and laboratory findings. Clinically, the patient has symptoms that are consistent with alveolar-capillary block. Other mechanisms of hypoxemia are usually also present. If only a diffusion defect is present, the arterial carbon dioxide levels would be below 40 mm Hg and the A-a oxygen gradient at rest 15 to 20 mm Hg. Any conditions that produce an increased cardiac output produce an increased A-a oxygen gradient. In the critical care situation,

diffusion defects have minimal clinical relevance, because they cannot be defined at the bedside and differentiated from ventilation-perfusion imbalances and shunts (unless the diffusion defect is enormous; that is, most of the lung is destroyed).

Ventilation-Perfusion Inequality

Impaired gas exchange related to an inequality or a mismatch in the ventilation-perfusion ratio is the most common mechanism of arterial hypoxemia. In the usual clinical situation, the extent of arterial desaturation due to hypoventilation and shunt is determined, and all otherwise unexplained hypoxemia is attributed to an uneven distribution of the lung functioning. Actually, all the mechanisms are alterations of the ventilation-perfusion ratio, but they are not so categorized.

Under normal circumstances, the pattern of air ventilation does not follow the pattern of blood perfusion in all regions of the lung. For example, the volume of air ventilating the lung apices is less than that ventilating the other lung regions. The amount of blood perfusing the apices is comparatively small. However, the amount of blood perfusing the apices is even less than the amount of air ventilating the apices. A different condition is found in the lung bases. There, proportionally more blood is perfused than air is ventilated.

Because of gravity, changes in position produce changes in ventilation and perfusion. For example, in dependent lung areas, blood flow per unit volume increases more rapidly than does ventilation. Because the changes are not uniform, a multitude of inequalities is produced.

Although there are many possible combinations of $\dot{V}A/\dot{Q}$ ratios, the ratio that usually produces hypoxemia occurs when ventilation is less than perfusion in many areas of the lung. In the opposite case, when perfusion is less than ventilation, much of the effort expended in the ventilatory portion of gas exchange is wasted. The ventilation is described as wasted or dead space. Unless very severe, an increased $\dot{V}A/\dot{Q}$ ratio does not cause hypoxemia or hypercarbia. It does, however, cause a significant increase in the amount of ventilation necessary to maintain the PaCO$_2$ within normal range.

There are four possible ventilation-perfusion combinations in scattered groups of alveoli: well-ventilated and well-perfused alveoli, poorly ventilated and well-perfused alveoli, well-ventilated and poorly perfused alveoli, and poorly ventilated and poorly perfused alveoli (Fig. 19-9). In the poorly ventilated, well-perfused alveolus, the alveolar hypoxia produces vasoconstriction. For example, in atelectasis, because the alveolar oxygen pressure is decreased in the unventilated portion, the blood flow (perfusion) is redistributed to the parts of the lung that are better ventilated. In the well-ventilated, poorly perfused alveolus, gas exchange is impaired, and the physiologic dead space is increased.

"Good" regions of the lung where ventilation and perfusion are evenly matched cannot compensate for "bad" regions, where ventilation is poor but blood flow continues (low $\dot{V}A/\dot{Q}$ units). This concept is easy to understand when we recall that oxygen is carried in the blood mainly in combination with hemoglobin. Blood from areas of perfect $\dot{V}A/\dot{Q}$ can never have an arterial oxygen saturation (SaO$_2$) of more than 100% and therefore cannot make up for blood coming from areas of low $\dot{V}A/\dot{Q}$, where little or no increase in PaO$_2$ (and therefore no increase in SaO$_2$) over the venous level takes place. For example, if blood that is only 75% saturated (that corresponds

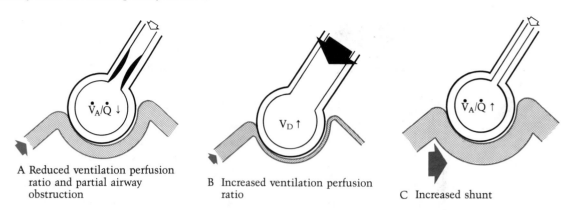

A Reduced ventilation perfusion ratio and partial airway obstruction

B Increased ventilation perfusion ratio

C Increased shunt

Figure 19–9

Nursing diagnoses: Impaired gas exchange related to possible ventilation-perfusion alterations. (*A*) Impaired gas exchange related to reduced ventilation-perfusion ratio and partial airway obstruction; the alveoli are more perfused than ventilated. This is the most common type of hypoxemia. Pulmonary toilet is usually indicated. Hypoxemia responds to an oxygen challenge and is corrected with supplemental oxygen. Antecedent conditions: airway spasm, retained secretions, bronchitis, chronic obstructive lung disease, asthma, congestion, and inspiratory obstruction. (*B*) Impaired gas exchange related to increased ventilation-perfusion ratio. The alveoli are ventilated but not well perfused and the alveolar dead space is increased. Oxygenation is satisfactory, and hypoxemia does not occur as long as ventilation continues to be increased. However, if ventilation is not increased to compensate for the increased dead space, the $PaCO_2$ rises. Antecedent conditions: hypovolemia, embolism, chronic obstructive lung disease, vasospasm, disseminated intravascular coagulation syndrome, and conditions causing increased intrathoracic pressure. (*C*) Impaired gas exchange related to right-to-left shunt. The alveoli are poorly ventilated and still perfused (although not well perfused). Hypoxemia does not respond to oxygen challenge alone, but it is improved by positive pressure with a sustained increase in airway pressure and alveolar reexpansion. Antecedent conditions: acute alveolar edema, aspiration, drowning, lung contusion, crush injury, adult respiratory distress syndrome, pneumonia, and obstructive atelectasis.

to a PaO_2 of 40 mm Hg—venous blood) mixes with the blood that is 100% saturated, the overall saturation for the blood returning to the left side of the heart has to be less than 100%. The actual saturation level depends on what portion of the total cardiac output was passing low $\dot{V}_A/\dot{Q}$ units. For example, in the situation just given, if 75% of the cardiac output goes to low $\dot{V}_A/\dot{Q}$ units and 25% to normal units, the result would be a saturation of approximately 80% (PaO_2 of 45 mm Hg).

The role of low $\dot{V}_A/\dot{Q}$ units in the production of hypoxemia is well recognized. It is less well known, however, that these same units cause hypercarbia. Because poorly ventilated units are unable to contribute to the elimination of carbon dioxide from blood passing these units, blood leaving these units still has near venous carbon dioxide levels. Why is it that at least in early stages of some diseases (*e.g.*, chronic obstructive pulmonary disease), hypoxemia is often seen without an elevation in the $PaCO_2$? It is because when carbon dioxide retention due to $\dot{V}_A/\dot{Q}$ inequality develops, there is an immediate response to the elevated $PaCO_2$, and alveolar ventilation promptly increases. The increase in alveolar ventilation results in a decrease of $PaCO_2$, usually to normal. The increase in ventilation also affects the PaO_2, which is raised slightly, but it cannot return to normal, since even overventilated lung units cannot raise the saturation of the blood above 100%.

Some patients with $\dot{V}_A/\dot{Q}$ abnormalities do not make the extra effort required to increase their ventilation when $\dot{V}_A/\dot{Q}$ inequality caused the $PaCO_2$ to increase. Or perhaps for a

time the patients do increase the ventilation, but later, with further increases in work or breathing, they abandon the effort, with the result that CO_2 retention develops. Why some patients let their $PaCO_2$ and hypoxemia increase rather than expend the energy required to increase their alveolar ventilation is not known. Central neurogenic and peripheral chemoreceptor respiratory drives are different from patient to patient. Patients are sometimes categorized as "pink puffers" or "blue bloaters." It is theorized that pink puffers have strong respiratory drives and consequently keep their PaO_2 and $PaCO_2$ at near normal levels despite large increases in the work of breathing and ventilation. Blue bloaters are thought to allow their $PaCO_2$ to rise and their PaO_2 to fall owing to a lower-than-normal respiratory drive (central hypoventilation). Blue bloaters become hypoxemic sooner and with equal or less derangement in pulmonary function because the blue bloaters are relatively insensitive to changes in blood gas levels.

The best measure of a ventilation-perfusion imbalance is a large or a widened A-a oxygen gradient on room air at rest that is almost completely corrected when high concentrations of oxygen are given. The hypoxemia is relieved by breathing oxygen. To determine the full effect of the therapy, one must allow time for the poorly ventilated areas of the lung to equilibrate to the new alveolar gas levels before the arterial blood gas levels are determined. This is the basis for the traditional 15- to 30-minute wait before drawing blood for arterial blood gas tests after the institution of or a change in oxygen therapy.

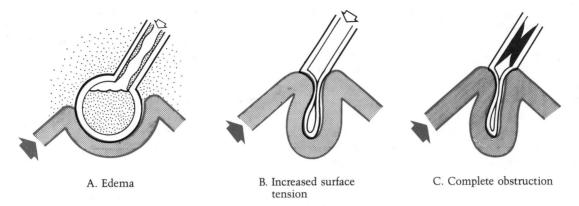

A. Edema
B. Increased surface tension
C. Complete obstruction

Figure 19–10

Right-to-left shunt. An unventilated or poorly ventilated region of the lung that still has a blood supply produces hypoxemia. Any one of three conditions can cause the shunt: (*A*) collapsed or fluid-filled alveoli, (*B*) increased surface tension, and (*C*) complete airway obstruction.

When the patient is given 100% oxygen, the widened alveolar-arterial gradient seen in $\dot{V}_A/\dot{Q}$ inequality is eliminated. Unless the lung disease is complicated by pneumonia or atelectasis, the hypoxemia is corrected by making small increases in inspired oxygen.

Shunt

Hypoxemia results when venous blood that has not come in contact with the ventilated lung mixes with arterial blood that has come in contact with the ventilated lung (Fig. 19-10). Blood reaches the arterial side of the heart without passing through ventilated regions of the lungs. It is shunted from the venous circulation to the arterial circulation. As previously discussed, a certain degree of mixing normally occurs—6 to 12% of the cardiac output. Abnormal mixing occurs with perfusion of nonventilated lung, an A-V fistula within the lung, a communication between the right and left sides of the myocardium, and an anastomosis between the systemic venous system and the pulmonary venous system. The most common cause of clinically important pulmonary shunting is an area (or areas) of the lung that is unventilated but continues to be perfused. Two clinical examples are areas of consolidated pneumonia or atelectasis.

The most common measure used to diagnose the presence of *impaired gas exchange related to a right-to-left shunt* is an increased A-a oxygen gradient, even with the administration of high concentrations of oxygen. The administration of 100% oxygen is the means to evaluate if a patient has a ventilation-perfusion imbalance or a right-to-left shunt. Any existing ventilation-perfusion imbalance is negated by the administration of 100% oxygen, because the partial pressure of oxygen is equalized in all ventilated alveoli. In shunting, the hypoxemia and A-a gradient remain, because the anatomical shunts remain. The arterial oxygen increases, but not to the levels to be expected from the elevated alveolar oxygen pressure. (The oxygen needed to saturate the hemoglobin is provided from the increased gas physically dissolved in the plasma.) Shunts can be thought of as the worst possible $\dot{V}_A/\dot{Q}$ inequality imaginable, but because the response of shunts to oxygen is so characteristic, it is useful to consider shunts separately from $\dot{V}_A/\dot{Q}$ inequality. A shunt is the only situation in which oxygen is ineffective in reducing the gradient. Even a lung with many

low $\dot{V}_A/\dot{Q}$ areas will eventually reach a normal alveolar-arterial oxygen gradient if enough time is given for oxygen to wash into the poorly ventilated areas of the lungs. However, when the blood passes totally unventilated portions of the lung, there is no way oxygen can reach the red blood cell.

Shunt Determination. At present, tests performed to measure the amount of pulmonary shunting do not separate out the normal anatomic pulmonary shunt from pathophysiologic pulmonary shunts. Any shunt greater than 25% that occurs despite respiratory therapy has a dire prognosis for the patient.

Several techniques to measure shunting have been used. One method for determining the degree of disturbance of ventilation-perfusion ratios is based on the infusion of a mixture of inert gases into the venous circulation with subsequent analysis of gas concentrations in the air exhaled and in the arterial blood. In the ^{133}Xe method, the xenon gas is injected intravenously and then arterial samples are drawn and assayed for xenon content. Xenon should be almost totally cleared from the blood by the first transit of blood through the lung. Any appearance of xenon in the arterial blood indicates that as perfusion occurred, some blood was passed through nonventilated alveoli and xenon was not removed by means of gas exchange in the lung. The higher the arterial blood content of ^{133}Xe, the greater the degree of shunt. However, the technique does not have widespread use for three reasons: an error of 2% to 3% remains, because all the ^{133}Xe is not removed in one passage of the lung; relatively elaborate measuring equipment is needed; and under some circumstances, ^{133}Xe and oxygen measure different shunt fractions due to solubility differences.

The oxygen challenge test for measuring pulmonary shunt flow is based on the fact that all causes of arterial hypoxemia, except shunting, are almost wholly reversible with the administration of 100% oxygen. Consequently, if a patient is permitted to breathe 100% oxygen for 15 to 30 minutes to the point of denitrogenation and the expected improvement in PaO_2 does not occur, the difference between the expected improvement and the actual measurement of PaO_2 indicates the degree of shunt. If a mixed venous blood sample is available, the shunt fraction can be calculated directly. First, oxygen content is determined for pulmonary capillary blood, arterial blood, and venous blood; second, simple computations give the shunt fraction. If mixed venous blood is not available, the shunt can be estimated by calculating the A-a gradient and estimating the shunt.

Although the 100% oxygen challenge is the accepted standard means of determining shunt and is the one accepted for both clinical and research use, the following disadvantages remain:

- The administration of an inspired oxygen concentration of 99.6% is essential in the oxygen challenge test. This can be achieved by placing an endotracheal tube or a tracheostomy tube in the patient or by using a special mouthpiece in the cooperative patient.
- Samples must be drawn from the pulmonary artery to obtain a true venous blood gas analysis. The procedure involves the placement of a pulmonary artery catheter.
- The effects of breathing 100% oxygen may result in an increase in any existing shunt.
- The administration of high concentrations of oxygen may abolish the hypoxic drive in patients with chronic obstructive pulmonary disease and result in respiratory arrest.
- Nitrogen washout (denitrogenation) that occurs secondary to 100% oxygen administration may cause alveolar collapse.
- Studies in experimental animals have shown that 100% oxygen administration for only 30 minutes causes anatomic changes in the lung.

Calculation of the Right-to-Left Shunt.   To calculate the right-to-left shunt, the nurse should do the following:

1. Administer 100% oxygen (for about 15 to 30 minutes or use a nitrogen analyzer to determine when less than 1% nitrogen remains).
2. Draw samples for arterial blood gas measurements.
3. Using the alveolar air equation, calculate the alveolar oxygen pressure.
4. Using peripheral arterial and mixed venous blood, use the following equation to calculate the shunt fraction (Qs/Qt):

$$Qs/Qt = \frac{Cc'O_2 - CaO_2}{Cc'O_2 - C\bar{v}O_2}$$

where

    Qs = quantity of blood shunted
    Qt = total CO
$Cc'O_2$ = O_2 content of the pulmonary capillary blood
CaO_2 = O_2 content of the systemic arterial blood
$C\bar{v}O_2$ = O_2 content of mixed venous blood

Oxygen content in the pulmonary capillary ($Cc'O_2$) is calculated from Equation 1 by using the P_AO_2, the solubility constant for oxygen in plasma (0.0031), the hemoglobin concentration (Hgb) in g/100 ml, the oxygen carrying capacity per gram of hemoglobin (1.39 ml/% saturation), and the percentage of oxygen saturation of the hemoglobin. An assumption is made because the pulmonary capillary oxygen pressure cannot be sampled and used to calculate the oxygen content in the capillary blood. It is assumed that the alveolar oxygen pressure is the same as the pul-

monary capillary oxygen pressure. During the inspiration of 100% oxygen, the amount of alveolar oxygen is more than enough for total saturation of hemoglobin, and so the pulmonary capillary partial pressure of oxygen is essentially equal to the alveolar partial pressure of oxygen. Therefore, the P_AO_2 is calculated from the alveolar air equation and used in equation 1:

$$Cc'O_2 = (P_AO_2 \times 0.0031) + (Hgb \times 1.39$$
$$\times \text{\%Hgb saturation}) \quad (1)$$

The content of arterial oxygen (CaO_2) is calculated from equation 2 by using the arterial oxygen pressure in the computation:

$$CaO_2 = (PaO_2 \times 0.0031) + (Hgb \times 1.39$$
$$\times \text{\%Hgb saturation}) \quad (2)$$

The content of mixed venous blood ($C\bar{v}O_2$) is calculated from equation 3, where the mixed venous oxygen pressure ($P\bar{v}O_2$) is used in the computation:

$$C\bar{v}O_2 = (P\bar{v}O_2 \times 0.0031) + (Hgb \times 1.39$$
$$\times \text{\%Hgb saturation}) \quad (3)$$

5. Realize that the different calculations for shunt used in critical care units across the country are all variations of the preceding equation. The variations have been derived by changing the form of the equation so that the measurements available in the particular critical care unit may be used directly in the equation, thus decreasing the computation required for the calculation. For example, the following is a modified shunt equation commonly used for patients who have an arterial oxygen pressure of more than 150 mm Hg:

Shunt

$$= \frac{\left(\begin{array}{c}\text{partial pressure of}\\ \text{alveolar oxygen}\end{array}\right) - \left(\begin{array}{c}\text{partial pressure of}\\ \text{arterial oxygen}\end{array}\right)0.0031}{\left(\begin{array}{cc}\text{arterial} & \text{mixed}\\ \text{oxygen} - \text{venous}\\ \text{content} & \text{oxygen}\\ & \text{content}\end{array}\right) + \left(\begin{array}{cc}\text{partial} & \text{partial}\\ \text{pressure} - \text{pressure}\\ \text{of alveolar} & \text{of arterial}\\ \text{oxygen} & \text{oxygen}\end{array}\right)0.0031}$$

6. Be able to estimate shunt. For simplicity and expedience, a reasonably good estimate of the degree of shunt may be made by comparing the difference between the P_AO_2 and PaO_2, the A-a gradient, before and after an oxygen challenge. For every 100 mm Hg difference, the shunt is 6%. In the normal patient, there is a 6% shunt. For example, a normal person breathing 100% oxygen for 15 minutes has a measured PaO_2 of approximately 550 or more mm Hg, a measured $PaCO_2$ of 40 mm Hg, and a calculated P_AO_2 of 673 mm Hg.

$$P_AO_2 = Pb - P_AH_2O)(FiO_2) - \frac{PaCO_2}{RQ}$$

$$= (760 - 47)(1.0) - (40/1)$$

[To facilitate computation in clinical situations, "1" is often used for the respiratory quotient.]

$$= 673 \text{ mm Hg}$$

$$\text{A-a gradient} = P_{A}O_2 - PaO_2$$

$$= 673 - 550$$

$$= 123 \text{ mm Hg}$$

Because there is a 6% shunt for each 100 mm Hg difference in pressure, it can be surmised that the person in question who is normal has a shunt of about 6%.

Example

Clinical example using A-a gradient to calculate shunt: Patient on ventilator with a tidal volume of 800 ml and a rate of 12 breaths/minute.

4:00 P.M.

Objective data:

ABG: $FiO_2 = 40\%$

$PaO_2 = 56$

$PaCO_2 = 51$

pH = 7.32

Assessment: Impaired gas exchange with hypoxemia and hypercarbia related to hypoventilation with acute carbon dioxide retention and other unidentified mechanisms.

Plan: Ventilation; increase tidal volume to 1000 ml and rate to 16/minute.

5:00 P.M.

Objective data:

ABG: $FiO_2 = 40\%$

$PaO_2 = 64$

$PaCO_2 = 38$

pH = 7.41

Assessment:

$$PaO_2 = (747 - 47)(.4) - 38/1$$

$$= 280 - 38$$

$$= 242 \text{ mm Hg}$$

Hypoxemia continues because of a ventilation-perfusion imbalance or a right-to-left shunt. A diffusion defect is not likely. The arterial oxygen pressure should be in the range of 220 to 240 mm Hg.

Plan: Differentiate a ventilation-perfusion mismatch from a right-to-left shunt. On 100% oxygen, the oxygen tension is uniform in all the alveoli so that any difference is due to shunting. Increase the oxygen to 100% for 15 minutes.

5:45 P.M.

Objective data:

ABG: $FiO_2 = 100\%$

$PaO_2 = 280$

$PaCO_2 = 26$

pH = 7.43

Assessment: Impaired gas exchange with hypoxemia related to right-to-left shunt.

Predicted value:

$$PaO_2 = (747 - 47)1 - 26/1$$

$$= 700 - 26$$

$$= 674 \text{ mm Hg}$$

$$\text{A-a } O_2 \text{ gradient} = 674 - 280$$

$$= 394$$

$$\text{Shunt} = \frac{394}{100} \times 6$$

$$= 4 \times 6$$

$$= 24\%$$

SUMMARY

Respiratory assessment is an important part of the critical care nurse's overall patient assessment. Each clinician should develop his or her own systematic technique using the principles of assessment outlined in the chapter. In addition to the bedside assessment, the critical care nurse can use information from diagnostic and pulmonary function tests to augment the pulmonary evaluation. The results of laboratory testing are useful for noting trends in acutely ill patients or in weaning a patient from mechanical ventilation. Pulmonary function tests also are used to evaluate lung volumes and forced exhalations and to evaluate obstructive and restrictive disease states. The principles of ventilation, perfusion, and oxygenation that were discussed and the nursing diagnoses that were identified examined some of the potential ventilation, perfusion, and oxygenation problems found in the critically ill patient.

REFERENCES

1. Bates, B. *A Guide to Physical Assessment and History Taking* (4th ed.). Philadelphia: J. B. Lippincott, 1987.
2. Cherniack, R. M., and Cherniack, L. *Respiration in Health and Disease* (3rd ed.). Philadelphia: W. B. Saunders, 1983.
3. Comroe, J. H. *Physiology of Respiration* (2nd ed.). Chicago: Year Book Medical Publishing, 1974.
4. Guyton, A. C. *Textbook of Medical Physiology* (7th ed.). Philadelphia: W. B. Saunders, 1986.
5. Kersten, L. D. *Comprehensive Respiratory Nursing*. Philadelphia: W. B. Saunders, 1989.
6. Loudon, R. and Murphy, R. L. H. State of the art: Lung sounds. *Am. Rev. Resp. Dis.* 130:663–673, 1984.
7. Mikami, R., Murao, M., Cugell, D. W., *et al.* International symposium on lung sounds. *Chest.* 92(2):342–345, 1987.
8. Murray, J. R. *The Normal Lung* (2nd ed.). Philadelphia: W. B. Saunders, 1986.
9. Pontoppidan, H., Geffln, B., and Lowenstein, E. *Acute Respiratory Failure in the Adult.* Boston: Little, Brown, 1973.

10. Ruppel, G. *Manual of Pulmonary Function Testing* (4th ed.). St. Louis: C. V. Mosby, 1986.

11. Rutherford, K. A. Principles and application of oximetry. *Crit. Care Nurs. Clin. North Am.* 1(4):649–657, 1989.

12. Sanchez, F. Fundamentals of chest x-ray interpretation. *Crit. Care Nurse* 6(5):41–61, 1986.

13. Shapiro, B. A., Harrison, R. A., Kacmarek, R. M., and Cane, R. D. *Clinical Application of Respiratory Care* (3rd ed.). Chicago: Year Book Medical Publishing, 1985.

14. Shapiro, B. A., Harrison, R. A., Cane, R. D., and Templin, R. *Clinical Application of Blood Gases* (4th ed.). Chicago: Year Book Medical Publishing, 1989.

15. Von Rueden, K. T. Noninvasive assessment of gas exchange in the critically ill. *AACN Clinical Issues in Critical Care Nursing* 1(2): 239–247, 1990.

16. West, J. B. *Respiratory Physiology* (4th ed.). Baltimore: Williams and Wilkins, 1990.

20

Acute Respiratory Failure: The Patient With Adult Respiratory Distress Syndrome

Susan F. Wilson

ARE YOU REALLY SPIRITUAL ENOUGH?

Equating spiritual and physical health is a notion that currently abounds in "holistic" health circles. We hear over and over that if one is "really" spiritual enough, perfect bodily health will follow. Cancers will be cured, heart disease and high blood pressure will fall away, and one can expect a long and healthy life. But this is not a holistic view, because it excludes certain things from the whole. It places certain qualities such as suffering or illness apart from the ultimate, and thus creates a dualism that is contrary to the principle of wholeness.

Another insidious problem crops up frequently when physical and spiritual health are seen as being the same. The problem manifests when one tries to "be more spiritual" with another agenda in mind—that of becoming physically healthier. Combining these two goals as if they are one frequently doesn't work. For example, as explored in Chapter 3, if a person engages in relaxation or meditation and tries to meditate with an overt reason in mind, it simply does not work. This point is also true when a person tries to warm hands and relax muscles. As long as there is an intentional, active, striving for a particular outcome, one is doomed to failure. However, when one puts personal agendas aside and learns to "let go" and not be attached to results, the real breakthrough occurs and the task is quickly learned. This passive volition, or doing nothing, is the key to the spiritual awareness necessary for peaceful living and peaceful dying.

LEARNING OBJECTIVES

After reading this chapter, the nurse should be able to do the following:

1. Define adult respiratory distress syndrome (ARDS).
2. State the incidence and mortality of ARDS.
3. List the medical diagnoses of patients who are at risk for developing ARDS.
4. Describe interrelationships among physiologic changes, the defining characteristics (symptoms), and the treatment modalities for ARDS.
5. Apply the nursing process to the patient with ARDS.

CASE STUDY

R. F., a 46-year-old man, underwent both an emergency laparotomy and surgery for fixation of a crushed femur. He had received multiple injuries in an automobile accident, and he suffered from hypovolemic hemorrhagic shock. The operation took 5 hours. Fluid replacement during surgery consisted of 6 U of whole blood and 3 L of lactated Ringer's solution. A postoperative chest radiograph showed correct placement of a central venous line in the superior vena cava and no pulmonary infiltrations.

Immediate Postoperative Period

After Mr. F.'s recovery from anesthesia, his respirations were spontaneous but guarded because of the pain from the abdominal trauma and laparotomy incision. This pain was controlled with intravenous morphine. His respiratory rate was 28 breaths/minute, and he did not complain of dyspnea or fatigue. His breath sounds were clear, with no adventitious sounds. The patient was encouraged to breathe deeply and to cough.

During the first 12 postoperative hours, Mr. F's cardiovascular parameters stabilized; his blood pressure was 110/70 mm Hg; pulse, 90/minute; hematocrit, 32%; hemoglobin, 10 g/100 ml; and central venous pressure, 9 to 13 cm H_2O. His urine output averaged 50 to 60 ml/hour; there was no evidence of red blood cells in the urine. The ratio of blood urea to urine urea was 1:20, which is normal. Neurologically, the patient appeared alert and oriented with regard to time, person, place, and circumstance. His cranial nerves and peripheral nerves seemed intact. Clinically, the patient seemed to be doing well.

Initial Respiratory Difficulty

During the next 12 to 24 hours, Mr. F. had persistent unexplained tachypnea not associated with pain or anxiety, and a slight hypocarbia ($PaCO_2$, 32 mm Hg) with mild respiratory alkalosis (pH of 7.47).

On the second postoperative day, he began to complain of progressive dyspnea and fatigue. Respiratory difficulty was manifested by increasing tachypnea and hyperventilation, use of accessory muscles of respiration with supraclavicular and suprasternal retractions, fine crackles audible in the dependent portions of both lungs, and radiographic suggestions of patchy irregular infiltrations.

Serial blood gas analyses showed a falling $PaCO_2$ (30 mm Hg), a rising pH (7.50), and a PaO_2 that had fallen to a borderline hypoxic value of 60 mm Hg on room air. Mr. F. seemed restless and agitated.

Respiratory Insufficiency

By the third to fourth postoperative day, Mr. F.'s unrelenting respiratory difficulty was manifested by tachypnea (35/minute), progressive dyspnea, moderate cyanosis of the tongue, decreased tidal volume (3 ml/kg), a minute volume of 8 L, an alveolar-arterial oxygen gradient of 520 mm Hg when 100% oxygen was inhaled for 10 minutes, a progressive hypoxia that was unresponsive to increasing fractions of inspired oxygen, and a deteriorating sensorium. Despite the patient's extreme hyperventilation, paradoxically his $PaCO_2$ level began to rise ($PaCO_2$, 49 mm Hg), his carbon dioxide content was 29, his base deficit was −1.0, his PaO_2 continued to fall (to 40 mm Hg), and his pH decreased to 7.36.

Fine-to-medium crackles were audible bilaterally and progressed to sibilant wheezes that were accentuated on expiration. A serial pulmonary radiograph revealed extensive progressive infiltrations with widespread areas of consolidation.

On the basis of Mr. F.'s clinical deterioration and the criteria for ventilatory support, a cuffed nasotracheal tube was inserted and the patient was placed on a positive-pressure volume ventilator adjusted to deliver a tidal volume of 1000 ml (15 ml/kg) at a rate of 18/minute, with a sigh volume of 1500 ml delivered at 6-minute intervals and an FiO_2 of 40%. Initially, the peak airway inspiratory pressure (PAIP) required to administer that selected tidal volume was 25 cm H_2O pressure, but it rose to 45 cm H_2O. Intravenous morphine sulfate was titrated to gain control during assisted ventilation.

Gram-stain microscopic smears made from the tracheal aspirate indicated the presence of *Klebsiella pneumoniae*, which is sensitive to gentamicin and cephalothin. Antibiotic therapy was initiated.

The patient's hematocrit was 33%, and his hemoglobin was 11 g/100 ml. One unit of packed red blood cells was given to enhance his oxygen-carrying capacity.

Terminal Stage

On the fifth postoperative day, the patient's PaO_2 was 35 mm Hg with an FiO_2 of 40%. Adequate PaO_2 was unobtainable even after

the FiO_2 was increased to 60%. An increasing lactic acidosis indicated by a rising lactate-to-pyruvate ratio occurred secondary to tissue hypoxia and was superimposed on the patient's respiratory acidosis ($PaCO_2$, 55 mm Hg, PaO_2, 40 mm Hg; pH, 7.12).

The PAIP required to deliver the same tidal volume had risen slowly to 60 cm H_2O. The patient was placed on 10 cm H_2O positive end-expiratory pressure (PEEP), and his blood pressure fell. His PEEP was reduced to 7.5 cm H_2O, his blood pressure returned to baseline, and his serial blood gas analysis showed a slight improvement in the PaO_2.

The PAIP continued to rise. The patient's static compliance was calculated to be 15 ml/cm H_2O. The administration of pancuronium bromide was ordered for respiratory control. After a loading dose of 7 mg, the patient was maintained on 2 mg as needed. Diazepam was ordered for sedation.

The chest radiographs showed excessive pulmonary infiltration and consolidation. The opacity of the chest film was termed a *white out* by the radiologist. The patient's sputum samples were mucopurulent, with rusty, blood-stained streaks.

On the fifth day, the patient died from a combined metabolic and respiratory acidosis that lead to bradycardia and asystole. On autopsy, gross examination revealed wet, dark, consolidated, and heavy lungs with scattered patches of necrosis and abscess formation. Histopathologic examination showed focal hemorrhage into the alveoli, hypertrophy of the alveolar lining cells, alveolar edema, cellular infiltration, and perivascular hemorrhage.

REFLECTIONS

Even though the critically ill patient with ARDS may present a poor prognosis, the nurse must strive to support the patient and family. Although the patient described in the case study died, many patients with ARDS survive. The mortality rate is about 50% despite therapy.[6] The mind and body are so closely related that hope and the will to live can influence the patient's outcome. The will to live seems to be associated with having someone or something for which to live. It is important for everyone concerned with the patient to maintain hope. Hope is a longing for something with the expectation of obtainment. At first the hope may be that the patient recover from the illness or injury without any disability. Then the hope may turn to recovery with minimal disability. If recovery is not possible and the patient is dying, then hope may be for a peaceful death.

Regardless of the patient's prognosis, the nurse demonstrates caring for the patient and family. Caring for the patient is demonstrated by talking to the patient even when he or she does not respond. Touching the patient is an important way to show caring for another. This is accomplished during activities such as bathing, turning, or suctioning. Caring toward the family is shown by providing information about the patient's condition and by allowing them to care for the patient if they desire. The nurse may need to accompany the family to the bedside and stay with them to demonstrate that it is permissible and desirable for them to touch and talk to the patient. Also, support for the family can be provided by requesting consultation from other family members, clergy, social workers, or psychiatric clinical nurse specialists.

DESCRIPTION

Acute respiratory failure is defined as a condition in which the arterial PCO_2 is above 50 mm Hg when the patient is at rest and breathing room air or in which the arterial PO_2 is less than 55 mm Hg.[8] *Respiratory failure* refers to the inability of the lungs to maintain normal oxygenation of the blood or elimination of carbon dioxide. In its most severe state, acute respiratory failure is referred to as *adult respiratory distress syndrome* (ARDS).[23] Adult respiratory distress syndrome is defined as a distinct form of acute respiratory failure that results from diffuse pulmonary injury of various causes and is characterized by diffuse alveolar-capillary wall injury, increased alveolar-capillary permeability, noncardiogenic pulmonary edema, hyaline membrane formation, and atelectasis.[6] The patient's primary medical diagnosis frequently is not related to the pulmonary system, but this progressive pulmonary syndrome develops as a complication of a variety of conditions.

ETIOLOGY

Adult respiratory distress syndrome is a type of respiratory failure that was described in World War I as posttraumatic pulmonary insufficiency. During World War II, it was called wet lung, and during the Vietnam War it was described as Da Nang lung. Table 20–1 provides some of the synonyms for ARDS.

Adult respiratory distress syndrome affects approximately 150,000 people each year and has a mortality rate of 50% despite therapy.[6] Identification of patients who are at risk for ARDS allows the use of early prophylaxis and aggressive therapeutic management to reduce the incidence. There seems to be no single exogenous or endogenous precipitating factor acting on pulmonary tissue that induces the altered function during ARDS. Table 20–2 provides a partial list of the disorders that may lead to ARDS.[6,24] Regardless of the cause, there does seem to be a common pathologic response of diffuse lung injury that occurs after a profoundly stressful event.

PATHOPHYSIOLOGY

Figure 20–1 illustrates a general concept of the pathogenesis and pathophysiology of ARDS. The physiologic reaction of all body tissues sometimes results in pathologic changes in the lung. Initially, a systemic insult causes low tissue perfusion and cellular hypoxia. Consequently, peripheral tissues are deprived of essential nutrients, and intracellular metabolic derangements result. The exact mechanisms by which ARDS develops from this low tissue perfusion state is unclear. It has been suggested that certain chemical factors, such as prostaglandins, clotting factors, lysosomal enzymes, activated

Table 20–1

Synonyms for Adult Respiratory Distress Syndrome

Adult respiratory insufficiency syndrome
Acute ventilatory insufficiency
Adult hyaline membrane disease
Centroneurogenic or noncardiogenic pulmonary edema
Congestive atelectasis
Progressive respiratory distress
Pump lung
Respirator lung
Shock lung
Stiff lung
White lung syndrome

Table 20–2

Disorders that Lead to Adult Respiratory Distress Syndrome

Trauma*
  Hypovolemic shock
  Thoracic trauma
  Lung or cardiac contusion
  Fat embolism
  Severe extrathoracic trauma, including head injury
  Extensive burns
Inhaled toxins
  Smoke
  Chemicals
  Oxygen toxicity
Liquid aspiration
  Gastric contents
  Near-drowning
Hematologic disorders
  Disseminated intravascular coagulation
  Massive transfusion of banked blood
Infections
  Gram-negative sepsis*
  Viral, bacterial, or fungal pneumonia
  Pneumocystis carinii
Drug overdose
Toxic metabolic disorders
  Pancreatitis
  Uremia
  Eclampsia

* Most common causes

complement, or histamine, are released into the systemic circulation.[10]

Prostaglandins contribute to vasodilation, capillary permeability, pain, and fever, which accompany cell injury. Changes in vessel walls and disturbances in blood flow increase platelet function, causing adhesiveness and aggregation. Lysosomal enzymes from neutrophils increase vascular per-

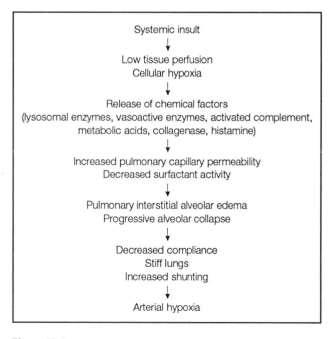

Figure 20–1

Pathogenesis and pathophysiology of adult respiratory distress syndrome.

meability and cause tissue damage. Activated complement has three outcomes: increased cell lysis, chemotaxis to attract phagocytic cells, and anaphylaxis causing degranulation of mast cells with release of histamine. Histamine also is released from platelets, mast cells, and basophils and causes arterial vasodilation and enhanced permeability of capillaries and venules.[16] These chemical factors are carried to the pulmonary microvasculature and cause diffuse pulmonary injury, which is characterized by an increase in the permeability of the pulmonary capillary endothelium and the alveolar endothelium.

To comprehend the significance of the progressive clinical changes occurring during ARDS, it is necessary to correlate the pathologic changes as they present themselves concurrently or sequentially. In the following pages, consideration is given to three pathophysiologic defects that exist to some degree at some point in ARDS: pulmonary capillary endothelial defects, alveolar epithelial defects, and alterations in gas exchange.

PULMONARY CAPILLARY ENDOTHELIAL DEFECTS

As the ARDS progresses, changes occur in the capillary endothelial cells and in the epithelial cells lining the alveoli. Figures 20–2 and 20–3 show lung architecture and fluid movement in the normal lung and in ARDS. They are useful to explain both the changes in the capillary cells (discussed in this section) as well as the alveoli (discussed in the next section).

The fluid-exchanging properties of the normal lung are shown in Figure 20–2. The capillary endothelial membrane is permeable to fluid and relatively impermeable to protein and solutes. Fluid filtered across the capillary basement membrane accumulates in the interstitial space. As with any capillary, the movement of water from the pulmonary vascular space into the lung tissue is governed by Starling forces. The intravascular hydrostatic pressure is the major force that promotes movement of water out of the intravascular space into tissue. In other vasculature, this pressure is opposed to some degree by the tissue hydrostatic pressure; however, this pressure is negligible in the lung and can be ignored for practical purposes. Thus, the net pressure across the vascular wall can be considered equal to the intravascular hydrostatic pressure, as shown by the wide arrow in Figure 20–2. The capillary oncotic pressure, which is caused primarily by serum proteins, is the major force promoting retention of water in the intravascular space (shown by the thin arrow). However, because tissue oncotic pressure is substantial, the net oncotic pressure promoting retention of water in the intravascular space is substantially less than the hydrostatic pressure across the capillary wall. This concept is shown in Figure 20–2 by the different widths of the arrows, which indicate fluid movement. The lymphatic channels absorb some interstitial fluid and return it to the vascular system, as shown by the horizonal arrow. Normally, none of this fluid gains access to the alveoli.[23]

In ARDS, the complement system is activated in response to antigen-antibody reactions.[6] There are two mechanisms by which complement affects pulmonary capillary permeability: directly by cell lysis and indirectly by release of mast cells, which liberate histamine, a potent vasodilator. The decreased blood flow through these capillaries causes stagnation of platelets and leukocytes in the pulmonary microvasculature.

Platelets release a platelet permeability factor, and leukocytes release additional histamine as well as bradykinin, collagenase, and elastase, which all increase capillary permeability. The increased permeability allows plasma, which is rich in large protein molecules, to leak from the intravascular spaces into the interstitial spaces. Also contained in the exudate are elastase and collagenase, which are proteolytic enzymes that cause disruption of the elastic and collagen fibers found in the interstitium. The plasma protein exudate and the breakdown products of interstitial fibers increase the tissue oncotic pressure of the interstitial space. The increase in tissue oncotic pressure tends to pull water from the blood into the interstitium, aggravating the interstitial edema. This interstitial edema causes decreased lung compliance (stiff lung), requiring more pressure to inspire air.

ALVEOLAR EPITHELIAL DEFECTS

In a normal lung, the alveolar epithelium membrane is relatively impermeable to fluid and protein, as shown in Figure 20–2. Surfactant is a surface-acting lipoprotein produced by alveolar type 2 epithelial cells that normally lines the alveoli and separates the air-water interface. Surfactant stabilizes the alveoli, decreases the surface tension of water, and decreases the tendency for alveoli to collapse. Normal production and release of surfactant from type 2 alveolar cells are stimulated by active ventilation, adequate tidal volume, and intermittent hyperventilation (sighing).

The fluid-exchanging properties of the lung in ARDS are shown in Figure 20–3. The integrity of the capillary endothelium and alveolar epithelium are compromised, leading to alveolar edema and atelectasis, as shown by the long, curved, wide arrow and the wide verticle arrow. The exact mechanisms contributing to this sequence of events have not been described completely.[23] In the early stages of ARDS, the interstitial edema can be removed by the lymphatic transport of the lungs. Serial chest radiographs appear essentially normal when early interstitial edema is present. As the paravascular and interstitial spaces become moderately edematous, the chest radiograph shows diffuse opacity, which is indicative of profuse pulmonary infiltration.

Late structural deterioration includes changes in the two types of epithelial cells that line the alveoli. These changes correlate with the symptoms in the respiratory insufficiency and the terminal stages of ARDS described in the case study. Alveolar type 1 epithelial cells are swollen. Reduction in surfactant production by the alveolar type 2 epithelial cells contributes to alveolar collapse. The alveoli become increasingly unstable and tend to collapse unless filled with interstitial fluid. With increasing pulmonary edema and progressive alveolar collapse, the alveoli can no longer participate in effective gas exchange.[12]

As fluid accumulates, the normally tight junctions between alveolar lining cells appear tortuous. The intra-alveolar spaces are filled with proteinaceous material, making alveolar ventilation difficult and compromising gas exchange. Red blood cells are found in the alveoli and account for the rust-colored sputum. Hyaline membranes form along the alveolar surface and represent coagulated protein. It is possible that fibrinogen exudate in the alveolar edema polymerizes to form intra-alveolar fibrin that cannot be reabsorbed in the fluid state but must be enzymatically lyzed or phagocytized. Proteinaceous

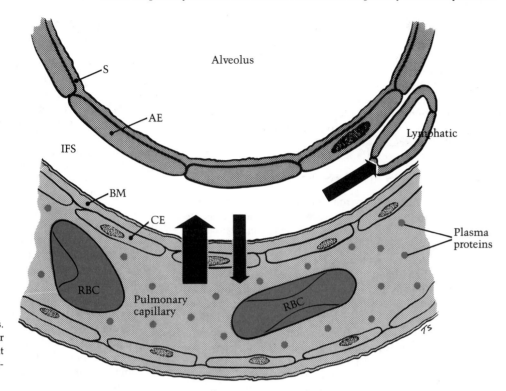

Figure 20–2

Fluid movement in normal lungs. S: surfactant layer; AE: alveolar epithelium; BM: capillary basement membrane; CE: capillary endothelium; IFS: interstitial fluid space.

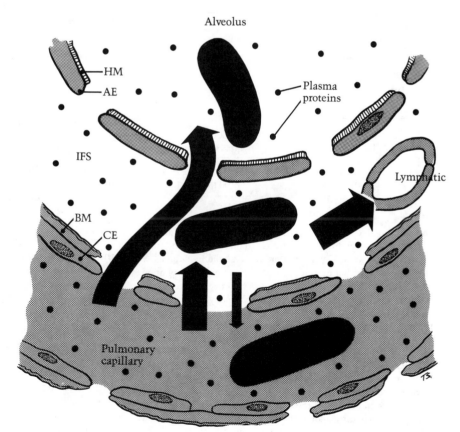

Figure 20–3

Fluid movement in adult respiratory distress syndrome. HM: deposition of hyaline membrane; AE: widened interalveolar epithelial junction; IFS: marked edema of the interstitial fluid space; BM: disruption of basement membrane; CE: capillary endothelium; RBC: red blood cells.

alveolar edema is a cultural medium for bacterial proliferation and is the reason that many patients die from a fulminating bronchopneumonia secondary to a bacterial infection.

As intra-alveolar edema and fibrosis occur, serial chest radiographs show progressive opacity until the x-ray film appears white; hence, the name *white lung* is often applied. Gross examination of the lung at autopsy shows a heavy, wet, boggy lung that is deep red in color and has areas of consolidation and focal abscesses.

ALTERATIONS IN GAS EXCHANGE

The stiff lung that results from interstitial edema decreases compliance, so that increased inspiratory pressure is required to overcome airway resistance and deliver adequate tidal volume for gas exchange. Figure 20–4 compares the normal pulmonary function tests with those found in patients with ARDS and defines the pulmonary function terms. For the ARDS patient who is breathing spontaneously, there is an increased work of breathing, as evidenced by increased respiratory rate and a decreased tidal volume. As compliance decreases, there is progressive reduction in the functional residual capacity. The lung volume may become so small that the alveoli collapse completely on deflation.[24] This collapse reduces the expiratory residual volume. In summary, the ventilation alterations can be determined by pulmonary function tests. The abnormal values found for patients with ARDS include a decreased tidal volume and a decreased functional residual capacity.

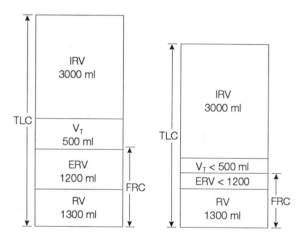

Figure 20–4

Pulmonary function test results in the normal lung (left) and in adult respiratory distress syndrome with decreased tidal volume and functional residual capacity. IRV: inspiratory reserve volume—the maximum amount of air that can be inspired after a normal inspiration. Normally, this amount is 3000 ml; V_T: tidal volume—the volume of air inspired or expired during each breath. Normally, this volume is 500 ml; ERV: expiratory residual volume—the maximum amount of air that can be exhaled after a resting expiration. Normally this amount is 1200 ml; RV: residual volume—the volume remaining in the lungs at the end of maximum expiration. Normally, this volume is 1300 ml; FRC: functional residual capacity—the volume of air remaining in the lungs at the end of normal expiration. This capacity is calculated by adding the ERV and the RV; TLC: total lung capacity—the volume of air contained in the lung at the end of a maximal inspiration. This capacity is calculated by adding the IRV plus the V_T plus the ERV plus the RV. Normally, this volume is 6000 ml.

Movement of Oxygen From Alveoli to Capillaries

In ARDS, several parameters change that could alter the rate of gas exchange. First, because of intra-alveolar edema, hyaline membranes, and a swollen alveolar-capillary unit, gases must diffuse across a greater distance. This results in a decreased diffusion capacity, which contributes somewhat to the severe hypoxemia seen in the later phases of ARDS, but it is not considered to be the major cause of hypoxemia. Second, a significant increase in the pulmonary shunt is the characteristic physiologic abnormality affecting gas exchange in ARDS. The pulmonary shunt occurs when alveoli receive blood flow but do not receive ventilation. The normal ventilation-perfusion relationship is shown in Figure 20–5. Oxygen in alveoli A and B diffuses into the pulmonary capillary to maintain normal oxygen tension in the pulmonary veins and arteries. The alveolar surface area across which the diffusion occurs in ARDS is reduced secondary to the degeneration of alveolar cells, the disruption of intra-alveolar septa, and the presence of atelectasis and fluid-filled alveoli. The reduced alveolar surface area causes underventilated alveoli. Consequently, a ventilation-perfusion imbalance occurs with "wasted perfusion" or intrapulmonary shunt as illustrated in Figure 20–6. The gas exchange of the blood that perfuses alveolus B is inadequate; therefore, its PaO_2 remains low, and its reduced hemoglobin remains high. Low oxygen tension and high reduced hemoglobin are characteristics of venous blood. When the venous blood of alveolus B and the arterial blood of alveolus A mix, the result is called a *venous admixture*.

Consequences of pulmonary shunting may be summarized as an increase in venous admixture leading to a decrease in systemic arterial oxygen content and a decrease in oxygen transport resulting in tissue hypoxia. The severity of the patient's condition depends on the degree of shunting and the subsequent degree of hypoxemia.

The normal amount of anatomic shunting is 3% to 5% of the cardiac output. The sum of the individual capillary shunt represents the total intrapulmonary shunt fraction. In ARDS, the shunt fraction usually represents 25% to 50% of the cardiac output.[23] Shunting is considered to be the major factor producing hypoxemia in ARDS.

During the progression of ARDS, there seems to be no alteration in the solubility of oxygen in plasma. The capacity of oxygen to dissolve in plasma remains constant, but the quantity of oxygen actually dissolved is reduced because less oxygen is moved across the alveolar-capillary membrane unit and into the pulmonary capillary blood. Patients with ARDS have decreased PaO_2 levels and decreased hemoglobin saturation. As the oxyhemoglobin dissociation curve in Figure 20–7 shows, at a PaO_2 of 60 mm Hg or less, the percentage of hemoglobin saturated with oxygen is reduced critically.

Although the cardiac output usually increases in the early phase of ARDS, it decreases in later stages owing to myocardial compromise. The decreased cardiac output and the inadequate oxygen exchange lead to severe hypoxemia and failure of adequate cellular oxygenation. This failure results in anaerobic cellular metabolism and an increased production of lactic acid and metabolic lactic acidemia. Declining perfusion of multiple organs with resulting hypoxia is manifested by a decreasing level of consciousness due to inadequate supply of oxygenated blood to the brain, a diminished urine output due to the de-

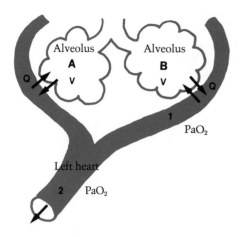

Figure 20-5

Normal ventilation-perfusion relationship. The *single arrow* shows direction of blood flow. The *double arrows* indicate normal gas exchange at the alveolar capillary membrane units. V: normal ventilation in alveolus A and alveolus B; Q: normal blood perfusion; $PaO_2(1)$: normal oxygen tension in the pulmonary veins; $PaO_2(2)$: normal oxygen tension in the systemic arterial blood.

creased cardiac output, and cardiac irregularities due to inadequate blood supply to the coronary arteries. The cardiac irregularities vary from ventricular fibrillation and sudden death to bradycardia that progresses to asystole.

Release of Oxygen at the Systemic Cellular Level

A patient with ARDS has several problems with oxygen release. The elevated arterial pH in early ARDS might reflect a mixed respiratory-metabolic alkalosis. The increased pH (decreased hydrogen ion level) shifts the oxyhemoglobin dissociation curve to the left, impeding the release of oxygen to the peripheral cells. In alkalosis, the bond of hemoglobin to

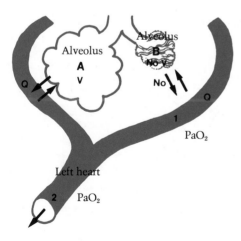

Figure 20-6

Abnormal ventilation-perfusion relationship of shunting. Alveolus A: a normally ventilated alveolus; Alveolus B: a fluid-filled atelectatic alveolus; No V: no ventilation; No ↕: no gas exchange; Q: normal perfusion; $PaO_2(1)$: decreased oxygen tension in the pulmonary veins; $PaO_2(2)$: decreased oxygen tension in the systemic arterial blood.

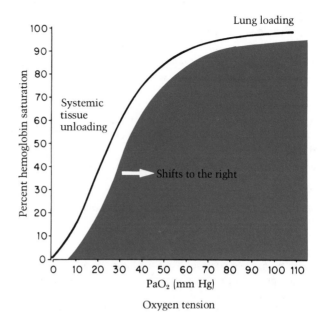

Figure 20-7

Oxyhemoglobin dissociation curve. The hemoglobin saturation is approximately 95% at a PaO_2 of 90 mm Hg. The slope of the curve is steep at a PaO_2 of less than 60 mm Hg. Shifts of the curve to the right release more oxygen at the systemic tissue level. Lung loading refers to the saturation of hemoglobin with oxygen that occurs in the pulmonary capillaries. The systemic tissue unloading refers to the movement of oxygen molecules from the hemoglobin to the plasma and then to the cells.

oxygen is stronger than normal, so that less oxygen is released. By contrast, in the later phases of ARDS, the $PaCO_2$ is abnormally high owing to hypoventilation and inadequate carbon dioxide exchange at the alveolar-capillary membrane. The retention of carbon dioxide together with the increased lactic acid production from the anaerobic metabolism produces a respiratory-metabolic acidosis. During acidosis, the oxyhemoglobin dissociation curve is shifted to the right, indicating that oxygen is released more readily from the hemoglobin; that is, the bond of hemoglobin to oxygen is weaker in acidosis. In this sense, the acidosis is beneficial to the patient, because more oxygen is released, although the amount of oxygen available to the tissues is decreased.

NURSING PROCESS

The ideal situation is to identify ARDS before symptoms occur by closely monitoring serial arterial blood gases. The onset of respiratory distress typically lags behind the initial insult by 24 to 48 hours. The symptoms that indicate ARDS are described in the following section.

ASSESSMENT

Respiratory Assessment

Subjective Findings. Patient complains of breathlessness and air hunger. This progresses to reports of increased effort required for breathing.

Objective Findings. Patient has tachypnea, but decreased respiratory rate in later stages, decreased breath sounds, crackles (rales), dyspnea, cough, and cyanosis of nail beds. Increased work of breathing is evidenced by use of accessory muscles and intercostal and supracostal retractions.

Laboratory Findings. Serial arterial blood gases indicate a sudden hypoxemia (PaO_2 < 55 mm Hg) before other symptoms are identified. Beginning in the respiratory-insufficiency stage, the patient has hypoxemia as well as hypercapnea ($PaCO_2$ > 50 mm Hg) and acidosis (pH < 7.35).

X-ray Findings. Early diagnostic changes include thickened or blurred margins of the bronchi and vessels. Diffuse pulmonary infiltrates are noted later.

Pulmonary Function Findings. Decreased tidal volume, vital capacity, minute volume, and functional residual capacity. It is now possible to measure a patient's forced vital capacity and peak flow at the bedside. When the forced vital capacity falls below 20 ml/kg, the patient is in a range bordering on respiratory failure.[6]

Cardiovascular Assessment

Objective Findings. Patient has decreased cardiac output as evidenced by restlessness, lethargy, tachycardia, hypotension, decreased urinary output, and elevated pulmonary capillary wedge pressure.

Psychosocial Assessment

Subjective Findings. Patient has anxiety, fear of suffocation, fear of being out of control if using a ventilator, fear of unknown, and frustration about not being able to communicate as a result of intubation.

NURSING DIAGNOSES, PATIENT OUTCOMES, AND PLAN

The preceding material on anatomy, physiology, nursing assessment, and diagnostic tests guides the nurse in establishing nursing diagnoses, patient outcomes, and the plan for the patient with ARDS.

NURSING CARE PLAN SUMMARY *Patient With Adult Respiratory Distress Syndrome*

NURSING DIAGNOSIS

1. *Impaired gas exchange related to alveolar-capillary membrane changes (from ARDS or fat emboli from fractures) (exchanging pattern)*

Patient Outcome	*Nursing Orders*
Patient will maintain adequate gas exchange as demonstrated by normal arterial blood gases and clear breath sounds.	The following are assessment interventions 1. Auscultate lungs for crackles (rales). 2. Evaluate arterial and mixed venous blood gas analyses. 3. Assess pulmonary artery pressure, pulmonary capillary wedge pressure, and jugular vein distention. 4. Observe for changes in awareness, orientation, and behavior. 5. Monitor electrocardiogram and cardiac status for dysrhythmias. The following are therapeutic interventions: 6. Administer oxygen as ordered. 7. Maintain mechanical ventilation as indicated (tidal volume, 10–15 ml/kg; PEEP for PaO_2 < 60 mm Hg on FiO_2 > 0.50). 8. Administer medications (diuretics, sedatives, neuromuscular blockers, steroids) as ordered. 9. Pace activities to patient's tolerance. 10. Position patient to allow maximum gas exchange.

NURSING DIAGNOSIS

2. *Ineffective breathing pattern related to decreased compliance (exchanging pattern)*

Patient Outcome	*Nursing Orders*
Patient will maintain a normal respiratory rate, rhythm, and tidal volume.	The following are assessment interventions: 1. Observe changes in respiratory rate and depth. 2. Measure tidal volume.

(continued)

NURSING CARE PLAN SUMMARY *Patient With Adult Respiratory Distress Syndrome*
Continued

Patient Outcome	Nursing Orders
	The following are therapeutic interventions: 3. Maintain ventilator settings as ordered. 4. Assist patient to use relaxation techniques. 5. Sedate patient as ordered.

NURSING DIAGNOSIS

3. *Ineffective airway clearance related to pulmonary and interstitial edema (exchanging pattern)*

Patient Outcome	Nursing Orders
Patient's airways will be patent, with clear breath sounds. Sputum will be thin and clear.	The following are assessment interventions: 1. Auscultate lungs for rhonchi, crackles, or wheezing. 2. Assess characteristics of secretions such as quantity, color, consistency, and odor. 3. Assess patient's hydration status by monitoring skin turgor, mucous membranes, tongue, and intake and output over 24 hours. 4. Monitor sputum, Gram stains, and culture and sensitivity reports. The following are therapeutic interventions: 5. Assist patient with coughing as needed. 6. Perform nasotracheal or tracheostomy tube suctioning as needed. 7. Administer mucolytic agents as indicated. 8. Position patient in proper body alignment for optimal breathing pattern. 9. Assist patient to turn from side to side every 2 hours. 10. Perform chest physiotherapy (postural drainage, percussion, vibration) as ordered. 11. Assist patient with oral hygiene as needed.

NURSING DIAGNOSIS

4. *High risk for infection related to decreased pulmonary function, possible steroid therapy, and ineffective airway clearance (exchanging pattern)*

Patient Outcome	Nursing Orders
Patient will have no infection, as evidenced by normal body temperature and leukocytes within normal limits.	The following are assessment interventions: 1. Monitor temperature. 2. Monitor leukocytes and albumin. 3. Assess nutritional status. 4. Monitor pulmonary function tests. The following are therapeutic interventions: 5. Assist with nebulizer treatments and physiotherapy. 6. Administer prophylactic antimicrobials as ordered. 7. Use aseptic technique in giving care. 8. Follow hospital protocol for changing dressings.

(continued)

NURSING CARE PLAN SUMMARY   *Patient With Adult Respiratory Distress Syndrome*
Continued

NURSING DIAGNOSIS

5. *Altered nutrition: less than body requirements related to inadequate intake secondary to hypoxia and fatigue (exchanging pattern)*

Patient Outcome	Nursing Orders
Patient will maintain adequate nutritional status.	The following are assessment interventions: 1. Assess dietary habits and needs. 2. Weigh patient weekly. 3. For patient with tracheostomy, inspect tracheal aspirate for food particles at each feeding. Add food coloring to tube feeding so that aspiration can be detected easily if suctioned from airway. Stop feedings if aspiration is found. 4. Auscultate bowel sounds. 5. Measure fluid intake and output. 6. Monitor albumin and lymphocytes. 7. Measure mid-arm circumference and triceps skinfold. The following are therapuetic interventions: 8. Administer total parenteral nutrition or enteral tube feeding as ordered.

NURSING DIAGNOSIS

6. *Fear related to suffocation, being on mechanical ventilation, uncertainty of prognosis, and inability to verbally communicate (feeling pattern)*

Patient Outcome	Nursing Orders
Patient will report a decrease in fear.	The following are assessment interventions: 1. Validate sources of fear with patient. Assess patient's perception of unmet needs and expectations. 2. Assist patient to identify coping skills used successfully in the past. The following are therapeutic interventions: 3. Encourage patient to ask questions and express feelings. 4. Explain ARDS, the intensive care unit regimen, and equipment. 5. Explain all procedures. If giving pancuronium bromide for respiratory control, explain skeletal muscle paralysis effects of the drug. Give sedatives with pancuronium to allay anxiety. 6. Provide oxygen as ordered. 7. Explain that some fear or anxiety is normal and expected. 8. Provide alternate forms of communication when patient is unable to speak (see Impaired Verbal Communication, Chap. 8).

NURSING DIAGNOSIS

7. *Knowledge deficit related to follow-up and home care (knowing pattern)*

Patient Outcome	Nursing Orders
Patient and family will verbalize plan for follow-up treatment and home care.	Teach patient the following: 1. Adaptive breathing techniques 2. The importance of turning, coughing, and deep breathing 3. The importance of not fighting the ventilator, and relaxing to permit maximum ventilation 4. The importance of periodic rest periods 5. The name, dosage, time of administration, and side effects of all medications

IMPLEMENTATION AND EVALUATION

The therapeutic goals related to ARDS are to achieve gas exchange, and to treat the initiating pathophysiologic process and the systemic responses caused by the altered pulmonary function. These goals are accomplished by fluid therapy, oxygenation, nutrition, drug therapy, reduction of fear, and education.

Fluid Therapy

Fluids are monitored carefully in the patient with ARDS. The type of fluid used may be colloids or crystalloids. Hypoalbuminemic patients should receive colloids, whereas all other patients should receive crystalloid fluids. To decrease pulmonary congestion, the patient's pulmonary capillary wedge pressure (PCWP) is kept as low as possible as long as the cardiac output and tissue perfusion can be maintained at normal levels. Maintenance of the PCWP at 10 to 15 mm Hg provides adequate, but not excessive, intravascular volumes. Additional assessment parameters include the quality of pulse, urine output, and blood pressure.[24]

Oxygenation

The goal of oxygen therapy is to administer the lowest possible oxygen concentration to sustain a mixed venous oxygen greater than 40 mm Hg. Oxygen may be delivered by mask in the first stages of ARDS, but when a mask is no longer sufficient, the patient is intubated and ventilated mechanically.

Positive end-expiratory pressure is indicated for use in patients who are being ventilated mechanically with high FiO_2 (>0.50) and who have a PaO_2 of less than 65 mm Hg or a venoarterial shunt that is greater than 20%. Positive end-expiratory pressure maintains positive pressure in the patient's alveoli at all times, even during exhalation. The purpose of PEEP in ARDS is to minimize alveolar collapse and small airway closure, and reduce interstitial edema and total extravascular lung water. Initial levels of PEEP should be in the range of 5 to 10 cm H_2O. Small increments of PEEP are added until the optimal level is reached. Optimal PEEP is characterized by normal PCWP, adequate arterial blood pressure, increased PaO_2, increased functional residual capacity, increased compliance, decreased shunting, and improved clearing of the lung fields.

Although PEEP is beneficial, it is not without complications. Positive end-expiratory pressure adds more pressure to the already high mean intrathoracic pressures caused by mechanical ventilation of stiff, noncompliant lungs. Part of this high pressure is transmitted to the pleural space and large vessels of the chest. This increased intrathoracic pressure can compress these vessels, causing decreased venous return to the heart, decreased cardiac output, and increased pulmonary vascular resistance. Complications include peripheral vasoconstriction, hypotension, and increased PCWP greater than 15 mm Hg. A PEEP in excess of 15 cm H_2O increases the incidence of barotrauma and pneumothorax.[20]

Once the patient is stabilized, the ventilation parameters should be decreased in small increments, such as decreasing the tidal volume from 10 to 5 ml/kg, decreasing the FiO_2 to 0.50, and decreasing the PEEP every 8 to 12 hours as tolerated. Patients who have achieved the desired outcomes for impaired gas exchange will be found to have no difficulty breathing and will achieve arterial blood gases within normal ranges (*i.e.*, PaO_2, 80–100 mm Hg; $PaCO_2$, 35–45 mm Hg; pH, 7.35–7.45). Likewise, patients who are able to achieve effective breathing patterns will be observed to have a normal respiratory rate, rhythm, and tidal volume. Such patients will have no cough and clear breath sounds on auscultation when demonstrating achievement of successful outcomes for the nursing diagnosis of ineffective airway clearance. Patients who have achieved the outcomes for the nursing diagnosis of infection will be found to be afebrile, will have negative cultures, and will have a normal white blood cell count.

Nutrition

Nutrition is maintained to support the work of the respiratory muscles and promote healing. External alimentation with a small feeding tube is best, but intravenous hyperalimentation (total parenteral nutrition) is instituted if enteral alimentation is not possible. The use of antacids and H_2 blockers to maintain the gastric pH at levels greater than 4 is warranted to prevent stress ulcers. Patients who are able to achieve the desired patient outcomes for altered nutrition: less than body requirements will demonstrate weight gain, an albumin of 3.2 to 4.5 g/dl, a triceps skinfold of 12.0 mm for men or 23.0 mm for women, and a mid-arm circumference of 32.7 cm for men or 29.2 cm for women.

Drug Therapy

Although there are no specific drugs to treat ARDS, several drugs are used to improve ventilation.

Morphine (3–5 mg/hour intravenously) may be used for sedating mechanically ventilated patients who are restless, fearful, and are experiencing tachypnea.

Pancuronium bromide (Pavulon) may be used as a neuroblocking agent to paralyze completely the voluntary respirations of the patient. Dosage must be calculated carefully and individually. The initial dose range for adults is 0.04 to 0.1 mg/kg. Although this drug paralyzes the patient, it does not alter the patient's level of consciousness or relieve pain.

Corticosteroid use is controversial. It is believed by some that corticosteroids help reduce pulmonary edema and stabilize pulmonary membranes by interfering with the inflammatory process and stabilizing lysosomes.

Diuretics are used to keep the patient's PCWP as low as possible without impairing cardiac output. Fluid therapy was discussed previously.

Reduction of Fear and Education

Fearful patients should demonstrate lower levels of fear after instituting nursing measures such as facilitating an effective means of communication; explaining the illness, equipment, and routines; encouraging and supporting the patient; and administering sedative medication as indicated. To evaluate the patient outcomes for the nursing diagnosis of knowledge deficit, patients and their families should be able to verbalize knowledge of the disease process, follow-up treatment, and home care management.

SUMMARY

The adult respiratory distress syndrome is a response of the lung to a variety of severe pulmonary or systemic insults. It is characterized by pulmonary shunting and increasingly stiff, noncompliant lungs. The result is a severe hypoxemia that requires high fractions of inspired oxygen. Successful management of a patient with ARDS depends on early detection of pulmonary abnormalities and prompt treatment. This can be accomplished by identifying patients who are at risk and recognizing the early signs and symptoms. The critical care nurse works within a team of health care providers to implement treatments to assist the patient to recovery or a peaceful death.

DIRECTIONS FOR FUTURE RESEARCH

Nursing is developing into a research-based profession. Research studies are being replicated to develop a practice based on scientific outcomes rather than tradition. This effort has a long way to go, but it must continue to move in this positive direction. Research questions about patients with ARDS that nurses may consider are as follows:[13]

1. What are the effects of patient positioning on the pulmonary functioning of the patient with ARDS?
2. What are the effects of nursing care procedures on the oxygen saturation of patients with ARDS?
3. What are effective nursing interventions for the patient with impaired communication (*e.g.*, related to intubation) to minimize anxiety, helplessness, and pain?
4. What are the most effective, least anxiety-producing techniques for weaning patients with ARDS from ventilators?
5. Can the complications of prolonged use of heparin flush solutions be reduced in arterial lines and intravenous catheters by using saline alone?

REFERENCES

1. Bernard, G. R., and Bradley, R. B. Adult respiratory disease syndrome: Diagnosis and management. *Heart Lung* 15:250, 1986.
2. Bradley, B. R. Adult respiratory distress syndrome. *Focus Crit. Care* 14:48, 1987.
3. Celentano-Norton, L. Mechanical ventilation strategies in adult respiratory distress syndrome. *Crit. Care Nurs.* 6:71, 1986.
4. Cherniack, R. M. *Current Therapy of Respiratory Disease* (2nd ed.). Philadelphia: B. C. Decker, 1986.
5. Fallat, R. J. Respiratory monitoring. *Clin. Chest Med.* 3:181, 1982.
6. Farzan, S. *A Concise Handbook of Respiratory Diseases* (2nd ed.). Reston, VA: Reston Publishing, 1985.
7. Fowler, A. A., Hamman, R. F., and Zerbe, G. O. Adult respiratory distress syndrome: Prognosis after onset. *Am. Rev. Respir. Dis.* 132:472, 1985.
8. George, R. B., Light, R. W., and Matthay, R. A. (eds.). *Chest Physiology.* New York: Churchill-Livingstone, 1983.
9. Gettrust, K. V., Ryan, S. C., and Engelman, D. S. (eds.). *Applied Nursing Diagnosis: Guides for Comprehensive Care Planning.* New York: John Wiley & Sons, 1985.
10. Holloway, N. M. *Nursing the Critically Ill Adult* (3rd ed.). Menlo Park, CA: Addison-Wesley Publishing Co., 1988.
11. Hudak, C. M., Gallo, B. M., and Lohr, T. *Critical Care Nursing* (5th ed.). Philadelphia: J. B. Lippincott, 1990.
12. Kinney, M. R., Packa, D. R., and Dunbar, S. B. *AACN's Clinical Reference for Critical-Care Nursing* (2nd ed.). New York: McGraw-Hill Book Co., 1988.
13. Lewandowski, L. A., and Kositsky, A. M. Research priorities for critical care nursing. *Heart Lung* 12:35, 1983.
14. Martin, L. *Pulmonary Physiology in Clinical Practice: The Essentials for Patient Care and Evaluation.* St. Louis: C. V. Mosby, 1987.
15. Mayo, J. M., and Hamner, J. B. A nurse's guide to mechanical ventilation. *RN.* 50:18, 1987.
16. McCance, K. L., and Huether, S. E. *Pathophysiology: The Biologic Basis for Disease in Adults and Children.* St. Louis: C. V. Mosby, 1990.
17. McDonald, R. B. Validation of three respiratory nursing diagnoses-ineffective airway clearance, ineffective breathing pattern, and impaired gas exchange. *Nurs. Clin. North Am.* 20:697, 1985.
18. Miller, L. G., and Kazemi, H. *Manual of Clinical Pulmonary Medicine.* New York: McGraw-Hill Book Co., 1983.
19. Rieman, M. D., and Wagner, Y. L. Acute respiratory failure. In B. M. Dossey, C. E. Guzzetta, and C. V. Kenner (eds.), *Essentials of Critical Care Nursing: Body-Mind-Spirit.* Philadelphia: J. B. Lippincott, 1990:239–255.
20. Shapiro, B. A., Harrison, R. A., and Trout, C. A. *Clinical Application of Respiratory Care* (3rd ed.). Chicago: Year Book Medical Publishers, 1985.
21. Stevens, J., and Raffin, R. Adult respiratory distress syndrome—etiology, mechanisms, and management. *Postgrad. Med.* 60:505, 1984.
22. Thompson, J. M., McFarland, G. K., Hirsch, J. E., *et al. Mosby's Manual of Clinical Nursing* (2nd ed.). St. Louis: C. V. Mosby, 1989.
23. Whitcombe, M. E. *The Lung: Normal and Diseased.* St. Louis: C. V. Mosby, 1982.
24. Wilson, S. F., and Thompson, J. M. *Respiratory Disorders.* St. Louis: C. V. Mosby, 1990.

21

Acute Respiratory Failure: The Patient With Chronic Obstructive Lung Disease

Martha L. Tyler

TELLING YOUR STORY AS A HEALING RITUAL

Your continuous inner dialogue creates stories. These stories assign meaning to your experiences in life and how you perceive the world. Learning to listen in a new way to the stories that you tell yourself creates the potential for opening new dialogue with yourself. The following are some guidelines to enhance your ability to use your stories as healing events:

- Listen for the themes that bridge one story to the next; listen for the threads of information that weave from one story to the next.
- Learn to listen, and try to recognize if you tell only one side of a story.
- If you tell only one side of a story, can you tell yourself the other side of the story? Often it is viewing the other side of the story that gives new context to your life. It is very easy to identify what is wrong in your life, but when you find the strengths in the current situation, you often gain a new meaning and inner wisdom about your present situation.
- Listen to the stories that your patients, family, colleagues, and friends tell. As you listen to them, become aware of the stories that you construct from what you hear. Also be aware of the insights that are revealed to you. Then if it seems right, have the courage to tell your story and listen to the additional patterns that are revealed to you.

LEARNING OBJECTIVES

After reading this chapter, the nurse should be able to do the following:

1. Define acute respiratory failure.
2. List and explain the physiologic basis of the signs and symptoms of acute respiratory failure.
3. Describe four major pathophysiologic mechanisms of hypoxemia.
4. Describe two pathophysiologic mechanisms of hypercapnia.
5. Compare and contrast methods of oxygen therapy.
6. Describe methods of facilitating secretion clearance.

7. Describe a safe suctioning technique.
8. Assess the success or failure of therapy by interpretation of arterial blood gas values.
9. Assess and intervene appropriately to increase the level of comfort of dyspneic patients.

CASE STUDY
Current Problems

Ms. C., a 59-year-old woman, was admitted to the hospital with a diagnosis of deteriorating chronic obstructive pulmonary disease (COPD). She had been seen in the hospital's chest clinic the day before her admission. Her complaints included increased weakness, fatigue, loss of appetite, and decreased activity tolerance due to short-

Table 21-1
Ms. C.'s Pulmonary Function Test Values

TEST	PERCENT PREDICTED	PERCENT PREDICTED AFTER BRONCHODILATOR
Vital capacity (VC)	52	68
Residual volume (RV)	216	
Total lung capacity (TLC)	111	
Forced expiratory flow (FEF) 25%–75%	8	23
Forced expiratory volume in 1 second (FEV$_1$)	24	28
FEV$_1$/VC ratio	35 (normal > 76%)	
Nitrogen elimination rate	9 (normal < 2.5%)	
Blood gases		
pH 7.48		
PaCO$_2$ 42 mm Hg		
HCO$_3^-$ 28 mEq/L		
PaO$_2$ 51 mm Hg		
SaO$_2$ 86%		
Base excess + 2.8 mEq/L		

ness of breath. She also felt that her secretion clearance was not as effective as usual despite the use of inhaled bronchodilators and steam.

Two weeks before her admission she had attended the clinic, where a recent, sudden weight gain (from 88 to 95 pounds in 2 weeks) and ankle edema (3+) were noted. Although her neck veins were not distended, chest films showed some evidence of pulmonary artery dilatation. Pulmonary heart disease (cor pulmonale) was suspected, and the patient was given digoxin (0.25 mg/day), along with furosemide (40 mg) and potassium chloride (2 teaspoons) daily. On the day before her admission, Ms. C. basically felt no better despite the institution of these medications. Her weight, however, was down to her usual 87 pounds. It was decided that she should be admitted to the hospital the following day for reevaluation of her current medication regimen, possible institution of continuous (home) oxygen therapy, a more thorough workup of her peripheral edema and increased shortness of breath (SOB), and evaluation of her decrease in appetite.

Past Medical History

Ms. C. has a long history of chronic cough with sputum production and progressively worsening shortness of breath. For 4 years she has been observed in the chest clinic for these symptoms. The results of her most recent pulmonary function test are shown in Table 21-1.

Ms. C.'s cough has been productive of approximately 1 cup of grayish mucoid sputum per day; the cough is worse in the morning, but it continues throughout the day. Periodically, she wakes at night with paroxysms of coughing and sputum production. She has a total of 80 to 90 "pack years" of smoking and continues to smoke about 1 pack per day. Until recently she had been able to keep up with her daily housework and had dyspnea only after walking three level blocks. Now, even minimal exertion, such as walking a few yards, makes her so short of breath that she must sit down. Her usual medications and therapies have been theophylline and bronchodilator inhalation every 4 hours and steam inhalation twice daily after the bronchodilator therapy (to loosen secretions).

Family and Social History

Ms. C. was married (once), but she has been separated from her husband for 12 years. She has no children. She has not worked in the past 6 years. Her financial support comes from Medicaid and Supplemental Security Income programs. Her brother lives directly across the street from her and helps her with shopping and heavy household tasks.

Clinical Presentation

Ms. C. was ambulatory when she was admitted to a general medical nursing unit. She was in "no acute distress." The arterial blood gas values, determined on her admission, were a pH of 7.48, a PaCO$_2$ of 41 mm Hg, a bicarbonate (HCO$_3^-$) level of 30 mEq/L, *and a PaO$_2$ of 27 mm Hg on room air.* Apparently, these blood gas values were not believed, because a half hour later a second blood gas analysis was made, again on room air, with the following results: pH 7.48, PaCO$_2$ 45 mm Hg, HCO$_3^-$ 33 mEq/L, and PaO$_2$ 36 mm Hg. On confirmation of the extent of her hypoxemia, Ms. C. was transferred to the medical intensive care unit (MICU). After institution of oxygen therapy at 2 L/minute by nasal cannula, the pH was 7.48, PaCO$_2$ 39 mm Hg, HCO$_3^-$ 28 mEq/L, and PaO$_2$ 47 mm Hg.

Physical Examination

Physical examination revealed a temperature of 36.5°C, blood pressure of 120/70, and a pulse of 88 without postural change. The head, eyes, ears, and throat were remarkable only for bluish mucous membranes. She had clubbing of the fingers and toes and 1 to 2+ ankle edema. Her weight was 87 pounds. Her lungs had significantly decreased breath sounds; there were no crackles, wheezes, or rhonchi. The diaphragm was low and did not move on percussion. There was increased tympany on percussion over the lung fields. A cardiovascular examination showed no venous distention and no murmurs.

Laboratory Data

The pertinent laboratory data were

Hematocrit	63%	Sodium	116
White blood count	9800	Potassium	4.4
Blood urea nitrogen	8	Chloride	70
Glucose	151	CO$_2$	36

The chest film showed hyperinflation compatible with COPD. There were no acute infiltrates. The ECG showed a normal sinus rhythm at a rate of 80 beats/minute. The axis was positive at 102 degrees, P-pulmonale and loss of R-wave forces in leads V$_2$ through V$_6$ were present.

Hospital Course

Ms. C. was transferred to the MICU because of extreme hypoxemia, for monitoring and for institution of a vigorous bronchial hygiene routine. The routine consisted of the inhalation of a bronchodilator from a gas-powered, small volume nebulizer, followed by inhalation of warm, moist air from a heated nebulizer. These procedures were followed by postural drainage and chest percussion to facilitate secretion removal. The treatments were done every 3 hours throughout the day and night in the hope of improving oxygenation by bringing the patient to optimal ventilation-perfusion status and preventing the need for assisted ventilation. Oxygen therapy was increased to 3 L/minute, resulting in a pH of 7.48, a $PaCO_2$ of 54 mm Hg, a HCO_3^- of 39 mEq/L, and a PaO_2 of 76 mm Hg. A subsequent and final adjustment of flow rate to 2.5 L/minute resulted in a pH of 7.47, a $PaCO_2$ of 52 mm Hg, a HCO_3^- of 37 mEq/L, and a PaO_2 of 56 mm Hg. A sputum Gram stain showed numerous polymorphonuclear leukocytes with many gram-negative diplococci. Ms. C. was given penicillin (250 mg four times a day). A phlebotomy was done (300 ml whole blood), lowering her hematocrit to 53. The furosemide and digoxin had been discontinued on her admission. With the bronchial hygiene regimen she was able to bring up large amounts of sputum, and her general condition improved significantly. After 3 days, she was moved from the MICU to a general medical nursing unit. Her bronchial hygiene treatments were reduced to four times a day because of a decrease in sputum production, but her oxygenation did not improve substantially despite what appeared to be optimal therapy. Therefore, it was decided that she would require continuous oxygen therapy to control or prevent further episodes of right-sided heart failure and possibly to permit her to be more active.

During her hospitalization, Ms. C. was examined by the physical medicine and rehabilitation service and was started on a graduated exercise tolerance program that she was to continue as an outpatient. She was told how to do postural drainage at home, and arrangements were made for oxygen to be delivered to her house. The visiting nurse service was contacted to supervise her medications, help in the use of continuous home oxygen therapy, and instruct a family member in chest percussion therapy to be done while the patient was in postural drainage positions. One week after her admission, Ms. C. was discharged ambulatory with oxygen and, once again, with information about the benefits of stopping smoking.[38]

REFLECTIONS

Gas exchange is basic to life. Therefore, the critical care nurse must be completely familiar with the components of normal respiratory function. When the lungs fail, the whole body fails. Patients know this as well as do the medical and nursing personnel caring for them. One needs to have been held under water only once by a too aggressive friend to know the panic that occurs when one's breathing is disrupted. The nurse can simulate the discomfort of the patient who has pulmonary emphysema or asthma by inhaling a large breath and exhaling only part of the breath, keeping the chest fixed at a partially inflated position. The technique simulates air trapping. The nurse should then breathe from the new end-expiratory position. To do so is uncomfortable and anxiety-producing. In fact, it can cause feelings of panic. Respiratory patients are often described as "crabby" and "difficult." Is it any wonder?

Dyspnea, or "shortness" of breath, is, like pain, a subjective symptom.[8,9,26,27,37,60] However, unlike with pain, we are now just beginning to try to find *specific* treatments for dyspnea. Almost all our current therapies for dyspnea are actually therapies for the underlying lung or heart conditions that most often are associated with this noxious symptom. Just as pain signals that something is wrong, so does dyspnea. We do not expect patients to bear pain without therapy while we figure out the basic cause of the pain.

Although some pain therapy is directed primarily at the underlying cause, analgesic and anesthetic medications and other therapies (cutaneous stimulation, biofeedback) focus directly on the control and management of the pain *per se*. In contrast, the treatment of dyspnea has not been widely studied, despite the fact that it is just as devastating as chronic pain in terms of loss of ability to carry out the activities of daily living and, perhaps more important, loss of the joy of life.[19,33,37] We *have* tried for years to alter the breathing pattern of dyspneic patients,[42,50] assuming that because the pattern was not normal[5,11,53] it was dysfunctional, and perhaps contributed to the dyspnea.

It now appears that the majority of dyspneic patients adopt a breathing pattern that results in the least work of breathing and is the least noxious for them.[5] Nurses should assist patients in using their chosen pattern of breathing while attempting to relieve any additional components of anxiety that may add to the patient's distress. Stress-reduction or relaxation techniques may be helpful in individual patients.[19] However, critical care nurses must be careful not to introduce any such technique without first verifying the patient's blood gas status. Intense anxiety and dyspnea often accompany, and are the primary way we recognize, severe, life-threatening hypoxemia.[1] The major concern is the hypoxemia; it must be treated first and promptly with oxygen, ventilation, or both. Then we can turn our efforts to relieving any remaining anxiety and dyspnea.

PHYSIOLOGY

A brief review of respiratory physiology is presented in the following sections.

Functions of the Lung

The major purpose of the respiratory system is to provide oxygen for the combustive process of metabolism and to remove carbon dioxide, a waste product of metabolism, from the body. The secondary functions of the respiratory system are acid–base balance, speech, the expression of emotion (laughing, crying, sighing), and, in a relatively minor way, maintenance of body water and heat balance.

Ventilation

To provide oxygen and remove carbon dioxide, air must be moved into and out of the lungs. The movement of air is properly termed *ventilation*, and the term *respiration* refers to the exchange of gases.[43] Ventilation can occur without effective gas exchange taking place. This is the case in severe ventilation-perfusion mismatch or intrapulmonary shunt. It is also true that only a minimal amount of gas exchange (respiration) can occur without ventilation. In such a situation (ventilatory arrest), gas exchange occurs by passive diffusion until equilibrium is reached between the gases (oxygen and carbon dioxide) in the alveoli and those in the blood. Life can be sustained for only four to six minutes under these circumstances. Therefore, ventilation and respiration are practically synonymous in the clinical setting, although they are defined differently and are separate concepts.

Movement of air into and out of the lung requires coordinated action of the diaphragm and intercostal muscles against a relatively fixed chamber, the rib cage. In addition, the pathway for airflow—the upper and lower (large and small) airways—must be patent. The alveolar-capillary membrane is the site of gas exchange. It must be of adequate size and normal structure for normal diffusion of oxygen and carbon dioxide into and out of the blood.

Control of Breathing

The muscular pump of ventilation is controlled by the central nervous system (CNS), which, in turn, responds to the metabolic needs of the body. Voluntary control of ventilation is also possible and can override metabolically set respiratory rates, resulting, at times, in grossly abnormal blood gases. The CNS receives its input from central and peripheral chemoreceptors that respond to $PaCO_2$, through its effect on brain extracellular fluid pH; and PaO_2 and pH, respectively. The ventilatory response to these humoral stimulants is determined by their combined effect. For example, a decrease in PaO_2 increases ventilation, which, in turn, decreases $PaCO_2$ and raises the pH, thus limiting the overall response to hypoxia. Under usual circumstances, CO_2 is the primary determinant of minute ventilation, and PaO_2 is a secondary determinant.

Perfusion

Another major factor in normal gas exchange is perfusion of the lung by blood that contains normal hemoglobin in adequate amounts. Not only must blood flow through the lungs, there must also be a reasonable match between the distribution of ventilation and perfusion within the lungs. There are different gradients for perfusion and ventilation in the lung owing to the different effects of gravity on lung tissue and blood flow. This phenomenon results in wasted ventilation at the top of the lung and excess perfusion at the bottom.[34,35,61] Nevertheless, overall there is a fairly good match of ventilation and perfusion, resulting in efficient gas exchange.

Measurement of Lung Function

The definitive physiologic indicator of overall pulmonary function is the arterial blood gas values. It is vital that the critical care nurse know the range of normal values for PaO_2, $PaCO_2$, and pH and be able to interpret blood gas test results. Priority must always be given to the PaO_2 value, because hypoxemia is the major cause of the morbidity and mortality associated with respiratory dysfunction. Next, in order of importance, is the pH. A high $PaCO_2$ level is a problem only if it is causing, or is associated with, severe acidemia.

Other tests of pulmonary function are measurements of lung volumes, flow rates, and the distribution and diffusion of gases within and through the lungs. The patient's test results are compared with "normal" or predicted values established for people of the same sex, age, and height. The pattern and degree of deviation from normal and the improvement (if any) after bronchodilator therapy are indications of the pathology that underlies any changes observed.[10]

For example, the pulmonary function tests in Table 21–1 show only a small improvement after bronchodilators were given, indicating that bronchospasm is not a major component of Ms. C.'s airflow obstruction. Additionally, the residual volume (RV) is greatly increased because of air trapping. Together these two facts are evidence that the obstruction is due to parenchymal destruction (emphysema) and airway collapse rather than asthma. The implication for nursing is that there is very little that is reversible about Ms. C.'s condition and that nursing care should emphasize what the patient can do to maintain current levels of function, to decrease symptoms, and enhance life within new and narrowing limits.

DEFINITIONS OF ACUTE RESPIRATORY FAILURE

Acute respiratory failure (ARF) is defined as a rapidly occurring inability of the lungs to maintain adequate oxygenation of the blood with or without impairment of carbon dioxide (CO_2) elimination. ARF is present when there is hypoxemia *with or without* hypercapnia. A clear understanding of ARF results in an ordering of priorities of management and therapy that best protects the patient from permanent damage, disability, or death due to tissue hypoxia in vital organs. The definition is also important because many nurses do not consider the possibility of ARF unless there is gross alteration in ventilation. Closer observation of patients with acute hypoxemia would reveal that many patients actually have an increased minute ventilation and hypocapnia due to hypoxic stimulation of respiratory chemoreceptors.

The arterial blood gas levels that have been used to define ARF objectively are an arterial oxygen tension (PaO_2) of 50 mm Hg or less with or without an elevation of the arterial CO_2 tension ($PaCO_2$) to 50 mm Hg or more.[33,51]

When the major blood gas derangement is an increase in $PaCO_2$, the descriptive terms *acute ventilatory failure* or *hypercapnic respiratory failure* are used. Acute ventilatory failure results in acute respiratory failure if the level of ventilation is so decreased that hypoxemia occurs. *Pulmonary failure* sometimes is used to indicate respiratory failure due specifically to lung disorders. Pulmonary insufficiency is another term that is used as a synonym for acute respiratory failure. *Pulmonary insufficiency* is properly defined, however, as altered function of the lung that produces clinical symptoms, such as dyspnea.[43]

Incidence, Etiologies, and Related Factors

A review of the number and variety of clinical conditions associated with ARF, listed in Table 21–2, reminds us of the high incidence of this potentially life-threatening complication and the vulnerability of patients in the critical care setting. Etiologies and related factors are numerous, but they often include conditions that increase the work of breathing. Examples are bronchospasm and secretion retention, both of which increase the resistance to airflow; and pulmonary edema, which decreases the compliance of the lungs. These conditions also result in poor matching of ventilation and perfusion and intrapulmonary shunting, often requiring an overall increase in ventilation. If energy demands for increased ventilation exceed the supply of oxygen and nutritional substrates, the respiratory muscles will become fatigued and be unable to maintain the level of ventilation necessary to support normal gas exchange; ARF will occur.[2,5,44,49] As a corollary, clinical conditions causing malnutrition, anemia, and low cardiac output put critically ill patients at added risk for ARF, particularly if their underlying lung function is abnormal.[13]

Psychopathophysiology

Mechanisms of Hypoxia and Hypercapnia

From the definition of acute respiratory failure it is evident that any cause of hypoxemia or hypercapnia is potentially a cause of ARF. There are four major pathophysiologic mechanisms causing hypoxemia: hypoventilation, diffusion (or gas transfer) impairment, ventilation-perfusion ($\dot{V}A/\dot{Q}$) mismatch, and right-to-left shunt. It is impossible to separate diffusion impairment from $\dot{V}A/\dot{Q}$ mismatch in the clinical setting. Diffusion impairment is seldom a cause of hypoxemia at rest. Therefore, there are only three pathophysiologic causes of hypoxemia that are of practical importance: hypoventilation, $\dot{V}A/\dot{Q}$ mismatch, and intrapulmonary shunt.[34,35,61] The two mechanisms that produce hypercapnia are hypoventilation and $\dot{V}A/\dot{Q}$ inequality. In clinical practice hypoventilation is the major cause of hypercapnia; however, $\dot{V}A/\dot{Q}$ inequality does add to the carbon dioxide retention seen in the later stages of diseases associated with low $\dot{V}A/\dot{Q}$ ratios.

In addition to the four primary causes of a low PaO_2, a fifth cause of hypoxemia is possible. At high altitudes, the inspired oxygen tension or pressure (PIO_2) is reduced owing to the lower barometric pressure. The reduction results in a low alveolar oxygen tension (PAO_2), which in turn lowers the PaO_2, and hypoxemia results. The clinical effect of this phenomenon is that patients living at high altitudes are more at risk of ARF than those at sea level, because they start at an already lowered PaO_2. The PIO_2 is also reduced when the person breathes mixtures with a low oxygen concentration. This circumstance occurs infrequently and is usually the result of an error in valving systems during the administration of anesthetic gases.

Oxygen Transport

Although hypoxemia and hypoventilation are major factors in acute respiratory failure, the critical care nurse must not forget that oxygen transport to the tissues also requires an adequate supply of hemoglobin that has normal oxygen-carrying characteristics, as well as an adequate cardiac output for distribution of oxygenated blood to the tissues. Anemia is a particularly serious problem in the patient who has a low PaO_2 due to lung disease. In such a patient, both the oxygen-carrying capacity and the ability to load oxygen are impaired. If there is also a low cardiac output (circulatory failure), tissue oxygen delivery is even more impaired. Such patients require skillful management in a critical care unit.

Emotions and Respiration

The respiratory system is intimately involved with emotional expression. Without the ability to breathe, we cannot laugh, shout, scream, or communicate in the way that makes us unique among animals. The physiologic consequences of intense emotions—anger, hatred, love, sorrow—include an increase in oxygen consumption due to catecholamine-induced

Table 21–2
Clinical Conditions Associated With Acute Respiratory Failure

Central nervous system (CNS) depression
  Drug overdose—self-administered or iatrogenic
    Barbiturates, narcotics, tranquilizers
    Uncontrolled high-flow oxygen therapy
  CNS infection
  Cerebral vascular accidents
  Head injury
Chest wall and respiratory muscle dysfunction
  Trauma
    Flail chest, diaphragmatic rupture, phrenic nerve transection
  Defect in neuromuscular transmission
    Disease states:
      Myasthenia gravis, muscular dystrophy, Guillain-Barré syndrome, poliomyelitis, spinal cord injury, amyotrophic lateral sclerosis, multiple sclerosis, botulism, tetanus
      Postoperative diaphragm dysfunction[18]
    Drug effects or side effects:
      Aminoglycosides, curare-like drugs
  Thoracic surgery
  Subdiaphragmatic abscess
  Fatigue of inspiratory muscles
Restrictive defect:
  Pulmonary: generalized:
    Interstitial fibrosis
    Infiltrative lung disease
    Diffuse atelectasis or acute respiratory distress syndrome (ARDS)
    Pulmonary edema (cardiogenic or noncardiogenic, ARDS)
  Pulmonary: localized:
    Pleural space alteration (pneumothorax, hemothorax, effusion, emphysema)
    Pulmonary embolism
    Pneumonia
    Local atelectasis (focal, segmental, lobar)
  Extrapulmonary:
    Kyphoscoliosis
    Ascites
    Intestinal distention (ileus)
    Obesity
    Pain
    Immobility
Obstructive defect:
  Upper airway:
    Severe maxillofacial injury
    Neoplasia
    Laryngeal edema
    Prolapsed tongue
    Foreign objects
  Lower airway:
    Foreign objects
    Tracheal stenosis or collapse
    Bronchoconstriction
    Retained secretions, mucus plugging
    Bronchial wall edema
    Airway collapse
    Neoplasia

increases in metabolism. Patients with severe respiratory dysfunction, particularly those with *chronic* dysfunction who cannot increase ventilation in response to such challenges, soon learn to control and limit their emotional repertoire, often by isolating themselves emotionally.[14,15] Families need reassurance that the patient has not stopped caring but is now less able to demonstrate affection. Nurses must also recognize that these patients often will not respond to them in an open, grateful manner. The emotion costs them too much. Also, we often cannot relieve them of the burden of dyspnea—a frustrating situation for both patient and caregiver. Mutual withdrawal frequently is the result.

Loss of self-esteem due to changes in life-style imposed by dyspnea often results in or is associated with significant depression.[14,15] Accurate diagnosis and treatment of the depression may be confounded by the restlessness, confusion, and anxiety that accompany the sudden changes in oxygenation that occur when ARF is superimposed on long-standing respiratory dysfunction. However, all patients deserve relief of depression if possible, and nurses should alert physicians to patients who exhibit symptoms.

NURSING PROCESS

ASSESSMENT

The assessment of patients with acute respiratory failure requires a systematic approach so that all signs, symptoms (defining characteristics), and related factors are identified.[22] If a careful assessment is done and recorded, the selection of *appropriate* interventions is both facilitated and documented in one step. Arterial blood gas levels are the major defining characteristics of this condition and give immediate objective information about the ability of the lungs to provide oxygen and remove carbon dioxide from the arterial blood.[1,33,35] The degree and possible mechanisms of ARF are immediately apparent from the direction and amount the PaO_2 or the $PaCO_2$ deviates from normal. If the $PaCO_2$ is elevated, hypoventilation is at least a partial cause of the hypoxemia. Calculation of the alveolar gas equation permits a quick estimate of the contribution of hypoventilation to any hypoxemia present. If hypoventilation is not the sole cause of hypoxemia, the alveolar-arterial oxygen ($P[A - a]O_2$) difference will be larger than normal. Increased $P(A - a)O_2$ values can be caused by either shunt of low $\dot{V}A/\dot{Q}$ ratios. The response of the PaO_2 to oxygen therapy allows one to separate shunt from $\dot{V}A/\dot{Q}$ abnormalities as the cause of hypoxemia. One hundred percent oxygen breathing is not needed to get a clinical indication of the presence of shunt. If the PaO_2 remains below 100 mm Hg when the inspired oxygen fraction is 0.3 to 0.4, shunted blood is contributing significantly to the hypoxemia.[6,7,34,35]

Sorting out the contribution of the various pathophysiologic causes of hypoxemia allows formulation of a more specific plan of care. For instance, if there is little response to oxygen therapy, intrapulmonary shunt is the mechanism, perhaps caused by a localized pneumonia. Since pneumonia is not primarily an airway disease, secretion-clearance therapies, such as chest physical therapy, are unnecessary in most patients with pneumonia.[21] Instead, nursing actions should center on accurate administration of antibiotic drugs and positioning the patient to maximize blood flow to the most normal areas of the lung. In the case of a unilateral pneumonia in the right lung, this means placing the normal, or left, lung down.[35,62]

Clinical Signs and Symptoms of ARF

More important than the mechanics of the assessment is the ability to recognize the clinical signs and symptoms or defining characteristics of ARF. ARF cannot be diagnosed unless its presence is suspected. The clinical signs and symptoms of ARF fall into three categories: pulmonary, cardiovascular, and neurologic.

Pulmonary Signs and Symptoms

Pulmonary symptoms can be misleadingly mild or even absent. Dyspnea, usually assumed to be a classic symptom of ARF or hypoxemia, is often absent despite marked hypoxemia. Remember the *blue bloater*, or *type B*, patients with COPD. Blue bloaters seldom complain of dyspnea or "look" short of breath because they may have a blunted respiratory drive. The reverse can also be true—marked dyspnea (with close to normal blood gas levels) is often observed in *pink puffer, or type A*, patients. Dyspnea is a subjective symptom that appears to correlate more frequently with disturbances in the stretch receptors of the lung or with a person's feeling that the work of breathing is inappropriate to the situation than with blood gas disturbances. To illustrate, people expect to be "short of breath" after having run hard to catch a bus, and they seldom consider the feeling a particularly noxious one. However, patients who have increased work of breathing even while at rest (*e.g.*, during chronic COPD or an asthmatic attack) interpret the symptom as undesirable and uncomfortable, even though their minute ventilation during the attack may be less than that required to run for a bus.

An increased respiratory rate, a paradoxical breathing pattern, and respiratory alternans all have been described as signs of respiratory muscle fatigue and impending ventilatory failure.[11] Other authors contend that these signs are a response to an increase in inspiratory load or work of breathing and that they do not imply respiratory muscle fatigue is also present.[55] Nevertheless, these signs do indicate an abnormal condition that should be corrected, making them important in assessment and monitoring. A respiratory rate over 25 is unusual in adults[51,52,53,56] and rates over 35 should be investigated immediately with blood gases, as should paradoxical breathing and respiratory alternans. *Paradoxical breathing* is a pattern in which the abdomen sinks rather than rises during inspiration. During *respiratory alternans*, the intercostal (and accessory) muscles and the diaphragm work alternately rather than synchronously. Normally, the diaphragm is the largest contributor to ventilation; however, when it becomes fatigued, the inspiratory intercostals, with the help of the accessory muscles of breathing, take over for several breaths, apparently to rest the diaphragm.[47]

The presence of cough and sputum production are often thought of as defining characteristics of ARF or hypoxemia, but, more logically, they should be considered etiologies or related factors. If sputum *retention* occurs, the nursing diagnosis is ineffective airway clearance (IAC).[1] Cough and sputum production may increase, or they may decrease. A sudden *decrease* in sputum production in patients who have chronic bronchitis with daily sputum expectoration is often a more serious indication of impending ARF than is a sudden increase in cough and sputum production. Decreased sputum expectoration may indicate that secretion retention is occurring, which in turn will cause hypoxemia due to an increase in $\dot{V}A/\dot{Q}$ inequality. The retained secretions fill the airways and decrease airflow, creating areas of low $\dot{V}A/\dot{Q}$ throughout the lung and causing an increase in the work of breathing.

Cardiovascular Signs and Symptoms

The presence or absence of cardiovascular signs of acute respiratory failure is determined by the amount of tissue hypoxia present. When arterial oxygenation falls, the usual response is to increase cardiac output to bring more oxygen to the myocardium and other vital tissues. Therefore, tachycardia and bounding pulses are often seen in hypoxemia. Dysrhythmias may develop if hypoxemia is severe and cardiovascular compensation is inadequate to prevent myocardial hypoxia. Both supraventricular and ventricular dysrhythmias occur as frequently in ARF complicating COPD as they do in myocardial infarction.[24] Changes in the transmembrane action potential in cardiac conducting tissue can result from hypoxemia, increased $PaCO_2$, and changes in pH (not associated with changes in $PaCO_2$). In this setting, dysrhythmias can be caused by a change in automaticity of the conducting tissue, the development of a reentry circuit, or both.[24]

Coldness of the extremities is another cardiovascular sign of hypoxemia. Peripheral vasoconstriction is a homeostatic mechanism by which blood is shunted from the extremities to vital organs. In contrast (but equally homeostatic), cerebral arteries dilate as hypoxemia and hypercapnia increase, often resulting in the symptom of headache. If acidemia occurs in addition to hypoxemia, then peripheral, renal, and coronary artery dilatation result. Diaphoresis is seen in this setting.

Cyanosis is an unreliable sign of hypoxemia. Many patients in ARF are severely hypoxemic without evidence of cyanosis. Cyanosis does not appear until at least 5 g of hemoglobin per 100 ml of blood are reduced (deoxygenated). This means that even with severe hypoxemia the anemic patient may not appear cyanotic, whereas the patient with polycythemia may appear cyanotic when his or her PaO_2 is normal. Added to these physiologic variables is the subjective nature of the observation. Central cyanosis is a more reliable sign of low PaO_2, but it also may be a result of low cardiac output independent of a low PaO_2. The principle should be to investigate (by analyzing an arterial blood gas sample) any patient with generalized cyanosis while remembering that the *absence* of cyanosis does not guarantee normoxemia.

Fatigue is a symptom that many persons with COPD report as they slip into ARF. Whether fatigue appears depends on the ability of the cardiovascular system to compensate for the low PaO_2.

Neurologic Signs and Symptoms

Central nervous system signs of ARF include restlessness, agitation, confusion, somnolence, and coma. Headache is also frequent, as noted. Sometimes families report subtle personality changes in the patient as the first sign of decreasing cerebral oxygenation. Any patient exhibiting changes in mentation should be assessed carefully.

NURSING DIAGNOSES, PATIENT OUTCOMES, AND NURSING ORDERS

The preceding material on physiology, nursing assessment, and diagnostic tests guides the nurse in establishing nursing diagnoses, patient outcomes, and plans for the patient with ARF.

NURSING CARE PLAN SUMMARY   Patient With ARF

NURSING DIAGNOSIS

1. Impaired gas exchange: Hypoxemia (demonstrated by PaO_2 or SaO_2 values) related to hypoventilation (demonstrated by increased $PaCO_2$) or absence of ventilation (apnea) (exchanging pattern)

Patient Outcomes	Nursing Orders
1. Hypoxemia will be absent or improved.	1. Encourage and help the patient to cough and clear mucus.
2. Excessive secretions will not obstruct the upper or lower airways.	2. Use suctioning as needed to stimulate cough and clear upper and lower (central) airway secretions.
3. The tongue will not obstruct the comatose patient's airway.	3. Position the comatose patient in a way that helps prevent aspiration.
4. The $PaCO_2$ will be maintained in a range normal for the patient.	4. Change the position of comatose and ventilated patients every hour to promote the clearance of secretions from the peripheral airways.
5. If ventilatory failure is present, the patient will respond appropriately to mechanical ventilation.	5. Auscultate the patient's breath sounds regularly to assess the need for and effectiveness of suctioning (indicated by presence or absence of rhonchi), any development of or change in wheezing, the sudden absence of breath sounds (for example, pneumothorax), and any development of or change in rales (also termed *crackles*), e.g., pulmonary edema.
	6. Record the objective measures of ventilation: $PaCO_2$, rate, minute ventilation.

(continued)

NURSING CARE PLAN SUMMARY   *Patient With ARF   Continued*

Patient Outcomes	*Nursing Orders*
	7. Note and record regularly the character of respirations (paradoxic, alternans, shallow, pursed lips).
	8. Support the patient in the position that best facilitates respiration and relieves dyspnea.
	9. Check ventilator settings for accuracy and check the *alarm system* every hour.
	10. Ensure *constant* observation of patients who are apneic without ventilatory support (*e.g.*, head injury, paralysis, respiratory muscle fatigue).
	11. Monitor and record changes in patient's response to mechanical ventilation.
	12. Relieve anxiety by explaining the purpose and expected outcomes of mechanical ventilation to patient and family.
	13. Provide intubated patients with a means of communication.

NURSING DIAGNOSIS

2. *Impaired gas exchange: Hypoxemia related to ventilation-perfusion mismatch or intrapulmonary shunt (blood gas data) (exchanging pattern)*

Patient Outcomes	*Nursing Orders*
1. The patient will be free of the signs and symptoms of tissue hypoxia.	1. Observe patients constantly for changes in mental, cardiac, or pulmonary status that indicate hypoxemia: confusion, restlessness, disorientation, headache, unconsciousness, tachycardia, peripheral vasoconstriction, diaphoresis, central cyanosis, hypotension, increased dyspnea.
2. The breath sounds will be free of wheezing, crackles (rales), and gurgles (rhonchi).	2. Assume responsibility for recording blood gas values, *including* the corresponding FiO_2 or liter flow, PEEP level, patient position (right or left lateral decubitus, sitting, supine, or prone).
3. If hypoxemia is refractory to usual therapies, the patient will respond appropriately to end-expiratory pressure, with mechanical ventilation (PEEP) or without (CPAP).	3. Check patient's hemoglobin/hematocrit level.
	4. Monitor O_2 therapy equipment to ensure that the necessary liter flow or concentration is maintained.
	5. Observe patients regularly for correct placement of O_2 cannula, catheter, mask, or T-piece connection.
	6. Observe the ventilator pressure dial to ensure maintenance of PEEP.
	7. Turn and reposition patients frequently to promote ventilation of dependent areas of the lung.
	8. Prevent unnecessary increases in the work of breathing and O_2 consumption by limiting or requiring patients to be active only to their tolerance level and by promoting emotional stability by explaining procedures and offering reassurance frequently.
	9. Ensure delivery of bronchodilator medications:
	A. Administer at scheduled intervals.
	B. Make sure patients receive the entire dose when drugs are given by nebulizer.
	C. Monitor and record response to therapy (*e.g.*, decreased wheezing, improved breath sounds or improved FEV_1, or peak flows) after bronchodilator administration.
	10. Maintain adequate hydration to facilitate liquefaction of secretions.
	A. Observe skin, mucous membranes, and sputum viscosity for signs of dehydration.
	B. Record total system intake and output (oral, parenteral, urinary, upper and lower gastrointestinal tract).
	C. Weigh patients and record weight daily.
	D. Monitor equipment used to hydrate the respiratory tract (humidifiers and nebulizers).

NURSING CARE PLAN SUMMARY Patient With ARF Continued

NURSING DIAGNOSIS
3. *Self-care deficit related to dyspnea and hypoxemia (and possibly depression)*
(moving pattern)

Patient Outcomes	Nursing Orders

1. Patient will gradually resume self-care.
2. Dyspnea will be resolved, or patients will report dyspnea has been reduced to usual levels.
3. Hypoxemia will be improved or absent.
4. Patient will report a decrease in anxiety.
	1. Confirm or introduce pursed-lip breathing; otherwise make *no* attempt to change the rate or pattern of breathing (inspiratory-to-expiratory time ratio, abdominal-diaphragmatic breathing).
	2. Maintain adequate cardiac output. Support cardiac function as necessary to ensure O_2 delivery to tissues.
	3. Maintain adequate nutrition.
	  A. Monitor weight, skinfold thickness, and midarm circumference for true tissue weight loss or gain.
	  B. Provide dyspneic patients with small, frequent, high-calorie, high-protein feedings.
	  C. Institute supplemental (gastric or parenteral) feedings *early* if patient is too fatigued to eat.
	  D. Do not give *excess* calories as this will increase CO_2 production and add to the ventilatory load.
	  E. If patients have trouble swallowing after prolonged intubation, arrange for speech therapist to evaluate and help reestablish proper swallowing sequence.
	4. Prevent loss of physical function.
	  A. Use proper positioning and footboards as necessary.
	  B. Make sure patients do (or receive) full range of motion exercises as indicated.
	  C. Help patients to ambulate as soon as possible; ventilatory support can be maintained with self-inflating bag (oxygen-enriched) for short walks.
	  D. Assist patients to chair if they cannot walk.
	5. Support psychologic function.
	  A. Limit sensory stimulation for dyspneic patients.
	  B. Support the coping mechanisms the patient has developed.
	  C. Reduce stress and anxiety by talking often with patients about procedures, dates, time, place, and names of staff and their specific roles and functions.
	  D. Allow patients to express anger, frustration, and fear without withdrawing from them.
	  E. Provide uninterrupted periods for family visits.

IMPLEMENTATION AND EVALUATION

Critical care nurses have a direct role, often shared with respiratory therapists, in the management of patients with ARF. Rapid changes in status are common in this condition, requiring continuous, knowledgeable surveillance by the nurse and frequent adjustment of both medical and nursing orders.

Emergency Care

The priorities set for the treatment of acute respiratory failure are based on the severity and duration of hypoxemia or hypercapnia. If the PaO_2 is less than 20 mm Hg, death due to cardiorespiratory arrest will usually occur within minutes. Oxygen must be administered immediately. In this situation, do not be concerned about low-flow versus high-flow oxygen in any patient, even the patient with COPD. Cerebral and myocardial hypoxia causes death in minutes. If hypoventilation is also present or becomes a problem during therapy, ventilation must be assisted. Resuscitation without oxygen is, of course, less satisfactory than assisted ventilation using a well-fitting bag-mask resuscitator with an oxygen reservoir, but time should not be wasted getting one. Mouth-to-mouth resuscitation should be begun immediately. However, if oxygen is available and attempts at mouth-to-mouth breathing are unsuccessful (or endotracheal intubation attempts are prolonged), the highest possible concentration of oxygen should be delivered to the patient's nose and mouth. Diffusion of gases is possible even if ventilation is not taking place, provided the upper airway is not occluded by foreign objects, edema, or a prolapsed tongue.

If hypoxemia is severe, there is almost always an increase in $PaCO_2$ due to hypoventilation caused by hypoxia of the respiratory centers or $\dot{V}_A/\dot{Q}$ inequality. Acute CO_2 retention causes profound acidemia. In addition, lactic acid is produced during anaerobic metabolism, which occurs when tissue hypoxia is severe and prolonged. The result is a combined metabolic and respiratory acidosis. Correction of the ventilation and oxygen defects will reverse the acid–base abnormalities. When correction of hypercapnia and hypoxemia is delayed, bicarbonate is sometimes administered to control acidemia.[3,20] One can "buy time" in acidemia but not in hypoxemia—the hypoxemia must be corrected with supplemental oxygen, improved ventilation, or both.

General Principles of Management

Once life-threatening alterations in blood gas tensions have been controlled or if the presenting situation is less critical, the general rules for management of ARF are to maintain or provide an open airway, to maintain an adequate PaO_2 at the lowest possible fraction of inspired oxygen, to maintain acid–base status within a clinically acceptable range, usually a pH of 7.35 to 7.45, to support cardiac output as necessary, to ensure adequate hemoglobin, and to give appropriate therapy to the underlying disease process.[4,28,34,42,48]

Blood gas levels not only are diagnostic in acute respiratory failure, but also are the basis of monitoring the efficacy of treatment and resolution of the underlying disease process. The cause of hypoxemia in ARF is often bronchospasm, inflammatory edema of the airway, or retained secretions. These conditions usually are at least partially reversible and require relatively simple methods of treatment. With therapy there is often an improvement in oxygenation; however, the *primary* treatment for hypoxemia is the administration of oxygen.

Oxygen Therapy

The basic rule for oxygen administration is to use the lowest amount of oxygen enrichment (FiO_2 or liter flow) that produces an acceptable SaO_2. Adhering to this rule prevents pulmonary oxygen toxicity, a time- and dose-related phenomenon. Oxygen toxicity should never occur as a result of oxygen therapy in the treatment of hypoxemia due to hypoventilation or $\dot{V}A/\dot{Q}$ inequality, since in these situations hypoxemia can be corrected with low FiO_2. The conditions with the highest risk for pulmonary oxygen toxicity are those associated with large intrapulmonary shunts (severe pneumonia, ARDS), because they are much less responsive to oxygen administration.[4,7,28,34,35,61]

A patient's response to a particular FiO_2 can be used to determine roughly the amount of shunt present or, conversely, if the percentage of shunt is known, to predict the FiO_2 required to obtain, if possible, an adequate PaO_2.[6]

For example, if the PaO_2 is less than 100 mm Hg when the FiO_2 is 0.3 to 0.4—around 6 L/minute by nasal cannula—a significant part of the hypoxemia is due to shunt. Also, if an increase in FiO_2 to 1.0 produces little increase in PaO_2, the shunt is 50% (or greater).[6] Despite the threat of oxygen toxicity, sometimes very high inspired oxygen tensions are required and *must be used* to preserve life until the underlying process is resolved.

Ventilatory maneuvers such as continuous positive airway pressure (CPAP) or positive end-expiratory pressure (PEEP) that are helpful in allowing a reduction in FiO_2 in ARDS (see Chap. 20) are seldom helpful in COPD because of the differences in the underlying disease process. However, it is unusual for COPD patients to require a high FiO_2 although it may be required when such patients have severe pneumonia. Resolution of the pneumonia usually occurs quickly enough that oxygen toxicity is not a concern, even though a high FiO_2 must be used for a while.

Nearly complete oxygen saturation (90% to 94%) is desirable, but this goal is not possible in some patients. The patient with pre-existing carbon dioxide retention who "can't" or "doesn't" respond to increased carbon dioxide levels is often, but not always, the patient who retains carbon dioxide when given oxygen.[35,42] These patients rely on hypoxic stimuli to drive ventilation instead of carbon dioxide. In most people, the hypoxic stimulus to ventilation is not very strong until the PaO_2 falls below 60 mm Hg.[34,35] When high concentrations of oxygen are administered to patients depending on a low PaO_2 to stimulate ventilation, the PaO_2 may be raised past their threshold of hypoxic stimulation. Blunting of the hypoxic drive occurs, alveolar ventilation falls, and carbon dioxide retention increases. The problem is avoided in almost all COPD patients with carbon dioxide retention by the administration of low doses of oxygen. A safe starting point is 2 liters per minute by nasal cannula or 24% to 28% oxygen by Venturi mask. The PaO_2 need be raised only to 60 mm Hg, since this level will provide a saturation of about 90% to 92%.

Careful monitoring of blood gases during the institution of oxygen therapy in the COPD patient with chronic carbon dioxide retention is mandatory, but often the benefits gained from the relief of hypoxemia (*e.g.*, increased mental ability and, therefore, increased cooperation with treatment) offset modest increases in $PaCO_2$.

Increases in $PaCO_2$ are clinically insignificant *unless* acidemia with a pH less than 7.3 occurs. Oxygen therapy should *never* be discontinued abruptly if unacceptable acidemia due to carbon dioxide retention does occur. This is so because ventilation will have decreased with relief of the hypoxemia, and before it can pick up again (when the oxygen is removed), the alveolar oxygen concentration and, consequently, the PaO_2 will fall rapidly as oxygen consumption exceeds the oxygen being supplied by the reduced ventilation. Reducing the oxygen flow to 1 to 1.5 L/minute will usually maintain a safe PaO_2 and reverse the rise in $PaCO_2$.

Oxygen Delivery Methods

Oxygen delivered by nasal cannula results in a varied FiO_2, depending on the flow rate used and the patient's rate, depth, and pattern of inspiration. Rapid, gasping inspirations result in a lower inspired FiO_2, at the same oxygen flow rate, than that achieved during a "quieter," less tachypneic respiratory pattern. This is so because the inspired oxygen is diluted by more room air in the first situation than in the second.[4,7,35] It is tempting for nurses to tell such patients to inspire slowly and deeply. However, studies have shown that patients cannot or will not maintain this kind of breathing pattern because it increases the work of breathing[5] and brings them closer to respiratory muscle failure. A calm, supportive presence while assisting the patient to a position of comfort, usually seated with arms supported on the overbed table, is recommended.

Despite the variations in FiO_2 obtained with the cannula, it is usually possible to achieve satisfactory levels of oxygenation in the majority of hypoxemic patients. In addition, it is easier for the patient to cough out secretions, eat, and communicate when a cannula is used rather than a mask.[4,30,42] Mouth breathing is not a contraindication for use of a nasal cannula to deliver low-flow oxygen. Studies have shown that the inspired PO_2 is at least as high in "mouth breathers" as in those breathing through the nose (if not higher).[30] Nasal oxygen catheters are capable of delivering approximately the same FiO_2 as are cannulas, but because of associated discomfort and the possibility of misplacement into the esophagus and resultant gastric distention, catheters should be avoided. A possible candidate for their use is the restless patient who frequently dislodges the cannula.

In cases in which a cannula does not provide adequate oxygenation, the use of oxygen masks or even intubation is required. These modes of delivery are usually necessary when shunt is the underlying mechanism of hypoxemia. Examples of disease processes causing shunt are pneumonia and ARDS (see Chap. 20). When a mask is used, the oxygen flow must be high enough to wash exhaled carbon dioxide from the mask; usually flows greater than 6 liters per minute are necessary. The adequacy of the washout can be monitored by following the $PaCO_2$. A mask with a reservoir bag (rebreathing or nonrebreathing) provides higher concentrations of oxygen than does the simple mask because it has 100% oxygen "stored" in the reservoir. For efficient use of such a mask, the oxygen flow into the mask must be high enough to prevent the reservoir bag from collapsing on inhalation. When a patient requires extremely high percentages of oxygen, no external system is stable enough to guarantee consistent oxygen therapy, and intubation becomes necessary, even though assisted ventilation may not be contemplated. Heated, moisturized, and oxygen-enriched gas can then be delivered *directly* to the lungs from a nebulizer. Most nebulizers are equipped with a diluter that, without modification, provides 40%, 70%, or 100% oxygen through a large-bore tube and a T-piece adapter attached to the endotracheal or tracheostomy tube. It should be remembered that at high concentrations of oxygen (70% to 100%), little air is entrained through the diluter. Thus, the patient's inspiratory flow rates may exceed the flow capabilities of the nebulizer. In a tachypneic patient, the inspiratory flow rate may sometimes be in the range of 50 or 60 L/second, and so even running the nebulizer at flush will not prevent dilution of the inspired gas with room air drawn in from the open (exhalation) side of the T connector. The dilution can be controlled by adding tubing on the exhalation side of the T piece. The extra tubing is filled with gas from the constant flow of the nebulizer and acts as an oxygen reservoir.[35] It does not act as dead space, because the flow of gas through the tubing from the nebulizer also flushes exhaled carbon dioxide out of the tubing and prevents the patient from rebreathing the carbon dioxide.

Adjunctive Therapies

Elimination of retained secretions often results in improved oxygenation. However, some methods used to clear airway secretions are themselves associated with falls in PaO_2. It has been known for several years that endotracheal suctioning can cause serious hypoxemia.[16] It is less well known, however, that nasotracheal (NT) suctioning causes similar falls in oxygenation. These falls have been observed to occur despite a preoxygenation regimen (100% oxygen by way of bag-mask resuscitator) that prevents hypoxemia when used in conjunction with endotracheal (ET) suctioning.[41] NT suctioning probably interrupts ventilation longer than does ET suctioning because of the difficulty in passing the catheter through the larynx, coughing and gagging, and the patient's tendency to hold his or her breath when the airway is being manipulated. To eliminate or lessen some of these problems, a nasopharyngeal airway is useful in guiding the catheter more consistently to the glottis and in protecting the nasal mucous membranes from repeated trauma.[35,59] The airway is lubricated with anesthetic jelly before it is inserted; it can be left in place for several days. In addition to the use of the nasopharyngeal

airway and preoxygenation, the patient's usual oxygen therapy should not be discontinued; in fact, it should be increased temporarily during suctioning so that any air that is inspired contains a high percentage of oxygen. The duration of suctioning should also be controlled strictly and limited to no more than 15 seconds.[45]

One of the common fallacies in the management of secretion problems in ARF is that once a patient is intubated, there need be no more concern about secretion retention because suctioning is "easy" and "effective" when an artificial airway is in place. *A good cough is always better than suctioning.* Suction catheters reach only the central airways, frequently only the right side. Also, cough is less effective when the patient is intubated. For these reasons, intubation for secretion control should always be a last resort unless a patient is completely obtunded, has no gag reflex, and must have the airway protected.

Postural Drainage

When secretion retention is a problem, drainage of secretions from peripheral airways is facilitated by changes in position that elevate the usually gravity-dependent portions of the lung (*e.g.*, the posterior basal segments of both lower lobes of the supine patient). Probably the best drainage of these segments occurs when the patient lies prone with the hips raised or with the bed in Trendelenburg's position; however, side-lying positions often appear equally effective. Changes in amount and location of air in the lung at end expiration (FRC) are thought to be mechanisms associated with the increased flow of secretions during postural drainage.[35,36]

Frequent position changes to prevent pressure sores have long been a part of nursing management. That frequent position changes are also effective in secretion management and gas exchange in the lung is less well known. However, "routine" position changes or "routine" postural drainage may also be associated with falls in oxygenation. Falls in PaO_2 were seen in almost all the subjects receiving routine postural drainage in two studies done in seriously ill patients.[12,57,58] One explanation for the fall in PaO_2 is that when a patient with a unilateral lung infiltrate (*e.g.*, the patient with single lobe pneumonia) is turned so that the affected lung is dependent, an increase in venous admixture and a consequent fall in the PaO_2 can occur.[62] This is so because blood flow is increased in the dependent lung owing to gravity; therefore, more blood passes the area of the infiltrate, where there is poor or no ventilation, resulting in an increase in venous admixture. This physiologically predictable result was seen in one of the studies just cited[58]; however, because some of the subjects without localized infiltrates also had falls in PaO_2 during postural drainage, other mechanisms of hypoxemia must also have been operative. Because drainage is definitely not facilitated when a lung with a unilateral infiltrate is dependent, use of this position should be minimized. Simply increasing the FiO_2 may not overcome the problem, because the fall in PaO_2 is often due to increased intrapulmonary shunt, which, by definition, is minimally responsive to oxygen therapy. Patients who have signs of hypoxemia or who are significantly distressed during postural drainage or when they are in a particular position should have their blood gases analyzed while in that position.

Commentary on Case Study

Some of the principles of nursing and medical management are illustrated in the following discussion of the case study presented earlier in this chapter. Therapy for ARF is always adapted to the particular cause of the failure, so this case highlights those aspects of ARF therapy pertinent to patients with underlying COPD.

Pulmonary Function Tests

Ms. C.'s pulmonary function tests were typical of severe COPD, with striking decreases in FEV_1, FEV_1/VC, and FEF 25% to 75%. The apparent restriction noted in the vital capacity (51% of predicted) is not true restrictive lung disease, because the total lung capacity is 111% of that predicted. Although restrictive and obstructive diseases can occur together, more often the small vital capacity seen in COPD is a function of the significant increase in the residual volume (in this case 216% of predicted) due to air trapping (see Chap. 19). Further evidence of air trapping is seen in the nitrogen elimination rate, which is prolonged. Slow washout of nitrogen from the lung indicates that there are areas of lung with very poor communication with the outside.[10] These areas of low $\dot{V}A/\dot{Q}$ are also responsible for the patient's hypoxemia.

The FEV_1 is also greatly reduced. Patients with this degree of airflow obstruction have a very limited ability to increase their ventilatory rate to meet increased metabolic demands. They cannot be hurried through procedures; simple activities of daily living, such as bathing, require more time than usual because the patients must pace themselves.[1,28,48,51]

Arterial Blood Gases

Without any knowledge of Ms. C.'s history, one would conclude from the evaluation of her blood gas levels (on admission and those reported earlier in conjunction with her pulmonary function tests) that Ms. C. had mild alkalemia due to metabolic alkalosis. Diuretics taken without sufficient chloride replacement result in metabolic alkalosis and a compensatory elevation of the $PaCO_2$. However, Ms. C. also has severe airflow obstruction (FEV_1 24% of predicted), so it is more likely that the HCO_3^- level is elevated in compensation for a *usually* more elevated $PaCO_2$. Acute hyperventilation often occurs because of discomfort while blood is being drawn for tests. Ms. C.'s $PaCO_2$ may have been suddenly lowered to 42 mm Hg, resulting in a temporary increase in pH to the limits of the normal range on the alkalemic side. Because Ms. C.'s admission electrolyte tests showed a low chloride value, a combination of these two mechanisms seems to be the cause of her alkalemia.

Electrolyte Imbalance

The low serum sodium and chloride values are apparently secondary to diuretic therapy and an inappropriate antidiuretic hormone level. Hyponatremia was resolved by fluid restriction during part of Ms. C.'s hospital stay. Potassium chloride supplement had been ordered when digoxin and diuretics were started 2 weeks before admission (but may not have been taken). In addition, there can be an obligatory loss of Cl^- ion when HCO_3^- is retained to compensate for respiratory acidosis.

Signs and Symptoms of ARF in COPD

The nonspecific symptoms of decompensation seen in Ms. C.—increased shortness of breath, difficulty with raising sputum, decreased effectiveness of cough, generalized fatigue, and anorexia—are typical of the patient with chronic obstructive disease.[42,48] It is often difficult to know when to hospitalize a patient with longstanding COPD, because it is difficult to assess what aspects of the disorder will be amenable to therapy. Also, prolonged and gradual deterioration of oxygenation blunts the usual symptoms of hypoxemia. Some patients develop an amazing tolerance for "anaerobia." Ms. C., however, had indications of right ventricular failure, which is potentially reversible, in addition to the nonspecific complaints just mentioned. Her admission blood gas levels were remarkable in that she had a strikingly low PaO_2 (27 mm Hg). According to an admission note, 45 minutes before blood for the test was drawn, the patient said that it was hard for her to breathe and that she had been unable to eat solid food of any kind. Despite her condition, Ms. C. was ambulatory. This amazing adaptation to tissue hypoxia is possible only in slowly developing hypoxemia. Oxygen administration was finally started after the severe hypoxemia was confirmed. Ms. C. had clubbing, an unusual finding in COPD even with longstanding hypoxemia. When clubbing is present, it is usually associated with coexisting cancer or bronchiectasis. The latter is more likely in Ms. C.'s case.

Polycythemia

Polycythemia is one of the adaptations to hypoxemia. It occurs as a result of hypoxic stimulation of the erythropoietin system, which in turn stimulates red blood cell production by the bone marrow. Ms. C. had a hematocrit of 63%. This was one reason she was able to "tolerate" the extremely low PaO_2. An increase in the amount of hemoglobin enables more oxygen to be carried per unit volume of blood. However, the increased "thickness" of the blood also causes increased resistance to blood flow, a particularly negative side effect in patients who also have increased pulmonary vascular resistance due to hypoxic vasoconstriction of the pulmonary capillary bed.[17,32] The two mechanisms produce an additive effect in terms of cardiac work, particularly for the right ventricle. For these reasons, Ms. C. had a phlebotomy, which in conjunction with hydration, lowered her hematocrit to 53%. A similar reduction in hematocrit would also have occurred, although more gradually, after the institution of oxygen therapy alone, because the stimulus for excessive production of red blood cells would have been removed.

Cardiovascular Compensation and Decompensation

Remarkably, Ms. C.'s extremely low PaO_2 was not accompanied by an increase in her cardiac rate. An increase in cardiac output, usually by an increase in rate, is one of the mechanisms that prevents tissue hypoxia in the face of extreme arterial hypoxemia. Failure of the heart rate to increase is unusual with such a degree of hypoxemia; however, in Ms. C.'s case the metabolic requirements were very low. She had virtually stopped eating and moving and had increased her oxygen-carrying capacity (hematocrit 63%). She sought help only when she was completely unable to meet the demands or perform the activities of daily living.

Pulmonary Heart Disease

Pulmonary heart disease (cor pulmonale) is a frequent complication of hypoxemic COPD.[17,42] The primary therapy for right-sided heart failure is relief of pulmonary artery hypertension. Increased pulmonary vascular resistance due to alveolar hypoxia is the major mechanism of pulmonary hypertension.[32] In this setting, pulmonary hypertension is usually responsive to increases in PaO_2 (alveolar oxygen pressure). If therapy such as inhalation of a bronchodilator and postural drainage improves ventilation enough to normalize the alveolar gases, cor pulmonale is reversible. If therapy is not successful, supplemental oxygen must be given to raise the PaO_2 to control hypoxic vasoconstriction.[17,39] It is of interest that Ms. C. had no signs or symptoms of left-sided heart failure. The two sides of the heart can, and do, fail independently. Ms. C.'s digoxin therapy was discontinued on her admission to the hospital; the efficacy of digoxin therapy when right-sided heart failure is the only cardiac problem has been questioned.[42] In addition, digoxin is well known for its toxicity when the myocardium is hypoxic.

Anorexia and Weight Loss

Anorexia and weight loss are frequent complaints in patients with severe COPD.[40,42] The symptoms are apparently due to poor digestion and absorption associated with hypoxia of the digestive tract. Decreased dietary intake is not always the cause of the weight loss and protein-calorie malnutrition found in some patients, since some patients exhibiting these problems have intakes equal to those who maintain their weight.[25] Differences in the work of breathing have been implicated, and inverse correlations have been found between increased work of breathing and failure to maintain weight.[13,25,40] Additionally, patients who have less body mass have lower values on certain ventilatory tests.[2,29] Clearly, there is a negative-feedback system that must be interrupted by treating hypoxemia and using every nursing skill to enhance an adequate intake. Recent true tissue weight loss was difficult to document in Ms. C.'s case, because her weight fluctuated frequently owing to right-sided heart failure and diuretic therapy. Her anorexia and general well-being improved after oxygen therapy was instituted.

Respiratory Care

Ms. C. was given intensive bronchial hygiene therapy designed to improve ventilation and oxygenation by enhancing secretion clearance. The regimen included inhalation of a bronchodilator from a gas-driven, small-volume nebulizer, followed by inhalation of warm, humidified air from a heated nebulizer, followed by chest physical therapy (percussion and coughing) in various postural drainage positions.[35,36] Positions suitable for general drainage of the right and left posterior lung bases were used because localized infiltrates were not seen on the chest film.

It has been customary to administer inhaled bronchodilator medications from gas-powered, small-reservoir nebulizers; however, there is no evidence that this method of delivery produces greater bronchodilation than having the patient inhale the medication from a metered-dose inhaler during a voluntary deep breath.[54] In addition, Ms. C. had significant air trapping (residual volume 216% of predicted). Her problem is getting the air *out* of the lungs. She does not need assisted inhalation. But this does not mean, of course, that no patient needs intermittent positive-pressure breathing (IPPB) assistance. The modes of therapy are selected on the basis of the pathophysiology to be treated.

Oxygenation

Oxygen therapy at 2 L/minute resulted in a PaO_2 of 47 mm Hg. Later the oxygen flow rate was adjusted to 2.5 L/minute, resulting in a PaO_2 of 56 mm Hg. At this level of oxygenation there was also an increase in carbon dioxide retention (15 mm Hg) to 54 mm Hg. However, it was not associated with a fall in pH. Ms. C. had a compensatory alkalosis that acted as a buffer for the carbon dioxide retention. The point to be stressed is that carbon dioxide retention should be tolerated unless there is a significant fall in pH (usually pH < 7.3), because the benefits of improved oxygenation outweigh the disadvantages of mild acidemia. During Ms. C.'s hospitalization, it was decided that even with optimum therapy her hypoxemia would not be resolved and that she met the criteria for continuous home oxygen therapy. These criteria include a PaO_2 of less than 55 mm Hg during the day, control of right ventricular failure and polycythemia, and a significant improvement in exercise tolerance.[39]

Antibiotic Therapy

Penicillin (250 mg four times a day by mouth) was used to treat the gram-negative diplococci seen on Gram stain. The most common organisms seen on culture in COPD are *Diplococcus pneumoniae* and *Hemophilus*. But in this setting, patients are often treated without waiting for culture results. In addition, because the *Hemophilus* strains frequently are not type B, penicillin is a satisfactory choice, although the use of broad-spectrum antibiotics, such as tetracycline and ampicillin, is more common.

Discharge Planning

The visiting nurse was contacted for supervision of Ms. C.'s medications, including the patient's use of oxygen in the home, and her secretion clearance regimen. The visiting nurse instructed the patient's brother in percussion and postural drainage.

Ms. C.'s therapy on discharge was a bronchial hygiene program consisting of the use of an inhaled bronchodilator, inhaled steam for moisturizing the airways, followed by postural drainage (with percussion when possible). Theophylline was given, and oxygen therapy was continued at 2 L/minute for as much of 24 hours as was practical. To facilitate continuous oxygen therapy, the patient was given 50 feet of extension tubing to enable her to walk freely around her house.

Adjusting to chronic oxygen therapy is difficult for most patients. Wearing nasal cannulas, or "prongs," is a sign of their disease that cannot be disguised. And storing five or six oxygen tanks or an oxygen concentrator in the home is often a problem. Ms. C.'s hospitalization was successful not only because she got "better," but also because she accepted her need for continuous oxygen therapy. Also, Ms. C. and her family understood the proper use of oxygen *as a medication*. These outcomes were due to careful teaching by the hospital nursing staff and coordination and continuity of care with the home care nurses.

SUMMARY

ARF is a rapidly occurring inability of the lungs to maintain adequate oxygenation of the blood. Carbon dioxide elimination may or may not be impaired. Arterial oxygen tension is 50 mm Hg or less. Nurses must be constantly alert to the possibility of ARF in all patients, and when the syndrome is seen, nurses must work diligently with other members of the team to return the patient to as high a level of functioning as possible.

DIRECTIONS FOR FUTURE RESEARCH

Did Ms. C. need to be admitted to a critical care unit? This question will have to be answered as health care availability is altered in response to changes in health care financing. However, careful monitoring is required when a patient has acute hypoxemia. Dysrhythmias are as likely to occur in patients with ARF as in patients with acute myocardial infarction.[24] Also, the frequency and intensity of the treatments needed for sputum clearance are not known but are thought to be sufficient indications that such patients should be treated in a critical care unit until their condition is stable.[36,42] Overall, there is a great need for nurses to study and determine just which of the many therapies we currently use in the treatment of the underlying causes of ARF and its consequences, particularly dyspnea and respiratory muscle fatigue, are most beneficial and cost effective.[23,31,46]

REFERENCES

1. American Association of Critical-Care Nurses. *Outcome Standards for Nursing Care of the Critically Ill.* Laguna Niguel, CA: American Association of Critical Care Nurses. 1990.
2. Arora, N. S., and Rochester, D. F. Respiratory muscle strength and maximal ventilation in undernourished patients. *Am. Rev. Respir. Dis.* 126:5, 1982.
3. Ayus, J. C., Krothapalli, R. K. Effect of bicarbonate administration on cardiac function. *Am. J. Med.* 87:5, 1989.
4. Beck, B. Oxygen therapy in acute and chronic pulmonary disease. In I. Ziment (ed.), *Practical Pulmonary Disease.* New York: Wiley, 1983.
5. Bellemare, F., and Grassino, A. Force reserve of the diaphragm in patients with chronic obstructive pulmonary disease. *J. Appl. Physiol. and Respirat. Environ. Exercise Physiol.* 55:8, 1983.
6. Benatar, S. R., Hewlett, A. M., and Nunn, J. F. The use of iso-shunt lines for control of oxygen therapy. *Br. J. Anaesthesiol.* 45: 711, 1973.
7. Braun, H. A., Cheney, F. W., Jr., and Loehnen, J. *Introduction to Respiratory Physiology.* Boston: Little, Brown, 1980.
8. Burki, N. K. Dyspnea. *Clin. Chest Med.* 1:47, 1980.
9. Carrieri, V. K., Janson-Bjerklie, S., and Jacob, S. The sensation of dyspnea: A review. *Heart Lung* 13:436, 1984.
10. Chusid, E. L. (ed.). *The Selective and Comprehensive Testing of Adult Pulmonary Function.* Mount Kisco, NY: Futura, 1983.
11. Cohen, C. A., Zagelbaum, G., Gross, D., Roussos, C., and Macklem, P. T. Clinical manifestations of inspiratory muscle fatigue. *Am. J. Med.* 73:308, 1982.
12. Connors, A. F., Jr., Hammon, W. E., Martin, R. J., and Rogers, R. M. Chest physical therapy: The immediate effect on oxygenation in acutely ill patients. *Chest* 78:559, 1980.
13. Driver, A. G., McAlevy, M. T., and Smith, J. L. Nutritional assessment of patients with chronic obstructive pulmonary disease and acute respiratory failure. *Chest* 82:568, 1982.
14. Dudley, D. L., and Sitzman, J. Psychosocial and psychophysiologic approach to the patient. *Semin. Respir. Med.* 1:59, 1979.
15. Dudley, D. L., Glaser, E. M., Jorgensen, B. N., and Logan, D. L. Psychological concomitants to rehabilitation in chronic obstructive pulmonary disease. Parts 1, 2, and 3. *Chest* 77:413, 544, 677, 1980.
16. Fell, T., and Cheney, F. W., Jr. Prevention of hypoxemia during endotracheal suction. *Ann. Surg.* 174:24, 1971.
17. Fishman, A. P. Pulmonary Hypertension and Cor Pulmonale. In A. P. Fishman (ed.), *Pulmonary Diseases and Disorders* (2nd ed.). New York: McGraw-Hill, 1988.
18. Ford, G. T., Whitelaw, W. A., Rosenal, T. W., Cruse, P. J., and Guenter, C. A. Diaphragm function after upper abdominal surgery in humans. *Am. Rev. Respir. Dis.* 127:431, 1983.
19. Freedberg, P. D., Hoffman, L. A., Light, W. C., and Kreps, M. K. Effect of progressive muscle relaxation on the objective symptoms and subjective responses associated with asthma. *Heart Lung* 16: 24, 1987.
20. Graf, H., Leach, W., and Arieff, A. I. Evidence for a detrimental effect of bicarbonate therapy in hypoxic lactic acidosis. *Science* 227:754, 1985.
21. Graham, W. G. B., and Bradley, D. A. Efficacy of chest physiotherapy and intermittent positive-pressure breathing in the resolution of pneumonia. *N. Engl. J. Med.* 299:624, 1978.
22. Guzzetta, C. E., Bunton, S. D., Prinkey, L. A., Sherer, A. P., and Seifert, P. C. *Clinical Assessment Tools for Use with Nursing Diagnoses.* St. Louis: Mosby, 1989.
23. Harver, A., Mahler, D. A., Daubenspeck, J. A. Targeted inspiratory muscle training improves respiratory muscle function and reduces dyspnea in patients with chronic obstructive pulmonary disease. *Ann. Intern. Med.* 111:117, 1989.
24. Hudson, L. D. Significance of arrhythmias in acute respiratory failure. *Geriatrics* 31:61, 1976.
25. Hunter, A. M., Carey, M. A., and Larsh, H. W. The nutritional status of patients with chronic obstructive pulmonary disease. *Am. Rev. Respir. Dis.* 124:376, 1981.
26. Janson-Bjerklie, S., Carrieri, V. K., and Hudes, M. The sensations of pulmonary dyspnea. *Nurs. Res.* 35:154, 1986.
27. Kinsman, R. A., Yaroush, R. A., Fernandez, E., Dirks, J. F., Schockert, M., and Fukuhara, J. Symptoms and experiences in chronic bronchitis and emphysema. *Chest* 83:755, 1983.
28. Kersten, L. D. *Comprehensive Respiratory Nursing: A Decision-Making Approach.* Philadelphia: Saunders, 1989.
29. Knowles, J. B., Fairbarn, M. S., Wiggs, B. J., Chan-Yan, C., and Pardy, R. L. Dietary supplementation and respiratory muscle performance in patients with COPD. *Chest* 93:977, 1988.
30. Kory, R. C., Bergmann, J. C., Sweet, R. D., et al. Comparative evaluation of oxygen therapy techniques. *J.A.M.A.* 179:767, 1962.
31. Larson, J. L., Kim, M. J., Sharp, J. T., and Larson, D. A. Inspiratory muscle training with a pressure threshold breathing device in patients with chronic obstructive pulmonary disease. *Am. Rev. Respir. Dis.* 138:689, 1988.
32. Lloyd, T. C., Jr. Effect of alveolar hypoxia on pulmonary vascular resistance. *J. Appl. Physiol.* 19:1086, 1964.
33. Liss, H. P., and Grant, B. J. B. The effect of nasal flow on breathlessness in patients with chronic obstructive pulmonary disease. *Am. Rev. Respir. Dis.* 137:1285, 1988.
34. Luce, J. M., and Pierson, D. J. *Critical Care Medicine.* Philadelphia: Saunders, 1988.
35. Luce, J. M., Tyler, M. L., and Pierson, D. J. *Intensive Respiratory Care,* Philadelphia: Saunders, 1984.
36. Mackenzie, C. F. (ed.), Ciesla, N., Imle, P. C., and Klemic, N.

Chest Physiotherapy in the Intensive Care Unit. Baltimore: Williams & Wilkins, 1981.

37. Mahler, D. A. (ed.). *Dyspnea.* Mount Kisco, NY: Futura, 1990.

38. McMahon, A., and Maibusch, R. M. How to send quit-smoking signals. *Am. J. Nurs.* 88:1498, 1988.

39. Nocturnal Oxygen Therapy Trial Group. Continuous or nocturnal oxygen therapy in hypoxemic chronic obstructive lung disease: A clinical trial. *Ann. Intern. Med.* 93:391, 1980.

40. Openbrier, D. R., Irwin, M. M., Rogers, R. M., Gottlieb, G. P., Dauber, J. H., Van Thiel, D. A., and Pennacle, B. E. Nutritional status and lung function in patients with emphysema and chronic bronchitis. *Chest* 83:17, 1983.

41. Peterson, G. M., Pierson, D. J., and Hunter, T. Arterial oxygen saturation during naso-tracheal suctioning. *Respir. Care* 23:68, 1978.

42. Petty, T. L. *Intensive and Rehabilitative Respiratory Care* (3rd ed.). Philadelphia: Lea & Febiger, 1982.

43. Pulmonary terms and symbols. A report of the AACP-ATS joint committee on pulmonary nomenclature. *Chest* 67:583, 1975.

44. Respiratory Muscle Fatigue Workshop Group. NHLBI workshop summary: Respiratory muscle fatigue. *Am. Rev. Respir. Dis.* 142: 474, 1990.

45. Rindfleisch, S. H., and Tyler, M. L. Suction duration: An important variable. *Respir. Care* 28:457, 1983.

46. Robin, E. D. Single-patient randomized clinical trial: Opiates for intractable dyspnea. *Chest* 90:888, 1986.

47. Rochester, D. F., and Arora, N. S. Respiratory muscle failure. *Med. Clin. North Am.* 67:573, 1983.

48. Sexton, D. L. *Nursing Care of the Respiratory Patient.* Norwalk, CT: Appleton & Lange, 1990.

49. Sharp, J. T. Therapeutic considerations in respiratory muscle function. *Chest* 88(suppl.):1185, 1985.

50. Sharp, J. T., Danon, J., Druz, W. S., Goldberg, N. B., Fishman, H., and Machrach, W. Respiratory muscle function in patients with chronic obstructive pulmonary disease: Its relationship to disability and to respiratory therapy. *Am. Rev. Respir. Dis.* 110(6, part 2):154, 1974.

51. Standards for nursing care of adult patients with pulmonary dysfunction. A report of the Nursing Standards Subcommittee of the ATS Section on Nursing—Scientific Assembly on Clinical Problems. *Am. Rev. Respir. Dis.* (in press).

52. Tobin, M. J., Chadha, T. S., Jenouri, G., Birch, S. J., Gazeroglu, H. B., and Sackner, M. A. Breathing patterns: 1. Normal subjects. *Chest* 84:202, 1983.

53. Tobin, M. J., Chadha, T. S., Jenouri, G., Birch, S. J., Gazeroglu, H. B., and Sackner, M. A. Breathing patterns: 2. Diseased subjects. *Chest* 84:286, 1983.

54. Tobin, M. J., Jenouri, G., Danta, I., Kim, C., Watson, H., and Sackner, M. A. Response to bronchodilator drug administration by a new reservoir aerosol delivery system and a review of other auxiliary delivery systems. *Am. Rev. Respir. Dis.* 126:670, 1982.

55. Tobin, M. J., Perez, W., Guenther, S. M., Lodato, R. F., and Dantzker, D. R. Does rib cage-abdominal paradox signify respiratory muscle fatigue? *J. Appl. Physiol.* 63:851, 1987.

56. Tobin, M. J. Respiratory monitoring in the intensive care unit. *Am. Rev. Respir. Dis.* 138:1625, 1988.

57. Tyler, M. L. *Arterial Blood Gases, Arterial Oxygen Saturation, Heart Rate and Blood Pressure During Chest Physiotherapy.* Master's thesis, University of Washington, 1977.

58. Tyler, M. L., Hudson, L. D., Grose, B. L., and Huseby, J. S. Prediction of oxygenation during chest physiotherapy in critically ill patients (Abstr.). *Am. Rev. Respir. Dis.* 121(4, part 2):218, 1980.

59. Wanner, A., Zighelboim, A., and Sackner, M. A. Nasopharyngeal airway: A facilitated access to the trachea. *Ann. Intern. Med.* 75: 593, 1971.

60. Wasserman, K. Dyspnea on exertion: Is it the heart or the lungs? *J.A.M.A.* 248:2039, 1982.

61. West, J. B. *Pulmonary Pathophysiology—The Essentials* (3rd ed.). Baltimore: Williams & Wilkins, 1987.

62. Zack, M. B., Pontoppidan, H., and Kasemi, H. The effect of lateral positions on gas exchange in pulmonary disease: A prospective evaluation. *Am. Rev. Respir. Dis.* 110:49, 1974.

22

Chest Trauma

Kathleen MacKay White   *Cornelia Vanderstaay Kenner*

FEAR

What is fear and where does it come from? Fear only comes in relationship to something else. Then what is fear in relationship to? Is it in relationship to the unknown? If fear is unknown, how can you fear it?

Is it possible that the origin of the fear is loss of the known? The known is when you acknowledge you don't know enough about the technology, procedures, or drugs, loss of a job or pleasures, not knowing the right thing to say, knowing that at some time you will die, or a family member or friends will die. These are known conditions that cause the fear. If this is so, how can you gain freedom from the fear? This is the healing journey—learning more about the relationship with all things. As you become more mindful of creating a space for fear and confusion to emerge, you can greet these experiences with peacefulness and openness.

Fear somehow can get a hold of your spirit, lodging somewhere within your physical body. Fear makes you feel separate and alone, but fear can become a path that will lead deeper into the present moment. It does not have to be a barrier to the moment. Fear states always create more of what you fear. However, every time fear surfaces, it can become a moment to learn about another level of life's journey.

Fear is useful in that it alerts you to areas in which you have resistance and are not ready to move through a certain event. To release the fear always returns you to your unconditional core of love so that you release the "shoulds." If you approach an event with the notion that you should behave a certain way, then you further distance yourself from your core of being present in the moment.

LEARNING OBJECTIVES

After reading this chapter, the nurse should be able to do the following:

1. Use physical examination of the chest to identify compromise of airway, breathing, and circulation.
2. Elicit and interpret information important to the mechanism and severity of injury.
3. Objectively communicate findings to the health care team.
4. Anticipate necessary treatment and quickly formulate a plan of action.
5. Carry out or assist other health team members in carrying out the plan of action to restore cardiorespiratory function.
6. Anticipate, assess, and detect delayed developments that can later threaten the patient.

CASE STUDY

Mr. R. T., a 35-year-old retail store manager, was brought to the emergency room because of injuries he sustained in a high-speed car accident. Witnesses claimed that Mr. T. lost control of his car, which was traveling at 50 to 60 mph, and crashed it into a telephone pole. At the scene of the accident, Mr. T. was found pinned against the steering wheel, but he was awake and responsive. The paramedics who were present at the scene of the accident said that Mr. T. was in obvious respiratory distress and that he complained of chest pain and shortness of breath. Examination of his chest revealed a right chest deformity. His right chest was immediately splinted with a sandbag. The patient's vital signs at the scene of the accident were blood pressure, 98/60; pulse, 110; respirations, 32 and labored. The patient's skin was pale, cool, and clammy. An intravenous infusion of 1000 ml of Ringer's lactate solution was begun. The patient had received 700 ml by the time of his admission to the hospital.

In the emergency room, Mr. T. was found to be in acute respiratory distress, with a blood pressure of 82/40, pulse of 150, and respirations of 26, with obvious right-sided paradoxical motion of a portion of his chest (flail chest). His respiratory pattern was also characterized by severe intercostal and sternal retraction. Air exchange could be felt at his mouth or nares. His breath sounds were absent. Airway maneuvers and suctioning failed to open his airway. Therefore, a no. 8 French endotracheal tube was inserted, and Mr. T. was ventilated with 100% oxygen for 20 breaths. He was placed on a mechanical ventilator.

Assessment of Mr. T.'s condition after intubation revealed improvement in his cardiopulmonary status. A stat upright portable chest radiograph showed multiple rib fractures, including a clavicular fracture on the right. The mediastinum appeared widened.

Mr. T.'s condition stabilized, with blood pressure of 102/80, pulse of 100, respirations of 12, and central venous pressure of 4 cm H_2O. A Foley catheter was connected to straight drainage; it drained clear, yellow urine. A nasogastric tube was placed and connected to low suction; it drained a small amount of blood and then normal gastric contents. A complete physical examination was then carried out. It revealed no abnormalities other than minimal abdominal tenderness and hypoactive bowel sounds. No masses were palpable, and there was no rebound tenderness or distention. Peritoneal taps were negative bilaterally, and peritoneal lavage was also negative. The rest of the physical examination was essentially negative.

After Mr. T.'s condition had stabilized sufficiently, he was taken to the operating room, where an aortogram was done. The aortogram revealed an intact aorta with no intimal tears or lacerations. Mr. T. was then taken to the trauma critical care unit and placed on a volume ventilator with a tidal volume at 1000 ml and an FiO_2 of 40%.

Clinical Presentation of Case Study

On Mr. T.'s arrival in the critical care unit, the primary care nurse made an assessment of him and recorded findings on the assessment sheet. The following notes, a synopsis of Mr. T.'s pulmonary management based on his hospital record, document the care he received during his first hours in the critical care unit:

3/1
4:30 PM

Arterial blood gases (ABG) on FiO_2 of 40%: PaO_2, 146; pH, 7.37; $PaCO_2$, 34; HCO_3^-, 19.6; delta base, −5. Central venous pressure was less than 3 cm H_2O. For increasing restlessness and pain, diazepam (5 mg intravenously) and meperidine (75 mg, one half intravenously and one half intramuscularly).

5:00 PM

Arterial blood gases on FiO_2 of 100%: PaO_2, 264; pH, 7.32; $PaCO_2$, 42; HCO_3^-, 21; delta base, −4. Vital signs: BP 110/74, P 96, R 10. For hyperventilation and restlessness, morphine sulfate (5 mg intravenously). Urine 50 ml/hour. Laboratory reports serum potassium of 3.1 mEq/L; 30 mEq potassium added to each peripheral intravenous line per physician order.

8:00 PM

Blood pressure, 76/42; pulse, 146; respirations, 40; central venous pressure less than 3 cm H_2O. Physician notified, Ringer's lactate solution opened wide, and patient's legs elevated. Arterial specimen to lab for blood gas analysis. X-ray technician and blood bank notified. Patient progressively more agitated and tachypneic. Chest examination by the primary care nurse revealed dull percussion note and absent breath sounds in the right lower base. Equipment for chest tube placement assembled.

8:05 PM

Doctor here. Right posterior chest catheter inserted, with the immediate return of 800 ml of gross blood. Right anterior tube placed. Two units whole blood started. Twelve-lead electrocardiogram showed sinus tachycardia.

8:15 PM

Stat portable chest film. Blood sent for complete blood count.

8:20 PM

Arterial blood gases on FiO_2 of 40%: PaO_2, 103; pH, 7.34; $PaCO_2$, 37; HCO_3^-, 19; delta base, −6. Vital signs: blood pressure, 92/60; pulse, 104; respirations, 26. Chest tubes connection to Pleurevac with wall suction.

10:00 PM

Vital signs: blood pressure, 108/70; pulse, 96; respirations, 12; central venous pressure, 15 cm H_2O. Hemoglobin, 8 g/100 ml, and hematocrit, 22.7%. Urine 25 ml/hour. Alert. Two units whole blood completed. Ringer's lactate solution slowed and foot elevation discontinued. Patient asked to see his wife. Seemed more relaxed in her presence.

10:45 PM

Lasix, 25 mg intravenous push.

11:15 PM

Vital signs: blood pressure, 110/70; pulse, 90. Alert. Urine output increased.

3/2
12:30 AM

Alert. Urine output 60 ml/hour. Arterial blood gases on FiO_2 of 40%: PaO_2, 80; positive end-expiratory pressure (PEEP) of 4 cm H_2O started. Vital signs stable. Anterior chest tube oscillating; posterior tube shows minimal increase in drainage (25–30 ml). Both tubes stripped. Turned. Gastric pH maintained at 7. Anti-embolism stockings applied.

2:00 AM

PaO_2 79 on FiO_2 of 50%. Morphine sulfate, 4 mg, given intravenously for hyperventilation and restlessness.

3:30 AM

PaO_2 122 on FiO_2 of 50%. Alert. Urine output 50 ml/hour. Vital signs stable. Demerol (50 mg intramuscularly) for pain.

8:00 AM

Alert. Urine output 60 ml/hour. Vital signs stable. Posterior chest tube drainage total 875 ml (anterior 75 ml). Both tubes connected to suction. Diazepam (10 mg intramuscularly) given. Forced vital capacity 1400 ml. PEEP decreased to 2 cm H_2O. Visited by family; seemed less tense during visit.

Mr. T. remained in the critical care unit until March 10th, when he was transferred to the intermediate care unit. During the time in the critical care unit, a pulmonary artery catheter and an arterial catheter were placed for monitoring purposes. Although his clinical course changed frequently, overall improvement could be seen on a daily basis. He began moving about in bed and consistently remembered to do all the bed exercises his primary care nurse recommended. He was out of bed twice a day. He enjoyed longer visits with his family and seemed to derive a lot of support and encouragement from their visits. During family visits, the primary care nurse remained in close proximity to answer questions, offer information, and help in communication.

Interpretation of Case Study

The process of assessing and managing Mr. T.'s injury was begun by the ambulance team. From the information gathered at the scene, the team learned that the accident occurred at high speed. That clue to the possible mechanisms of injury warned the health care team to consider the severe internal injuries that can result from the tearing, torsional forces of rapid deceleration. The aorta is vulnerable to this type of injuring mechanism. Next, the team learned that the patient had been thrown against the steering wheel, information that alerted them to the possibility of blunt chest injury with rib fracture or lung damage. The patient's complaint of shortness of breath and chest pain narrowed the injury to chest involvement. Inspection of the chest revealed the presence of flail chest. Splinting the flail segment with a sandbag was the best available first-aid method of stabilizing the segment. The paradoxical motion of the flail segment was stabilized to some degree, and the patient's ability to expand his chest on inspiration and recoil on expiration was somewhat improved. This improvement helped to reduce the work of breathing and to maintain minimal respiratory function with adequate gas exchange while the patient was being transported to the hospital.

En route, Mr. T.'s falling blood pressure, a sign that another problem was developing, was detected by the ambulance crew. Considering the force of the blow that caused the patient's severe chest injury, the possibility of shock due to internal bleeding from intrathoracic or intra-abdominal injury had to be considered. Because the blood pressure remained lower than 90 mm Hg despite the administration of 700 ml of Ringer's lactate solution, the hypotension most likely had hypovolemic causes. Little or no response to the rapid infusion of 500 to 2000 ml of Ringer's lactate solution indicates that greater than 30% of the blood volume has been lost—unless, of course, the problem is decreasing cardiac output secondary to mediastinal shift seen in tension pneumothorax, which also would not respond to Ringer's lactate solution.

Had Mr. T.'s condition remained the same in the emergency room as it had been before transport, with his airway, breathing, and cardiac function maintained, attention would have been directed toward assessing his injuries quickly, treating the shock and uncovering and correcting its cause, and ensuring adequate oxygenation. This would have been followed by a complete and orderly examination to detect the less serious or occult injuries that might have been overlooked in the initial assessment. This course of management, however, had to be set aside temporarily when a more serious problem, airway obstruction, demanded a rearrangement of priorities. Management of this problem proceeded from the simple to the complex; that is, when simple airway maneuvers failed to establish an airway, the more complex maneuver of endotracheal intubation became necessary. Had intubation also failed, cricothyrotomy would have been appropriate, because at that point failure to correct the obstruction could have led to Mr. T.'s death.

Once Mr. T.'s condition had been stabilized, a thorough physical examination was done. It is important to conduct a systematic examination after the crises have been resolved so that minor or occult injuries that may have gone unseen or unattended can be found and evaluated.

Because Mr. T. had undergone rapid deceleration, and was found to have a widened mediastinum, the possibility of aortic injury had to be considered. Therefore, additional radiographic studies were necessary to determine if aortic injury was present. Mr. T. was taken to the operating room, not the x-ray department, for an arteriogram, because operative repair of an aortic tear must be done immediately. Having the patient in the operating room prevents unnecessary delay and avoids the risk of the aorta rupturing in the x-ray department, where immediate surgical intervention is not available. Also, the arteriographic study itself might cause a torn aorta to rupture, and it should not be undertaken without operative interventions being immediately possible. After Mr. T.'s arrival in the trauma unit, he showed agitation, tachypnea, and tachycardia, which signaled that his hypoxia had become worse. The person with a thoracic injury is usually in shock primarily because of hemorrhage or pericardial tamponade and only secondarily because of respiratory distress or pain. Mr. T.'s continued shock, absent breath sounds, and dullness to percussion of the

right lower lobe pointed to hemothorax. Again, the history of injury strongly warned of intrathoracic vessel tear and bleeding. The ineffectiveness of the positive pressure suggested a space-occupying lesion of the chest—hemothorax. Positive pressure would also have been ineffective with tension pneumothorax, but that condition was ruled out on physical examination, when hyperresonance was not found. An immediate chest radiograph confirmed the suspicion of hemothorax, and a blood gas analysis documented the hypoxia and hypercapnia already suspected. Continued hypoventilation, followed by acute respiratory failure and death, would occur inevitably if the space-occupying blood was not removed.

Once the chest tubes were inserted (the posterior tube was placed first, because evacuation of the pleural blood took priority over the evacuation of air by the anterior tube), Mr. T.'s condition quickly stabilized. Administration of 2 U of whole blood helped replace the volume loss and increase the circulating red blood cells so that the oxygen-carrying capacity of the blood was adequate for tissue demands (see Chap. 19). The chest tubes were connected to underwater seal drainage, with suction. Although rarely necessary, suction was ordered for Mr. T. to help evacuate the intrapleural air. This degree of negative pressure safely evacuates intrapleural air without damage to the delicate pulmonary structures near the end of the chest tube. Pressures greater than -30 cm H_2O can create potentially such great transpulmonary pressure gradients that fluid is literally suctioned into the pleural spaces out of the pulmonary vasculature.

Although Mr. T.'s initial chest drainage was 800 ml, the rate of continued blood loss after chest tube insertion is the usual factor that determines whether open thoracotomy is necessary. Because Mr. T.'s bleeding slowed soon after insertion of the tube, it was assumed that the bleeding was venous and capillary in origin and that hemostasis could be maintained by the chest tube's expansion of the injured lung. Had the rate of bleeding exceeded 100 ml/hour or had the first episode of bleeding been more than 1500 ml, however, exploratory thoracotomy would have been indicated for repair of the larger intercostal and internal mammary arteries.

Pulmonary artery and radial artery catheters were placed so that cardiopulmonary function could be monitored closely (see Chap. 17). Pulmonary complications in particular are likely to occur in trauma patients who have been in shock, have had direct pulmonary injury, have had transfusions, or have been hypoxic. In severe cases or in cases detected and treated too late, refractory hypoxemia, hypercapnia, acidosis, pulmonary failure, and death may result. The danger to the patient from pulmonary complications is reflected in the fact that respiratory failure is one of the leading causes of death after blunt chest trauma. The majority of deaths are caused by respiratory failure due to a ventilatory problem or inadequate gas exchange, hemorrhage from injury to the heart or great vessels (or both), or an associated injury.[29]

REFLECTIONS

Often in the hustle and bustle of the emergency environment, the patient and how he can cooperate are forgotten. For example, once Mr. T. became aware of his environment, he could either cooperate or, in his fear, fight treatment. It is important for the nurse to help orient and relax the patient. The nurse must remember that a patient can often hear the communications of the health team members even though the team may think the patient is unconscious.

As much as possible, the nurse should explain what is going to happen to the patient, as seen in Figure 22–1. Naturally, in some situations, time is of the essence, and there is not enough time for explanations. However, such complex situations are relatively infrequent; it is much more ordinary that there is sufficient time for simple explanations. How much more at ease will the patient be who has some

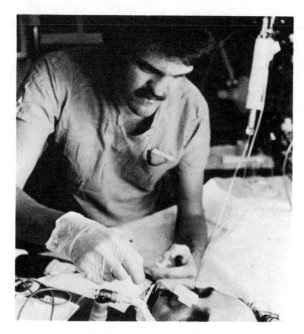

Figure 22–1

Even the simplest nursing act should be performed with skill and understanding, because it is never a neutral event.

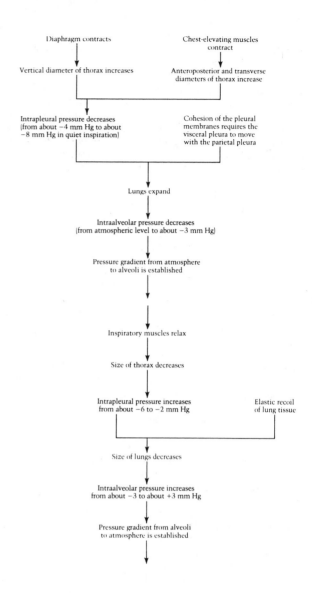

Figure 22–2

Inspiration-expiration.

idea what a procedure will feel like? For too long, nurses have hidden behind the "emergency situation" and made excuses for not helping the person because they were too "busy" with the emergency. How many nurses have spoken with patients after emergency events and found out what they remembered? Much can be learned by simply asking.

The anxious, fearful, and uncomfortable patient experiencing chest trauma is acutely aware of the rhythm of the breath. Often they have a feeling of not being able to breathe. When doing routine procedure, in an emergency, or working with complicated technology attached to the patient, breathing and imagery exercises can be easily integrated to help the patient relax and regain a sense of control and hope (see Chap. 3 for details). Self-regulation interventions allow critical care nurses to use their expertise and share their humanity—their compassion, touch, caring, warmth, and sense of humor.

ANATOMY AND PHYSIOLOGY

The thoracic cavity is divided into three compartments: the pleural space, which is occupied by the lungs; the mediastinum, which is occupied by the trachea, esophagus, and great vessels; and the pericardial space, which is occupied by the heart. The parietal pleura separates each compartment from the other and partitions off the three compartments by lining the entire thoracic cavity (*i.e.*, the internal surface of the chest wall), part of the superior surface of the diaphragm, and the mediastinum. The lungs are covered by the visceral pleura and are thus separated from the rest of the thoracic structures. In fact, the lungs are attached to the body only at their hila.

To understand the mechanics of many types of chest injuries, it is important to understand the normal mechanics of respiration (Fig. 22–2). The outer surface of the lungs, the

visceral pleura, is a smooth, moist membrane that lies in complete contact with the smooth, moist parietal pleura that lines the inner thoracic wall. These two layers slide over one another during inspiration and expiration. Between these two layers of pleura is a "potential space"; that is, the presence of any type of fluid or air will create a space between the thoracic wall and the lung. The membranes, however, constantly absorb any fluid or gas that enters the potential space. In other words, the visceral and parietal pleural membranes are in an apposition that is maintained by the surface tension of a thin layer of fluid between them. Furthermore, a partial vacuum exists between the two membranes, partly as a result of the constant resorption of fluid or air, but largely as a result of two opposing forces: the natural elastic recoil of the lungs and the outward expansion of the chest wall. Together these forces establish a constant vacuum in the pleural space that not only keeps the lung from collapsing but also is the mechanism by which negative pressures (pressures less than that of the atmosphere) are produced within the thorax. Intrapleural pressure is always less than (negative to) atmospheric pressure.

Air moves into and out of the lungs for the same reason blood flows through vessels—a pressure gradient exists. Air moves from an area of greater pressure to an area of lesser pressure. At the end of expiration, the intrapleural pressure is −4 mm Hg (because of a naturally occurring vacuum). Because of the connection to the atmosphere through airways, the pressure within the lungs (intra-alveolar or intrapulmonic pressure) is 0 mm Hg. At the end of expiration, no pressure gradient exists between the airways and the atmosphere; thus, there is no movement of air into the airways. When the size of the thorax is increased by chest expansion, however, intrapulmonic pressure drops and produces a pressure gradient between alveoli and the atmosphere. As volume increases, pressure decreases (Boyle's law).

Thoracic size and volume are increased by the downward movement of the diaphragm and the elevation of the ribs, which increases the anteroposterior diameter of the chest cavity. Although normal inspiration is caused principally by contraction of the diaphragm, 70% of the expansion and contraction of the lungs is caused by the anteroposterior movement of the chest cage and only 30% by movement of the diaphragm. In normal breathing, the diaphragm contracts and descends several centimeters, so that approximately 500 ml of air enters the lungs. If the body needs more air, additional muscles are needed for inspiration, and the external intercostals contract and move the ribs outward.[49]

Once the size of the thorax is increased, the pressure in the potential pleural space (the intrapleural or intrathoracic pressure) falls from its end-expiratory pressure of −4 mm Hg to the more negative pressure of −8 mm Hg, and the pressure in the intra-alveolar space is lowered from atmospheric pressure to −3 mm Hg. At this point, the pressure gradient between the airways and the atmosphere produces air movement into the airways.

In expiration, the muscles of inspiration (the diaphragm and the external intercostals) relax and spring back to the resting position. If for some reason (*e.g.*, airway obstruction) one has to use muscles to help in expiration, one cannot use the diaphragm, because it is a muscle of inspiration. Instead, the abdominal and internal intercostal muscles must be recruited to assist expiration. As the expiratory muscles contract, the intra-alveolar pressure and the intrapleural pressure increase. The intra-alveolar pressure is now +3 mm Hg (*i.e.*, higher than atmospheric pressure), so air moves out of the lungs. The following pressure cycles are repeated with each respiration.

Intra-alveolar Pressures for Normal Quiet Breathing (All Are Variable, Depending on the Force of Inspiration and Expiration)

Inspiration	−3 mm Hg
Expiration	+3 mm Hg
Pressure at the end of expiration before inspiration begins	0 mm Hg

Intrapleural Pressures

During inspiration	−8 mm Hg
During expiration	−2 mm Hg
At the end of expiration	−4 mm Hg
At the end of inspiration	−6 mm Hg

ETIOLOGY

Chest injuries frequently are lethal. Approximately 25% of people who die as a result of trauma have sustained significant chest trauma.[32,42] Chest trauma follows head injury as the second most common cause of death due to injury.[6] If the chest alone is injured, the mortality is approximately 6%. If one or more organ systems is involved, the mortality increases to 15%. If two systems are involved, the mortality rate approaches 30% to 35%.[43] For every person who dies as a result of trauma, there are at least two who become permanently disabled.[46]

More than 26 million drivers and 15 million passengers are involved in motor-vehicle accidents each year, and 9% sustain significant disability or death. Thirty-five to 50 percent suffer from a chest injury.[46]

Automobile accidents are the leading cause of hospitalization for blunt chest injury, and the incidence ranges from 40% to 75%. Falls are the next leading cause of hospitalization; the incidence is from 15% to 25%. With penetrating injuries, stab wounds are by far the leader, with an incidence range of 70% to 80%. However, the mortality rate is not high: Only 2% to 4% of patients with a stab wound die as a result of their injury.[32] Although gunshot wounds account for an incidence of 20% to 30%, the mortality rate approximates 15% to 20%. Blunt trauma is responsible for 35% to 40% of lung injuries, 15% to 20% of cardiac injuries, and 12% to 20% of cases of hemothorax.[34] In penetrating trauma, the organs injured most frequently are the lung (65%–70%), the diaphragm (15%–20%), the heart (10%–15%), and the major vessels (5%–10%).

PATHOPHYSIOLOGY

Blunt Trauma and Penetrating Trauma

When caring for the patient with chest trauma, consideration should be given to the type of injury sustained. The patient may be suffering from blunt (nonpenetrating) trauma to the chest or may have sustained a penetrating injury. *Blunt trauma* is defined as closed injury without communication to the outside (unless a fractured rib has penetrated the chest wall). Direct impact causes the greatest injury to the chest wall. Injuries to the structures within the chest may result from the forces of acceleration-deceleration, shearing, and compression-decompression. Direct impact with severe force may grossly deform the chest, pressing the sternum almost against the spinal column.[69] Sudden compression increases intravascular pressure and may result in vascular damage and bleeding. Because the glottis is usually closed during injury, the chest acts as a closed system, and pressure is transmitted anywhere in the system. Pulmonary contusion may result. Thus, injuries after blunt trauma may occur anywhere in the chest, and the injuries can be severe even though there are few external signs. Compression injuries commonly occur to the chest wall, pleura, trachea, bronchi, lung (pneumothorax or hemothorax), heart, great vessels, esophagus, or diaphragm.[43] The forces of acceleration-deceleration cause the greatest injury to the vascular system. Rapid deceleration from a high speed, as in a highway accident, can cause major vessels to undergo extreme stretching and bowing. Stretching forces that exceed the elasticity of these vessels can produce shearing damage to the vessel walls, which then tend to tear, dissect, rupture, or form an aneurysmal deformity. For example, with deceleration, the arch of the aorta does not move as much as the more mobile descending aorta. This difference produces a strong shearing force on the aortic isthmus. Most ruptures of the intrathoracic aorta caused by blunt trauma occur at the isthmus. Also, shearing damage occurs in vessels that decelerate at a rate different from that of the structures they perfuse. Hence, organs may be torn from the source of their blood supply.

Penetrating chest injuries usually are less of an assessment problem than are blunt injuries. The presence of entrance and exit wounds helps greatly in determining the site of injury. A line plotted between an entrance wound and an exit wound allows the trauma team to determine what structures lie in the path and, hence, what types of pathology are likely to occur.

When penetrating injuries are encountered, consideration must be given to the injuring instrument:

- Gunshot wounds have special injuring mechanisms in that the ballistics of certain missiles can produce injury beyond just the missile's tract.
- Missiles do not always travel in a straight line, so they can injure more than just the structures lying beneath the entrance wound.
- Missiles do not always exit; thus, it is not always possible to plot the path between entrance and exit and to estimate the extent of injury.
- Missiles are not sterile, and they expose the chest wound to considerable contamination.
- All apparent gunshot wounds of the chest are not always *just* gunshot wounds of the chest. Owing to the extreme mobility and upward excursions of the diaphragm, a missile to the fifth intercostal space can cut a path through not only the chest but also the dome of the diaphragm and the structures that lie beneath it—the spleen and the liver. What may initially appear to be chest trauma may actually be complicated thoracoabdominal trauma.[24]

With regard to knife-blade–type injuries, the following considerations must be kept in mind:

- If the patient is admitted to the hospital with the instrument (*e.g.*, knife, arrow, or screwdriver) in place, it must not be removed. In most cases, the blade, despite the lacerating injury produced, provides "mechanical" hemostasis for the lacerated vessels. Removing the instrument may release the temporary hemostasis and precipitate instant hemorrhage. In such a situation, the blade must be *immobilized*, and nothing, not even a sheet, must be allowed to exert its weight on the blade. Even the slightest movement could disturb the tamponade and result in internal bleeding and death before operative intervention could be undertaken.
- Stab wounds can have amazing depth, and they may contain pieces of broken blade or other foreign material.
- Stab wounds are usually low-velocity, localized wounds, with injury occurring to structures directly in the path of the weapon. Stab wounds do not necessarily produce a significant injury. As a matter of fact, asymptomatic patients with minimal injury may be treated on an outpatient basis.[12,70]
- It is important to obtain information about the size of the knife and about the angle at which it was thrust. Estimating the angle of entry can help determine what structures are likely to be involved in the trauma.

Rib Fracture

Fractured ribs are overlooked frequently as a sign of potential chest trauma. The medical advice to the patient with a fractured rib often is "Strap it, take aspirin for the pain, and don't cough too much. The pain will go away in about 2 weeks." However, even though most people with uncomplicated fractured ribs have relatively minor injuries and can be treated as outpatients, the nurse must remember that serious associated injuries do occur with rib fracture. Among people with severe rib fractures, as many as 20% have an associated hemothorax, 25% have a pneumothorax, and 30% have both.[2,54] The frequency of potential underlying complications should be remembered whenever the staff assesses a fractured rib as a matter of little importance. When the chest radiograph indicates a rib fracture, nurses should remember that more serious problems may be present, and they should observe the patient for underlying internal chest trauma.

Rib fractures usually are accompanied by pain that can lead to shallow breathing and an ineffective cough (Fig. 22–3). Particularly in patients with pre-existing lung disease or advanced age, the threat of pneumonia or respiratory failure is significant.

Flail Chest

When multiple adjacent rib fractures or costosternal separations result in the "floating" of a segment of the rib cage, a *flail chest* is said to exist (Fig. 22–4). The segment, having lost continuity with the rest of the chest wall, moves paradoxically. On inspiration, when the chest wall is expanding in an attempt to establish the negative intrathoracic pressures necessary for air to enter the lungs, the free (floating) segment sinks inward. This phenomenon negates some of the chest expansion

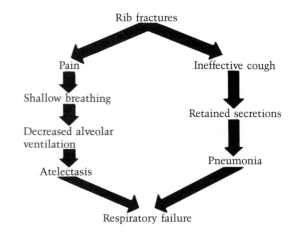

Figure 22–3

Rib fracture can lead to ineffective coughing and shallow breathing, which in turn may lead to respiratory failure.

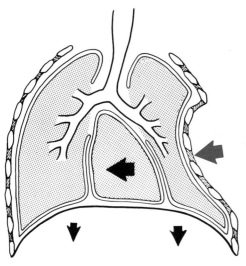

Inspiration

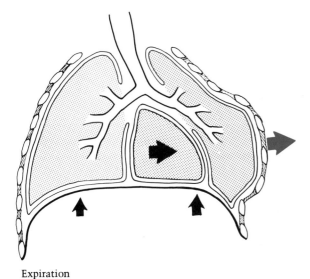

Expiration

Figure 22–4
Flail chest.

brought about by anteroposterior and diaphragmatic movement and begins to abolish the pressure gradients essential for inspiration. Consequently, movement of air during inspiration is diminished.

During expiration, when the diaphragm relaxes or accessory respiratory muscles contract and the compression of the chest cavity works to increase intrapulmonic pressure, the flail segment bulges out. This "paradoxical" movement of the flail segment prevents effective chest compression and reduces the positive-pressure gradient necessary for complete expiration. Furthermore, decrease of the cough mechanism results in retained secretions.[52] In all probability, the respiratory distress, hypoxemia, and increased intrapulmonary shunt associated with flail chest are made more extreme by the pulmonary contusion and resulting parenchymal insult. The alveolar-capillary interface is disrupted and results in hemorrhage and edema, both interstitial and intra-alveolar. The end result may

be a decreased functional residual capacity, decreased arterial oxygenation, decreased lung compliance, and increased work of breathing. Because the patient must work harder to maintain minute ventilation, the oscillations (inspiratory and expiratory extremes) of pleural pressure are increased, and the paradoxical movement of the flail segment is thereby exaggerated.[52]

The fundamental problem in flail chest is pulmonary, not orthopedic. The patient suffers from a form of acute respiratory failure with pulmonary contusion.[14] It was once thought that one of the problems associated with flail chest was that a large segment of air moved back and forth between the lungs, resulting in increased dead-space ventilation. Now the movement of air back and forth (sometimes called *pendelluft*) is not considered significant.

A flail chest may result in the movement of other structures within the chest. There may be a shift of the mediastinal structures toward the uninjured lung, with a concomitant reduction in the amount of gas going to the normal lung. This reduction may further impair gas exchange. Furthermore, the shifting of the mediastinal structures may cause the great vessels to kink and obstruct, thus decreasing the venous return to the heart. This would decrease the cardiac output and produce a shock of cardiac origin.

A sternal flail, in which fractured ribs or costochondral separations around the sternum result in the sternum itself becoming a free-floating segment, is also a potential threat to the patient's cardiac function. If the condition is severe enough, the sternum may compress the mediastinum and the heart at the time of initial injury, resulting in myocardial contusion or pericarditis. Heart failure due to myocardial injury, pericarditis, blood in the pericardial space, or mechanical compression of the heart as the sternal segment flails may result.

Pneumothorax

Pneumothorax may accompany blunt trauma or penetrating trauma. In *pneumothorax*, an injury to either pleural membrane through the chest wall or through a punctured lung will allow air from the atmosphere to enter the pleural space.[51,52] When the normal negative intrapleural pressure is lost, there is nothing to counteract the elastic recoil of the lung. Consequently, the lung collapses. Both circulatory and respiratory functions are affected to a degree dependent on the volume of air accumulated. Small amounts of air may cause no symptoms and few, if any, physical signs. Massive accumulations, however, can lead to rapid respiratory and circulatory failure. The pathophysiology of the two most serious forms of pneumothorax, open pneumothorax and tension pneumothorax, usually accounts for the grave condition of patients with pneumothorax.

An *open pneumothorax* is the result of air entering the pleural space through a chest wall defect, usually one caused by a penetrating injury from a stab wound, a gunshot wound, or an explosion (Fig. 22–5). On inspiration, a characteristic swishing or sucking noise can be heard as air rushes from an area of greater pressure (the atmosphere) to an area of lesser pressure (the pleural space). Atmospheric and intrapleural pressures rapidly equilibrate. Negative intrapleural pressure is then lost, resulting in collapse of the lung, shift of the mediastinal structures toward the unaffected side, and impairment of the lung's ventilation. On expiration, as pressure on the

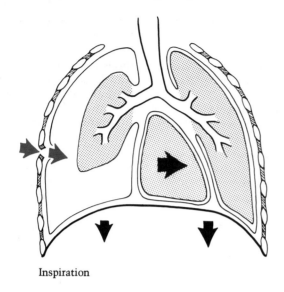

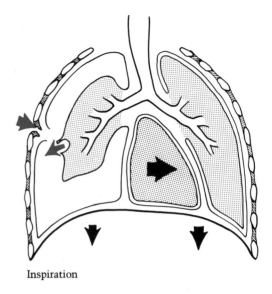

Inspiration

Inspiration

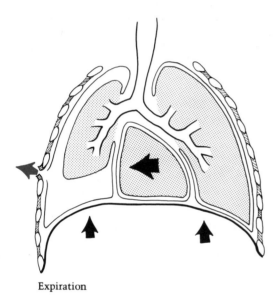

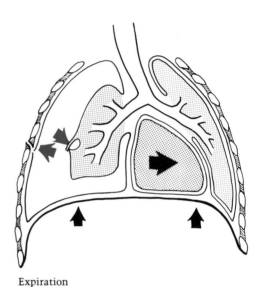

Expiration

Expiration

Figure 22–5
Open pneumothorax.

Figure 22–6
Tension pneumothorax.

unaffected side increases, the mediastinal structures shift to the area of lesser pressure (*i.e.*, the side of the collapsed lung). As it does in flail chest, the mediastinal shift results in kinking of the great vessels, with reduced venous return and cardiac output. The problem with reduced venous return is compounded because negative intrathoracic pressure is no longer present to facilitate the flow of venous blood into the thorax. The degree of seriousness of open pneumothorax depends on the size of the opening; air enters the chest wound in preference to the trachea when the wound is larger than the upper airway.

A *tension pneumothorax* results when the volume of air accumulating in the pleural space continues to increase in size with each breath, adding more and more air to a pleural space that has no outlet (Fig. 22–6). Air enters the pleural space during inspiration and cannot escape during expiration through the wound in the trachea, bronchus, lung, or chest wall. For several reasons, the effects of a tension pneumothorax

are more severe and more pronounced than in any other type of pleural involvement. As the size of the pneumothorax increases, pressure begins to build, which forces the mediastinal structures toward the unaffected side. Each breath adds to the expanding volume and exerts more pressure on the mediastinum. If the patient is receiving positive-pressure breathing, this process is accelerated. If the situation is allowed to continue, a progressive mediastinal shift occurs that impairs the function of the uninjured lung. Venous return is reduced by the rising positive intrathoracic pressure to a much greater extent than in even an open pneumothorax. Because there is no escape for the accumulating air and no mediastinal flutter, the progressive shift to the uninjured lung continues unabated.

Hemothorax

Hemothorax, the accumulation of blood in the pleural space, involves not only the cardiorespiratory impairments of chest

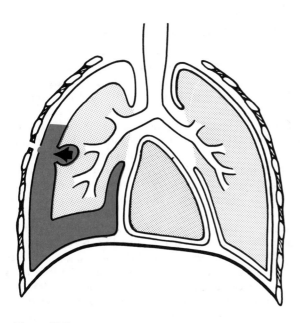

Figure 22–7
Hemothorax.

trauma but also the problems of shock from blood loss (Fig. 22–7). As much as 2 L of blood, enough to induce profound levels of hemorrhagic shock, may accumulate in the chest cavity. Furthermore, the amount and severity of the "internal chest bleed" cannot be seen but only estimated by the signs produced. Detection is a key part of the management of this type of chest involvement.

Hemothorax may occur in both blunt and penetrating trauma. Although more common in penetrating trauma, it must also be considered in severe blunt or decelerating accidents, both of which may rupture intrathoracic vessels by pressure and torsional mechanisms. Rapid deceleration is particularly notorious for producing aortic tears, which bleed into the chest slightly at first, dissect through the intimal layers of the aorta, and eventually end in a ruptured aneurysm. The association of hemothorax with traumatic pneumothorax suggests laceration of the pulmonary parenchyma. Additional sources of bleeding may be lacerated intercostal muscles and vessels, torn pleural adhesions, and injury to the heart or great vessels and at the site of fractured ribs.

There are four usual sources of bleeding in hemothorax:

1. The pulmonary parenchyma and vessels. Because the pulmonary artery pressure is one third that of systemic pressure, bleeding from the pulmonary artery branches seldom continues.
2. The intercostal and internal mammary arteries. Bleeding from these sites is usually longer and greater than bleeding from the lung. However, the bleeding may be massive and continuous, requiring thoracotomy and ligation owing to the high flow in the internal mammary artery (the flow is similar to that in the radial artery). If the vessel is torn, but not transected completely, bleeding will be greater. Transected vessels undergo retraction into the tissue and vasospasm, both of which thrombose the vessel and reduce or stop the bleeding. Torn vessels, however, cannot retract and are therefore more likely to continue to bleed.

3. The mediastinum—heart, aorta, and great vessels. Bleeding from these sites is not difficult to detect; the patient will be moribund, in profound shock, and unresponsive to even the most vigorous resuscitative measures. The bleeding may be occult initially and clinically apparent only later, when the traumatic aneurysm ruptures into the pleura.
4. The spleen or liver. Because of their vascularity, these subdiaphragmatic organs are potential sources of bleeding when the chest injury is accompanied by diaphragmatic trauma.

Hemothorax impairs cardiorespiratory function much as does any other space-occupying lesion of the thorax. As the size of the accumulation increases, greater and greater pressures are exerted on the lung of the involved side, leading to compression atelectasis. Eventually, the growing mass encroaches on the mediastinal structures, which progressively shift away from it, toward the unaffected side, thus impairing the function of the good lung. Again, the mediastinal shift produces kinking of the great vessels, which, with the obstructing pressure of the blood mass, reduces venous return and cardiac output. Therefore, shock of both cardiac and hemorrhagic origin occurs in hemothorax. The rate at which the shock occurs, as well as its severity, depends on the source and rate of the bleeding.[50,52]

Tracheal and Bronchial Injuries

Tracheal rupture and bronchial rupture are rare problems caused more often by a crushing than by a penetrating injury.[53,56] They usually occur as a result of the victim's hitting the steering wheel in a motor-vehicle accident. Patients with tracheal rupture frequently are dead before they arrive at the hospital. The tears may vary from small lacerations to complete rupture of the cervical and intrathoracic trachea and even avulsion of the bronchi. Rupture is more likely to result from a blow to the anterior chest when the glottis is closed.

Injuries involving the intrathoracic trachea or the right and left main-stem bronchi may be caused by one or more of three types of disruptive forces: avulsion of the bronchus near the trachea caused by a sudden and forceful lateral movement of the lungs away from the fixed tracheal rings (this sudden lateral movement occurs when the anteroposterior diameter of the chest is decreased rapidly by a blow to the anterior chest that widens the thorax horizontally and produces a lateral force on the lungs); rupture of the intrathoracic trachea or bronchi produced by the sudden, large increase in air pressure related to glottal closing; and shearing of the mobile trachea or bronchi away from the fixed portions because of rapid deceleration.

Cardiovascular Injuries

Penetrating Injuries

Penetrating injuries of the heart are the gravest of injuries, and most victims die instantly at the scene of the accident or crime.[11,15,45] For the few who live long enough to reach the hospital, the mortality is greater than 50%.[36] Death is the result of major cardiac injury involving large atrial, ventricular, or aortic disruption followed by sudden and massive hemorrhage.

Pericardial Tamponade

In less severe cardiac injuries, such as ones inflicted by a small knife, immediate death from massive blood loss may be averted by the development of a pericardial tamponade. The pericardial sac is a tough, fibrous, inelastic membrane surrounding the heart. With small knife wounds and (rarely) with small-caliber, low-velocity gunshot wounds, the wound in the pericardial sac may seal, trapping the blood that escapes from the myocardial wound. Blood trapped by the pericardial sac can exert enough pressure to arrest, or *tamponade*, the hemorrhage. The pericardial tamponade, which can last from several minutes to several hours, provides the patient with a temporary, life-saving reprieve from massive blood loss from the cardiac wound, often allowing time to reach emergency care and to take an orderly approach to the management of the injury. The inelasticity of the pericardial sac, however, does not allow much trapped blood to accumulate without the development of excessively high intracardiac pressure. Eventually, the tamponading effect of a small amount of trapped blood gives way to the restrictive effects of a pericardium full of a large amount of trapped blood. Compression of the atria and ventricles prevents adequate cardiac filling.[31] As the mounting intracardiac pressure begins to exceed the pressure within the thin-walled venae cavae and pulmonary veins, it impedes venous return to the heart. Increasing intrapericardial pressure begins to impede coronary artery blood flow. Eventually, the stroke volume and cardiac output fall, and the patient develops profound shock. If the situation is not remedied, pressure continues to build within the pericardial sac until the fibrous membrane tears. At this point, the patient is in the same situation as the victim who dies of massive blood loss at the scene of the accident.

Cardiac Contusion

Blunt chest trauma results in myocardial injury much more often than is recognized clinically.[64] If one considers the anatomy of the heart and the surrounding structures, it becomes obvious that the heart's position behind the sternum is a vulnerable one. The heart may be damaged severely from an external force without any visible injury to the chest wall. Myocardial damage may be slight or severe. The injury may be forgotten in the initial assessment, particularly if there are other injuries. Interestingly, myocardial injuries seem to be well tolerated by most patients. However, one fifth of patients with crushing chest injuries have cardiac damage.[8]

The myocardium, pericardium, endocardial structures, and coronary arteries may be contused, lacerated, or ruptured, resulting in myocardial contusions and pericardial effusion, rupture of the cardiac wall, tears of the valves and chordae tendineae, rupture of the interventricular septum, coronary artery injury, rupture of the pericardium and formation of a left ventricular aneurysm, and rupture of the aorta or great vessels.[5] Injury results from a direct blow, a transmitted blow, compression, deceleration, or blast effects. Using the technique of high-speed cinecardiography with a simulated deceleration model, Cooper[16,17] determined that significant cardiac motion and distortion occurred within milliseconds of the deceleration.

Aortic Injury

About 10% to 15% of patients who die in traffic accidents sustain an aortic rupture. Death is instantaneous in 80% to 90%, and the remaining 10% to 20% live long enough to reach the hospital.[1]

Blunt trauma subjects the thoracic aorta and the great vessels to a variety of forces. Sudden acceleration or deceleration may create shearing forces between different parts of the aorta, between the heart and the aorta, and between the aorta and the great vessels. Compression of the aorta or of the great vessels over the vertebral column may cause an aneurysm or rupture.

Aortic trauma must be suspected in all patients surviving a motor-vehicle accident that occurred at speeds greater than 45 mph. Aortic injury occurs with sudden deceleration, typically a head-on collision and when the victim is wearing a seat belt. Because of the sudden deceleration, the descending aorta literally bows forward in a whiplash movement and undergoes severe bending and shearing stress.[24] This segment of the aorta is relatively mobile and unrestrained by attachments to nearby structures, whereas the arch of the aorta is relatively fixed. The points at which the stresses most commonly produce damage are the aortic isthmus just distal to the origin of the left subclavian artery, distal descending aorta at the aortic hiatus, mid-thoracic descending aorta, and the origin of the left subclavian artery.[1,35,36] The sudden whiplash stress results in extensive stretching, shearing, and tearing of the aorta wall. Blood then escapes through the transverse, linear tears, producing a traumatic aneurysm. The aortic rupture is contained temporarily by adventitia, pleura, and surrounding mediastinal tissue. This false aneurysm may rupture within hours or days.

When the patient arrives at the hospital, the outer layer of the aneurysm may be all that is keeping the aorta intact (Fig. 22–8). Blood escaping through the tears into the vessel wall may exert great pressure on that outer layer as the aneurysm expands, leaving the patient vulnerable to spontaneous rupture and death from severe intrathoracic hemorrhage.

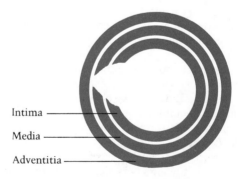

Intima

Media

Adventitia

Figure 22–8
Aortic laceration.

Fear and Anxiety

Refer to Nursing Diagnosis 2 in Chapter 8, page 111 for details.

NURSING PROCESS

ASSESSMENT

If patients are to be cared for properly, their presenting signs and symptoms must be assessed and their problems managed. The question arises: What should the nurse do to help the patient on his arrival in the emergency room? The nurse must know how to assess the patient and how to set the priorities of care (see Chap. 40 for primary and secondary surveys).

Certain historical information should be gathered to help estimate the location and extent of injury. As much information as possible should be obtained by radio from the paramedics in the ambulance or the helicopter before the patient arrives at the hospital. Once the patient is in the emergency room, emphasis is on the examination, but the staff continues to try to gather as much information as possible about the injury. Firefighters, police, eyewitnesses, other less severely injured victims, and family members are possible sources of information. The information they supply is often invaluable in the patient assessment.

Certain questions should be asked. If the injury was a penetrating one, what was the weapon? Was it a knife? A gun? What was the length of the knife or the caliber of the gun? What was the angle from which the assailant attacked the patient? If the injury involved blunt chest trauma, was rapid deceleration a factor? Was the patient sitting in the driver's seat or in the front passenger's seat, where the energy from the impact against the steering wheel or dashboard was absorbed by the body? All the details of the accident and any treatment given after it are important.

The examination begins even while the patient is being brought into the emergency room (Table 22–1). Level of consciousness, any obvious blood loss, color, and the appearance of any distress should be noted. A systematic examination should follow, with relevant questions being asked and answered as the examination proceeds. Respiratory and cardiac status should be evaluated. Is the airway patent? If not, emergency room personnel should perform the airway maneuvers (airway insertion, endotracheal intubation, or cricothyrotomy) as indicated. Is the patient exchanging air? If not, artificial ventilation should be instituted. Is the trachea in the midline? If not, does the patient have a mediastinal shift from a pneumothorax or hemothorax, and should chest tube(s) be inserted? Is the carotid pulse palpable? It is important to remember that the ABCDs of resuscitation have first priority. Are the patient's neck veins distended? If so, there should be further evaluation for cardiac tamponade and preparation for pericardiocentesis. Does the patient have a penetrating chest injury? If so, where are the entry and exit wounds? Does the patient have a blunt chest injury? Is there a flail segment? What are the respiratory rate and depth? Does the patient retract or use accessory muscles? Does the patient have stridor? Does the chest expand equally on both sides, or is one side larger than the other? Does the patient show paradoxical motion? Is there hemoptysis? Does the chest expand equally on palpation? Does the

Table 22-1

Initial Assessment: Priority Approach

A Airway
B Breathing
　　Chest wall and neck vein inspection
　　Breath sounds, percussion note
C Circulation
　　Presence of significant external bleeding
　　Pulse and blood pressure
　　Heart rate, rhythm, and sounds
　　Abdominal inspection, palpation, percussion
D Determine neurologic status
　　Level of consciousness, pupils
　　Motor movement
E Extremities
　　Inspection for deformity
　　Pulses
　　Movement
F Follow-up assessments
　　Vital signs, urinary output, central venous pressure,
　　　level of consciousness
　　Arterial blood gases, chest radiograph, pulmonary
　　　artery pressures
　　Electrocardiogram, cardiac output
　　Hemoglobin, hematocrit
G Get
H History, and
I Immunize

examiner feel rib movement, crepitation, or a deformity? Does the patient complain of a painful or tender area? Where is the point of maximal impulse? Are there areas of hyperresonance or dullness on percussion? What are the pattern and quality of breath sounds on auscultation? Are the sounds diminished or absent? Are adventitious sounds present? Is there a difference in pulse amplitude between the upper and lower extremities?

Additional information about the patient is essential to assessment and management. The patient's response to the treatment for shock must be determined. It is important to remember that Military Anti-Shock Trousers (MAST) are contraindicated in chest injuries. Laboratory reports of the arterial blood gas determinations must be evaluated. The chest radiograph must be examined. As soon as possible, the data base should be completed by the addition of a complete history of the injury, pertinent points in the patient's past medical history, and the findings from a thorough physical examination. Throughout the emergency phase, the health team should continue to monitor and reassess the patient to determine his condition and response to resuscitation.

The data obtained from the assessment must be used. If the nurse does not know what the assessment data mean, she should give them to someone who can interpret them. The nurse's ability to describe is of the utmost importance. If the physician is not present, the nurse can transmit a description of the patient that may give the physician a basis for decision making. The tools of assessment are essential to the nurse.

Clinical Manifestations

Rib Fracture

The patient may have an uncomplicated rib fracture, with the major data obtained by a positive history, pain with point tenderness, and confirmation by chest radiograph, or the patient may have a much more complicated injury with a lateral or sternal flail chest.

Lateral Flail Chest

The patient is examined for obvious deformity of the chest wall with associated paradoxical movement. The examiner should be aware that the paradox may not be apparent initially. Damage to the chest wall musculature may cause spasm and initially conceal the severity of the underlying injury. Also, the patient may splint his respirations in an effort to reduce the pain associated with the fracture. As the patient becomes exhausted from the work of breathing, the paradoxical movement becomes apparent. Respiratory difficulty increases, and the patient tries to increase the rate and depth of breathing (as carbon dioxide increases and oxygen decreases). Later cyanosis, noisy breathing, and a moribund appearance complete the clinical picture.[52] Chest radiographs are used to obtain a baseline evaluation and serial assessments. Not only will the extent of injury to the ribs be documented, but the presence of a pneumothorax, hemothorax (or hemopneumothorax), or heart and great vessel injury will be detected.

Such patients should be examined for the presence of other clues. They may be tachypneic and have painful respirations; they may be apprehensive, anxious, or dyspneic; or they may have diastolic hypertension. If the person was previously normotensive, diastolic hypertension suggests carbon dioxide retention. Particularly in younger persons, progressive skin changes from red to white may be seen. First, the skin is flushed from carbon dioxide retention and vasodilatation; next, it is pale from diastolic hypertension; and then it has a bluish hue from cyanosis. The patient may have decreased air flow on expiration, suggesting ventilatory inadequacy. Ventilation can be grossly evaluated by having the patient expire forcefully against the examiner's hand. The patient must also be observed for any signs that indicate the degree of respiratory embarrassment. The signs of hypoxemia are irritability, restlessness, confusion, cyanosis, and tachycardia. The signs of hypercapnia are headache, dizziness, lethargy, stupor, confusion, and disorientation.

Using palpation, the examiner may find point tenderness, crepitus indicative of rib fracture, changing site of the apex beat, and tracheal deviation. Using percussion, the examiner may find pronounced tenderness, hyperresonance due to pneumothorax, and decreased resonance due to an associated hemothorax. Using auscultation, the examiner may hear noisy respirations.

Sternal Flail Chest

To detect a sternal flail, the patient should be examined for paradoxical movement of the sternum during respirations and the following signs of cardiac involvement: weak and slow pulse, falling blood pressure, rising central venous pressure, and dysrhythmias.[52] The examiner should palpate the area around the sternum for rib fracture and the trachea for normal positioning (no deviation is present with a sternal flail). In addition, the patient may exhibit the signs of traumatic asphyxia. Forceful compression of the chest can increase intrathoracic pressure to the extent that venous blood is suddenly forced out of the chest and into the neck and face. The visible

signs are edema of the face, lips, tongue, and conjunctivae, and gross cyanosis of the face and neck.

Pneumothorax

In assessing patients for the presence and seriousness of open pneumothorax, the patient should be examined for chest wall defect, cyanosis, dyspnea, and hyperpnea. Using palpation, the examiner should note any deviation of the trachea as a result of mediastinal shift. Using percussion, the examiner should listen for hyperresonance on the affected side. Using auscultation, the examiner should listen for a sucking sound audible to the unaided ear or for decreased or absent breath sounds detectable with the stethoscope.

In assessing patients in order to determine the presence of tension pneumothorax, the patient should be examined for severe agitation and apprehension accompanied by cyanosis and air hunger (signs of hypoxia); an intact chest wall but a history of crushing, blunt, or blast injury to the chest; a thorax that appears larger on one side than the other; asymmetric chest excursion (the affected side lags behind the unaffected side during inspiration); deviation of the trachea toward the unaffected side; and circulatory embarrassment, with falling blood pressure, weak rapid pulse, cold, clammy skin, distended neck veins, and rising central venous pressure. Using palpation, the examiner should note any deviation of the trachea toward the unaffected side, shifting of the apex beat away from the affected side, and subcutaneous emphysema. Using percussion, the examiner should note any resonance (which could reach extreme hyperresonance) on the affected side. Using auscultation, the examiner should listen for diminished or absent breath sounds on the affected side with absent voice sounds and vocal fremitus.

Hemothorax

If the accumulation of blood is less than 350 ml, the patient is usually asymptomatic. Also, accumulations of less than 300 ml are not seen commonly on chest radiograph. If the accumulation of blood is greater than 350 ml but less than 1500 ml, the patient probably is short of breath and has distant breath sounds, dullness on the affected side, and decreased arterial oxygen tension. A chest radiograph with the patient in the upright position shows a shadow curving upward and laterally on the involved side. An accumulation of more than 1500 ml of blood may produce deviation of the trachea toward the unaffected side; dullness, absence of breath sounds, limited excursions on the affected side, and an even further decreased arterial oxygen tension; profound shock, from both blood loss and compression; tightness and severe pain in the chest, shortness of breath, faintness, and pain radiating to the neck, shoulder, and upper abdomen; and cyanosis and cardiopulmonary compromise.[10]

Tracheobronchial Injuries

Two basic types of rupture of the intrathoracic trachea and mainstem bronchi are seen—free communication of the tracheobronchial rupture with the pleural cavity and no free communication.[6,9,19] With free communication, the most common clinical manifestations are increased respiratory distress when suction is applied to the chest tube; persistent lung collapse; large air leak; cervical and mediastinal emphysema with Hamman's sign (on auscultation, a "crunching" sound heard synchronously with the heartbeat); and a chest radiograph showing the lung has lost the anchoring support provided by the bronchus and has dropped down into the chest cavity (related to a complete bronchial transection). The diagnosis is confirmed by bronchoscopy.[53]

With little or no communication with the pleural cavity, the clinical manifestations differ and may be few in number. The most common signs are minimal or moderate signs of respiratory distress, small pneumothorax, re-expansion of the lung after insertion of a chest tube, little or no mediastinal or subcutaneous emphysema, and complete atelectasis of the involved lung 1 to 3 weeks after the injury (develops when granulation tissue obstructs the disrupted ends of a bronchial rupture).

Fracture of the first rib alerts the examiner to the possibility of bronchial rupture. Because the first rib is short and broad and well protected by adjacent musculoskeletal structures, it has long been thought that only a significant force would produce a fracture. Therefore, first-rib fractures were considered a hallmark of severe trauma (i.e., if the force was strong enough to fracture the first rib, there was an increased possibility of associated injury to the bronchus as well as to the subclavian artery/vein, myocardium, and brachial plexus). However, present data have not confirmed this increased incidence.[39,54] It remains to be seen if further study will confirm the significance. In any event, the nurse should be cognizant of the fact that the physician will observe the patient closely for any associated injuries and will consider the use of arteriography for further assessment of the patient's condition.

Cardiovascular Injuries

Pericardial Tamponade

Assessing pericardial tamponade is a challenge. Initially, the tamponade produces only the most subtle of changes in the patient's condition, changes that can easily go unnoticed. A typical example is the patient with cardiac injury who presents with an obvious penetrating injury in the vicinity of the heart but no apparent signs of cardiac compromise. The patient may be alert, his vital signs may be within normal limits, and the wound may even be dismissed as superficial. If the need for continued close monitoring is not appreciated, the potentially lethal nature of the patient's injury may go undetected. To prevent this from happening, early detection is needed.

Severe, imminent compromise can be detected by use of the "rule of 20s": central venous pressure increased by more than 20 cm H_2O, pulse increased by 20 beats/minute, systolic blood pressure decreased by 20 mm Hg, and pulsus paradoxus greater than 20 mm Hg. The finding of blood (nonclotted or clotted) on pericardiocentesis is considered a diagnostic aid for pericardial tamponade and cardiac trauma. The following parameters are the ones generally accepted for assessment of cardiac tamponade from any cause. They should be committed to memory, because any one or more may be seen in the patient with accompanying chest injury.

- Distended neck veins
- Deep shock that seems out of proportion to the severity of the wound and the amount of apparent blood loss
- Falling arterial pressure
- Narrowing pulse pressure
- Rising central venous pressure
- Pulsus paradoxus—more beats palpated on expiration than on inspiration, loss of the palpated pulse on inspiration, or a fall in systemic arterial blood pressure greater than 10 mm Hg during inspiration. During inspiration, the limited output from the right heart may pool in the lungs and thus reduce the amount of blood delivered to the left heart. The descent of the diaphragm on inspiration pulls on the pericardium to further decrease its volume and further constrict the venae cavae. Expiration, however, pumps blood out of the lungs to augment left ventricular filling and cardiac output.[36,63]
- Tachycardia with distant heart sounds
- Reduced cardiac pulsation shown by fluoroscopic examination and cardiac enlargement shown by physical examination and chest radiograph.

A cardiac injury with possible accompanying tamponade should be suspected in any patient with a wound in the cardiac area. The four key signs of pericardial tamponade are detected easily by the nurse. They are falling arterial pressure, rising central venous pressure, distant heart sounds (Beck's triad), and distended neck veins. Unfortunately, all four signs do not usually appear in every patient with pericardial tamponade. One study showed that the first three signs acted as a diagnostic indicator in two thirds of the patients.[21] The admission mean blood pressure was 58 mm Hg, with one third of the patients admitted without an obtainable blood pressure. The survival rate was 63%. Fourteen percent of the patients were admitted with fixed pupils and survived with normal neurologic function. The most common causes of death were exsanguination and refractory dysrhythmias. A high mortality was associated with shotgun wounds, left ventricular injuries, thoracotomies in the emergency room, presence of coma on admission, and no blood pressure obtainable on admission.

Cardiac Contusion

The most reliable technique to assess cardiac contusion or blunt trauma to the myocardium is serial electrocardiography (ECG) on a daily basis.[26] The most common abnormalities are seen in the ST segment and T wave; QRS abnormalities and conduction defects are also seen.[37] Serial isoenzymes are used in many institutions, but elevation can be caused by several other problems. Many physicians also use radionuclide imaging or echocardiography within the first 24 hours of injury.[27,38]

In assessing the degree of myocardial damage, the injury is described usually as mild, serious, or critical. With a mild injury, the patient shows such findings as pericardial friction rub, benign dysrhythmias, and ST-T wave abnormalities on the ECG. Pre-existing cardiac disease makes determination of cardiac contusion difficult, if not impossible. With a serious injury, the likely findings are pericardial or angina-type pain, persistent sinus tachycardia, systolic or diastolic murmurs consistent with valvular regurgitation, atrial or ventricular dysrhythmias on serial ECGs, bundle branch block, enlarged heart on serial chest radiographs, abnormal uptake with radionuclide imaging with a tracer substance, and (rarely) myocardial infarction (e.g., one demonstrated by transient abnormal Q waves with an intraventricular conduction defect). With a critical injury, the findings include low cardiac output, severe ventricular dysrhythmias, progressive tamponade, congestive heart failure, ventricular aneurysm, and mural thrombi with systemic or pulmonary embolism.[22]

If a new systolic murmur is heard, the physician should be notified and the possibility of interventricular septal damage investigated. The holosystolic murmur is best heard at the left third to fourth intercostal space and is usually accompanied by a thrill. The murmur can usually be differentiated from that of valvular injury, because the latter is best described as a regurgitant murmur and often is accompanied by the signs of congestive heart failure.

Aortic Injuries

In the assessment and monitoring of all patients with chest trauma, a high index of suspicion must be maintained with regard to the possibility of aortic damage.[1,35] Prompt investigation and surgical repair by the physician will avert a potential catastrophe. The important signs and symptoms to look for are mediastinal widening of more than 8 cm on chest radiograph, difference in pulse amplitude between the upper and lower extremities, and systolic murmur over the precordium or posterior infrascapular area. Other possible assessment parameters are chest pain, dyspnea, dysphagia, hoarseness from pressure on the laryngeal nerve, an enlarged neck, severe back pain, paraplegia, hemothorax, feelings of apprehension, the patient's involvement in a motor-vehicle accident at a speed greater than 45 mph, a patient in adolescence or young adulthood (possibly because the physical stamina of people in that age range is such that they are able to survive the initial injury), and positive findings on arteriography. Although it occurs only in about one quarter of patients, the most common symptom is retrosternal or infrascapular pain.

One third of all patients with an aortic rupture have little or no evidence of chest trauma on first examination.[35] Serial monitoring is mandatory. The most ominous sign is a widened mediastinum shown by chest radiograph, a finding that is reason enough for further diagnostic study involving arteriography to identify and locate the site of the lesion.[25] (Anteroposterior chest radiographs occasionally give the impression that the mediastinum is widened slightly when it is normal.) Because the aortic wall is elevated by the blood stream, the aortic tear usually is seen as a filling defect. Other radiographic signs associated with thoracic rupture are tracheal shift to the right, blurring of the normal sharp outline of the aorta, obliteration of the medial aspect of the apex of the left upper lobe, opacification of the clear space between the aorta and pulmonary artery, and depression of the left main-stem bronchus below 40°.

Diagnostic Studies

Initial blood work includes arterial blood gas analysis, hemoglobin/hematocrit determination, blood typing and cross matching, electrolytes, blood urea nitrogen, amylase, glucose, toxicology assay, platelet count, and partial thromboplastin time. Because many patients are hypoxic, the A-a gradient is usually determined. A urinalysis is obtained.

A chest film is obtained as early as possible. Many specific chest injuries, such as tension pneumothorax, hemothorax, and cardiac tamponade, are diagnosed clinically and treated before the chest film is obtained. The initial films obtained are usually suboptimal, but important information for assessment can still be derived. Films taken with the patient supine are anteroposterior projections, so that the mediastinal shadows seem more prominent than when chest films are taken in the posteroanterior projection. With the patient supine, it is hard for the physician to see small fluid accumulations and lateral rib fractures. Information that can be obtained include mediastinal displacement, tracheal deviation, air or fluid accumulations, and retained missiles.

Based on an assessment of the patient's condition, the physician may order other diagnostic studies, including arteriography, bronchoscopy, esophagoscopy, computed tomographic (CT) scanning, and water-soluble contrast esophagography.

NURSING DIAGNOSES, PATIENT OUTCOMES, AND PLAN

The preceding material on anatomy, physiology, nursing assessment, and diagnostic tests guides the nurse in establishing nursing diagnoses, patient outcomes, and plan for the patient with chest trauma.

NURSING CARE PLAN SUMMARY Patient With Chest Trauma

NURSING DIAGNOSIS

1. *Fluid volume deficit related to third-space loss during shock and incomplete replacement of isotonic fluid and blood loss or loss of adequate circulating volume related to shock or blood loss (exchanging pattern)*

Patient Outcome	Nursing Orders
1. The patient will maintain normal cardiopulmonary function.	1. See Chapters 40 ("Trauma Assessment") and 41 ("Abdominal Trauma"). A. Restore an adequate circulating volume by crystalloid and blood therapy as

(continued)

NURSING CARE PLAN SUMMARY   Patient With Chest Trauma   Continued

Patient Outcome	Nursing Orders
	ordered. Ringer's lactate solution is given initially in amounts up to 2 L and then continued at a rate to keep systolic blood pressure at least 100 mm Hg, urinary output at least 0.5 ml/kg/hour, central venous pressure at least 5 mm Hg, and pulmonary capillary wedge pressure at least 8 mm Hg. Blood is replaced as packed red cells according to the estimate of blood loss and to keep hemoglobin at least 10 g and hematocrit at least 30%. If capillary leak syndrome has resulted from severe shock or hypoxemia, colloid solutions are usually held for 24 to 48 hours until the syndrome has abated. B. Monitor peripheral tissues for edema. Check capillary refill in all extremities. Elevate extremity if necessary. Protect skin from injury during edematous states. C. Maintain intravenous flow rates, checking for kinks in tubing or catheter, obstructions, and improper connections. D. Weigh the patient every day. E. Monitor the patient's nasogastric drainage and urinary output, determining the amount of both and the loss of electrolytes. F. Maintain the patient's intake by mouth (when able to take nourishment by mouth).

NURSING DIAGNOSIS

2. *Decreased cardiac output related to myocardial compromise (exchanging pattern)*

Patient Outcome	Nursing Orders
The patient will demonstrate hemodynamic stability.	1. Prepare for chest tube placement, periocardiocentesis, emergency open thoracotomy, or surgery, as indicated by patient assessment and per physician order. A. Monitor cardiovascular functioning by measuring blood pressure, pulse, pulmonary capillary wedge pressure, pulmonary artery pressures, central venous pressure, sensorium, urinary output, cardiac output, capillary refill, ECG results, and hemoglobin and hematocrit levels. B. Provide volume replacement as ordered. C. Administer therapy as ordered to prevent acid-base imbalance and hypoxemia. D. Monitor and replace electrolytes as ordered. E. Administer diuretics if ordered.

NURSING DIAGNOSIS

3. *Impaired gas exchange related to hemopneumothorax (exchanging pattern)*

Patient Outcomes	Nursing Orders
The patient should demonstrate the return of adequate pulmonary function.	1. Monitor the patient's pulmonary status as evidenced by the assessment. The nurse should do the following: A. Perform a respiratory examination, including percussion notes and breath sounds. B. Measure the patient's temperature and respiration every 2 to 4 hours. C. Measure the central venous pressure and pulmonary artery pressure. D. Calculate compliance if the patient is mechanically ventilated. E. Draw an arterial blood sample and send it to the laboratory for the determination of PaO_2, pH, $PaCO_2$, HCO_3^-, and delta base. F. Order a chest radiograph daily as directed by the physician.

(continued)

NURSING CARE PLAN SUMMARY   *Patient With Chest Trauma*   *Continued*

Patient Outcomes	Nursing Orders

Nursing Orders

G. Send specimens to the laboratory for a white blood cell count with a differential count and a sputum smear or culture.

H. Monitor for altered behavior or increased restlessness.

2. Encourage maximal diaphragmatic excursion by placing patients in a semi-Fowler's position, repositioning frequently, and using maximal inspiratory maneuvers. Apply and maintain the chest-tube drainage system for hemothorax.

A. Strip, or milk, the tubes every 5 minutes until the flow significantly decreases (an accepted nursing procedure, but one whose validity has not been established by research).

B. Measure the amount of drainage at 5 minute intervals until the flow of blood begins to slow, and then measure it at 15-minute intervals.

C. Encourage the patient initially to lie with the affected side down so that the chest tube, which is now dependent, can collect the intrathoracic blood more efficiently.

D. Evaluate the entire chest tube drainage system for proper assembly every 4 hours. Starting at the patient's chest, the nurse should make certain that of the following:
    (1) The airtight dressing is in place.
    (2) The tubing is free of kinks, loops, and obstructions.
    (3) The air outlet is open (unless attached to suction).
    (4) The waterseal is intact.
    (5) The reservoir is kept at a level lower than the chest.

E. Check the chest tube drainage system every hour to make sure of the following:
    (1) The oscillations in the column occur with respiration (up on inspiration, down on expiration, except during positive-pressure ventilation, when the opposite is true). If the work of breathing is increased, the oscillations will be seen at a greater level.
    (2) Bubbles occur on expiration or cough only (with positive pressure, on inspiration). Any continuous bubbling should be investigated because it usually means that there is a leak in the system.
    (3) The level, consistency, color, and rate of drainage have not changed significantly.
    (4) The blood loss is not greater than 100 ml/hour. If it is, the physician should be notified.

F. Maintain the proper functioning of the chest tubes. The nurse should do the following:
    (1) Strip the tubes every hour. Gently compress the tube in the direction of the drainage apparatus (away from the patient to remove fluid, air, or blood clots). Clasp the tube and slide the hand over the tube in a direction away from the chest and toward the drainage. Use alcohol sponges or a water-soluble lubricant to facilitate sliding. Be gentle—the procedure can be painful.
    (2) Reconnect any tube that is disconnected and do not clamp it.
    (3) Do not clamp the tube if the patient is to be moved to another unit.
    (4) Monitor the patient closely if the physician orders the tubes clamped.
    (5) Position the patient on the affected side for hemothorax and in the semi-Fowler's position for pneumothorax.
    (6) Keep the tubes hanging straight from the bed to the bottles; the tubes should not be left in a dependent position.
    (7) Observe the following procedure for chest tube removal: Have petrolatum gauze and a sterile dressing ready for the physician. The tube should be removed with a steady, quick motion during expiration or following a deep inspiration, and the dressing should then be applied. Follow-up chest radiographs are mandatory.

G. Apply added suction as ordered.
    (1) When using a disposable, controlled suction chest drainage unit, fill the

(continued)

NURSING CARE PLAN SUMMARY   *Patient With Chest Trauma*   *Continued*

Patient Outcomes	*Nursing Orders*
	suction control chamber to the prescribed level (cm of H_2O). Keep the air vent in the suction control chamber open to atmosphere.
	(2) Add suction by connecting to the air vent at the water seal chamber, and increasing the suction until a small amount of constant bubbling can be seen in the suction control chamber.
	(3) Observe the water seal chamber and determine if air is being evacuated from the patient's pleural space (bubbles will appear in the water seal chamber).
	(4) Because of water evaporation from the suction control chamber, disconnect from suction and refill to the prescribed level. Reapply suction.
	(5) Check for constant bubbling in the suction control chamber, a sign of proper functioning.
	(6) If the suction equipment ever fails (no bubbling present in the suction control chamber), disconnect the patient from it to provide the means of venting air trapped in the pleural space.
2. The patient will demonstrate no signs of an air embolism. A. Patients will not perform any excessive Valsalva maneuvers.	2. Identify all patients at high risk for air embolism—those having sustained penetrating thoracic trauma with lung involvement. The best treatment is prevention. A. Caution patients against excessive Valsalva maneuvers, such as forceful coughing, sneezing, or straining. 　(1) Maintain fluid volume and central venous pressure. 　(2) Have patients lie initially with the injured side of the chest in a dependent position to minimize the drainage of blood into the trachea or the uninjured lung and to increase pulmonary venous pressure. 　(3) Do not attempt endotracheal intubation in the awake or straining patient. 　(4) Avoid vigorous manual ventilatory assistance. B. If loss of consciousness, shock, or ventricular fibrillation ensue, assess for air embolism by using the following methods: 　(1) History 　(2) Cardiac irregularities or ischemia on ECG 　(3) Visualization of intracapillary air on funduscopic examination. C. When necessary, use the following emergency care measures: 　(1) Place the patient in a head-down position, increase pulmonary venous pressure, and minimize coronary artery and cerebral access. 　(2) Prepare for resuscitative thoracotomy with direct air aspiration from the aorta and left ventricle. 　(3) Prepare for surgery.

NURSING DIAGNOSIS

4. *Ineffective breathing pattern related to pulmonary contusion (exchanging pattern)*

Patient Outcomes	*Nursing Orders*
1. The patient will maintain adequate arterial oxygen levels.	1. Maintain oxygen as ordered. A. Monitor respiratory rate and depth; measure tidal volume and vital capacity hourly with Wright's spirometer. B. Maintain regional anesthesia and pain relief as ordered.
2. The patient's lungs will re-expand, as demonstrated on auscultation and chest radiograph.	2. Coordinate chest physiotherapy, incentive spirometry, and postural damage with periods of maximal pain relief. A. Maintain artificial airway. B. Maintain mechanical ventilation.

(continued)

NURSING CARE PLAN SUMMARY   *Patient With Chest Trauma*   Continued

NURSING DIAGNOSIS

5. *Ineffective airway clearance related to retained secretions (exchanging pattern)*

Patient Outcomes	Nursing Orders
1. The patient should exhibit good pulmonary toilette.	1. Maintain the patient's pulmonary hygiene. The nurse should do the following: A. Have the patient breathe deeply every hour. The nurse should remain with the patient and remind the patient to inhale slowly and evenly, hold the breath for 3 seconds, and exhale normally. The procedure should be repeated five times.

2. The patient's lungs will re-expand, as demonstrated on auscultation and chest radiograph.	2. Coordinate chest physiotherapy, incentive spirometry, and postural damage with periods of maximal pain relief.
	    A. Maintain artificial airway.
	    B. Maintain mechanical ventilation (see Chap. 16).

NURSING DIAGNOSIS

6. *Pain (altered comfort) related to chest trauma (feeling pattern)*

Patient Outcomes	Nursing Orders

1. The patient will maintain relative comfort.	1. Provide initial splinting for flail chest with a small weight (*e.g.,* intravenous bag or sandbag) or by turning the patient toward the affected side. Help the patient concentrate on abdominal breathing.
	    A. Strip the chest tubes carefully.
	    B. Stabilize chest tube so that tube does not move excessively.
	    C. Splint the patient's chest with the hands or with pillows to make deep breathing and coughing easier.
	    D. Assist the physician with nerve blocks.
	        (1) Work efficiently and quickly so that the patients will feel they are in competent hands.
	        (2) Stabilize chest tube so that tube does not move excessively.
	        (3) Splint the patient's chest with the hands or with pillows to make deep breathing and coughing easier.
	        (4) Give the patients information about what will happen to them. Include sensations to be experienced.
	        (5) Use pain medication as ordered in conjunction with other measures that have been effective for the individual patient. Remember that the patient paralyzed for respiratory control still has pain and requires pain relief.
	        (6) Assist the physician with nerve blocks.

2. The patient will experience no inordinate amount of pain.	2. Use deep breathing and other relaxation techniques.
	    A. Strip the chest tubes carefully.
	    B. Give the patient a chance to talk about any pain and what makes it better or what makes it worse.
	    C. If possible, relieve any other sources of discomfort, including worry.
	    D. If possible, involve the family in the patient care.
	    E. Use the established nursing techniques for making the patient comfortable: changing the bed linens, giving back rubs, and changing positions.

(continued)

NURSING CARE PLAN SUMMARY   *Patient With Chest Trauma*   *Continued*

NURSING DIAGNOSIS

7. *Impaired physical mobility related to chest injury (moving pattern)*

Patient Outcome	Nursing Orders

The patient will perform exercises adequately and will maintain the full range of motion.	1. Use active, active-assisted, and passive range-of-motion exercises for each joint three to four times each day.
	  A. Maintain appropriate body alignment when doing positioning techniques. Think carefully about each body part and whether or not it has been positioned for ultimate functioning.
	  B. Instruct the patient concerning breathing and shoulder, arm, and lower extremity exercises.
	  C. Encourage ambulation.
	  D. Institute comfort measures.
	  E. Use a footboard or a commercial device, such as Bunny Boots or Space Boots, to maintain the lower extremity positioning.
	  F. Use a trochanter roll, which can often prevent hip and leg abduction.
	  G. Remember that contracture complications are much more easily prevented than treated.
	  H. Consult with physical and occupational therapists as needed.
	  I. Provide an overhead bar or rope on the end of the bed to facilitate the movement of the patient in bed.

NURSING DIAGNOSIS

8. *Sensory/perceptual alterations related to confinement in a small area with inadequate stimulation (perceiving pattern)*

Patient Outcome	Nursing Orders
The patient will return to and maintain psychologic equilibrium.	1. Explain to the patient in simple terms what has happened and what is happening. Provide the patient with some means of communication.

NURSING DIAGNOSIS

9. *Anxiety related to difficulty in breathing and possibility of dying (feeling pattern)*

Patient Outcome	Nursing Orders
The patient (and family) will demonstrate decreased levels of anxiety.	See Nursing Diagnosis: Anxiety, page 111.

NURSING DIAGNOSIS

10. *Knowledge deficit related to limited understanding of therapy (knowing pattern)*

Patient Outcome	Nursing Orders

The patient will demonstrate understanding by explaining why therapeutic measures are employed, will show decreased levels of anxiety, and will participate in care planning.	1. Explain the disease process and how therapy alters the process and allows for healing.
	  A. Describe diagnostic procedures, including sensations, the patient will encounter.
	  B. Encourage questions.
	  C. Ask for feedback on the care plan and its implementation.
	  D. Communicate with other members of the health team.

IMPLEMENTATION AND EVALUATION

Approximately 85% of patients with chest trauma can be managed with a large-bore chest tube. About 15% of patients require surgery.[46] Patients with penetrating injuries are managed according to their presenting injuries and stability of condition. For example, asymptomatic patients with stab wounds may now be managed as outpatients in many institutions,[70] whereas patients with transmediastinal gunshot wounds who are unstable on admission are transferred immediately to surgery.[57] Open thoracotomy in the emergency room is performed in patients who are too unstable or whose condition is too precarious for transfer to the operating room.

Clinical criteria vary, but there are several well-accepted management strategies. In hemothorax, hemopneumothorax, and tension pneumothorax, chest tubes usually are placed immediately based on clinical evidence, rather than waiting for diagnostic studies. Chest tubes are prophylactically placed in patients with small pneumothoraces when other injuries require surgery in order to prevent a tension pneumothorax from occurring while the patient is being ventilated mechanically under anesthesia.[46] Indications for thoracotomy include hemodynamically unstable patient;[57] pericardial tamponade or penetrating wounds that may have reached the heart in association with acute loss of vital signs or shock that does not respond to blood replacement; continued hemothorax (*i.e.,* immediate egress of 1500 ml blood after chest tube placement or increased or continued rate of bleeding at a rate greater than 100 ml/hour); massive air leak that prevents the lung from re-expansion or constitutes a significant portion of the tidal volume when the patient is on the ventilator; hypovolemic cardiac arrest; radiographic evidence of tracheobronchial, vascular, or esophageal injury; traumatic thoracotomy with loss of chest wall substance; parasternal entrance wound; vascular injury to the thoracic outlet; bullet embolus to the heart or pulmonary artery; retained hemothorax; and injury to the diaphragm.[24]

Rib Fracture

Uncomplicated Rib Fracture

Management for the patient with uncomplicated rib fracture with no associated injury basically is pain relief and the prevention of complications.

Several techniques for pain relief may be chosen by the physician: chest strapping, intercostal nerve block, local infiltration, or paravertebral block. Chest strapping is not commonly recommended, except in selected cases of very minor injury. Increased splinting may be fostered by strapping, and the risk associated with shallow respirations is thus compounded. Also, local skin irritation may result from the tape. The intercostal nerve block is considered effective and is generally recommended. The usual procedure is that the physician injects an anesthetic proximal to and including the intercostal spaces below and above the injured rib. Usually the injections are given every 4 to 6 hours for 8 to 24 hours. Occasionally, plastic cannulas are inserted and used for intermittent injections. The major potential complication is pneumothorax.

The nurse can greatly assist patients by explaining to them the very real danger of the complications of inadequate pulmonary ventilation as well as signs and symptoms. It is important for the nurse to remember that ventilation is restricted, which predisposes the patient to atelectasis and pneumonia.

Patients should be instructed about deep-breathing exercises, coughing with support, and reporting any clinical signs. Analgesics should be used carefully and supplemented with relaxation therapy or other measures to make patients as comfortable as possible while keeping them alert and participating actively in their care. Patients must remain mobile, turn and move frequently, inspire deeply, and cough.

Flail Chest

Emergency Care

The objective of whatever type of emergency treatment is used is maintenance of adequate pulmonary oxygenation and ventilation. Splinting the mobile flail segment is followed by drainage of the pleural space and maintenance of respiratory excursion.[52]

As an immediate first-aid measure, the palm of the hand may be used to exert firm but gentle pressure against the flail segment and thus stabilize it. The chest does not have to be stabilized in an outward position; an inward position will suffice. Other measures are use of a small weight, such as a sandbag or intravenous bag, or turning the patient toward the affected side. Stabilization of the chest wall will relieve respiratory distress.

If a patient with a severe flail chest and respiratory distress enters the hospital and a physician is not available and the nurse is not skilled in endotracheal intubation, a temporary means of stabilization employing traction may be instituted. The effectiveness of external splinting is questionable, but in such a situation, it may be the only alternative. Traction can be applied with the use of towel clips. First, either side of the ribs is anesthetized with 0.5 ml of a 1% lidocaine solution, and the towel clips are applied through the skin to the ribs. A cord is tied to the clips and attached to an intravenous pole with enough traction (5 lb–15 lb) to reduce retraction of the flail on inspiration. With a sternal flail, mechanical compression of the mediastinal structures may be treated by elevation of the flailing sternal segment. A uterine tenaculum may be used to grasp the mobile sternum and lift it off the pericardium. Later, the towel clips or tenaculum may be replaced with a Kirschner wire placed behind the ribs or sternum. Certain potential problems exist with external splinting: difficulty in identifying the appropriate ribs, inadequate control of the paradox, infection, necrosis, hemothorax, pneumothorax, and subsequent bony deformity.

Management in the Critical Care Unit

The most common method to improve respiratory exchange and decrease shunting is internal stabilization with endotracheal intubation and controlled positive-pressure breathing. The outcomes to be achieved are full expansion of both lungs and adequate alveolar ventilation. Most important, adequate ventilation averts the complications of hypoxemia because the rate and depth of respiration may be controlled. Abnormalities in ventilation and perfusion are produced by the underlying pulmonary parenchymal contusion and splinting of the chest wall. Splinting inhibits coughing and allows tracheobronchial secretions to accumulate and atelectasis to develop. Also, because positive pressure is applied within the lung on inspiration, it is not necessary to create negative pressure on inspiration. The paradoxical motion of the flail segment is thus prevented. Stabilization of a flail chest requires several weeks;

the positive pressure "splints" the flail segment during that time. However, it is generally agreed that, in many patients, internal stabilization is associated with a prolonged hospitalization and some degree of morbidity. Therefore, many patients today are being managed without internal stabilization and mechanical ventilation. If this protocol is selected, nursing management must include incentive spirometry, humidification, effective coughing or endotracheal suctioning, cupping, and postural drainage. Pharmacologic control of pain includes small doses of intravenous narcotics and intercostal nerve blocks. Nonpharmacologic control of pain includes imagery, sensory information, and relaxation. Patient monitoring is critical to determine if and when the patient will need ventilatory assistance.

In an important documentation of the selective use of ventilatory therapy, Shackford et al[61] prospectively studied patients with flail chest injuries. They made one of the first attempts to quantitate the severity of injury, and they have helped substantiate the premise that patients should not be ventilated on the basis of abnormalities in the chest wall. Depending on the degree of pulmonary dysfunction on admission, patients were assigned to one of three groups. Group 1 consisted of those with clinically apparent respiratory distress (tachycardia, dyspnea, arterial oxygen tension less than 60 mm Hg on room air, arterial carbon dioxide tension greater than 60 mm Hg, or an intrapulmonary shunt greater than 25%). These patients were intubated and received ventilatory assistance with continuous positive airway pressure alone or combined with intermittent mechanical ventilation. Group 2 patients consisted of those who required temporary respiratory support for associated injuries but had no pulmonary dysfunction (based on clinical assessment and arterial blood gas analysis). Group 3 patients consisted of those who had no evidence of pulmonary dysfunction and no indication for respiratory support. Review of the patients showed that the number of ribs fractured in each group was similar; that the number of associated injuries were greater in groups 1 and 2; that the incidence of pulmonary contusion was 100% in group 1, 28% in group 2, and 25% in group 3; that arterial oxygenation on admission was lowest and intrapulmonary shunt was highest in group 1; and that the complication (pneumonia and adult respiratory distress syndrome) and mortality rates were greatest in group 1. By using a respiratory protocol with intermittent mechanical ventilation and continuous positive airway pressure, adequate pain relief, and good pulmonary toilets, the patients were extubated in 10 days. For many, this occurred even before the chest wall had stabilized.[52]

Pneumothorax

Open Pneumothorax

Because open pneumothorax can be quickly lethal, management of the patient entails immediate closure of the wound with an occlusive dressing by any means available. Petrolatum gauze is best, but if nothing else is available, the palm of the hand can be used to prevent further pneumothorax and mediastinal shift. An additional 100 ml to 200 ml of air can be evacuated from the pleural space if the occlusive dressing is applied after the patient coughs or exhales forcibly. The edges of the wound should not be approximated with tape or suture at this time, because subcutaneous air may invade the area. Care must be taken not to convert the open pneumothorax into a more lethal condition, tension pneumothorax. An

emergency dressing of petrolatum gauze will close the open wound. The dressing is applied to cover the wound and extend 6 inches to 8 inches beyond the wound edges. It is then covered with gauze and 3-inch adhesive tape. A new dressing must be applied when the old dressing becomes saturated with blood, is stiff, and stands away from the chest. A "flutter valve" dressing that closes the open pneumothorax but allows air to escape from a tension pneumothorax can be made by taping only three sides of the dressing. The dressing acts as a valve, letting air out but not in.

After the emergency care, decompression and drainage of the pleural space are achieved by the use of chest tubes. Because the wounds are inevitably contaminated, attention to the details of asepsis is needed to prevent further infection.

Tension Pneumothorax

Management of the patient with tension pneumothorax requires providing a route for the escape of air from the pleural space. Introduction of a chest tube or needle aspiration is the technique generally used to remove the air.

An emergency maneuver that offers temporary relief involves the insertion of a 16-gauge intravenous catheter or a large needle attached to a large syringe with a stopcock into the second intercostal space in the midclavicular line on the affected side. Intercostal vessels and nerves may be avoided by entering at the midpoint in the intercostal space. When the tension inside the chest is encountered, the high intrapleural pressure will suddenly push the plunger out of the syringe. In using the intravenous catheter, the inner needle stylet is removed from the catheter so that the air will have a larger pathway through which to escape, and the slowly re-expanding lung will not be further traumatized by a needle present at the chest wall. The soft plastic catheter will not harm the re-expanding lung.

Pleural decompression can be maintained by attaching a flutter valve to the end of the catheter so that air will continue to escape on expiration but not enter the thorax on inspiration, as would happen with an open pneumothorax. Pleural decompression can be improvised by taping a perforated finger cot to the hub of the intravenous catheter. The finger cot, which is pliable, will allow air to escape through the perforation on expiration, and it will collapse and seal on inspiration. Commercially prepared flutter valves are available under the trade name Heimlich valve.

Hemothorax

Management depends in part on the size of the hemothorax. If less than 350 ml has accumulated, no treatment is indicated; the clot will be defibrinated by normal respiratory excursions and absorbed in 10 to 14 days.[35] Serial chest radiographs are needed to rule out continued bleeding if a chest tube is not placed. With accumulations of up to 1500 ml, thoracentesis or tube thoracostomy is indicated, and with accumulations of more than 1500 ml, immediate chest tube drainage, possibly followed by emergency surgery, may be indicated.[66]

As an emergency measure, when the accumulation of blood in the chest begins to produce both circulatory and respiratory impairment, needle aspiration may be performed. The procedure is similar to that used in tension pneumothorax, except that the site is different. One of two sites is usually used: the fifth or sixth intercostal space, or the seventh or eighth intercostal space between the anterior and posterior axillary lines. Insertion of the needle into a lower intercostal space may injure a high-lying diaphragm and an underlying organ, such as the liver or spleen. Thoracentesis may be repeated or even continued intermittently through the use of stopcock maneuvering as long as the bleeding continues and until tube thoracostomy can be performed.

Chest tube drainage should be instituted as soon as possible, because it is the only really effective method of maintaining and monitoring the drainage. Serial chest radiographs are essential in monitoring the effectiveness of treatment and the success in evacuating the blood from the pleural space. While the dangerous level of intrathoracic blood is reduced, attention is directed to restoring the blood volume. Thoracic blood loss of less than 1000 ml requires replacement with Ringer's lactate solution in an amount two to three times the volume of blood loss.

Autotransfusion is a technique gaining acceptance for patients suffering from hemothorax. Up to 5 L may be collected and reinfused. Commercial systems that are simple to use are now available. Risks are low, and advantages include the rapid provision of warm, fresh, matched blood at a substantially decreased cost and certainly without all the elaborate processing needed by the blood bank.

Cardiovascular Injuries

Pericardial Tamponade

When the amount of blood in the pericardial space is so great that myocardial compression is apparent, immediate aspiration of the pericardial sac is mandatory to prevent death. If aspiration is not performed immediately, the patient will die either as the tamponade's mechanical compression restricts cardiac filling, resulting in shock, or from the exsanguination that follows the eventual rupture of the sac and release of the tamponade. With pericardiocentesis, however, the removal of as little as 10 ml to 20 ml of blood may be enough to relieve the pressure and revive even a moribund patient. The procedure is as follows:

1. Unless contraindicated by the patient's condition, the patient is placed in a semi-Fowler's position (so that accumulated blood will be dependent), and the patient is monitored continuously with a 12-lead ECG.
2. An area to the left of the fifth or sixth intercostal space at the sternal margin or a few centimeters below the left intercostal margin and to the left of the midline is prepared antiseptically.
3. A large-bore (18-gauge), short-beveled spinal needle attached to a 50-ml syringe with a three-way stopcock is directed superiorly and posteriorly at a 30° to 45° angle to the subxyphoid area of the chest wall. The chest lead is attached to the needle by an alligator clamp. If the needle touches the epicardium, ST-segment elevation occurs. If the needle is in the pericardial space, the ECG reading, including the ST segment, is normal. The needle is inserted by the physician upward through the diaphragm and then gently into the pericardial sac. Because the pericardium is much less compliant than the ventricular muscle, as little as 10 ml blood may reverse the hypotension.

Emergency open thoracotomy with a midsternal incision is used by some physicians. Data are being collected to determine the incidence and ultimate patient outcome for open thoracotomy in the emergency room.[9,29,59] The protocol varies from physician to physician. Many physicians do the pericardiocentesis procedure once or twice, and if bleeding continues, they turn quickly to the surgical approach.[11] Many others consider surgery to be the treatment of choice and use pericardiocentesis as a means to provide a safe time until surgery can be performed.

In the treatment of penetrating cardiac trauma, Evans *et al*[21] outlined four principles: rapid diagnosis, relief of cardiac tamponade by pericardiocentesis, control of hemorrhage, and repair of cardiac defects and restoration of blood volume. They emphasize that pericardiocentesis should not be considered definitive therapy, but rather should be used as an assessment technique for diagnosis and as a helpful temporizing procedure before surgery.

Cardiac Contusion

Management depends largely on the actual injury. A surgical or medical approach is chosen according to the ramifications of the injury and the clinical prognosis. Anticoagulant therapy may be instituted if the danger of mural thrombi is present or if musculoskeletal injuries and prolonged immobilization are associated. In selected patients, the injury may not be diagnosed for weeks or even years after the trauma, so repeated follow-up examinations are mandatory.

Treatment of cardiac contusion resembles that of myocardial infarction: continuous cardiopulmonary monitoring, prevention of hypoxemia, maintenance of normal fluid volume levels, and prevention and management of dysrhythmias.[22] Life-threatening complications (cardiogenic shock, heart block, dysrhythmia, pericardial effusion, and constrictive pericarditis) are most likely to occur in patients with multiple associated injuries (*e.g.*, flail chest and hypoxemia). Most commonly, ECG abnormalities disappear in 2 to 3 weeks, but there are numerous case reports of patients who later develop several complications (*e.g.*, coronary artery occlusion, ventricular septal defect, or ventricular aneurysm).

Tube Thoracostomy

In the critical care unit, all supportive measures to prevent the complications of injury must be given the patient. Unless the nursing measures are comprehensive and detailed, the patient may suffer from the side effects of immobility, pulmonary dysfunction, psychologic alterations, sepsis, and altered metabolism. These complications are discussed in other chapters of this text.

Patients in critical care units frequently have problems that require the placement of chest tubes. There are some variations in the type of drainage system, but the basic principles remain the same. Chest tubes are used primarily to return the lung to functioning at normal pressure and dynamics. Various types of injury allow air or fluid to enter the pleural space so that the normal negative pressure (−8 mm Hg intrapleural pressure and −3 mm Hg intra-alveolar pressure during inspiration) is lost and proper lung inflation cannot occur. Chest tubes are used to evacuate the pleural space so that the negative pressure may be re-established. The fluid or air removed may be monitored and changes noted. Coughing, deep breathing, and the removal of secretions are mandatory for the adequate re-expansion of the lung.[28]

The drainage system that is connected to the chest tube includes the safety feature of an underwater seal. The water functions as the flutter valve, permitting air or fluid to escape from the chest on expiration and preventing its re-entrance into the pleural space on inspiration. Also, the device permits persistent air leaks, as well as continuing hemorrhage, to be evaluated. Other problems are prevented: compression of the trachea, mediastinal shift, and compression of the unaffected lung.

A person who has been injured naturally positions himself to decrease pain and restrict movement of the affected part. When the injury is a lung injury, the inadequate lung expansion due to the restricted movement results in stasis, with the accumulation of secretions and the occlusion of lung passages. Atelectasis progresses rapidly, and the entire lung can be involved. Atelectatic areas are perfused but not ventilated, and right-to-left shunting results in hypoxia and hypercarbia. These problems must be prevented.

Insertion Sites

Various sites are used for chest tube insertion. The more common site for the anterior tube is the second intercostal space in the midclavicular line, and the posterior tube is placed in an intercostal space from the fifth to eighth intercostal space between the anterior and the posterior axillary lines. Tubes are usually used in both sites for a hemopneumothorax. However, it must be noted that an increasing number of surgeons place chest tubes in the fourth to fifth intercostal space in the mid-axillary line in a posterosuperior direction, because this site has been seen to be clinically effective in treating pneumothorax after trauma.

The second intercostal space in the midclavicular line is chosen for many reasons. Because air gravitates upward in the chest cavity, use of the anterior site commonly results in quick, complete re-expansion. Few injuries are associated with insertion, because there are no major anatomic hazards. The mammary artery is close to the sternal border, and the subclavian artery and vein are near the first intercostal space. If the patient is lying in the supine or semi-Fowler's position, the area is easily accessible. Last, but not least, the tube is out of the way during many procedures (*e.g.*, cardiopulmonary resuscitation).

The posterior tube is placed in a dependent position for drainage. Although the tube is posterior, a site is chosen so that the patient in the supine position will not compress the tube or be uncomfortable. The lowest position possible is chosen; the seventh or eighth intercostal space is the lowest usually used, because the diaphragm bulges into the thoracic cavity at the eighth or ninth intercostal space. In cases in which the tube is lower, it is usually placed as a drain rather than as a chest tube.

Chest tubes are inserted in patients with pneumothorax to re-establish normal chest functioning, to relieve the dyspnea, and to correct imbalances of the arterial blood gases. Repeated needle aspiration, an alternate method, is used rarely because of the ease of inserting a chest tube and because a tube allows for continuous evacuation. When the potential for tension pneumothorax exists, chest tubes are mandatory.

Chest tubes are also used for patients with hemothorax; they allow for continuous evacuation so that the lung is expanded more quickly and completely. The amount the patient is bleeding can be seen and monitored. The blood in the chest cavity remains liquid if it is not mixed with air. However, when it is mixed with air, a clot forms that is difficult to remove with a chest tube. If a large amount of clotted blood forms, the lung will not re-expand. The thrombus progresses and forms a fibrothorax, which then physically restricts expansion. Usually a no. 34 or no. 36 tube (large-bore, to allow the passage of blood clots) is placed posteriorly to drain the dependent regions of the thorax, where the blood accumulates. The chest tube is connected to underwater seal drainage, which serves as a collection system for the blood drained from the thorax while it keeps atmospheric air from entering the thoracotomy wound and thus compounding the hemothorax with a pneumothorax.[18,72] The tube—or tubes, because two may be inserted beside each other in case severe bleeding occurs or one tube clots—must be managed scrupulously in order to maintain position and patency, encourage evacuation of the blood from the thorax, and determine the amount and extent of the bleeding.

Chest Tube Drainage System

The chest tube drainage system has several components. Essentially, a chest tube (catheter) drains the pleural space and is attached to a valve arrangement. The valve arrangement can be a one-way valve, a waterseal drainage system, or a waterseal drainage system with suction.

The one-way valve is a simple, unidirectional system, such as the Heimlich flutter valve, in which a latex-type material is used in the tube so that the tube collapses on inspiration and opens on expiration. Thus, air and fluid drain from the chest. The thin, wide rubber tube is open at the end of the valve proximal to the chest tube and compressed at the end distal to the chest tube so that the flat sides remain in contact with each other. The apparatus is encased in clear plastic, making it possible to see what is draining through the valve. A relatively new approach for patients with a simple pneumothorax is to treat them as outpatients with the Heimlich flutter valve. For these selected patients, outpatient care costs only one fifth that of inpatient care.[12]

The most common drainage system is a water-sealed valve arrangement (Fig. 22–9). The chest tube drains the pleural

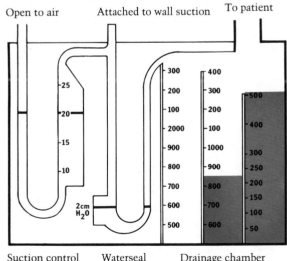

Figure 22-9

Disposable chest drainage unit.

space and is connected to another system that remains under water (usually saline solution is used). The water acts as a seal. Because the chest tube system essentially remains under water and the intrapleural pressure is negative, water rises in the tube. Thus, the underwater seal valve must remain at a level sufficiently below the chest to prevent the column of water from re-entering the pleural space. Any intrapleural pressure that is greater than the valve pressure forces air or fluid through the system. Thus, the waterseal is important because it seals the chest so that the air cannot leak back. The waterseal drainage system is sufficient if the fluid or air that has collected is well localized and in a walled space. Any accumulation that exerts more than 3 to 4 cm H_2O will be drained. The patient is instructed to cough forcefully and frequently to help evacuate the trapped air. How successful the patient is in coughing out the air can be monitored by watching the system: Bubbles will escape on forced expiration.

The tubing must always hang straight from the patient to the drainage system, because any fluid in the dependent tubing will alter pressures and obstruct flow. The intrapleural pressures will have to be higher to force air or fluid from the chest.

The compartmentalized chamber system is also important because it allows for gravity drainage of fluid and permits air to escape from the pleural space. Although disposable chest units are now used in most critical care units, the chest bottle system should not be condemned. It offers a great deal of flexibility and is by far the more economical system.

In an alternate—but still simple—drainage system, the drainage chamber or reservoir is used. The first chamber of the disposable chest apparatus is for drainage and the second chamber is for the waterseal (the open air vent at the top of the well makes it a simple drainage system). The volume of drainage can be measured accurately, and the waterseal valve is maintained. Drainage accumulates in the first reservoir, displacing air in the second reservoir. When intrapleural pressure is higher than atmospheric pressure, air escapes through the second reservoir into the atmosphere. Instead, if a two-bottle chest drainage system is in use (Fig. 22–10), the drainage bottle is placed between the patient and the waterseal bottle.

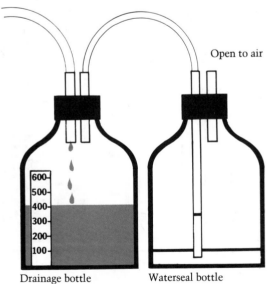

From patient

Open to air

600
500
400
300
200
100

Drainage bottle   Waterseal bottle

Figure 22–10
Water-sealed drainage system with added drainage bottle.

In the third type of system, controlled suction is added in order to apply negative pressure to the chest. Suction is necessary if the flow of air and fluid must be increased (as it must be when there is a large air leak or a large amount of fluid that reaccumulates) or when the negative intrathoracic pressure must be re-established. For example, the egress of air is thus increased in order to evacuate the continued pneumothorax if the tear in the lung is large. The third chamber in the disposable plastic chest system is used. Suction is connected to the air vent and maintained between −15 and −30 cm H_2O pressure, because higher degrees of subatmospheric pressure may result in large transpulmonary pressure gradients with the precipitation of acute pulmonary edema. Negative pressure applied to the thorax may be adjusted from 1 to 15 cm H_2O by varying both the level of fluid and the inflow of atmospheric air. The principles remain the same when the chest bottle system is used (Fig. 22–11).

Even after the chest tubes have ceased to function, they are left in place another 24 or so hours. If the air leak is persistent, or if the possibility of recurrence remains, the amount of time is increased to 48 hours. Serial radiographs are the primary determining factor.

Complications

Many problems can arise with chest tubes. The nurse must think through whatever problem situations arise. If, by some accident, the chest tube is pulled out, the problem is rarely life-threatening (unless the danger of tension pneumothorax is present). The patient is asked to cough, and the area is covered with petrolatum gauze and a dry sterile dressing. The physician is notified, and a stat portable chest radiograph is ordered from the x-ray department.

If the chest tube is accidentally disconnected from the chest tube drainage, the tube should be reconnected in the patient who has a continuing air leak. It is best not to clamp the chest tube but to reconnect it to avoid a tension pneumothorax. If reconnection is not possible, it is better to let the chest tube act as an open pneumothorax.

When the patient with a tension pneumothorax who still has a continuing air leak is to be transferred from the emergency department, or if the bottles break, the chest tubes should not be clamped. If the tubes are clamped, by the time the transfer is complete the patient has arrived on the next service, a tension pneumothorax may not only have redeveloped but be worse if positive-pressure ventilation is being used. However, if the air leak has ceased and the chest tube has stopped functioning before disconnection, there is no danger in clamping the tube next to the chest wall. Also, when a continuing air leak is not present and the chest tube is pulled loose from the connector (or if the bottle breaks), the chest tube may be clamped close to the chest while the connector is replaced quickly (or the bottle is changed).

There can also be problems with the drainage system. One simple problem is that the chest tube is connected to the air vent. In such a case, air in the pleural space cannot leave and room air will enter the pleural space. A persistent air leak may be present in the apparatus rather than in the patient. Usually, the leak is caused by a loose connection. Replacement of the tubing may be necessary. If it is, the chest tube is clamped at the patient's chest wall, and the system is evaluated inch by inch. If the bubbling is due to a leak in the tubing, it can be pinpointed by putting a clamp distal to each connection. Each

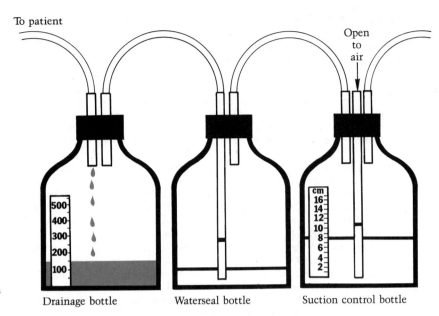

To patient

Open to air

500
400
300
200
100

Drainage bottle

Waterseal bottle

cm
16
14
12
10
8
6
4
2

Suction control bottle

Figure 22–11
Water-sealed drainage with added suction with chest bottle system.

portion is observed closely because the leak is often difficult to find. However, the problem may be obvious but overlooked. If no leak is found in the tubing, the leak is in the patient or at the insertion site.

SUMMARY

Chest trauma may be one of the most complicated forms of trauma the nurse will encounter. It is imperative that the nurse be able to function as a member of the health team and work appropriately with other team members. Actual actions may vary from site to site, but the responsibility and accountability for knowledgeable actions continue. Nurses must be able to foresee potential problems and either notify someone who can take action or take action themselves.

DIRECTIONS FOR FUTURE RESEARCH

There are many researchable questions concerning the nursing of the patient who has incurred chest trauma. Nurses have been taught lore for many years, and it is time to investigate the lore and ferret out the truth. It is difficult to reason out answers even if logic is used unless sufficient data are present to validate the findings.

Nurses have been taught to strip chest tubes and do so religiously. Why? Investigations concerning pressures obtained, pain imposed, drainage obtained, criteria to begin and to stop, and a tested protocol for the procedure are only at beginning stages. Every nurse blithely writes "turn, cough, deep breathe" on the care plan, but have nurses systematically looked at the best way to assist the patient in coughing or determined whether coughing is needed when inspiratory movements are maintained on a regular schedule? Nurses have relegated much of respiratory investigation as well as respiratory care to therapists rather than assuming a collaborative role. The challenge is there for nurses to begin studying clinical patient care delivery at the bedside.

REFERENCES

1. Akins, C. W., Mortimer, J. B., Daggegett, W., *et al*. Acute traumatic disruption of the thoracic aorta: A ten-year experience. *Ann. Thorac. Surg.* 31(4):305, 1981.

2. Alyono, D., and Perry, J. F. Impact of speed limit: I. Chest injuries, review of 966 cases. *J. Thorac. Cardiovasc. Surg.* 83(4):519, 1982.

3. American College of Surgeons Committee on Trauma. *Advanced Trauma Life Support*. Chicago: American College of Surgeons, 1984.

4. Atkinson, J. H., Stewart, N., and Gardner, D. The family meeting in critical care settings. *J. Trauma* 20:43, 1980.

5. Baxter, B. T., Moore, E. E., Synhorst, D. P., *et al*. Graded experimental myocardial contusion: Impact on cardiac rhythm, coronary artery flow, ventricular function, and myocardial oxygen consumption. *J. Trauma* 28:1411, 1988.

6. Belling, D., Kelley, R., and Simon, R. Use of the swivel adaptor aperture during suctioning to prevent hypoxemia in the mechanically ventilated patient. *Heart Lung* 7:320, 1978.

7. Benfeld, J. R. Chest Trauma. In J. P. Hardy (ed.), *Critical Surgical Illness*. Philadelphia: W. B. Saunders, 1980.

8. Beresky, R., Klingler, R., and Peake, J. Myocardial contusion: when does it have clinical significance? *J. Trauma* 28:64, 1988.

9. Bodai, B. I., Smith, J. D., Ward, R. L., *et al*. Emergency thoracotomy in the management of trauma. *J.A.M.A.* 249(14):1891, 1983.

10. Borne, J. *Management of Emergencies in Thoracic Surgery*. New York: Appleton-Century-Crofts, 1972.

11. Breaux, E. P., Dupont, J. B., Albert, H. M., *et al*. Cardiac tamponade following penetrating mediastinal injuries: Improved survival with early pericardiocentesis. *J. Trauma* 19:461, 1979.

12. Cannon, W. B., Mark, J. B. D., and Jamplis, R. W. Pneumothorax: A therapeutic update. *Am. J. Surg.* 142(1):26, 1981.

13. Chulay, M. Arterial blood gas changes with a hyperinflation and hyperoxygenation suctioning intervention in critically ill patients. *Heart Lung* 17:654, 1988.

14. Clark, G. C., Schecter, W. P., and Trunkey, D. D. Variables affecting outcome in blunt chest trauma: Flail chest vs. pulmonary contusion. *J. Trauma* 28:298, 1988.

15. Cogbill, T. H., Moore, E. E., Millikan, J. S., *et al*. Rationale for selective application of emergency department thoracotomy in trauma. *J. Trauma* 23(6):453, 1983.

16. Cooper, G. J., Pearce, B. P., Stainer, M. C., *et al*. The biochemical response of the thorax to nonpenetrating impact with particular reference to cardiac injuries. *J. Trauma* 22(12):994, 1982.

17. Cooper, G. J., Maynard, R. L., Pearce, B. P., *et al*. Cardiovascular distortion in experimental nonpenetrating chest impacts. *J. Trauma* 24(3):188, 1984.

18. Cornwall, P., Gortner, D., and Bodar, B. Suctioning induced hypoxia in patients with severe respiratory failure. *J. Burn Care Rehab.* 2:216, 1981.

19. Deslauriers, R. T., Beaulieu, M., Archambault, G., et al. Diagnosis and long-term follow-up of major bronchial disruption due to nonpenetrating trauma. Ann. Thorac. Surg. 33(1):32, 1982.
20. Dunham, C. M., and LaMonica, C. Prolonged tracheal intubation in the trauma patient. J. Trauma 24(2):120, 1984.
21. Evans, J., Gray, L. A., Rayner, A., et al. Principles for the management of penetrating cardiac wounds. Ann. Surg. 189:777, 1979.
22. Fabian, T. C., Mangiante, E. C., Patterson, C. R., et al. Myocardial contusion in blunt trauma: Clinical characteristics, means of diagnosis, and implications for patient management. J. Trauma 28: 50, 1988.
23. Flynn, A. E., Thomas, A. N., and Schecter, W. P. Acute tracheobronchial injury. J. Trauma 29:1326, 1989.
24. Gay, W. A., and McCabe, J. C. Trauma to the Chest. In Shires, G. T. (ed.). Principles of Trauma Care. New York: McGraw-Hill Book Co., 1985.
25. Gundry, S. R., Burney, R. E., Mackenzie, J. R., et al. Assessment of mediastinal widening associated with traumatic rupture of the aorta. J. Trauma 23(4):293, 1983.
26. Harley, D. P., Mena, I., Miranda, R., et al. Myocardial dysfunction following blunt chest trauma. Arch. Surg. 118(12):1384, 1983.
27. Helling, T. S., Duke, P., Beggs, C. W., et al. A prospective evaluation of 68 patients suffering blunt chest trauma for evidence of cardiac injury. J. Trauma 29:961, 1989.
28. Helling, T. S., Gyles, N. R., Eisenstein, C. L., et al. Complications following blunt and penetrating injuries in 216 victims of chest trauma requiring tube thoracostomy. J. Trauma 29:1367, 1989.
29. Horner, T. J., Oreskovich, M. R., Copass, M. K., et al. Role of emergency thoracotomy in the resuscitation of moribund trauma victims: 100 consecutive cases. Am. J. Surg. 142(1):96, 1981.
30. Hoyt, K. S. Chest trauma. Nursing '83 13(5):34, 1983.
31. Ivatury, R. R., and Rohman, M. The injured heart. Surg. Clin. North Am. 69:93, 1989.
32. Jones, K. W. Thoracic trauma. Surg. Clin. North Am. 60(4):957, 1980.
33. Kaunitz, V. H. Flail chest. J. Thorac. Cardiovasc. Surg. 82(3):463, 1981.
34. Kern, C. Creating an intensive care unit: A nurse manager's perspective. Crit. Care Q. 2:27, 1982.
35. Kirsh, M. M., and Sloan, H. Blunt Chest Trauma. Boston: Little, Brown, 1980.
36. Kite, J. H. Cardiac and great vessel trauma: Assessment, pathophysiology, and intervention. J. Emerg. Nurs. 13:346, 1987.
37. Kron, I. J. Cardiac injury after chest trauma. Crit. Care Med. 11(7): 524, 1983.
38. Kumar, S. A., Puri, V. K., Mittal, V. K., et al. Myocardial contusion following non-fatal blunt chest trauma. J. Trauma 23(4):327, 1983.
39. Lazrove, S., Harley, D. P., Grinell, V. S., et al. Should all patients with 1st rib fractures undergo arteriography? J. Thorac. Cardiovasc. Surg. 83(4):532, 1982.
40. Lewis, F. Chest trauma. Surg. Clin. North Am. 60(6):1541, 1980.
41. Lewis, F. Thoracic trauma. Surg. Clin. North Am. 62(1):97, 1982.
42. Levison, M., and Trunkey, D. D. Initial assessment and resuscitation. Surg. Clin. North Am. 62(1):9, 1984.
43. Locicero, J., and Mattox, K. L. Epidemiology of chest trauma. Surg. Clin. North Am. 69:15, 1989.
44. Mann, R. L., Graziano, C. C., and Turnbill, A. D. Comparison of electronic and manometric central venous pressures. Crit. Care Med. 9:98, 1981.
45. Marshall, W. G., Bell, J. L., and Kouchouskos, N. T. Penetrating cardiac trauma. J. Trauma 24(2):147, 1984.
46. Mattox, K. L. Thoracic injury requiring surgery. World J. Surg. 7(1):49, 1983.
47. Merlotti, G. Penetrating thoracic trauma. Trauma Q. 1:42, 1985.
48. Morris, J. A., MacKenzie, E. J., and Edelstein, S. L. Effect of pre-existing conditions on mortality in trauma patients. Crit. Care Med. 17:A145, 1989.
49. Murray, J. The Normal Lung. Philadelphia: W. B. Saunders, 1976.
50. Naigow, D., and Powaser, M. The effect of different endotracheal suction procedures on arterial blood gases in a controlled experimental model. Heart Lung 6:808, 1977.
51. Parker, J. G. Thoracic trauma: Nursing assessment and management. Nurs. Clin. North Am. 21:685, 1986.
52. Pate, J. W. Chest wall injuries. Surg. Clin. North Am. 69:59, 1989.
53. Pate, J. W. Tracheobronchial and esophageal injuries. Surg. Clin. North Am. 69:111, 1989.
54. Poole, G. V., and Myers, R. T. Morbidity and mortality rates in major blunt trauma to the upper chest. Ann. Surg. 193(1):70, 1981.
55. Powers, S. R. The use of PEEP for respiratory support. Surg. Clin. North Am. 54:1125, 1974.
56. Ramzy, A. I., Rodriguez, A., and Turney, S. Z. Management of major tracheobronchial ruptures in patients with multiple system trauma. J. Trauma 28:1353, 1988.
57. Richardson, J. D., Flint, L. M., Snow, N. J., et al. Management of transmediastinal gunshot wounds. Surgery 90(4):671, 1981.
58. Richardson, J. D., Polk, Jr., H. C., and Flint, L. M. Trauma. Clinical Care and Pathophysiology. Chicago: Year Book Medical Publishers, 1987.
59. Rohman, M., Ivatury, R. R., Steichen, F. M., et al. Emergency room thoracotomy for penetrating cardiac injuries. J. Trauma 23(7): 570, 1983.
60. Scanlon-Schilpp, A. M., and Levesque, J. Helping the patient cope with the sequelae of trauma through the self-help group approach. J. Trauma 21:135, 1981.
61. Shackford, S. R., Virgilio, R. W., and Peters, R. M. Selective use of ventilator therapy in flail chest. J. Thorac. Cardiovasc. Surg. 81: 194, 1981.
62. Shires, G. T. Principles of Trauma Care. New York: McGraw-Hill Book Co., 1985.
63. Sulzbach, L. M. Measurement of pulsus paradoxus. Focus Crit. Care 16:142, 1989.
64. Sutherland, G. R., Calvin, J. E., Driedger, A. A., et al. Anatomic and cardiopulmonary responses to trauma with associated blunt chest injury. J. Trauma 21(1):1, 1981.
65. Thompson, D. A., Rowlands, B. J., Walker, W. E., et al. Urgent thoracotomy for pulmonary or tracheobronchial injury. J. Trauma 28:276, 1988.
66. Trunkey, D. D., and Lewis, F. R. Chest trauma. Surg. Clin. North Am. 60(6):1541, 1980.
67. Trunkey, D. D., and Lewis, F. R. Current Theory in Trauma 1984–85. Philadelphia: B.C. Decker, 1984.
68. Trunkey, D. D. Cervicothoracic Trauma. In Blaidsell, R. W., and Trunkey, D. D. (eds.), Trauma Management, (vol. 3). New York: Thieme, 1986.
69. Viano, D. C., and Lau, V. K. Role of impact velocity and chest compression in thoracic injury. Aviat. Space Environ. Med. 54(1): 16, 1983.
70. Weigelt, J. A., Aurbakken, C. M., Meier, D. E., et al. Management of asymptomatic patients following stab wounds to the chest. J. Trauma 22(4):291, 1982.
71. Woodson, R. Physiological significance of oxygen dissociation curve shifts. Crit. Care Med. 7:368, 1979.
72. Yee, E. S., Verrier, E. D., and Thomas, A. N. Management of air embolism in blunt and penetrating thoracic trauma. J. Thorac. Cardiovasc. Surg. 85(5):661, 1983.

23

Acute Pulmonary Embolism

Elaine Kiess Daily   *Barbara Montgomery Dossey*

PRAYERS AND MANTRAS

Prayers and mantras (the repetition of special phrases or words) can break many lonely hours for patients while in critical care. Often patients will ask you to pray for them. Assess which prayers or repeated phrases they wish to use. It is recommended that patients choose a focus word from their own personal belief system. Combining guided relaxation and imagery experiences with a patient's prayers or mantras creates a state of healing and well-being.

You might be asking and wondering what the intent of the prayer should be. It might be helpful to pray for the highest good for yourself or others rather than to pray for what your or the patient wants. If you are praying for another, hold the person in your conscious thought.

Prayers and mantras also give you and other family members and friends meaningful moments during long hours, particularly when sleep is necessary or when the critically ill person shifts into different states of awareness depending on drugs or severity of illness. Prayers and words also take on a different level of importance at the time of death and afterwards.

LEARNING OBJECTIVES

After reading this chapter, the nurse should be able to do the following:

1. Recognize the urgent symptoms of acute pulmonary embolism.
2. Construct a problem list for the patient with acute pulmonary embolism.
3. List the precipitating factors of acute pulmonary embolism.
4. Identify the factors that constitute a high risk for acute pulmonary embolism.
5. Write appropriate nursing orders for a patient with acute pulmonary embolism.
6. Teach the patient self-care during convalescence.
7. Identify prophylactic measures used to prevent pulmonary embolism.
8. Discuss the necessary precautions in patients undergoing thrombolytic therapy.

CASE STUDY

Ms. J. C., aged 25, was hospitalized for elective cholecystectomy. Her chief complaint was increasingly frequent episodes of right upper quadrant abdominal pain over the preceding year, with the recent onset of nausea and vomiting. The pain was associated most often with the evening meal.

In the patient's profile and social history, Ms. C. was described as a 5 foot 8 inches tall, 220-lb white, married housewife, and a mother of 6-month-old female identical twins. Ms. C.'s husband, aged 27, was an unemployed automobile mechanic. Ms. C. was a Roman Catholic. Her hobbies were baking and sewing. Her alcoholic intake consisted of an occasional beer. She smoked half a pack of cigarettes a day. She was not nursing her infants.

Ms. C.'s current medical history included diabetes mellitus (since age 19) and significant varicose veins in her lower extremities (3 years duration). She had no history of pulmonary disease. She had never had complications of diabetes mellitus. Her medications included NPH insulin (25 U daily), Valium (5 mg as needed), and occasionally, aspirin for tension headaches. She had no known drug allergies. She was using oral contraceptives.

Ms. C.'s medical history listed an appendectomy at age 12. Her family history noted that her mother had adult-onset diabetes mellitus that was controlled with diet. She had two sisters and one brother, and they were alive and well.

The physical examination disclosed no abnormalities of the pulmonary, cardiovascular, renal, or nervous system. The abdominal examination revealed tenderness of the right upper quadrant.

The initial diagnostic studies included tests of renal and hepatic function, a complete blood count, a platelet count, a prothrombin time determination, and radiographic examinations of the chest and abdomen. All the tests were normal. An oral cholecystogram confirmed the diagnosis of cholelithiasis.

On the morning after Ms. C.'s admission, a cholecystectomy with operative cholangiography (revealing no choledocholithiasis) was performed. Multiple stones and chronic inflammatory changes were found in the gallbladder. After the operation, which was uncomplicated, thigh-length stockings were put on Ms. C., and she was given 5000 U of heparin subcutaneously every 8 hours because she was felt to be at high risk for pulmonary embolism. Because Ms. C. had pain from her incision, she refused to get out of bed or cough and deep breathe on her own. Only when a nurse or physician insisted did she perform these activities—and then only minimally.

Superficial thrombophlebitis on the inner aspect of the left thigh appeared on the second postoperative day. Ms. C. complained of anterior chest pain, which was attributed to her recent surgery. She had a fever of 100°F. She did not complain of calf tenderness. By late afternoon, the nurse detected an increase in left-leg circumference at the calf and ankle.

Late on the third postoperative day, Ms. C. complained of shortness of breath of sudden onset. Her blood pressure was 130/90, her pulse was 120, and her respiration was 30/minute. Coarse rales were heard at both lung bases, and a pleural friction rub was present in the right anterolateral chest. Arterial blood gas analysis on room air revealed a PO_2 of 74 mm Hg (normal is 80 to 100 mm Hg), a PCO_2 of 34 mm Hg (normal is 35 to 45 mm Hg), and a pH of 7.48 (normal is 7.35 to 7.45). A chest radiograph revealed a density in the right lateral lung base that was not present preoperatively and elevation of the right hemidiaphragm. The heart size was normal and the left lung appeared normal. A lung scan revealed perfusion defects at the right base and in the right upper lobe. The diagnosis of pulmonary embolism was made, and the patient was transferred to the critical care unit.

The patient remained in the critical care unit for 4 days, and she had an uncomplicated recovery thereafter. She received a total of 14 days of intravenous heparin therapy, and when she was discharged, she was taking the oral anticoagulant warfarin. Her physician prescribed a weight-reduction diet.

REFLECTIONS

Feelings of loneliness were a major hurdle in Ms. C.'s recovery and required some skillful nursing interventions. Loneliness is a person's conscious experience of separation from something or someone desired, required, or needed.[41] With loneliness, a person experiences a desire for human contact, a need, and an inability to bring it about. Loneliness is a felt psychophysiologic experience that moves a person to look inward, see who he or she is, what he or she needs, and what the meaning of life and relationships is about. Loneliness is such an all-consuming experience that there is no space for any other perceptions.[41] Two types of loneliness may be felt by the critical care patient. *Existential loneliness* is that state in which both psychophysiologic pain and the threat of illness are experienced. *Loneliness anxiety* is that state of loneliness in which vague anxiety feelings of self-alienation and self-rejection occur. Either or both occur in critical care patients.

Ms. C.'s complaints were seen in her threat of acute illness after a routine surgical procedure. The psychophysiologic pain was a separateness from her children and husband, as well as feelings of separation from her body. She referred to her acute crisis as "those lungs." She refused to follow routine postoperative exercises. She felt out of control and detached from everything around her. Her pain was very real to her, and her pain tolerance was practically nonexistent. She overreacted to her pain. Everything that the nurses wanted her to do, such as turn, cough, and deep breathe, were drastically painful. Her constant retort was

"This is awful. You just don't know how bad it is. I need my family. They need me. I'm such a burden to them. I need my babies. I wish I could just curl up and die."

Critical care nurses have heard these comments many times. Their goals must be to recognize this common situation as either existential loneliness or loneliness anxiety and minimize the state. Nurses can overcome these situations by minimizing the threat of illness and decreasing psychophysiologic pain. The threat of illness can be dealt with by nurses by helping the patient let go of feelings of guilt about being ill and the stresses that the illness places on significant others. Nurses can help the patient identify the strengths of family members and how they can take over household or business responsibilities during the patient's acute illness.

The patient gets locked into clock time during acute crisis. The acute illness seems like it will last forever. The nurse can help the patient expand the constricted boundaries of the acute illness by assessing readiness to learn and then repeatedly teaching about the stages of illness and recovery. Psychologic pain can be decreased if the nurse has an awareness of the three components of psychologic pain: separateness from contact with significant others, separateness from the body, and separateness from personal values and beliefs.[41] These can all be decreased when the nurse actively listens and actively sets aside 10 to 20 minutes per shift to really be with the patient. Whether performing a procedure or simply spending an extended period of time with the patient, the nurse must attempt to help the patient feel real-life connections with significant others and get the patient to identify strengths, optimal health, and body-mind connections. Visiting hours should be assessed. If possible, have family members or children around when appropriate. Significant others can tape record messages or conversations that can be played back when they are not at the hospital or between visiting periods. Photographs, letters, and children's drawings help strengthen a patient's awareness of support systems.

When patients talk about "that monitor," "that IV system," or "that procedure," the nurse can help them increase their sense of relatedness to their body by referring to these as the patient's, which personalizes the strange feelings and critical care environment to the patient. The values and beliefs of patients are reinforced when patients are encouraged to participate in their own care. Emphasis should be placed on the ideas of "can" rather than "cannot." When the nurse and patient together discuss the limits or constricted boundaries that exist because of the acute illness, the patient will most frequently respond with ideas, and this will help decrease the patient's thoughts of loneliness.

PATHOPHYSIOLOGY

Pulmonary embolism refers to an embolus carried to the pulmonary vasculature that results in some occlusion of the pulmonary artery with partial or complete interruption of blood flow to a portion of the lung.[43] Almost all (approximately 95%) pulmonary emboli result from a deep venous thrombosis in the legs, usually from the veins above the knees.[2] (Frequently, the deep venous thrombosis is not clinically evident.) Other sources of pulmonary emboli include atrial thrombus, septic

MECHANISM	PRECIPITATING CAUSE
Venous stasis	Immobility
	Obesity
	Congestive heart failure
Hypercoagulability	Polycythemia
	Malignancy
	Pregnancy
	Oral contraceptive
	Thrombocytosis
	Nephrotic syndrome
	Antithrombin III deficiency
	Protein C deficiency
	Protein S deficiency
	Thrombocytopenia purpura
Vascular injury	Trauma
	Surgery
	Intracardiac catheters

emboli, and intracardiac catheters. Table 23-1 lists the mechanisms and associated conditions responsible for pulmonary embolism. The acute events of pulmonary embolism are subject to rapid change as resolution of the embolism proceeds. The clinical picture varies from subclinical presentation to acute cor pulmonale according to the size and location of the embolus. A variety of factors predispose one to intravascular thrombosis[4,31,48] and have the potential of causing pulmonary embolus.[43]

ACUTE EMBOLIZATION

Once a thrombus has developed, it may loosen and break from its attachment. A flowing clot is known as an *embolus.* An embolus travels from the venous circulation through the right side of the heart and into the pulmonary arterial system. There it eventually reaches a branch too small for it to pass through, and it becomes impacted, obstructing the flow of blood in that vessel. The amount of circulation that is compromised is directly related to the size of the embolus (Fig.

23-1). A *massive* pulmonary embolism refers to a more than 50% occlusion of the pulmonary vasculature, whereas a *submassive* pulmonary embolism refers to occlusion of less than 50% of the pulmonary circulation. The pathophysiologic consequences of the obstruction are of two types—pulmonary and hemodynamic.

Pulmonary Consequences

Acute pulmonary embolism almost always results in abnormal gas exchange. The three major respiratory effects of pulmonary embolism are the development of alveolar dead space, reduced lung volume, and loss of alveolar surfactant. Pulmonary embolism produces alveolar dead space because areas of the lung are fully ventilated but not perfused. In the physiologic sense, such ventilation is "wasted" because the lung zone involved fails to participate in gas exchange. Overall ventilation in the uninvolved lung zones must be increased to maintain normal gas exchange. For this reason, dyspnea and tachypnea, with resultant hypocapnia, are common in patients with pulmonary embolism. If a large volume of the lung is affected, the patient may not be able to compensate adequately and acute ventilatory failure occurs. This is particularly true if underlying pulmonary disease is also present.

A reduction in lung volume occurs with pulmonary embolism because of decreased or absent pulmonary perfusion and associated bronchoconstriction and pneumoconstriction caused by the release of substances by the platelets in response to the presence of thrombin on fresh emboli. Local hypoxia also contributes to pneumoconstriction. The result of these responses is a shifting of ventilation away from the underperfused lung areas, so less ventilation is wasted. Pulmonary embolism also causes a loss of alveolar surfactant. Surfactant, the lipoprotein material that stabilizes and prevents the collapse of alveoli, is produced by type 2 alveolar cells. When the perfusion of nutrients to these cells ceases, the production of surfactant terminates. When surfactant decreases, alveoli collapse, causing atelectasis and transudation of interstitial fluid into alveoli, which results in pulmonary edema. Loss of surfactant develops later in the course of pulmonary embolism (approximately 24 hours).

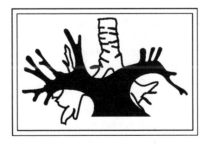

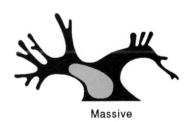

Massive

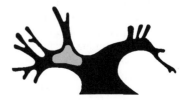

Peripheral   Submassive

Figure 23-1

Types and extent of obstruction in pulmonary embolism. (Tsapogas, M.J. Pulmonary embolism. Part I. Incidence, pathophysiology, and diagnosis. *Ala. J. Med. Sci.* 24:405, 1987; with permission.)

Hypoxemia is found in the majority (>80%) of patients with pulmonary embolism and represents both a pulmonary and hemodynamic consequence of the obstruction. Alveolar dead space as well as loss of surfactant and decreased cardiac output are all causative factors of hypoxemia.

Hemodynamic Consequences

The patient's previous physical condition and the number and size of emboli determine the severity of the acute hemodynamic events. Patients without existing cardiopulmonary disease may suffer submassive pulmonary embolism with little or no hemodynamic consequences, whereas an embolus of the same size may be fatal in a patient with underlying cardiopulmonary disease such as congestive heart failure, aortic or mitral valve disease, or chronic obstructive pulmonary disease.

The cardiovascular response to a sudden reduction in blood flow through the lung is a rise in pulmonary vascular resistance with a concomitant rise in pulmonary artery pressure. Elevations of the mean pulmonary artery pressure greater than 40 mm Hg are associated with massive pulmonary embolism and usually are accompanied by decreases in the cardiac output.[46] However, pulmonary hypertension may not develop in patients in whom pulmonary vascular resistance is not significantly increased, or in whom right ventricular stroke volume falls significantly. In patients without existing cardiopulmonary disease, elevations in the pulmonary artery pressure are usually associated with a greater than 25% obstruction of the pulmonary vasculature.[46]

The fundamental structure and design of the right ventricle limit the amount of pressure the right ventricle can develop on an acute basis. Studies show that in patients without prior cardiopulmonary disease and right ventricular hypertrophy, a maximum mean pulmonary artery pressure of 40 mm Hg can be produced without development of acute right ventricular failure and tricuspid regurgitation.[29] As right-heart afterload increases, the right ventricular stroke volume falls, resulting in decreased filling of the left ventricle, with consequent diminished left ventricular stroke volume and cardiac output. Decreased left ventricular preload results in a normal or low pulmonary artery wedge pressure despite elevations in the pulmonary artery pressure. (Fig. 23–2) Pressure in the right atrium also becomes elevated, reflecting the increased pulmonary vascular resistance and dilatation of the right-heart chambers. If acute tricuspid regurgitation develops in response to right ventricular dilatation, a prominent v wave may be present in the right atrial waveform. Pulsus paradoxus, with an exaggerated (>10 mm Hg) decline in the arterial systolic pressure during spontaneous inspiration, may be observed.

A rare but often serious complication of pulmonary embolism is *pulmonary infarction,* the necrosis of lung tissue that results from the interference of blood supply. Approximately 80% to 90% of occlusive emboli fail to cause infarction because the involved lung continues to receive adequate blood perfusion through the bronchial arterial system.[1] Pulmonary infarction appears to result from embolism to middle-sized vessels when pulmonary congestion due to systemic hypotension or to left ventricular failure interferes with bronchial collateral circulation.[1] This complication is more likely to occur in patients with left ventricular failure or obstructive lung disease.[35]

Natural History

The body's response to the acute single event of pulmonary embolism results in restoration of patency through progressive fibrinolysis and organization of the embolus. The rate and degree of resolution depend on the severity of the occlusion, the presence of coexisting disease states, and the timing and appropriateness of therapy. Spontaneous resolution of pulmonary embolism can occur in as little as 30 hours, with complete resolution usually occurring over several weeks.[14,45] Most patients with pulmonary embolism recover completely without obvious sequelae. Data from the Urokinase in Pulmonary Embolism Trial showed that 55% of patients with pulmonary embolism had evidence of increased perfusion at 13 days after treatment with urokinase.[43] If untreated, pulmonary embolism is prone to recur and become potentially fatal.

CLOTTING AND LYSIS

Clotting and lysis are well-balanced mechanisms in humans, and when either mechanism is unbalanced, the patient may demonstrate hemorrhage or thrombosis.

The Clotting Mechanism

The clotting mechanism can be initiated by an extrinsic mechanism or by an intrinsic mechanism (Fig. 23–3).[23] After trauma, a normal clotting sequence occurs that results in clot formation. When a blood vessel is damaged, the extrinsic mechanism goes into effect. The intrinsic mechanism goes into effect when blood has been traumatized directly (*e.g.,* when it has been removed from the body by venipuncture).

The clotting of blood involves 13 well-defined factors. An inactive proenzyme is converted into an active factor, which initiates the next step. Calcium is required at many points. Three major stages occur in coagulation: procoagulants (from platelets, plasma proteins, and tissue factors) combine in the presence of calcium to form thromboplastin; thromboplastin activates prothrombin to form thrombin; and thrombin enzymatically converts fibrinogen to insoluble fibrin. The fibrin clot is stabilized by a factor, and it can be broken down by fibrinolysins.[21]

The following is a summary of the basic concepts of clotting (see Fig. 23–3):[22]

- Inactive factor XII is the first factor to be activated. Factor XIIa is the active enzyme of factor XII.
- Next, factor XIIa acts on inactive factor XI. Factor XIa is the active enzyme of factor XI. The process continues in the same manner.
- Factor X requires factor VIII for activation.
- Prothrombin requires factor V for activation.
- Platelet cofactor-3 (a fatty lipid substance from platelets) must be present to activate factors VIII and V.
- The activation of factor X through the effects of thrombin on factor VIII perpetuates the cycle.
- Thrombin converts fibrinogen to soluble fibrin, which is stabilized by factor XIII.

The Fibrinolytic System

The fibrinolytic system functions through the conversion of enzymes that are capable of dissolving fibrin clots.[21] Plasmin-

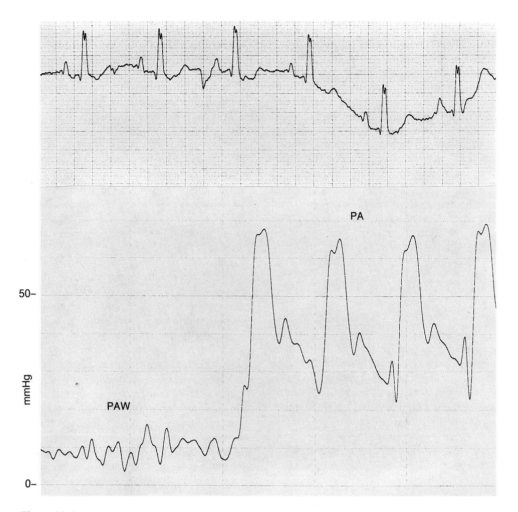

Figure 23–2

Pulmonary artery wedge (PAW) and pulmonary artery (PA) pressures in a patient with pulmonary embolism. Note the low normal PAW pressure of approximately 9 mm Hg and the high PA pressure of 65/25 mm Hg, with a mean of approximately 40 mm Hg.

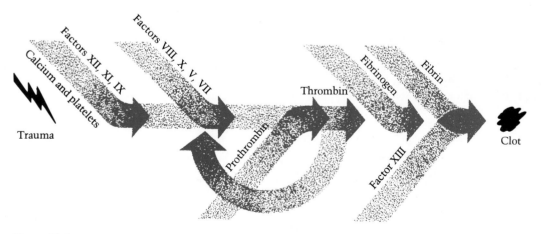

Figure 23–3

Clotting factors.

ogen is one such proenzyme normally found in whole blood that may be converted to plasmin, a major lytic (dissolving) enzyme that can dissolve fibrin.

Because of the normal turbulence of blood flow, the endothelial surface of blood vessels constantly undergoes wear and tear. Whenever an area is denuded, platelets adhere to the damaged area. Platelets, produced by megakaryocytes in the bone marrow, are important factors in hemostasis. Platelets not only plug the injured vessel site, they also release vasoactive substances that cause local vasoconstriction. They also contribute several factors to promote coagulation. Eddy currents that are set up by the adhered platelets may activate the intrinsic clotting mechanism, causing further clot formation. If it were not for the fibrinolytic system, total vessel occlusion might occur; however, the fibrinolytic system keeps a normal balance between clotting and lysis.

NURSING PROCESS

ASSESSMENT

The nurse should assess the patient for signs and symptoms of hypoxia: restlessness, headache, apprehension, euphoria, hallucinations, delirium, unconsciousness, and color (pallor cyanosis). The nurse should also assess the lung functioning of the patient suspected of having pulmonary arterial embolism. This assessment should include the following:

- Inspection. Does the patient show splinting, supraclavicular, suprasternal, or intercostal retractions; tachypnea; or dyspnea?
- Palpation. Does the patient show decreased chest excursion unilaterally, nonsymmetric diaphragmatic excursion, rubs (thrills), an accentuated point of maximal impulse (PMI), or a decrease in vocal fremitus?
- Auscultation. Does the patient have abnormal breath sounds (whispered pectoriloquy, bronchial or bronchovesicular sounds), abnormal voice sounds, or a friction rub (an accented pulmonic second sound)?

The nurse should also assess the right-sided heart functioning of the patient suspected of having pulmonary arterial embolism by doing the following:

- Inspection. Does the patient have peripheral edema or distended neck veins?
- Palpation. Does the patient have an enlarged liver?
- Auscultation. Does the patient have abnormal heart sounds, such as accented pulmonic sounds, pulmonic murmurs, gallop rhythms, or tachycardia?

The nurse should also assess for superficial thrombophlebitis and deep venous thrombosis.[13] Superficial thrombophlebitis (which usually follows a benign course) is diagnosed by the early signs of inflammation at the affected site—rubor, dolor, calor, and swelling. If lightly palpated, the vein may feel firm; however, deep venous thrombosis presents an increased risk of complications, because 15% of deep venous thrombi migrate above the popliteal vein, which increases the risk of pulmonary embolism. A first sign of deep venous thrombosis is swelling in the circumference of the affected limb at the ankle, calf,

and lower thigh. Therefore, the nurse should measure the size of each leg. The patient may complain of tenderness, pain, warmth, and heaviness. Palpation may reveal increased tissue turgor. Both superficial thrombophlebitis and deep vein thrombosis may reveal a positive Homan's sign (calf pain on dorsiflexion of the foot).

Clinical Manifestations

The clinical manifestations associated with pulmonary embolism are nonspecific and can be attributed to numerous other causes, including congestive heart failure, pneumonia, myocardial ischemia or infarction, chronic obstructive lung disease, and pleurisy. Symptoms (Table 23–2) range from mild respiratory alterations to acute right-heart failure, depending on the size of the obstruction and presence of pre-existing disease states.

The characteristic presentation of sudden pleuritic pain, dyspnea, and tachypnea in the presence of one or more predisposing factors (see Table 23–2) should always make one suspect pulmonary embolism. Occasionally, however, the chest pain is nonpleuritic and can mimic angina. Apprehension is another nonspecific finding in many patients with pulmonary embolism. Crackles and tachycardia are common. Hemoptysis is less common (Fig. 23–4). The triad of cough, hemoptysis, and pleuritic pain suggests pulmonary infarction that has occurred hours or days after formation of a submassive embolus. Acute right-heart failure is evidenced by tachycardia, distended neck veins, Kussmaul's sign (distended neck veins on inspiration), accentuated and split pulmonic sounds, and pulsus paradoxus. Circulatory collapse with syncope or shock is associated with more extensive embolization and occurs in less than 20% of the patients with acute pulmonary embolism. Although the clinical findings associated with pulmonary embolism are nonspecific and found in a wide variety of other disease states, a careful history and physical assessment are essential tools in the detection of the underlying pathology.

Diagnostic Tests

The diagnosis of pulmonary embolism is based on clinical manifestations and the results from a variety of diagnostic tests.

Chest Radiographs

Although many patients with documented pulmonary embolism have a normal chest radiograph, abnormalities of this

Table 23–2
Signs and Symptoms Associated with Pulmonary Embolism

SIGNS	SYMPTOMS
Tachypnea	Dyspnea
Rales	Chest pain
Tachycardia	Jugular venous distention
Loud pulmonic S_2	Cough
Fever	Hemoptysis
Thrombophlebitis	Diaphoresis
S_3 and S_4	Palpitations
Pleural friction rub	Syncope
Hypotension	
Cyanosis	

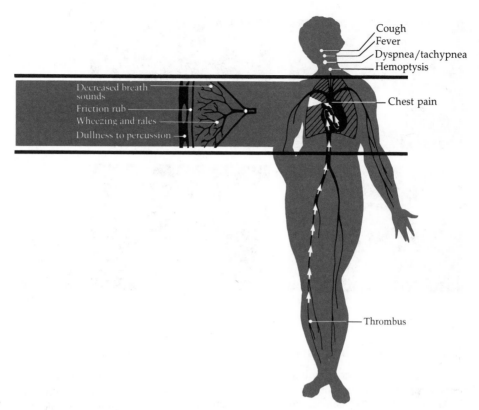

Figure 23–4
Clinical features.

test are a common finding in patients with pulmonary embolism. Radiographic manifestations are nonspecific, and they frequently include atelectasis and pleural effusion. An elevated hemidiaphragm may occur on the side of the embolus as a result of decreased lung volume. Pulmonary infarction may be evidenced by a peripheral wedge-shaped infiltrate (Hampton's hump) whose base is contiguous with the pleura. Dilatation or prominence of the pulmonary outflow tract with either an obvious cut-off or an area of decreased perfusion distal to it is termed the *Westermark sign* and is specific for pulmonary embolism, but it is not a common finding.[35]

Electrocardiogram

Changes in the electrocardiogram (ECG) due to pulmonary embolism usually appear early after the embolic episode and may be transient in nature.[4] Although the ECG is usually abnormal in pulmonary embolism, changes are often nonspecific (T-wave abnormalities, ST depression) and are associated with pre-existing cardiopulmonary conditions. The majority of patients present with sinus rhythm or, more commonly, sinus tachycardia. Evidence of acute right ventricular strain, including right-axis deviation, right bundle branch block, and an $S_1Q_3T_3$ pattern (prominent S wave in lead 1, with a Q wave and an inverted T wave in lead 3), are associated with massive embolism.[48] Other findings include a late R wave in aV_R and, in severe embolism, T-wave inversion in leads V_1 and V_2.[36] ST changes consistent with myocardial ischemia or infarction may occur with massive pulmonary embolism secondary to reduced cardiac output and elevated right ventricular pressures, which compromise coronary perfusion. The primary value of the ECG in patients with pulmonary embolism is elimination of myocardial infarction as the cause of the patient's clinical manifestations.

Arterial Blood Gases

Acute pulmonary embolism is almost always associated with abnormalities in gas exchange, and the majority of patients have abnormalities of their arterial blood gases, although normal blood gases in patients breathing room air do not preclude the existence of pulmonary embolism.

Severe perfusion/ventilation inequality in the affected lung secondary to pulmonary embolism usually results in hypoxemia with PaO_2 levels less than 80 mm Hg on room air.[43] In addition, the corresponding reduction in cardiac output results in a low venous oxygen saturation (SvO_2), which further contributes to hypoxemia.

Compensatory increases in minute ventilation associated with pulmonary embolism cause hypocapnia and respiratory alkalosis, with $PaCO_2$ levels less than 40 mm Hg in most patients.

A more specific finding associated with pulmonary embolism appears to be the measured or calculated alveolar-arterial oxygen gradient (A-aO_2) or ratio.[11] Normally, PO_2 equilibrates between the alveoli and arterial blood, resulting in an A-aO_2 difference of approximately 10 mm Hg. The mismatch between perfusion and ventilation that occurs secondary to pulmonary embolism results in an increase in the PO_2 gradient between the alveoli and arterial blood greater than 20 mm Hg in patients breathing room air. The A-aO_2 gradient normally widens with increases in inspired oxygen (FiO_2), making interpretation of the A-aO_2 gradient in patients receiving oxygen more complex. A better assessment of gas exchange in patients receiving oxygen supplement is the calculation of the ratio between alveolar and arterial PO_2 (the a/AO_2 ratio). Normally, the a/AO_2 ratio is greater than 0.75. Values below 0.75 represent true shunt, ventilation/perfusion imbalance, or diffusion abnormalities.[16]

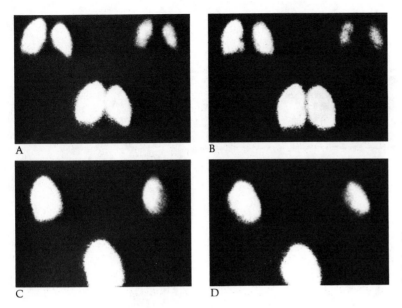

Figure 23–5

A normal lung scan. (*A*) Anterior view. (*B*) Posterior view. (*C*) Right lateral view. (*D*) Left lateral view. The lungs are smooth and regular in outline, without evidence of "perfusion defects."

Deep Venous Thrombosis

Although not diagnostic of pulmonary embolism, the determination of the presence of deep venous thrombosis in association with strong clinical findings may prompt some clinicians to treat the patient for pulmonary embolism empirically. Clinical evidence of deep venous thrombosis is present in less than 50% of patients with pulmonary embolism and is extremely difficult to diagnose.

It may or may not be detected with safe, noninvasive procedures, such as the ^{125}I-labeled fibrinogen test, which is frequently used to detect deep vein thrombosis in the calf and lower thigh; the Doppler ultrasound technique, which is used to detect deep vein thrombosis in the popliteal and iliofemoral veins; and phlebography, which is used for visualization of the deep venous system.[1,32] Venography may be performed at the time of pulmonary angiography to visualize the venous system.

Lung Scan

Noninvasive assessment of the perfusion of the lung can be determined with a perfusion scan, which can provide information about blood flow in vessels as small as 20 μm in diameter.[6] This is done by imaging the passage of radioactively tagged particles from a peripheral venous injection through the capillaries of the lung (Fig. 23–5). Any blockage within the pulmonary vasculature preventing blood flow will cause an abnormality in the lung scan, or a perfusion defect (Fig. 23–6). Unfortunately, numerous pathologic disorders other than pulmonary embolism also can cause perfusion defects. Such a defect may appear in a variety of pulmonary disorders, such as pneumonia, pulmonary edema, chronic bronchitis, and emphysema. In the absence of these other conditions, however, the lung scan may be a reliable diagnostic tool for pulmonary embolism. Frequently, combined perfusion/ven-

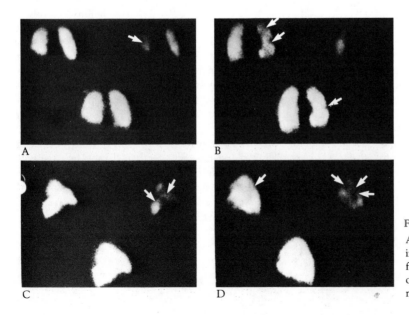

Figure 23–6

An abnormal lung scan. The views are the same as those in Figure 23–5. There are a number of dark areas, or "perfusion defects," mostly in the middle and lower regions of the right lung (*arrows*.) These defects represent pulmonary emboli.

tilation scans are done in order to detect perfusion/ventilation mismatch.

Assessment of ventilation is performed through imaging of the uptake of a radioactive gas (xenon[133]) in the lungs. When combined with a perfusion lung scan, any inequalities or mismatch between perfusion and ventilation can be determined. In the presence of pulmonary embolism, a defect will be present on the perfusion scan but not on the ventilation scan.

Pulmonary Angiography

Definitive and precise detection of pulmonary embolism can be obtained with pulmonary angiography, which involves right-heart catheterization and injection of radiolucent contrast material into the pulmonary arterial system. To prevent excessive administration of contrast material and reduce associated risks, selective injection is carried out in those vessels previously identified through the lung scan as possessing perfusion defects (Fig. 23–7).

Diagnostic tests such as pulmonary angiography can differentiate between non–life-threatening and life-threatening embolism. Life-threatening massive pulmonary embolism is said to occur when there is a sudden mechanical obstruction of 50% or more of the pulmonary arterial bed.[48] Pulmonary angiography usually provides a definitive diagnosis.

The lung scan and pulmonary angiography are complementary, not competitive, procedures for arriving at a sometimes difficult diagnosis. The less invasive procedures are done first, and the physician proceeds to more complicated diagnostic procedures, depending on the clinical evidence shown by each patient suspected of having pulmonary embolism.

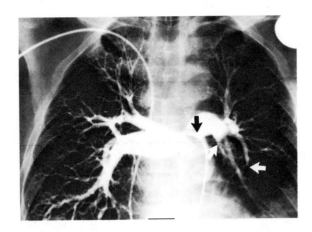

Figure 23–7

A pulmonary angiogram. The catheter enters from the right arm, and the contrast medium is being injected into the pulmonary artery, filling its right and left branches to give a treelike appearance. The main trunk of the left pulmonary artery appears shorter and more irregular than normal ("cut off"), and it has several areas that are poorly opacified ("filling defects") (*arrows*). These abnormalities represent pulmonary emboli.

NURSING DIAGNOSES, PATIENT OUTCOMES, AND PLAN

The preceding material on anatomy, physiology, nursing assessment, and diagnostic tests guides the nurse in establishing nursing diagnoses, patient outcomes, and plan for the patient with acute pulmonary embolism.

NURSING CARE PLAN SUMMARY   *Patient with Acute Pulmonary Embolism*

NURSING DIAGNOSIS

1. (Acute Phase) Impaired gas exchange related to ventilation/perfusion inequality or pulmonary edema as a result of pulmonary embolus (exchanging pattern)

Patient Outcome	**Nursing Orders**
The patient will experience adequate oxygenation and ventilation, as evidenced by normal pulmonary function parameters (arterial blood gases, A-aO$_2$ gradient or ratio, normal respiratory rate and pattern).	1. Initiate bed rest. 2. Administer oxygen by way of nasal cannula or face mask. 3. Elevate head of bed 30° to 40°.

NURSING DIAGNOSIS

2. High risk for decreased cardiac output related to increased pulmonary vascular resistance due to embolism, tachycardia, and dysrhythmias (exchanging pattern)

Patient Outcome	**Nursing Orders**
The patient will have normal hemodynamic parameters and normal sinus rhythm.	See Nursing Diagnosis: Decreased Cardiac Output (electrical factors), page 426.

(continued)

NURSING CARE PLAN SUMMARY   *Patient with Acute Pulmonary Embolism   Continued*

NURSING DIAGNOSIS

3. *High risk for decreased cardiac output secondary to recurrent pulmonary embolism (exchanging pattern)*

Patient Outcome	Nursing Orders
The patient will experience no recurrent pulmonary embolism.	1. Initiate heparin therapy (a bolus followed by continuous infusion) as ordered.
	2. Apply graded compression stockings or intermittent pneumatic compression to lower extremities.
	3. Slightly elevate the foot of the bed without a bend at the knee.
	4. Change patient's position frequently (every 30 minutes).
	5. Instruct the patient regarding active leg exercises; have the patient perform these exercises at least twice a shift. Perform passive leg exercises if patient is unable to do them.
	6. Instruct the patient regarding coughing and deep-breathing exercises; have the patient perform them hourly.

NURSING DIAGNOSIS

4. *Fluid volume deficit related to bleeding due to anticoagulation and thrombolytic therapy (exchanging pattern)*

Patient Outcome	Nursing Orders
The patient will experience no internal or external bleeding episodes.	1. Obtain PTT or activated clotting time values approximately 1 hour after initiation of heparin therapy. Notify the physician if not within desired range (two to three times control value). Adjust heparin dosage, or administer heparin bolus as ordered. Once therapeutic anticoagulation is achieved, obtain PTT or activated clotting time values on a daily basis.
	2. Check the patient regularly for signs of bleeding (petecchiae, ecchymosis, gingival oozing, oozing from puncture sites).
	3. Measure the circumferences of extremities to detect evidence of slow accumulation of blood in tissues.
	4. Monitor all emesis, nasogastric contents, stool, and urine for presence of fresh or occult blood.
	5. If severe bleeding occurs, discontinue therapy. Administer neutralizing agent if bleeding continues (protamine sulfate for heparin therapy; amicar or cryoprecipitate plasma for thrombolytic therapy).
	6. If hemodynamic monitoring is required, prepare patient for catheter insertion (before thrombolytic therapy) in upper extremity to allow for direct compression in the event of bleeding.
	7. If thrombolytic therapy is administered, initiate the following procedures:
	A. Start peripheral intravenous line. Avoid subclavian, jugular, or femoral veins where bleeding would be difficult to control.
	B. Insert arterial line in peripheral artery to obtain repeated blood gas samples.
	C. Obtain baseline blood studies, including coagulation studies, hematocrit, and platelet count.
	D. Discontinue anticoagulants and antiplatelet agents. Obtain PTT results after discontinuation.
	E. When PTT values return to normal, administer thrombolytic agent as ordered.
	F. Closely monitor patient for evidence of adverse reaction to thrombolytic agent (fever, chills, dermatitis).

(continued)

NURSING CARE PLAN SUMMARY   *Patient with Acute Pulmonary Embolism*   *Continued*

Patient Outcome	*Nursing Orders*
	G. Closely monitor patient for evidence of reperfusion pulmonary edema (elevated pulmonary artery wedge pressure, dyspnea, rales, increased hypoxemia).
	H. Avoid all intramuscular, intravenous, or skin punctures during thrombolytic therapy.
	I. Keep patient at bed rest with minimal handling during thrombolytic therapy.
	J. Establish flow sheet for medication administration, laboratory results, and vital signs.
	8. After completion of thrombolytic infusion, do the following:
	A. Obtain PTT values. Begin heparin administration when PTT is less than two times the control value.
	B. Avoid intravenous or intramuscular injections for 24 hours.
	C. Continue monitoring for evidence of bleeding.
	9. If anticoagulants or thrombolytic agents are not effective, prepare patient for pulmonary embolectomy or placement of a vena caval filter.

NURSING DIAGNOSIS

5. *(Recovery Phase) High risk for knowledge deficit regarding long-term anticoagulation therapy for prevention of recurrent pulmonary embolism (knowing pattern)*

Patient Outcome	*Nursing Orders*
The patient will be able to describe the medication regimen, the necessary precautions to be observed while on anticoagulation therapy, the activities and exercises to be performed as well as the symptoms that require immediate reporting to the physician.	Instruct the patient and family regarding the following:
	1. The need to take medication regularly as prescribed
	2. The need for regular measurement of prothrombin time (preferably on a monthly basis)
	3. Signs of excessive anticoagulation to be reported, such as the following:
	A. Easy bruising
	B. Minor cuts that stop bleeding initially, but begin bleeding later
	C. Severe nosebleeds
	D. Black stools
	E. Evidence of blood in the urine or stool
	F. Coughing up blood
	G. Joint swelling and pain
	H. Severe headaches
	I. Visual disturbances
	J. Confusion, disorientation
	4. Avoidance of trauma that could cause bleeding:
	A. Using an electric shaver for shaving
	B. Using a soft toothbrush
	5. The need to apply ice immediately to any bumped or bruised areas
	6. Avoidance of any drugs that affect the action of anticoagulation
	7. The need to avoid large intakes of foods that are high in vitamin K (*e.g.,* cauliflower, dark-green vegetables, bananas, and tomatoes)
	8. The need to report being on oral anticoagulants to the dentist or physician before undergoing any procedure
	9. The importance of reporting signs of redness or swelling in any extremities, sudden dyspnea or chest pain, cough, or hemoptysis

(continued)

NURSING CARE PLAN SUMMARY   Patient with Acute Pulmonary Embolism   Continued

Patient Outcome	Nursing Orders

	10. Ways to enhance venous return and avoid venous stasis, such as the following:
	   A. Avoid constricting stockings and clothing.
	   B. Avoid prolonged sitting and standing positions.
	   C. Avoid crossing legs while sitting.
	   D. Perform regular exercise of legs.
	   E. Wear elastic stockings.
	   F. Maintain adequate hydration.
	11. The need for the patient to carry a card or wear a bracelet indicating that the patient is taking an anticoagulant

---

IMPLEMENTATION AND EVALUATION

Recognition and Prevention of Deep Venous Thrombosis and Pulmonary Embolism

The high incidence of sudden death in patients with clinically unsuspected pulmonary embolism supports the importance of efforts aimed at prevention rather than cure. Because almost all pulmonary emboli arise from deep venous thrombosis, preventive measures are predominantly directed toward this entity. The goals of preventive techniques are directed at the mechanisms associated with pulmonary embolism, specifically a decrease in venous stasis and alteration of the patient's state of coagulability.

Prophylactic interventions aimed at the prevention of a primary or initial embolic episode are suitably applied to all patients who are identified as being at high risk for the development of pulmonary embolism (see Table 23–1). The two general categories of prophylactic interventions include nonpharmacologic (or physical) measures and pharmacologic measures. Physical assessment is the easiest and most effective way for nurses to screen patients who are at risk for pulmonary embolism (see Assessment and Nursing Diagnoses).

Nonpharmacologic Measures

In patients who are determined to be at mild to moderate risk for pulmonary embolism, nonpharmacologic methods to decrease venous stasis may be sufficient to prevent this complication. The primary focus of this approach is the immobilized postoperative patient. Until ambulation can occur, venous stasis can be prevented by the application of graded elastic compression stockings or intermittent pneumatic calf compressors to the lower extremities. Until early, active mobility occurs, passive flexion and extension leg exercises and frequent turning should be carried out by the nurse. Slight elevation (10°–15°) of the legs may also enhance venous return; however, excessive elevation could, potentially, result in venous congestion in the inguinal area and, thus, should be avoided. With adequate instruction and preparation, even the bedridden patient can usually carry out some flexion and extension exercises of the lower extremities. Isometric exercises should be avoided because they increase left ventricular end-diastolic pressure and myocardial oxygen consumption.

Frequent deep-breathing exercises to increase venous return and prevent atelectasis can be carried out by most patients if they are given instruction and an occasional reminder. Ensuring adequate pain relief is necessary for the patient to do the exercises. Inclusion of the family when teaching the principles and practice of these simple exercises can provide another important reminder for the patient to do these exercises.

Maintenance of adequate hydration to decrease blood viscosity and stasis is another important nonpharmacologic measure the nurse can carry out in all patients at risk for pulmonary emboli.

The patient's legs should be inspected routinely for tenderness, redness, swelling, or pain, especially in the calf and popliteal areas. Measurement of the circumference of the extremities should be done if there is any suspicion of thrombosis.

Pharmacologic Measures

Prevention of pulmonary embolism in patients who are at higher risk consists of anticoagulation or antiplatelet therapy in addition to the physical measures to decrease venous stasis.

Low-dose heparin (5000 U) administered subcutaneously every 8 to 12 hours for 7 days has been shown to decrease significantly the incidence of thrombosis in postoperative patients without associated increased bleeding complications.[50] Small amounts of heparin decrease thrombogenicity by enhancing the activity of antithrombin III to inhibit factor X. Another reported benefit of low-dose heparin is a reduction in blood viscosity.[6]

A new pharmacologic agent, Embolex, has been recently used successfully to reduce the incidence of deep venous thrombosis in postoperative patients.[3] This drug combines dihydroxyergotamine mesylate, 0.5 mg, with heparin, 5000 U, and 1% lidocaine hydrochloride. Like heparin, it is administered subcutaneously into the abdominal wall 2 hours before surgery and then every 12 hours for 5 to 7 days postoperatively or until the patient is ambulatory. The addition of dihydroxyergotamine selectively exerts a constrictive effect on the capacitance vessels (veins and venules), thus counteracting venous stasis. Contraindications to use of this drug include patients with peripheral vascular disease, coronary artery disease, cerebrovascular disease, and hepatic dysfunction.

Low molecular weight dextran (70 and 40) has antithrombotic actions through alterations in factor VII that impair platelet function and decrease platelet aggregability through polymerization and hemodilution. Complications associated with administration of Dextran include volume overload, anaphylaxis, and kidney damage.

Antiplatelet therapy with the use of aspirin appears to have limited value in prophylaxis of pulmonary embolism. Some protection has been reported in male patients undergoing major orthopedic procedures.[23]

In general, prevention of pulmonary embolism involves physical, nonpharmacologic measures in low-risk patients. Pharmacologic measures are used in patients who are at higher risk. Table 23–3 outlines appropriate preventive measures in certain subgroups of patients.[10]

Treatment

The objectives in the treatment of patients with acute pulmonary embolism are to maintain cardiopulmonary function until resolution of the embolus[43] occurs and to prevent recurrent embolization. Initial treatment is directed at general support and maintenance of homeostatic function with administration of oxygen by a nonbreather mask to combat hypoxemia, and control of pain with small doses of morphine sulfate, taking care to assess for any respiratory changes. Intubation and mechanical ventilation may be necessary if oxygenation cannot be improved. In patients without evidence of pulmonary congestion, volume administration may be helpful to increase preload and, thus, augment ventricular ejection. If patients are hypotensive, vasopressors and inotropic agents may be necessary to maintain adequate perfusion pressure. Dobutamine or isopreterenol may be used in patients with moderate reductions in cardiac output. The patient's blood pressure should be monitored carefully, because hypotension secondary to decreased vascular resistance can occur with either of these agents. Recent evidence indicates that norepinephrine may be very effective in patients with more marked decreases in cardiac output.[39]

Anticoagulation

Drug therapy for patients with pulmonary embolism is based on the dynamics of the coagulation system. After embolism and damage to the pulmonary vessel wall, secondary sites of thrombus formation occur in the lung. Thrombi may continue to form at the site of origin in the legs or in the lungs. The pulmonary arterial endothelium damaged by the embolus releases fibrinolysins, which lyse the primary clot. However, there may be a continuous formation of a secondary thrombus in response to the primary embolus. The major components of the secondary thrombus are platelets and fibrin. High levels of fibrinogen contribute to the fibrin formation.

Because the majority of patients who die rapidly with pulmonary embolism do so as a result of recurrent embolization, anticoagulation therapy with intravenous heparin is usually begun immediately after the diagnosis of pulmonary embolism is strongly suspected (except in patients with massive pulmonary embolism who may be undergoing thrombolytic therapy). A careful history is necessary to determine the presence of any contraindications to heparin therapy (see Table 23–4).

Heparin is a naturally occurring mucopolysaccharide that

Table 23–3
Prophylactic Measures Against Deep Venous Thrombosis and Pulmonary Embolism

CONDITION	INTERVENTION
Bedridden with severe cardiopulmonary disease, thrombotic stroke, cancer, or inflammatory bowel disease	Low-dose heparin Intermittent pneumatic calf compression Frequent turning
Hemorrhagic stroke	Intermittent pneumatic calf compression Frequent turning
Head or spinal trauma	Intermittent pneumatic calf compression Frequent turning
Hip, pelvis, or lower extremity trauma	Low-dose heparin Warfarin Frequent turning
Orthopedic surgery	Low-dose heparin Intermittent pneumatic calf compression Warfarin Frequent turning
Neurosurgery	Intermittent pneumatic calf compression Frequent turning
General and obstetric/gynecologic surgery Age <30–40 yr Surgery <30 min Minimal postoperative immobilization	Early ambulation Graded compression Flexion/extension leg exercises Frequent turning
Age > 40 yr Prolonged surgery Prolonged immobilization Abdominal surgery	Low-dose heparin Intermittent pneumatic calf compression Frequent turning

Table 23–4
Contraindications to Anticoagulation Therapy

ABSOLUTE CONTRAINDICATIONS	RELATIVE CONTRAINDICATIONS
Active internal bleeding	Recent major surgery
Known hypersensitivity	Recent gastrointestinal bleed
Recent hemorrhagic stroke	Coagulation disorders
Recent surgery of brain, eyes, or spinal cord	Hematuria
	Intracranial neoplasm

is found in most cells of many tissues, including the liver, lung, and intestine. Commercially prepared heparin is extracted from beef lung and pork gut tissue and purified for use as an anticoagulant.

Heparin inhibits activation of thrombin, inactivates already formed thrombin, and inhibits the aggregation of platelets on the surface of thrombin.[1]

Heparin is used to arrest an active thrombotic state.[24,48] Heparin is given intravenously by continuous drip or by intermittent intravenous doses, preferably through a heparin lock every 4 hours. Heparin should not be administered through intramuscular or subcutaneous routes in patients with acute pulmonary embolism due to unpredictable absorption with variations in systemic blood pressure and tissue perfusion. To achieve immediate anticoagulation, a loading dose of 10,000 U to 15,000 U is given, followed by sufficient heparin to prolong the clotting time to two to three times the control level.

The heparin dosage required to achieve therapeutic anticoagulation depends on the patient's weight, but generally, it is in the range of 800 U to 1500 U/hour by intravenous infusion. Such large doses are necessary to reverse changes such as bronchoconstriction and pulmonary vascular constriction, in addition to fibrinolysis. Frequently, heparin requirements decrease during the first 2 or 3 days of therapy, especially in patients with right-heart failure.[15] Increased resistance to heparin may occur in patients with fever, thrombosis, thrombophlebitis, myocardial infarction, and cancer. Increased dosages are necessary in these cases.

Anticoagulant therapy should continue for at least 7 to 10 days after acute pulmonary embolism to allow the necessary time for thrombi to adhere to the vessel wall and be covered with endothelium.

The primary complications associated with heparin therapy are hemorrhage and thrombocytopenia. Bleeding occurs in approximately 15% to 20% of patients who receive heparin therapy and is the leading cause of adverse drug effects in hospitalized patients.[17] Major bleeding, defined as a decrease in hemoglobin greater than 2 g/dl, or hemorrhage into a vital organ, or a fatal bleed, occurs infrequently (in 5%–10% of patients), whereas "minor" bleeding (hematoma, hematuria) occurs more often. Risk factors associated with hemorrhage in patients receiving heparin include the female gender, age above 60 years, the presence of severe intercurrent illness, heavy use of alcohol, and concomitant use of aspirin.[17,52] The risk of bleeding secondary to this agent is reportedly greatest on the third day of heparin therapy.[52]

Bleeding complications secondary to heparin can be reduced by avoiding concomitant administration of aspirin and aspirin-containing products and dipyridamole; avoiding intramuscular injections; avoiding all elective invasive procedures; and care-

fully monitoring the patient's clotting time with appropriate adjustments in the heparin dosage. Early ambulation is discouraged during heparin therapy to prevent the possibility of embolization from venous thrombi that have not become firmly adhered to the vein wall.[44] Should major bleeding occur, discontinuation of heparin causes elimination of its effects within a few hours. More serious bleeding may require immediate neutralization with protamine sulfate. This drug should always be available for emergency use when a patient is given heparin. It is a low–molecular-weight protein that contains large amounts of arginine, an amino acid. It combines with heparin to form a stable compound that has no anticoagulant properties. Each 1 mg of protamine sulfate neutralizes approximately 100 U of heparin. Usually no more than 50 mg is infused slowly over a 10-minute period. Rapid infusion can result in severe hypotension and bradycardia. Anaphylactoid reactions also may occur.

A paradoxic heparin-associated thrombocytopenia occurs in 4% to 30% of patients who receive heparin therapy.[5,38] A higher incidence occurs with bovine (beef) heparin versus porcine (pork) heparin preparations. The severity of this complication ranges from a moderate reduction in the patient's platelet count to life-threatening arterial thrombosis. Although the pathophysiology is poorly understood, an immune-mediated mechanism that triggers platelet aggregation, which lowers the platelet count and initiates thrombosis, is believed to be the underlying mechanism.[28] Thrombocytopenia rarely develops until 6 days of heparin therapy, unless the patient has had prior exposure to heparin.[17] Laboratory measurement of the platelet count should be performed every few days while the patient is receiving heparin. Discontinuation of heparin therapy should immediately reverse platelet reductions and normalize their value.

Hypersensitivity to heparin is infrequent and can be manifested as fever, chills, bronchoconstriction, urticaria, and, rarely, anaphylactic shock. Obtaining a careful history is essential to determine prior heparin usage and the development of any complications from it.

Laboratory Monitoring. The partial thromboplastin time (PTT) and the activated partial thromboplastin time (APTT) measure the clotting time of plasma and are used to monitor heparin therapy. Patient values should be compared with normal laboratory values to assess therapeutic heparinization. The normal PTT is 60 to 70 seconds, whereas a normal APTT is 35 to 50 seconds. Because the half-life of heparin is 60 to 90 minutes, the first APTT is usually measured after approximately 30 to 60 minutes of therapy. Numerous measurements are determined within the first 24 hours (approximately every 4 hours), followed by appropriate adjustments in infusion as well as boluses of heparin until full therapeutic levels are obtained, with the APTT ranging approximately two to three times the control level. Thereafter, daily PTTs are monitored.

Measurement of the activated clotting time is a recent technique that is easily performed at the bedside for rapid determination of the patient's clotting time. The test is performed on small amounts (<0.5 ml) of fresh whole blood and reportedly provides a more accurate evaluation of the patient's intrinsic coagulation status, particularly over wide ranges of heparin concentration levels.[51] In addition, the rapidity with which clotting information is available allows prompt adjustments in heparin dosage and, potentially, better maintenance of therapeutic levels.

Thrombolysis

Although heparin has remained the cornerstone of therapy in pulmonary embolism to prevent further embolic recurrences, it has little or no effect on existing thrombus.[43] Although spontaneous dissolution of thrombus may occur over a period of days or weeks, it may be desirable to hasten this process in patients who are experiencing cardiopulmonary compromise secondary to massive pulmonary embolism.

Streptokinase and urokinase are two thrombolytic agents (Fig. 23-8) approved by the Food and Drug Administration for treatment of acute pulmonary embolism since 1977. Their use, however, has been relegated to those patients suffering massive pulmonary embolism with severe cardiovascular collapse. This approach may be changing, however, with the availability of newer, clot-specific thrombolytic agents.[18] Thrombolytic therapy has also received strong endorsement by a consensus development conference of the National Institutes of Health.[47] Observations from several studies suggest that thrombolytic therapy of acute pulmonary embolism causes more complete resolution of pulmonary emboli than heparin therapy and may reduce the associated long-term morbidity of this complication.[43] Other potential advantages include the prevention of chronic pulmonary hypertension, reduction in the frequency of recurrent pulmonary embolism, and reduction in the overall mortality rate associated with acute pulmonary embolism.[18]

Before initiation of thrombolysis, a careful history must be obtained to determine the presence of any contraindications to thrombolytic therapy (Table 23-5). If anticoagulation therapy has been started, it should be discontinued and a laboratory coagulation profile obtained.

The currently available or experimental types of pharmacologic agents that initiate thrombolysis differ in their pharmacologic actions and mechanisms as well as in their fibrin specificity.

Streptokinase is a protein purified from beta-hemolytic streptococci that complexes with circulating plasminogen to form plasmin, a clot-lysing agent. It may cause severe febrile and other allergic reactions in some patients that may be prevented by pretreatment administration of hydrocortisone, diphenhydramine, and acetaminophen. Its antigenic nature prevents repeated treatment for about 6 to 12 months.[27,42] Patients with prior streptococcal infections may have a relative resistance to streptokinase. Streptokinase is usually initiated

with a bolus of 250,000 U intravenously over 30 minutes that is followed by a 24-hour infusion at a rate of 100,000 U/hour.

Urokinase is obtained from purified human urine or human fetal kidney cell cultures. Urokinase differs from streptokinase in that it directly activates plasminogen to generate plasmin (the lysing agent) and, therefore, does not produce such significant systemic lytic effects. Allergic reactions to this agent are rare, and it can be administered on repeated occasions without inducing an antibody response that will cause drug resistance. Urokinase is usually given as a bolus of 4400 U/kg that is followed by an infusion of 4400 U/kg/hour for 12 hours.

Tissue plasminogen activator, originally isolated from human melanoma cells, is produced through recombinant DNA technology and represents a major advance in thrombolytic therapy. Tissue plasminogen activator is more fibrin-specific, joining plasminogen on the fibrin surface of the clot and subsequently producing fibrinolysis. For this reason, tissue plasminogen activator produces greater reduced systemic lytic effects than streptokinase or urokinase, and it has the ability to lyse other potentially dangerous thrombi in the legs. Investigations of tissue plasminogen activator in patients with acute pulmonary embolism report both high efficacy and safety.[20] Tissue plasminogen activator is administered as an intravenous infusion of 100 mg over 2 hours.

Thrombolytic therapy may be life-saving for the hemodynamically compromised patients because it can rapidly reverse pulmonary hypertension and resultant right ventricular dysfunction and dilatation.[9]

The degree of lysis achieved by any of the thrombolytic agents depends on numerous factors, including the location, size, and duration of the embolus, the activatability of the patient's fibrinolytic system; the concentration of plasminogen on the thrombus; and the patient's body temperature. Thrombolysis is most effective with emboli that have been located in large vessels for less than 7 days. Extremes in body temperature (either direction) decrease the efficiency of the fibrinolytic system and can diminish the effects of thrombolytic agents.

The major complication seen in patients treated with thrombolytic agents is bleeding, which occurs approximately two to four times more often than in patients treated solely with heparin. However, increased clinical experience with these agents appears to reduce the overall incidence of serious bleeding to less than 5%.[27] Careful patient selection that is based on a thorough history and physical examination can help reduce the risk of bleeding. Absolute and relative contraindications to thrombolytic therapy are listed in Table 23–

Table 23-5

Contraindications to Thrombolytic Therapy

ABSOLUTE CONTRAINDICATIONS	RELATIVE CONTRAINDICATIONS
Active internal bleeding	Pre-existing hemorrhagic diathesis
Cerebrovascular process	Thrombocytopenia
Neoplasm	Severe uncontrolled hypertension
Recent intracranial surgery or trauma	Chronic renal failure
Recent intraspinal surgery	Chronic liver failure
Recent cerebrovascular accident	Intrapartum and immediate postpartum state
Arteriovenous malformation	Recent major surgery, trauma, or deep biopsies (<10 days)
Severe blood dyscrasia (hemophilia)	

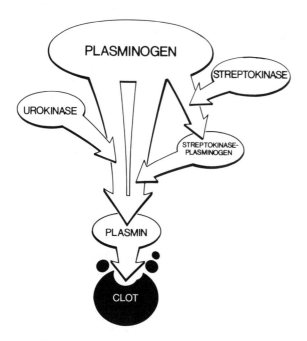

Figure 23–8

Thrombolytic enzyme activation of the fibrinolytic system. Streptokinase joins plasminogen and forms a complex that then reacts with plasminogen to form plasmin. Urokinase reacts directly with plasminogen, creating plasmin. The lysing agent, activated plasmin, then dissolves the clot.

5. To avoid the risk of cerebral hemorrhage, patients with severe uncontrolled hypertension should be excluded from this therapy; however, the degree of hypertension should be determined from blood pressure readings obtained when the patient is not in extremis from associated pain and anxiety.

The most common bleeding sites associated with thrombolytic therapy include puncture sites (needles and catheters), the urinary tract, the gastrointestinal tract, and, in postpartum patients, the uterus.[12] However, thrombolytic therapy does not appear to enhance menses and can be given safely to menstruating women.[12]

The incidence of bleeding has been correlated to the duration of lytic therapy and to the concomitant use of antiplatelet aggregation agents and heparin.[19,27] Heparinization is instituted after discontinuation of any thrombolytic agent to prevent rethrombosis. A continuous infusion at 1000 U/hr, without a preceding bolus, is begun when the thrombin time decreases to 1.5 to 2 times the control level. The optimal duration of thrombolytic therapy has yet to be determined. Currently, studies are assessing the efficacy of short, bolus administration of these agents.[26]

Careful monitoring for signs and symptoms of bleeding is essential in caring for patients who are undergoing thrombolytic therapy. All elective invasive procedures should be avoided during treatment. Blood samples should be drawn from an in-line catheter or a heparin lock. Previous puncture sites should be assessed closely for evidence of hematoma formation or oozing. Any evidence of bleeding at the puncture sites should be controlled with manual pressure for 15 minutes, followed by the application of a pressure dressing. Patient handling and excessive movement should be avoided during thrombolytic therapy. One should analyze all urine and stool samples for evidence of bleeding. A baseline and repeated neurologic assessment are essential to determine alterations associated with intracranial hemorrhage.

If severe bleeding occurs, the thrombolytic agent should be discontinued immediately and the lytic state reversed with infusions of fresh frozen plasma or cryoprecipitate. If bleeding persists, a 3-g to 5-g intravenous bolus of epsilon aminocaproic acid (Amicar) over 30 minutes, followed by an infusion of 1.0 g/hr, will prevent further plasmin generation and plasmin lysis.[27] Other adverse effects of thrombolytic therapy include fever (most common with streptokinase), allergic dermatitis, and, rarely, reperfusion pulmonary edema.[53]

Recent and current studies investigating the synergistic combinations of various thrombolytic agents as well as reduced dosages of thrombolytic agents combined with systemic heparinization provide promising evidence of the ability to achieve successful thrombolysis with a reduced number of complications associated with bleeding.[30]

Laboratory Monitoring. Before initiation of thrombolytic therapy, laboratory evaluation of the patient's complete blood count, chemistry profile, and coagulation profile is essential to determine contraindications to therapy as well as to determine baseline values.

During and after therapy, the patient's hemoglobin and hematocrit levels should be determined daily to assess for evidence of occult bleeding.

Documentation of the lytic state can be obtained by measurement of fibrinogen levels or fibrinogen degradation products. Complete lysis causes decreases in the amount of circulating fibrinogen and increases in the fibrinogen degradation products.

Measurements of the prothrombin time and partial thromboplastin time are less sensitive to the lytic state, whereas prolongation of the thrombin time usually accompanies thrombolysis.

Long-Term Therapy

After initial treatment of acute pulmonary embolism with thrombolytic agents or heparin, long-term prevention of the recurrence of an active thrombotic process is begun.

This is achieved by coumarin derivatives, of which warfarin is the one most commonly used after the acute phase of pulmonary embolism, during the recovery phase, and after discharge from the hospital.[31] Warfarin interferes with the biochemical reactions that cause the liver to synthesize several clotting factors (prothrombin and factors VII, IX, and X). It acts as a competitive inhibitor of vitamin K, which is essential for the production of these factors. Increasingly large doses of warfarin are given until the prothrombin time rises to a therapeutic range (2 to 2.5 times the control time). Because of its slow onset of action, oral administration of warfarin should begin during heparin therapy. Approximately 3 to 5 days are required to reduce sufficiently the circulating levels of factors IX and X, the key factors for the antithrombotic effects.[31] Therefore, heparin is continued for that length of time after the initiation of oral anticoagulants. The dosage of heparin need not be tapered before discontinuation.

Several factors determine how long a patient should take oral anticoagulants. The physician considers the events that occurred with the embolism, whether the patient has a predisposition to further thromboembolism, how well the patient tolerates anticoagulants, and how reliable the patient is about taking medications. The exact length of anticoagulation therapy is debatable, but most patients remain on oral anticoagulants for a 3-month to 6-month period. Bleeding episodes represent the primary complication associated with warfarin therapy. Major bleeding complications, including intracerebral bleeding, hematemesis, and retroperitoneal bleeding, occur in approximately 5% to 10% of patients receiving warfarin.[25,37] The patient should be checked regularly for signs of bleeding. Bleeding secondary to the deficiency or inhibition of clotting factor generally presents as deep dissecting hematomas. Therefore, the circumference of the extremities should be measured. Other common signs of bleeding are large, often solitary ecchymoses, gingival oozing, and delayed bleeding from puncture wounds. Discharged patients taking oral anticoagulants should know the signs of over-anticoagulation, such as easy bruising, minor cuts that stop bleeding normally (in the platelet phase of bleeding) but begin bleeding later, black stools, blood in the urine or stool, coughed-up blood, swelling and pain in the joints, and severe headaches. They should be told to avoid foods that are high in vitamin K. If the patient taking an anticoagulant requires dental surgery or other minor surgery, he should tell the dentist or physician about the anticoagulant therapy.

A rare, although serious, complication of warfarin therapy is skin and soft-tissue necrosis due to thrombosis secondary to rapid declines in levels of protein C. This is usually manifested within 5 to 7 days of initiating therapy and begins as an area of painful erythema that evolves rapidly into hemorrhagic necrosis. Patients with pre-existing deficiencies in protein C are at increased risk for skin necrosis.[33] Treatment includes discontinuation of warfarin, followed by the administration of vitamin K, which rapidly neutralizes its effects, and heparin to maintain anticoagulation. The necrotic process may resolve spontaneously or continue, requiring surgical debridement or amputation.

Other less common complications of warfarin therapy include alopecia, urticaria, erythema, dermatitis, and hypersensitivity. These complications usually occur later in the course of treatment.

Contraindications to warfarin therapy are the same as those to heparin therapy (see Table 23–4). An additional contraindication includes patients with hereditary deficiencies in protein C. Special caution is required in patients with liver disease or vitamin K deficiency.

When the patient is taking coumarin, particular attention should be given to the other medications he or she takes. Many medications can increase or decrease the effect of coumarin anticoagulants by altering the bioavailability of vitamin K, by displacing coumarin from its binding sites on serum albumin, and by altering the concentration of prothrombin complex. The most common medications that increase the effect of coumarin anticoagulants are salicylates, indomethacin, phenylbutazone, diphenylhydantoin, quinidine, clofibrate, chloral hydrate, thyroxine, bowel-sterilizing antibiotics, chloramphenicol, dipyridamole, amiodarone, ethacrynic acid, sulfonamides, and anabolic steroids. Drugs that decrease the effect of coumarin anticoagulants include most antacids, barbiturates, adrenocorticosteroids, estrogen, oral contraceptives, griseofulvin, meprobamate mercurial and thiazide diuretics, and cholestyramine.

Certain phenomena are contraindications to anticoagulant therapy. Among them are an actively bleeding or symptomatic gastrointestinal or genitourinary lesion that may bleed, acute cerebrovascular accident, severe systemic hypertension, recent surgical procedures in which bleeding may constitute a risk, renal or hepatic insufficiency, and platelet or coagulation factor abnormalities. When any of those phenomena are present, the physician must consider inferior vena caval interruption to prevent recurrent pulmonary embolism.

During pregnancy, anticoagulant therapy presents special problems. Because heparin does not cross the placental barrier, it is the safest drug for the patients and the fetus; in addition, heparin is not present in breast milk of nursing mothers.[34] Coumarin derivatives do cross the placental barrier, and not much is known about the extent and duration of resulting fetal clotting derangements. Oral anticoagulants should be avoided during the first trimester of pregnancy because of their possible teratogenic effects and during the last 3 weeks of pregnancy because of the increased risk of perinatal hemorrhage.

Laboratory Monitoring.   The prothrombin time is probably the most common routine test of blood coagulation. It is used to monitor anticoagulation therapy with warfarin (Coumadin). This drug suppresses the vitamin K–dependent factors produced by the liver. Warfarin is given until the prothrombin time rises to a therapeutic range of 2 to 2.5 times control, which is the range that seems necessary to prevent most venous thrombotic complications.[31]

In determining a prothrombin time, a sample of venous blood is drawn from the patient and a sample of plasma is placed in an anticoagulated tube. Next, calcium and tissue thromboplastin are added. Usually a clot forms in 11 to 14 seconds. Thromboplastin activity varies with each test, so a control must be done on normal plasma with each test. The values that are recorded give the number of seconds for clot formation in the test blood and the number of seconds for clot formation in the normal blood.

Surgical Procedures

In view of the high mortality rate associated with untreated pulmonary embolism, patients who are not suitable for anticoagulant or thrombolytic therapy, or in whom the appropriate therapy has failed, may benefit from interruption of the inferior vena cava.[24] Other indications for this procedure include recurrent episodes of embolization despite therapeutic anticoagulation, bleeding or other contraindications to anticoagulation, massive pulmonary embolism, or septic embolism. A number of techniques have been used to narrow the lumen of the inferior vena cava, resulting in occlusion of the flow of blood, reduced venous return, and, unfortunately, compromised cardiac output. The high morbidity and mortality associated with these interrupting procedures have severely limited their use.

Filtering of blood returning to the heart from the legs successfully prevents recurrence of pulmonary embolism in the majority of patients, with less impairment of venous return. Placement of a specially designed stainless steel filter within the lumen of the inferior vena cava can be performed under local anesthesia using the transvenous approach from the jugular or femoral vein. The filter, which is folded about the catheter tip during insertion, is then opened like an umbrella to obstruct the flow of emboli (Fig. 23–9).[48] The wires of this filter are spaced to entrap emboli larger than 3 mm. Although use of the vena cava filter is associated with a significant reduction in the rate of recurrent emboli, lower extremity sequelae are frequently present, including peripheral edema, stasis dermatitis, and ulceration.[40] However, none of these procedures for vena caval interruption is completely effective in preventing the recurrence of emboli.

Pulmonary Embolectomy

Pulmonary embolectomy, in the appropriate clinical situation, may be a life-saving procedure.[31] However, because of its emergent nature and associated high mortality rate, it is reserved for a select group of patients who show evidence of severe hemodynamic compromise due to embolism that does not respond to other measures. These patients must show clear evidence of massive pulmonary embolism to the main pulmonary artery or its major branches involving more than 60% of the pulmonary vasculature.[31] When therapy or circulatory assist procedures do not bring dramatic improvement, emergency cardiopulmonary bypass and pulmonary embolectomy must be considered.[31] Indications for surgical embolectomy include contraindications to anticoagulation or thrombolysis,

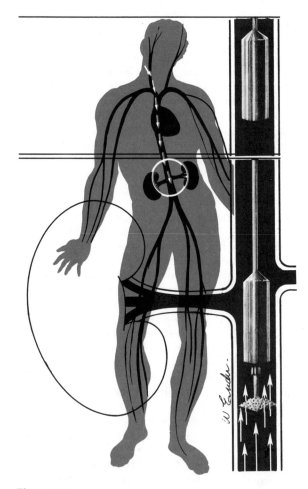

Figure 23–9
An umbrella filter.

recurrent pulmonary embolism despite adequate anticoagulation, massive pulmonary embolism that is not responsive to thrombolysis, septic thromboembolism, and chronic pulmonary embolism with secondary pulmonary hypertension.

Prognosis in Acute Pulmonary Embolism

Most patients recover from the acute event of pulmonary embolism; with appropriate treatment, the prognosis of patients experiencing an acute pulmonary embolism is good, with reported mortality rates of 5% to 8%.[34] If residual thromboemboli continue to accumulate, chronic pulmonary hypertension with right-heart failure may result, with associated high morbidity and mortality.

SUMMARY

The frequency with which pulmonary embolism occurs in hospitalized patients demands that everyone caring for hospitalized patients be thoroughly familiar with the causative and high-risk factors in pulmonary embolism. The signs and symptoms of pulmonary embolism are usually nonspecific. Routine laboratory studies, chest radiographs, arterial blood gas analyses, and ECGs are helpful but not diagnostic. The lung scan and pulmonary angiograms are the best diagnostic techniques. Treatment is aimed at preventing further embolism by anticoagulation. Rapid dissolution of the embolism with thrombolytic therapy is useful in those patients suffering massive pulmonary embolism with severe cardiopulmonary compromise.

Because this complication can occur in a variety of clinical settings, a high degree of suspicion should be maintained when caring for all patients who are at increased risk for pulmonary embolism. The nursing and medical professions are concerned with the prevention of deep venous thrombosis and early recognition of the occurrence of pulmonary embolism.

DIRECTIONS FOR FUTURE RESEARCH

Research questions that nurses may consider for improving the care of patients with acute pulmonary embolism are as follows:

1. What is the most effective teaching format for educating patients and their families about anticoagulants?
2. How does long-term anticoagulation affect the patient's quality of life?
3. What are the most effective relaxation techniques for patients with acute pulmonary embolism?
4. What is the best way to monitor patients receiving thrombolytic agents?
5. How will the effects of thrombolytic therapy be monitored?
6. What is the best protocol for administration of thrombolytic therapy?

REFERENCES

1. Albrechtsson, W., Anderson, J., and Einarsson, E. Streptokinase treatment of deep venous thrombosis and the post thrombotic syndrome. *Arch. Surg.* 116:33, 1981.
2. Ansari, A. Acute and chronic pulmonary thromboembolism:

Current perspectives. Part II. Etiology, pathology, pathogenesis and pathophysiology. *Clin. Cardiol.* 9:449, 1986.

3. Ansari, A. Acute and chronic pulmonary thromboembolism: Current perspectives. Part IV. Differential diagnosis and prophylaxis. *Clin. Cardiol.* 9:567, 1986.

4. Ansari, A. Acute and chronic pulmonary thromboembolism: Current perspectives. Part VI. Course and prognosis and natural history. *Clin. Cardiol.* 10:40, 1987.

5. Bell, W. R., Tomasulo, P. A., Alving, B. M., et al. Thrombocytopenia occurring during the administration of heparin. *Ann. Intern. Med.* 85:155, 1976.

6. Bell, W. R., and Simon, T. L. Current status of pulmonary thromboembolic disease: Pathophysiology, diagnosis, prevention, and treatment. *Am. Heart J.* 103:239, 1988.

7. Bullas, J. B. Fibrinolytic therapy: Nursing implications. *Crit. Care Nurs.* 1:43, 1981.

8. Collen, D. Synergism of thrombolytic agents: Investigational procedures and clinical potential. *Circulation* 77:731, 1988.

9. Come, P. C., Kim, D., Parker, A., et al. Early reversal of right ventricular dysfunction in patients with acute pulmonary embolism after treatment with intravenous tissue plasminogen activator. *J. Am. Coll. Cardiol.* 10:971, 1987.

10. Coon, W. W., Hirsh, J., and Rubin, L. J. Preventing deep venous thrombosis. *Patient Care* February 15:82, 1987.

11. Cvitanic, O., and Marino, P. L. Improved use of arterial blood gas analysis in suspected pulmonary embolism. *Chest* 95:48, 1989.

12. Donovan, B. C. How to give thrombolytic therapy safely. *Chest* 95:290S, 1989.

13. Fahey, V. Deep vein thrombosis. *Nursing '84* 14:33, 1984.

14. Fred, H. L., Axelrod, M. A., Lewis, J. M., et al. Rapid resolution of pulmonary thromboembolism in man. *J.A.M.A.* 196:1137, 1966.

15. Genton, E. Guidelines for heparin therapy. *Ann. Intern. Med.* 80:77, 1984.

16. Gilbert, R., and Keighley, J. F. The arterial/alveolar oxygen tension ratio: An index of gas exchange applicable to varying inspired oxygen concentrations. *Am. Rev. Respir. Dis.* 109:142, 1974.

17. Glenny, R. W. Pulmonary embolism: Complications of therapy. *South Med. J.* 80:166, 1987.

18. Goldhaber, S. Z., Meyerovitz, M. F., Markis, J. E., et al. Thrombolytic therapy of acute pulmonary embolism: Current status and future potential. *J. Am. Coll. Cardiol.* 10:96B, 1987.

19. Goldhaber, S. Z., Kessler, C. M., Heit, H., et al. Randomized controlled trial of recombinant tissue plasminogen activator versus urokinase in the treatment of acute pulmonary embolism. *Lancet* 2(8606):293, 1988.

20. Goldhaber, S. Z. Tissue plasminogen activator in acute pulmonary embolism. *Chest* 95:282S, 1989.

21. Guyton, A. C. *Textbook of Medical Physiology* (5th ed.). Philadelphia: W. B. Saunders, 1981.

22. Hardaway, R. M. Pathology and pathophysiology of disseminated intravascular coagulation. In R. A. Calley and B. Trump (eds.), *Pathophysiology of Shock, Anoxia, and Ischemia.* Baltimore: Williams & Wilkins, 1982.

23. Harris, W. H., Salzman, E. W., Athanasoulis, C. A., et al. Aspirin prophylaxis of venous thromboembolism after total hip replacement. *N. Engl. J. Med.* 97:146, 1977.

24. Huffman, M. H. Acute care of the patient with a pulmonary embolism due to venous thromboemboli. *Crit. Care Nurs.* 3:70, 1983.

25. Husted, S., and Andreasen, F. Problems encountered in longterm treatment with anticoagulants. *Acta Med. Scand.* 200:379, 1976.

26. Kessler, C. M., Druy, E., and Goldhaber, S. Z. Acute pulmonary embolism treated with thrombolytic agents: Current status of tPA and future implications for emergency medicine. *Ann. Em. Med.* 17:1216, 1988.

27. Kessler, C. M. Anticoagulation and thrombolytic therapy: Practical considerations. *Chest* 95:245S, 1989.

28. King, D. J., and Kelton, J. G. Heparin-associated thrombocytopenia. *Ann. Intern. Med.* 100:535, 1984.

29. Knapp, R. S., and Mullens, C. B. Progressive tricuspid regurgitation as a limit to right ventricular output in acute pulmonary hypertension. *Clin. Res.* 20:69, 1972.

30. Leeper, K. V., Popovich, J., Lesser, B. A., et al. Treatment of massive acute pulmonary embolism: The use of low doses of intrapulmonary arterial streptokinase combined with full doses of systemic heparin. *Chest* 93:234, 1988.

31. McFadden, E. R., and Braunwald, E. Cor pulmonale and pulmonary thromboembolism. In E. Braunwald (ed.), *Heart Disease.* Philadelphia: W. B. Saunders, 1980.

32. McGregory, J., and Roach, A. Unusual complications in a patient receiving streptokinase treatment for deep venous thrombosis. *Crit. Care Nurs.* 1:53, 1981.

33. Mannucci, P. M., and Vigano, S. Deficiencies of protein C, an inhibitor of blood coagulation. *Lancet* 2(8296):463, 1982.

34. Melillo, E., DiRicco, G., Rindi, M., et al. Short-term follow-up of patients with pulmonary embolism. *Chest* 96:144S, 1989.

35. Moser, K. M. Pulmonary embolism. *Am. Rev. Respir. Dis.* 115:89, 1977.

36. Petruzzelli, S., Palla, A., Pieraccini, F., et al. Routine electrocardiography in screening pulmonary embolism. *Respiration* 50:33, 1986.

37. Pollar, J. W., Hamilton, M. J., Christensen, N. A., et al. Problems associated with long term anticoagulant therapy: Observation in 139 cases. *Circulation* 25:311, 1962.

38. Powers, P. J., Kelton, J. G., and Carter, C. J. Studies on the frequency of heparin-associated thrombocytopenia. *Thromb. Res.* 33:439, 1984.

39. Prewitt, R. M. Hemodynamic management in pulmonary embolism and acute hypoxemic respiratory failure. *Crit. Care Med.* 18:S61, 1990.

40. Richenbacher, W. E., Atnip, R. G., Campbell, D. B., et al. Recurrent pulmonary embolism after inferior vena caval interruption with a Greenfield filter. *World J. Surg.* 13:623, 1989.

41. Roberts, S. *Behavioral Concepts and the Critically Ill Patient.* Englewood Cliffs, NJ: Prentice-Hall, 1976.

42. Rubin, R. N. Fibrinolysis and its current usage. *Clin. Ther.* 5:211, 1983.

43. Sasahara, A. A., Hyers, T. M., Cole, C. M. et al. The Urokinase Pulmonary Embolism Trial: A national cooperative study. *Circulation* 47 (suppl 2):1, 1973.

44. Sasahara, A. A., and St. Martin, C. C. Update of the treatment of pulmonary embolism. *Prim. Cardiol.* (Nov):41, 1989.

45. Sautter, R. D., Fletcher, F. E., Ousley, J. L., et al. Rapid resolution of a pulmonary embolus. *Dis. Chest* 5:85, 1967.

46. Sharma, G. V. R. K., McIntyre, K. M., Sharma, S., et al. Clinical and hemodynamic correlates in pulmonary embolism. *Clin. Chest Med.* 5:412, 1984.

47. Thrombolytic Therapy in Thrombosis. A National Institutes of Health Consensus Development Conference. *Ann. Intern. Med.* 93:141, 1980.

48. Thomas, M. N. Acute pulmonary embolism. *Focus Crit. Care* 10:21, 1983.

49. Tsapogas, M. J. Pulmonary embolism. Part I. Incidence, pathophysiology and diagnosis. *Ala. J. Med. Sci.* 24:405, 1987.

50. Wessler, S., and Yin, E. T. Theory and practice of minidose heparin in surgical patients. *Circulation* 47:671, 1973.

51. Varah, N., Smith, J., and Baugh, R. F. Post-PTCA heparin monitoring in the CCU. *Heart Lung* (in press).

52. Walker, A. M., and Jick, H. Predictors of bleeding during heparin therapy. *J.A.M.A.* 44:109, 1980.

53. Ward, B. J., and Pearse, D. B. Reperfusion pulmonary edema after thrombolytic therapy of massive pulmonary embolism. *Am. Rev. Respir. Dis.* 138:1308, 1988.

V

The Critically Ill Adult With Cardiovascular Problems

NEEDED: A COMPLEMENTARY APPROACH

Even someone who has a mechanistic orientation to nursing would agree that patients who are critically ill have enormous psychologic reactions to their illness and that it is the duty of the critical care nurse to help such patients cope. Critical care nurses must not only understand the disease process, know how to operate sophisticated equipment, and render basic patient care; they must also help patients cope with the emotional responses to their illness.

But patients' psychologic responses to their illness are generally regarded as somehow less real than their so-called purely physical derangements. That fact can be verified by reviewing the literature on acute myocardial infarction. The most detailed discussions are generally of the physical complications of myocardial infarction, such as dysrhythmias, congestive heart failure, pulmonary embolism, and ventricular septal rupture. The psychosocial complications, such as fear, stress, rage, and depression, are mentioned, one feels, as a gesture toward completeness, the implication being that the psychologic complications are distinct from the physical complications, which are somehow more real.

24

Cardiovascular Assessment

Cathie E. Guzzetta   *Patricia E. Casey*

LAUGHTER, HUMOR, AND JOY

Laughter is often said to be the shortest distance between two people. The stress in critical care nursing can be lessened by laughter and humor because joy and sadness pathways cannot operate simultaneously. Laughter and humor literally increase our production of endorphins. They serve as healthy ways to relieve tension, help manage pain, and act as distractors. A sense of being in control, new hope, and alternatives to fear, anger, and grief also emerge as moments of the lighter side of life are explored.

You cannot stay in stressed states continuously without sadness and depression. Moments of laughter and humor have a way of bringing a sense of balance, helping you to be more objective, and releasing tension and unexpressed emotions. Laughing at yourself and the situation allows you to contact your inner core of joy and to lighten the load of being human.

Healing moments in which you spend time with patients and others talking, actively listening, and sharing times of life experienced together bring about humor and joy. Laughter and humor can come from telling stories or listening to the stories of others. Reflecting on laughter shared can ease stress long after the story. Often laughing can break the barriers for you or others to speak from your heart.

LEARNING OBJECTIVES

After reading this chapter, the nurse should be able to do the following:

1. Discuss the importance of a systematic approach to the cardiovascular nursing assessment.
2. Discuss the specific variables within each human response pattern to be assessed for the cardiovascular patient.
3. Identify the components of the cardiovascular assessment.
4. Adapt the Critical Care Response Pattern Assessment Tool (see Chap. 5) specifically for the critically ill cardiovascular patient by changing and adding the assessment variables that are discussed in this chapter.
5. Assess a cardiovascular patient using the adapted Response Pattern Assessment Tool.
6. Explain the procedure, rationale, and nursing implications for noninvasive techniques of assessment such as the electrocardiogram, atrial electrogram, Holter monitoring, chest radiograph, echocardiogram, phonocardiogram, graded exercise test, transesophageal atrial pacing, and nuclear scans.
7. Explain the procedure, rationale, and nursing implications for invasive techniques of assessment such as a cardiac

catheterization, electrophysiologic studies, and endomyocardial biopsy.

COMPONENTS OF THE CARDIOVASCULAR ASSESSMENT

When assessing and caring for cardiovascular patients, nurses should review and incorporate the Standards of Cardiovascular Nursing Practice from the American Nurses' Association and the American Heart Association Council on Cardiovascular Nursing.[1] The seven standards include information and criteria related to collection of data; nursing diagnoses; observable goals, written as outcomes; plan for nursing care; implementation; evaluation; and reassessment. The standards are specific for cardiovascular patients and are useful in guiding the nurse in the assessment phase and the remaining steps of the nursing process.

When assessing cardiovascular patients, nurses need to use a data-base format that ensures that all of the patient's body-mind-spirit problems are assessed. As discussed in Chapter 5, such a holistic assessment can be accomplished by evaluating the patient's nine human response patterns. The knowing and feeling patterns are particularly important to assess in the cardiovascular patient. The data obtained from these patterns must be carefully interrelated and synthesized with the data obtained from the exchanging pattern and the results of cardiac diagnostic testing procedures. Such synthesis is necessary to understand the unique psychophysiologic patterns that characterize the patient's state of health and to facilitate the identification of nursing diagnoses.

The following sections discuss the components of a cardiovascular assessment using the nine human response patterns as a framework (see Chap. 5).[14,15] This chapter was developed to illustrate how the Critical Care Response Pattern Assessment Tool (see p. 59) can be adapted specifically for the cardiovascular patient. The physical assessment discussion under the exchanging pattern reflects how assessment variables are rearranged from a medical to a nursing framework. Also, variables that have relevance for the cardiovascular patient have been added or expanded and are the focus of this chapter. The reader should refer to Chapter 5 for assessment of other generic variables that can be applied to most adult patients regardless of their dysfunction.

COMMUNICATING PATTERN

Evaluate the patient's ability to understand, speak, read, and write English. Determine if there is any physiologic or psychologic reason for such difficulty. Document if the patient is intubated and whether any alternate form of communication has been established with the patient (see Chap. 5).

KNOWING PATTERN

Current Health Problem

Ask patients to describe their symptoms and their reason for seeking medical assistance. The history of the current health problem is reviewed and recorded in chronologic order, including changes in symptoms over a period of time; circumstances that predisposed, precipitated, aggravated, prolonged, or alleviated the problem; and the patient's response to medical, self-prescribed, or drug therapy (for details, see Chap. 5).

Risk Factors

Determine whether the patient has any coronary artery disease risk factors, and assess the patient's perception and level of understanding of each. Determine if the patient is aware of how the risk factors affect the heart and whether he or she considers the risk factors to be a significant risk to health.

Identify any history of hypertension or hyperlipidemia. Determine when it was diagnosed, and refer to current medications, diet, and rest for how the hypertension or hyperlipidemia is being treated. Query the patient about a history of smoking, and identify the type of tobacco (e.g., cigarettes, cigars, pipe, chewing tobacco). Determine the amount smoked per day or per week, the age the patient began smoking, and the age the smoking habit increased, decreased, or ceased. Inquire whether the patient has attempted to quit smoking in the past and whether there is a current interest to stop.

Identify whether the patient is obese and how long this condition has existed. (Refer to ideal body weight under nutrition in the exchanging pattern to determine the number of pounds overweight). Investigate whether the obesity is being treated with exercise, diet, or medications. Explore whether the patient has a history of diabetes mellitus and, if so, at what age it was diagnosed. Determine if the diabetes currently is being treated with diet, pills, or insulin injections (refer to current medications and diet).

Explore whether the patient has a daily history of sedentary living or whether the patient's daily activities involve any type of exercise (also refer to the moving pattern). Identify major stressors in the patient's life. Determine if work or family interactions are highly stressful (also refer to recent stressful life events under the feeling pattern; see Chap. 5). Document any substance abuse such as *alcohol or cocaine* use in terms of the type, amount, and pattern of use.[34] Explore whether such substance abuse has interfered with the patient's job, marriage, or health, and whether the patient has been hospitalized for this problem. Identify the date and time the patient last used or ingested such substances.

Determine any family history of heart disease. Document the age, sex, and health status of living family members, including parents, siblings, children, and spouse. Record the age, sex, and cause of death of deceased family members. Determine any family history associated with the coronary artery risk factors discussed in the preceding paragraphs.

Previous Illnesses, Hospitalizations, and Surgeries

The history of previous illnesses, hospitalizations, and surgeries is explored. The history is assessed to elicit any information related to congenital abnormalities, heart enlargement, heart failure, heart murmurs acquired in infancy or adulthood, myocardial infarction, arthritis, rheumatic fever, or heart infection. Bacterial, viral, and fungal infections are identified, especially those associated with pneumonia, influenza, tuberculosis, mumps, chicken pox, venereal disease, acquired immunodeficiency syndrome, dental extractions, or invasive genitourinary manipulations (e.g., cystoscopy).

Determine any history of peripheral vascular disease, such as intermittent claudication (calf cramping or pain when walking that is relieved by rest) or varicosities. Identify any history of cerebrovascular disease (such as dizziness, fainting, or strokes) or lung, liver, gallbladder, gastrointestinal, or kidney disease.

Injuries and accidents are recorded, particularly those involving chest trauma, thrombophlebitis, or arterial problems. Any history of cardiovascular disease, cardiovascular surgery, or invasive cardiovascular tests should be elicited. Metabolic abnormalities, such as gout, hypothyroidism, or hyperthyroidism should be investigated.

Family History

Elicit information about any family history of congenital heart disease, cardiac disease, heart murmurs, premature or sudden death caused by cardiovascular disease, cerebrovascular disease, peripheral vascular disease, gout, rheumatic fever, respiratory or renal disease, nervous or mental conditions, epilepsy, arthritic conditions, hematologic abnormalities, sickle cell anemia, and thyroid disorders.

Additional Data

Elicit information to assess current medications, the patient's perceptions and knowledge of the illness, expectations of therapy, misconceptions, readiness to learn, orientation, and memory (see Chap. 5).

VALUING PATTERN

Spiritual and Cultural Practices and Concerns

Identify the patient's religious preference and any religious beliefs or practices that might affect how the patient will be treated during the hospitalization and influence compliance with the plan of care at home. Also assess the patient's cultural orientation, and identify any special family customs that are practiced when family members become ill. Explore whether there are any medical treatments the patient will not accept because of cultural beliefs. Investigate the patient's cultural beliefs surrounding cardiovascular illness.

RELATING PATTERN

Role Performance

Explore how this current illness will affect the patient's ability to return to his or her roles at work and home. Assess the patient's occupational role to determine physical workload, satisfactions, disappointments, degree of stress, and exposure to toxins, chemical, or fumes. Also evaluate the patient's sexual and social relationships and any patient concerns regarding how this current illness will alter such relationships (see Chap. 5).

FEELING PATTERN

Pain or Discomfort

When assessing pain or discomfort, gather data that are particularly pertinent to the cardiovascular system, keeping in mind the cardinal symptoms of chest pain, palpitations, and dyspnea.[1,5,13]

When information about *chest pain* is elicited from the patient, it is necessary to categorize the quality of the pain as crushing, squeezing, aching, heavy, tight, dull, burning, pleuritic, or associated with a feeling of indigestion.[24] The patient should be asked to describe the location of the pain by pointing exactly to where it occurs and to identify if the pain radiates or travels to other parts of the body. Ask the patient to describe the severity of the pain on a scale of 1 to 10 and any associated symptoms such as nausea, vomiting, diaphoresis, and shortness of breath. Also determine the onset of the pain, its duration, and any precipitating factors, such as the classic "4E" factors that produce angina pectoris (*i.e.,* exertion, eating, exposure to extreme temperatures, and excitement).

Palpitation is the term used when patients describe an unpleasant awareness of the heart beat. The phenomenon is commonly caused by changes in heart rate, rhythm, or hemodynamic states. Patients may use such terms as *stopping, jumping, skipping, pounding,* and *turning over* to describe their heart action. It is valuable to have the patient describe sensations of rhythm, rate, and forcefulness of the heart beat.

Ask the patient to describe the experience at the time of onset and termination of the episode as well as precipitating and terminating factors (*e.g.,* coughing, gagging, and vomiting). Because emotional states often can cause dysrhythmias, it is important to explore what the patient was doing at the onset of symptoms. Questions should be phrased to determine whether the patient experienced any associated congestion, cyanosis, dizziness, syncope, dyspnea, diaphoresis, or chest pain. Often it is helpful to ask relatives or others who witnessed the event to describe the details surrounding it.

Dyspnea is a symptom described by the patient as shortness of breath. The history should explore the time of onset, duration, and frequency of the attacks, along with any associated symptoms, such as dizziness, syncope, diaphoresis, nausea, or vomiting. Ask the patient to describe any factors that aggravate or precipitate the discomfort (*e.g.,* breathing, lying down, walking, or climbing steps) and any factors that alleviate it (*e.g.,* resting, walking, or sitting up).

Dyspnea is characterized according to type, degree, progression, and duration. Dyspnea may be associated with congestive heart failure or chronic lung disease or both. It is generally referred to as one of three types: dyspnea on exertion, orthopnea, or paroxysmal nocturnal dyspnea.

Exertional dyspnea, a common complaint, may be associated with both heart failure and lung disease. Common precipitating factors include climbing a hill or stairs, upper extremity exercise, and sexual intercourse. Exertional dyspnea, produced by either heart or lung disease, may also be accompanied by wheezes. It is important to determine the degree of activity in a normal day that is necessary to produce the symptom (*e.g.,* the number of flights of stairs climbed or blocks walked) and the length of time it has increased in severity.

Orthopnea is a form of dyspnea that occurs within a few minutes after the patient assumes the supine position and is relieved when the patient sits, stands, or is propped up. The patient often sleeps elevated on two or three pillows to improve breathing. Orthopnea is most frequently associated with congestive heart failure, but occasionally it is associated with severe lung disease.

Paroxysmal nocturnal dyspnea is specific for left ventricular failure. The patient characteristically has little difficulty going to sleep in the recumbent position but is awakened from sleep 1 to 2 hours later with severe shortness of breath. In contrast to orthopnea, paroxysmal nocturnal dyspnea is not relieved immediately when the patient assumes an upright position. It requires a number of minutes to subside.

Emotional Integrity States

Patients who enter the critical care unit find themselves in a foreign and technical environment filled with threatening equipment, tests, procedures, and professional jargon. Thus, assess the patient's level of anxiety and fear by noting any verbal complaints and physical manifestations of anxiety or fear. The patient's level of anxiety or fear must be taken into consideration when gathering physical data, because severe anxiety can increase blood pressure, heart rate, and cardiac output, and it can cause dysrhythmias, pain, and episodes of myocardial ischemia.[2,9,26] Because anxiety and fear levels fluctuate in critical care patients, continuous assessment of those problems is necessary on a day-to-day basis (see Chap. 5).

MOVING PATTERN

Activity

Assess the patient for any history of physical disability such as difficulty moving or walking, or limitations in movement. Query the patient regarding any pain, discomfort, or shortness of breath when performing normal daily activities. Determine whether there are any normal daily activities that the patient is no longer able to perform because of the current illness (*i.e.,* activity intolerance). Assess the patient's response to activities (*i.e.,* do heart rate and blood pressure return to preactivity levels within 3 minutes).

Explore any verbal complaints of fatigue or weakness. Fatigue is a subjective feeling that is commonly experienced by the elderly patient and is particularly associated with congestive heart failure. Investigate whether the patient verbalizes a lack of energy or a feeling of exhaustion, or whether he or she feels tired constantly during the day despite appropriate amounts of rest and sleep.

Determine if the patient is involved in any type of exercise program. Document what type of program, how many times per week the exercise is performed, and for how long. Investigate the amount of exercise involved with the patient's job and household or outside activities.

Assess the patient's usual sleep/rest pattern and any current manifestations of sleep pattern disturbance (see Chap. 5). Also evaluate the patient's involvement in leisure and social activities. Assess the patient's commitment to health maintenance (*i.e.,* does the patient routinely visit a physician and dentist for checkups) and whether the patient demonstrates an understanding of basic health practices.

PERCEIVING PATTERN

Perception of Self and Body Functioning

Discover how patients view their personality type (A or B). Assess how patients view themselves with cardiovascular disease and to what degree the illness has impacted on their self-esteem and body image and feelings of hopelessness or powerlessness (see Chap. 5).

CHOOSING PATTERN

Evaluate the patient's individual coping behaviors (see Chap. 5), such as exercising, listening to music, or practicing relaxation techniques.[17] Determine the patient's level of acceptance and adjustment toward the illness. Discover if the patient is denying the current health problem. Explore the patient's decision-making ability, compliance with past medical regimens, and willingness to comply with the future health care regimen (see Chap. 5). Evaluate the patient's willingness to incorporate healthy behaviors in daily activities. For example, do patients express a desire to stop smoking; lose weight; reduce cholesterol, saturated fats, and calories in their diet; begin an exercise program; or reduce stress in their lives?

EXCHANGING PATTERN

Cerebral Circulation

When assessing the cerebral circulation, determine if the patient reports any dizziness, falls, weakness, or numbness (see Chap. 5). Explore whether the patient describes any episodes of syncope. *Syncope,* which is caused by an inadequate oxygen supply to the brain, is a temporary loss of consciousness that may be due to heart blocks, severe sinus bradycardia or arrest, ventricular tachydysrhythmias, or cardiac asystole.[13] Determine the patient's Glasgow Coma Scale score (see Chap. 29).

Peripheral Circulation

Arterial Pulses

The arterial pulse is a propagated wave of arterial pressure caused by left ventricular contraction. The arterial pulses are palpated for rate, rhythm, character, contour, amplitude, and bilateral equality. Each carotid pulse is palpated separately, so that cerebral blood flow is not compromised. To avoid the carotid sinus at the bifurcation of the common carotid artery just below the mandible, palpate the carotid gently at the base of the neck. All peripheral pulses, which include the brachial, radial, femoral, popliteal, posterior tibial, and dorsalis pedis pulses, are assessed.

The radial pulse is the most frequently used peripheral pulse. It should be palpated for 30 seconds in the presence of a regular cardiac rhythm and for 1 minute if an irregular rhythm exists. If an irregularity exists, the apical and radial pulses should be checked for a deficit. An apical-radial deficit is present if the apical rate (counted by auscultation) exceeds the radial rate (counted by palpation). A deficit occurs in the presence of cardiac irregularities, such as premature extrasystoles, or with atrial fibrillation, when some cardiac contractions are not forceful enough to produce a palpable peripheral pulse. An Allen test is performed to assess radial and ulnar patency, particularly before an arterial catheter is placed in a radial artery (see Chap. 17).

When palpating the arterial pulse, the character of the arterial wall is assessed. Normally, it will feel soft and pliable to the touch, whereas with atherosclerotic changes, the wall will be resistant to compression and feels much like a hard rope.[13] The pulse is also evaluated for contour by lightly compressing the artery with a finger. Normally, it will be smooth and rounded, with a sharp upstroke and a more gradual downstroke. Large, bounding pulses may be encountered in patients during exercise or under such conditions as fear, hyperthyroidism, hypertension, or aortic regurgitation, or in the elderly patient with significant arteriosclerosis of the arterial wall.[13] In contrast, small, weak pulses are found in patients with decreased stroke volumes, such as those with left ventricular failure, cardiogenic shock, or severe cases of aortic stenosis. The amplitude of the arterial pulses is compared bilaterally and categorized into levels according to the following scale:[24]

0 = not palpable
1+ = faintly palpable (weak and thready)
2+ = palpable (normal)
3+ = bounding

Auscultation of the arteries normally reveals no sound. With occlusive arterial disease, however, a blowing sound called a *bruit* can be heard because the arteriosclerosis interferes with the normal blood flow through the artery. When auscultating the carotid arteries, ask patients to hold their breath so that any carotid bruits can be differentiated from respiratory sounds. The abdominal aorta and femoral arteries are also auscultated for the presence of bruits. Frequently, the abnormal arterial vibrations are detected not only as audible bruits but also as palpable thrills.

Arterial Blood Pressure

The arterial blood pressure is measured to evaluate the patient's systolic and diastolic blood pressures. The arterial blood pressure is an overall reflection of the patient's ventricular function. In the aorta and brachial arteries, normal blood pressure ranges between 110 mm Hg to 140 mm Hg systolic and 60 mm Hg to 90 mm Hg diastolic. Because wide variations of the normal blood pressure exist in the healthy adult and also vary with age, sex, and race, normal blood pressures can fall outside this given range. A blood pressure of 90/56 mm Hg may be hypotensive for one individual but normal for another. Thus, one should evaluate and treat trends in blood pressure rather than place any clinical significance on an isolated individual blood pressure reading.

Arterial blood pressure is measured by indirect or direct methods. Indirect blood pressure monitoring is accomplished by either manual or automated devices. The manual indirect blood pressure, obtained by use of a stethoscope and a sphygmomanometer, is the most convenient and noninvasive technique. It is necessary to listen carefully for more than just the appearance and disappearance of the arterial sounds below the blood pressure cuff. During the procedure, pay attention to the changes in sounds and be aware of using the equipment properly and doing the procedure correctly. The indirect blood pressure is usually measured with the patient sitting or lying down. In some cases, the pressure may change with body positioning, and in such a case, it should be recorded with the patient lying, sitting, and standing. If the pressure decreases severely when the patient shifts from the lying position to the sitting or standing position, this indicates postural hypotension; assess the patient for the cause (*e.g.*, dehydration, hemorrhage, medication).

On the initial evaluation, the patient's blood pressure is taken in both arms. Normally, there may be a 5 mm Hg to 10 mm Hg difference between the two arms. For an accurate blood pressure recording, patients should be comfortable, with their arms slightly flexed at the elbow and the brachial artery at heart level. The inflatable sphygmomanometer cuff is applied snugly over the brachial artery, with the lower cuff border approximately 2.5 cm above the antecubital crease. The width of the cuff should be about 40% of the circumference of the arm, and the length of the bladder should encircle half of the arm.

The cuff is inflated to about 30 mm Hg above the level where the radial pulse disappears. The diaphragm of the stethoscope is placed firmly over the brachial artery in the antecubital space, avoiding contact with the cuff or clothing. The cuff is slowly deflated about 3 mm Hg per heart beat. When a mercury sphygmomanometer is used, the readings are noted with the meniscus at the operator's eye level. Blood pressure in the arterial system varies with the cardiac cycle. As the pressure falls and intermittent blood flow returns, the examiner begins to hear Korotkoff sounds, which normally consist of five phases (Fig. 24–1), as discussed in the following paragraphs[4]:

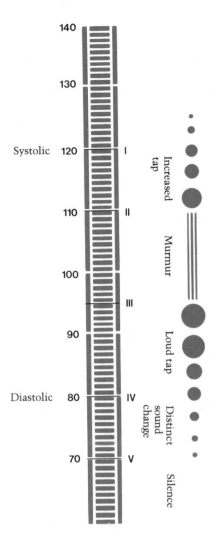

Figure 24–1
Korotkoff sounds.

- *Phase 1* is characterized by the appearance of faint, clear, tapping sounds that gradually increase in intensity. The sounds are produced by the quick distention of the collapsed artery walls as the pulse wave becomes greater than the cuff pressure. Blood suddenly enters the collapsed artery. The force of blood determines the intensity of the tap. Phase 1 represents the systolic pressure.
- *Phase 2* is marked by the beginning of a murmur sound. The murmur sound is thought to be caused by blood flow produced from the narrowed artery under the blood pressure cuff into a wider artery distal to the inflated cuff. This change of artery width creates eddy currents that, in turn, cause the blood and vessel walls to vibrate.
- *Phase 3* is identified by a crisper and more intensified tapping sound than that of phase 1. It is louder and higher pitched than the sound of phase 2. During phase 3, there is no audible murmur.
- *Phase 4* is marked by a distinct change in sound that is muffled, less intense, and lower pitched than the sounds of the other phases. Phase 4 represents the diastolic pressure.
- *Phase 5* is the point at which the sound disappears.

Phase 1 is identified as the systolic pressure, or the greatest pressure of blood against the vessel wall reached at the end of the rapid ventricular ejection phase. The cuff pressure should continue to be lowered until the muffled sound of phase 4 is heard that denotes the diastolic pressure. There is conflict, however, as to whether phase 5 (the point at which the sound disappears) is a more accurate indicator of diastolic pressure.[16] The diastolic pressure is the lowest pressure that occurs just before the next ventricular ejection. The cuff pressure is then completely released until no sounds are heard (phase 5). All three points, the onset of phase 1, 4, and 5, are recorded (*e.g.,* 120/80/70 mm Hg). In aortic regurgitation, the diastolic sound can continue until 0 mm Hg. In such a case, the systolic, muffled, and zero values are all recorded (*e.g.,* 140/100/0 mm Hg).

In some patients who are hypertensive, an auscultatory gap is present. It is a silent gap between the systolic and diastolic pressures. If the gap is not recognized, incorrect systolic and diastolic pressures may be recorded. When phase 1 is heard and phase 2 is absent, the silent period is called an *auscultatory gap.* The usual length of this gap is 20 mm Hg to 40 mm Hg. The complete recording of the blood pressure in this situation would be 210/110/100 mm Hg, with an auscultatory gap from 180 mm Hg to 140 mm Hg.

The difference between the systolic and diastolic readings is called the *pulse pressure;* it represents the range of pressure in the arteries, normally 30 mm Hg to 40 mm Hg. A widened pulse pressure of greater than 40 mm Hg may indicate ventricular enlargement due to coronary artery disease or aortic regurgitation. Conversely, a narrow pulse pressure of less than 30 mm Hg may indicate diminished cardiac output due to aortic stenosis or heart failure. The *mean arterial pressure* (MAP), in contrast, is the average pressure that exists in the aorta and its major branches during the cardiac cycle. The MAP is calculated using the following equation:

$$MAP = P_d + \tfrac{1}{3}(P_s - P_d),$$

where P_d is the diastolic pressure and P_s is the systolic pressure. If a patient had a blood pressure of 120/80 mm Hg, for example, the MAP is 93 mm Hg.

The examiner taking a blood pressure reading may encounter one or more problems. If the patient's arm is obese, a wider cuff should be used for an accurate measurement. In obese patients, arterial sounds often are higher than the simultaneous intraarterial pressure. A normal-sized cuff may give a false hypertensive reading, because the force applied by the cuff is lost in the subcutaneous layers of the patient's arm.

On occasion, the nurse may have difficulty hearing the blood pressure sounds. The most severe problem that causes an inaudible blood pressure is shock. Shock should be immediately recognized and treated. If the blood pressure cannot be heard by auscultation, then the systolic blood pressure can be evaluated by means of palpation. Because the diastolic pressure cannot be obtained by palpation, the pressure would be recorded as, for example, 90/p. Use of the ultrasound (Doppler) device in situations of low blood pressure will provide more accurate systolic measurements. Such devices are applied with conduction gel over the brachial artery and use amplified reflected ultrasound to determine the systolic pressure audibly.

In some clinical situations, the leg pulses must be evaluated and an indirect blood pressure in the lower extremities must be assessed. If necessary, the volume and timing of the radial and femoral pulses should be determined and a comparison of arm and leg pressures should be made, especially when coarctation of the aorta is suspected. Normally, an 18-cm to 20-cm blood pressure bladder and a wide cuff are used for the thigh recordings. The patient should lie on his or her abdomen, if possible. The compression bag of the blood pressure cuff should be placed over the posterior aspect of the patient's midthigh. The nurse then places the stethoscope in the popliteal fossa over the popliteal artery and uses the techniques for measuring arm pressure. If patients cannot lie on their abdomen, they should lie in the supine position. The patient should flex his or her knee enough to permit the stethoscope to be placed in the correct position in the popliteal fossa. Thigh recordings usually reveal a systolic pressure from 10 mm Hg to 40 mm Hg higher than that in the arm, but the diastolic pressure is approximately the same as that in the arm.

Indirect blood pressures may also be measured by noninvasive automated blood pressure monitors, which have become popular in critical care units. One type of automated monitor detects infrasound waves that occur with arterial wall motion. Another type of monitor detects arterial wall oscillations by means of a double air bladder cuff that is applied like a conventional cuff. The proximal bladder is inflated to occlude arterial blood flow and then deflated slowly. The distal bladder senses the point at which maximum arterial wall oscillations occur (recording the systolic pressure) and the point at which the oscillations disappear (recording the diastolic pressure).

Direct blood pressure monitoring is accomplished by inserting a catheter or needle into an artery and attaching the catheter to a plastic tubing filled with a heparinized saline solution. The tubing is connected to a transducer, which converts the mechanical energy exerted by the blood on the transducer membrane to electrical voltage or current that can be calibrated in millimeters of mercury. The electrical signal is then transmitted to an electronic recorder and an oscilloscope for continuous recording and display of the pressure waves (see Chap. 17).

In some situations, there are major discrepancies between the measurements obtained from indirect blood pressure auscultation and those obtained directly from the arterial line. Such discrepancies may occur because the direct and indirect methods measure two different phenomena.[16] Arterial line pressures reflect the normal physiologic changes occurring in the pressure pulse as it travels to the periphery, whereas auscultatory measurements are dependent on blood flow. Thus, if blood flow is diminished (*e.g.,* in patients with high peripheral vascular resistance, those in shock, or those who are hypothermic or edematous), arterial line monitoring should be employed because auscultatory methods, which are influenced by low flow states, may be unreliable. In such situations, discrepancies are likely to occur between the two methods, leaving the nurse to wonder which is the most accurate reflection of the true blood pressure. Thus, the routine of obtaining and comparing both direct arterial line and auscultatory blood pressure readings should be discouraged.[16] Therefore, when a high degree of accuracy is required, such as in low blood flow states or when titrating intravenous drugs, especially those used for hypertension or hypotension, arterial line monitoring is recommended. Arterial lines are also beneficial in providing continuous monitoring without disturbing the patient or interrupting sleep and can be used for frequent blood gas and serum electrolyte sampling.

Venous Pulse

The external (superficial) jugular veins and the internal (deep) jugular veins are inspected to assess venous pulse, venous pressure, right atrial pressure, and right ventricular function. They are located just above the clavicle and the sternocleidomastoid muscle. When evaluating the venous waveform, the right internal jugular vein generally is selected for observation.[4,8]

The contour of the jugular venous pulsations reflects pressure changes that occur during the cardiac cycle. Normally, they are seen when the patient is supine, however, if the patient's venous pressure is elevated, the head must be raised so that the top of the blood column in the veins can be observed. The two pulsations that are visible are the *a* wave and the *v* wave (Fig. 24–2A). The *a* wave is produced by right atrial contraction that occurs just before ventricular systole. When the nurse palpates the carotid pulse on the opposite side of the neck, the *a* wave is seen to precede the carotid

pulsation slightly. If the *a* wave is exaggerated, it indicates elevation of the right atrial pressure. The *a* wave disappears in the presence of atrial fibrillation because of the loss of coordinated atrial contractions. In atrial flutter, venous *a* waves may be seen to occur at a rapid rate.

The tricuspid valve then closes, and the atrium relaxes during the start of ventricular systole. As a result, right atrial pressure is reduced and can be observed by a fall in the jugular venous blood column height, the *x* descent (see Fig. 24–2A). The *v* wave is a consequence of continued atrial filling during the latter part of ventricular systole, when the tricuspid valve is closed. If the *v* wave is exaggerated, it suggests tricuspid insufficiency or right ventricular overloading. At the beginning of ventricular diastole, the tricuspid valve opens and rapidly empties blood into the right ventricle. As the right atrial pressure falls again, the *y* descent is formed. The *c* wave, not generally visible in the neck veins, is caused by a slightly backward deflection of the tricuspid valve during early ventricular systole.

Venous Pressure

The pressure exerted by the blood within the venous system, referred to as the *venous pressure*, reveals information about right-heart functioning. Venous blood flow is continuous rather than pulsatory.[12] The venous pressure in the arm ranges from 5 cm H_2O to 14 cm H_2O; in the inferior vena cava, it ranges from 6 cm H_2O to 8 cm H_2O.

When estimating venous pressure, the internal jugular veins are preferred for observation because the external jugular veins do not tend to transmit changes in pressure well.[8] Normally, the right atrium is the zero point at which venous pressure is measured. During physical examination, however, that landmark is difficult to determine. Instead, the sternal angle of Louis (located at the junction of the sternum with the second rib) is used, because it maintains a fairly constant position 5 cm above the right atrium for all positions between supine and 90°. When venous pressure is assessed at the bedside, the patient's head is elevated to a 45° angle. The patient's head is turned to the side so the neck veins can be observed tangentially. (The use of tangential lighting is helpful.) The venous pressure level is determined by finding the point above which the internal jugular vein collapses. The venous pressure is recorded using a ruler by measuring the vertical distance in centimeters, from the top of the distended jugular vein to the sternal angle. Normally, neck veins will become distended when the patient is lying down (Fig. 24–2B). When the patient is placed at a 45° angle, the neck veins should collapse or become visible only 1 cm or 2 cm above the clavicle. Pressures greater than 3 cm above the sternal angle are considered to be elevated (Fig. 24–2C).

The venous pulses are affected by respiration; deep inspiration lowers the pulsation level, whereas deep expiration increases the pulsation. Increased jugular venous pressure is observed during inspiration in congestive heart failure, cardiac tamponade, and restrictive cardiomyopathies. Both the right and the left jugular veins should be inspected. Pressure elevation on only one side may indicate a local abnormality.

When precise venous pressures are needed, such as when monitoring the critically ill patient, direct measurement of central venous pressure (CVP) is indicated. The CVP reflects right atrial pressure, which, in turn, reflects alterations in right

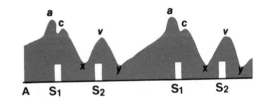

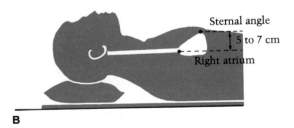

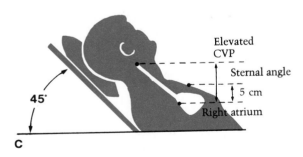

Figure 24–2

(*A*) Jugular venous pulsations, illustrating *a*, *v*, and *c* waves and the *x* and *y* descents. (*B*) Neck veins are normally distended when the patient is in the supine position. (*C*) Measurement of jugular venous pressure.

ventricular pressure but only secondarily reflects changes in the pulmonary venous pressure or left-sided heart pressures. After cannulating a vein with a catheter and threading the catheter into the vena cava, the CVP is then measured by a water manometer in centimeters of water or by a pressure transducer in millimeters of mercury (see Chap. 17). Mercury is 13.6 times heavier than water. To convert millimeters of mercury to centimeters of water, the number of millimeters of mercury is multiplied by 1.36 (*e.g.*, 8 mm Hg $\times$ 1.36 = 10.88 cm H_2O). The normal CVP ranges from 4 cm H_2O to 15 cm H_2O or 3 mm Hg to 11 mm Hg.[5] Elevated CVPs can indicate fluid overload or hypervolemia, right ventricular failure, cardiac tamponade, or pulmonary hypertension or embolism. Low CVPs may indicate hypovolemia.

Hepatojugular Reflex

The hepatojugular reflex is also evaluated, especially in patients who are suspected of having right ventricular failure but who have normal jugular venous pressures. It is demonstrated by positioning the patient at the point at which the highest venous pulsation can be visualized in the middle of the patient's neck. Firm pressure is placed over the right upper quadrant of the patient's abdomen for 30 to 40 seconds. An increase in jugular venous pressure of more than 1 cm during this period is abnormal. If the patient tenses the abdominal muscles or performs a Valsalva maneuver during the procedure, a false-positive response may be observed.

Tissue and Skin Integrity

Assess whether the patient's skin temperature is normal, warm, hot, moist, cool, or clammy. Evaluate the coloring and observe for pallor, jaundice, mottling, abnormal pigmentation, blanching, or cyanosis.

Cyanosis is divided into peripheral and central cyanosis.[8] *Peripheral*, or cold, *cyanosis* is more common than central cyanosis and is caused by reduced peripheral blood flow, allowing the peripheral tissues (capillaries) to extract increased amounts of oxygen, which results in reduced oxygen saturation of the *venous blood*. The arterial saturation of oxygen is normal. Because the tissues use more oxygen because of blood stasis, the arteriovenous oxygen difference is much greater than normal. Peripheral cyanosis occurs in dependent and peripheral regions of the body, such as the distal extremities and the face. The skin temperature of those areas is usually cold to the touch. Peripheral cyanosis can be caused by exposure to cold, excessive vasomotor stimulation, increased venous pressure (*e.g.*, right-sided heart failure), left-sided heart failure, and shock.

In contrast, *central*, or warm, *cyanosis* represents an excessive amount of unsaturated arterial hemoglobin. It is detectable when there is 5 g or more of unsaturated hemoglobin per 100 ml of blood. The arteriovenous oxygen difference is usually normal. Central cyanosis can affect not only the extremities and face but also the mucous membranes in the mouth, the earlobes, and skin of the trunk. The skin temperatures of those areas are usually warm or hot to the touch. Central cyanosis usually reflects cardiopulmonary disease and can occur in patients with right-to-left venous-arterial shunts, pulmonary edema, and chronic bronchitis.

Also assess the patient for capillary refill (see Chap. 5) and

for clubbing of the nail beds and splinter hemorrhages (see Chaps. 5 and 28). Evaluate the patient's skin turgor by pinching the skin over the elbow. If the patient is dehydrated, the skin will remain pinched, a phenomenon known as tenting.[6]

Fluid retention and edema, often documented by a sudden weight gain, frequently indicate cardiac failure. Because edema tends to accumulate in the dependent areas of the body, inspect the feet and ankles (especially for the ambulatory patient) as well as the sacrum, thighs, and abdomen (in the patient on bedrest).[32] Evaluate the degree of pitting edema by pressing the skin with the fingertips. The degree of pitting can be quantified and described by noting the depth of the finger indentation in the skin and the length of time necessary for it to disappear by using the following scale:[34]

```
0   =  none present
1+  =  0 to ¼ inch (trace); indentation disappears rapidly
2+  =  ¼ to ½ inch (moderate); indentation disappears in 10
       to 15 seconds
3+  =  ½ to 1 inch (deep); indentation disappears in 1 to 2
       minutes
4+  =  more than 1 inch (very deep); indentation present after
       5 minutes
```

When evaluating the skin and mucous membranes, assess the patient for *xanthelasmas,* a yellow lipid plaque on the eyelids and elbows that may be associated with hyperlipidemia and a predisposition to atherosclerosis. Also assess the patient for a whitish opaque ring surrounding the iris, which is called *arcus senilis* in the elderly patient. If this phenomenon occurs in the younger patient, it is termed *corneal arcus* and is an abnormal finding associated with hyperlipidemia. While assessing the mucous membranes of the eyes, also look for conjunctival petechiae associated with infective endocarditis and for pale conjunctiva, which may indicate anemia.[6,34]

Cardiovascular Circulation

Assessment of the cardiovascular circulation begins by inspecting the patient's chest. Note the gross appearance of the chest, looking for distortions of the thoracic cage, bulges, lack of symmetry, skin lesions, scars, abnormal pigmentation, and petechiae. The following topographic areas are defined (Fig. 24–3):

- The *primary aortic area,* located in the second intercostal space at the right sternal border (2ICS, RSB)
- The *pulmonic area,* located in the second intercostal space at the left sternal border (2ICS, LSB)
- The *secondary aortic area,* or Erb's point, located in the third intercostal space at the left sternal border (3ICS, LSB)
- The *tricuspid area,* located in the fifth intercostal space at the lower left sternal border (5ICS, LLSB). It is also called the *septal* or *right ventricular area.*
- The *mitral area,* located in the fifth left intercostal space at the midclavicular line (5ICS, MCL). The mitral area is sometimes referred to as the *apical* or *left ventricular area* or the point of maximal impulse.

Inspection and palpation should proceed in an orderly manner, from the primary aortic, pulmonic, secondary aortic, tricuspid, and mitral areas. First locate the apical impulse and

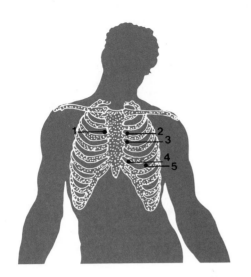

Figure 24–3
Topographic areas of the chest. (1) Aortic area, (2) pulmonic area, (3) Erb's point, (4) tricuspid area, and (5) mitral area.

then examine the rest of the precordium for other pulsations or thrills.

The apical impulse is caused by the forward and rightward rotation of the heart at the onset of ventricular systole that brings the apex of the heart closer to the chest wall. The apical impulse, also known as the *point of maximal impulse* is normally found near the fifth intercostal space, 7 cm to 9 cm from the midsternal line. It may, however, be absent in the normal person who is obese or muscular. Palpation is done by placing the hand over the anterior precordium and shifting the second and third fingers until the apical impulse is located. It is normally the size of a penny or a nickel. If the apical impulse is as large as a quarter and is displaced to the left, left ventricular enlargement is suspected. In addition to the location, the contour of the apical impulse is also assessed. The duration of the apical impulses' outward movement can be prolonged in patients with ventricular hypertrophy, producing a *sustained apical impulse.*

The nurse continues inspecting and palpating the precordium for other pulsations or thrills. Thrills are palpable vibratory sensations generally produced by the turbulent flow created by heart murmurs. (One palpates for thrills and listens for heart murmurs.) The flat portions of three fingers are used for systematic palpation of the precordium for thrills. Palpable pulsations in the second or third intercostal space to the left or right of the sternum are abnormal findings; they suggest pulmonary hypertension, aortic aneurysm, or systematic hypertension. Palpation of a right ventricular lift (a diffuse impulse causing the palpating hand to rise) along the left sternal edge is indicative of possible right ventricular hypertrophy, because the right ventricle normally does not produce a palpable pulsation. The nurse should also palpate for friction rubs. They also are located over the precordium and are caused by the two pericardial layers rubbing together (the visceral and parietal pericardium [and pleura]) (see Chap. 27).

The next step of cardiovascular assessment is precordial percussion to define the cardiac borders. It is often not done because it is not always reliable. Furthermore, the cardiac size is more accurately assessed by means of a chest radiograph. When percussion is used, the patient is placed in the supine position. The left border of cardiac dullness can be defined by percussing the third, fourth, and fifth left intercostal spaces, beginning over resonant lung tissue near the axilla and moving medially until relative cardiac dullness is heard. Those distances usually are around 4 cm, 7 cm, and 10 cm in each of the three intercostal spaces, respectively.

Heart Sounds and Murmurs

All heart sounds and murmurs are assessed thoroughly in cardiovascular patients. Several theories attempt to explain the generation of heart sounds. Heart sounds may arise from energy sources within the heart or the great vessels, or both, or they may be produced by the acceleration and deceleration of blood in the cardiac chambers. Cardiac sounds do occur after the closure of heart valves, however, and they are related to various pressure gradients within the heart and great vessels.

The point of maximum intensity in the chest wall may be closest to the points where the sounds are produced, although those sounds can often be heard in other areas. Many heart sounds may be heard best over the auscultatory areas (the places where vibratory sounds radiate) rather than over the anatomic locations (the places where the sounds originate) (see Fig. 24–3).

Auscultation must proceed systematically. The nurse should concentrate on one sound at a time rather than try to take in all the sounds at once. For example, identify the first heart sound and then the second heart sound. Count the heart rate. Determine whether the rhythm is regular or irregular. If it is irregular, is it "regularly irregular," or is it totally irregular? Listen to the heart sounds by "inching" the stethoscope over the precordium from the aortic auscultatory area to the pulmonic area to Erb's point and, finally, to the tricuspid and mitral areas. Individually identify the first and second heart sounds by appraising the intensity, pitch, splitting, and respiratory changes of each sound. Listen for extrasystolic sounds (such as ejection clicks) and for extradiastolic sounds (such as the third heart sound, the fourth heart sound, or a mitral-opening snap). Finally, listen for murmurs or rubs, and evaluate the timing, configuration, pitch, quality, intensity, location, and radiation.

The diaphragm of the stethoscope filters out low frequencies and should be used to identify high-pitched sounds, such as the first and second heart sounds and the murmurs of aortic and mitral insufficiency, friction rubs, and clicks. The bell of the stethoscope is then used to identify low-pitched sounds, such as the third and fourth heart sounds and the murmurs of aortic and mitral stenosis.

First Heart Sound

The first heart sound (S_1) is associated with closure of the tricuspid and mitral valve at the time when ventricular pressures exceed atrial pressures. It corresponds to the onset of ventricular contraction and therefore indicates the beginning of systole (Table 24–1). It is heard shortly after the QRS complex on electrocardiogram (ECG).

Right-sided events usually follow left-sided events because of the higher pressures found in the left heart. Accordingly, the mitral valve closes slightly before the tricuspid valve. The first heart sound is, therefore, split into two components—mitral (M_1) and tricuspid (T_1) (Fig. 24–4A). The louder M_1 is

Table 24–1
Heart Sounds

SOURCE	CAUSE	STETHOSCOPE	LOCATION
S_1 (M_1T_1)	Closure of tricuspid and mitral valves	Diaphragm	Entire precordium (apex)
S_2 (A_2P_2)	Closure of pulmonic and aortic valves	Diaphragm	A_2 heard at 2RICS; P_2 at 2LICS
S_3 Ventricular gallop	Rapid ventricular filling	Bell	Apex
S_4 Atrial gallop	Forceful atrial ejection into distended ventricle	Bell	Apex
Ejection clicks	Distention of great vessels or opening of deformed aortic or pulmonic valve	Diaphragm	2RICS, 2LICS, or apex
Midsystolic clicks	Prolapse of mitral valve leaflet	Diaphragm	Apex
Opening snaps	Abrupt recoil of stenotic mitral or tricuspid valve	Diaphragm	LLSB

followed immediately by T_1. The first heart sound can be differentiated from other heart sounds because it closely corresponds to each carotid pulsation. Palpation of the carotid artery during auscultation helps the nurse to identify S_1 which may be particularly difficult to distinguish from other heart sounds when the patient has a fast heart rate. The first heart sound is usually a lower-pitched and longer sound than the second heart sound. It is heard best with the diaphragm of the stethoscope over the entire precordium, although it is generally loudest at the apex. The sounds may become softer during inspiration because expansion of the lungs increases the distance between the heart and the chest wall. In the presence of atrial fibrillation, S_1 may assume a variable intensity. Exercise, excitement, or drugs, such as amyl nitrite, epinephrine, or atropine sulfate, intensify the sound. The splitting of S_1 into M_1T_1 may often be easy to hear in young children but difficult to hear in adults.

The first heart sound may be abnormally split and, therefore, audible in adults as a result of mechanical or electrical problems, causing the ventricles to contract at different times. In right bundle branch block, for example, right ventricular stimulation, tricuspid valve closure, and right ventricular contraction are delayed abnormally, producing a longer time period between M_1T_1. Mechanical delay problems, on the other hand, such as in mitral stenosis, may produce a reverse split of S_1 in which the tricuspid valve closes before the mitral valve (T_1M_1).

Second Heart Sound

The second heart sound (S_2) is associated with closure of the pulmonic and aortic valves when the pressures in the pulmonary artery and aorta exceed right and left ventricular pressures, respectively (see Table 24–1). The second heart sound corresponds with the onset of ventricular relaxation and indicates the beginning of ventricular diastole. Because of the higher pressure in the left side of the heart, left-sided events precede those on the right. The phenomenon is accentuated during inspiration, when increased venous return to the right heart occurs as a result of a more negative intrathoracic pressure. During inspiration, the right ventricle needs a

longer time to eject blood than does the left ventricle because of augmented right-sided filling volumes. That causes the pulmonic valve to close after the aortic valve, thereby producing a *physiologic split* of S_2. The split may also be a result of blood pooling in the inflated lung during inspiration that causes a reduced flow of blood into the left atrium and earlier aortic valve closure. Physiologic splitting of S_2, composed of a louder aortic component (A_2), followed by a softer pulmonic sound (P_2), is a normal event during inspiration in the adult (Fig. 24–4B). The disparity between right- and left-sided filling volumes is normally reversed during expiration, causing A_2 and P_2 to narrow and occur about the same time to produce a single sound. The physiologic split is often accentuated in people with thin chest walls or during exercise.

The second heart sound is generally a higher-pitched sound and of shorter duration than S_1. It is best heard with the diaphragm of the stethoscope and with the patient in either the sitting or the supine position. The aortic component (A_2) is loudest over the second to third right intercostal space; the pulmonic component is heard best over the second to third left intercostal space.

An abnormal variation in the splitting pattern of S_2 is known as a *fixed S_2 split*. In that phenomenon, the split of the two components is unaffected by respiration or blood volume changes, causing A_2P_2 to be heard with equal intensity during both inspiration and expiration. Fixed splitting suggests problems related to pulmonary stenosis or atrial septal defect.

Other pathophysiologic states may produce variations in the normal splitting pattern of S_2. *Paradoxic* or *reversed splitting* of S_2 occurs when left ventricular systole is delayed, causing the aortic valve closure to follow pulmonic valve closure instead of to precede it. As a result, the pulmonic sound occurs before the aortic sound during expiration (P_2A_2). (Normally, during expiration, the two components of S_2 fuse.) During inspiration, however, when pulmonic valve closure is normally delayed as a result of augmented right-sided filling, P_2 moves closer to the abnormally delayed A_2 to produce a fusion of the two components. That occurrence produces a reversal of the normal splitting pattern and may be caused by patent ductus arteriosus, left bundle branch block, aortic stenosis, severe left ventricular disease, or uncontrolled hypertension.

PITCH	RESPIRATIONS	POSITION	VARIATIONS
High	Softer on inspiration	Any position	Increased with excitement, exercise, amyl nitrite, epinephrine, atropine
High	Expiration produces fusion of A_2P_2; inspiration produces physiologic split	Sitting or supine	Increased in thin chest walls and with exercise
Low	Increased on inspiration	Supine or left lateral	Increased with exercise, fast heart rate, elevation of legs, and increased venous return
Low	Increased on forced inspiration	Supine or left semilateral	Same as for S_3
High		Sitting or supine	
High	Increased on expiration	Sitting or supine	
High		Any position	May be confused with S_3

LICS: left intercostal space; RICS: right intercostal space; LLSB: lower left sternal border.

Third Heart Sound

A normal physiologic third heart sound (S_3) is heard frequently in children and young adults, and it usually disappears completely if the patient stands or sits up. A pathologic S_3 is synonymous with such terms as *ventricular gallop* and *protodiastolic gallop*, and an early diastolic ventricular filling sound. The third heart sound is caused by the vibrations of a noncompliant ventricle that occur during the period of rapid ventricular filling in early diastole after closure of the aortic and pulmonic valves and the opening of the mitral and tricuspid valves (see Table 24–1).

The third heart sound is a low, faint sound that is heard best with the bell of the stethoscope applied lightly to the apex and with the patient in the left lateral or supine position. It occurs immediately after S_2. The rhythm and pattern of S_1, S_2, and S_3 somewhat resemble the sounds produced by saying Ken-tuc-ky (Fig. 24–4C).

The third heart sound is an abnormal sound found in the adult, and it is associated with any condition that increases early diastolic pressures or rapid ventricular filling. The third heart sound is generally an early sign of congestive heart failure. A left-sided S_3 may be produced by mitral regurgitation or left ventricular failure caused by myocardial ischemia or infarction, hypertension, or aortic valvular disease. A right-sided S_3 may be the result of right-heart failure, pulmonary embolism, or pulmonary hypertension. The third heart sound is accentuated by exercise, inspiration, elevation of the legs, or any other factor that increases the rate of blood flow to the heart. Conversely, the sound is diminished by phenomena that decrease venous return, such as assuming an upright posture or using venous tourniquets.

Fourth Heart Sound

The fourth heart sound (S_4) is often referred to as an *atrial gallop* or a *presystolic gallop*. Generally, it is an abnormal finding in the adult, but it may be heard normally in infants or small children and it may occasionally be heard in the athlete and in the "normal" person. It is a soft, low-pitched diastolic sound heard best with the patient in the supine or the left semilateral position, with the stethoscope bell placed at the apex (see Table 24–1). The fourth heart sound closely precedes S_1, so that the cadence of S_4, S_1, and S_2 is similar to the sound produced by saying Ten-nes-see (see Fig. 24–4D). The fourth heart sound may indicate increased resistance to ventricular filling; it is produced after atrial contraction as a result of the forceful ejection of blood into an overdistended ventricle. It is caused by any condition that impairs ventricular compliance, such as hypertensive cardiovascular disease, coronary artery disease, or aortic stenosis. The fourth heart sound becomes intensified and diminished by the same maneuvers that accentuate or diminish S_3.

Quadruple Rhythms

Quadruple rhythms refer to the cadence of the normal S_1 and S_2 plus S_3 and S_4. When the heart rate is slow, all four components may be heard separately, and they have been described as sounding like a cogwheel or a locomotive (see Fig. 24–4E).

In the presence of tachycardia or delayed atrioventricular conduction time, S_3 and S_4 may fuse together in middiastole to form a single sound that is almost as loud as S_1 and S_2. Instead of a quadruple rhythm, a triple rhythm is heard to produce what is known as a *summation gallop* (see Fig. 24–4F). That rhythm sounds much like a horse cantering on a dirt track.

Ejection Clicks

Ejection clicks (early systolic ejection clicks) are sounds that occur during the onset of early ventricular systole (see Table 24–1). The sound may be produced either by vibrations resulting from the sudden distention of the great vessels or by the movement of stiff and deformed valves. Ejection clicks are commonly heard in association with pulmonic or aortic stenosis and in pulmonary or systemic hypertension. They are sharp, high-pitched sounds heard immediately after S_1 (Fig. 24–5A) in the pulmonic or aortic auscultatory areas. They are best heard with the diaphragm of the stethoscope and with the patient in the sitting or supine position.

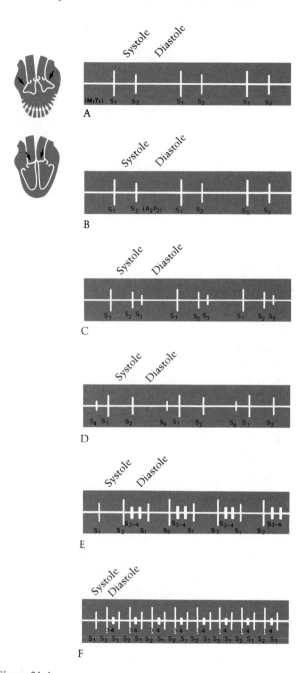

Figure 24–4

(*A*) First heart sound (S₁). (*B*) Second heart sound (S₂). (*C*) Third heart sound (S₃). (*D*) Fourth heart sound (S₄). (*E*) Quadruple rhythm. (*F*) Summation gallop.

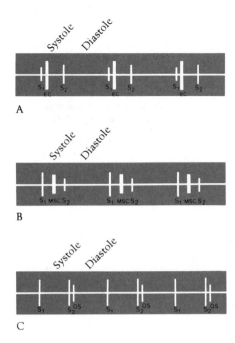

Figure 24–5

(*A*) Ejection click (EC). (*B*) Midsystolic click (MSC). (*C*) Opening snap (OS).

Opening Snaps

In the normal setting, the opening of the mitral and tricuspid valves is inaudible. In the presence of mitral and tricuspid stenosis, opening snaps may be heard as a result of the abrupt recoil or cessation of opening movement of the valve during ventricular diastole (see Table 24–1). The high-pitched, snapping sound is heard shortly after S₂ (Fig. 24–5C) with the diaphragm of the stethoscope over the mitral and tricuspid areas, and it is often followed by a diastolic rumbling murmur. The timing frequently overlaps with an S₃, making it difficult to distinguish.

Murmurs

During auscultatory assessment of the heart, each area must be checked carefully for the presence of murmurs. Murmurs are audible vibratory sounds. Several mechanisms are responsible for heart murmurs. The to-and-fro flow of blood over diseased heart valves creates turbulence and eddy currents, producing vibrations and resultant murmurs. Other conditions, such as increased blood flow (the flow murmur of hyperthyroidism or of fever), an abnormal communication between intracardiac chambers, or blood flow in a dilated great vessel may also generate vibrations and produce murmurs. In some people with normal heart valves, a functional murmur may be heard that is caused by normal hemodynamic factors rather than disease states. Murmurs are identified and assessed with regard to their timing, configuration, pitch, quality, location, radiation, and intensity.[6]

Timing in the Cardiac Cycle. Murmurs are classified according to their timing in the cardiac cycle as systolic, diastolic, or continuous. A systolic murmur begins with or after S₁ and ends at or before S₂. A diastolic murmur begins with or after

Midsystolic Clicks

Midsystolic clicks, also known as middle or late systolic sounds, are most commonly associated with prolapse of the mitral leaflet into the left atrium in patients with Barlow's syndrome. Midsystolic clicks often may be followed by a systolic murmur, representing mitral regurgitation (see Table 24–1). They are sharp, high-pitched sounds heard during the midportion of ventricular systole (Fig. 24–5B). They are best heard during expiration, with the diaphragm of the stethoscope placed at the apex and with the patient in the sitting or supine position.

S_2 and ends at or before S_1. A continuous murmur begins in systole and extends through S_2 into part or all of diastole.

Systolic murmurs may be subdivided further according to their time of onset and duration. An early systolic murmur begins with S_1 and ends about the middle of systole. A midsystolic ejection murmur begins in the middle of systole and ends before S_2. A late systolic murmur begins in the middle or late systole and ends with S_2. Likewise, diastolic murmurs may be subdivided into early, middle, and late diastolic murmurs.

Configuration.   Murmurs frequently have an identifiable configuration. A crescendo murmur is one that progressively increases in loudness. A decrescendo murmur progressively decreases in sound (such as the murmur of aortic regurgitation). A crescendo-decrescendo, or diamond-shaped murmur (such as the murmur of aortic stenosis), is one that peaks to intensity and then progressively decreases in sound. A holosystolic (pansystolic, sustained, or plateau) murmur is one that remains constant throughout systole.

Pitch and Quality.   Murmurs may be classified as high, medium, or low pitched. A high- or medium-pitched murmur, such as that in aortic regurgitation, is heard best with the diaphragm of the stethoscope; it sounds much like the forceful expiration of air through an open mouth. A low-pitched murmur, such as that in mitral stenosis, makes a rumbling noise, and it is best heard with the bell. Murmurs may be further identified by their quality of sound; they may be described as harsh, rumbling, musical, blowing, or whooping.

Intensity (Grading).   Murmurs are usually graded on a scale of one to six according to the intensity of sound. A grade I murmur is barely audible (it is sometimes thought that only the instructor can hear a grade I/VI murmur). A grade II murmur is faint but audible. A grade III murmur is moderately loud. A grade IV murmur is a loud murmur associated with a thrill. A grade V murmur is the loudest murmur heard that requires the use of a stethoscope. A grade VI murmur is so loud that it can be heard with the stethoscope slightly removed from the chest.

Location and Radiation.   Each murmur is generally heard the loudest at a specific area or location over the precordium (*e.g.*, the aortic, pulmonic, mitral, and tricuspid locations), as discussed earlier. Radiation of a murmur refers to the transmission of the sound to the sites other than the primary anatomic location of the murmur. Sound may be transmitted through the vascular wall, soft tissues, bone, and blood stream. The radiation of sound is dependent on the quality and pitch of the murmur, as well as on its anatomic proximity to adjacent structures. The direction of radiation gives important information about the origin of the murmur. If a valve leaks, for example, the murmur may be best heard in the direction of the leak rather than in the auscultatory region.

Types of Murmurs.   Using the characteristics of timing, configuration, quality, pitch, location, and radiation, murmurs associated with abnormalities of the atrioventricular and semilunar valves will be classified in the following paragraphs. (Aortic and mitral valvular disease, the most common

abnormalities found in the adult, are discussed in detail in Chap. 26).

Aortic Stenosis (Fig. 24–6A)
   Cause: Forward flow of blood from the left ventricle to the aorta through an obstructed aortic valve
   Timing: Systole
   Configuration: Crescendo-decrescendo
   Quality and pitch: Harsh and low pitched
   Location: Aortic auscultatory area
   Radiation: Into the neck or carotid vessels
Aortic Regurgitation (Fig. 24–6B)
   Cause: Backward flow of blood from the aorta to the left ventricle through an incompetent (leaky) aortic valve
   Timing: Diastole
   Configuration: Decrescendo
   Quality and pitch: Blowing and high pitched
   Location: Aortic auscultatory area
   Radiation: Left sternal border
Mitral Stenosis (Fig. 24–6C)
   Cause: Forward flow of blood from the left atrium to the left ventricle through an obstructed mitral valve
   Timing: Diastole
   Configuration: Crescendo-decrescendo
   Quality and pitch: Rumbling and low pitched
   Location: Apex
   Radiation: Usually none

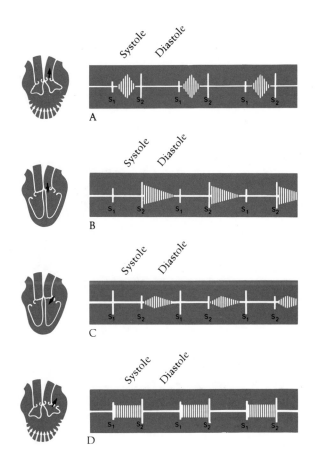

Figure 24–6
(*A*) Aortic stenosis. (*B*) Aortic regurgitation. (*C*) Mitral stenosis. (*D*) Mitral regurgitation.

Mitral Regurgitation (Fig. 24–6D)
   Cause: Backward flow of blood from the left ventricle to the left atrium through an incompetent mitral valve
   Timing: Systole
   Configuration: Holosystolic
   Quality and pitch: Blowing and high pitched
   Location: Apex
   Radiation: Left axillary line
Pulmonary Stenosis (Fig. 24–7A)
   Cause: Forward flow of blood from the right ventricle to the pulmonary artery through an obstructed pulmonic valve
   Timing: Systole
   Configuration: Crescendo-decrescendo
   Quality and pitch: Harsh and medium pitched
   Location: Pulmonary auscultatory area
   Radiation: Usually none
Pulmonary Regurgitation (Fig. 24–7B)
   Cause: Backward flow of blood from the pulmonary artery to the right ventricle through an incompetent pulmonic valve
   Timing: Diastole
   Configuration: Decrescendo, increases in intensity with inspiration
   Quality and pitch: Blowing and high (or low) pitched
   Location: Third and fourth left intercostal spaces
   Radiation: Usually none

Tricuspid Stenosis (Fig. 24–7C)
   Cause: Forward flow of blood from the right atrium to the right ventricle through an obstructed tricuspid valve
   Timing: Diastole
   Configuration: Crescendo-decrescendo
   Quality and pitch: Rumbling and low pitched
   Location: Lower left sternal border and tricuspid auscultatory area
   Radiation: Usually none
Tricuspid Regurgitation (see Fig. 24–7D)
   Cause: Backward flow of blood from the right ventricle to the right atrium through an incompetent tricuspid valve
   Timing: Systole
   Configuration: Holosystolic, increases in intensity with inspiration
   Quality and pitch: Blowing and high pitched
   Location: Tricuspid auscultatory area
   Radiation: Usually none
Pericardial Friction Rub (Fig. 24–8)
   Pericardial friction rubs sound similar to and may be confused with heart murmurs. Rubs are characterized by the following:
   Cause: Roughening and irritation of pericardial surface
   Timing: Systole, diastole, or both (may have systolic, early diastolic, and presystolic components)
   Quality and pitch: Usually loud, leathery, scratchy, and high pitched
   Location: Third intercostal space at left sternal border
   Radiation: Usually none

Oxygenation

Explore any complaints of cough, sputum production, or hemoptysis (associated with pulmonary embolism or pulmonary edema). Evaluate the patient's respiratory pattern, breath sounds, and blood gases (see Chap. 19).

Physical Regulation

Assess the patient lymph nodes, and evaluate the white blood cell count (see Chap. 5). Assess the patient's temperature. Rectal temperatures are the most accurate and range from 36.1°C (97°F) to 37.0°C (99.6°F) (where Fahrenheit = 1.8°C + 32 or Centigrade = °F − 32/1.8). In the past, it was believed that rectal temperatures should be avoided in cardiac patients,

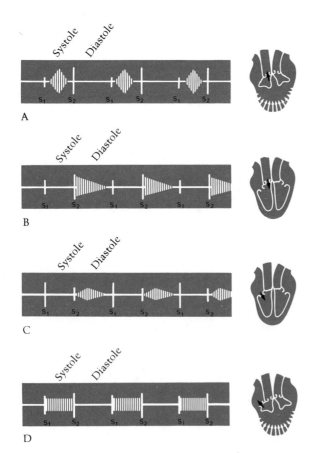

Figure 24–7

(A) Pulmonary stenosis. (B) Pulmonary regurgitation. (C) Tricuspid stenosis. (D) Tricuspid regurgitation.

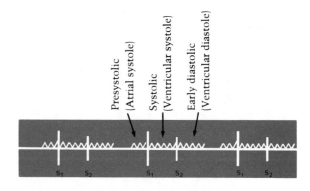

Figure 24–8

Pericardial friction rub.

especially those with acute myocardial infarction, because of the possibility of excessive vagal stimulation. Recent studies have found that obtaining rectal temperature in cardiac patients is not contraindicated; thus, it is not necessary to avoid this route when precise measurements are indicated.[18]

Nutrition

Eating Pattern

Assess the patient's nutritional pattern (see Chap. 5). Specifically evaluate the level of cholesterol, saturated fats, salt, and caffeinated beverages (*i.e.*, coffee, tea, or caffeinated sodas) consumed each day, including the amount of chocolate intake. Query the patient regarding any changes in appetite or drinking patterns.

Urinary Pattern

Assess the patient's urinary pattern (see Chap. 5). Specifically explore any problems with burning, frequency, hematuria, nocturia, or polyuria.

NONINVASIVE TECHNIQUES OF ASSESSMENT

Electrocardiogram

The standard ECG records the electrical activity of the heart from 12 different leads. It is a routine diagnostic procedure used to evaluate patients with possible cardiovascular disease, and it provides baseline data for comparison when a patient's condition changes. It can be used in the diagnosis and management of acute myocardial infarctions, myocardial contusions, dysrhythmias, conduction disturbances, atrial and ventricular hypertrophy, cardiac drug therapy, and electrolyte or metabolic disturbances.

It is important that the patient is provided privacy and is informed that the test will not hurt (*i.e.*, the purpose of the ECG is only to "listen" to the electricity generated by the heart; it does not send electricity into the patient.) (See Chap. 12 for assessment of electrical activity of the heart, dysrhythmias, and conduction disturbances.)

Atrial Electrogram

By placing electrodes on or near the atrium, an electrogram that emphasizes atrial depolarization is obtained. Atrial electrodes may be placed in the esophagus at the bedside or on the epicardium intraoperatively. Because atrial activity is clearly demonstrated, the atrial electrogram is useful in differentiating atrial from ventricular dysrhythmias (see Fig. 24–9).

Holter Monitor

Holter monitoring is a method used to obtain a continuous ECG over a period of time while the patient performs normal activities. The period of time is usually 24 hours. Electrodes are placed on the patient and are connected to a small battery-operated tape recorder. The patient carries the recorder and documents in a diary all activities (*e.g.*, meals, position changes, exercise, and stress), symptoms (*e.g.*, chest pain, palpitations,

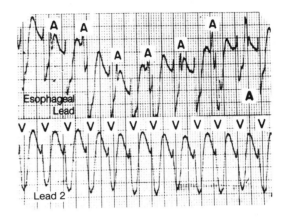

Figure 24–9
Unipolar esophageal recording during ventricular tachycardia that is displayed with simultaneous surface electrocardiogram lead 2. The esophageal recording shows atrioventricular dissociation, which cannot be recognized from the surface electrocardiogram. (Platia, E.V. Electrocardiography and cardiac arrhythmias. In E.V. Platia, *Management of Cardiac Arrhythmias*. Philadelphia: J.B. Lippincott, 1987.)

or dizziness), and the time of occurrence. The tape is then returned and electronically reviewed for abnormalities. Rhythm disturbances are then correlated to the patient's activities and symptoms to determine possible precipitating events and resulting effects. The results of Holter monitoring facilitate the diagnosis of intermittent dysrhythmias, the correlation of a dysrhythmia to the patient's symptoms, the quantification of diagnosed dysrhythmias, identification of potential or silent dysrhythmias, and the evaluation of response to treatment for dysrhythmias.[11]

Chest Radiograph

A chest radiograph is also a routine part of the cardiovascular examination. It is more reliable than percussion for determining the exact size and contour of the heart. Chest radiographs provide data about the size and location of the heart and cardiac chambers, the size of the great vessels, presence of calcium in the heart or coronary vessels, changes in the lung or other thoracic structures (*e.g.*, pulmonary congestion, pleural effusion, and so forth), and the location of invasive catheters and wires. The best films are taken with the patient standing or sitting erect. The patient is instructed to take a deep breath and hold it while the chest radiograph is taken. If a cardiac series can be obtained, that series includes posteroanterior, lateral, right anterior oblique, and left anterior oblique views. Frequently, however, the critical care patient must remain in bed, so the radiograph is usually obtained with a portable machine, using an anteroposterior view, which does not give as accurate an estimation of heart size.[27]

Echocardiogram

The echocardiogram is a safe and painless technique that uses ultrasound, a high sound frequency that is above the audible range, to diagnosis various cardiac disorders. It is used to identify abnormalities of valves (*e.g.*, mitral stenosis, mitral valve prolapse, and vegetations of bacterial endocarditis), cardiac tumors, pericardial effusions, mural and atrial thrombi,

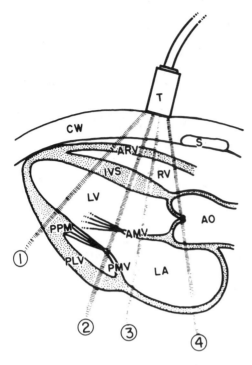

Figure 24–10

Cross section of the heart showing structures traversed by the ultrasonic beam transmitted by the echocardiogram's transducer (T). CW: chest wall; S: sternum; ARV: anterior right ventricular wall; RV: right ventricular cavity; LV: left ventricular cavity; IVS: intraventricular septum; AO: aortic root; LA: left atrium; AMV and PMV: anterior and posterior mitral valve leaflets; PPM: posterior papillary muscle; PLV: posterior left ventricular wall. (Greisler, H.P., Bahler, A.S., and Hayes, A.C. Noninvasive cardiovascular techniques. In J.I. Lamb and V. Carlson (eds.), *Handbook of Cardiovascular Nursing.* Philadelphia: J.B. Lippincott, 1986).

abnormal aortic size (*e.g.,* dilatation and aneurysm), aortic dissection, congenital cardiac lesions, hemodynamic alterations (*e.g.,* pulmonary hypertension), and abnormal ventricular size and wall movement (*e.g.,* due to infarctions, aneurysms, and cardiomyopathies).[10]

During the procedure, the patient is awake and is in a recumbent position. An ultrasound transducer is coated with conductive gel to assure airless skin contact and is placed on the patient's chest. The transducer emits a high-frequency sound wave in a short burst or pulse that is neither heard nor felt. When the ultrasound wave passes through the various tissues, a portion of the wave is reflected back. The amount of reflection varies with the degree of difference in the densities of the interfacing tissues. The transducer then receives the reflected sound waves or echoes. As the ultrasound echoes are received, they are amplified on an oscilloscope and recorded on paper.

Two recording techniques (unidirectional M mode and two-dimensional) are currently in use. Both techniques are employed routinely during an echocardiographic study. The M-mode echocardiogram provides an "ice-pick" like view of the heart (*i.e.,* it assesses those structures directly in line with the column of ultrasound from the transducer). Figures 24–10 and 24–11 illustrate M-mode echocardiography. It allows the physician to assess the motion of different cardiac structures as they change position and shape in relation to the transducer position during the cardiac cycle. M-mode echocardiography is most useful for measuring chamber size and for careful timing of cardiac motion (*e.g.,* detecting systolic anterior motion of the mitral valve in hypertrophic cardiomyopathy).

Two-dimensional echocardiography provides more information by assessing a "pie-slice" or 80° sector view of the heart.[30] Its advantage is that it displays the spatial orientation of cardiac structures to each other, as compared with an M-

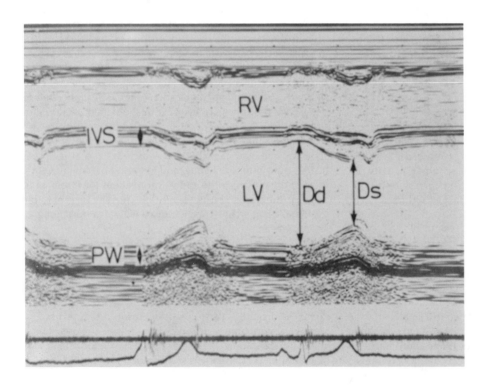

Figure 24–11

M-mode echocardiogram of normal left ventricle (transducer position 1). Dd: end-diastolic left ventricular internal dimension; Ds: end-systolic left ventricular internal dimension; PW: left ventricular posterior wall; RV: right ventricular cavity; LV: left ventricular cavity; IVS: intraventricular septum. (Modified from Tei, C., and Shaw, P.M. Echocardiography. In E.K. Chung, *Quick Reference to Cardiovascular Diseases* (2nd ed.) Philadelphia: J.B. Lippincott, 1983).

mode display.[30] An example of spatial orientation is both leaflets of the mitral valve viewed at one time. The recording displays correct anatomic configurations, as opposed to the wavy lines in the M-mode recording. Figures 24–12 and 24–13 illustrate two-dimensional echocardiography.

Doppler echocardiography records the direction and velocity of blood flow through the heart, across intracardiac shunts, and in the great vessels. In this type of echocardiography, the transducer continuously or in a short burst (pulse) transmits the ultrasound at a known frequency. The transducer then detects the reflected echoes and their frequency. Based on the Doppler principle, if the object that reflects the echoes is moving toward the transducer, it will cause an increase in frequency of the reflected sound waves, like the sound of a train moving toward you.[10] Just the opposite occurs if the object is moving away from the transducer. The results can be plotted out as a spectral recording on paper, or they may be displayed in color, called a color flow Doppler, which can be superimposed on a M-mode or two-dimensional echocardiogram. Doppler echocardiography may be used to assess intracardiac pressure gradients and ventricular function, and to calculate cardiac output.[25] It can be used for assessing regurgitant lesions and intracardiac shunts. Although usually noninvasive, a transducer may be placed in the esophagus to obtain high-resolution two-dimensional assessments of cardiac function (*e.g.*, during and after cardiac surgery).[25]

Phonocardiogram

The phonocardiogram records heart sounds and murmurs during the cardiac cycle. Its major value is in identifying the timing and configuration of heart sounds (*e.g.*, murmurs, splits, ejection sounds, and extra sounds) and their relation to each other.[27] The phonocardiogram assists in differentiating heart sounds and in estimating the severity of valvular diseases.

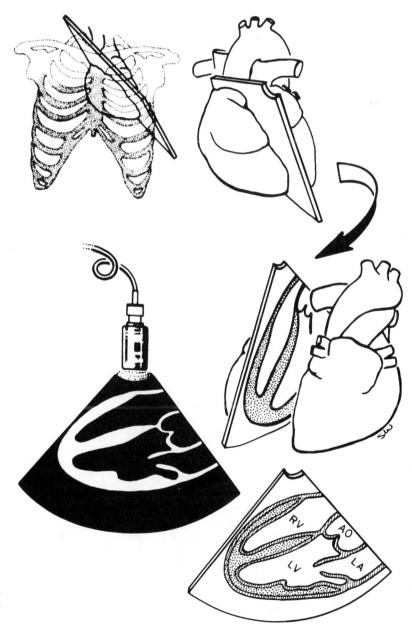

Figure 24–12

Derivation of the two-dimensional echocardiogram. Unlike the M-mode single-dimensional echocardiogram, which provides an "ice-pick" view, two-dimensional echocardiography simultaneously detects all cardiac structures lying within the plane of examination and displays the images on a video screen. (Fowles, R.E. Interpretation of Cardiac Catheterization. In A.K. Ream and R.P. Foghall (eds.), *Acute Cardiovascular Management: Anesthesia and Intensive Care.* Philadelphia: J.B. Lippincott, 1982).

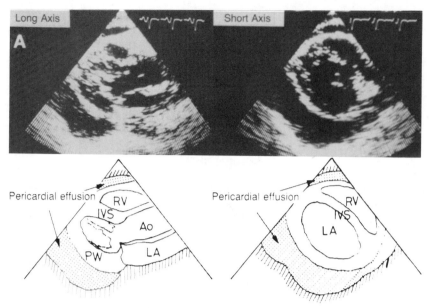

Figure 24–13

Two-dimensional echogram from a patient with massive pericardial effusion. (*A*) shows long-axis and short-axis two-dimensional echograms. In the long-axis view, massive pericardial effusion is observed behind the left ventricular posterior wall (PW), but it is not seen behind the left atrium (LA). In the short-axis view, the pericardial effusion is observed around the heart. RV: right ventricle; IVS: intraventricular septum; Ao: aorta root. (Modified from Tei, C., and Shaw, P.M. Echocardiography. In E.K. Chung, *Quick Reference to Cardiovascular Disease* (2nd ed.). Philadelphia: J.B. Lippincott, 1983).

The phonocardiogram is obtained with the patient in a comfortable position, such as for an ECG. The patient is awake during the procedure. The patient should be assured that there are no risks and that the procedure does not cause discomfort. Conduction gel is placed on the patient's chest, and microphones are placed over the heart in various positions. Some patients also have their carotid, apex, or venous pulse wave recorded. Heart sounds are amplified and recorded along with simultaneous ECG and pulse wave recordings.

These recordings are assessed for exact timing of multiple sounds and their relation to each other.

Graded Exercise Test

A stress, or graded exercise, test is an important noninvasive means of evaluating the cardiovascular function of patients with or without known heart disease. By increasing the oxygen demands of the heart with physical exertion, the heart's ability to increase the oxygen supply to the myocardium can be assessed. The heart's response is evaluated by monitoring changes in the patient's heart rate and rhythm, blood pressure, ECG waveform (especially the ST segment), and symptomatology. The graded exercise test is generally accomplished by the use of one of three types of procedures: the Master's double two-step test, bicycle ergometry, or a multistage treadmill test. The Master's test, the oldest of the techniques, involves having the patient walk up and down a set of 9-inch steps. Bicycle ergometry involves dynamic leg or arm exercises applied against a calibrated amount of resistance. The treadmill stress test, which is the most common, subjects the patient to walking on a motor-driven belt at increased stages of exercise. The exercise is increased every 2 or 3 minutes by adjusting the walking speed and the incline of the treadmill.

The nature of the test and procedure should be thoroughly explained to the patient. The patient should also be instructed to wear comfortable clothes and rubber-soled walking shoes, and not to eat, smoke, or drink alcohol for 3 to 4 hours before the test. If the patient is anxious, the test may be postponed until the source of the patient's fear is identified and reduced.

High levels of anxiety may alter the results of the test or produce serious complications during the procedure.

Before the graded exercise test is done, a complete history and physical examination must be completed. Patients who are found to have an acute myocardial infarction, new or changing chest pain, uncontrolled hypertension, uncontrolled heart failure, uncontrolled dysrhythmias, severe valvular disease, acute myocarditis or pericarditis, or other life-threatening cardiovascular disease are not candidates for stress testing.[28] Patients who are severely limited by noncardiac illnesses, such as those that produce neurologic, peripheral vascular, or musculoskeletal disease (*e.g.*, arthritis, acute hepatitis, pneumonia, amputation, or mental illness), also may not be eligible for stress testing.[5]

Electrocardiograms and blood pressure measurements are obtained at the onset, during each stage of exercise, and at least 5 to 10 minutes after the test. The testing is continued until the patient reaches a target heart rate (determined by sex and age) or until the subjective or objective endpoints are reached (Table 24–2). Although rare, the graded exercise test may cause serious complications, such as lethal dysrhythmias (*e.g.*, ventricular tachycardia, atrioventricular block, or asystole), acute myocardial infarction, cerebral vascular accident, or even sudden death. Emergency equipment, including a resuscitation mask, medications, intravenous fluids, and a defibrillator, should be at hand in the exercise laboratory. Physicians and other staff members should be trained in both basic and advanced life support.

A 1-mm depression of the ST segment is the most reliable indicator for a positive graded exercise test, indicating ischemia and coronary artery disease.[7] The ECG changes that occur in specific leads during the test indicate the exact area of the heart that is vulnerable. The specific level of exercise at which the symptoms appear indicate the patient's safe functional capacity. The graded exercise test can be used in diagnosing coronary artery disease, in the differential diagnosis of chest pain, in evaluating the efficacy of current therapy, in assessing the prognosis and severity of diagnosed coronary artery disease (*i.e.*, identifying those at high risk for an acute myocardial

Table 24–2
Endpoints for Graded Exercise Testing

SUBJECTIVE ENDPOINTS	OBJECTIVE ENDPOINTS
Severe chest pain	Target heart rate
Severe fatigue	ST-segment depression $\geq$ 1 mm
Dizziness, visual disturbances, or syncope	Onset of the following:
Loss of coordination	Supraventricular tachycardia
Leg pain	Frequent premature ventricular contractions
Patient asks to stop (even if none of the above is present)	Ventricular tachycardia
	Bradycardia
	Atrioventricular blocks
	Systolic blood pressure $\geq$ 220 mm Hg
	Fall in systolic blood pressure of $\geq$10 mm Hg after rising
	Rise in diastolic blood pressure
	Signs of circulatory insufficiency pallor, cold and clammy skin

infarction or sudden death), in objectively classifying the patient's functional ability and symptoms (*e.g.*, after cardiac surgery or acute myocardial infarction, or before beginning an exercise program), and in evaluating exercise-induced dysrhythmias.[28] False-positive tests can occur (*e.g.*, in patients with bundle branch blocks or ventricular hypertrophy, or those on digitalis), as can false-negative tests (*e.g.*, in patients on beta-adrenergic receptor blockers).[5,7,28]

Transesophageal Atrial Pacing

Transesophageal atrial pacing with stress echocardiography has been used recently as an alternative to the graded exercise test, especially in patients with noncardiac illnesses that interfere with their ability to exercise.[3] A pacing catheter is placed in the esophagus. A baseline ECG and echocardiogram are obtained. The patient is then atrially paced at increasing rates to 85% of the patient's maximum heart rate; an echocardiogram is obtained at each pacing stage. The ECG and echocardiogram results at rest and during pacing are compared, which will assist in the detection of significant coronary artery disease and abnormal ventricular wall motion. The procedure is discontinued at the same objective endpoints as the graded exercise test. The subjective endpoints include severe chest pain and intolerable pacing-induced discomfort (see Table 24–2).

Nuclear Cardiovascular Scans

Nuclear scans (*e.g.*, thallium scans, technetium-99 pyrophosphate scans, and multiple-gated acquisitions) have dramatically changed the manner in which cardiovascular illness is diagnosed and monitored. The tests are safe and cause little discomfort. Refer to Chapter 23 for information on lung imaging and radioactive fibrinogen scans, to Chapter 25 for myocardial imaging, and to Chapter 27 for blood-pool scans.

INVASIVE TECHNIQUES OF ASSESSMENT

Cardiac Catheterization

Cardiac catheterization is a procedure in which a catheter is placed in the heart in order to diagnose and quantify the se-

verity of coronary artery, valvular, and congenital heart disease and to evaluate ventricular dysfunction.[31] Generally, cardiac catheterization is an elective procedure and may be performed on an outpatient basis. It may be performed on an emergency basis to evaluate unstable angina that is potentially correctable by various interventions (*e.g.*, surgery, percutaneous transluminal coronary angioplasty, or thrombolytic agents). Before the catheterization, a complete history is taken, and a physical examination, 12-lead ECG, chest radiograph, and blood work (*e.g.*, hemoglobin, hematocrit, coagulation studies, and serum potassium level) are done. When indicated, a graded exercise test, phonocardiogram, and echocardiogram may be done.

Because most of the contrast media that are injected during the procedure contain iodine, it should be established whether the patient is allergic to iodine-containing substances (*e.g.*, shellfish). Antihistamines or steroids may then be administered before the study. The assessment of the peripheral pulses is documented in order to provide a baseline for postprocedural comparison. In some institutions, the best site for palpation of the distal peripheral pulses may be marked with ink or magic marker before the test.

An important precatheterization nursing responsibility is patient teaching. The physician generally is responsible for explaining the procedure to the patient and informing the patient about the indications, benefits, and risks of the study. The nurse should be present during the explanation and reinforce the information given by the physician, clarify the instructions, and discuss the patient's anxieties or concerns. Booklets and videotapes on cardiac catheterization are available and can assist with the implementation of the patient and family teaching plan.

The specific teaching plan for the patient and family is determined by the nurse's assessment of their present level of knowledge, emotional status, and desire for further information. The nurse also identifies available time and resources. All or part of the following information may be included in the plan. The patient is made familiar with the catheterization laboratory environment (*e.g.*, the room, the equipment, and the personnel) and with the requests that will be asked of the patient during the catheterization (*e.g.*, holding the breath, coughing, and deep breathing). The patient is told that the catheterization site, usually the groin or antecubital area, will be washed and shaved. The sensations that may occur during the catheterization (*e.g.*, the injection of the contrast medium which may cause the patient to feel flushed, hot, or nauseous) are discussed. These feelings dissipate within a minute. The patient may also experience a pressure sensation at the insertion site as the physician manipulates the catheter. Although sedated, the patient will be awake and should communicate any concerns to the staff. The patient also is instructed to report any chest pain or its equivalent immediately. The standard postcatheterization procedures, which include frequent vital signs and assessments, restriction of activity, application of a leg restraint, and administration of pain medication, are reviewed with the patient and family. The patient should not have anything to eat or drink for about 6 hours before the study. The patient and family are informed of the average length of the study (usually, 2 to 4 hours) and when they may expect to discuss the results with the physician.

Approximately one-half hour before the beginning of the procedure, the patient is brought to the catheterization laboratory. The laboratory is considered a sterile area and contains a hard x-ray table, a fluoroscope, cameras with recording capabilities, and a television screen. The table may be stationary and the cameras mounted on a large device that rotates over the table, or the camera may be stationary over the table and the table may rotate from side to side. The fluoroscopic image is displayed on the television screen to assist with monitoring of catheter movement. The videotaping allows for instant playback and review of the image. Emergency equipment and medications are readily available in the room. Personnel are in sterile garb and include the physician and two or three nurses or cardiopulmonary technicians.

The patient may be heparinized at the onset of the procedure to prevent thrombus formation. This may be reversed with protamine after completion of the test. Depending on the procedure, the patient's history, and the physician's preference, the catheter may be inserted directly into the right basilic vein and brachial artery or percutaneously into the femoral vein and artery after the site is anesthetized locally. During catheterization, the patient is monitored continuously.

Cardiac catheterization may include a right-heart study, a left-heart study, coronary angiography, ventriculography, or all those procedures. The heart studies involve measuring and recording intracardiac pressures and taking blood samples to determine oxygen saturation levels. Cardiac output also is determined. The studies identify myocardial dysfunction, inappropriate oxygen saturation differences (indicating intracardiac shunts), and pressure differences, called gradients, across the valves (indicating valvular disease).[27]

Right-heart catheterization is performed by advancing the catheter through the vein, right atrium, right ventricle, and pulmonary artery. Left-heart catheterization is usually performed by advancing the catheter retrograde through the artery and across the aortic valve. In certain conditions (*e.g.*, severe aortic stenosis or aortic valve prosthesis), it may also be done by transseptal entry from the right atrium. Blood samples and pressure measurements are taken from the various areas. Coronary angiography is done by injecting a contrast medium (that is opaque to x-rays) into the coronary arteries to visualize any narrowing or obstruction. The camera records serial pictures of the coronary artery as the contrast medium passes through it. Angiograms of the left and right coronary arteries are obtained and recorded from several different views.

A ventriculogram may also be done by injecting contrast dye into the ventricle to delineate areas of poor ventricular contractility (see Fig. 24–14). There are different types of altered contractility: hypokinesis, a reduction in wall movement; akinesis, an absence of wall movement; and dyskinesis, the paradoxic expansion of the ventricular wall with contraction (*e.g.*, due to aneurysm). A ventriculogram also helps to determine the degree of valvular incompetence or regurgitation by observing the amount of reflux into the atrium and to determine whether the valve is thickened, stenotic, or prolapsed. The stroke volume and ejection fraction are also determined. Cardiac output is determined by using the thermodilution, or Fick, method.

The common complications of cardiac catheterization in-

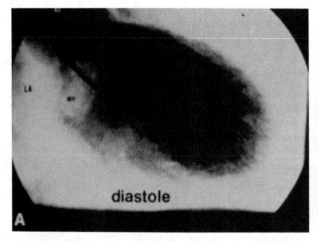
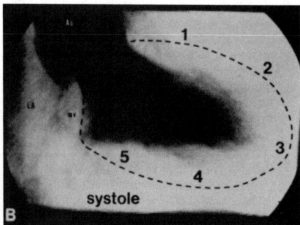

Figure 24–14

(*A* and *B*) Normal left ventriculogram, 30° right anterior oblique (RAO) projection. The diastolic ventricular outline is shown (*dashed line*) with the wall segments labeled as follows: (1) anterobasal, (2) anteroapical, (3) apical, (4) posteroapical, and (5) posterobasal. AO: aortic root; LA: left atrium; MV: mitral valve. (Fowles, R.E. Interpretation of Cardiac Catheterization. In A.K. Ream and R.P. Foghall (eds.), *Acute Cardiovascular Management: Anesthesia and Intensive Care*. Philadelphia: J.B. Lippincott, 1982).

clude vessel spasm and dysrhythmias.[31] Bradycardia and hypotension may develop as a result of injection of contrast medium or as a vasovagal response. The patient is instructed to cough, which helps to clear the contrast medium and return the blood pressure to normal. Atropine also may be administered. Ventricular tachycardia also may develop as a result of catheter manipulation. If sustained, the patient is treated with antidysrhythmic medications or immediate countershock. Infrequently, the procedure may also be associated with such serious complications as acute myocardial infarction, cerebrovascular accidents, dissection, perforation of the heart or great vessels, systemic or pulmonary embolism, pulmonary edema, and sudden death.[31] Other complications include nausea and vomiting, back pain, hypotension, hematoma, hemorrhage, infection, allergic reaction, including contrast medium–induced acute tubular necrosis, and arterial thrombosis.

After the procedure, the patient's vital signs are checked every 15 minutes for 1 to 2 hours and then in decreasing frequency. A small decrease in systolic blood pressure from baseline is not unexpected owing to volume depletion and effects of medications given during the procedure (*e.g.*, nitroglycerin and protamine). A slight increase in the heart rate may be seen for the same reasons. The distal pulse of the extremity used during the procedure is checked for pulsation, the extremity is checked for color, sensation, and temperature, and the insertion site is checked for bleeding or swelling. These assessments are compared with the previous and preprocedural assessments.

The patient is generally instructed to stay in bed and not to move or bend the extremity until the time specified by the physician (usually 6 to 8 hours). If the femoral arterial site was used, the head of bed is not elevated for the first few hours and the patient is instructed to log roll. Frequently, a soft restraint is applied to the leg as a gentle reminder. If the brachial site was used, an ace bandage is applied. Because eating a regular meal is difficult, a tray of finger foods (*e.g.*, a sandwich and fresh fruit) is usually obtained. The patient is also encouraged to drink plenty of fluids to counteract the significant diuresis caused by the contrast medium. Intravenous fluid replacement may also be ordered. Because of the diuretic effect of the contrast medium, urine output is usually increased initially. If the patient has not voided within 4 hours of the procedure, the bladder is assessed and bladder catheterization is considered. If the patient is being discharged, instructions are given on actions to take if chest pain, infection, or bleeding develops.

Electrophysiology Study

Electrophysiology study is an invasive procedure that uses intracardiac pacing and electrocardiography. It assists in the diagnosis and differentiation of potentially lethal or symptomatic tachydysrhythmias and conduction abnormalities, the determination of the most appropriate therapy (medical and surgical), and the assessment of the efficacy of therapy.[19,22] Patients with a pre-excitation syndrome (*e.g.*, Wolff-Parkinson-White syndrome), those who have survived a sudden death event, those who have had an unexplained syncopal episode, or those who have had recurrent tachycardias are usually referred for electrophysiology study.[33] To diagnose the dysrhythmia accurately and to assess the effectiveness of therapy, the clinical dysrhythmia that occurred must be documented

and reproduced by electrophysiology study. Sustained ventricular tachycardia can be reproduced in over 90% of the patients with documented clinical ventricular tachycardia.[33] However, some patients (up to 35%) will not have an inducible sustained dysrhythmia.[33]

Electrophysiology study involves cardiac catheterization, so the preparation of the patient is similar. One of the major differences is that induction of a dysrhythmia is a planned and controlled event. This may heighten the patient's level of anxiety and therefore warrant more careful assessment and support. Inducing a potentially lethal dysrhythmia, especially in patients who have survived a sudden death event, often causes a high level of anxiety that can interfere with the patients' ability to learn and to participate in decisions about their care.[20] Although most patients are not sedated before the study because of the possible altered electrophysiologic effects, some patients may require psychotherapy and psychopharmacologic agents.[21] For the initial electrophysiology study, all antidysrhythmic medications are discontinued at least 4 half-lives before the study to prevent them from affecting the results. During this time, patients usually are placed on a cardiac monitor. After surgical or medical therapy has been determined and implemented, the patient will return for another electrophysiology study. The efficacy of the therapy is determined by the inability to induce the same causative dysrhythmia. The patient may undergo the electrophysiology study several times before satisfactory control of the dysrhythmia is achieved, which further emphasizes the need for emotional support.

Catheters with pacing and recording capabilities are inserted percutaneously through the femoral or brachial vein and, under fluoroscopy, are positioned in the right atrium near the sinoatrial node, in the coronary sinus (to access the left atrium), across the tricuspid valve in the right ventricular septum (near the atrioventricular node and His bundle), and in the right ventricular apex. Arterial catheterization is done if left ventricular recordings are needed. The exact number and site of catheters used depends on the information needed.[19] The catheters are connected to a multichannel recorder that simultaneously displays and records at least three surface ECG leads and four intracardiac ECG leads. With the catheters in place, a baseline intracardiac ECG is obtained, producing atrial (A), His bundle (H), and ventricular (V) deflections. The ECG is analyzed to determine P-A interval (intra-atrial conduction), A-H interval (atrioventricular nodal conduction), and H-V interval (His bundle conduction). The catheter may be programmed to pace at incremental rates to evaluate sinus node function and atrioventricular conduction. The catheter may also be programmed to deliver premature paced stimuli (identified as S_2, S_3, and so forth), to initiate and define the mechanism of a tachydysrhythmia, and to measure the refractory periods.[33] The induced dysrhythmia may terminate spontaneously. If conversion does not occur, the physician may terminate it by programming another series of properly timed stimuli, rapid pacing, or administering medications. If hemodynamically indicated, cardiopulmonary resuscitation and countershock may be initiated. Patients have a 25% chance of requiring defibrillation.[23]

Analysis of the intracardiac ECG reveals the sequence and timing of electrical activation. For example, if the impulse originates below the common bundle, the A deflection may be absent or follow the V deflection, and the H-V interval will be less than normal. A prolonged PR interval on a surface ECG indicates a block between the atria and ventricles, whereas a prolonged H-V interval on an intracardiac ECG indicates that the block is located in the His-Purkinje system.

In a tachydysrhythmia, the site of earliest activation is the place of its origin. Locating the specific site of origin for the ectopic focus that initiates the dysrhythmia is called *ventricular mapping*. It may be done during electrophysiology study by using multipolar endocardial catheters. Endocardial mapping may also be done intraoperatively. Electrocardiographic recordings are taken from several endocardial sites and then analyzed for similarity in morphology to the clinical dysrhythmia and identification of the site of earliest activation (Fig. 24–15). If indicated, the specific site of ectopic focus may be rendered inoperative by extreme cooling (cryoablation), electrical ablation, or surgical resection.[19,23,29]

When the test is finished, the catheters are usually removed. However, if the patient is to undergo a series of electrophysiologic studies within a short period of time, the catheters may be left in place for a week or longer.[23] The postprocedural care depends on whether arterial catheterization occurred and is similar to postcardiac catheterization care.

Relatively few contraindications are associated with electrophysiologic study, other than the potential for difficulty in terminating the induced dysrhythmia (*e.g.*, altered electrolytes, acute myocardial infarction).[33] Most of the complications are related to the catheterization procedure.[33] Active discharge planning can begin on admission and should include assessment of the patient's and family's knowledge of the dysrhythmia and associated symptoms, risk factors, risk-factor modification, electrophysiologic study, when and how to seek medical assistance, and cardiopulmonary resuscitation.

Endomyocardial Biopsy

An endomyocardial biopsy is an invasive procedure in which a small amount of tissue is extracted from the right or left ventricle. It is most often indicated to identify cardiac transplant rejection.[5] It also may be used to evaluate myocarditis and adriamycin-induced cardiomyopathy, and to differentiate restrictive from constrictive cardiac disease.[5] Because endomyocardial biopsy involves cardiac catheterization, nursing care before and after the procedure is similar to that for catheterization. The care after the procedure is also determined by whether arterial catheterization occurred or not. The procedure usually is performed in a cardiac catheterization laboratory.

A bioptome, a catheter with a jaw-like tip that is controlled

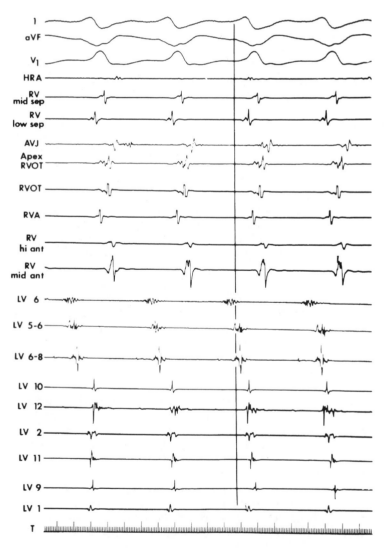

Figure 24–15

Catheter endocardial map of ventricular tachycardia. From top to bottom are surface electrocardiographic leads and intracardiac electrograms. HRA: high right atrium; RV: right ventricle; sep: septum; AVJ: atrioventricular junction; RVOT: right ventricular outflow tract; RVA: right ventricular apex; hi ant: high anterior; mid ant: mid anterior; LV: left ventricle; T: time (at 10-msec intervals). The numbers represent different electrode sites on the left ventricle. The *solid line* marks the onset of the QRS complex. The site of origin is site 6, from which presystolic activity is recorded during ventricular tachycardia. (Modified from Marchlinski, F.E., and Josephson, M.E. Surgical Treatment of Ventricular Tachyarrhythmias. In E.V. Platia, *Management of Cardiac Arrhythmias.* Philadelphia: J.B. Lippincott, 1987).

by a forceps-like handle, is introduced percutaneously into the femoral or internal jugular vein. If samples are needed from the left ventricle, the femoral artery is used. The bioptome is advanced under fluoroscopy into the right ventricle. Echocardiography may also be used to confirm proper positioning of the bioptome. The bioptome takes a 1-mm to 3-mm tissue sample from the ventricular septum. Three to five samples may be obtained during the procedure.

Complications due to endomyocardial biopsy (*e.g.*, cardiac perforation, hemopericardium, and cardiac tamponade) are rare. The nursing implications include frequent monitoring for the development of chest pain, hypotension, pulsus paradoxsus, and an increase in jugular venous distention. New onset of mitral or tricuspid murmur could indicate inadvertent biopsy of the papillary muscle or chordae tendineae. Other complications (*e.g.*, embolization, arterial thrombosis, hematoma, and dysrhythmias) are due to the catheterization.

NURSING DIAGNOSES

The nursing diagnoses are derived from the specific areas of patient assessment and specific diagnostic tests. Common cardiovascular nursing diagnoses are as follows:

1. Alteration in comfort related to the following:
   A. Chest pain (caused by angina, extension of infarction, or pericarditis), thromboembolism, Dressler's syndrome, or cardiac surgery
2. Decreased cardiac output related to the following:
   A. Electrical factors (rate, rhythm, or conduction)
   B. Mechanical factors (preload, afterload, or inotropic state of the heart)
   C. Structural factors (interventricular septal rupture, papillary muscle dysfunction, or ventricular aneurysm)
3. Anxiety related to the following:
   A. Acute illness
   B. Fear of death
   C. Critical care unit environment and monitoring equipment
   D. Pain
   E. Difficulty in communication
   F. Helplessness
4. High risk for noncompliance related to inadequate knowledge about acute illness and discharge regimen for health maintenance

SUMMARY

Cardiovascular assessment is an ongoing process. Critical care nurses must continue to increase their knowledge and skills in order to formulate the appropriate nursing diagnoses, which lead to high-level performance in using the remaining steps of the nursing process.

REFERENCES

1. American Nurses Association Division on Medical Surgical Nursing Practice and American Heart Association Council on Cardiovascular Nursing. *Standards of Cardiovascular Nursing Practice.* Kansas City, MO: American Nurses Association, 1981.
2. Barry, J., Selwyn, A. P., and Nabel, E. G. Frequency of ST-segment depression produced by mental stress in stable angina pectoris from coronary artery disease. *Am. J. Cardiol.* 61:989, 1988.
3. Barta, K. J. Transesophageal atrial pacing with stress echocardiography. *Focus Crit. Care Nurs.* 16:1, 1989.
4. Bates, B. *Guide to Physical Examination* (3rd ed.). Philadelphia: J. B. Lippincott, 1983.
5. Braunwald, E. *Heart Disease* (3rd ed.). Philadelphia: W. B. Saunders, 1988.
6. Dennison, R. Cardiopulmonary assessment: How to do it better in 15 easy steps. *Nursing 86* 16(4):34, 1986.
7. Detrano, R., Gianrossi, R., and Froelicher, V. Diagnostic accuracy of the exercise electrocardiogram: A meta-analysis of 22 years of research. *Prog. Cardiovasc. Dis.* 32:3, 1989.
8. DiBianco, J. B. Cardiovascular Assessment. In C. E. Guzzetta and B. M. Dossey, *Cardiovascular Nursing.* St. Louis: C. V. Mosby, 1984.
9. Dossey, B. M., Keegan, L., Guzzetta, C. E., *et al. Holistic Nursing: A Handbook for Practice.* Rockville, MD: Aspen, 1988.
10. Feigenbaum, H. *Echocardiography* (4th ed.). Philadelphia: Lea & Febiger, 1986.
11. Greenspoon, A. J. Detection of Potential Serious Cardiac Arrhythmias in Coronary Artery Disease: Use of the Signal-Averages Electrocardiogram. In D. David, E. Michelson, and L. Dreifus (eds.), *Ambulatory Monitoring of the Cardiac Patient.* Philadelphia: F. A. Davis, 1988.
12. Guzzetta, C. E. Physiology of the Heart and Circulation. In C. E. Guzzetta and B. M. Dossey, *Cardiovascular Nursing.* St. Louis: C. V. Mosby, 1984.
13. Guzzetta, C. E. Cardiovascular Assessment. In M. Kinney and D. Packa (eds.). *Comprehensive Cardiac Care* (7th ed.). St. Louis: C. V. Mosby, 1991.
14. Guzzetta, C. E., Bunton, S. D., Prinkey, L. A., *et al.* Unitary person assessment tool: Easing problems with nursing diagnosis. *Focus Crit. Care.* 15:12, 1988.
15. Guzzetta, C. E., Bunton, S. D., Prinkey, L. A., *et al. Clinical Assessment Tools for Use with Nursing Diagnoses.* St. Louis: C. V. Mosby, 1989.
16. Hanneman, E. A., and Henneman, P. L. Intricacies of blood pressure measurement: Reexamining the rituals. *Heart Lung* 18:263, 1989.
17. Jollings, C. Nursing interventions with the family of the critically ill patient. *Crit. Care Nurs.* 1:27, 1981.
18. Kirchhoff, K. T. An examination of the physiologic basis for "coronary precautions." *Heart Lung* 10:874, 1981.
19. Kowey, P., and Friehling, T. Uses and limitations of electrophysiology studies for the selection of antiarrhythmic therapy. *Pace* 9:231, 1986.
20. Main, C. Nursing care of the dysrhythmia patient hospitalized for electrophysiology testing. *J. Cardiovasc. Nurs.* 3:1, 1988.
21. Menza, M., Stern, T., and Cassem, N. Treatment of anxiety associated with electrophysiologic studies. *Heart Lung* 17:5, 1988.
22. Mercer, M. The electrophysiology study: A nursing concern. *Crit. Care Nurs.* 7:2, 1987.
23. Miccolo, M. Management of patients with sudden cardiac death caused by ventricular dysrhythmias. *J. Cardiovasc. Nurs.* 3:1, 1988.
24. Quinless, F. Assessing the client with acute cardiovascular dysfunction. *Topics Clin. Nurs.* 8(1):45, 1986.
25. Reynolds, T. Noninvasive hemodynamic assessment of intracardiac pressures and assessment of ventricular function with cardiac doppler. *Crit. Care Nurs. Clin.* 1:3, 1989.
26. Rozanski, A., Bairey, C. N., Krantz, D. S., *et al.* Mental stress and the induction of silent myocardial ischemia in patients with coronary artery disease. *N. Engl. J. Med.* 319:1005, 1988.
27. Sanderson, R. Diagnostic Techniques. In R. Sanderson and C. Kurth, *The Cardiac Patient* (2nd ed.). Philadelphia: W. B. Saunders, 1983.
28. Schlant, R., Blomqvist, C., Brandenburg, R., *et al.* Guidelines for exercise testing. A report of the American College of Cardiology.

American Heart Association Task Force on Assessment of Cardiovascular Procedures. (Subcommittee on exercise). *J. Am. Coll. Cardiol.* 8:725, 1986.

29. Stevens, L., Redd, R., and Buchingham, T. Emergency catheter ablation of refractory ventricular tachycardia. *Crit. Care Nurs.* 9:5, 1989.

30. Swanson-Kauffman, K. Echocardiography: An access route to the heart. *Crit. Care Nurs.* 1:5, 1981.

31. Tilkian, A., and Daily, E. Cardiac Catheterization and Coronary Arteriography. In A. Tilkian and E. Daily (eds.), *Cardiovascular Procedures: Diagnostic Techniques and Therapeutic Procedures.* St. Louis: C. V. Mosby, 1986.

32. Underhill, S. L., Woods, S. L., Sivarajan-Froelicher, E. S., *et al. Cardiac Nursing* (2nd ed.). Philadelphia: J. B. Lippincott, 1989.

33. Wiener, I. Electrophysiologic Studies. In A. Tilkian and E. Daily (eds.), *Cardiovascular Procedures: Diagnostic Techniques and Therapeutic Procedures.* St. Louis: C. V. Mosby, 1986.

34. Yacone, L. A. Cardiac assessment: What to do, how to do it. *R.N.* 43:May, 1987.

25

Acute Myocardial Infarction

Barbara Riegel   *Barbara Montgomery Dossey*

HEALING INTO PAIN

Freedom from most pain or relief of pain is possible. The worst of pain can be shifted in many ways. Even though the physical body can experience various levels of pain, the mind's fear of the pain is often more intense.

Your presence and how you give pain medication can be a healing moment. When giving pain medication, be aware of the words you use. Using phrases such as "The pain medication is in your body and is working" helps patients evoke their own endorphin supply and helps them relax. It is also important to let the patient know the moment that you are giving the medication in order to enhance their own inner resources. It is so easy to give a medication intravenously without the patient knowing that they are receiving it. If the patient's eyes are closed, this is even more reason to tell them they are receiving the medication. Learn to give medication while simultaneously teaching the patient relaxation and imagery exercises, as explored in Chapter 3.

Different levels of physical and emotional pain emerge around and during illness. With a calm and healing tone, suggest that the patient allow himself to be open to pain. This often allows the patient to feel a deep level of trust in you that may enable him to share his worries or fears without holding back. The worries and fears are often linked with the pain.

Sometimes when you are caring for the patient in pain, you might feel frustrated or guilty because the pain remains in spite of the potent drugs or other modalities that you deliver. You do not have to take someone's pain, anger, or fear away to be therapeutic. Your physical presence is very powerful, and giving the medication, doing accupressure or a gentle massage and touch, and then doing nothing can help the person's pain to become manageable. Often a patient will ask what will happen next. Be honest and say "I don't know." Encourage this person to trust the "I don't know," so that his inner wisdom may come forward with answers.

As you guide the person in pain, suggest that he or she be with the pain that emerges in the body or thoughts. Each patient will enter pain in a way that is available to them, and each will know how far to go in exploring the pain.

Let pain images and the different felt experiences emerge. Common expressions of pain include "The pain attaches," "It has a grip on me and takes my breath away," "Its pulsation is loud and deafening," "It's violent and unrelenting." These ideas or words create active images that, when stayed with long enough, may allow either positive or negative symbolic images to come forth for patients dealing with the pain. Negative imagery indeed must be shifted for the patient to be open to the pain, as discussed in Chapter 3.

Continued gentle exploration of opening and releasing into the pain can cause it to begin to float and diminish. For moments when the pain seems to intensify, suggest that the patient imagine stepping aside and watching the pain to see how it might be changed to release some of the pressure and resistance and to relinquish the hold on the pain. Your presence and guidance over time will help the patient to stay focused to open and soften into the pain. Your repeated words have a healing way of releasing any resistance around the pain.

LEARNING OBJECTIVES

After reading this chapter, the nurse should be able to do the following:

1. Identify the urgent problems of patients with acute myocardial infarction. (Time should not be used for history taking until the urgent problems are alleviated.)

2. Plan nursing care designed to limit infarct size.
3. Describe the pathologic changes in acute myocardial infarction and be aware of the specific complications.
4. List the most common complications of acute myocardial infarction.
5. Carry out rapidly the nursing care for each complication as it occurs.
6. Evaluate nursing care based on established outcome criteria.

CASE STUDY

Mr. C.V., aged 44, was admitted to the coronary care unit. He was wearing tennis clothes. In the initial assessment, the nurse described Mr. V. as an anxious man of medium build who was in acute distress. Mr. V. stated, "I have chest pain going down my left arm and up into my left jaw. I'm short of breath." The pain was graded by the patient as 8 on a 10-point scale of severity.

Mr. V.'s wife stated that Mr. V. had been playing tennis and had complained of a dull, pressing heaviness in his chest that forced him to stop his tennis game. His tennis partner called an ambulance, and Mr. V. was taken to the hospital. Mr. V.'s wife stated that Mr. V. had been very healthy and that he had no history of heart disease. Two weeks before his admission, the patient had had a routine health examination that was normal.

In the patient's profile and social history, it was noted that Mr. V. was an attorney, that he was 6 feet 2 inches tall, and that he weighed 185 pounds. His wife, aged 40, was well. She seemed very apprehensive and spoke of her fear that her husband would die. Mr. and Mrs. V. had three children, ages 17, 18, and 20; they were alive and well. The youngest son was with his mother at the hospital; the other children were away at school. The wife stated that her husband was active in community, church, and professional organizations. She said that this was an unfortunate time for him to be sick because he had several lawsuits pending in which he was the trial lawyer. Mr. V. did not smoke. He drank socially, consuming three drinks at the most at parties.

Mr. V.'s past medical history indicated that he had no heart disease, hypertension, or diabetes mellitus. He had never been hospitalized. He had no known allergies, and he was not taking any medications.

Mr. V.'s family history was positive in that his father died of a heart attack at age 54 and that his two brothers, aged 46 and 50, were taking antihypertensive medication. His mother, aged 72, was alive and well.

A physical examination showed that Mr. V.'s blood pressure was 80/50 mm Hg, his pulse 140 and irregular, his respirations 28, and his temperature 98.6°F. Lateral motion of his chest wall showed that he used accessory muscles for respiration. His breath sounds were normal. His skin was warm and moist. Examination of his cardiovascular system showed the point of maximal impulse (PMI) at the fifth intercostal space in the left midclavicular line. He had no murmurs or thrills. His peripheral pulses were full and equal. He had no abdominal tenderness or masses.

Mr. V.'s initial diagnostic tests, which were done approximately 3 hours after his chest pain began, showed that his total serum creatine kinase (CK) was borderline elevated to 265, suggesting myocardial infarction (MI). (Enzymes released from damaged or infarcted muscle elevate the serum levels, but maximum elevation does not occur this early.) His electrolytes and urine were normal. The 12-lead electrocardiogram (ECG) showed ST-segment elevation in leads V_1 through V_4 (Fig. 25–1). These leads reflect the electrical activity of the anterior wall of the left ventricle. The occlusion was most probably in the anterior descending branch of the left coronary artery. Both lead 1 and lead 2 were used to monitor Mr. V. because lead 1 reflects the anterior surface of the left ventricle and lead 2 helps discriminate among possible sites of premature ventricular contractions (PVCs).

The bedside monitor showed that he had tachycardia (140 beats/ minute), with occasional multifocal PVCs and elevated ST segments.

Mr. V. was first given intravenous morphine sulfate (5 mg slow intravenous push) for his chest pain, then lidocaine (a 50 mg/2.5 ml intravenous bolus), and then a continuous intravenous infusion of lidocaine (4 mg/ml) for his persistent multifocal PVCs. He continued to complain of chest pain after the initial dose of morphine, and he was given 2 mg of morphine sulfate every 15 to 30 minutes for the next 2 hours while the nurse frequently assessed his blood pressure and respirations.

About 24 hours after admission, Mr. V.'s condition changed suddenly and cardiogenic shock was diagnosed. His skin became cool and clammy. His blood pressure dropped to 50/0 mm Hg, and his pulse was rapid (140) and thready. Mr. V.'s physician ordered that Mr. V. be given dopamine (2 to 4 μg/kg/minute) to keep systolic pressure at 100 mm Hg. Arterial blood gases were measured. A Foley catheter was inserted, and 50 ml of urine was drained. A pulmonary artery catheter was inserted with an initial pulmonary artery wedge pressure (PAWP) of 25 mm Hg (normal is 8 to 12 mm Hg; patients with acute MI optimize cardiac contraction at 14 to 16 mm Hg). Intravenous furosemide (80 mg) was given. Third-degree heart block developed with a rate of 35 beats/minute. To treat the heart block, an external pacemaker was used.

Cardiogenic shock occurred owing to widespread necrosis of the anterior surface of the left ventricle that caused left ventricular dysfunction. The extent of the infarct was evident by the extremely elevated CK, which peaked at 2135 (16% CK-MB) a day after the onset of chest pain.

Mr. V. showed no clinical improvement over the next hour, and his physician decided to use intra-aortic balloon counterpulsation (IABC) (see Chap. 18). Intra-aortic balloon counterpulsation was used in Mr. V. to decrease the workload of the left ventricle, to support coronary artery perfusion during diastole, and thus to restore the balance between the myocardial oxygen supply and demand and improve peripheral tissue perfusion. The balloon was inserted percutaneously into Mr. V.'s descending thoracic aorta through the femoral artery to a position just distal to the left subclavian artery.

After approximately 36 hours, Mr. V.'s condition had stabilized, and he was weaned from balloon support. His vital signs and urine output were normal.

REFLECTIONS

Patients with acute MI commonly experience anxiety, severe pain, and fear of death and disability. Although the pain is understood to be the result of ischemic heart muscle, fear and anxiety accentuate the pain experience.

The pain of an MI is one of the most severe and debilitating pains experienced by human beings. Patients may describe their pain as "a tight band squeezing the very life out of me" of a "vice gripping my chest in two pieces." Alternately, patients may describe their pain in terms of pressure (*e.g.*, "I feel like an elephant (or a truck) is crushing my chest"). Listening to such expressions helps the nurse

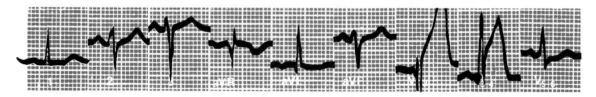

Figure 25–1

The electrocardiogram (ECG) reveals elevated ST segments of acute anterior wall myocardial infarction, illustrating infarction of the anterior wall of the left ventricle.

determine not only the severity but the significance of the patient's pain. The negative images evoked by such expressions clue the nurse regarding fears of an unpleasant death.

Pain stimulates the sympathetic nervous system, causing a reflex increase in heart rate, blood pressure, and cardiac output due to epinephrine release.[46] Fear and anxiety also stimulate the sympathetic nervous system, thereby increasing the work of the heart. Normally, such stimulation is well tolerated by a healthy heart. However, when coronary occlusion limits the amount of available oxygen supply, increases in oxygen demand caused by stimulation of the sympathetic nervous system may extend infarct size and cause complications.

The pain of MI is frightening not only to the patient but to the nurse as well. Understanding that pain must be relieved rapidly, the nurse may rely entirely on pharmacologic modalities. However, realizing that fear and anxiety are extremely potent stimulators of the sympathetic nervous system, the nurse must incorporate techniques designed to decrease patient fear and anxiety. Such techniques are described in detail in Chapter 3. Treating pain of acute MI with only relaxation techniques, however, is dangerous and unacceptable. Relaxation techniques are adjuncts to pharmacologic analgesia.

ANATOMY AND PHYSIOLOGY OF THE HEART

The heart is located in the lower anterior mediastinal space of the thoracic cavity. When one is standing, the left ventricle of the heart lies on the superior aspect of the diaphragm, anterior to the trachea, esophagus, and thoracic aorta and posterior to the sternum. The heart is surrounded by the inferior and middle (right) lobes of the lungs, and it is separated from the lungs by the pericardium. Because the right and the left sides of the heart differ in musculature, vascular structure, and function, the left side and the right side are discussed separately in the material that follows.

The heart is a complex muscle with the sole function of pumping blood. It is composed of four chambers that act as a double pump with four one-way valves (Fig. 25–2). The function of the right atrium and the right ventricle is to pump venous blood to the lungs. The function of the left side of the heart is to pump oxygenated blood into the systemic circulation. The pumps operate simultaneously. In the normal heart, the atria are separated by the thin, muscular interatrial septum, and the ventricles are separated by the interventricular septum. These structures prevent communication between the right and the left sides of the heart. The movement of blood in and out of each chamber of the heart is determined by the cardiac cycle. Diastole is the time during which the ventricles relax and fill with blood. Systole is the time during which the ventricles contract and eject blood.

Blood from the superior vena cava, inferior vena cava, coronary sinus, and thebesian veins enters the right atrium, a thin-walled, muscular structure. Blood enters the right atrium under low pressure. It then passes through the tricuspid valve (the three-leaflet atrioventricular valve).

The right ventricle is a crescent-shaped, thin-walled, muscular structure. Blood flows forward through the heart chambers owing to changes in pressure. As the pressure in one

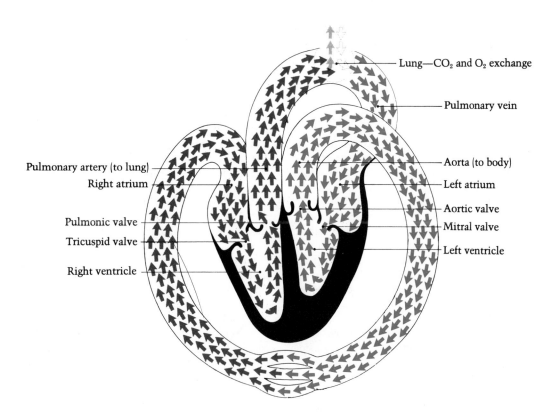

Pulmonary artery (to lung)
Right atrium
Pulmonic valve
Tricuspid valve
Right ventricle

Lung—CO_2 and O_2 exchange
Pulmonary vein
Aorta (to body)
Left atrium
Aortic valve
Mitral valve
Left ventricle

Figure 25–2
Normal circulation.

chamber exceeds pressure in the next, the valve opens and blood moves forward. A slightly greater pressure in the right atrium moves blood into the right ventricle during diastole. During atrial contraction and right ventricular relaxation, additional blood enters the ventricle because of a pressure gradient. The right ventricle receives about 85% of its unoxygenated blood passively through the open tricuspid valve during diastole. Atrial contraction contributes the remaining 15% of unoxygenated blood. Blood leaves the right ventricle under low pressure through the pulmonic semilunar valve and the pulmonary artery to the lungs. Contraction of the right ventricle is a bellows-like action. A healthy tricuspid valve keeps blood from regurgitating into the right atrium; a healthy pulmonic valve keeps blood from regurgitating into the right ventricle.

Within the right ventricle are papillary muscles that are attached to the ventricular wall. The chordae tendineae are attached at one end to the apex of the papillary muscles and at the other end to the free edges of the three leaflets of the tricuspid valve. As venous blood enters the right atrium, the leaflets of the tricuspid valve move downward; during right ventricular contraction, the chordae tendineae pull on the tricuspid valve, causing the valve to close. During closure of the tricuspid valve, pressure exerted in the contracting right ventricle is reflected onto the three semilunar leaflets of the pulmonic valve, causing the leaflets to flap open and back against the pulmonary artery wall as blood is sent to the lungs.

The main pulmonary artery bifurcates into the right and left branches, which go to the right and left lungs, respectively. The right pulmonary artery has branches that supply the three lobes of the right lung, and the left pulmonary artery has branches that supply the two lobes of the left lung. Unoxygenated blood in the lungs becomes oxygenated in the pulmonary circulatory system. Carbon dioxide is exchanged for oxygen at the alveolar capillary level. Oxygenated blood is returned to the left side of the heart, specifically the left atrium, through the four pulmonary veins.

The left atrium has a thicker musculature than the right atrium. During ventricular systole, the major portion of oxygenated blood enters the left atrium. This occurs at the same time as the onset of atrial diastole, during which the left atrium expands to accept blood from the pulmonary circulation. The pressure difference between the blood-filled left atrium and the relaxed left ventricle in diastole forces the oxygenated blood through the mitral valve (the two-cusp atrioventricular valve), which opens during the filling of the left ventricle.

The left ventricle is approximately two to three times thicker than the right ventricle owing to the difference in workload. Greater force is required to move blood from the left ventricle to the systemic circulation than to move blood from the right ventricle to the lungs. The left ventricle, a high-pressure chamber, contracts in a corkscrew action as it propels blood through the outflow tract and the aortic valve to the aorta and the systemic and cerebral circulation.

At the beginning of ventricular systole, the mitral valve closes with the help of two papillary muscles on the left side of the heart. As ventricular pressure increases, the only exit for blood is through the ascending aorta, which originates at the outflow tract of the left ventricle. The aortic valve, a three-leaflet valve, opens as a result of increased ventricular pressure during systole, just as does the pulmonic valve on the right

side. At the end of systole, the pressure in the aorta exceeds the pressure in the left ventricle. The aortic valve closes, preventing regurgitation of blood into the left ventricle.

Anatomy of the Coronary Arteries

Critical care nurses can anticipate the complications of acute MI more accurately if they know the anatomy of the coronary arteries (Fig. 25–3). This knowledge is useful, although the anatomy of the arteries may vary in each patient.

Left Coronary Artery

The main left coronary artery originates in the left sinus of Valsalva and branches into the left anterior descending artery and the circumflex artery immediately below the level of the pulmonary artery. The left anterior descending artery travels in the anterior intraventricular sulcus to the apex and, typically, wraps around it. It terminates in the inferior third of the posterior interventricular sulcus. Branches of the anterior descending artery perforate into the right half of the interventricular septum toward the posterior interventricular sulcus. The first large branch is referred to as the major septal branch. The other branches supplying the anterior left ventricular wall are referred to as the diagonal branches because of their position on the free wall of the left ventricle.

The left anterior descending artery has five segments: the proximal segment, the portion from its origin to the beginning of the first major septal branch; the midsegment, the portion from the first major septal branch to the midpoint of the midsegment and the apex; the apical segment, the portion from the midsegment to the apex of the heart; the first diagonal branch; and the second diagonal branch.

Circumflex Artery

The left circumflex artery runs along the left posterior atrioventricular groove to the crux of the heart (the crossing of the interatrial and the interventricular septa in the atrioventricular plane). In approximately 10% of people, the circumflex artery continues past the crux of the heart and then turns downward to form the posterior descending artery. In these people, the left coronary artery supplies the entire left ventricle and the interventricular septum. The circumflex artery supplies part of the left ventricular, anterior, lateral, and, in some cases, the posterior parts. The largest branch of the circumflex artery is the obtuse marginal branch. The posterolateral branch supplies a part of the posterior part of the left ventricular wall. The circumflex artery has branches to the atria that are called the atrial circumflex branches. Forty-one percent to 45% of people have a branch of the circumflex artery that goes to the sinus node; 12% of people have a branch of the circumflex artery that goes to the atrioventricular node.[1]

The circumflex artery also has five segments: the proximal segment, the portion from the artery's origin to the beginning of the obtuse marginal branch; the obtuse marginal branch; the distal segment, the portion between the origin of the obtuse marginal and the posterior descending artery; the posterior descending artery (not always present); and the posterolateral branch.

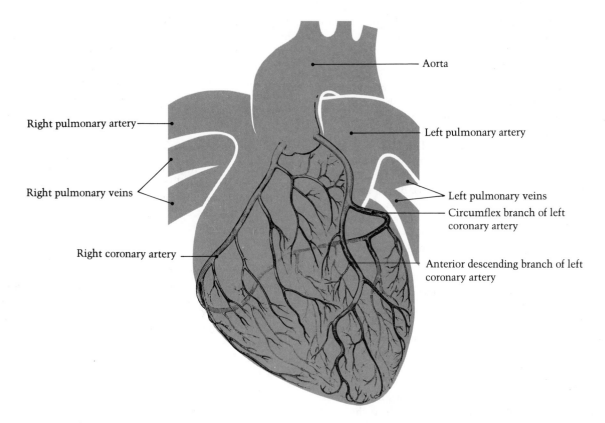

Right pulmonary artery

Right pulmonary veins

Right coronary artery

Aorta

Left pulmonary artery

Left pulmonary veins

Circumflex branch of left coronary artery

Anterior descending branch of left coronary artery

Figure 25–3
Anatomy of the coronary arteries.

Right Coronary Artery

As the right coronary artery leaves the wall of the ascending aorta in the right anterior sinus of Valsalva, it enters the right atrioventricular sulcus toward the diaphragmatic surface of the heart. At this point, the posterior portions of the interatrial and interventricular septa meet, forming the crux of the heart.

The right coronary artery has anterior branches that spread to the right ventricle. It has branches that spread superiorly and posteriorly and supply the atria. The anterior branches of the right coronary artery are the conus branch, the sinus node branch, two or more right ventricular branches, the posterior descending branch, and a branch or branches to the left ventricle. The important superior and posterior branches of the right coronary artery are those to the sinus node. The right coronary artery provides blood supply to the sinus node in about 59% of people. In 38% of people, the branch to the sinus node originates in the circumflex artery, the intermediate atrial artery, or the atrioventricular node branch.[31] It can also originate from the right coronary artery. The right coronary artery has three segments: the proximal segment, the portion from the ostium to the right ventricular branch; the midsegment, the portion from the right ventricular branch to the acute margin of the heart; and the distal segment, the portion from the acute margin to the crux of the heart. The right coronary artery has a fourth segment, the posterior descending artery.

Coronary Artery Circulation

The heart receives its blood supply from the coronary arteries, which are perfused primarily during ventricular diastole. Decreased blood flow to coronary arteries may produce myocardial ischemia, which causes a variety of problems such as poor contraction and conduction abnormalities. Diseases such as polyarteritis nodosa, lupus erythematosus, and hereditary disorders associated with cardiomyopathies also affect the small arteries of the heart and can cause dysrhythmias and conduction disturbances. These diseases are not discussed here.

The left coronary artery supplies the right bundle branch, the anterosuperior division of the left bundle branch, part of the posteroinferior division of the left bundle branch, and the anterior two thirds of the ventricular septum. Knowing the relevant anatomy suggests that the most common complications of anterior wall MI will be pump failure, atrial and ventricular dysrhythmias, and intraventricular conduction disturbances (Mobitz type II, bundle branch blocks, and hemiblocks).[42]

Patients with inferior wall MI usually have occlusion of the right coronary artery. In most people, the right coronary artery supplies the sinoatrial node, the atrioventricular junctional tissue, the His bundle, the posterior one third of the ventricular septum, and the posteroinferior division of the left bundle branch. People who have had an acute inferior wall MI often have either bradydysrhythmias caused by an ischemic sinus or atrioventricular node, and Wenckebach phenomenon (Mobitz type I heart block).

Collateral Circulation

There are few connections between the large coronary arteries, but there are many anastomoses between the small ones. When coronary arteries occlude progressively, many people develop a collateral blood supply that functions when the coronary arteries are completely occluded. Usually, the collateral blood supply becomes well developed only after complete occlusion. At the time of occlusion, the arterioles reach their maximum diameters within seconds. Blood flow at that time, however, is only half that which is needed to keep cardiac muscle alive. Over the next 8 to 24 hours, the collateral vessels enlarge further, and collateral flow begins to increase over the next several days, sometimes reaching a near-normal coronary supply within a month. Collateral intercoronary anastomoses increase the patient's chances of surviving a coronary occlusion. For unknown reasons, some people do not develop collateral vessels.

ETIOLOGY AND RISK FACTORS FOR ATHEROSCLEROSIS

Etiology

The most common cause of acute MI is coronary artery disease (CAD) or atherosclerosis in the arteries that feed the heart. This same process occurs in the arteries feeding all other organs and body parts, especially the brain, kidneys, and extremities. Atherosclerosis begins early in childhood, with fatty streaks becoming apparent as early as age 10. These fatty streaks progress over time to form plaques that obstruct blood flow in middle life and older years. Atherosclerosis is characterized by atheromas, which are lipid plaques within and beneath the intimal layer of the arterial wall. This atherosclerotic plaque formation occurs where blood flow is turbulent, and coronary arteries are particularly vulnerable. Besides interfering with blood flow and oxygen supply, the plaquing of atherosclerosis may cause the following: blood clot formation around atheromas, mechanical destruction of blood cells from contact with rough surfaces, obstruction from blood-clotting substances or thrombi from plaques, hemorrhage within the intima of the arterial wall, and plaque rupture.

The exact cause of atherosclerosis is as yet unknown. The major current theory explaining intimal plaque development is the response-to-injury hypothesis.[51,52] This theory combines the major earlier theories of plasma lipid infiltration and mural thrombosis.[1] According to this theory, injury to the intimal endothelium may begin the process of atheromatous formation. Injury to the lining of the artery exposes the endothelium to growth factors, stimulates plaque formation, and promotes platelet adherence. Injurious agents include cigarette smoke, hypertension, and increased blood viscosity associated with the lipid-laden macrophages of hyperlipidemia. Another theory of atherosclerosis, the monoclonal hypothesis, suggests that plaques are benign neoplasms derived from a single cell transformed by toxins, viruses, or chemicals.

Major Risk Factors

The data that have accumulated over the last decade on multiple risk factors for coronary atherosclerosis are impressive.

The major modifiable risk factors are hypercholesterolemia, hypertension, and cigarette smoking.[3] The contributing risk factors consistently associated with coronary atherosclerosis are heredity, age, physical inactivity, obesity, glucose intolerance, and stress. The relative contribution of each risk factor is difficult to determine, however, because of their interrelationships (Fig. 25–4).

Hypercholesterolemia

Hypercholesterolemia is one of the major modifiable risk factors for CAD. Isolated treatments directed at lowering blood cholesterol levels through medication have been shown to lower the risk of CAD dramatically. Cholesterol is the most important sterol normally present in all cells. Cholesterol levels increase in both sexes until the fourth decade, at which time they decline in men; in women, the decline occurs around the sixth decade. Cholesterol is synthesized endogenously and consumed in dairy and animal food products. Current data indicate that levels above 180 mg/dl are associated with an increased risk of CAD when other risk factors are present. In countries where total cholesterol levels are below 150 mg/dl routinely, CAD is rare. Specific fractions of cholesterol have been found to be either atherogenic (*i.e.*, low-density lipoproteins [LDL]) or antiatherogenic (*i.e.*, high-density lipoproteins [HDL]).

Hypertension

Hypertension has been well established as a major cause of CAD. High blood pressure is defined as a systolic pressure greater than 140 mm Hg or a diastolic pressure greater than 90 mm Hg. The risk associated with elevations of blood pressure is continuous; no threshold at which blood pressure is entirely safe is known. The risk of CAD increases with increases in blood pressure in both genders, all races, and all ages.

Approximately one quarter of the American population has hypertension, but many fewer are treated or controlled.[27] Hy-

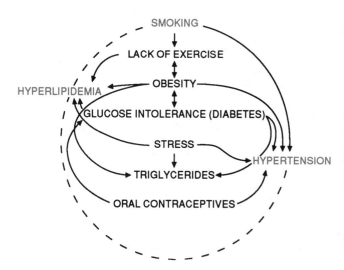

Figure 25–4

Depiction of the major and associated modifiable risk factors of coronary artery disease. (Riegel, B. From the editor. *J. Cardiovasc. Nurs.* 1:4, vi–viii, 1987; with permission.)

pertension is deadly, not just as a cause of CAD, but as a major cause of stroke and renal disease. The extreme force exerted with each heart beat appears to damage the arteries, making them more susceptible to the formation of atheroma. Hypertension also increases the turbulence of blood flow, another factor associated with atheromatous formation.

Cigarette Smoking

Cigarette smoking has been called the most modifiable risk factor by the Surgeon General. Smoking is associated statistically with accelerated atherosclerosis and acute MI. The exact mechanism by which smoking accelerates atheroma formation is not known. However, infarction may occur as a result of stimulation of the sympathetic nervous system, displacement of oxygen from hemoglobin, and perhaps increased platelet adhesiveness and coronary spasm. Catecholamines, liberated in response to nicotine, increase systolic blood pressure, heart rate, and cardiac output. Dysrhythmias caused by hypoxia and catecholamine release may be fatal in vulnerable persons. Most prospective studies indicate that the risk of developing CAD is related directly to the number of cigarettes smoked per day. In those patients who quit smoking, the excess risk declines 50% 1 year after discontinuing the habit.[21] Cigarette smoking has been found to have an independent, dose-related association with decreases in HDL cholesterol in both genders.

Contributing Risk Factors

Age

Hypertension is more prevalent in the later decades of life. Although atherosclerosis is more prevalent in older persons, it does occur in younger persons. Children with hyperlipidemias of type II or type III are known to develop severe atherosclerosis, as do young people with insulin-dependent (type I) diabetes mellitus. It is thought that in each person the flexibility of the artery and the effect of aging on metabolism affect the rate of atheroma formation.

Gender

Coronary artery disease is the leading cause of death in men after the age of 40; it is the major cause of permanent disability among workers under the age of 65.[21] Coronary artery disease is also the leading cause of death in women, although most attacks occur after the age of 65 years.[39] Women of childbearing age have a lower incidence of atherosclerosis than have men of corresponding age perhaps because of the effect of estrogen. Estrogen is thought to cause a decrease in the ratio of beta- to alpha-lipoprotein at given serum cholesterol levels, a beneficial effect. Estrogen also appears to stimulate the resistance of the coronary arteries to atheroma formation. Surprisingly, however, a study of estrogen therapy in men was halted early for ethical reasons after estrogens were found to increase rather than decrease the incidence of MI in men.

Heredity

People with familial hyperlipidemias, which are heredity disorders, have a high rate of coronary atherosclerosis. Other genetically transmitted traits associated with CAD include A-I/C-III deficiency, homocystinuria, hypertension, glucose intolerance, and obesity. These factors are discussed elsewhere in this chapter and in other sources. Although clinical lore suggests that earlobe configuration is a marker of CAD, no correlation has been found.[21]

Physical Inactivity

Physical activity has been shown to influence some of the major risk factors for CAD. Long-term, regular exercise has been shown to maintain body weight and muscle tissue, lower blood pressure and triglyceride levels, and raise HDL cholesterol fractions and glucose tolerance. Clinical practice suggests that a program of regular exercise can help people attain and maintain smoking cessation, but research is needed on this topic. The data are inconsistent regarding the relationship between exercise and sudden cardiac death. Therefore, some authors[21] suggest that persons over 35 years of age consult a physician before beginning a program of vigorous physical exercise.

Obesity

Atherosclerosis is more prevalent among obese persons than among people of normal weight; however, fat distribution is a more important predictor of CAD than body weight. High waist-to-hip circumference is a strong predictor of CAD. Epidemiologic evidence shows that as a group obese people have hypertension and hypercholesterolemia more often than thin individuals. Obesity also appears to be the major determinant of glucose intolerance and type II diabetes mellitus.[10]

Glucose Intolerance

The elevations of circulating insulin associated with glucose intolerance are thought to damage the intima and begin the process of atherosclerosis. Glucose intolerance is associated with obesity, hypertriglyceridemia, uremia, oral contraceptives, and prolonged stress. People who are obese and glucose intolerant have a small but definite risk of developing diabetes mellitus. Diabetics have a higher incidence of atherosclerosis than nondiabetics. Besides damaging the intima, insulin modifies lipid metabolism. Diabetics often have increased levels of cholesterol and other circulating fats, which increase their risk of atherosclerosis.

Behavior and Stress

Researchers believe that there is a relationship between CAD and emotions and behavior.[12] Two major behavior patterns have been described, type A and type B. Type A individuals are described in terms of hard-driving aggressiveness, competitiveness, free-floating hostility, and time urgency.[24] Type B persons are more introverted, patient, relaxed, and nonhostile. People with type A behavior are more likely to develop CAD than are people with type B behavior.[18]

It should be noted that there are those who believe that behavior and stress have no influence on CAD. This is because how and to what degree stress and behavior affect immunity, circulation, lipid metabolism, and coagulation are not fully understood. It is known that some people respond to stressful situations by overeating[10] and becoming frustrated, whereas other people turn stressful situations into positive experiences. The relationship between stress and CAD is also not fully understood and is currently being widely investigated.

Other Risk Factors

In men, gout is associated with a twofold risk of developing CAD. This may be explained by the fact that hypertension, obesity, hyperlipidemia, and glucose intolerance are associated with gout.

The use of oral contraceptives by women increases blood pressure in susceptible persons. It also worsens the major atherogenic traits such as hyperlipidemia. Oral contraceptives also are associated with increases in blood coagulability, which can cause thrombosis. Studies have shown that the risk of CAD and MI is increased by the use of oral contraceptives, particularly in women over the age of 35 years who smoke.

MYOCARDIAL ISCHEMIA AND INFARCTION

Myocardial ischemia and infarction can best be understood as an imbalance of oxygen supply and demand. When oxygen supply is limited by partial or total physical obstruction of the coronary arteries, increases in oxygen demand will result in ischemia or infarction. Causes of obstruction include atheromatous plaquing, thrombus, and coronary spasm. Spasm occurs primarily in people with atherosclerotic CAD. Naturally occurring vasoconstrictors such as prostaglandins released with ischemia may cause spasm, platelet aggregation, and coronary occlusion.[42]

Myocardial ischemia is defined as oxygen deprivation accompanied by inadequate removal of metabolites.[9] Ischemia occurs when the blood and oxygen supply available to the tissues is not sufficient to meet the demand for oxygen and waste removal. This occurs typically after atherosclerotic plaquing occludes at least 70% of the arterial area.

Myocardial infarction occurs when a coronary artery is totally occluded long enough to cause irreversible tissue death. Acute MI was thought until recently to occur when the atheromatous plaque grew to occlude the coronary artery. It is now known that acute MI occurs in the vast majority of cases as a result of disruption of the intima covering the plaque. Following that disruption, thrombus forms, coronary spasm may occur, and blood flow ceases, causing tissue death. Thrombus is the final occluding event in 80% to 90% of cases (Fig. 25–5).[14] Based on this information, patients with acute MI are treated frequently with thrombolytic therapy in an attempt to re-establish blood flow to the ischemic tissue.

The event precipitating thrombus formation appears to be rupture of the plaque into the vessel lumen. Recent research has been directed toward determining the causes of plaque rupture. Based on data that acute MI is most likely to occur between 6 AM and noon, it has been suggested that plaque rupture may occur as a result of the normal morning rise in systemic blood pressure and catecholamine release associated with assuming the upright posture after sleeping.[38] This is an intriguing line of research with implications for nursing management of the patient with acute MI.

Myocardial infarction is not a static event. In fact, 10% of patients with acute MI extend the amount of damage incurred during the first 10 days.[55] Limitation of infarct size and pre-

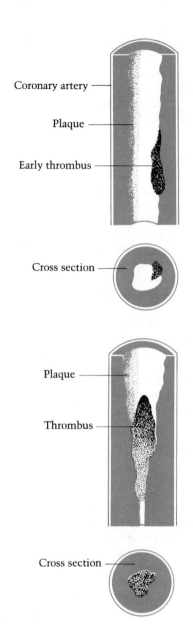

Figure 25–5

The arterial thrombus most frequently begins at the areas of luminal narrowing caused by atherosclerotic plaques. The chief thrombus components are platelets and then platelets and fibrin.

vention of extension is accomplished by maintaining a balance of oxygen supply and demand during the evolution of the acute occlusion, *i.e.*, throughout hospitalization.[54]

Myocardial Oxygen Supply and Demand

Myocardial oxygen supply is dependent on the amount of oxygen extracted from the blood, coronary blood flow, and the oxygen content of the blood. However, the heart normally extracts the majority of the oxygen available from the circulating blood. When coronary occlusion limits the oxygen supply available, the only method of increasing oxygen supply is to increase the oxygen content of the blood. Oxygen therapy is an effective method of increasing oxygen supply in hypoxic individuals.[6]

Myocardial oxygen demand is a function of wall tension (preload and afterload), contractility, and heart rate. Preload, or resting muscle length, is determined by the volume and pressure in the ventricle at the end of diastole. Afterload is defined as the force or stress developed in the ventricular wall during cardiac ejection.[53] Afterload is strongly influenced by resistance to systole such as systemic blood pressure or aortic stenosis and aortic compliance. Afterload, however, is *not* synonymous with resistance to ejection. Contractility is a function of preload as determined by the Frank-Starling mechanism. Finally, heart rate influences myocardial oxygen demand because conservative increases in heart rate increase contractility and the frequency of wall-tension development.[8]

Many nursing interventions designed to prevent or limit infarct size are based on recognition of the variety of factors influencing myocardial oxygen supply and demand. For instance, severe exhaustion or emotional stress may increase heart rate and contractility owing to catecholamine release. Surgical procedures that are associated with blood loss can precipitate an MI because of the decrease in myocardial oxygen supply associated with anemia. Serum sickness, respiratory infections, pulmonary embolism, allergic reactions, hypoglycemia, and hypoxia from any cause have been documented to cause acute MI. These seemingly diverse causes can all be understood as factors influencing the balance of myocardial oxygen supply and demand. Physical states such as hypotension may reduce myocardial perfusion and decrease myocardial oxygen supply. Tachycardia, fever, and agitation are all causes of increases in myocardial oxygen demand.

NURSING PROCESS

ASSESSMENT

Chief Complaint and History

When a patient is suspected of having an acute MI, a brief description of the chief complaint and a history of the present illness are obtained (see Chap. 24). Details can be elicited after the initial admission. A brief assessment should also include a patient self-report on the present level of anxiety on a scale of 1 to 10, with 10 as the highest level, as well as a description of the patient's usual (preinfarction) anxiety level on the same scale; previous medical therapy for anxiety and depression; and self-prescribed treatment for anxiety or depression.[64]

Chest Pain

The appearance and behavior of people just after they have an acute MI vary tremendously. Some people clutch their chests with pain. They may be pale, restless, diaphoretic, and nauseous, and may vomit. Most people are apprehensive and have pain. They may change their position frequently or sit absolutely still. Some patients belch or walk to try to relieve the pain.

Angina pectoris usually lasts for 3 to 5 minutes. It can be relieved by removing the precipitating factor or by taking sublingual nitroglycerin, which should relieve the pain within minutes.[28] The pain of acute MI is usually continuous; it commonly radiates to the arms, fingers, shoulders, and jaw. The radiation of the pain suggests that the visceral afferent nerve fibers have central connections in common with the somatic afferent system. The persistence and severity of the pain of acute MI helps to differentiate it from angina pectoris. Narcotics are usually necessary to relieve the pain of acute MI.

With luminal occlusion, a patient may die suddenly, apparently without pain. The usual cause of sudden death is thought to be a lethal dysrhythmia. Approximately 20% of the people with acute MI have actual cardiac muscle damage without pain.

Assess all patients often to see if they are in pain. Some patients may be reluctant to report pain, or may not interpret "heaviness" or "indigestion" as "pain").

Vital Signs and Physical Findings

After an acute MI, the patient may have a rapid and irregular pulse, or may be profoundly bradycardic. If the pulse is rapid, it is usually due to the patient's pain and anxiety. Irregularity typically results from premature atrial or ventricular contractions or second-degree heart block.

After acute MI, systolic blood pressure may fall below 90 mm Hg, but it will return to preinfarction levels during recovery. However, hypotension must be assessed in relationship to the signs of hypoperfusion, which are indicative of impending cardiogenic shock. As a consequence of catecholamine release secondary to pain, anxiety, and agitation, some patients may be hypertensive. If a patient is hypertensive, frequently a history of hypertension can be elicited. Patients who have systolic blood pressures below 125 mm Hg in the early stages of hospitalization have higher mortality than those with high blood pressures.[40] Lower blood pressures reflect lessened ability of the left ventricle to generate an adequate systemic pressure.

As a result of pain and anxiety, the patient's respiratory rate may be elevated after acute MI. The respiratory rate will return to normal with relief of the psychophysiologic stress unless heart failure is present; then the increased respiratory rate usually correlates with the degree of left ventricular failure.

Within the first 24 to 48 hours after MI, most patients have a low-grade fever resulting from tissue damage. Temperatures may reach 101°F orally. If a patient develops pericarditis, temperature elevations are then usually secondary to pericardial inflammation.

The patient's jugular venous pulse is usually normal after the acute event, because this pulse reflects right atrial and right ventricular activity. However, if a right ventricular infarct is present, significant jugular venous distention may be found. With papillary muscle necrosis of the right ventricle, there are tall v waves of tricuspid regurgitation on right atrial pressure waveforms. If cardiogenic shock develops, the jugular venous pressure is most often elevated. In addition, the patient's carotid pulse should be assessed because it gives data on left ventricular stroke volume. A small pulse indicates a reduced stroke volume, and a sharp, brief pulse upstroke suggests left-to-right shunt, aortic insufficiency, mitral regurgitation, or ruptured ventricular septum.

Baseline assessment of the patient's lung and heart sounds is essential. It is common for a patient to have no early symptoms of left-sided heart failure in the early stages of acute infarction. With a large infarct, varying symptoms of decreased cardiac output will appear over time. In patients with left ventricular failure, moist crackles at the lung bases are usually heard. Rhonchi, wheezes, and poor air exchange may also be heard if a patient has severe left ventricular failure and pulmonary edema. If a patient expectorates blood-tinged mucus plugs when left ventricular failure is present, pulmonary edema should be suspected. Left ventricular failure may predispose the patient to pulmonary embolus. This should be suspected if blood-tinged mucus plugs are expectorated and there is an abrupt decrease in oxygen saturation, negative chest x-ray findings and acute shortness of breath.

On chest palpation, the precordial pulse may be normal in patients with uncomplicated MI. If patients have a history of previous infarction or if left ventricular failure is persistent, an abnormal precordial pulse that is displaced laterally may occur as a sign of left ventricular enlargement.

Heart sounds are frequently muffled and may be inaudible after acute MI or cardiac tamponade. Heart sounds are more easily heard during the recovery phase. A fourth heart sound is considered universal with ischemic heart disease and is best heard between the left sternal border and the apex. A fourth heart sound can also be due to reduced left ventricular compliance and is associated with elevated left ventricular end-diastolic pressure even when acute heart failure is absent. A third heart sound in an adult is pathologic and demonstrates decreased compliance, extensive left ventricular dysfunction, and ventricular dilation. It is most common in patients with transmural anterior wall MI. With the patient positioned in the left lateral recumbent position, the third heart sound is best heard with the bell of the stethoscope at the apex. When a third heart sound occurs in the acute phase of infarction, the mortality rate increases to 40%, as compared with 15% in patients without a third heart sound.

A systolic murmur of mitral regurgitation secondary to papillary muscle dysfunction may also occur. A transient pericardial friction rub is most common in patients with transmural infarction and is best heard along the left sternal border or just inside the PMI. Pericardial friction rub appears most frequently on the second or third day after infarction, is usually intermittent, and occurs in over 20% of patients with acute MI.

Diagnostic Tests

Electrocardiogram

Several diagnostic studies may be done to confirm the presence of acute MI. In some patients, the ECG may be normal, or the serum enzymes may be negative. If the history and physical examination suggest MI, however, the patient should be observed closely and considered for thrombolytic therapy if he or she presents within 4 hours after the onset of pain.

A definitive diagnosis of acute MI can be made when the signs of myocardial necrosis appear on the ECG. These signs

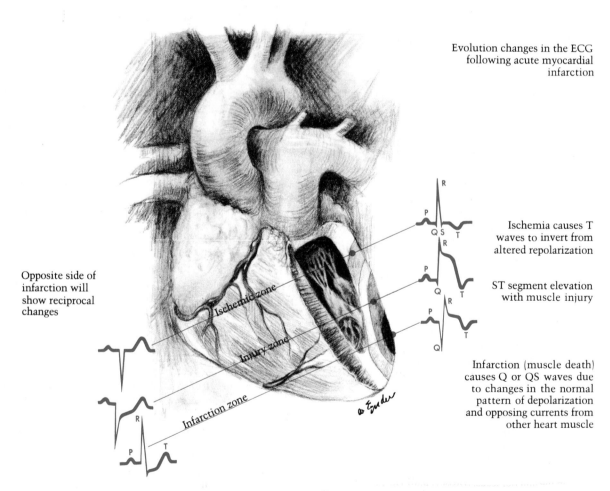

Evolution changes in the ECG following acute myocardial infarction

Ischemia causes T waves to invert from altered repolarization

ST segment elevation with muscle injury

Opposite side of infarction will show reciprocal changes

Infarction (muscle death) causes Q or QS waves due to changes in the normal pattern of depolarization and opposing currents from other heart muscle

Figure 25–6

The effects of cardiac ischemia, injury, and infarction.

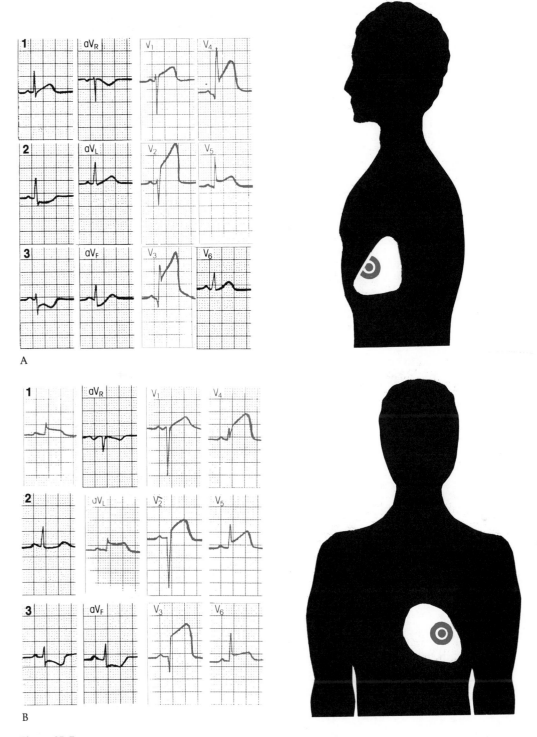

Figure 25–7

(*A*) Hyperacute phase of acute anterior myocardial infarction. ST-T wave elevation in leads V_1 to V_5 with appearance of diagnostic Q waves in V_3 and V_4. Reciprocal changes are seen in leads 2, 3, and aV_F. (*B*) Hyperacute phase of acute anterolateral myocardial infarction. Elevated ST segment in leads 1, Av_L, V_2, V_3, V_4, V_5, and V_6 with diagnostic Q waves in V_2 and V_3. Reciprocal changes are seen in leads 2, 3, and aV_F. (*C*) Hyperacute phase of acute inferior myocardial infarction. Elevated ST segments in leads 2, 3, and aV_F with Q waves in 2, 3, and aV_F. Reciprocal changes are seen in leads 1, aV_L, V_1, V_2, V_3, V_4, and V_5. (*D*) Hyperacute phase of acute posterolateral myocardial infarction. Increased R waves are seen in leads V_1 and V_2 with wider T waves in V_1, V_2, and V_3. Reciprocal changes are seen in the anterior leads. (Dossey, B.M. The person with acute myocardial infarction. In Guzzetta, C.E., and Dossey, B.M., *Cardiovascular Nursing: Bodymind Tapestry*, St. Louis: C.V. Mosby, 1984; with permission.)

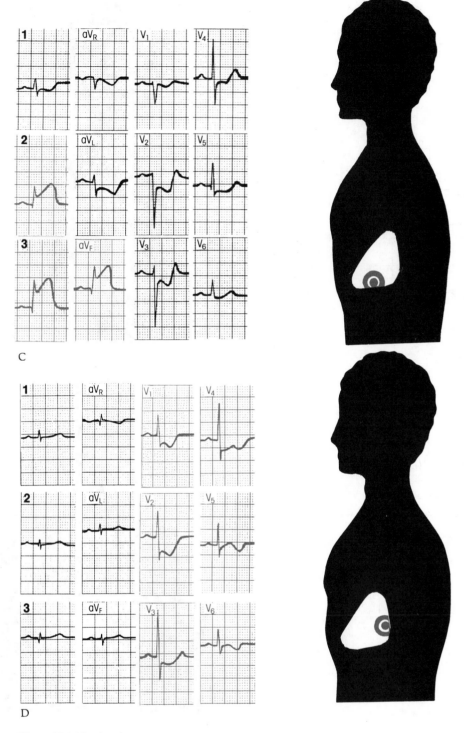

C

D

Figure 25-7 (*Continued*)

can appear within several days of the infarction or as late as a week after it.[42]

In acute MI, three ECG changes can be observed. There is T-wave inversion, indicating an ischemic pattern; ST-segment elevation, showing injury; and diagnostic Q waves (0.04 seconds) over the area of infarction, showing myocardial necrosis (Fig. 25–6). Myocardial necrosis means that the cells in the affected area are electrically dead. Once the Q wave has evolved, it usually remains. Electrocardiographic ischemia suggests that cellular metabolism is interrupted, thus causing the classic ECG pattern of electrical instability. The injury pattern records cell membrane damage, which indicates more serious electrical instability. The T wave and ST segment usually return to normal after the acute event.

Because the left ventricle is the primary pumping chamber of the heart, an acute MI affects primarily the left ventricle. The left ventricle is divided into anterior, inferior, lateral, and posterior walls (Fig. 25–7A to D). Acute MI is classified according to the place in the left ventricular wall at which it occurs. An insult can involve several places in the wall, as shown in Figure 25–8.

Right ventricular infarction can occur as a complication of inferoseptal left ventricular infarction. Electrocardiographic abnormalities of a right ventricular MI include Q waves in leads 2 and 3, and aV_F and ST-segment elevation in V_3R.[41] Right ventricular involvement occurs in approximately 33% to 66% of inferior wall transmural infarctions, although isolated right ventricular MI occurs in only 3% to 5% of cases.[2]

Inferior wall infarction carries a better prognosis than anterior infarction because the right ventricle has less effect on the primary pumping function of the heart. However, severe or extensive right ventricular infarction is difficult to treat because traditional therapies, such as inotropic medications and IABC, influence primarily the left ventricle. Treatment of right ventricular dysfunction is aimed primarily at maintaining adequate fluid volume to maximize the Frank-Starling mechanism.

Left ventricular function and prognosis are usually worse after anterior infarcts than after posterior infarcts of equal size. This may occur because posterior infarcts typically involve the right ventricle, whereas anterior infarcts typically involve the major pump, the left ventricle. Therefore, anterior MI compromises cardiac output more than posterior MIs.[2]

Location of Infarction in the Ventricular Wall

An acute MI can be subendocardial, subepicardial, intramural (confined to the interior of the myocardium), limited to the endocardium, limited to the layer below epicardial tissue, or transmural (involving the full thickness of the myocardium) (see Fig. 25–8). A nontransmural subendocardial or non–Q-wave infarction typically produces a depressed ST segment without a QRS-complex alteration or permanent Q waves.

An MI that destroys the entire thickness of the myocardium is called a transmural myocardial infarction. A significant Q wave (one that lasts at least 0.04 seconds) is produced in the lead overlying the infarction.

Cardiac Enzymes

The major serum enzyme measurements that are used to confirm the presence of acute MI are creatine kinase (CK), and lactic dehydrogenase (LDH). The usual time sequence of serum enzyme changes after acute MI is characteristic. Creatine kinase rises 4 to 8 hours after occlusion and lasts 3 or 4 days. Lactic dehydrogenase rises 24 to 48 hours after the event and stays elevated 8 to 14 days.

The fractionation of CK into its various isoenzymes provides additional information about the presence or absence of MI.[48] Creatine kinase can be fractionated into BB, which is present in the brain; MM, which is found in skeletal and cardiac muscle; and MB, which is specific for myocardium. Determination of the CK-MB level is the best laboratory parameter for the diagnosis of acute MI. People who have not had an acute MI but who have muscle damage in other body areas (*e.g.*, massive trauma, fractures) have elevated levels of either BB or MM. Levels of CK-MB are useful in estimating the size of an infarct, but they may be falsely elevated after cardiac surgery, cardiopulmonary resuscitation, thrombolytic therapy, and balloon angioplasty.

As in other acute injuries, the leukocyte count and sedimentation rate are elevated in the early phase of an acute MI.[42] The degree of elevation depends on the degree of damage sustained as a result of the infarct and the associated inflammatory process.

Chest x-rays are usually obtained on admission to collect baseline information; the incidence of atelectasis and congestive heart failure after acute MI is high and an indicator of prognosis.[40] Other diagnostic studies may include serum electrolytes, blood sugar, clotting profiles and an echocardiogram. Estimates of left ventricular wall function obtained with two-dimensional echocardiography correlate well with angiography.[42] Serum lipids should not be tested during acute hospitalization because they may be falsely elevated.[61]

NURSING DIAGNOSES, PATIENT OUTCOMES, AND PLAN

The preceding material on anatomy, physiology, nursing assessment, and diagnostic tests guides the nurse in establishing nursing diagnoses, patient outcomes, and a plan for the patient with acute myocardial infarction.

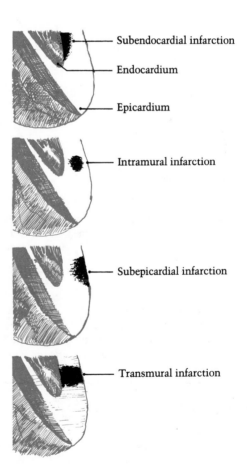

Figure 25–8

Location of various types of infarctions in the ventricular wall.

NURSING CARE PLAN SUMMARY *Patient with Acute Myocardial Infarction*

NURSING DIAGNOSIS

1. *Altered comfort (chest pain) related to inadequate myocardial tissue perfusion (e.g., angina, infarction, thromboembolism), inflammation (e.g., pericarditis, Dressler's syndrome), or irritation (e.g., chest wall myalgias, hiccupping, gastrointestinal problems) as evidenced by patient report of pain, guarded position, increased pulse, blood pressure, and respiration (feeling pattern)*

Patient Outcomes	Nursing Orders
1. The patient will notify the nurse immediately of recurrence of pain.	1. Evaluate patient's chest pain. A. Assess the following: (1) Type (squeezing, constrictive, steady, heavy, dull, intermittent, or crescendo) (2) Location (midsternal, radiating, or left precordial) (3) Whether relieved by meperidine hydrochloride, morphine, or small or large doses of sublingual nitroglycerin (4) Severity (have patient grade pain on scale of 1–10) (5) Effects (diaphoresis, nausea and vomiting, or anxiety) B. Assess all patients often to see whether they are in pain. Some patients may be reluctant to tell the nurse they are in pain. C. Watch for signs and symptoms of extension of myocardial infarction with recurrence of chest pain after initial relief. D. Check the patient's vital signs before giving narcotics (narcotics cause hypotension due to venous pooling of blood). E. Reassure patients often and help them during periods of pain. These kinds of support may help them feel positively about recovery.
2. The patient will be free of pericardial pain.	2. Assess for pericarditis during acute hospitalization as follows: A. Listen with diaphragm of the stethoscope for a friction rub. B. Be aware of the following persistent clinical symptoms: (1) Pain in the precordial area (mild to sharp or severe). The pain may be relieved when the patient leans forward and may increase with deep breathing or chest rotation. (2) Dyspnea or tachypnea (3) Fever, chills, sweating (which may be masked by salicylates) (4) Four stages of ECG changes (Table 25–1)
3. The patient will be free of pain caused by thromboembolism.	3. Watch for the following signs of thromboembolism: A. Loss of pulses in the lower extremities (if pulses were present when the patient was admitted) B. Cold, mottled, painful extremities
4. The patient will demonstrate no signs and symptoms of Dressler's syndrome.	4. Watch for signs and symptoms of chest pain related to Dressler's syndrome: pericarditis or pericardial friction rub, fever, pleuritis, pneumonitis, chest-wall tenderness.

NURSING DIAGNOSIS

2. *Decreased cardiac output related to electrical factors (dysrhythmias), mechanical factors (infarct extension, preload, afterload, inotropic factors), and structural factors (papillary muscle dysfunction, or tear and aneurysm) evidenced by low blood pressure, rapid pulse, restlessness, cyanosis, dyspnea, angina, dysrhythmia, oliguria, fatigability, vertigo, edema (exchanging pattern)*

Patient Outcomes	Nursing Orders
Electrical Factors 1. The patient will demonstrate no electrical complications of heart rhythm	1. Assess carefully every patient who has a dysrhythmia. Look for the following: A. A change in the patient's heart rate, respirations, and blood pressure

(continued)

NURSING CARE PLAN SUMMARY *Patient with Acute Myocardial Infarction* *Continued*

Patient Outcomes	*Nursing Orders*

Patient Outcomes

that would alter cardiac output (bradydysrhythmias; tachydysrhythmias; bundle branch blocks; sustained ectopy; aberrancy; first-, second-, or third-degree heart blocks; or atrial, junctional, or intraventricular conduction disturbances). Should electrical abnormalities occur, the patient will be diagnosed early. Early treatment will prevent decompensation.

Nursing Orders

B. A change in the patient's temperature and color of the skin

C. A change in the patient's mental state

D. The development of left ventricular failure. (Tachydysrhythmias shorten ventricular filling time and thus decrease the cardiac output and coronary blood flow. Bradydysrhythmias decrease the cardiac output, and they can allow dangerous tachydysrhythmias to take over.)

  (1) Give medications as ordered for ventricular dysrhythmias (*e.g.*, lidocaine, quinidine, digoxin, procainamide, diphenylhydantoin, tocainide, flecainide, and bretylium). Be aware of potential toxicity if cimetidine and lidocaine are used together.

  (2) Be aware of the patient's ECG pattern and be on the alert for changes in the ST segment and for dysrhythmias. (The "emergency" dysrhythmias are ventricular fibrillation, ventricular tachycardia, asystole, and complete heart block. They should be treated according to the standing coronary care unit orders.) Report any significant changes or persistent dysrhythmias to the physician.

    a. Maintain a patent IV line at all times.

    b. Know what antidysrhythmia drugs need to be given for specific dysrhythmias.

    c. Know the effects that antidysrhythmia drugs have on the patient and on the QRS complex, as shown on the ECG.

    d. Give atropine only if essential for bradyarrhythmia and treat it with an external pacemaker if necessary.

    e. Give medications for ventricular dysrhythmias as ordered.

    f. If atrioventricular block appears first with anterior myocardial infarction, watch for first-degree heart block and Mobitz type II heart block or for the development of intraventricular conduction disturbances.

    g. If Mobitz type II heart block appears, have available a functioning temporary pacemaker and an isoproterenol drip.

    h. Anticipate third-degree heart block if the patient has an idioventricular rhythm.

    i. If a temporary pacemaker must be inserted, follow these steps:

      (i) Explain the procedure to the patient.

      (ii) Have the procedure permit signed by the patient or a member of the family.

      (iii) After the insertion of a pacemaker, evaluate the pacemaker's functioning and the patient's rhythm. Record the rate, mode, and milliampere setting of the pacemaker on the patient's chart and on the care plan as ordered by the physician. Confirm placement with x-ray.

    j. If cardioversion is necessary in an emergency or for a dysrhythmia not corrected by medication, prepare for cardioversion.

    k. In preparing for cardioversion, follow these steps:

      (i) Explain the procedure to the patient in simple terms.

      (ii) Prepare the patient for sedation or anesthesia.

      (iii) If possible, discontinue digoxin for 1 to 2 days before the procedure. Give quinidine or another antidysrhythmia drug as ordered.

      (iv) Have the procedure permit signed.

      (v) Make sure that the patient is fasting.

      (vi) Have emergency drugs available.

E. When cardioversion is to be performed, follow these steps:

  (1) Place the patient in a supine position.

  (2) Remove the patient's dentures.

  (3) Secure the electrodes to the patient's chest and obtain a rhythm strip before cardioversion. (It is preferable to get a rhythm strip from a 12-lead ECG.)

(continued)

NURSING CARE PLAN SUMMARY **Patient with Acute Myocardial Infarction** *Continued*

Patient Outcomes	*Nursing Orders*

Nursing Orders

(4) Place conductive pads on the paddles.

(5) Set the cardiovertor on synchronization.

(6) Set the cardiovertor to the desired voltage.

(7) Charge the cardiovertor to the desired voltage.

(8) Position the paddles, using two anterior paddles or an anterior paddle and a posterior paddle.

(9) Apply firm pressure to the paddles.

(10) Avoid contact with wet areas and make sure no one is in contact with the patient or bed while the physician performs the cardioversion.

(11) Obtain a 12-lead ECG after the cardioversion.

(12) Anticipate the possible complications—further instability and systemic or pulmonary embolism.

(13) Remain until the patient is stable and fully awake.

(14) Observe the patient closely for 2 to 3 hours after the cardioversion.

(15) Allow the patient to resume oral intake and drugs 1 hour after the cardioversion.

(16) If defibrillation for ventricular dysrhythmia is necessary, follow the steps for cardioversion, except turn off the synchronizer circuit and turn on the defibrillator circuit. (Because the patients are unconscious, the procedure is not explained to them.)

2. The patient will experience no complications of antidysrhythmics, medications, cardioversion, or pacemaker when needed.

2. If pacemaker is required:
   A. Assess function
   B. Continue to assess patient's vital signs, ECG, anxiety, fear.

Mechanical Factors

1. The patient will demonstrate normal mechanical function, normal vital signs, and hemodynamic stability with normal preload, afterload, and myocardial contractility.

1. Protect ischemic myocardium to prevent infarct extension by minimizing myocardial oxygen demand by the following:

   A. Avoid increases in heart rate and contractility from medications, exercise, fever, pain, fluid volume deficit, tachydysrhythmias, and anxiety.

   B. Avoid increases in ventricular wall tension, especially afterload related to hypertension, epinephrine, hypothermia, and stress.

   C. Be prepared to initiate thrombolytic therapy if the infarct began 4 or fewer hours previously.

   (1) Screen for the following contraindications:
       a. Active internal bleeding
       b. History of cerebrovascular accident
       c. Intracranial or intraspinal surgery or trauma within 2 months
       d. Intracranial neoplasm, atrioventricular malformation, or aneurysm
       e. Known bleeding diathesis
       f. Severe uncontrolled hypertension[17]

   (2) Prepare for agent administration as follows:
       a. Start two intravenous lines using a minimum of venous punctures.
       b. Draw coagulation parameters.
       c. Obtain a baseline ECG.

   (3) Administer the following prophylactic medications:
       a. Lidocaine to prevent reperfusion dysrhythmias
       b. Steroids and antihistamines to avoid anaphylaxis with streptokinase
       c. Heparin to prevent acute reocclusion

   (4) Administer 1.25 mg/kg recombinant t-PA over 3 hours.
       a. Administer 10% of the total dose as an intravenous bolus over 1 to 2 minutes to open the occluded artery.
       b. Administer 60% of total dose in first hour.
       c. Administer 20% in second hour.
       d. Administer remainder in third hour.

   (5) Administer intravenous streptokinase dose of 1.5 million U over 30 to 60 minutes. Intracoronary dose of 25,000 to 50,000 U bolus is followed by 2000 to 4000 U/minute infusion over 60 minutes.

   (6) Administer 2 to 3 million units of urokinase as an intravenous bolus over 30 minutes. If given as intracoronary dose, 4000 to 8000 U/minute is the maintenance infusion.

(continued)

NURSING CARE PLAN SUMMARY   *Patient with Acute Myocardial Infarction*   Continued

Patient Outcomes	Nursing Orders

Nursing Orders

(7) Assess for the following evidence of reperfusion:
   a. Return of elevated ST segments toward baseline (most reliable indicator)
   b. Angiographic evidence of patency
   c. Resolution of chest pain
   d. Reperfusion dysrhythmias

(8) Monitor closely for following complications:
   a. Hypotension (in 15% of patients receiving streptokinase)
   b. Anaphylaxis, which may occur with streptokinase
   c. Major and minor bleeding:
      (i) Assess for changes in neurologic status and level of consciousness that suggest intracerebral bleeding.
      (ii) Assess blood pressure and heart rate frequently as measures of internal bleeding.
      (iii) Surface bleeding from puncture and invasive sites is common and can often be controlled with pressure.

(9) Be prepared to initiate other approaches to protect ischemic myocardium:
   a. Nitrates optimize preload and decrease afterload.
   b. Beta-blockers decrease myocardial contractility.
   c. Diltiazem may prevent reinfarction.
   d. Glucocorticoids increase infarct size and are contraindicated in the early stages of acute MI.[42]

Patient Outcomes

2. The patient will show no signs of hypotension, hypoxemia, pain, shortness of breath, dyspnea, tachycardia, orthopnea, rales, S_3 gallop, diffuse PMI, neck vein distention, hepatic enlargement, or peripheral edema (congestive heart failure).

Nursing Orders

2. Watch for signs of CHF and treat it early if it occurs.
   A. Assess for the following:
      (1) Diminished first heart sound and second heart sound. The development of a third heart sound may be a sign of CHF.
      (2) The development of a murmur or a change in an existing murmur
      (3) Gallop rhythms
      (4) Coughing
      (5) Dyspnea
   B. Provide cardiac rest for the patient: semi-Fowler's position.
   C. Give oxygen via a face mask or cannula.
   D. Give diuretics as ordered and watch for side effects.
   E. Anticipate further complications of CHF and the onset of pulmonary edema:
      (1) Check the patient's vital signs.
      (2) Observe the patient for an increase in dyspnea or coughing.
      (3) Place the patient in a high Fowler's position. (Preload is reduced quickly by pooling blood peripherally without significantly reducing the stroke volume. Afterload is reduced by dilating the peripheral arteries and thus reducing the left ventricular end-diastolic pressure.)
   F. Anticipate the need for the following items and have them available:
      (1) Vasodilators
      (2) Diuretics
      (3) Morphine sulfate
      (4) Aminophylline
      (5) Advanced life-support equipment
   G. Optimize preload by administering diuretics as ordered:
      (1) Assess effectiveness:
         a. Weigh the patient at the same time each day.
         b. Maintain accurate records of intake and output.
         c. Monitor fluid restrictions.
      (2) Watch for side effects:
         a. Weakness and muscle cramps
         b. Hypovolemia
         c. Electrolyte depletion, especially hypokalemia
      (3) Use caution when giving digitalis due to increased risk of toxicity associated with CHF.

(continued)

NURSING CARE PLAN SUMMARY *Patient with Acute Myocardial Infarction* Continued

Patient Outcomes	*Nursing Orders*
	H. Decrease afterload by giving vasodilators (*e.g.*, IV nitroglycerin or nitroprusside): (1) Watch for hypotension (2) Prepare for hemodynamic monitoring to regulate drugs.
3. The patient will show no signs of hypotension, tachycardia, urine output below 30 ml/hour, mental confusion, decreased peripheral perfusion, or abnormal blood gas analysis (cardiogenic shock).	3. Be alert to the following signs of cardiogenic shock: A. A systolic pressure below 90 mm Hg (or unobtainable). (A drop of 20 to 40 points in systolic pressure in a patient who has been hypertensive is significant.) B. Pallor or cyanosis C. A rapid, thready pulse or an imperceptible pulse D. Cool, clammy skin E. Collapsed, constricted peripheral veins F. Mental dullness, restlessness, agitation, or confusion G. Decreased urinary output H. Oliguria (a urinary output of less than 30 ml in 1 hour) I. Anuria (no urinary output) J. If cardiogenic shock is present, follow these steps: (1) Establish and maintain an airway. (2) Give oxygen by nasal cannula or face mask. Before giving oxygen, find out if the patient has a history of chronic respiratory disease. If the history is positive, give oxygen at low-flow rates (2 to 3 L/min) to maintain the hypoxic drive to breath. (3) Coordinate and maintain mechanical ventilation if needed. (4) Obtain filling pressures hourly. (5) Maintain the patient's arterial blood pressure with vasopressors (*e.g.*, dobutamine dopamine) as ordered. (6) Establish and maintain a fluid and electrolyte balance, using a crystalloid solution, volume expanders, or an electrolyte infusion. (7) Administer medications to correct rhythm disturbances as needed. (8) Anticipate the patient's needs by providing quiet and efficient care, by relieving anxiety, and by positioning the patient comfortably. (9) Anticipate the need for IABC (see Chap. 18 for the care of these patients). K. Evaluate the effectiveness of treatments given for CHF and cardiogenic shock by systematically assessing the patient as follows: (1) Listen to the lungs for air movement, crackles, rhonchi. (2) Assess arterial blood gases. (3) Assess cardiac output. (4) Assess urinary output.
4. The patient will show no signs of tachycardia, hypotension, muffled heart sounds, pulsus paradoxus, or ECG evidence of electrical alternans tachycardia, or decreased QRS complex voltage (cardiac tamponade).	4. Be alert to the possibility of cardiac tamponade. A. If cardiac tamponade is suspected, check for Kussmaul's sign, distention of the neck veins on inspiration. B. Check for pulsus paradoxus. If it is greater than 10 mm Hg, pericardial tamponade should be suspected. C. If pericardial effusion develops rapidly, watch for signs of a decreased cardiac output. D. Watch for ECG changes (electrical alternans, tachycardia, or a decrease in QRS complex voltage). E. Watch for muffled heart sounds, hypotension, and orthopnea. F. Have emergency equipment at hand.
Structural Factors 1. The patient will maintain structural integrity without sudden signs of heart failure.	1. Assess for signs of heart failure (listed under Mechanical Factors, Patient Outcome, number 2).
2. The patient will demonstrate no systolic murmur, left-sided heart failure, or pulmonary edema (papillary muscle rupture or dysfunction).	2. Assess for the following signs of papillary muscle dysfunction or papillary muscle rupture: A. Transient systolic murmur at apex (papillary muscle dysfunction) B. Sudden onset of pulmonary edema with sudden loud holosystolic murmur (papillary muscle rupture) and hypotension

(continued)

NURSING CARE PLAN SUMMARY *Patient with Acute Myocardial Infarction* *Continued*

Patient Outcomes	*Nursing Orders*
	C. Prepare for hemodynamic monitoring and administration of vasodilators. D. Prepare for intra-aortic balloon counterpulsation and cardiac surgery, if necessary.
3. The patient will demonstrate no pansystolic murmur, hypotension, or heart failure (ventricular septal rupture).	3. Assess for the following signs of ventricular septal rupture: A. Loud holosystolic murmur at lower left sternal border with palpable thrill B. Varying degrees of CHF to extreme of pulmonary edema C. Hypotension D. Prepare for cardiac catheterization and intra-aortic balloon counterpulsation.
4. The patient will demonstrate no persistent ST-segment elevation in precordial leads, no outward systolic impulse medial or superior to PMI, or no activity intolerance (ventricular aneurysm).	4. Assess for the following signs of ventricular aneurysm: A. Persistent ST segment elevation in precordial leads B. Prolonged palpable outward systolic impulse medial to PMI C. Persistent ventricular dysrhythmias D. Persistent asymptomatic or symptomatic heart failure E. Prepare for cardiac catheterization or cardiac surgery, if indicated.

NURSING DIAGNOSIS

3. *Anxiety (mild, moderate, severe) related to CCU regimen, acute illness, or fear of death as evidenced by stated feelings of apprehension, helplessness, nervousness, fear, tension, irritability, angry outbursts, crying, criticism, withdrawal, inability to concentrate, ruminating, insomnia, and restlessness (feeling pattern)*

Patient Outcome	*Nursing Orders*

1. The patient and family will verbalize feelings, learn relaxation and imagery techniques to reduce anxiety, and show a reduction in anxiety.	1. Prevent and treat potential anxiety by doing the following:
	A. Establish rapport with the patient.
	B. Explain the CCU regimen.
	C. Evaluate the patient's emotional response to the illness.
	D. Evaluate the patient's understanding of the information given. Allow time for questions and feedback.
	E. Be aware of any distress or depression that the patient shows, and respond to these feelings.
	F. Allow 60- to 90-minute periods of uninterrupted sleep to decrease sleep deprivation[58] and facilitate coping. Encourage naps in the morning so that afternoon naps with predominately stage 4 deep sleep do not interfere with night-time sleep.
	G. When explaining physical limitations, avoid being overly cautious and frightening patients.
	H. Explain the CCU regimen (*e.g.*, bed rest, monitoring, IV lines, light diet) to decrease the unknown.
	I. Talk freely with the patient about anxieties.
	  (1) Allow time for the patient to give the nurse information about routines and daily activities.
	  (2) Ask open-ended questions about the patient's feelings and knowledge of MI.
	  (3) Be aware of the patient's mental state as concerns are expressed. The patient may reveal one of the following states:
	    a. Denial: ignores symptoms (*e.g.*, avoids discussing the MI)
	    b. Isolation or repression: seems unafraid or unconcerned about the illness
	    c. Displacement: complains about relatively unimportant matters (*e.g.*, noise, food, or air conditioning)
	    d. Projection: talks about the anxieties of relatives but not about his own anxieties
	    e. Rationalization: blames the MI on hard work rather than on smoking, obesity, high blood pressure or cholesterol levels, or other risk factors

(continued)

NURSING CARE PLAN SUMMARY   *Patient with Acute Myocardial Infarction*   *Continued*

Patient Outcomes	*Nursing Orders*
	f. Hallucinatory or delusional behavior: shows symptoms of delirium, agitation, hallucination, delusion, or mania (accuses the staff of trying to poison him or her).
	J. Help the patient to develop trust in the nursing staff.
	(1) Include the patient in routine decisions when appropriate.
	(2) Give frequent explanations to the patient about progress and give specific information about present condition. Do not make polite, evasive remarks (*e.g.*, "You're okay").
	(3) Spend some time alone with the patient each day so that he or she can express thoughts and feelings as soon as they occur. The extra time allows the nurse to learn more about the patient's concerns, whether verbalized or expressed without words.
	(4) Allow time to receive feedback from the patient.
	(5) Allow the patient's spouse or significant others to help the patient with some daily activities or to give special instructions. Be aware of family hierarchies and allow family and significant others to be helpful.
	(6) Make sure that the patient understands the rehabilitation program.
	K. Help the patient work through the common responses to MI: anxiety, denial, withdrawal or depression, aggressive sexual behavior.
	(1) Teach relaxation and imagery techniques. Use music tapes, relaxation tapes, and drawing materials to enhance the experience.

NURSING DIAGNOSIS

4. *Activity intolerance related to myocardial ischemia, illness, physical deconditioning from bed rest as evidenced by dyspnea on exertion, shortness of breath, excessive increase or decrease in heart rate, blood pressure, and respiratory rate with activity that fails to return to normal after 3 minutes, rhythm change, weakness, pallor or cyanosis, confusion, vertigo (moving pattern)*

Patient Outcomes	*Nursing Orders*
1. The patient will experience minimal activity intolerance.	1. Encourage patients to perform the following activities of daily living as tolerated: A. Allow men to stand to void unless specifically contraindicated by physical condition or femoral support lines. B. Allow patients to use bedside commode or the bathroom rather than the bedpan. Using the bedpan puts more strain and workload on the heart than getting out of bed to use the commode or bathroom. C. Explain the need to avoid sudden physical effort and isometrics. D. Teach the patient how to turn from side to side in bed without overexerting. E. Adhere to principles of progressive activity. Explain the need for graduated, supervised levels of activity.
2. The patient will experience no adverse effects of early mobilization (infarct extension).	2. Note factors influencing the ability to be active (Refer to Box 25-1 following Nursing Care Plan Summary), such as the following: A. Medications B. Body weight C. Time on bed rest D. Size of the infarct (note maximum CK level and MB-CK percentage) E. Age F. Time since a meal or procedure 3. Evaluate the patient's tolerance of activity by monitoring the following: A. Blood pressure response B. Dysrhythmias C. Pain D. ECG changes E. Dyspnea

(continued)

NURSING CARE PLAN SUMMARY *Patient with Acute Myocardial Infarction* Continued

NURSING DIAGNOSIS

5. *Knowledge deficit related to acute and chronic illness as evidenced by a verbalized deficiency in knowledge or skill, expressions indicating inaccurate perceptions of health status, incorrect performance of a health behavior, noncompliance with prescribed health behavior (knowing pattern)*

Patient Outcome	*Nursing Orders*

1. The patient and family will demonstrate self-care knowledge and skills of risk factors, how to take pulse, medications, progressive activity schedule, and compliance with medical regimen and self-care.	1. Assess readiness to learn by evaluating stress responses and ability to retain information given.
	2. Evaluate present knowledge level and adjust instructional level to meet needs of the individual.
	3. Encourage experiential input from patient and family during instruction.
	4. Teach the patient and family about the following:
	  A. Basic anatomy and physiology of the heart
	  B. Risk factors and reduction
	  C. Activity schedule and pulse record
	  D. Return to sexual activity
	  E. Diet
	  F. Stress management and stress-reduction techniques
	  G. Medications (name, dosage, frequency, action, side effects)
	  H. Symptoms requiring immediate attention
	  I. Follow-up information
	5. Evaluate potential compliance problems.
	6. Implement a system of follow-up.

IMPLEMENTATION AND EVALUATION

Hospital Care of the Patient With Acute Myocardial Infarction

Nursing and medical management in the coronary care unit after acute MI are aimed at limiting infarct size by reducing the workload on the heart, anticipating and treating complications, treating emergencies, and promoting psychological adjustment and optimal rehabilitation (see Nursing Orders for details). Coronary care unit nurses must determine individually what their patients find stressful and intervene effectively.

Patients who experience an uncomplicated MI can be discharged 7 to 9 days after the acute event.[25] Recent experience suggests some patients can be discharged safely at 5 days. Those who have significant complications after the infarction, such as frequent ventricular dysrhythmias, advanced heart block, symptomatic congestive heart failure, pulmonary edema associated with cardiogenic shock, or infarct extension may require a longer length of stay.

Complications of Acute Myocardial Infarction

A number of complications can occur after an acute MI. The most important ones are psychological distress, dysrhythmias, congestive heart failure, cardiogenic shock, pericarditis, papillary muscle dysfunction, ventricular aneurysm, Dressler's syndrome, and pulmonary embolism.

The medical or surgical treatment of each of these complications is discussed in the pages that follow. For specific nursing care with regard to these complications, refer to the Nursing Care Plan Summary.

Psychological Distress

Patients in the coronary care unit often go through stages of denial, anxiety, anger, and depression. Although these stages can be predicted after an acute MI, the intensity of the response as well as the duration of the stages varies with each patient. Because an acute MI is often a sudden event, many patients initially experience shock and disbelief; this stage is commonly characterized by denial. Anxiety with agitation and hypervigilance is also an early response, lasting for the first 24 to 48 hours. Several days after the MI, patients usually develop an awareness of what has occurred. Anger and depression are frequent responses as the patient realizes the significance of the event. Aggressive sexual behavior may occur in some patients. Such behavior is rarely what it seems; patients are usually expressing a need or anxiety through the sexual comments. The final stage of resolution may begin before or after hospital discharge. Resolution is typically characterized by fluctuations

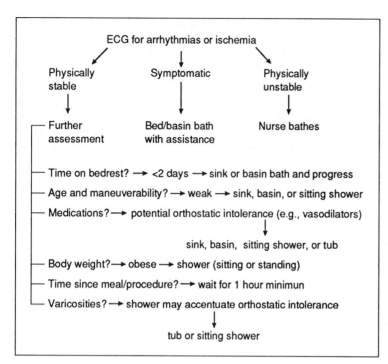

ECG for arrhythmias or ischemia

Physically stable → Further assessment

Symptomatic → Bed/basin bath with assistance

Physically unstable → Nurse bathes

Time on bedrest? → <2 days → sink or basin bath and progress

Age and maneuverability? → weak → sink, basin, or sitting shower

Medications? → potential orthostatic intolerance (e.g., vasodilators) → sink, basin, sitting shower, or tub

Body weight? → obese → shower (sitting or standing)

Time since meal/procedure? → wait for 1 hour minimun

Varicosities? → shower may accentuate orthostatic intolerance → tub or sitting shower

Box 25–1

Decision tree for bathing. This decision tree can be used to evaluate patient variables known to affect activity response. This assessment facilitates prescription of an appropriate method of bathing. *Note:* Response to bathing can be evaluated during the activity by leaving the monitoring unit on the patient and covering it with a rubber glove.

in all the behaviors just described. As the patient begins to assume responsibility during recovery, behavior may change from day to day.

Nurses must listen to and observe their patients and try to understand how their patients perceive what is happening to them. Keep in mind that everyone is unique and that everyone responds differently to stress. When the patient seems very anxious, maintain continuous contact to help develop trust in the staff so that the patient's condition can be accurately assessed. Learn about the patient's previous experiences with illness, hospitalization, and severe stress and how the previous experience relates to the present condition. What does the illness mean to the patient? Ask for and listen to comments about feelings. Respond when necessary. Determine whether the patient's denial hinders treatment. Is the denial verbal, or does the patient act it out?[63] Assess the "threat" that has caused the patient's denial or sexual comments. If sexual aggressiveness makes the nurse uncomfortable, tell the patient so, simply and directly.[37] Let the patient know that it is normal to feel depressed while one is ill.[15]

Members of the patient's family often react to the patient's illness with depression, fear, anxiety, hostility, and overprotective behavior. The health care team must address any psychological problems that the patient and family might experience during hospitalization as well as in the rehabilitative phase and try to help them adjust to the changes brought on by the illness.

Dysrhythmias

Dysrhythmias occur in 72% to 96% of patients who have had an acute MI.[42] It is of the utmost importance for the nurse to remember that she or he is observing and treating a person with a dysrhythmia, not the dysrhythmia itself, because each person responds differently to a dysrhythmia.

Patients admitted with the diagnose of massive MI, obesity,

congestive heart failure, or a history of anxiety should be considered at high risk for occurrence of dysrhythmias after an MI.[64]

Ventricular Dysrhythmias. Early and late-phase ventricular dysrhythmias are the most common of all the rhythm disturbances after an acute MI.[42] Within the first 12 to 48 hours after an MI, early phase dysrhythmias are usually due to the immediate ischemic effects on the ventricular muscle, slowing the initial phase of depolarization in the ischemic myocardium. This results in a disparity between the injured and healthy tissue that allows the re-entry mechanism to stimulate ventricular extrasystoles, tachycardia, and fibrillation. Late-phase ventricular dysrhythmias are a result of enhanced automaticity of ventricular cells.

Ventricular tachycardia and ventricular fibrillation are "emergency" dysrhythmias. Tachydysrhythmias shorten ventricular filling time and thus decrease cardiac output and coronary blood flow. The prophylactic use of lidocaine is recommended before the occurrence of ventricular dysrhythmias. Multiple studies have shown that the warning dysrhythmias occur just as frequently in the patient who does not develop primary ventricular fibrillation as in the patient who does develop it.[67] The occurrence of primary ventricular fibrillation is greatest in the first few hours after acute MI. It has been calculated that the incidence of ventricular fibrillation in the first 4 hours after infarction is 15 times that in the next 8 hours.[4] Because primary ventricular fibrillation and sudden death are major problems in patients after acute MI, routine lidocaine prophylaxis is both safe and practical (see Appendix II for details). Ventricular ectopy may also be a symptom of hypokalemia.

Sinus Bradycardia. Sinus bradycardia occurs more frequently after inferior wall infarction as a result of decreased blood flow to the sinoatrial node or enhanced vagal stimulation. The increased vagal activity can be protective or detrimental. It may be a protective mechanism because, with a decreased sinoatrial node discharge rate, there are reduced myocardial oxygen demands. It can also be a detriment because a slow rate allows more possibility for ventricular premature contractions, ventricular tachycardia, and ventricular fibrillation. Continued bradycardia decreases cardiac output and the available oxygen supply. Atropine is used for only symptomatic bradycardia because it may cause tachycardia, increase myocardial oxygen demand, and extend infarct size.

Conduction Disturbances. Conduction system disturbances are common in patients with acute MI. Conduction abnormalities can interfere with the normal sinus impulse transmission to the ventricles, resulting in decreased cardiac output, slow ventricular response, hypotension, and, in the extreme, complete ventricular standstill and death.

In patients with acute MI, 4% to 14% experience first-degree block. Four percent to 10% of patients with acute MI experience Mobitz type I second-degree heart blocks. A Mobitz type I block occurs in up to 90% of all second-degree blocks reported.[1]

Conduction problems are usually in the atrioventricular node after inferior infarctions but below the bundle of His in anterior infarctions. A complete heart block that involves the bundle branches is more common after anteroseptal MI. With inferior wall MI, Mobitz type I first-degree and second-degree atrioventricular blocks are most common. Mobitz second-degree atrioventricular block accounts for 10% of the total oc-

currences of second-degree block. These occur more frequently in patients with acute anterior, rather than inferior, infarction. Complete heart block occurs in approximately 5% of patients with acute MI. Conduction disturbances can occur within the intraventricular conduction system and do occur in 10% to 20% of patients with acute MI.

Left anterior hemiblock occurs in 3% to 5% of patients with acute MI and is usually benign. Right bundle branch block occurs in 2% of patients. This block is frequently associated with complete heart block and carries a high mortality.

Left posterior hemiblock occurs in 1% of patients with acute MI and usually those with a large anterior infarction. If blocks occur in two fascicles after MI, patients have an increased risk of developing complete heart block. Temporary pacing measures should be available in the acute period.

Supraventricular Dysrhythmias. Atrial premature beats, atrial fibrillation, sinus tachycardia, atrial flutter, and paroxysmal supraventricular tachycardia are frequent in the patient with acute MI. Most often these are associated with congestive heart failure, pericarditis, and cardiogenic shock.

Congestive Heart Failure

Congestive heart failure (CHF) is a common complication of acute MI (Fig. 25–9). Heart failure causes one third of the deaths of these patients. When acute MI involves the large muscle of the left ventricle and normal reserve mechanisms of the heart are exceeded, left-heart failure occurs.

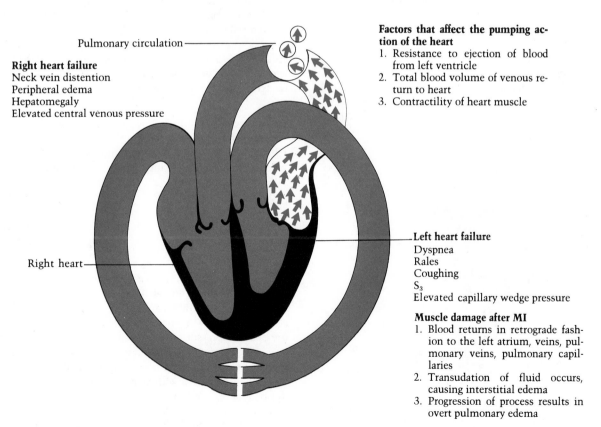

Right heart failure
Neck vein distention
Peripheral edema
Hepatomegaly
Elevated central venous pressure

Pulmonary circulation

Factors that affect the pumping action of the heart
1. Resistance to ejection of blood from left ventricle
2. Total blood volume of venous return to heart
3. Contractility of heart muscle

Right heart

Left heart failure
Dyspnea
Rales
Coughing
S_3
Elevated capillary wedge pressure

Muscle damage after MI
1. Blood returns in retrograde fashion to the left atrium, veins, pulmonary veins, pulmonary capillaries
2. Transudation of fluid occurs, causing interstitial edema
3. Progression of process results in overt pulmonary edema

Figure 25–9
Congestive heart failure. MI: myocardial infarction.

It is common for a patient to have no early symptoms of left-sided heart failure. The patient may develop symptoms of decreased cardiac output when the heart fails to pump enough blood into the systemic circulation. At that time, the pressure in the left ventricle increases, and it is transmitted in a retrograde path to the left atrium, the pulmonary veins, and the pulmonary capillaries. When pulmonary capillary pressure exceeds the oncotic pressure of plasma proteins, fluid transudates and causes interstitial edema. If fluid moves into the alveoli, dyspnea, frequent coughing, and crackles may develop. If the condition progresses, the patient may develop overt pulmonary edema.

In pure left ventricular failure, there is no peripheral edema or neck vein distention. On radiograph, the left ventricle may or may not be seen to increase in size. Third and fourth heart sounds in acute MI are probably secondary to changes in ventricular compliance rather than to enlargement.

Treatment of acute CHF following MI should begin with bed rest, sedation, and oxygen. Preload and afterload reduction can be accomplished with diuretics with or without the addition of vasodilators.

Intravenous nitroglycerin may also be used with CHF.[65] Hemodynamic monitoring, discussed elsewhere in this text, may be required in order to regulate appropriate drug therapy. In patients who exhibit CHF and elevated PAWP, nitroglycerin reduces right and left ventricular filling pressures. There is a reduction in cardiac work because of a lower preload and afterload. Reduced preload occurs as a result of a decrease in the blood volume returning to the right ventricle as well as to the pulmonary system and left ventricle. Nitroprusside may also be used. It has a balanced effect of decreasing both preload and afterload.[13]

Cardiogenic Shock

Cardiogenic shock is another major complication of acute MI that occurs in approximately 10% of patients (Fig. 25–10).[8] In cardiogenic shock, the heart fails to pump effectively, decreasing the stroke volume. Eventually, general tissue ischemia

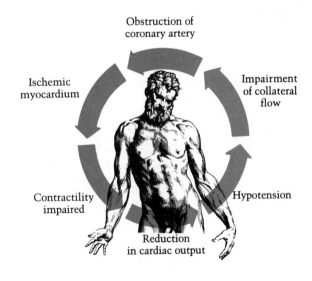

Figure 25–10
The vicious cycle of cardiogenic shock.

and hypoxia occur. A hypotensive state due to low cardiac output exists.

Statistics show that patients who die from cardiogenic shock have acute necrosis of at least 40% of the left ventricle.[35] Cardiogenic shock is difficult to treat because the biochemical and physiologic changes associated with shock change constantly and the exact mechanisms of shock are not fully understood. Owing to inadequate tissue perfusion, anaerobic metabolism ensues, causing lactic acidosis. Treatment is aimed at improving myocardial contractility without increasing the workload of the heart and raising the mean arterial pressure to obtain adequate coronary blood flow and increased peripheral vascular resistance without decreasing blood flow to the kidneys.

Early manifestations of cardiogenic shock must be recognized by the nurse and reported to the physician. Research has shown that effective communication between the critical care nurse and physician may decrease the incidence of cardiogenic shock. Pyles[44] reported that manifestations of early shock were more frequently recognized by experienced critical care nurses. Regardless of whether early warning signs of shock were discovered, patient outcomes depended on communication skills of the nurse in reporting the findings and then obtaining an appropriate response from physicians.[44] It is recommended that critical care nurses implement identified assessment criteria, have guided experiences to help the new critical care nurse, have regular patient care conferences to discuss responses to illness and treatment modalities, and have in-service education classes on effective communication and power strategies to enhance autonomy and nurse-physician collaborative relationships.

The following classification is helpful when cardiogenic shock is associated with acute MI.[19,22] Filling pressure refers to left atrial pressure (LAP), PAWP, or pulmonary artery end-diastolic pressure (PAEDP). Left atrial pressure is the most accurate measure of the filling pressure available to the left ventricle, but LAP is not usually available. Pulmonary artery wedge pressure is preferred to the PAEDP.

Filling pressure group 1: Low; no pulmonary edema. Intravenous fluids are indicated.
Filling pressure group 2: Low; pulmonary edema is present. Intravenous fluids are indicated to increase filling pressures.
Filling pressure group 3: High; no pulmonary edema. Vasodilator drugs are indicated. Mechanical circulatory devices can be used.
Filling pressure group 4: High; pulmonary edema is present. Treatment is similar to that for group 3.

Hemodynamic Monitoring and Intravenous Fluid Challenge.
The most helpful and reliable way of determining if fluid challenge is needed in cardiogenic shock is to obtain serial readings of LAP, PAWP, or PAEDP. The PAWP approximates the diastolic pressure within the left ventricle. It can also determine if the circulating blood volume needs expanding. Low filling pressures indicate that intravenous fluids are needed. Low filling pressures with signs of pulmonary congestion in the patient still indicate that intravenous fluids are needed (Fig. 25–11).

Correct intravenous fluid amounts can be determined by using the following intravenous fluid challenge and response guidelines:[19]

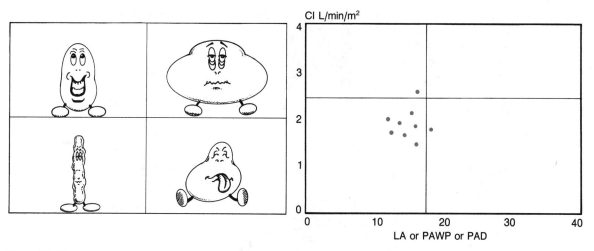

Figure 25–11

Shock box pictorally and graphically representing the four hydration states of normal, hypovolemia, hypervolemia, and heart failure. In the right graph, a patient's filling pressures—left atrial (LA) pressure, pulmonary artery wedge pressure (PAWP), or pulmonary artery end-diastolic (PAD) pressure—have been graphed in relation to the cardiac index over time. The trend demonstrates that the patient is hypovolemic and would benefit from a fluid challenge. (Modified from figures drawn by Diane E. Moore, Sharp Memorial Hospital, San Diego, CA; with permission.)

1. Filling pressures less than 15 mm Hg
   Give: 100 ml intravenous fluid over 5 minutes
   Response: Good (increased blood pressure, urine flow, rise in PAWP no more than 2 mm Hg above initial level)
2. Filling pressures remain stable, do not rise above 2 mm Hg or exceed 16 mm Hg; no signs of pulmonary congestion or a worsening of pulmonary congestion
   Give: 500 to 1000 ml/hour until low blood pressure and other clinical signs disappear. Check vital signs and lung sounds and PAWP every 15 minutes.
   Response: 16 to 18 mm Hg satisfactory
3. Filling pressures initially 15 to 18 mm Hg
   Give: 100 ml intravenous fluid over 10 minutes. Further challenge depends on PAWP and clinical signs.
4. Filling pressures 20 mm Hg or higher; low blood pressure
   Give: First, give a vasopressor (*e.g.,* dopamine) and then cautiously give a vasodilating drug before use of the intravenous fluid challenge.
5. Filling pressures: A rise of initial PAWP to 16 mm Hg or higher when an intravenous fluid challenge is done suggests that predominant cause of shock is not inadequate circulating blood volume but pump failure. Fluid challenge is discontinued only when PAWP reaches optimum (16-18) levels.
6. Filling pressures rise to 25 mm Hg (indicates moderate pulmonary edema); rises to 25 to 30 mm Hg indicate severe pulmonary congestion.
   Stop: Intravenous fluid challenge
   Give: Intravenous vasodilator may be helpful; supportive low-dose dopamine; mechanical circulatory assist. Assess oxygenation to evaluate need for mechanical ventilation.

If the patient does not respond to these drugs, mechanical assist may be necessary (see Chap. 18).

Pericarditis

Pericarditis is a troublesome complication after acute MI (Fig. 25–12), occurring in approximately 15% of patients.[1] The clinical hallmark of pericarditis is a friction rub, which sounds like cellophane crunched in the fingers. Although often transitory, a friction rub is most easily heard on forced expiration while the patient leans forward or is in the left lateral position. Diffuse ST-segment elevations may be seen on the 12-lead ECG as the condition worsens. Bleeding from an inflamed pericardium may occur, leading to hemorrhagic tamponade and shock due to myocardial compression, which severely limits myocardial filling. Tamponade is an uncommon but life-threatening complication.[45] Respiration may be painful if the surrounding pleura is involved. With splinting, atelectasis may occur and oxygen saturation may fall, predisposing to dysrhythmias or possible infarct extension. The most obvious symptom of pericardial inflammation is pain, which is often aggravated by swallowing, coughing, inspiring, and rotating or moving the trunk. The treatment of pericarditis is aimed at relieving the pain and inflammation. Table 25–1 gives the four stages of ECG evolution of acute pericarditis.

Papillary Muscle Dysfunction

Many disease processes can cause left ventricular papillary muscle dysfunction (see Fig. 25–12A). The most common ones are MI and coronary insufficiency. The papillary muscles receive their blood supply from the terminal portions of the large penetrating branches of the coronary arteries. If flow to the coronary arteries is impaired, the papillary muscles become susceptible to injury. Papillary muscle dysfunction in the

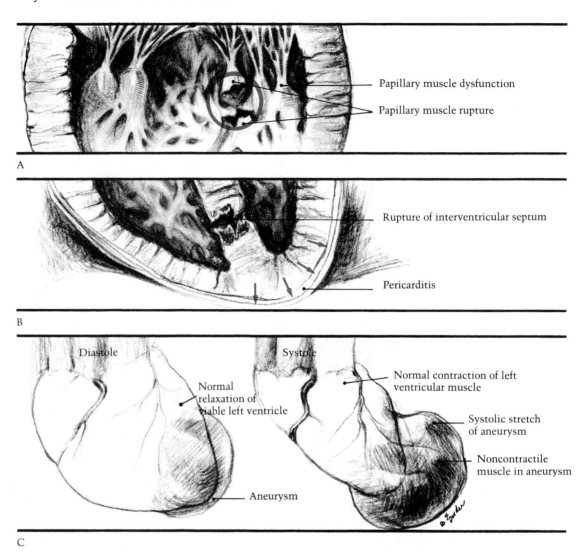

A

B

C

Figure 25–12

(A) Papillary muscle dysfunction and rupture. (B) Rupture of the interventricular septum and pericarditis.
(C) Ventricular aneurysm.

presence of acute MI is suggested by the presence of an apical systolic murmur that may radiate to the axilla and occasionally is associated with a thrill.

If acute MI involves the papillary muscle to the point of necrosis, papillary muscle rupture may occur, although it is uncommon. If papillary muscle rupture does occur, it usually does so within the first week after infarction. A pansystolic murmur may be heard, and a thrill is usually present. Typically, the patient has worsening of heart failure or sudden onset of heart failure, often with dysrhythmias, cyanosis, and marked reduction in cardiac output. Papillary muscle rupture interrupts the normal pattern of forward flow through myocardial chambers. Afterload reduction may optimize flow and stabilize the patient by decreasing impedance to left ventricular ejection. Immediate surgical intervention is required to prevent death in most patients. Mechanical support with cardiopulmonary support of IABC may stabilize cardiac status while the patient is being prepared for surgery.

Ventricular Aneurysm

The incidence of ventricular aneurysm accompanying acute MI is not well established (see Fig. 25–12C). Variations in the literature appear to be related to how aneurysm was defined in the study and whether patients were studied clinically or at autopsy. The term *aneurysm* is used to refer to an area of the ventricle that is both akinetic and dyskinetic during systole. Dyskinesis varies from full-thickness muscle to scarred, thin muscle.

The paradoxical motion of the ventricular wall (systolic stretch) interferes with the overall pumping action of the heart. As the normal portion of the ventricular muscle mass contracts, the area of aneurysm is forced outward by the increasing pressure inside the ventricle; thus, much of the pumping force of the ventricle is lost because of the ischemic or nonfunctional cardiac muscle. Ischemic bulges of the myocardium occur frequently during the clinical course of infarction. Many of these

Table 25-1
Four-Stage ("Typical") Electrocardiographic Evolution of Acute Pericarditis

SEQUENCE	LEADS OF "EPICARDIAL" DERIVATION (I, II, AVL, aV_F, V_{3-6})			LEADS REFLECTING "ENDOCARDIAL" POTENTIAL AVR, OFTEN V_1, SOMETIMES V_2		
Stage	J-ST	T waves	PR segment	ST segment	T waves	PR segment
I	Elevated	Upright	Depressed or isoelectric	Depressed	Inverted	Elevated or isoelectric
II early	Isoelectric	Upright	Isoelectric or depressed	Isoelectric	Inverted	Isoelectric or elevated
II late	Isoelectric	Low to flat to inverted	Isoelectric or depressed	Isoelectric	Shallow to flat to upright	Isoelectric or elevated
III	Isoelectric	Inverted	Isoelectric	Isoelectric	Upright	Isoelectric
IV	Isoelectric	Upright	Isoelectric	Isoelectric	Inverted	Isoelectric

J-ST: junction of S (or T) wave with the end of the QRS complex.
(Modified from Spodick, D. H. Electrocardiographic changes in acute pericarditis. *Am. J. Cardiol.* 33:470, 1974; with permission.)

bulges disappear and cannot be identified at autopsy because systolic pressure is needed to identify them. Aneurysms involve the left ventricle in 95% of cases and the right ventricle in 5% of cases.[1] Ventricular dysrhythmia (primarily ventricular tachycardia), impaired ventricular function, and arterial embolism are complications of aneurysm.

Systemic arterial embolism due to mural thrombus formation in the left ventricle may occur at the site of an aneurysm. Patients suspected of embolization should be observed for any changes in sensorium, specifically any decreased or absent pulse or a change in temperature in the involved extremity. Cerebral embolism may also occur, with changes in mental status and level of consciousness as the primary signs. Any of these changes must be brought to the attention of the physician immediately. Anticoagulant therapy with heparin should be instituted quickly if it is not contraindicated. If the problem is not resolved by medical therapy, surgical intervention may be considered.

Dressler's Syndrome

Dressler's syndrome, the postmyocardial infarction syndrome, occurs in 3% to 4% of the patients who have had an acute MI. Dressler's syndrome is thought to be attributed to a hypersensitivity reaction to the products of the necrotic myocardium. Typically, the syndrome causes pleuritic-type chest pain, fever, and an elevated sedimentation rate. It begins 10 days to 3 months (usually 3 to 4 weeks) after the acute MI. Dressler's syndrome is distinguished from a new MI by the fact that the pain is pleuritic and there are no changes in the EGG or the cardiac enzymes. Dressler's syndrome is usually benign, although uncomfortable and perhaps frightening, and it lasts for 1 to 2 weeks.

Pulmonary Embolism

Pulmonary embolism (PE) is uncommon, but it can be a life-threatening complication of acute MI. Pulmonary emboli usually originate in the deep veins of the lower extremities (see Chap. 23). Atrial fibrillation, transmural MI, or non–Q-wave infarction of the right ventricle predispose a patient to thrombus formation and subsequent pulmonary emboli. Morbidity from PE varies according to the size of the embolus.

Anticoagulants decrease the risk of bed-rest complications such as PE. Some patients may be placed on low-dose heparin schedules, 5000 U every 8 to 12 hours, until 2 to 3 days before discharge. Patients at high risk for embolization, such as those with atrial fibrillation, obesity, present or past thrombophlebitis, ventricular aneurysm, or cardiogenic shock, may be placed on full-dose anticoagulation, 10,000 to 20,000 U infused continuously or intermittently to maintain the clotting time and partial thromboplastin time (PTT) at 1.5 to 2.5 normal. Depending on each patient's history, 5 to 7 days of such therapy may then be followed by oral anticoagulants after hospitalization. The effectiveness of oral anticoagulants following acute MI to reduce morbidity or mortality has not been clearly shown.[1] However, low-dose aspirin (one baby aspirin a day) has been shown to decrease the incidence of reinfarction.

Thigh-high antiembolic hose are used commonly in patients with moderate risk imposed by bed rest and immobility. Those immobilized for longer periods of time because of mechanical ventilation or mechanical ventricular assistance may benefit from pneumatic pulsatile compression hose in addition to antiembolic stockings.

PROTECTION OF ISCHEMIC MYOCARDIUM

Thrombolysis

Thrombolysis is the most effective treatment available for limiting infarct size[51] based on the knowledge that 80% to 90% of infarctions are the result of thrombus.[14] Thrombolytic agents are recommended for patients in whom acute MI is documented or strongly suspected who present to the hospital without contraindications within 3 or 4 hours after the onset of chest pain. Specific nursing care for the patient receiving thrombolytics is covered in the Nursing Care Plan. It should be noted that dosing schedules are evolving and changing frequently. Only guidelines are given in the care plan.

Thrombus recanalization or lysis by thrombolytic agents such as t-PA, streptokinase, and urokinase continues to be widely investigated. To date, t-PA appears to have the best reperfusion rates, but the reocclusion rate of 9% to 13% is equal among the agents.[51] The debate surrounding intravenous versus intracoronary administration continues, although, to save time, most thrombolytics now are administered by the intravenous route. Heparin sodium and aspirin are often used in conjunction with thrombolytics to maximize their effectiveness. The specific effects of the thrombolytics on the clotting cascade can be found in Chapter 23 of this text.

The major complication of thrombolytic therapy is bleeding. Careful screening for contraindications (included in the Nursing Care Plan) and close assessment of coagulation profiles (PTT, prothrombin time [PT], fibrinogen, platelets, hemoglobin, and hematocrit) are essential.

Percutaneous Transluminal Coronary Angioplasty

Percutaneous transluminal coronary angioplasty (PTCA) is a nonsurgical alternative to coronary artery bypass surgery. Performed in the cardiac catheterization laboratory under local anesthesia, the technique involves inflation of a balloon catheter in the coronary artery at the site of stenosis. The atheromatous lesion is compressed and split, expanding the arterial lumen to improve distal coronary blood flow.

Just a few years ago, PTCA was considered an experimental procedure. It is now estimated that 400,000 PTCAs/year will be performed in the early 1990s.[51] Approximately 50% of the cases of CAD previously sent to surgery can now be treated with PTCA. Where early guidelines specified single-vessel disease, cardiologists are now performing multivessel dilations with a wide variety of steerable, dual-balloon, and reperfusion catheters.

After routine angiography, angioplasty catheters are threaded into the coronary arteries, where the atheromatous plaque is dilated using up to 14 or sometimes greater atmospheres of pressure. The availability of reperfusion catheters now allows lengthy dilation without distal myocardial anoxia due to interference with blood flow. Patients are pretreated with antiplatelet agents, usually aspirin, which are continued after hospital discharge. Use of these agents has greatly influenced the success of PTCA.

Teaching the patient with PTCA is similar to teaching patients about cardiac catheterization. Research has demonstrated that information about visual, auditory, and tactile sensations experienced by the patient are most effective in decreasing anxiety.[26] The patient should also receive basic anticipatory preparation for coronary artery bypass surgery in case of complications. Most patients considered as candidates for PTCA should also be acceptable candidates for coronary artery bypass surgery. Although much less common than in years past, emergent coronary artery bypass surgery may be indicated for complications arising during PTCA. In high-risk cases, the surgical team is on call during the procedure.

Little is known about the behavioral recovery process of patients with PTCA. Portu and colleagues[43] found PTCA patients less anxious than bypass surgery patients 7 months after treatment. Patients with PTCA returned to a normal life approximately 11 weeks sooner than bypass patients, but bypass patients were more likely to perceive that their overall health was improved. Clinical experience suggests that PTCA patients may be less adherent to life-style modifications than bypass surgery patients perhaps because the procedure is less traumatic. Research is needed in this area.

Lasers

Lasers are now being used experimentally to open occluded coronary arteries, diffuse lesions, tandem lesions, and discrete lesions distal to a graft site.[16] Used in conjunction with balloon angioplasty, laser primarily is used to recanalize totally occluded vessels so that a dilating balloon can be inserted. Laser is being used intraoperatively and during percutaneous procedures performed in the catheterization laboratory under local anesthesia.

Argon, carbon dioxide, and neodymium-yttrium-aluminum garnet (Nd:YAG) lasers are used most commonly in medicine. Alternating-current lasers, such as the excimer, also are being investigated because the continuous-wave lasers, such as those used routinely, cause secondary tissue damage. A new argon "hot-topped" catheter is being investigated as a method of avoiding thermal injury.

Intracoronary Stents

Intravascular stents have been devised in an attempt to deal with the still high (20% to 40%) reocclusion rate after PTCA. Stents are placed percutaneously in the coronary artery, bridging an area that has reoccluded or will not remain open immediately after PTCA. At this time, three devices are being investigated for use in coronary arteries. The nitinol coil stent, the spring-loaded, self-expanding stent made of stainless steel or polyester, and the balloon-expandable stent.

Placement of the stent is accomplished in the catheterization laboratory. Patient preparation is identical to that for patients undergoing PTCA, except that informed consent must be obtained for this experimental procedure. Postprocedural care is identical to that for patients with PTCA.

Atherectomy Devices

A variety of cutters, grinders, shavers, and extractors are in clinical trials and close to approval for general usage. The principle common to all of these devices is the actual removal of atheromatous plaque and thrombus from the artery. All of these devices have been used on peripheral vascular disease with success. However, the technical refinements required to allow their use in the coronary arteries have slowed the progress toward using them in CAD.

At this time, atherectomy devices have only an adequate success rate in carefully chosen patients. Further, restenosis rates appear to be comparable to those for standard balloon angioplasty. Vascular wall smooth muscle cell proliferation in response to any mechanical intervention in atheromatous disease causes a restenosis rate averaging 30%. The vascular smooth muscle cell remains the nemesis of percutaneous intervention in coronary artery disease.

Beta-Adrenergic Blockade

Administration of beta-adrenergic blockers may be used to protect the ischemic myocardium from increased sympathetic stimulation after acute MI. Intravenous metoprolol is administered in three doses of 5 mg each over 5-minute intervals.[42] Heart rate and arterial pressure (either by cuff or indwelling catheter) should be measured frequently. If no side effects occur, 50 mg of metoprolol is given orally 8 hours later. If the patient is hemodynamically stable a day later, 100 mg is administered daily. A heart rate between 50 and 65 beats/minute is acceptable. All patients given beta-blockers should be assessed carefully for a lengthening PR interval, second- or third-degree heart block, lung crackles, wheezes, or increased filling pressures.

Calcium Antagonists

Calcium channel blockers have been studied as potentially limiting infarct size because intracellular calcium accumulation causes cellular dysfunction and cell death.[20] Animal studies suggest that diltiazem protects myocytes but that nifedipine and verapamil are ineffective. Diltiazem was found to prevent reinfarction for 2 weeks in patients with acute MI.[49]

CARDIAC REHABILITATION

Cardiac rehabilitation after acute MI should include instruction, counseling, and activity.[7,18,59,60] The best results are achieved by using a multidisciplinary team approach. Rehabilitation begins as soon as the patient's condition is stable, and it continues throughout the hospital stay and after discharge. The level of activity after a patient's discharge from the hospital must be tailored to the individual patient. Patients who have had an acute MI should be able to perform their daily activities at about 3 metabolic equivalents (METs). (One MET is the energy a person expends sitting quietly in a chair, or about 3 to 4 ml of oxygen/kg of body weight/minute.)[1]

The goals of cardiac rehabilitation are to help the patient achieve the highest possible level of wellness and to stabilize the disease process. The multidisciplinary team must view themselves as facilitators as they help the patient reorder his or her life. Along with exercise and diet prescriptions, cardiac rehabilitation programs must also include behavioral counseling, relaxation skills, and stress-management strategies to help the patient and family learn new life-style skills, thus helping to reduce the occurrence of major cardiac events and behavioral dysfunctions, particularly in the area of social interaction with family, spouse, and friends.

SUMMARY

Myocardial infarction is the single most important cause of death in the United States. Diagnosis is accomplished through physical examination and evaluation of the results of laboratory tests. The clinical manifestations of acute MI include chest pain and its variations, nausea and vomiting, diaphoresis, dyspnea, and characteristic physical findings. Acute MI is diagnosed and quantified by ECG and cardiac enzyme tests. Thrombolytic therapy is used routinely to dissolve the thrombus and open the occluded coronary artery if the patient arrives at the hospital within approximately 4 hours after the onset of symptoms.

The most frequently occurring complications of acute MI are psychological distress, dysrhythmia, congestive heart failure, cardiogenic shock, pericarditis, and papillary muscle dysfunction. Nurses caring for patients who have had an acute MI must understand the disease process, be able to assess symptoms suggesting complications, relate those complications to the physiologic causes, and initiate or anticipate the appropriate treatment with the goal of limiting infarct size. Expert assessment skills are needed to prevent complications. When complications occur, the nurse must be capable of implementing decisive action. The condition of these patients is unpredictable and, therefore, a great challenge to the nurse.

DIRECTIONS FOR FUTURE RESEARCH

Based on the American Association of Critical Care Nurses' research priorities and studies, research questions that nurses may consider for improving the care of patients with acute MI are as follows:[32]

1. What nursing interventions most effectively minimize stress in the patient with MI?
2. What are the effects of various visiting policies for critical care units on the psychophysiologic responses of patients with MI and their families?
3. What is the effect of patient education on the readmission rate of patients after infarction?
4. What combination of content and teaching method is most effective in preparing the patient with MI to return to a nonhospital situation and function without fear?
5. Which nursing interventions are most useful in helping the cardiac patient cope with an altered self-image and fears regarding sexuality?
6. What effect does the use of biofeedback have on the treatment of patients with MI during rehabilitation?

REFERENCES

1. Alpert, J. S., and Braunwald, E. Pathological and clinical manifestations of acute myocardial infarction. In E. Braunwald (Ed.), *Heart Disease.* Philadelphia: WB Saunders, 1980.
2. Anderson, H. R., Falk, E., and Nielsen, D. Right ventricular infarction: Frequency, size and topography in coronary heart disease: A prospective study comprising 107 consecutive autopsies from a coronary care unit. *J. Am. Coll. Cardiol.* 10(6):1223–32, 1987.
3. American Heart Association. *Heart Facts 1989.* Dallas: American Heart Association, 1988.
4. Barnaby, P., Barrett, P., and Lvoff, R. Routine prophylactic lidocaine in acute myocardial infarction. *Heart Lung* 12:362, 1983.
5. Berg, R., Selinger, S. L., Leonard, J. J., et al. Immediate coronary artery bypass for acute evolving myocardial infarction. *J. Thorac. Cardiovasc. Surg.* 81:493, 1981.
6. Berne, R. M., and Levy, M. N. *Cardiovascular Physiology* (5th ed.). St. Louis: CV Mosby, 1986.
7. Berra, K. Cardiac rehabilitation update. *Crit. Care Update* 9:30, 1982.
8. Braunwald, E., Sonnenblick, E. H., and Ross, J. Mechanisms of Cardiac Contraction and Relaxation. In E. Braunwald (Ed.), *Heart Disease* (3rd ed.). Philadelphia: WB Saunders, 1988.
9. Braunwald, E., and Sobel, B. Coronary Blood Flow and Myocardial Ischemia. In Braunwald, E. (Ed.), *Heart Disease* (3rd ed.). Philadelphia: WB Saunders, 1988.
10. Brownell, K. D., and Venditti, E. M. The Etiology and Treatment of Obesity. In Fasin, W. E., Kararan, I., Pokorny, A. D., et al. (Eds.). *Phenomenology and Treatment of Psychophysiological Disorders,* Bridgeport, CT: Luce Publishers, 1982.
11. Carpenito, L. J. *Nursing Diagnosis: Application to Clinical Practice.* Philadelphia: JB Lippincott, 1983.
12. Chesney, M. A., and Rosenman, R. H. Type A behavior: Observation in the past decade. *Heart Lung* 11:12, 1982.
13. Cohn, J. N. Vasodilator therapy: Implications in acute myocardial infarction and congestive heart failure. *Am. Heart J.* 103:773, 1982.
14. Dewood, M. A., Spores, J., Notske, R., et al. Prevalence of total coronary occlusion during the early hours of transmural myocardial infarction. *N. Engl. J. Med.* 303:897, 1980.
15. Dossey, L. *Space, Time and Medicine.* Boulder, CO: Shambhala, 1982.
16. Eagan, J. S. Lasers: Applications in cardiovascular atherosclerotic disease. *Crit. Care Nurs. Clin. North Am.* 1:2, 311–326, 1989.

17. Emde, K. L., and Searle, L. D. Current practices with thrombolytic therapy. *J. Cardiovasc. Nurs.* 4:1, 11–21, 1989.
18. Friedman, M., Thoresem, C. E., Gill, J. J., *et al.* Feasibility of altering type A behavior pattern after myocardial infarction. *Circulation* 66:83, 1982.
19. Goldberger, E. *Textbook of Clinical Cardiology,* St. Louis: CV Mosby, 1982.
20. Genton, R. E., and Sobel, B. E. Early intervention of interruption of acute myocardial infarction. *Mod. Concepts Cardiovasc. Dis.* 56: 7, 35–41, 1987.
21. Gotto, A. M., and Farmer, J. A. Risk Factors for Coronary Artery Disease. In E. Braunwald (Ed.), *Heart Disease* (3rd ed.). Philadelphia: WB Saunders, 1988.
22. Guzzetta, C., and Dossey, B. *Cardiovascular Nursing: Bodymind Tapestry.* St. Louis: CV Mosby, 1984.
23. Halfman-Franey, M., and Levine, S. Intracoronary stents. *Crit. Care Nurs. Clin. North Am.* 1:2, 327–337, 1989.
24. Helgeson, V. The origin, development, and current state of the literature on type A behavior. *J. Cardiovasc. Nurs.* 3:2, 59–63, 1989.
25. Hlatky, M. A., Cotugno, H. E., Mark, D. B., *et al.* Trends in physician management of uncomplicated myocardial infarction, 1970–1987. *Am. J. Cardiol.* 61:8, 515–518, 1987.
26. Johnson, J. E. Effects of accurate expectations about sensations on the sensory and distress components of pain. *J. Pers. Soc. Psychol.* 27:261–275, 1973.
27. Kaplan, N. M. Systemic Hypertension: Mechanisms and Diagnosis. In E. Braunwald (Ed.), *Heart Disease* (3rd ed.). Philadelphia: WB Saunders, 1988.
28. Kim, Y. I., and Williams, J. F. Large dose sublingual nitroglycerin in acute myocardial infarction: Relief of chest pain and reduction of Q wave evolution. *Am. J. Cardiol.* 49, 842, 1982.
29. Krieger, D. *Foundations for Holistic Health Nursing Practices: The Renaissance Nurse.* Philadelphia: JB Lippincott, 1981.
30. Leavitt, M., and Minarik, P. The agitated, hypervigilant response. In B. Riegel and D. Ehrenreich (Eds.), *Psychological Aspects of Critical Care Nursing.* Rockville, MD: Aspen, 1989.
31. Levin, D. C., and Gardiner, G. A. Coronary Arteriography. In E. Braunwald (Ed.), *Heart Disease* (3rd ed.). Philadelphia: WB Saunders, 1988.
32. Lewandowski, L., and Kositsky, A. Research priorities for critical care nursing: A study by the American Association of Critical Care Nurses. *Heart Lung* 12:35, 1983.
33. Luna-Raines, M. The Confused Response. In B. Riegel and D. Ehrenreich (Eds.), *Psychological Aspects of Critical Care Nursing.* Rockville, MD: Aspen, 1989.
34. Mautner, R., and Phillips, J. Coronary arteriography prior to hospital discharge after first myocardial infarction. *Heart Lung* 12: 171, 1983.
35. Meador, B. Cardiogenic shock: Help break the vicious circle. *RN* 45:38, 1982.
36. Medical news: Lidocaine-cimetidine interaction can be toxic. *J.A.M.A.* 247:3174, 1982.
37. Miller, N. Acute Myocardial Infarction. In B. Riegel and D. Ehrenreich (Eds.), *Psychological Aspects of Critical Care Nursing.* Rockville, MD: Aspen, 1989.
38. Muller, J. E., and Tofler, G. E. Circadian variation in onset of cardiovascular disease. In E. Braunwald (Ed.), *Heart Disease: Update.* Philadelphia: WB Saunders, 1988:13–24.
39. Murdaugh, C. Coronary heart disease in women. *Prog. Cardiovasc. Nurs.* 1:1, 2–8, 1986.
40. Norris, R. M., Brandt, P. W. T., Caughey, D. E., *et al.* A new coronary prognostic index. *Lancet* 1:274–278, 1969.
41. Ornish, D. Effects of stress management training and dietary changes in treating ischemic heart disease. *J.A.M.A.* 249:54, 1983.
42. Pasternak, R. C., Braunwald, E., and Sobel, B. E. Acute myocardial infarction. In E. Braunwald (Ed.), *Heart Disease* (3rd ed.). Philadelphia: WB Saunders, 1988.
43. Portu, J. B., Mooney, J. F., Kilber, L. A., *et al.* Differences in psychological status and risk factor modification at follow-up between patients undergoing coronary angioplasty and bypass surgery (abstract 0749). *Circulation* (Suppl. II) 80:4, 1989.
44. Pyles, S. H. Role of the critical care nurse in the early detection and prevention of cardiogenic shock: Discovery of the weak link (abstract). *Heart Lung* 12:428, 1983.
45. Randall, E. Recognizing cardiac tamponade. *J. Cardiovascular. Nurs.* 3:3, 1989, 42–51.
46. Riegel, B. Acute Myocardial Infarction: Nursing Interventions to Optimize Oxygen Supply and Demand. In L. Kern, *Cardiac Critical Care Nursing.* Rockville, MD: Aspen, 1988.
47. Robbins, M., and Schacht, T. Family hierarchies. *Am. J. Nurs.* 82: 284, 1982.
48. Roberts, R. Diagnostic assessment of myocardial infarction based on lactate dehydrogenase and creatine kinase isoenzymes. *Heart Lung* 10:486, 1981.
49. Roberts, R. Results of calcium antagonist trials in the management of acute myocardial infarction. Presented at the American College of Cardiology Conference at Snowmass, CO, January, 1987.
50. Roberts, R. Calcium antagonists in the prevention of reinfarction. Presented at the American College of Cardiology Conference at Snowmass, CO, January, 1989.
51. Ross, R. The Pathogenesis of Atherosclerosis. In E. Braunwald (Ed.), *Heart Disease* (3rd ed.). Philadelphia: WB Saunders, 1988.
52. Ross, A. M. Thrombolysis and angioplasty in acute myocardial infarction—1988. Presented at the American College of Cardiology: Future Directions in Interventional Cardiology, Santa Barbara, CA, September 16–18, 1988.
53. Ross, J. Role of vasodilator therapy. In J. S. Karliner and G. Gregoratos, *Coronary Care.* New York: Churchill Livingstone, 1981.
54. Rude, R. E., Muller, J. E., Braunwald, E., *et al.* Efforts to limit the size of myocardial infarcts. *Ann. Intern. Med.* 95:736, 1981.
55. Rude, R. E., and MILIS Study Group. Myocardial infarct extension: Incidence and clinical significance in MILIS. *Circulation* (Suppl. III) 72:55, 1985.
56. Sarkar, A. Myocardial rupture in myocardial infarction: Case report and review of the literature. *Heart Lung* 12:88, 1983.
57. Saunders, J., and Valente, S. The Withdrawn Response. In B. Riegel and D. Ehrenreich (Eds.), *Psychological Aspects of Critical Care Nursing.* Rockville, MD: Aspen, 1989.
58. Sebilia, A. J. Sleep deprivation of biological rhythms in the critical care unit. *Crit. Care Nurse* 1:19, 1981.
59. Seger, H., and Schlesinger, Z. Rehabilitation of patients after acute myocardial infarction: An interdisciplinary, family-oriented program. *Heart Lung* 10:841, 1981.
60. Sivarajan, E., Newton, K., Almes, M. J., *et al.* Limited effects of outpatient teaching and counseling after myocardial infarction: A controlled study. *Heart Lung* 12:65, 1983.
61. Smith, A. Physiology, diagnosis, and life-style modification for hyperlipidemia. *J. Cardiovasc. Nurs.* 1:4, 1987, 15–27.
62. Spence, M. E., and Lemberg, L. Glucose-insulin-potassium in acute myocardial infarction. *Heart Lung* 9:905, 1980.
63. Thomas, S., Sappington, E., Gross, H. S., *et al.* Denial in coronary care patients—an objective reassessment. *Heart Lung* 12:74, 1983.
64. Trevino, S. Risk factors for arrhythmias after myocardial infarction. *Heart Lung* 12:74, 1983.
65. Valladares, B., and Lemberg, L. Intravenous nitroglycerin in acute infarction. *Heart Lung* 11:383, 1982.
66. Winslow, E. H., Lane, L., and Gaffney, A. Oxygen uptake and cardiovascular response in patients and normal adults during in-bed and out-of-bed toileting. *J. Cardiac Rehab.* 4, 348, 1984.
67. Wyman, M., and Gore, S. Lidocaine prophylaxis in myocardial infarction: A concept whose time has come. *Heart Lung* 12:358, 1983.

26

Cardiac Surgery

Gayle R. Whitman   *Cathie E. Guzzetta*

HEALING IN THE MIDST OF DYING

When technology cannot reverse the death process, how often are you aware of creating a place for peace, love, compassion, and openness for the patient and family? Can you remember seeing people die surrounded by their families and friends in the midst of love and life because they were fully present in the moment? The following are a few examples of times when nurses helped facilitate dying in peace for patients and their families:

- Lynn, a 30-year-old mother of three children, was dying with end-stage heart failure. She asked her nurse whether guitar music could be played in her critical care room. The nurse spoke from her heart and arranged to meet Lynn's last request. Three hours before her death, the nurse tended to Lynn, her family, and friends. Her friends sang her favorite songs as one played a guitar. Lynn died with her children, husband, parents, and three friends surrounding her in the critical care unit.

- Jack, a 14-year-old boy in end-stage pulmonary failure, never made it off of the ventilator. However, while on the ventilator, when he was still conscious, he wrote a note to his nurse. The note read, "Call mom and have her bring my collection of bandanas and my country music tapes."

  Nothing else could be done. The physician and nurses felt that death was imminent. As the nurse continued to care for Jack, she let the family remain in the room at all times. Jack's mother, father, brother, and sister surrounded him during his last 3 hours. During his dying time, Jack and his family were listening to his favorite music while he wore a brightly colored bandana across his forehead. The last gesture Jack made was to smile as he tied another bandana around the palm of his hand; he made a fist and raised his arm, indicating being a winner. With a smile on his face, he lapsed into a coma, his heart beat dropped, and he died within minutes.

  Jack's critical care bed was needed for another patient from the emergency room. However, the nurse realized this family needed more time to be with Jack. All life-support equipment and intravenous lines were removed, and the family and Jack's body were moved to a private room at the end of the critical care unit. The family stayed for another hour with their deceased son. When the nurse discussed the steps necessary in preparing their son for transport to the funeral home, the mother asked if she could help. Indeed, this was an unusual happening, but the nurse had an inner knowing that this is what the mother wanted. Tears fell down the mother's cheeks as she stroked her son's upper body, and held him on his side for the nurse to finish his care. Tears also flowed down the nurse's cheeks as she completed her work. When the work was finished, the mother and nurse held each other while crying together. The room was filled with immense love and healing.

LEARNING OBJECTIVES

After reading this chapter, the nurse should be able to do the following:

1. Describe the pathophysiology of coronary artery disease and valvular heart disease.
2. Discuss the major indications for coronary artery bypass surgery.
3. Compare and contrast mechanical versus biologic prosthetic heart valves.
4. Outline the steps involved in the patient's preparation for cardiac surgery.
5. Describe the management of patients during the immediate postoperative phase.
6. Identify and describe the management of postoperative complications.
7. Outline the nursing diagnoses, patient outcomes, and nursing orders for patients undergoing cardiac surgery.
8. Describe the management of patients during the rehabilitation phase.

CASE STUDY

Mr. G. H., a 64-year-old white shoemaker, was admitted to the telemetry unit for evaluation of chest pain. He was free of symptoms despite his moderately strenuous job until about 6 months ago, when he began experiencing chest pain during physical exertion (about one or two times a week). The dull, tight chest pain was retrosternal and radiated to his neck and left arm. The pain was relieved promptly by rest and nitroglycerin. It was not associated with dyspnea or diaphoresis, and it never lasted more than 5 minutes.

During the past 2 months, the pain had increased in frequency and severity, occurring three or four times a day with minimal exertion (e.g., walking short distances) or excitement. Occasionally, it occurred when Mr. H. woke up or when he was at rest. He was given sublingual isosorbide dinitrate (5 mg every 6 hours) in addition to his usual nitroglycerin, but his condition did not improve. Because the attacks continued to become more frequent and severe, Mr. H. was hospitalized for further assessment and observation.

Mr. H. had a nervous, restless personality. Divorced once, he was currently married. He had a son, aged 36, from his first marriage. He had smoked two packs of cigarettes a day for 30 years, and he drank moderately on weekends (four or five cocktails). His interests were bass fishing and bowling. He said that he was allergic to sulfa drugs. He was Catholic.

Mr. H.'s past medical history included an appendectomy in 1952 and a hemorrhoidectomy in 1960. His mother had a history of diabetes mellitus, and his father died at age 60 of a myocardial infarction. His older brother, aged 66, had an acute myocardial infarction 2 years ago. The rest of Mr. H.'s family history was not relevant.

Mr. H.'s physical examination showed that he was a well-developed, well-nourished, middle-aged man who was not in acute distress. His blood pressure was 160/110. He had grade II hypertensive changes in his fundi. Examination of his neck was normal with no jugular venous distention. Examination of his lungs revealed bilateral rhonchi that cleared when he coughed. His heart was regular at 110 beats/minute. He had a normal first and second heart sound and no third heart sound, murmurs, or rubs. He had an atrial gallop at the fifth intercostal space, midclavicular line. His abdomen, back, genitourinary system, and extremities were normal.

Mr. H.'s electrocardiogram (ECG) showed a regular sinus tachycardia, and his chest x-ray was normal. His lung fields were clear. His electrolyte values, serum cholesterol, and triglyceride levels were within normal limits. A graded exercise test was performed. The results were clearly positive, with the simultaneous development of angina pectoris.

Coronary angiography was performed. The results revealed that the high lateral branch of the proximal circumflex coronary artery was narrowed 80% to 85% by a number of nondiscrete lesions. The first third of the proximal anterior descending branch of the left coronary artery was narrowed 70% to 80%. Both arteries appeared to have good distal runoff. The right coronary artery was found to be normal. A left ventriculogram revealed a normal ejection fraction and normal contractility. There were no valvular defects or ventricular aneurysms.

Because of the information gathered from Mr. H.'s history, exercise testing, and coronary angiography, myocardial revascularization was recommended. Discussion of the risk factors, surgery, and preoperative teaching were done by a nurse-physician team. The next day, Mr. H. was taken to surgery.

REFLECTIONS

Cardiac surgery has a profound impact on the psychobiologic unity of the patient. In many cultures, the heart is popularly regarded as the center of life. A disease of the heart can seriously disrupt one's adaptation capacity, perhaps more than can a disease of most other organs. The nurse and the patient participate together in an important role; together they work to help the patient achieve an acceptable level of psychobiologic adaptation during the preoperative and postoperative phases. The nurse might ask "Why is that process beneficial in helping patients to adapt?" The following paragraphs discuss this issue.

The idea of the patient as a psychobiologic unit (see Chap. 1) can be enormously fruitful when applied to patient education. As a psychobiologic unit, patients are not divisible into body and mind; they are inseparably both. Mind and body operate on a continuum. If the mind is educable, so is the body; thus, to educate the mind is to educate the body.

The idea of psychobiologic unity increases the nurse's opportunities for providing effective care. Because of the body-mind continuum, therapy can be more than drugs, treatments, and surgical procedures. The nurse's contributions to patient education can result in "body effects" that are as real as those achieved by traditional forms of therapy. Because of its importance in affecting the body-mind continuum, patient education should be viewed as a mandatory goal, not an elective one. The critical care nurse must come to view the teaching-learning process as an indispensable part of the therapeutic process, one that is applicable to all patients and all illnesses.

What about teaching a patient who is in crisis or who has been admitted to a critical care unit because of a sudden illness? Most of the research done in this area has led us to believe that teaching critically ill patients is not effective because patients are too anxious and too sick. Under such conditions, we say that teaching is not effective because patients usually do not remember or understand much of the information or do not comply with what has been taught. When we measure the effectiveness of teaching in terms of how much patients remember or change their behavior, we are evaluating only the products of the teaching-learning process. It has been suggested that it is inappropriate to evaluate the *products of teaching* when dealing with critically ill patients. In such patients, we should be more concerned about evaluating the immediate impact that the teaching has on the patient or the *process of the teaching*.[98]

Evaluating the process is very different from evaluating the products (outcomes) of teaching because it implies that each nurse-patient encounter has therapeutic value and worth. Each time the patient and nurse interact, the nurse meaningfully affects the patient's physiologic and psychologic status. Each time a nurse answers a patient's question regarding the illness or diagnostic tests or procedures or identifies a patient's need, such intervention is viewed as a teaching encounter that produces a body-mind-spirit response in the patient. Each time a nurse provides physical care, the intervention affects much more than the patient's physical status. The immediate teaching exchange can be viewed as effective because of the process, or the body-mind-spirit impact, that the exchange had on the patient at that moment. This exchange may not be remembered by the patient hours or even minutes later, and the effects (outcomes) of the exchange may be subtle and unmeasurable, but there is no doubt that it was effective in meeting the momentary body-mind-spirit needs of the patient at the time. Examining the value of the teaching process permits us to view all teaching-learning experiences as successful. It permits us to focus our attention on teaching exchanges that are therapeutic and have meaning for the patient, rather than being concerned about evaluating inappropriate outcomes for critically ill patients.[98]

When dealing with patients who are not in extreme crisis and who are assessed to be ready to learn, the nurse may ask "How do I begin? What should I teach?" A starting point for any type of patient education program is standardizing the information to be presented. The content should be developed and approved by nurses, physicians, dietitians, psychiatrists, members of the clergy, and occupational, physical, and respiratory therapists. The input from the health team members helps in deciding what should be taught, prevents the omission of necessary information, and ensures that the material is presented consistently by everyone.

Standardization, however, does not imply formalization of patient education. The patient's needs, concerns, level of learning, and anxiety and other factors that inhibit or promote the teaching-learning process are individually assessed and incorporated into the body-mind-spirit approach. During preoperative and postoperative teaching periods, nurses also identify and evaluate what areas the patient feels are important. They should encourage the patient to ask questions and to participate actively in the process. Nurses who are involved in the preparation of written teaching materials might also identify other areas of concern by sending the materials to patients who have been discharged and asking them for their recommendations and suggestions.

An important objective in educating cardiac surgical patients is reduction of their anxiety and fear. Descriptions of procedures, treatments, and methods of care are usually included in the teaching. It has also been discovered,[112] however, that the usual practice of explaining the meaning or need for a test, procedure, or surgery in detail is not as effective in reducing the patient's stress as is giving the patient accurate descriptions of how and what will be felt (*i.e.,* during a cardiac catheterization, with an endotracheal tube, while on a ventilator, or when being suctioned). Thus, the patient wants to know the "how" and "what" of an experience before the "why."

MYOCARDIAL REVASCULARIZATION

Vineberg developed the first operative approach for myocardial revascularization in 1946.[236] This approach involved tunneling the left ventricular wall and implanting the internal mammary artery in the myocardium (Fig. 26–1). Vineberg be-

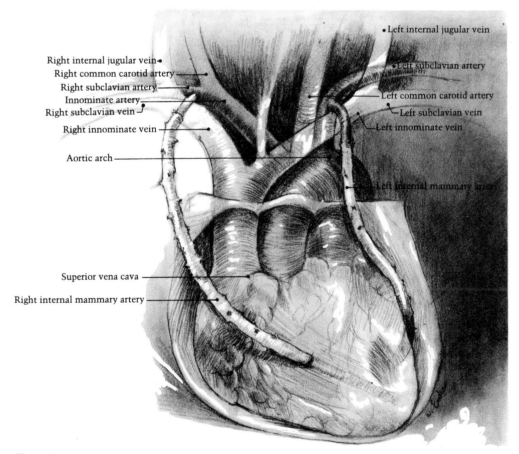

Figure 26–1

Internal mammary artery implant (Vineberg procedure). The Vineberg procedure is the older method of myocardial revascularization.

lieved that the implanted artery would anastomose with the arteriolar network of the cardiac muscle and form channels supplying blood to the main coronary circulation. Vineberg's indirect revascularization approach was reported to have had excellent clinical results. But because methods to evaluate the approach objectively were lacking, it did not become popular until the early sixties.

In 1962, Sones developed a safe and reliable procedure for coronary angiography.[216] The procedure enabled the location and extent of the atherosclerotic coronary obstruction to be visualized, and it also provided a method to evaluate the results of cardiac surgery. Consequently, new interest was created in the Vineberg procedure,[74,173] and in developing techniques for direct myocardial revascularization.[67,199,207]

Investigators began exploring the feasibility of direct revascularization using the saphenous vein for grafts. Aortocoronary bypass surgery was first performed in 1965,[86] and the initial trials were reported on by Favalaro and associates[75,76] and Johnson and associates.[113] Although there have been minor changes in the techniques of cardiopulmonary bypass, the basic procedure, aortocoronary saphenous vein bypass, has remained one of the important methods of revascularization.

In addition to aortocoronary saphenous vein bypass, the use of one of the branches of the internal mammary or thoracic artery has accelerated over the past few years and in some centers accounts for at least half of the conduits used to achieve revascularization.[2,44,146] With this technique, the internal mammary artery is anastomosed to the coronary artery rather than being implanted in a tunnel in the myocardium, as was done in the past.

Occasionally, endarterectomy is done, which involves removing the arterial endothelium and cholesterol plaques attached to the coronary artery.[139] Percutaneous transluminal coronary angioplasty (PTCA) also can be used as a nonsurgical alternative to aortocoronary bypass surgery in a select group of patients (see p. 440).

INDICATIONS FOR MYOCARDIAL REVASCULARIZATION

In coronary artery disease, atherosclerotic plaques are primarily composed of cholesterol, other lipids, and fibrous tissue that are deposited along the intimal wall of the coronary artery (see Chap. 25). Typically, the atherosclerotic plaques are found in the larger portions of an artery, resulting in proximal narrowing or occlusion with little involvement in the smaller distal sections. The amount of involvement of one or more branches of the coronary arteries depends on the patient's individual disease process. When the atherosclerotic process impairs the coronary blood flow to the myocardium, serious hemodynamic disturbances and clinical manifestations are observed.[167]

The selection of a patient for myocardial revascularization surgery is based on the belief that revascularizing the myocardium will improve the patient's symptoms and will lengthen the patient's survival, particularly in those patients with left main or triple-vessel coronary artery disease.[139] Not all patients with coronary artery disease are candidates for surgery. Myocardial revascularization is frequently recommended for patients with angina pectoris, signs of ischemia, or an increased risk of myocardial infarction or death based on angiographic findings.[139] Moreover, it is recommended, that it be performed before or done simultaneously with other needed operations

to protect the myocardium and prevent the occurrence of cardiac complications, particularly the development of acute myocardial infarctions.[140,156] The following pages discuss the indications for aortocoronary bypass surgery.

Intractable Angina Pectoris

Patients with severe, or intractable, angina pectoris find their lives greatly limited or crippled because their disease imposes great psychobiologic and socioeconomic problems.[68] Medically, such patients are treated first by controlling hypertension or other coexisting medical problems, stopping smoking, and giving long-acting nitrates, beta-adrenergic blocking drugs, or calcium channel–blocking drugs alone or in combination.[211] If a patient continues to have intractable pain that is easily precipitated by emotional or physiologic stressors despite adequate medical therapy, surgery (or PTCA) is considered. In patients with mild to moderate angina, surgical intervention is also more likely to provide relief of symptoms than medical therapy,[33,73] with two thirds of patients still reporting themselves asymptomatic 5 years after surgery.[146]

High-risk Pathoanatomic Lesions

The increased risk of developing an acute myocardial infarction or death with severe stenotic lesions in specific anatomic locations has been proved. A significant lesion is illustrated in Figure 26–2. Conclusive findings from several groups have shown increased survival after myocardial revascularization in patients with left main coronary artery lesions when compared with those patients treated medically.[44,73,107,169,175,228] Survival has also been shown to be increased after myocardial revascularization in patients with significant triple-vessel disease[33,73] and, perhaps, double-vessel disease, provided that the patient's left ventricular function is not severely impaired. Patients with single-vessel disease and less severe double-vessel disease are particularly controversial groups with regard to their treatment, although recently PTCA has been used to treat significant lesions for these patients to improve the quality of life and reduce dependence on medications.[211]

Although survival has not been shown to be different in medically versus surgically treated patients with single-vessel disease (with the exception of left main coronary artery lesions), stenoses of the proximal left anterior descending coronary artery (just below the bifurcation of the left main coronary artery) are more serious lesions than those in the right or circumflex coronary artery.[139] Such patients are considered for myocardial revascularization or PTCA because proximal lesions in the left anterior descending coronary artery affect a larger portion of the myocardium, thereby placing a larger segment of the myocardium in jeopardy than do more distal lesions.[114,139,211]

Unstable Angina Pectoris

Unstable angina pectoris, another indication for myocardial revascularization, has been called a number of different names (Table 26–1). The term *unstable angina pectoris* is probably the best one to describe patients with a broad spectrum of disorders.[51,188] It is characterized by the following phenomena:[67,85]

- Recurring progressive episodes of angina pectoris lasting longer than 15 minutes and poorly relieved by rest or nitroglycerin.

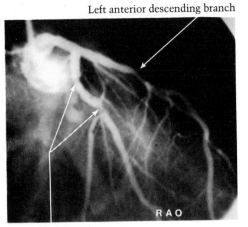

Left anterior descending branch

Circumflex branch

A

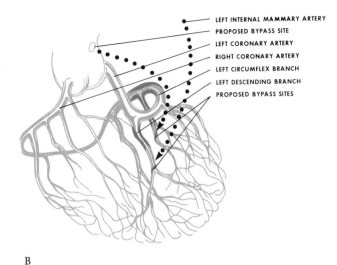

LEFT INTERNAL MAMMARY ARTERY
PROPOSED BYPASS SITE
LEFT CORONARY ARTERY
RIGHT CORONARY ARTERY
LEFT CIRCUMFLEX BRANCH
LEFT DESCENDING BRANCH
PROPOSED BYPASS SITES

B

Figure 26–2

(*A*) Selective coronary angiography prior to surgery, showing a right anterior oblique projection of the left coronary artery and demonstrating significant occlusive lesions (>50% narrowing of the luminal diameter) in the circumflex and anterior descending branches of the left coronary artery (*arrows*). (*B*) Proposed bypass of severe stenosis of the circumflex and anterior descending branches of the left coronary artery. The *arrows* indicate the routes taken in placing a saphenous vein graft in the circumflex and the internal mammary artery in the left anterior descending branch.

- Deteriorating chronic angina pectoris (which was previously stable) that has become more easily provoked, increased in frequency, intensity, and duration, and less readily relieved by nitroglycerin or rest.
- No diagnostic evidence of serum cardiac enzyme changes.
- No ECG evidence that is consistent with acute myocardial infarction.
- ST- or T-wave changes associated with myocardial ischemia.

Physiologically, the condition suggests that the coronary blood supply relative to the demand is deficient, even at rest. Hemodynamically, unstable angina pectoris is associated with a rise in heart rate and blood pressure that precedes the onset of pain. Because heart rate and blood pressure are the chief determinants of coronary blood flow demand, increasing these parameters can create a relative ischemia.

As its name states, the condition is unstable and associated with a higher morbidity and mortality than is stable angina

pectoris. In medically treated patients, the incidence of myocardial infarction is high,[129,142,174,196] and the mortality rate at 1 year from the onset of symptoms is 10%, with about half these deaths occurring within 1 month.[188] Aspirin therapy is useful in reducing myocardial infarction in this group of patients.[132,192]

Because unstable angina pectoris usually responds well to aggressive medical treatment, the patient is stabilized for several days to weeks with bed rest, a quiet environment, oxygen, sedation, intravenous nitroglycerin, vasodilators, beta-adrenergic receptor blocking drugs, calcium channel–blocking drugs, and, perhaps, anticoagulation or antiplatelet therapy (to prevent myocardial infarction), and the intra-aortic balloon pump. After stabilization, coronary angiography, thrombolysis therapy, or PTCA or aortocoronary bypass surgery are then performed.[71,187,193] Control of the ischemia thus allows the surgeon to operate on a stable patient who is at low risk. If the pain does not subside in 48 to 72 hours, however, emergency coronary angiography and aortocoronary bypass surgery are seriously considered.[109,217]

Acute Myocardial Infarction

Many new interventions are available for patients with acute myocardial infarction. Because the balance between myocardial oxygen demand and supply appears to determine the fate of the ischemic area, various pharmacologic and mechanical interventions have been used to improve this relationship in patients with evolving acute myocardial infarctions.

Intravenous nitroprusside and nitroglycerin can be used to reduce left ventricular afterload. Beta-blocking agents such as timolol and propranolol have been shown to have not only antianginal effects but also a secondary preventative effect on

Table 26-1

Terms Used to Describe the Syndrome Between Stable Angina Pectoris and Acute Myocardial Infarction

Unstable angina pectoris
Intermediate coronary syndrome
Acute coronary syndrome
Preinfarction angina pectoris
Crescendo angina pectoris
Accelerated angina pectoris
Impending myocardial infarction
Threatening myocardial infarction
Prethrombotic syndrome
Preocclusive syndrome
Coronary failure
Rest angina

the myocardium and when given intravenously can decrease the mortality and rate of infarction.[15,108,177] Mechanical circulatory-assist devices, have also been effective in decreasing the ischemic process in this group of patients.[18,71,100]

Thrombolytic therapy using intracoronary or intravenous infusions of *streptokinase* or tPA (recombinant tissue plasminogen activator) can restore blood flow in patients with transmural myocardial infarctions and decrease the size of the infarction (see Chap. 25). Percutaneous transluminal coronary angioplasty or coronary artery bypass surgery may need to be performed in patients with unstable angina pectoris or persistent stenosis to ensure continued myocardial reperfusion after thrombolysis therapy.[140]

In the past, aortocoronary bypass surgery was contraindicated in the presence of acute myocardial infarction. Current evidence suggests that emergency revascularization performed on selected patients may be effective in interrupting the ischemic process or in reducing the size of the infarct.[20,24,25,118,140,244]

It is known that infarcted muscle is surrounded by a "twilight zone" of ischemic tissue after an acute myocardial infarction. Such a zone, which is destined to become necrotic, remains viable for several hours after the acute infarct.[70] It can be salvaged if emergency revascularization is performed in 3 to 6 hours.[85,118] Thus the success of emergency surgery for an evolving myocardial infarction depends largely on the timing of the operation, and only patients who arrive at the hospital early after the onset of symptoms are considered as candidates. Because preparing the patient for coronary angiography and surgery is generally time-consuming, emergency surgery is frequently not feasible.

The question of whether to recommend cardiac angiography and possible myocardial revascularization in patients who have recently suffered an acute myocardial infarction is an important one. In patients who survive acute myocardial infarction, 10% to 15% will die in the first year.[72,139] Of those who survive the initial insult, 20% will have severe left ventricular impairment (ejection fraction < 30%), and from this subgroup, mortality ranges from 25% to 45% in the first year[61,169] and as high as 60% at two years.[172] In the remaining 80%, the mortality rate is very low.[61,139]

It is therefore important to determine the patient's risk status after acute myocardial infarction. Patients at high risk include those with persistent or recurrent angina pectoris, congestive heart failure, or intractable ventricular dysrhythmias.[139,190] These patients may be considered for coronary angiography and cardiac catheterization to determine the extent of coronary artery disease and to evaluate the presence of ventricular aneurysm, ventricular septal defects, or mitral regurgitation.[72,139] In contrast, exercise testing has been recommended to help identify high-risk patients who have no clinical postinfarction pain, ventricular failure, or dysrhythmias.[61,72] It has also been recommended that patients who develop pain and electrocardiographic evidence of myocardial ischemia during exercise should undergo coronary angiography to determine whether they are candidates for PTCA or surgical revascularization.[72,139] Recent evidence has shown, however, that when compared with medical therapy, myocardial revascularization does not appear to improve the 5-year survival nor prevent myocardial infarction in patients who are free of angina pectoris or who have mild angina pectoris after acute myocardial infarction.[32]

Congestive Heart Failure

The indications for myocardial revascularization in the treatment of congestive heart failure are controversial.[174] Ventricular dysfunction is generally the result of an extensive area of infarcted myocardium, and it is reasonable to believe that revascularization may not be beneficial in reversing the damage.

Candidates for surgery are those who have angina pectoris as their major symptom, an acceptable ejection fraction, bypassable coronary arteries, and not more than two dyskinetic left ventricular wall segments (*i.e.*, segments that show paradoxical systolic expansion).[174] The use of early postoperative mechanical circulatory assistance has been helpful in this group of patients.[104]

Incremental risk factors for operative mortality in patients with congestive heart failure undergoing surgery are age, ejection fraction, presence of mitral regurgitation, and presence of left main coronary artery disease.[237] Generally, the poorer the left ventricular ejection fraction is the higher the mortality. However, recent studies indicate, that despite operating on patients with lower ejection fractions than in the past, the operative survival rates have remained the same or improved in spite of the increasing risk of these patients.[44,52,183] This is largely attributed to improved pre-, intra-, and postoperative management and acumen.

Congestive heart failure may also develop secondary to an aneurysm, rupture of the intraventricular septum, or mitral insufficiency. In patients who develop an aneurysm that is refractory to medical therapy, excision of the ventricular aneurysm and semiemergent myocardial revascularization may be considered.[118] Patients who develop a systolic murmur and heart failure after myocardial infarction may have intraventricular septal rupture or mitral insufficiency. Patients with septal rupture should undergo immediate operation to close the defect, and myocardial revascularization is usually not performed.[118] Depending on the severity of the problem, patients with mitral insufficiency may be treated medically or valve replacement surgery may be considered.

Cardiogenic Shock

Cardiogenic shock after an acute myocardial infarction has an 85% to 95% mortality in patients treated medically.[143,174] Intra-aortic balloon pumping with its ability to unload the left ventricle and augment coronary blood flow has been effective in reversing the shock state for several hours or days. In some instances, as many as 75% of these patients have been stabilized.[19] Once stabilized, these patients can proceed to coronary angiography and more definitive therapy over the next few days or weeks. Long-term survival is about 80%.[19] If stabilization does not occur, then immediate coronary angiography, closure of an intraventricular septal rupture, excision of a ventricular aneurysm, mitral valve replacement, or myocardial revascularization is required. Operative survival rates in these patients can be as high as 45% to 84%.[19,20,136,231]

Refractory Ventricular Irritability

Myocardial revascularization has been indicated for other complications of acute myocardial infarction. Recurrent, symptomatic ventricular dysrhythmias that are refractory to medical management pose a serious problem. If the ventricular dysrhythmias are induced by ischemia, myocardial revascularization can be helpful. Most frequently, however, these dysrhythmias arise as a result of re-entry pathways that exist along the rim of an aneurysm or infarcted tissue. When this is the case, extensive endocardial and epicardial mapping is performed to identify the precise areas of arrhythmogenesis (see Chap. 24). Surgical resection of the endocardium or catheter ablation of the tissue is then carried out to destroy the re-entry pathways. Although quite successful, antidysrhythmic drugs or an automatic implantable cardioverter-defibrillator (AICD) may still be required.[28,96,102,116,154,159]

PATIENT SELECTION

To determine whether a patient is a candidate for surgery, the findings from the history, physical examination, and laboratory and diagnostic tests must be evaluated (see Assessment).

OPERATIVE TECHNIQUE: MYOCARDIAL REVASCULARIZATION

In addition to the parameters usually monitored, most patients undergoing cardiac surgery have continuous monitoring of systemic and pulmonary arterial pressures, venous pressures, urinary output, the ECG, and blood gas measurements. Depending on the hospital's policy and the availability of equipment, left atrial pressure monitoring may also be done. The anesthetic drugs used may include narcotic anesthetics (*e.g.*, morphine sulfate, fentanyl, or sufentanil) with supplemental inhalation agents (*e.g.*, halothane, enflurane, or isoflurane).

The surgery is performed through a median sternotomy incision to allow good exposure of the heart and to avoid entering the pleural spaces. The pericardium is opened to expose the heart. The patient is prepared for cardiopulmonary bypass or extracorporeal circulation used to oxygenate the blood, remove carbon dioxide, and provide peripheral blood flow to meet the metabolic needs of the body. A cannula is placed in a vein and artery to direct blood flow from the heart to the bypass machine and then return it to the patient. Arterial cannulas can be placed in the femoral artery, iliac artery, or ascending aorta. Venous cannulas are placed in the venae cavae or the right atrium. The specific sites for vessel cannulation are determined by the type of surgery performed and the preference of the surgical team. Generally, the left ventricle is vented with a cannula to aspirate intracardiac blood and to avoid overdistention of the chamber.

The bypass machine is equipped with a mechanical pump that substitutes for left ventricular pumping action and an oxygenator that performs the work of the lungs by creating a blood-gas exchange. There are several kinds of good oxygenators. The bubble oxygenator and the membrane oxygenator are the ones most commonly used.[66]

Before the patient is placed on cardiopulmonary bypass, the machine is completely primed with varying amounts of fluid (*e.g.*, dextrose, balanced salt solutions, albumin, or blood) to replace the venous blood that is diverted to the machine. The primer solution dilutes the patient's blood volume, and attempts are made to limit this degree of hemodilution so that the patient's hematocrit does not fall lower than 25%.[66,139]

Hemodilution is advantageous because it reduces the need for additional units of blood and lowers the elevated blood viscosity levels that occur with hypothermia, thereby facilitating perfusion to the microcirculation.[125,135]

The concept of blood conservation has been used in recent years to reduce the risks of hepatitis, acquired immunodeficiency syndrome (AIDS), transfusion reactions, coagulation problems, and hemolysis as well as to promote better pulmonary function.[139] In some centers, patients do not receive any blood or blood products. Blood conservation techniques are discussed in Box 26-3.

The patient is given heparin for anticoagulation, and cardiopulmonary bypass is begun. The venous reservoir is connected to the oxygenator, where venous blood is oxygenated and carbon dioxide is removed. The arterialized blood enters the heat exchanger, where it is cooled to hypothermic levels (25 to 30°C) to reduce the metabolic rate and the oxygen demands of the tissues. Cooling further protects the major organ systems from the effects of anoxia and ischemia. The blood is returned to the patient via the arterial cannula. A filter or bubble trap is used to prevent clots, fat debris, air, or other particulate matter from entering the patient's blood. The mean blood pressure is maintained during bypass by adjusting the rate of perfusion and blood volume or by administering vasopressor drugs.

Both the formed elements (red blood cells, white blood cells, and platelets) and the unformed elements (plasma proteins) of blood are traumatized by the direct contact they have with the surfaces of the pump, its mechanical action, the resultant turbulent flow, and the intracardiac suction systems. Free hemoglobin, which can generally be cleared from the blood by using mannitol or some other diuretic, clinically demonstrates its presence with transient hematuria or hemoglobinuria. The damage incurred by the other elements is tolerated well by the majority of patients; consequently, clinical symptoms do not prevail. In a small number of patients, particularly those whose perfusion times extend beyond 3 hours, blood element damage is not as well tolerated. Postoperatively, these patients develop bleeding dyscrasias, permeability pulmonary edema, and transient neurologic alterations.[125,135]

Once the patient's temperature has been lowered to 25 to 30°C, the aorta is cross-clamped and the heart is arrested and cooled by the infusion of a cold hyperkalemic cardioplegic solution into the aortic root or directly into the ostium of the coronary arteries.[205] This maneuver quickly produces an electromechanical arrest during diastole, thereby providing a quiet operative field. Additionally, the pericardium may be filled with 1 to 2 L of 4°C Ringer's lactate solution to maintain the myocardium's temperature below 15°C.[191] These myocardial preservation techniques (hypothermia and chemically induced arrest) tremendously lower the metabolic demands of the myocardium, thereby limiting the amount of myocardial cellular damage that can occur during the surgical procedure and reducing the incidence of perioperative infarctions.[139] Use of these techniques can afford the surgeon a 90- to 120-minute interval of safe myocardial protection in the majority of patients.[218]

The two most common graft conduits selected for use in myocardial revascularization are the saphenous vein and the internal mammary artery. A segment of the saphenous vein is removed from the patient's lower leg or thigh. One long incision is used or multiple short incisions are used to gain access to the vein. Once removed, the tributaries on the vein are ligated and the vein is irrigated to check for leaks. Care is taken to avoid excessive manipulation and stretching of the vessel, because this can induce spasm and cause contraction of the internal elastic membrane with resultant initiation of a thrombolic process that can affect early and late graft patency rates.[13]

The veins are grafted to the myocardium in a reversed position to avoid impedance of flow through the graft by the venous valves. Owing to their anatomic locations, the internal mammary arteries, both right and left, can also be used as grafts and are suitable for anastomosis to the right coronary artery and the left anterior descending branch of the left coronary artery. These vessels normally arise from the subclavian artery, and for revascularization purposes, they are dissected off the chest wall distally and left attached to the subclavian artery proximally. Their distal portions are then grafted to the coronary vessels.

Sequential anastomoses of a single internal mammary artery to multiple coronary artery branches can further expand the use of the internal mammary artery. In addition, difficult-to-reach posterior coronary vessels can be reached by using the internal mammary artery as a free graft with attachments at the aorta and the coronary artery.[62,149] The right gastroepiploic artery can also serve as a conduit for revascularization. Partially dissected from its omental origin, this vessel is then extended upward and serves as an *in situ* graft to the right coronary artery and its branches and the anterior descending coronary artery.[151,226] Other vessels suitable for use in revascularization include the cephalic vein and specially processed human umbilical veins. Figure 26–3 depicts a vein graft after completion of the distal anastomosis. The vein is brought upward over the right ventricle and is then proximally connected to the aorta.

Another technique still considered experimental is the use of laser energy to vaporize the occlusion. Presently, the procedure is being done in combination with traditional grafting. Follow-up on these patients and improvements in technology may demonstrate laser revascularization to be a useful technique.[87,168]

After the bypass grafts have been completed, the rate of blood flow is measured with a flowmeter. Optimal basal flow rates should exceed 40 ml/minute, and peak rates should be greater than 80 to 100 ml/minute depending on the caliber of the graft and the vessel grafted.[218]

Before removing the patient from bypass, anesthetics are discontinued, the patient is ventilated with 100% oxygen, suctioned, and the blood is rewarmed. Perfusion is discontinued slowly by reducing the venous flow over a period of several minutes. The cannulas are not removed until satisfactory arterial pressure and cardiac functioning are achieved. Atrial and ventricular pacing wires and mediastinal chest tubes are placed. Protamine sulfate is given to neutralize the effects of heparin. The sternum is sutured with wire, and the skin is closed.

OPERATIVE MORTALITY

The overall operative mortality for patients with chronic stable angina pectoris undergoing coronary bypass surgery is under 3%.[85,88] The percentage varies somewhat from institution to

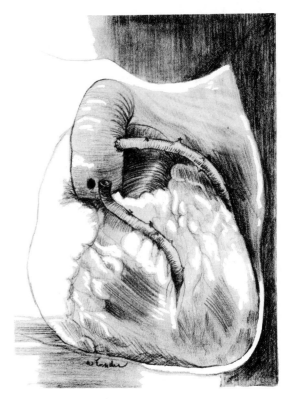

Figure 26–3
Nearly completed aortocoronary saphenous vein bypass of the circumflex and anterior descending branches of the left coronary artery.

institution, and it depends primarily on the skill of the surgeon, anesthesiologist, and cardiology team, including the skill in selecting patients.[3]

A number of risk factors have been found to affect the operative mortality. The most important factor is the patient's resting left ventricular function,[64,139] as measured by the ejection fraction. A normal ejection fraction of greater than 55% indicates an excellent operative risk, whereas an ejection fraction of 30% to 35% would be considered to be high risk. Ejection fractions of 20% to 25% or less are associated with very high risks. Other risk factors include age, urgent surgery, and reoperations. Although success rates have continued to improve in the elderly over the past few years, the increasing number of septuagenarians and octogenarians undergoing surgery has counterbalanced this improvement, still allowing age to remain as a risk factor.[44,54,64,121,171]

Emergent operations[44,54] and reoperations[44,80] are also viewed as high-risk factors. Some studies suggest that a higher risk is also evident in women.[54,77] This is generally thought to be related to their small physical size and associated small coronary artery caliber. Other studies suggest that improved microvascular surgical techniques and preoperative management have negated the effects of gender.[163,247] The same diversity of opinion exists in viewing left main trunk disease as a risk factor, with some studies indicating that it is not a risk factor because of better preoperative management and myocardial protection techniques[44,80] and others viewing it as a major risk factor.[54]

The operative mortality for patients undergoing myocardial revascularization has been reduced in recent years because of better preoperative stabilization of the patient, better adjustment of hemodynamic parameters during surgery, improved preoperative monitoring and management, and blood conservation (see Box 26-3). The most significant improvement, however, is related to the use of cold chemical cardioplegic solutions and more complete revascularization of the myocardium.

More recently, it has been demonstrated that the use of blood cardioplegia with warm induction[196] and a terminal warm cardioplegic infusion,[229] the addition of substrates,[230] Krebs-cycle intermediates,[179] or calcium antagonists[143] may decrease the incidence of postoperative low cardiac output syndrome and operative mortality.

POSTOPERATIVE COMPLICATIONS

Physiologic and psychologic complications may occur as a result of cardiopulmonary bypass, prolonged surgery time, and preoperative risk factors or disease.[188] The occurrence of perioperative myocardial infarction, which is associated with a higher hospital mortality, has been reduced to approximately 5%[85,137] for patients undergoing myocardial revascularization. Other complications are listed in Table 26–2 and are discussed on pages 450 to 495.[50]

RESULTS OF MYOCARDIAL REVASCULARIZATION

The most impressive results of myocardial revascularization are improvement in survival in selected subgroups of patients, reduction in the number of cardiac events and preoperative symptoms, and general improvements in the patient's quality of life. Myocardial revascularization has been shown to improve short-term and long-term (5 to 12 years) *survival* in patients with a significant stenosis of the left main coronary artery, triple-vessel disease, and perhaps double-vessel disease.[27,33,73,140,211,233]

The factors that influence late survival in myocardial revascularization patients are outlined in Table 26–3.[140,145] Of these factors, *left ventricular function* is the most important. A predictor of late survival is also related to the number of *un-*

Table 26-2
Postoperative Complications of Myocardial Revascularization

COMMON COMPLICATIONS	LESS COMMON COMPLICATIONS
Acute myocardial infarction	Renal failure
Vein graft closure	Stress ulcer
Dysrhythmias	Respiratory failure
Hemorrhage	Cardiac tamponade
Pneumonia	Cardiogenic shock
Pericarditis	Endocarditis
Postpericardiotomy syndrome	Gastrointestinal bleeding
Embolism	
Postcardiotomy delirium syndrome	Infection, mediastinitis
Atelectasis	Paralytic ileus
Pneumothorax	
Hemothorax	

Table 26-3
Factors That Influence Late Survival in Myocardial Revascularization Patients

Preoperative left ventricular function
Completeness of the revascularization
Age at operation
Perioperative morbidity and mortality
Graft patency
Number of ungrafted diseased vessels

grafted diseased vessels, which may, in turn, depend on the completeness of the revascularization.[140] *Complete revascularization* refers to grafts performed to all major coronary arteries (*i.e.,* greater than 1 mm in diameter) that supply viable myocardium and have 50% or greater narrowing of their luminal diameters.[140] Those patients who are completely revascularized experience less postoperative angina and have an increased length of survival.[56]

Myocardial revascularization also reduces the number of *cardiac events* in the first 5 years after operation.[35,145] One study has reported a 26% decrease in the number of cardiovascular-related hospital admissions (patients primarily admitted for acute myocardial infarction) in surgically versus medically treated patients.[99] The incidence of acute myocardial infarction in the surgically treated group was 1.1%/year, whereas the incidence in the medically treated group was 2.6%/year.

When considering a quality-of-life issue, improvement in preoperative *symptoms* may be equally important to the patient and almost as impressive as the statistics related to survival and cardiac events. There is no doubt that surgical revascularization is superior to medical therapy in improving angina pectoris.[73,165,222,239] Eighty to 90% of patients have total relief of chest pain 1 year after surgery.[50] At 5 years after surgery, about 70% of patients remain pain-free, although the recurrence of angina increases more rapidly after the 5-year period.[22,60,104,204] Unfortunately, these statistics are extremely difficult to quantify because of the subjective criteria used to evaluate chest pain.

Aortocoronary bypass surgery improves oxygenation of the myocardium.[164] A patent bypass graft establishes a normal autoregulatory pattern of functioning. There are appropriate changes in coronary blood flow during exercise, for example, that are dictated by increases in coronary vascular resistance.[122] This mechanism can be objectively evaluated by excercise testing, and most patients show improvement of their exercise tolerance both postoperatively and up to 5 years after surgery.[33,73,235] Aortocoronary bypass patients also report fewer symptoms during sexual activity and use less antianginal medications than do angina patients treated medically.[139]

Preoperative left ventricular dysfunction resulting from ischemia is improved during exercise after myocardial revascularization,[50,164] but it is not changed if the dysfunction was a result of myocardial infarction.[188] Postoperatively, ejection fraction and ventricular wall motion abnormalities during exercise are also improved.[139] Thus, there is an increase in myocardial work capacity, allowing the patient to be physically able to engage in more activity and generally to experience a greater quality of life.[104,127]

Relief of angina pectoris usually does, although it may not, correspond with the effectiveness of the bypass graft. In some patients, one or more grafts may become occluded, but the patients still have relief from angina pectoris; whereas other patients may have patent grafts, but no improvement in symptoms. The rate of vein graft occlusion varies in patients from 5% to 20% within the first year after surgery, with an average yearly occlusion rate of 2.2% between 1 and 6 years.[145,211]

Postoperative atherosclerotic changes in vein grafts or in coronary arteries are much greater in patients who experience a recurrence of pain than in those who are asymptomatic. Additionally, vein graft patency is significantly lower in patients who have a positive-graded exercise test postoperatively than in patients who have a negative test.[139] Thus, it is important that patients routinely undergo such testing to help monitor graft patency.

Important variables that affect graft patency include preservation of the vein endothelium, the operative technique, the size of the vein, the extent of distal atherosclerosis affecting coronary arterial distribution and runoff, and the use of antiplatelet drugs.[139,145]

The use of internal mammary artery grafts is associated with a higher patency rate than saphenous vein grafts. Five-year patency rates for saphenous grafts is generally reported to be about 82% compared with a 97% patency rate with internal mammary grafts. Five to 12-year patency rates are 55% for saphenous vein grafts compared with 95% for internal mammary grafts.[2,146,147,149]

The causes of angina pectoris after surgery include initial hyperplasia or atherosclerotic changes of the venous graft, progressive coronary artery disease, or surgical iatrogenic narrowing of the coronary arteries.[50,145] In patients with recurrent pain within the *first year* after surgery, subintimal hyperplasia appears to play an important role. Subintimal injury occurring during the surgical preparation of the vein or postoperatively, when the vein is exposed to systemic arterial pressures, can produce localized or diffuse subintimal scarring.[50] Recurrent angina pectoris occurring after the *first year* of surgery is probably caused by progressive atherosclerotic changes within the vein grafts or the native coronary arteries.[210] This can lead to direct stenosis and occlusion. In addition, progression of atherosclerosis in the native circulation can decrease the outflow from the graft. This low velocity through the graft can lead to thrombus formation.[50,145] Furthermore, *competition* can occur between the bypass graft and the coronary artery after surgery because of reduced blood flow in the artery proximal to the graft. Competition may lead to progressive atherosclerotic obstruction in the proximal bypassed coronary artery.[139] Therefore, if a partially occluded coronary artery becomes completely obstructed after bypass, later graft occlusion can be a dangerous situation because, essentially, the patient has less coronary blood flow than before the surgery. This problem is a major drawback to aortocoronary bypass surgery.

There is now evidence to show that early and late vein graft occlusion can be reduced in patients receiving dipyridamole and aspirin. Dipyridamole and aspirin reduce platelet deposition, mural thrombosis formation, and smooth muscle cell intimal proliferation. It is recommended that dipyridamole be administered 2 days before surgery, that aspirin be given the day of surgery, and that dipyridamole-aspirin therapy be continued for 1 year after surgery.[38,39,181,188]

Patient variables have been correlated to whether angina will recur after surgery. Patients who are likely to be asymp-tomatic postoperatively are those who have typical preoperative angina pectoris relieved by rest or nitroglycerin; objective evidence of preoperative myocardial ischemia; focal high-grade lesions; good left ventricular function; complete myocardial revascularization; psychological motivation to improve; and current or recent employment.[124] In contrast, those patients who are likely to experience a recurrence of pain postoperatively include those who have atypical preoperative pain; no objective evidence of preoperative ischemia; single-vessel disease; poor left ventricular function; lesions in vessels perfusing a segment of noncontractile myocardium; anatomically small vessels or poor distal runoff; no psychological motivation to improve; and/or processed disability claims.[124] The recurrence of angina within the first 6 weeks postoperatively is generally a result of unsuccessful surgery.[139]

The benefits of myocardial revascularization on return to work are influenced more by socioeconomic rather than medical determinants.[26,43,134] Approximately 90% of patients undergoing surgery are medically improved, yet only 50% of these patients return to work. Patients who are likely to return to work are those who were employed preoperatively, are less than 55 years of age, have high incomes, are male, self-employed, white-collar workers, and have a college education, relief from angina, and good left ventricular performance.[140,141]

Although it has been recommended that postoperative aortocoronary bypass patients who are asymptomatic and who have good left ventricular function after successful surgery should not be advised to stop working, there is an increasing number of physically able patients who are currently unemployed. Nurses should assume the responsibility of investigating those socioeconomic factors that contribute to unemployment and research various types of intervention programs to favorably affect the decision of whether to return to work.[219] One study, for example, reports that the number of men returning to work postoperatively (who had been employed preoperatively) was increased after participation in an outpatient cardiac rehabilitation program.[97]

REOPERATION

Reoperation is being performed with increasing frequency, with estimates that 6% to 18% of all revascularization surgeries are reoperations.[23,138,150] The major indication for reoperation is the recurrence of angina from progressive coronary artery disease. Early mortality is reported to be 3.4% to 12% and is associated with patients over the age of 65 with left ventricular ejection fractions less than 40%. The incidence of perioperative myocardial infarction is 5.3% with 5-year actuarial survival at 87% to 90% and 10-year survival at 75%. The proportion of asymptomatic patients at 5 years is generally 50%, with only 13% complaining of severe angina.[23,148]

ACQUIRED VALVULAR DISEASE

Valve replacement began in 1960 when Harken and Starr independently replaced the aortic valve with a ball-valve prosthesis.[103,221] Since that time, advancement in the design and understanding of prosthetic valve replacements has been progressive. The development of valvular surgery has enabled many patients to lead active and useful lives. Valvular surgery is primarily recommended for adult patients with aortic stenosis or regurgitation and mitral stenosis or regurgitation.

These conditions will be discussed in detail in the following pages.

AORTIC STENOSIS

Etiology

Approximately 25% of all patients with chronic valvular disease have aortic stenosis.[22,185] Of these symptomatic patients, about 80% are men. Aortic stenosis causes left ventricular outflow tract obstruction at the supravalvular, valvular, or subvalvular level. Valvular aortic stenosis is the most common lesion. Aortic stenosis can be congenital in origin (producing a unicuspid, bicuspid, or multicuspid valve) or secondary to rheumatic inflammation or calcification.

The congenitally affected valve may be stenotic at birth and become progressively calcified over the next three decades of life. Calcification produces valvular rigidity and, hence, increases the obstruction already present. A history of rheumatic fever is present in 30% to 50% of patients with aortic stenosis.[185] Rheumatic endocarditis of the aortic valve produces stenosis, which leads to calcification and further narrowing. Idiopathic calcific aortic stenosis occurs most frequently in the older patient. It is generally a mild physiologic obstruction associated with "wear and tear" of the valve.

Pathophysiology

Aortic stenosis is observed during systole when blood is being ejected from the left ventricle to the aorta across a narrowed aortic valve. It is a hemodynamic abnormality caused by an obstruction to the left ventricular outflow tract, causing a high-pressure gradient between the left ventricle and the aorta during systolic ejection. Because of the increase in left ventricular systolic pressure over a period of time, the cardiac work load is increased, leading to a progressive ventricular hypertrophy and a rise in myocardial oxygen demands. These compensatory mechanisms generally permit cardiac output and stroke volume to be maintained within normal limits at rest. During exercise, however, these variables may fail to rise.

The normal aortic valve has a cross-sectional area of 2.5 to 3.5 cm^2. Severe aortic stenosis exists if the cross-sectional area is reduced to 0.5 to 0.7 cm^2, requiring a systolic pressure gradient of over 50 mm Hg to produce a moderate cardiac output.[22,185]

Clinical Manifestations

Generally, there is a prolonged latent period before the symptoms of aortic stenosis develop. Most patients do not become symptomatic until their forties or fifties. Cardiac output is generally maintained at rest until the late stages of the illness. Clinical disability depends on the patient's lifestyle, but generally it is not produced until the valve orifice has been narrowed to approximately one-third normal. The turning point in the disease is heralded by one or more of the three cardinal signs: angina pectoris, syncope, or exertional dyspnea. During late stages of the illness, fatigability, peripheral cyanosis, orthopnea, paroxysmal nocturnal dyspnea, pulmonary edema, and other symptoms of left ventricular failure appear.

Sudden death accounts for about 20% of the fatalities associated with the disease.[185] The average life expectancy for a patient with untreated aortic stenosis once angina pectoris or syncope appears is 3 to 4 years. Left ventricular failure, a grave development, demands immediate treatment. Death after the development of left-sided heart failure usually occurs within 1 to 2 years, but it may occur within a week.

Physical Findings

The systemic arterial pressure of a patient with aortic stenosis is usually normal. The arterial pulse tracing characteristically records a delayed systolic peak and an anacrotic notch (a small, abnormal, extra wave in the ascending limb of the pulse tracing).

A classic finding in aortic stenosis is a systolic diamond-shaped ejection murmur caused by the forced flow of blood through a stenotic orifice. The low-pitched, harsh murmur is best heard in the aortic region (the second intercostal space to the right of the sternum), and it is generally transmitted up to the neck and carotid vessels. It begins shortly after the first heart sound, increasing in intensity toward the middle of the ejection period and decreasing until aortic valve closure (see Chap. 24).

A systolic thrill is generally present at the base of the heart. The jugular venous pulse is normal in pure aortic stenosis. The cardiac rhythm is usually regular. In advanced stages, left ventricular systole may become so delayed that aortic valve closure comes after pulmonic valve closure (P_2A_2). The phenomenon is known as paradoxical splitting of the second heart sound. An atrial gallop (S_4) may be audible at the apex, signifying the presence of left ventricular hypertrophy. A ventricular gallop (S_3) frequently reflects left ventricular dilatation and failure (see Chap. 24).

The ECG reveals left ventricular hypertrophy. In advanced stages of the illness, there may be a "strain" pattern, with ST-segment depression and T-wave inversion in leads 1, aV_L, V_5, and V_6. The chest x-ray may show enlargement of the left ventricle and, in advanced cases, pulmonary congestion. The chest x-ray and echocardiogram may reveal valvular calcification, and radionuclide studies may be performed to assess ventricular function and myocardial perfusion.

A cardiac catheterization is performed to determine the pressure gradient between the left ventricle and aorta in order to estimate the severity of the stenosis. The cross-sectional area of the valve is also determined by measuring the pressure gradient and the cardiac output. The presence of aortic regurgitation or mitral valvular disease is also assessed. Coronary angiography is generally performed on patients who have anginal symptoms and on all patients over age 40 regardless of symptoms.

Treatment

The management of the patient depends on the symptoms and the degree of stenosis and cardiac hypertrophy. The patient with associated cardiac failure is treated with digitalis glycosides, a low-sodium diet, diuretics, and reductions in activity. Once the patient develops symptoms of heart failure, angina pectoris, or syncope, however, the mortality is high despite medical therapy. The outlook and symptomatic relief for such a patient is significantly improved by surgical replacement of the aortic valve.[185] In a patient who has both aortic stenosis and coronary artery disease, aortic valve replacement and aortocoronary bypass surgery frequently result in enhanced late survival and a striking hemodynamic improvement.[128]

The anesthetic drugs, monitoring lines, surgical incision, and cardiopulmonary bypass techniques used in aortocoronary bypass surgery (described under Operative Technique: Myocardial Revascularization) are also used in aortic valve replacement. In this operation, the ascending aorta is clamped and an incision is made in the aorta above the right coronary artery. The coronary arteries are cannulated and perfused with a cold cardioplegic solution. After removal of the entire aortic valve, sutures are inserted through the remaining annulus of the excised valve and then threaded through the sewing ring of the valve prosthesis. Using a valve holder, the prosthesis is lowered into place and the sutures are tied. The aorta is closed, the heart is filled with blood, the aorta is vented for air, and the patient is removed from bypass.

The average operative mortality for aortic valve replacement is in the range of 3%; it may be lower in patients without longstanding heart failure.[49,55] Most patients show a significant clinical improvement after surgery and little or no limitations in their physical activities.

AORTIC REGURGITATION (INSUFFICIENCY)
Etiology

Approximately 75% of all patients suffering from aortic regurgitation are men. Rheumatic fever is a common cause of aortic regurgitation. Infective endocarditis, dissecting aortic aneurysm, and dilatation of the aortic annulus can also produce the disease.[185] It may also be congenital in origin, or it can be produced by rheumatoid arthritis or connective-tissue degeneration, resulting in the "floppy valve" syndrome (see Mitral Regurgitation [Insufficiency]).

Pathophysiology

Aortic regurgitation is observed during diastole when the aortic valve is closed. Because the aortic valve is incompetent, blood is ejected forward in the aorta, but it also leaks back through the closed aortic valve into the left ventricle.

There is an increase in the total stroke volume ejected by the left ventricle in aortic regurgitation. Total stroke volume is the sum of the forward stroke volume and the volume of blood that regurgitates into the left ventricle. An increase in left ventricular end-diastolic volume is the major hemodynamic compensation in the disease. Progressive dilatation of the left ventricle occurs. A normal forward stroke volume may be observed even in patients with moderately severe aortic regurgitation and elevated left ventricular end-diastolic pressure and volume.[185] The cardiac output may be normal at rest but often fails to rise during exercise. Tachycardia may have a beneficial effect because the period of diastole is shortened and thus allows less time for the blood to regurgitate into the ventricle. Peripheral vasodilatation plays a compensatory role by reducing peripheral vascular resistance and the amount of regurgitant flow.

In advanced stages of the illness, left ventricular failure ensues, lowering cardiac output and bringing an associated rise in left atrial, pulmonary capillary, and right ventricular pressures. Because most coronary blood flow occurs during diastole, coronary perfusion may be significantly impaired owing to reduced diastolic perfusion pressures, which, coupled with tachycardia and augmented myocardial oxygen demands, may result in myocardial ischemia.

Clinical Manifestations

A person who has severe aortic regurgitation may be asymptomatic for many years. The earliest symptom may be palpitations produced by the forceful contractions of a dilated left ventricle. Sinus tachycardia or premature ventricular contractions may contribute to the uncomfortable phenomenon. Dyspnea on exertion is generally the first indication of diminished cardiac reserve. Symptoms of left ventricular failure or angina pectoris frequently follow.

Physical Findings

The patient with severe aortic regurgitation can be observed to have a bobbing motion of the head (de Musset's sign) or jarring of the body with each systole. A water-hammer (Corrigan's) pulse, which collapses suddenly during late systole as arterial pressure rapidly falls, is characteristic of the disease. Capillary pulsations (Quincke's pulse) may be demonstrated by applying pressure to the tip of the nail and observing alternate flushing and blanching at the nailbed root. A "pistol-shot" sound (Traube's sign) is heard with the bell of the stethoscope over the femoral arteries. A to-and-fro murmur (Duroziez's sign) can frequently be heard over the femoral artery. A diastolic thrill is often palpated along the left sternal border.

The arterial pulse is widened with an elevated systolic pressure. The diastolic arterial pressure is lowered and may even be heard when the sphygmomanometer cuff is completely deflated. The sound of aortic valve closure is generally reduced or absent. An atrial or ventricular gallop is commonly heard.

Three types of murmurs may be associated with aortic regurgitation:[185]

- The classic murmur of aortic regurgitation, produced by the backflow of blood from the aorta to the left ventricle, which is a blowing, high-pitched, decrescendo, diastolic murmur that is heard best in the third left intercostal space (see Chap. 24). When the murmur is soft, the diaphragm of the stethoscope should be applied to the chest with the patient holding the breath in forced expiration while sitting up or leaning forward. The murmur may radiate widely, especially to the lower sternal border.
- The systolic ejection murmur, which is caused by the increased volume of blood across the aortic valve. It has the following salient characteristics:
    It does not necessarily signify the presence of aortic stenosis.
    It is heard best at the base of the heart.
    It may radiate to the carotid arteries.
    It is generally higher pitched than the murmur of aortic stenosis.
- The Austin Flint murmur, which is a low-pitched, soft, diastolic bruit heard best at the cardiac apex. It is probably caused by the aortic regurgitant blood flow passing the an-

terior mitral valve leaflet, preventing it from fully opening and thereby creating a functional mitral stenosis.

The ECG may show left ventricular hypertrophy and ST-segment depression and T-wave inversion in leads 1, aV$_L$, V$_5$, and V$_6$. The chest x-ray frequently shows left ventricular enlargement. An echocardiogram is done to identify ventricular overload and enlargement. Radionuclide studies may be used to determine the patient's resting and exercise ejection fractions and to estimate left ventricular function. The best invasive method of measuring the severity of the disease is aortography, in which dye is injected into the aorta and the degree of reflux into the left ventricle is estimated. Cardiac catheterization and coronary angiography are usually performed on patients suspected of having other associated valvular lesions or coronary artery disease.

Treatment

When signs of heart failure are present, the patient is treated with digitalis glycosides, diuretics, vasodilating drugs, and sodium and activity restrictions. Because prolonged aortic regurgitation frequently leads to irreversible ventricular damage, however, aortic valve replacement is recommended for asymptomatic patients before the development of heart failure or angina pectoris. Cardiac dysrhythmias or infection are not well tolerated and must be treated promptly. The details of aortic valve replacement were discussed in this section on aortic stenosis.

MITRAL STENOSIS

Etiology

Mitral stenosis is frequency caused by rheumatic fever, which produces ulceration, fusion, and calcification of the mitral valve. Approximately two thirds of the patients are women. Congenital mitral stenosis is rare. It is called the parachute mitral valve because all the chordae are inserted into a single papillary muscle.

Pathophysiology

Mitral stenosis is observed during diastole when blood is being ejected from the left atrium across a narrowed mitral valve to the left ventricle.

The mitral valve orifice is approximately 5 cm^2 in the normal adult. When the orifice is less than one-half normal, significant obstruction is present. Mitral stenosis produces three significant events: an increase in left atrial mean pressure, an increase in pulmonary vascular resistance, and a decrease in cardiac output.

When the orifice is significantly narrowed, blood can flow from the left atrium to the left ventricle only as a result of a high left atrioventricular pressure gradient. The high left atrial mean pressure that develops is an important compensatory mechanism to maintain cardiac output despite the stenotic valvular lesion. The left ventricular diastolic pressure generally is maintained at normal levels.

A rise in left atrial mean pressure, however, is also accompanied by a rise in the pulmonary venous, capillary, and arterial pressures. When the pulmonary capillary pressure exceeds the oncotic pressure of the blood, pulmonary transudation occurs. If pulmonary transudation exceeds the rate of pulmonary lymphatic drainage, pulmonary congestion and edema develop.

The degree of pulmonary vascular resistance varies from patient to patient. Pulmonary hypertension is caused by the backward transmission of the elevated left atrial pressure, arteriolar constriction, and degenerative changes in the pulmonary vascular bed. Severe pulmonary hypertension is a serious complication of mitral stenosis; it produces tricuspid and pulmonic regurgitation and right-sided heart failure.

There is also considerable variation in cardiac output in patients with mitral stenosis. Exercise tends to increase left atrial, pulmonary venous, pulmonary capillary, pulmonary arterial, and right ventricular pressures. Patients with mild stenosis are usually able to maintain an effective cardiac output at rest that increases with exercise. Generally, however, the cardiac output is fixed at a low level by the rigid stenotic valve. In people who have severe mitral stenosis, the cardiac output may be normal at rest, but exercise may produce no change in or even a decrease in cardiac output. Right-sided heart failure and tricuspid regurgitation may further reduce cardiac output during exercise. Despite an associated rise in left atrial pressure, cardiac output may be lowered as a result of tachycardia. Accelerated heart rates shorten the period of diastole more than the period of systole. In mitral stenosis, the accelerated rate reduces the time available for blood flow across the mitral valve (the flow occurring from atrium to ventricle during ventricular diastole), thereby decreasing left ventricular filling and cardiac output.

Clinical Manifestations

The symptoms of mitral stenosis are related to the degree of valvular dysfunction and to disturbances in the cardiac rhythm. The most characteristic symptom is dyspnea. Dyspnea generally is precipitated by extreme exertion, excitement, severe anemia, sexual intercourse, pregnancy, fever, thyrotoxicosis, or paroxysmal tachycardia. As the stenosis becomes more severe, dyspnea is produced by lesser degrees of exertion or stressors, and the patient becomes progressively limited in daily activities.

Several other symptoms develop as a result of recurrent pulmonary congestion. Complaints of orthopnea, paroxysmal nocturnal dyspnea, or cough may be elicited. These problems are aggravated by recumbency or exercise. The degenerative pulmonary changes that occur in association with pulmonary hypertension include a reduction in vital capacity, diffusion capacity, and pulmonary compliance.

Hemoptysis that is not associated with pulmonary edema is a frequent complication. It is alarming, but it is almost never fatal. It is caused by the rupture of alveoli, and it may vary from a small amount of blood-tinged sputum to a large amount of bright-red blood.

Atrial dysrhythmias, such as premature atrial contractions, paroxysmal atrial tachycardia, and atrial flutter or fibrillation, occur frequently in mitral stenosis. Arterial embolism associated with ineffective left atrial contractions and with thrombus formation in atrial fibrillation can occur to the brain, kidney, spleen, or extremities.

Physical Findings

On physical examination, the patient may be found to have peripheral cyanosis and a classic malar flush. The jugular venous pulse may reveal a prominent *a* wave due to the powerful atrial systole in a person who has a normal sinus rhythm and pulmonary hypertension. In atrial fibrillation, the jugular pulse may be only a single pulsation (a *c-v* wave).

The size of the heart is generally normal; the apical impulse is normal but diminished in intensity. A diastolic thrill can be felt at the cardiac apex, particularly when the patient is turned on the left side. A right ventricular "lift" may be present along the left sternal border, resulting from a hypertrophied right ventricle.

The three significant auscultatory findings in mitral stenosis are a loud first heart sound, an opening snap (OS), and a diastolic murmur.[185] The loud first heart sound is generally accentuated because mitral valve closure is often delayed until the left ventricular pressure reaches the level of the elevated left atrial pressure.

The OS of the stenotic mitral valve (not heard when the valve is normal) is audible early in diastole along the lower left sternal border and apex (see Chap. 24). In mitral stenosis with an elevated left atrial pressure, the rigid valve snaps open during the period of diastole to allow blood to flow from the atrium to the ventricle. The OS is produced by a sudden stop in the opening movement of the stenotic valve. The higher the left atrial pressure, the more rapidly the valve is opened to produce the sound. Also, the more severe the mitral stenosis, the closer the OS is to the second heart sound. The OS is frequently mistaken for a ventricular gallop.

Following the OS, a low-pitched, rumbling diastolic murmur is heard best at the apex with the patient turned on the left side (see Chap. 24). The murmur is produced by the flow of blood passing through the stenotic mitral valve. The intensity of the murmur does not correlate with the severity of the stenosis. A soft systolic murmur is commonly heard at the apex, but it does not necessarily signify mitral regurgitation.

The ECG may show bifid P waves in leads 1, 2, and V_5 that are consistent with left atrial enlargement, right-axis deviation, and right ventricular hypertrophy. Atrial fibrillation is common. The chest x-ray may show dilatation of the left atrium with calcification of the mitral valve. The echocardiogram is useful in determining abnormal movement of the valve. Radionuclide studies performed at rest and during exercise are done to evaluate ventricular function. Cardiac catheterization is an important procedure used to evaluate the severity of the disease with regard to the transvalvular pressure gradient, the cardiac output, and the cross-sectional area of the mitral valve. Coronary angiography is often indicated.

Treatment

Symptomatic patients are treated medically with avoidance of strenuous activity, restriction of sodium intake, and diuretics. Although digitalis glycosides do not necessarily improve the hemodynamic functioning, they are indicated to slow the ventricular rate in patients with rapid atrial fibrillation.[186] Attention is directed toward the correction of anemia or infection and conversion of atrial fibrillation to normal sinus rhythm.

Surgery is recommended for patients who are symptomatic or who have minimal symptoms and evidence of pulmonary vascular disease. There are three major surgical approaches to correct mitral stenosis: closed commissurotomy, open commissurotomy, and mitral valve replacement.

A closed commissurotomy was indicated in the past for patients who had good valvular mobility, who had not had previous mitral valve surgery, and who did not show evidence of valvular calcification, regurgitation, or left atrial thrombosis.[186] An incision was made into the left atrium, and the valve was blindly opened by a finger or a dilator. If the closed commissurotomy did not open the orifice, the patient was put on cardiopulmonary bypass and an "open" repair was carried out. The procedure, however, is rarely used today in the United States, but it may be the procedure of choice in other parts of the world.

Open mitral commissurotomy is usually indicated for patients who have little or no mitral regurgitation and a pliable valve leaflet with no calcification or mural thrombi. It is done by using cardiopulmonary bypass and lowering the myocardial temperature to hypothermic levels. A median sternotomy or a right anterolateral thoracotomy is performed. An incision is made over the left atrium, the mitral valve is exposed, and the atrium is examined for mural thrombi. The fused commissures are exposed and carefully separated with a knife, while extreme caution is taken to ensure that the newly mobilized leaflets remain attached to the chordae tendineae. The competence of the restructured valve is evaluated by measuring the left atrial and ventricular pressures.

Recently, mitral valve reconstruction surgery has gained acceptance in the United States. With these techniques, a number of other options are available to patients with either mitral stenosis, regurgitation, or mixed lesions before complete valve replacement becomes necessary. Dilatation of the mitral valve annulus can be corrected by an annuloplasty ring, which is a flexible oval ring that can be sewn to the annulus, thereby reducing or reshaping the mitral orifice to assist with valve-leaflet coaptation. Ruptured chordae can be managed by transferring chordae from one leaflet to the other to prevent a "floppy" leaflet. Elongated chordae can be surgically shortened to allow the attached leaflets to coapt or can be shortened by transplanting their base to another area in the ventricle. These techniques have been associated with superior hemodynamic results and lower operative mortality than can be achieved with mitral valve replacement and fit sequentially into a spectrum of surgical treatment that can then place complete valve replacement as a final option.[29,37,53,101]

Replacement of the mitral valve with a prosthetic valve is particularly indicated for patients with more severe mitral stenosis and regurgitation or for patients with extensively calcified valves.[4,53] The patient is put on cardiopulmonary bypass. A median sternotomy or right thoracotomy is performed, and myocardial temperatures are lowered to hypothermic levels. An incision is made into the left atrium to expose the mitral valve. The mitral valve and papillary muscle are excised. Sutures are inserted into the remaining annulus of the excised mitral valve and then into the sewing ring of the prosthetic valve. The valve is lowered into place and the sutures are tied. Care is taken not to injure the conduction system or the circumflex coronary artery. The motion of the valvular prosthesis is determined. The ventricle and aorta are vented to remove air, and the patient is removed from cardiopulmonary bypass. The operative mortality is about 5%.[186] Many patients show symptomatic improvement after valve replacement, and they are able to resume their normal daily activities.

MITRAL REGURGITATION (INSUFFICIENCY)

Etiology

Rheumatic fever is the cause of mitral regurgitation in approximately 50% of the patients who have it. Unlike mitral stenosis, rheumatic mitral regurgitation occurs more frequently in men than in women. Mitral regurgitation is also caused by myocardial ischemia or infarction. It may be congenital, or it may be the result of the "floppy valve" syndrome, also called *mitral valve prolapse*, a connective-tissue degenerative disease in which the valve leaflets and chordae are thin and elongated and permit prolapse of the leaflets during systole.[12]

Pathophysiology

Mitral regurgitation is observed during ventricular systole when the mitral valve is closed and the ventricle is ejecting blood to the aorta. Because the mitral valve is incompetent, blood is ejected not only forward to the aorta, but also backward to the left atrium.

The regurgitant volume may be nearly as large as the forward stroke volume. The left ventricle attempts to compensate for the regurgitant blood flow by emptying more completely during systole to maintain an effective cardiac output. Progressively, the left ventricle dilates, producing a rise in left ventricular end-diastolic pressure, until eventually left ventricular failure appears. The regurgitant blood produces a rise in left atrial pressure and enlargement of the left atrium. Left atrial hypertension may eventually be the cause of increased pulmonary vascular resistance and right-heart failure.

Clinical Manifestations

Some patients with mitral regurgitation never have any symptoms or any loss of cardiac reserve. Symptomatic patients, however, experience fatigue, exertional dyspnea, orthopnea, nocturnal dyspnea, palpitations, and, less commonly, pulmonary congestion and edema.

Physical Findings

In patients with mitral regurgitation, the arterial pressure is normal, but the arterial pulse is characterized by a sharp upstroke. The jugular venous pulse may show an abnormally prominent *a* wave. A systolic thrill usually is palpable at the apex. A characteristic rocking motion of the chest during each cardiac cycle may be observed as a result of both left ventricular contraction and left atrial expansion during systole.

The first heart sound is soft or absent. The second heart sound is normal, but it may be widely split in a patient with severe regurgitation. Occasionally, both third and fourth heart sounds are present.

The characteristic feature of mitral regurgitation is a high-pitched blowing, holosystolic (throughout systole) murmur (see Chap. 24) that is heard best at the apex and radiating to the axilla. It is produced by the regurgitation of blood from the left ventricle to the left atrium after mitral valve closure. In patients with ruptured chordae tendineae, the murmur may have a "sea gull," or cooing, sound. A short rumbling diastolic murmur may also be present, resulting from increased blood flow across the mitral valve.

The chest x-ray usually shows enlargement of the left ventricle and atrium. Left ventricular hypertrophy and left atrial enlargement are frequently shown on the ECG. Atrial fibrillation is associated with chronic severe regurgitation. Echocardiography may be used to evaluate valvular thickening, prolapse, or calcification. Exercise testing is sometimes performed to assess symptoms associated with chronic mitral insufficiency. Radionuclide studies may be done to evaluate ventricular performance. Mitral regurgitation is best assessed by cardiac catheterization. The degree of insufficiency is estimated by injecting dye into the left ventricle and evaluating the amount of reflux into the left atrium.

Treatment

The management of the patient with mitral regurgitation depends on the symptoms and the severity of the valvular incompetence. Medical management of dyspnea and fatigue includes limiting physical activity, administering digitalis glycosides and diuretics, and restricting sodium. Atrial fibrillation should be converted to a normal sinus rhythm. Vasodilators may be used to reduce the amount of regurgitant blood flow into the left atrium by lowering systemic vascular resistance.

Mitral valve replacement has provided symptomatic improvement in patients with mitral regurgitation. Patients with progressive symptoms or with mild symptoms but an enlarging heart are urged to undergo surgery in an attempt to prevent irreversible ventricular failure.[186]

TYPES OF VALVE PROSTHESES

Two types of valve prostheses are currently available: mechanical valves and biologic valves. *Mechanical valves* are highly durable and able to withstand stress and wear over a long period of time. These valves are associated with a high incidence of thromboembolic complications, necessitating that patients be placed on a life-long regimen of anticoagulant therapy.

Three types of mechanical valves are currently being used or can be found in patients: the caged-ball, the caged-disc, or the tilting-disc valve.[243] The *caged-ball valve* consists of a ball housed in a cage which is attached to a sewing ring (Fig. 26–4). The ball rests on the sewing ring when the valve is in the closed position. As a pressure gradient develops, the ball moves forward in the cage and the valve opens. Examples of caged-ball prostheses are the Starr-Edwards, Smeloff, Braunwald-Cutter, and Magovern-Cromie.

Caged-disc valves are similar in design to caged-ball valves (Fig. 26–5). They consist of a sewing ring with an attached cage that houses a movable silicone disc. The disc sets in the sewing ring when the valve is closed and drops into the cage as blood flows through the open valve. Examples of caged-disc valves are the Hufnagel, Cross-Jones, Kay-Suzuki, Kay-Shiley, and Beall valves.

With the *tilting-disc valve* (Fig. 26–6), the disc sets against the sewing ring when the valve is closed. In the open position, the disc tilts at an angle so that semicentralized flow occurs through the valve orifice. The disc is held in place by hinges on the ring or struts. Examples include Wada-Cutter, Bjork-Shiley, and Medtronic-Hall. In the Wada-Cutter and the convex-concave model of the Bjork-Shiley, the incidence of strut failure and embolization of the disc have been significant

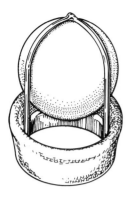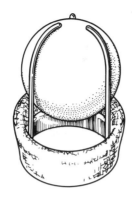

Figure 26-4

Schematic drawing of caged-ball valves. The closed-cage version on the left is an example of a Starr-Edwards valve. The open-cage on the right resembles the Smeloff, Braunwald-Cutter, and Magovern-Cromie valves. (Whitman, G. Prosthetic cardiac valves. *Prog. Cardiovasc. Nurs.* 2:116, 1987; with permission.)

enough to have them recalled from the market. Many patients still have these valves implanted.[157] The St. Jude valve, a bileaflet tilting-disc valve, consists of two semicircular discs that, when closed, occlude the valve orifice and, when open, pivot on hinges and allow centralized flow.

There are basically two types of tissue valves being implanted: porcine and bovine valves. The Hancock and Carpentier-Edwards valves are examples of porcine valves in which aortic porcine valves have been mounted on stents attached to a sewing ring to form a valve. The Ionescu-Shiley valve is made of bovine pericardium fashioned into valve leaflets (Fig. 26–7). Most recently human cadaver homografts have also been used with success.[155]

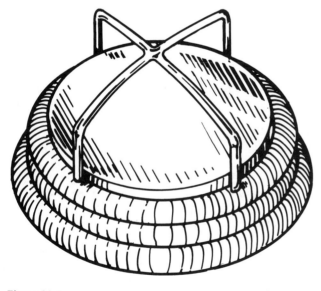

Figure 26-5

Schematic representation of a caged-disc valve. (Whitman, G. Prosthetic cardiac valves. *Prog. Cardiovasc. Nurs.* 2:116, 1987; with permission.)

COMPLICATIONS ASSOCIATED WITH VALVE REPLACEMENT

The incidence of thromboembolic complications is high for all the mechanical valves, ranging from 1.0% to 3.0%/patient-year, with the St. Jude valve achieving the lowest thromboembolism rate.[6,14,36,161] Life-long anticoagulation is required of all patients with mechanical valves. Because of this, elderly or confused patients who would be unable to adhere to a medication regimen or women of childbearing years are generally considered for tissue valves. With tissue valves, anticoagulation generally is recommended only for the first 3 to 5 months after surgery. In patients with a mitral valve bioprostheses and atrial fibrillation or an enlarged left atrium in which constant vigilance against embolization is required, longer periods of anticoagulation may be required. Other patients who might require long-term anticoagulation include those with large, dilated ventricles and histories of left atrial thrombus and embolic events.[222,243]

Prosthetic valve wear, and dysfunction can cause mechanical problems and severe valve failure. Symptoms can range from slight congestive failure to frank arrest due to catastrophic failure. Tissue leaflets from the bioprosthesis can develop tears or calcification, leading slowly to regurgitation or stenosis. The discs and balls can develop variances over a period of time owing to lipid infiltration, which can cause a ball to alter its size, or wear, which can develop on discs that constantly strike the same portion of a strut. In all these instances, valve dysfunction occurs and generally replacement is required.[21,25,152,248]

The incidence of endocarditis is relatively the same for all valve prostheses and has been reported to range from 1% to 4%. Approximately one third to one half of the cases develop within the first 2 months after surgery. Early prosthetic valve endocarditis generally is associated with wound and urinary tract infections or sepsis from invasive lines. Late prosthetic valve endocarditis generally is attributed to dental or genitourinary procedures (see Chap. 28).[195,243]

NURSING PROCESS

ASSESSMENT

The preoperative assessment of patients undergoing cardiac surgery involves a comprehensive biopsychosocial evaluation to determine physical problems and coexisting disease and to gather information that will serve as a baseline. The information collected is sent with the patient to the critical care unit. Pertinent information is written on the patient's care plan and communicated to all critical care unit personnel.

The history is especially important to determine the severity and frequency of the chest pain and to find out whether the patient had a previous myocardial infarction. Risk factors are evaluated, and particular attention is given to topics such as history of smoking, diabetes mellitus, obesity, hypercholesterolemia, any fluid and electrolyte imbalance, blood dyscrasias and clotting defects, or other vascular problems, such as hypertension and cerebrovascular disease.

The peripheral pulses are evaluated, and the extremities are assessed for varicosities, ulcerations, injuries, and edema. The saphenous veins are assessed for their suitability as grafts for surgery. Heart rate, rhythm, and regularity are determined, noting the presence of any extra sounds, clicks, rubs, or murmurs. Breath sounds are auscultated for normalcy. Renal

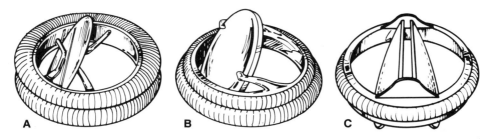

Figure 26-6
Schematic drawings of various tilting-disc valves. Parts (A) and (B) illustrate the Bjork-Shiley valve, which has one circular disc that tilts back and forth against metal struts. Part (C) depicts the St. Jude valve, which consists of two semicircular discs that pivot open on hinges. (Whitman, G. Prosthetic cardiac valves. *Prog. Cardiovasc. Nurs.* 2:116, 1987; with permission.)

function is evaluated. The patient is assessed for any neurologic deficits, particularly any history of stroke or transient ischemic attacks, and the carotids are auscultated for bruits.

An endocrine assessment is performed, noting any signs or symptoms of thyroid disorders and any history of adrenocortical abnormalities. The patient's level of anxiety, knowledge about the current situation, and readiness to learn are explored and evaluated.

The patient should be weighed daily—and at the same time each day. Information about the patient's weight is used to interpret any postoperative fluctuations. The evening before surgery, the patient should be weighed on the scales in the critical care unit so that the postoperative weight can be assessed accurately.

Diagnostic and Laboratory Tests

A detailed hematologic assessment is done and includes a coagulation panel (platelet count, prothrombin time, partial thromboplastin time, bleeding time, thrombin time, and clotting time), complete blood count, electrolyte panel, serum creatinine and blood urea nitrogen levels, serum glutamic oxaloacetic transaminase level, lactic dehydrogenase level, creatine phosphokinase level, alkaline phosphatase level, bilirubin level, lipoproteins, and a fasting blood sugar level. A urinalysis and sedimentation rate are done. Posteroanterior, lateral, right oblique, and left oblique chest x-rays and a portable upright chest x-ray (to be used as a baseline for postoperative evaluations) are done to evaluate the lungs and heart size and to detect any coexisting disease. Pulmonary function tests and arterial blood gases are usually ordered preoperatively. The patient is typed and cross-matched for blood and blood products.

A normal resting ECG and a graded exercise test are generally performed to determine the duration and intensity of exercise necessary to produce angina pectoris or electrocardiographic changes. Radionuclide imaging may also be useful (see Chap. 25) in determining which patients might be candidates for coronary angiography and future myocardial revascularization.[104,115]

The most important information is obtained from coronary angiography (see Chap. 24). Surgery is considered for the patient who has an atherosclerotic plaque that narrows the diameter of an artery more than 50% corresponding to a reduction in the cross-sectional area of greater than 75%.[139] The patient must have good distal runoff in the vessel to be bypassed, which is visualized on coronary angiography as a large segment of the artery that is minimally diseased beyond the

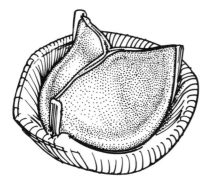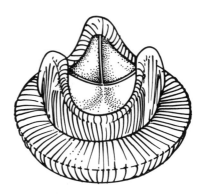

Figure 26-7
Schematic drawings of tissue valves. The valve on the left resembles the Ionescu-Shiley valve, which is constructed of bovine pericardium. The valve on the right depicts a Carpentier-Edwards valve, which is constructed of porcine tissue. The stent configuration varies for each design. (Whitman, G. Prosthetic cardiac valves. *Prog. Cardiovasc. Nurs.* 2:116, 1987; with permission.)

site of major obstruction. Also, a ventriculogram is performed to determine the functioning of the left ventricle. The preoperative and postoperative nursing diagnoses, patient outcomes, and nursing orders are discussed in the following sections.

NURSING DIAGNOSES, PATIENT OUTCOMES, AND PLAN

The preceding material on pathophysiology, nursing assessment, and diagnostic tests guides the nurse in establishing the

---

NURSING CARE PLAN SUMMARY *Patient Undergoing Cardiac Surgery Preoperative Period*

NURSING DIAGNOSIS

1. Knowledge deficit related to impending surgery and inadequate knowledge of preoperative and postoperative management (knowing pattern)

Patient Outcomes	Nursing Orders
1. The patient will be able to discuss the preoperative diet.	1. Teach the patient and family about the preoperative diet. For a patient with coronary artery disease, a low atherogenic diet (one low in cholesterol and saturated fat and high in polyunsaturated fat) may be ordered in the preoperative period. However, a regular diet may be maintained and the low-animal-fat diet not initiated until after surgery. For the volume-overloaded patient, sodium restrictions may be initiated to reduce fluid retention. For the cachexic patient, a nutritional assessment consisting of anthropometric body measurements and analyses of biochemical laboratory data may be obtained. Because cachexic patients have a higher risk associated with surgery than well-nourished patients,[16] surgery may be postponed in patients who are hemodynamically stable while nutritional supplements by enteral feedings or parenteral avenues may be initiated in an attempt to replete the patient's nutritional stores before the procedure.
2. The patient will verbalize an understanding of the following: A. The reason for cardiac surgery	2. Teach the patient and family the preoperative information they will need to prepare for surgery related to the following: A. The surgical procedure. The physician is responsible for explaining the type of surgery, risk factors, operative mortality, and complications. The nurse must also know these facts to reinforce them or further explain them to the patient. The use of heart models and drawings can be used to explain the procedure to the patient and family.
B. The tests, procedures, and restrictions, experienced in the preoperative period	B. Tests, procedures, and restrictions that the patient may experience in the preoperative period: (1) The how, what, and why of tests: ECG, bloodwork, chest x-rays, pulmonary functions, and so on (2) The need to restrict smoking (3) The implementation of the nothing-by-mouth status immediately preceding surgery (4) The procedure and rationale for the preoperative skin-preparation techniques, which usually include both skin-shaving procedures and showers with povidone-iodine or regular soap products. The physician's preference usually dictates the extent of the skin shave, which may range from a shoulders-to-toes, front-to-back shave to a limited shave involving only the area over the sternum and the inner aspects of the thighs. Depending on the extent of the skin shave and the patient's status, the patient may be allowed to perform all of or portions of the preparations, with the nurse serving as the final evaluator of their thoroughness.
C. The names and types of medications to be received in the preoperative period	C. Names and types of medications the patient will receive in the preoperative period. The nurse should know the following: (1) Nitroglycerin should be placed at the patient's bedside, and the patient should be told to tell the nurse when and how often the medication is taken. Prophylactic application of nitroglycerin ointment concurrently with administration of preoperative medications may also be ordered and should be anticipated. Both chronic oral and transcutaneous nitrate

(continued)

NURSING CARE PLAN SUMMARY *Patient Undergoing Cardiac Surgery Preoperative Period*
Continued

Patient Outcomes	Nursing Orders

administration should be continued up until the time of surgery because decreases in cardiac output and increases in systemic vascular resistance will occur after their discontinuation. In addition, withdrawal may increase the sensitivity of the systemic and coronary vasculature to vasoconstrictive stimuli.[1]

(2) Digitalis is generally discontinued in the immediate 12-hour preoperative period to reduce the possibility of ventricular dysrhythmias intraoperatively, but it may be continued in patients with supraventricular tachycardia or in those patients with severe cardiac failure. Preoperative administration of digitalis is generally unnecessary in patients on chronic therapy owing to the 40-hour half-life of digitalis. In addition, maintenance doses will be reduced in the early postoperative period until renal function normalizes.

(3) Oral or intravenous potassium chloride replacement may be ordered in the preoperative period to elevate or maintain the patient's serum potassium at levels greater than 3.5 to 4.0 mEq/L to avoid dysrhythmias.

(4) Diuretic therapy is usually discontinued several days before surgery to prevent the development of hypovolemic hypotension during the surgical procedure. In severely ill patients, diuretic therapy may be continued on schedule in the preoperative period as long as careful attention to the patient's fluid and electrolyte status is maintained and appropriate therapies are ordered for abnormalities that develop.

(5) Beta-blocker therapy is frequently administered to patients preoperatively to control hypertension as well as ischemic disease. These drugs are most frequently continued during the preoperative period because withdrawal has been associated with myocardial ischemia, infarction, hypertension, and tachydysrhythmias.[78,105,223]

(6) Efforts are made to discontinue aspirin and all anticoagulants 1 week before surgery. Currently, if anticoagulation from coumadin therapy needs to be maintained because of atrial fibrillation, heparin therapy can be substituted because its effects can be countered intraoperatively with protamine. Some studies suggest that preoperative administration of dipyridamole and administration of aspirin within the first few hours after surgery decrease the incidence of early and late graft closure.[38,39] However, controversy over the issue of long-term patency has been questioned recently by some authors.[90]

(7) Antidysrhythmic agents should be administered per schedule before surgery.

(8) Calcium channel–blocking agents such as nifedipine, diltiazem, and verapamil can also be safely continued preoperatively. Possible advantages to maintaining these agents include protection against myocardial injury, improvement in myocardial oxygenation, and possible prevention of post-cardiopulmonary bypass coronary spasm.[34,69,130]

(9) Antihypertensive agents are also routinely maintained on their administration schedules before surgery.

(10) Diabetic patients should omit their usual dose of insulin the morning of surgery, and they may be given 10 U of regular insulin with each 500 ml of a 5% dextrose in water solution. Insulin is usually administered intraoperatively in response to serum glucose levels.

(11) Patients who have been taking steroids must be given supplemental doses to prevent the complications induced by the stress of surgery.

(12) Prophylactic antibiotics (cephalothin, oxacillin) are administered generally 20 to 30 minutes before the surgical incision and maintained for no longer than 48 hours.[94]

(continued)

NURSING CARE PLAN SUMMARY   *Patient Undergoing Cardiac Surgery Preoperative Period*
Continued

Patient Outcomes	Nursing Orders
	(13) The use of other drugs, such as stool softeners, hypnotics, sedatives, and tranquilizers, may also be necessary before surgery. The nurse should identify the patient's normal strategies for maintaining adequate elimination and sleep/rest cycles, and attempts should be made to assist the patient in using these strategies before adjunctive pharmacologic therapies are used.
D. The sensations, equipment, and procedures experienced in the preoperative and immediate postoperative periods	D. Sensations, equipment, and procedures the patient may experience in the immediate postoperative period. (1) Preparing patients and their families for admission to the ICU. Before surgery, the ICU nurse should visit the patient and family to explain to them what will happen in the immediate postoperative period. The patient and family should be shown the critical care unit, the patient's room, and the family waiting area. Also, they should be told about noises, alarms, lights, visiting hours, approximate length of surgery and stay in the critical care unit, and what items the patient may bring to the unit. (2) What patients will experience when they awaken from surgery. Slides, booklets, videotapes, and preoperative teaching dolls (Fig. 26–8) can be used as aids in describing the endotracheal tube, ventilator, median sternotomy, chest tubes (and bloody drainage), cardiac monitor, intravenous lines, arterial and central venous pressure lines, Foley catheter, and elastic stockings. Related routines concerning this equipment and care should also be explained, such as suctioning and chest-tube stripping. Additionally, explaining and demonstrating a method of communication (such as "finger writing" key words on the nurse's hand) that can be used while the patient is intubated should also be emphasized. Often the first postoperative visit is a terrifying experience for the family, despite the best explanations. We have found teaching dolls useful in preparing members of the patient's family for their first visit.
3. The patient will demonstrate activities to be performed in the postoperative period.	3. Teach activities the patient can perform that will assist with recovery, such as the following:[178] A. Coughing and deep-breathing exercises B. Using the incentive spirometer

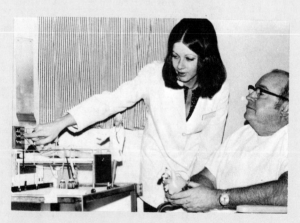

Figure 26–8

A cardiovascular clinical nurse specialist using teaching dolls and a heart model to explain to the patient what he can expect in the immediate postoperative period.

(continued)

NURSING CARE PLAN SUMMARY   Patient Undergoing Cardiac Surgery Preoperative Period
Continued

Patient Outcomes	*Nursing Orders*
	C. Performing leg and arm exercises, particularly "ankle pumps" (repeated extension and flexion of the foot), which enhance venous return and reduce edema
4. The patient will discuss the procedures and protocols concerning visiting hours and communication of information during the postoperative period.	4. Explain procedures and protocols concerning visiting hours and communicate information concerning the patient's status. A. When the physician will report the results of the surgery and the patient's immediate postoperative condition. It is advisable for the nurse to meet with the family during the intraoperative waiting period. Norheim[176] reported that the needs for honesty and information are the highest-ranked needs for families during the intraoperative waiting period and that they would like to receive more information at that time concerning the patient's progress. B. When the first postoperative visit will be allowed C. How ongoing information or emergency contacts will be made D. When the patient can be expected to transfer to the floor
5. The patient will learn and practice relaxation techniques twice a day for 20 minutes preoperatively.	5. Teach the patient and family self-regulation techniques that can be used to induce relaxation during the preoperative and postoperative periods. Music therapy or a head-to-toe relaxation technique (see Chap. 3) can be especially useful for such patients in reducing their psychophysiologic stress levels and in assisting them to achieve some degree of control over the situation. Relaxation techniques and controlled diaphragmatic breathing may also be helpful in reducing pain and in enhancing the effectiveness of pain medication. Patients should be taught such techniques prior to surgery, encouraged to practice them twice a day for 20 minutes, and reminded to continue to use the techniques in the early and late postoperative periods.

NURSING CARE PLAN SUMMARY   Immediate Postoperative Period

NURSING DIAGNOSIS

1. *High risk for physiologic and psychologic instability related to anesthesia, cardiopulmonary bypass, and cardiac surgery (exchanging pattern)*

Patient Outcomes	*Nursing Orders*
1. The patient will maintain respiratory stability.	1. Observe skin color and for presence of bilateral chest excursion as the patient is being ventilated with a bag-valve device. Auscultate both lung fields once the patient's endotracheal tube is attached to the ventilator. The respiratory therapist at this point will adjust the ventilator settings with regard to the oxygen concentration, respiratory rate, tidal volume, and appropriate pressures and will set the ventilator alarms.
2. The patient will maintain cardiac stability.	2. Maintain the patient's cardiac stability. A. Evaluate the ECG. Note the rate and rhythm. Monitor the ECG continuously. Set the upper and lower alarm limits. Obtain a rhythm strip on admission for documentation and then every 2 hours or as necessary. Record the heart rate every 15 minutes until stable. Lead selection varies but MCL_1 is commonly monitored (see Chap. 12). This placement does not interfere with the mediastinal or chest tube dressings and allows easy access to the left side of the chest if defibrillation is required.[242] B. Auscultate the apical pulse. Validate the rate with the ECG. Identify the

(continued)

NURSING CARE PLAN SUMMARY   *Immediate Postoperative Period   Continued*

Patient Outcomes	Nursing Orders
	quality of heart sounds for future comparison. Assess for extra sounds, murmurs, or rubs. C. If an artificial cardiac pacemaker is being used, note the type of pacing, the mode, the rate, and the milliamperage (mA), and determine if the pacemaker is functioning properly. If the patient is not being paced, ensure that the unused pacemaker wires are covered with gauze, placed in a plastic covering (finger cot), and secured to the patient's chest to protect the patient from electrical hazards. Usually two atrial and two ventricular wires are attached to the epicardium with absorbable suture before chest closure. The wires exit by way of a stab incision at the distal portion of the sternotomy incision; the atrial wires are usually on the right side, and the ventricular wires are on the left. These wires are usually removed within the first few days after surgery either by gentle traction or by clipping them at the level of the skin.

3. The patient will maintain hemodynamic stability.	3. Attach the intravascular lines to transducers or manometers. Ensure patency and establish wave tracing or digital recordings. The length of time these intravascular lines are left in varies from institution to institution. Pierson and Funk[184] recently reported, however, that as early as 18 hours after surgery, clinical parameters rather than parameters provided by hemodynamic monitoring are used to make fluid management decisions in post–bypass surgery patients. Early removal of these devices would most likely lessen the complications seen with these catheters. Specific intravascular parameters that are measured and assessed are outlined in Box 26-1.
	
	A. Calculate and obtain the hemodynamic parameters on admission and as often as necessary. These parameters include the following:
	    (1) Mean arterial pressure (MAP)
	    (2) Central venous pressure (CVP) or right atrial pressure (RAP)
	    (3) Pulmonary artery systolic (PAS), pulmonary artery diastolic (PAD), pulmonary artery mean (PAM), pulmonary capillary wedge pressure (PCWP)
	    (4) Left atrial pressure (LAP)
	    (5) Venous-oxygen saturation (SvO$_2$)
	    (6) Cardiac output (CO)
	    (7) Cardiac index (CI)
	    (8) Systemic vascular resistance (SVR)
	    (9) Pulmonary vascular resistance (PVR)
	
	B. Historically, it has been the practice to place patients in a supine position when obtaining their hemodynamic parameters; this practice interrupts rest and comfort. Studies suggest that hemodynamic parameters (*i.e.,* RAP, PAS, PAD, PCWP, LAP, and CO) are not affected by various supine backrest positions.[46,131,246] However, recent evidence indicates that some patients placed in a left lateral position will have significant changes.[30,119,241] Patients at greatest risk for these alterations seem to be those with a CI less than 2.3 L/minute/m^2, in whom time elapsed since surgery is less than 12 hours, and in those receiving vasoactive agents or mechanical ventilation.[65] In this group of patients, the bedside practitioner must make individual decisions concerning the patient's positioning, balancing comfort versus accuracy of readings.
	
	C. Whether or not to remove a patient from mechanical ventilation when obtaining hemodynamic parameters, particularly when obtaining the ventricular preload values of the RAP, PCWP, and LAP, still remains unanswered and, therefore, varies from patient to patient and institution to institution. In the presence of positive end-expiratory pressure (PEEP), hemodynamic parameters may be falsely elevated owing to the increase in intrathoracic pressure that PEEP creates. However, removing PEEP and allowing the intrathoracic pressure to fall abruptly may create a sudden increase in blood flow through the right side of the heart and toward the left atrium. In a failure state, this bolus of volume would be poorly handled by

(continued)

NURSING CARE PLAN SUMMARY   *Immediate Postoperative Period*   *Continued*

Patient Outcomes	*Nursing Orders*
	the left ventricle and consequently would also create a falsely high left atrial reading or could contribute to further left ventricular failure. Additionally, the ventilatory effects of abrupt discontinuation of PEEP should be considered, because discontinuation may create a transient state of ventilatory insufficiency and thus trigger or contribute to further hemodynamic instability.[59,89] In patients being ventilated without PEEP, data demonstrate that pressures can be measured accurately without disconnecting the patient from the ventilator.[95]
	D. Remember that isolated hemodynamic readings are generally not significant. Serial readings and trends should be monitored because they provide essential information about the patient's response to fluids, diuretics, and cardiovascular medications. Additionally, accurate interpretation and diagnosis of any one hemodynamic parameter require that it be correlated with the patient's clinical condition and simultaneously evaluated with other hemodynamic parameters.
	E. Review and assess with the anesthesiologist all intravascular lines and solutions with regard to type, drugs being infused, flow rates, patency, and expiration times if applicable. Ensure that all intravascular lines are securely anchored.
	F. Assess and document the patient's neurologic status on admission and every 30 to 60 minutes until the patient arouses from anesthesia. After arousal, neurologic checks can be decreased to every 2 hours as necessary. Neurologic checks should consist of assessment of pupillary, motor, cognitive, and verbal function. Total assessment of the last two cannot be performed completely until after extubation. Use of the Glasgow coma scale is recommended (see Chap. 29).
	G. Establish the chest tube drainage system. Note location, number, and types of chest tubes. Most patients will have one or two mediastinal chest tubes that will facilitate intrathoracic drainage after surgery. If the pleura was opened during the procedure or the patient's internal mammary artery was dissected off the chest wall, then pleural chest tubes will also be inserted to facilitate drainage and to prevent a pneumothorax.
	Attach the chest tubes to the drainage system, securely taping all connections. Drainage systems can include the following:
	(1) Water-seal drainage, in which the system may or may not be attached to 20 to 25 cm of suction
	(2) Autotransfusion systems, in which the patient's shed blood is reinfused as volume replacement when needed (see Box 26-3)
	H. Assess and record the amount and type of chest tube drainage every 30 to 60 minutes. Chest tube drainage should not exceed 100 cc/hour for longer than 4 hours. Normal chest tube drainage consists of a portion of blood not totally removed from the chest before sternal closing and a small amount of fresh blood. This will appear in the chest tube as bloody yet thin drainage. This drainage rarely clots in the chest tube because it has been defibrinogenated in the chest cavity by the movement of the lungs. When active bleeding is occurring, the drainage not only increases in amount but also tends to clot in the chest tube.
	I. Milk or gently strip chest tubes per unit routine to maintain patency. Chest tubes are usually removed within the first 12 to 48 hours after surgery, when the drainage is less than 200 cc for the previous 6 hours. Petrolatum gauze dressings are maintained for approximately 24 hours after removal.
4. The patient will achieve normothermia.	4. Obtain the patient's temperature on admission and every hour until the patient returns to and maintains normothermia for 2 hours; then obtain the temperature every 4 hours. The temperature can be measured rectally, from a pulmonary artery catheter thermistor, or from a commercially available thermistor attached to a Foley catheter. Although it is routine for the patient to be rewarmed to 36°C in the operating suite before transfer, frequently temperatures will drift back to

(continued)

NURSING CARE PLAN SUMMARY   *Immediate Postoperative Period*   *Continued*

Patient Outcomes	*Nursing Orders*
	as low as 33 to 34°C by the time the patient reaches the critical care area. Rewarming therapy should be immediately instituted. Current rewarming techniques include the following: A. Rewarming lights: Infrared or quartz lamps that are usually suspended over the patient's bed B. Blankets: Alcohol-circulating mattresses, reflective insulative blankets, or regular thermal blankets heated in a warmer Current evidence suggests that all these devices are equally effective in returning the patient to normothermia.[240] Rewarming should be discontinued once the patient reaches or is close to 37°C. Overaggressive rewarming can precipitate a hyperthermic overshoot, which will increase the patient's metabolic rate and myocardial workload.
5. The patient will achieve normal gastrointestinal functioning.	5. Assess the abdomen on admission and then every 2 hours or as necessary. A. Auscultate for bowel sounds. These are usually absent or hypoactive on admission but return within 24 hours or once the patient starts to take ice chips. B. Palpate and percuss the abdomen for distention and tympany, which may develop if the patient has a gastric air bubble. C. If a nasogastric tube is inserted, check the tube for correct placement and connect it to low intermittent suction or gravity drainage. Ensure that the tube is securely taped to the patient's nose or, if it is inserted orally, to the oral endotracheal tube. Observe the amount and type of nasogastric drainage. The nasogastric tube is usually removed when the patient is extubated.
6. The patient will achieve normal renal functioning.	6. Assess the catheter's patency and tape the catheter to the patient's thigh. Empty the urinary drainage bag on admission and begin measuring and recording hourly urinary outputs. Observe the color and consistency of urine. Initially, urinary output may exceed 3 to 4 L for the first few hours after surgery. This urine is usually pale and dilute and is a result of diuretics given as the patient is weaned from cardiopulmonary bypass. A transient hematuria may develop after cardiopulmonary bypass or administration of autotransfused blood. This is usually self-limiting or will clear after the administration of mannitol. Urine output should not fall to less than 30 cc/hour or 0.5 cc/kg/hour. The physician should be notified if these parameters cannot be maintained.
7. The patient will achieve normal peripheral circulatory functioning.	7. Assess and record the status of the peripheral circulation on admission and then every 2 hours or as necessary. A. Note the presence and grade the strength of carotid, radial, brachial, dorsalis pedis, posterior tibial, and femoral pulses. Pulses may initially be faint or absent owing to vasoconstriction and hypothermia. B. Obtain and record cuff blood pressures from both arms. These may also initially be absent. Auscultate for bruits. C. Observe the patient's skin color and temperature. Note capillary refilling in the nailbeds of both hands and feet. Observe the skin for any breaks, bruising, or reddened areas and for the presence of edema. Due to hypothermia, vasoconstriction, and prolonged immobility on the operating table, these patients are highly prone to developing skin breakdown. Attempt to reposition or turn the patient as soon as the patient is stable.
8. The patient will not experience postoperative complications.	8. Prevent postoperative complications as follows: A. Record locations and assess all incision and intravascular line insertion sites. B. Check dressings for bleeding, and outline the borders of the drainage and label with the date and time. Light palpation of saphenous incisions through the elastic leg wraps for hardened areas will assist in early identification of hematoma formation. Measuring thigh circumference is also beneficial. Dressings are usually removed once drainage has stopped. Incisions are then left open to air and cleansed with a solution such as povidone-iodine three times a day. In some settings, transparent dressings are used on both the sternal and leg incisions and are left on for 3 to 4 days as long as they remain intact. Transparent dressings for intravascular insertion sites are generally changed every 24 hours.

(continued)

NURSING CARE PLAN SUMMARY   *Immediate Postoperative Period*   *Continued*

Patient Outcomes	**Nursing Orders**
	C. Coordinate activities and allow technicians access to the patient as soon as possible in order to obtain a chest x-ray, 12-lead ECG, and laboratory work. Initial laboratory studies include arterial blood gases, hemoglobin and hematocrit, and coagulation and electrolyte profiles. Inspect the chest x-ray for positioning of the endotracheal tube, nasogastric tube, intravascular lines, and chest tubes, as well as the width of the mediastinum, the size of the heart, and the condition of the lung fields.
	D. Discuss with the surgeon and anesthesiologist any pertinent preoperative history or intraoperative events that will affect the patient's postoperative course. Review the nursing care plan from the preoperative area if it has not been previously reviewed.
	E. Document an admission assessment and begin to formulate a specific plan for nursing care.
	F. Allow the family to visit once the patient is stable and they have met with the surgeon to discuss the surgical procedure.

BOX 26-1.   Evaluation of Commonly Measured Hemodynamic Parameters

1. Mean arterial pressures (MAP) is obtained most often from either a radial, brachial, or femoral artery as follows:
   A. Monitor continuously with the lower and upper alarm limits set at 60 and 120 mm Hg, respectively, or at other parameters established by the physician or nurse.
   B. Record the parameters every 15 minutes as necessary until the patient is stable.
   C. Maintain the parameters at levels determined by the physician via ordered pharmacologic or fluid therapies. Notify the physician if the parameters cannot be maintained.
   D. Observe the contour of the arterial pressure curve. Obtain a strip recording on admission and then every 2 hours or as necessary. Alterations in arterial wave configurations can be indicative of physiologic alterations and complications in the postoperative period. The normal arterial curve consists of two waves separated by the dicrotic notch. The upstroke of the pressure curve ascends steeply corresponding with the QRS complex of the ECG, and it represents ventricular systole. The dicrotic notch indicates closure of the aortic valve. The final downstroke represents diastole; it is characterized by a fall in pressure. The highest point of the arterial pressure curve is the systolic pressure. The lowest point just before the next upstroke is the diastolic pressure (Fig. 26–9A).
2. Central venous pressure (CVP) or right atrial pressure (RAP) can be obtained from a catheter inserted directly through the right atrial wall during surgery; from the proximal port of a pulmonary artery flow-directed catheter; or from a catheter inserted in the brachial, external jugular, or subclavian veins. The tips of these catheters reside in the right atrial cavity and therefore serve as the volume measurement or the preload measurement of the right side of the heart. The RAP reflects the ability of the heart to pump the volume of blood being returned to it. The RAP measurement can be used to assess for hemoconcentration (hypovolemia) or hemodilution (hypervolemia). It is also used to determine complications, such as right-sided heart failure. The CVP or the RAP does not, however, necessarily indicate how well the left side of the heart functions. It does not, therefore, differentiate hypovolemia from poor venous return or hypervolemia from left-sided heart failure.

   The normal RAP ranges from 4 to 15 cm H_2O or 3 to 11 mm Hg. In the patient who has undergone open heart surgery, the RAP is allowed to be elevated, on the basis of the Frank-Starling law, which states that the greater the stretch of the muscle (the more volume), the greater the strength of contraction.

   The RAP may be measured in centimeters of water by a water manometer or in millimeters of mercury from a transducer. An understanding of the conversion factor is important. Mercury is 13.6 times heavier than water. To convert millimeters of mercury (from a transducer) to centimeters of water, the number of millimeters of mercury should be multiplied by the conversion factor 1.36 (*e.g.*, 8 mm Hg $\times$ 1.36 = 10.88 cm H_2O).

   The transducer, or the zero of the water manometer, must be positioned at the level of the right atrium, which is also known as the phlebostatic axis. The *phlebostatic axis* is defined as the junction between the transverse plane of the body passing through the fourth intercostal space at the lateral margin of the sternum and a frontal plane of the body passing through the midpoint of a line

   (continued)

BOX 26-1 *Continued*

from the outermost point of the posterior chest (the spine) to the outermost point of the anterior chest (the sternum).[245]

A. Monitor the RAP continuously if this line is not used as a primary volume or medication route.

B. Obtain and record the RAP every 30 to 60 minutes until the patient is stable. Because the right atrial wave is biphasic, these waves should be monitored on "mean" when using a digital display.

C. Maintain parameters at levels determined by the physician. Notify the physician if the parameters cannot be maintained.

D. Observe for alterations in the right atrial tracing. Obtain a strip recording on admission and then every 2 hours or as necessary. The normal right atrial wave is a low-pressure wave that consists of positive and negative deflections that are normally of the same amplitude. Alterations in these deflections can be indicative of physiologic changes and complications.

3. Pulmonary artery pressures consist specifically of pulmonary artery systolic (PAS), pulmonary artery diastolic (PAD), pulmonary artery mean (PAM), and pulmonary capillary wedge pressures (PCWP). These pressures are obtained via a flow-directed, balloon-tipped pulmonary artery catheter that can be inserted into a vein and passed through the vena cava, the right atrium, the tricuspid valve, the right ventricle, and the pulmonary valve and positioned in the pulmonary artery. The passage of the catheter through the heart can be observed by watching the coded distance markings on the catheter and the changes in the pressure waveforms displayed on the cardiac monitor.[58]

The PAS pressure represents the peak pressure of the right ventricle and ranges from 20 to 30 mm Hg. The lowest pressure generated in the pulmonary artery is the PAD, which ranges from 10 to 15 mm Hg. In patients without significant pulmonary disease, this parameter can serve as an indirect reflection of left atrial pressure (LAP) and left ventricular end-diastolic pressure (LVEDP). The PAM pressure represents the average of the systolic and diastolic pulmonary artery pressures. It ranges from 10 to 20 mm Hg. The PCWP is measured by inflating the balloon on the catheter to wedge it tightly in the small distal branch of the pulmonary artery. The pressures exerted distal to the inflated balloon are blocked so that the proximal tip of the catheter measures only the pressure in the pulmonary capillary system. The PCWP also indirectly reflects the LAP and LVEDP and normally ranges from 4 to 12 mm Hg.

A. Monitor the pulmonary artery tracing continuously to ensure immediate recognition in case the catheter drifts forward into the wedge position or falls backward into the right ventricle.

B. Obtain and record the PAS, PAD, or PAM pressure every 15 to 30 minutes until the patient is stable.

C. Maintain the parameters at prescribed levels, and notify the physician if they cannot be maintained.

D. Obtain a strip recording of all pulmonary artery pressures on admission and then every 2 hours or as necessary to assess for changes in the wave configuration that could indicate a slow drifting of the catheter or physiologic changes.

E. Obtain and record the PCWP per unit routine or physician's order. Particular care needs to be taken during balloon inflation in these patients because

many have pulmonary vessels that are stiff and nondistensible from a history of pulmonary hypertension or mitral valve disease. With these conditions, balloon inflation will more likely precipitate a pulmonary artery rupture. Other factors that may heighten the risk of pulmonary artery rupture include the patient's hypothermic state, which will cause the catheter to remain rigid and stiff for longer periods, thereby lengthening the exposure time of these highly susceptible vessels to a rigid catheter tip. Additionally, because the lungs are not fully inflated during the operative procedure, this may allow the stiff catheter to advance further in the vascular bed than it would if the lungs were totally inflated, thereby causing some resistance. Thus, the nurse should be particularly cautious when inflating the balloon and may frequently find the balloon "wedges" at volumes less than the balloon's normal filling volume. This occurrence or frequent self-wedging may be indicator that the catheter should be slightly withdrawn. For these reasons, some surgeons and anesthesiologists will either avoid using a flow-directed catheter in patients with mitral valve disease or pulmonary hypertension or will order that the catheter not be wedged in the postoperative period.[10]

An alternative method to measuring pulmonary artery pressures is by a pulmonary artery thermistor catheter. This is a single-lumen catheter with an attached thermistor apparatus. The catheter is inserted directly into the pulmonary artery at the conclusion of the operative procedure and exits the skin via a stab incision at the distal portion of the sternotomy. It may or may not be secured in the pulmonary artery with an absorbable suture. Although wedge readings cannot be obtained from this catheter, it allows recording of PAS, PAD, and PAM pressures. Additionally, because it has a thermistor attached to it, it can measure cardiac output.

4. Left atrial pressure is obtained via a catheter that is inserted into one of the pulmonary veins prior to chest closure. The tip of the catheter resides in the left atrium, and as with the pulmonary artery line, it exists by way of a stab wound at the distal portion of the sternal incision.

The LAP is the preload measurement for the left side of the heart because it directly reflects the filling pressure of the left ventricle just before contraction—the LVEDP. The normal range for LAP is 4 to 12 mm Hg. In normal situations, the LAP, PCWP, and PAD pressures all reflect LVEDP. In the postoperative period, in order to ensure maximal filling pressures and, hence, maximal stroke volume, the LVEDP is generally maintained at 15 to 20 mm Hg. To achieve this higher filling pressure, the physician will usually prescribe parameters for LAP, PCWP, and RAP that slightly exceed their normal ranges or are reflective of the upper portion of their normal ranges.

A. Monitor the LAP continuously to ensure immediate recognition should the wave become dampened. Left atrial lines are never irrigated but can be gently aspirated if the wave dampens.

B. Obtain and record the LAP every 30 to 60 minutes until the patient is stable. Because left atrial waves

(continued)

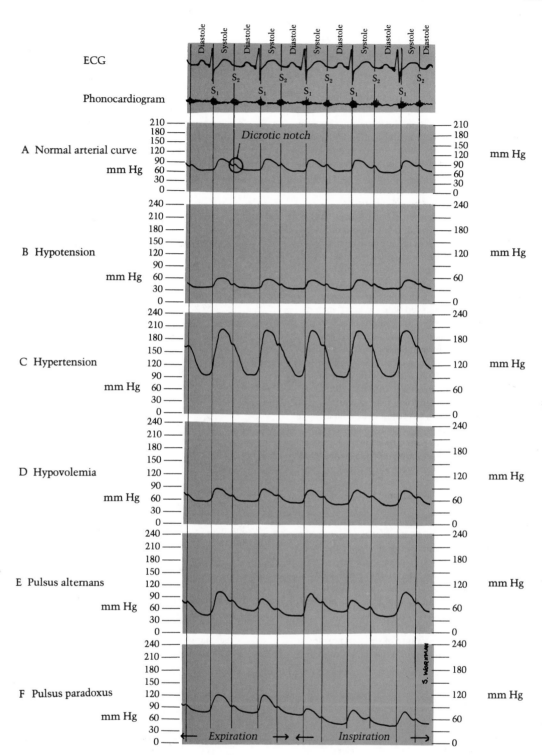

Figure 26–9

Arterial curves: (*A*) normal arterial curve; (*B*) hypotension; (*C*) hypertension; (*D*) hypovolemia; (*E*) pulsus alternans; (*F*) pulsus paradoxus.

BOX 26-1   *Continued*

are biphasic, these waves should be monitored on "mean" when using a digital display.

C. Maintain parameters at levels determined by the physician. Notify the physician if the parameters cannot be maintained.

D. Observe for alterations in the LAP tracing. Obtain a strip recording on admission and then every 2 hours or as necessary. The normal left atrial wave is a low-pressure wave that consists of positive and negative deflections that are normally of the same amplitude. Alterations in these deflections can be indicative of physiologic changes and complications.

5. SvO_2. Mixed venous-oxygen saturation results (SvO_2) can be obtained either by withdrawing a pulmonary arterial blood sample and sending it to the laboratory for evaluation or by using a pulmonary artery catheter with a fiberoptic photometric lumen that can supply continuous monitoring of SvO_2 results. A normal range for SvO_2 is 60% to 80%, which reflects that oxygen supply to the tissues is balanced with oxygen demand and, thus, tissue perfusion is adequate. A low SvO_2 (*i.e.* less than 60%) can develop in a cardiac surgery patient during shivering, when oxygen demand exceeds oxygen supply; during episodes of hypotension, hypovolemia, dysrhythmias or shock, when there is a decrease in cardiac output; or due to anemia from hemodilution or hemorrhage because of insufficient hemoglobin. It can also be low when there is a reduction in arterial oxygen saturation such as occurs with respiratory distress or atelectasis. A SvO_2 greater than 80% can develop in these patients when oxygen supply exceeds demand, as occurs in hypothermia, excessive inotropic therapy, or pharmacologic paralysis.[85,201]

6. Cardiac output (CO) can be measured by the following techniques:[58]

A. The thermodilution technique, which involves injection of an injectate solution into the right atrium and measuring the temperature change of the blood in the pulmonary artery by means of a thermistor-tipped catheter. Studies indicate that either iced (0 to 5°C) or room-temperature (21 to 26°C) injectate will yield valid readings and that, additionally, either 5- or 10-cc injectate boluses can be used.[11,209,234]

B. The indicator dilution technique, which involves injecting a measured quantity of some indicator (an isotope or contrast media) into the right atrium or pulmonary artery and drawing a blood sample from the peripheral arterial circulation. The cardiac output is calculated by an indicator dilution curve that measures the passage of the indicator over time from the venous blood to the arterial blood.

C. The oxygen-consumption technique, which is carried out by calculating the arteriovenous oxygen difference using systemic and pulmonary arterial samples

7. Cardiac index (CI) can be calculated by the following formula:

$$CI = \frac{CO \text{ (cardiac output)}}{BSA \text{ (body surface area)}}$$

Classification of cardiac index levels is as follows[79]:

2.7–4.3 L/minute/m² = normal perfusion
2.2–2.7 L/minute/m² = subclinical depression
1.8–2.2 L/minute/m² = onset of clinical hypoperfusion
<1.8 L/minute/m² = cardiogenic shock

8. Systemic vascular resistance (SVR) is calculated by the following formula:

$$SVR = \frac{MAP - \overline{RAP} \times 80}{CO}$$

where $\overline{RAP}$ is mean right atrial pressure. Normal SVR levels range from 900 to 1300 dyne-seconds/cm⁵ (absolute units). The SVR is usually elevated in the postoperative cardiac surgical patient as a result of the effects of cardiopulmonary bypass, hypothermia, sympathetic drive, and the vasoconstrictive effects of some pharmacologic agents. An elevated SVR increases the afterload of the left ventricle. This resistance to left ventricular ejection can create left ventricular failure and a low CO state.

9. Pulmonary vascular resistance (PVR) is calculated by the following formula:

$$PVR = \frac{PAM - (PCWP \text{ or } LAP) \times 80}{CO}$$

Normal PVR levels range from 80 to 240 dyne-seconds/cm⁵ (absolute units). An elevated PVR increases the afterload of the right ventricle. This resistance to right ventricular ejection can create right ventricular failure.

NURSING CARE PLAN SUMMARY   *Postoperative Period*

NURSING DIAGNOSIS

1. *Decreased cardiac output or tissue perfusion related to vasoconstriction (exchanging pattern)*

Patient Outcomes	Nursing Orders
1. The patient will exhibit signs of adequate cardiac output and tissue perfusion as evidenced by normotension, normothermia, normal SVR, adequate CO/CI, warm	1. The severe vasoconstriction seen in these patients is most often a direct reflection of their elevated SVR. Factors contributing to this increase in SVR include cardiopulmonary bypass, systemic hypothermia, vasoactive drugs, and the patient's own normal sympathetic drive, which is initiated by the surgical manipulation of the heart and great vessels and their attached pressor receptors.

(continued)

NURSING CARE PLAN SUMMARY   *Postoperative Period*   *Continued*

Patient Outcomes	*Nursing Orders*
vasodilated extremities, adequate peripheral pulses, and absence of tachycardia.	A. Monitor, assess, and record signs and symptoms of vasoconstriction: (1) Hypertension (MAP greater than 120 mm Hg). Hypertension is characterized on the arterial waveform by a steep and peaked systolic upstroke usually greater than 160 mm Hg and a diastolic downstroke greater than 90 mm Hg (Fig. 26–9C). (2) Elevated SVR (SVR greater than 1400 dyne-seconds/cm^5) (3) Hypothermia (rectal or Foley catheter temperature less than 37°C) (4) Decreased CO/CI (CO less than 5 L/minute or CI less than 2.7 L/minute/m^2) (5) Tachycardia (heart rate greater than 110 beats/minute) (6) Cold, pale extremities (7) Absent or diminished peripheral pulses
2. The patient will not develop complications related to vasoconstriction.	2. Identify and describe major complications that can develop as a result of postoperative vasoconstriction. A. Hemorrhage. Persistent elevation of arterial pressures can cause leaking or rupture of the newly anastomosed graft and cannulation sites. Critical levels of arterial pressure elevation can vary from patient to patient. Most commonly, attempts are aimed at maintaining the MAP at levels lower than 110 to 120 mm Hg. However, in patients with friable aortas due to extensive atherosclerotic changes, the upper pressure limits may be determined by the surgeon to be 80 to 90 mm Hg. (1) Monitor, assess, and record the amount and quality of chest tube drainage. Notify the physician if amounts exceed 100 cc/hour. B. Low cardiac output and myocardial ischemia. Persistent elevation of SVR causes impedance to left ventricular ejection and ultimately decreases stroke volume and cardiac output. Additionally, this high resistance can cause myocardial ischemia. (1) Monitor, assess, and record CO/CI.
3. The patient will respond to therapy to reverse vasoconstriction.	3. Implement strategies according to either the physician's orders or standing unit policies to reverse vasoconstriction. A. Identify commonly used pharmacologic agents to reverse vasoconstriction and control hypertension. Identify their routes of administration, their actions, and their dosages. These agents can include the following: (1) Sodium nitroprusside. A potent and rapidly reversible peripheral vasodilator, this drug causes an acute reduction in systemic vascular resistance by its action on both the peripheral venous and arterial musculature and can thereby lower the MAP within 2 minutes. Administered by way of a continuous intravenous infusion, doses are determined by the response in the patient's arterial pressure. Normal infusion rates usually range from 0.5 to 3.0 µg/kg/minute, although doses up to 8.0 µg/kg/minute can be used. (2) Nitroglycerin. Intravenous boluses of this agent (0.04 mg/cc) given a half cubic centimeter at a time can produce a fall in MAP within seconds owing to its ability to dilate venous capacitance vessels. This may be an effective technique to use during the period of time the sodium nitroprusside solution is being ordered and initiated or during acute transient situations such as after a procedure in which the patient may become acutely hypertensive. Because it has been demonstrated that nitroglycerin can increase blood flow in the coronary collateral vessels,[41,93] continuous infusions of nitroglycerin are also used frequently in patients after routine revascularization as well as in patients experiencing coronary artery spasm or postoperative ischemia. (3) Other vasoactive agents used less frequently include phentolamine, diazoxide, and trimethaphan. Primarily an alpha-adrenergic blocking agent, phentolamine also serves as a direct vascular smooth muscle relaxer. Diazoxide acts as a arteriolar dilator, and trimethaphan causes relaxation of vascular smooth muscle through its ganglionic blocking effects.

(continued)

NURSING CARE PLAN SUMMARY *Postoperative Period* *Continued*

Patient Outcomes	*Nursing Orders*

B. Administer the preceding pharmacologic drugs to maintain MAP and SVR between parameters determined by the physician. The usual levels are SVR less than 1400 dyne-seconds/cm[5] and MAP between 80 and 120 mm Hg. However, there is evidence that lowering the MAP to normotensive levels (*i.e.*, 80 mm Hg) will maintain adequate functional clinical parameters such as cardiac index and ejection fraction but may fail to maintain adequate myocardial metabolic indices and may increase cardiac lactate production.[81] This would seem to indicate that lowering the MAP to normotensive levels in the postoperative period could cause a mild amount of myocardial ischemia. From a nursing perspective, this reinforces the concern for careful manual titration of vasodilator drugs to avoid even moderate falls below the specified parameters.

More recently, a computerized closed-loop sodium nitroprusside titration system has been introduced into the market. Using the patient's MAP recording as a means of feedback, a computer regulates the infusion of sodium nitroprusside by an infusion pump. The desired MAP is determined by the nurse or physician. The system senses the patient's pressure every 1/100 second and adjusts the infusion rate every 10 seconds. Initial studies demonstrate that this device controls the blood pressure more quickly than the manual titration technique, requires less time spent on titration tasks, and produces less overall hypotensive and hypertensive blood pressure fluctuations.[110]

C. If manual administration of sodium nitroprusside or the other vasodilators is required, the nurse should perform the following:
   (1) Observe the MAP every 2 to 3 minutes until the desired pressure is achieved.
   (2) Record the MAP every 15 minutes on the flowsheet or more frequently to adequately reflect the patient's postoperative course.
   (3) Observe monitored filling pressures (RAP, PAD, and LAP) every 2 to 3 minutes.
   (4) Record filling pressures every 15 minutes or more frequently to reflect the patient's postoperative course adequately. Hypovolemic hypotension is the most frequent complication associated with vasodilator therapy and should be aggressively observed for and treated.
   (5) Administer volume replacement to maintain the patient's filling pressures to prevent hypovolemic hypotension.
   (6) If severe hypotension develops, immediately decrease or discontinue vasodilator infusion. If hypotension is due to hypovolemia, elevate the lower extremities either manually or by raising the foot of the bed. This supplies the patient with an autotransfusion of volume that is sequestered in the dilated lower extremities.
   (7) Avoid dramatic and precipitous falls in blood pressure due to rapid infusion of vasodilators and inadequate volume replacement. Lowering MAP to levels less than 60 mm Hg may precipitate graft closure or cause myocardial ischemia.
   (8) Attempt to discontinue vasodilators once the effects of vasoconstriction are reversed. This can usually be done 6 to 8 hours after surgery. In patients who were hypertensive before surgery, vasodilators may need to be continued until preoperative medications are resumed.

D. Initiate rewarming therapies to assist in vasodilatation.[182] During rewarming do the following:
   (1) Monitor the patient's temperature either continuously or every hour.
   (2) Protect the patient's skin during rewarming. If using a warming mattress, apply lotion or cream and place a sheet between the patient and mattress. Observe the skin frequently during rewarming.
   (3) Monitor filling pressures as described for vasodilator therapy, and observe for signs of hypovolemic hypotension.

(continued)

NURSING CARE PLAN SUMMARY *Postoperative Period* *Continued*

Patient Outcomes	Nursing Orders
	(4) Maintain optimum filling pressures by appropriate volume replacement. (5) Discontinue rewarming as the patient's temperature nears 37°C. (6) Continue to monitor the temperature continuously or hourly until the patient remains normothermic for 2 hours in order to identify and treat hyperthermic overshoots immediately.

NURSING DIAGNOSIS

2. *Decreased cardiac output related to a decrease in mechanical factors (contractility from myocardial depression) (exchanging pattern)*

Patient Outcomes

Nursing Orders

1. The patient will exhibit signs of adequate CO and contractility as evidenced by normal CO/CI, warm vasodilated extremities, adequate peripheral pulses, adequate urinary output, normal cardiac enzymes, normal ECG, and normal sensorium.

1. Identify and describe factors or conditions that directly affect myocardial contractility after cardiac surgery. Common factors include perioperative myocardial infarction or ischemia, metabolic disturbances, myocardial edema from surgical manipulation, faulty surgical repair, and myocardial depression from anesthesia and hypothermia.
   A. Although the incidence of perioperative infarction has been decreased in recent years, the nurse should be aware of risk factors associated with its development (see p. 451). Although they are becoming increasingly less predictive, preoperative and intraoperative risk factors are as follows:[162,200]
      (1) Severity of preoperative myocardial ischemia
      (2) Multivessel disease
      (3) Severe left ventricular function and decreased ejection fraction
      (4) Prolonged cardiopulmonary bypass and aortic cross-clamping time
      (5) Left main coronary artery disease
   B. Postoperative risk factors for myocardial infarction and ischemia that the nurse should observe for and avoid include the following:
      (1) Hypertension and tachycardia. These can disproportionately increase myocardial oxygen consumption over myocardial oxygen supply. Although these are normal sequelae after surgery owing to vasoconstriction, the nurse should particularly anticipate their development in patients with preoperative essential hypertension or with aortic stenosis lesions. These patients are at increased risk to develop a hyperdynamic left ventricular syndrome characterized by excessive postoperative contractility and difficult-to-control hypertension. Myocardial infarction and arrest can quickly ensue in these patients.
      (2) Hypovolemia, hypotension, and dysrhythmias. These can lower aortic root diastolic pressure to levels that supply inadequate coronary artery perfusion and hence lead to myocardial ischemia or infarction.
      (3) The remaining causes of decreased contractility are usually short-lived and resolve within hours after surgery or, in the case of faulty surgical repair, resolve on reoperation. The degree of myocardial depression associated with all these entities ranges from levels that are clinically imperceptible to the development of cardiogenic shock.
   C. Monitor, assess, and record the following signs and symptoms of decreased myocardial contractility and cardiogenic shock:
      (1) Decreased CO/CI (CO less than 5 L/minute or CI less than 2.7 L/minute/m^2)
      (2) Hypotension (systolic blood pressure less than 80 mm Hg or MAP less than 60 mm Hg)
      (3) Elevated SVR or PVR (SVR greater than 1300 dyne-seconds/cm^5 and PVR greater than 240 dyne-seconds/cm^5)

(continued)

NURSING CARE PLAN SUMMARY   *Postoperative Period*   *Continued*

Patient Outcomes	*Nursing Orders*
	(4) Elevated filling pressures
	(5) Urinary output less than 30 cc/hour or less than 0.5 cc/kg/hour
	(6) Presence of S$_3$ and S$_4$ heart sounds
	(7) Jugular venous distention
	(8) Pulmonary crackles
	(9) Hypoxemia and acidosis
	(10) Tachycardia (heart rate greater than 110 beats/minute)
	(11) Cyanosis
	(12) Rapid, shallow respirations
	(13) Cold, clammy, mottled skin
	(14) Decreased level of consciousness
	(15) Presence of pulsus alternans (Fig. 26–9E): A classic sign of left ventricular failure in which the pattern is characterized by alternating high and low arterial pressure curves.
	(16) Observe for other diagnostic signs of loss of myocardial contractility, such as the following:
	a. ST-segment changes or T-wave inversion lasting more than 48 hours on the ECG. These changes can be nonspecific and attributed to electrolyte imbalances, pericardial inflammation, or subendocardial infarction.
	b. New Q waves on the ECG. The presence of these are a fairly specific sign indicative of a perioperative myocardial infarction. However, in patients with pre-existing Q waves, left bundle branch block, intraventricular conduction defects, and after aneurysmectomy, the interpretation of new Q waves can be difficult.[212]
	c. New complete left bundle branch block. The presence of a new complete left bundle branch block postoperatively in a patient after myocardial revascularization has been shown to correlate with intraoperative myocardial damage.[31]
	d. Elevation in CPK determinations. CPK levels three to six times normal, peaking on day 2 with a CPK-MB fraction of 8% to 15% is a fairly specific and accurate indicator for the presence of a perioperative myocardial infarction.[91]
	e. Elevation in the SGOT in the immediate postoperative period that exceeds 50 U generally indicates myocardial injury either from ischemia or a long and difficult surgical procedure. If the SGOT is over 140 units, however, it usually indicates myocardial damage from an infarction. In some centers, a SGPT is also obtained if the SGOT is higher than 100 U to assist in differentiating myocardial from hepatic injury.

2. If decreased myocardial contractility occurs, the patient will respond to the appropriate therapy.	2. Implement strategies according to either the physician's orders or standing unit policies to improve myocardial contractility:
	A. Identify commonly used pharmacologic drugs to improve contractility. Identify their routes of administration, their actions, and their dosages as outlined in Box 26-2.
	B. Administer the pharmacologic agents outlined in Box 26-2 and titrate them to achieve parameters determined by the physician. Usual parameters might include MAP greater than 80 mm Hg and/or a CI greater than 2.7 L/minute/m². During administration of these vasopressors and inotropic agents, the nurse should perform the following:
	   (1) Observe MAP every 2 to 3 minutes when active titration is being performed.
	   (2) Record MAP every 15 minutes or more frequently to reflect the patient's postoperative course adequately.
	   (3) Observe for dysrhythmias that might be indicative of further myocardial ischemia from too much contractile drive.

(continued)

NURSING CARE PLAN SUMMARY *Postoperative Period* *Continued*

Patient Outcomes

Nursing Orders

(4) Monitor filling pressures for hypervolemic parameters. Observe hemodynamic tracings for presence of v waves that could indicate regurgitant blood flow back across either the mitral or tricuspid valves.

(5) Obtain CO/CI per unit routine or after changes in the patient's status or in the doses of the preceding drugs.

C. Identify and assist with initiating and maintaining other therapies used to improve the patient's myocardial contractile performance and cardiac output:

(1) Intra-aortic balloon pump. Positioned in the descending thoracic aorta,

---

BOX 26-2.   Pharmacologic Agents Used to Improve Myocardial Contractility

1. Dopamine. As an inotrope, dopamine increases cardiac contractility through its cardiac beta-adrenergic receptor activity. Additionally, in small doses (2 to 4 μg/kg/minute), it also induces peripheral vasodilatation. As doses exceed 6 μg/kg/minute, its effect on the peripheral beds becomes progressively more vasoconstrictive. At doses of 1 to 2 μg/kg/minute, its actions are exerted on dopaminergic receptor sites that can enhance renal and mesenteric blood flow.

2. Dobutamine. Dobutamine is a synthetic catecholamine that enhances contractility through its effects on cardiac beta-adrenergic receptors. Its chronotropic effects are minimal until doses greater than 10 to 15 μg/kg/minute are reached, at which point tachycardia may become problematic.

3. Isoproterenol. Isoproterenol has a significant inotropic effect due to its beta-adrenergic receptor–stimulating properties. It is particularly useful in treating patients with right ventricular dysfunction associated with pulmonary hypertension because it lowers pulmonary vascular resistance. It is also particularly useful in patients with low CO due to bradycardia. However, a major disadvantage of this drug centers on its tendency to create tachycardia and ventricular dysrhythmias that may contribute to cardiac failure.

4. Norepinephrine. In doses less than 0.02 to 0.2 μg/kg/minute, norepinephrine exhibits a moderate yet significant increase in contractility due to its beta-adrenergic receptor effects. Once doses exceed 0.3 μg/kg/minute, it becomes a strong peripheral vasoconstrictor due to its alpha-receptor actions. This increase in SVR can potentially negate its ability to improve cardiac output.

5. Amrinone. A phosphodiesterase inhibitor, amrinone allows higher levels of cyclic AMP to develop in the cells, which subsequently increases calcium transport and, thus, contractility and CO. In addition, it has vasodilator activity, which results in a decrease in filling pressure and systemic and pulmonary vascular resistance. Amrinone therapy is usually begun with a bolus dose of 0.75 to 1.5 mg/kg administered over 3 to 5 minutes and followed by a maintenance infusion of 5 to 10 μg/kg/minute.[92]

6. Epinephrine. Epinephrine's inotropic effect is attributed to its beta-adrenergic receptor activity. As with norepinephrine, low doses of epinephrine serve to decrease peripheral vascular resistance; conversely, high doses increase it. These actions can limit its use in patients with a severely failing myocardium unless concurrent vasodilator therapy is used.

7. Digoxin. As an inotropic agent, digoxin has a relatively rapid onset of action (5 to 30 minutes) and can enhance contractility for 2 to 6 days. Normal digitalization doses are 1.0 to 1.5 mg. This total dose is usually administered over a 24-hour period and then followed with a maintenance dose of 0.125 to 0.25 mg once or twice daily. The use of digoxin as an inotropic agent is generally indicated in settings of inadequate CO due to impaired systolic ventricular function. Diastolic ventricular dysfunction is best treated initially with vasodilators and diuretics.[214]

8. Glucagon. Glucagon stimulates non–beta-adrenergic sites in the myocardium and is usually used in conjunction with the previously mentioned catecholamines. It is particularly useful in patients who preoperatively were receiving beta blockers and who then experienced difficulty in being weaned from cardiopulmonary bypass.

9. Calcium chloride. Maintenance of sufficient ionized calcium levels is critical after surgery because cardiopulmonary bypass can reduce these levels and adequate levels of intracellular calcium are required to promote cardiac muscle contraction. For this reason, ionized calcium levels may be monitored, because this is the portion of calcium that is physiologically active. Low levels may be treated with calcium chloride administration.[49,63,201]

10. Oxygen. Adequate oxygenation and ventilation levels should be maintained. Evaluating arterial blood gas measurements will reflect the adequacy of this therapy.

11. Sodium bicarbonate. Because acidosis serves as a myocardial depressant, sodium bicarbonate may be given to return the blood pH to physiologic neutrality.

(continued)

NURSING CARE PLAN SUMMARY   *Postoperative Period*   *Continued*

Patient Outcomes	*Nursing Orders*
	the intra-aortic balloon sequentially inflates and deflates in diastole. At the beginning of diastole, the balloon inflates, causing an increase in aortic diastolic pressure that increases coronary artery perfusion and, hence, myocardial oxygenation. Immediately before systole, the balloon rapidly deflates, which assists in decreasing resistance to left ventricular ejection during systole. This decreases left ventricular workload and, hence, decreases myocardial oxygen demand. Nursing interventions with the intra-aortic balloon pump mainly center on establishing and maintaining optimum timing of deflation and inflation. (2) Hemopump. The hemopump is a temporary left ventricular assist device that uses axial flow to function. With this system, a special cannula is inserted through the femoral artery and is passed across the aortic valve so that its tip lies in the left ventricle. An axial flow pump is located on the cannula and lies at approximately the level of the descending thoracic aorta. Once activated, the pump begins to rotate, and this rotation causes blood to be lifted out of the ventricle through the tip of the cannula and to be ejected into the aorta. This pump can generate 0.5 to 3.0 L/minute of continuous flow. This decreases left ventricular workload and, thus, myocardial oxygen demand.[197] (3) Ventricular assist devices. Ventricular assist devices are indicated for patients who cannot be weaned from cardiopulmonary bypass after trials with pharmacologic therapies and the intra-aortic balloon pump. Ventricular assistance can be either univentricular (right- or left-sided heart assist) or biventricular (right- and left-sided heart assist). Both this device and the intra-aortic balloon pump are temporary devices and require that the ventricle will eventually regain its own function (see Chap. 18).

NURSING DIAGNOSIS

3. *Decreased cardiac output related to mechanical factors (cardiac tamponade) (exchanging pattern)*

Patient Outcome	*Nursing Orders*
1. The patient will exhibit signs of adequate cardiac output and absence of resistance to right-sided heart filling or fluid accumulation around the heart, as evidenced by adequate CO/CI, normotension, adequate heart rate, normal pulse pressure, absence of pressure plateau, absence of neck vein distention, pulsus paradoxus less than 10 mm Hg, normal cardiac and mediastinal silhouette on chest x-ray, normal heart sounds, adequate ECG voltage, and adequate level of consciousness.	1. Identify situations or risk factors for the development of cardiac tamponade. Cardiac tamponade occurs when there is a compression of the heart due to an accumulation of fluid in the pericardium. This compression limits ventricular filling and consequently causes a decrease in stroke volume and CO. Additionally, the compression creates resistance to right-sided heart filling, causing signs of right-sided heart congestion. If fluid accumulates quickly, tamponade can occur with as little as 150 to 200 cc being sequestered in the pericardium. If fluid accumulates slowly, a liter or more can sequester before signs and symptoms are apparent. Early tamponade usually occurs within the first 6 hours after surgery and can develop either from a slow oozing of blood secondary to a coagulopathy or from direct bleeding from a surgical suture line. Bleeding after removal of epicardial pacing wires or left atrial or pulmonary artery lines can also occur in the early postoperative period. Late tamponade can occur as late as 30 days after surgery. At this date, it is most often associated with anticoagulation or postpericardiotomy syndrome. A. Monitor, assess, and record the following signs and symptoms of cardiac tamponade: (1) Persistent low CO/CI (CO less than 5 L/minute and CI less than 2.7 L/minute/m²)

(continued)

NURSING CARE PLAN SUMMARY Postoperative Period *Continued*

Patient Outcome	Nursing Orders

Nursing Orders (continued):

(2) Hypotension (MAP less than 60 mm Hg or systolic arterial pressure less than 80 mm Hg)

(3) Tachycardia (heart rate greater than 110 beats per minute)

(4) Sudden cessation of previously heavy chest tube drainage. This occurs as a result of occlusion of chest tubes from clots. It should be remembered that blood immediately initiates its clotting processes once it exits the blood vessels. In situations in which bleeding and oozing from surgical sites are minimal, this drainage will clot in the chest but is quickly defibrinogenated or declotted by the motion of the lungs and then exits the chest tubes as thin, bloody drainage. In situations in which there is significant hemorrhage, this previously balanced ratio of bleeding, clot lysis, and chest tube drainage is altered. As fresh blood quickly accumulates in the chest and clots, it surpasses the ability of the chest tubes to drain it and the lung action to assist in declotting it. This leads to blockage of chest tubes with clots and accumulation of blood in the chest and, hence, cardiac tamponade.

(5) Narrowed pulse pressure

(6) Elevated RAP

(7) Neck vein distention

(8) Development of a sustained pressure plateau or equalization of RAP and LAP.[120,189] Normally, left-sided heart pressures exceed right-sided heart pressures. In the presence of tamponade, however, right and left pressures equalize, and clinically, this can be best observed in the atrial pressures. Sustained equalization or equalization of these measurements over a 2-hour interval is a good indicator for both early and late tamponade.[129,189]

(9) Elevated SVR (SVR greater than 1400 dyne-seconds/cm^5)

(10) Presence of a pulsus paradoxus (Fig. 26-9F): A pulsus paradoxus exists when there is a decrease in systolic blood pressure by more than 10 mm Hg during inspiration. Although normally there can be a 3 to 10 mm Hg decrease in systolic pressure during inspiration, the exaggerated decline occurring in pulsus paradoxus is due to the transmission of negative intrathoracic pressure to the great vessels and a decrease in left ventricular stroke volume. The presence of a pulsus paradoxus is not a consistent finding in tamponade; it can also occur in other constrictive processes, such as chronic obstructive lung disease, pericarditis, and pulmonary emboli. However, there is evidence that an increasing magnitude in the pulsus paradoxus is a specific indicator for cardiac tamponade.[49]

(11) Widening of the mediastinum or enlargement of the cardiac silhouette on the chest x-ray

(12) Muffled heart sounds. As fluid sequesters in the pericardial sac, it increases the distance between the epicardium and the chest wall and, hence, muffles the heart sounds. This finding may not be significant in the cardiac surgical patient if the anterior portion of the pericardium was removed during the surgical procedure.

(13) Diminished ECG voltage. This may also not be apparent in the surgical patient if the pericardium remains open.

(14) Decreased urinary output (urine output less than 30 cc/hour or less than 0.5 cc/kg/hour)

(15) Unexplained apprehension or anxiety or alteration in level of consciousness

B. Report the presence of any of these signs and symptoms to the physician.

C. Prepare the patient for possible return to the operating room.

D. Continue to observe the patient's vital signs closely.

E. Have emergency equipment readily available. The beginning signs of tamponade are usually insidious. Once they become apparent, however,

(continued)

NURSING CARE PLAN SUMMARY Postoperative Period *Continued*

Patient Outcome	Nursing Orders
	there is a very rapid progression to cardiac arrest if the situation is not rectified. The nurse should therefore be prepared to assist with an emergency opening of the chest in the critical care area. In situations of tamponade, once the chest is opened and the intrapericardial pressure is alleviated, the patient's vital signs immediately improve and the patient can then be transported to the operating suite under less emergent conditions for surgical repair.

NURSING DIAGNOSIS

4. *Decreased cardiac output related to electrical factors (dysrhythmias) (exchanging pattern)*

Patient Outcome	Nursing Orders
1. The patient will exhibit signs of adequate CO and absence of dysrhythmias as evidenced by adequate CO and CI; adequate peripheral, cerebral, and renal perfusion; normal sinus rhythm or return to a hemodynamically stable dysrhythmia.	1. Identify and describe major and contributing factors for the development of dysrhythmias. In the postoperative patient, the incidence of atrial and ventricular dysrhythmias can be as high as 25% to 30%, with dysrhythmias occurring within the first 7 days after surgery. The impact these dysrhythmias have on cardiac output is highly variable and ranges from clinically imperceptible effects to major hemodynamic consequences. Other consequences of dysrhythmias can include discomfort to the patient, prolonged hospitalization, and embolization.

Major etiologic causes of dysrhythmias include iatrogenic, ischemic, pharmacologic, or metabolic processes. Iatrogenically, surgical manipulation itself, with its potential consequences of injury, ischemia, or transient edema involving the electrical conduction system, is a major factor. Additionally, manipulation increases the sympathetic drive and, thus, increases endogenous catecholamine release with its dysrhythmogenic capabilities. Mechanical irritation from intravascular lines, such as pulmonary artery flow-directed catheters or right atrial lines, can also serve as iatrogenic causes.

Ischemia due to acute myocardial infarction, hypotension, or hypoxemia may cause dysrhythmias. Such dysrhythmias generally occur in the early postoperative period.

Inotropic drugs that increase contractility and, thus, myocardial oxygen demand can cause ectopic rhythms, as can chronotropic agents, which may precipitate undesirable tachycardias and thus cause myocardial ischemia.

Fear and anxiety can stimulate the sympathetic nervous system to release catecholamines, which can initiate dysrhythmias. The development of pericarditis, reperfusion injury, or an inflammatory response also can cause dysrhythmias, especially in the later stages of recovery.

Lastly, metabolic processes such as acidosis or alkalosis, either from metabolic or respiratory causes, or electrolyte imbalances, particularly hypokalemia, also contribute to dysrhythmia production. The myocardium is particularly sensitive to hypokalemia in the postoperative period. Hypokalemia develops as a result of diuresis during and after cardiopulmonary bypass surgery and in the presence of metabolic alkalosis, where potassium ions are excreted in the urine in exchange for hydrogen ions.

A. Identify the following commonly occurring postoperative dysrhythmias and their appropriate treatment strategies:
   (1) Sinus bradycardia (heart rate less than 60 beats/minute). Therapy consists of the following measures:
      a. Institute temporary atrial pacing. Performed by the atrial epicardial pacing wires, atrial pacing achieves a higher CO than ventricular pacing because it ensures that atrial contraction is coordinated with ventricular filling. Atrial contraction and emptying can account for 30% of ventricular volume. This increased volume ensures a larger stroke volume and consequently a larger CO.

(continued)

NURSING CARE PLAN SUMMARY *Postoperative Period* *Continued*

Patient Outcome	*Nursing Orders*
	b. Administer pharmacologic drugs such as atropine and isoproterenol.

(2) Sinus or atrial tachycardia (heart rate greater than 110 beats/minute). Therapy consists of the following measures:
   a. Treat the underlying cause. Usual causes are hypervolemia, hypovolemia, hypotension, fever, anxiety, or pain.
   b. Administer pharmacologic drugs such as verapamil to decrease the heart rate.

(3) Atrial fibrillation or atrial flutter. The overall incidence of atrial fibrillation ranges from 10% to 40%, with the major incidence occurring 2 days after surgery. The prevalence of the disorder is higher in older patients.[82,158]

   When the ventricular response in these dysrhythmias is extremely accelerated, it may be difficult to differentiate between atrial fibrillation and atrial flutter as well as atrial tachycardia or paroxysmal atrial tachycardia. Use of the atrial pacing wires to obtain an atrial ECG assists in this differentiation. With this technique, the atrial response is accentuated on the rhythm strip and can be easily identified as atrial flutter or fibrillation. One method of obtaining an atrial rhythm recording is to attach the lower limb leads as usual to the patient and then attach, with an alligator clamp, the atrial wires individually to the right and left lead cable connectors. With the ECG machine on lead 1, a rhythm strip can be obtained. Treatment for these dysrhythmias can consist of the following measures:
   a. Administer pharmacologic drugs such as digoxin, verapamil, or beta-blockers. Patients who experienced atrial fibrillation or flutter in the preoperative period will almost invariably return to that rhythm postoperatively. In these situations, digoxin is usually initiated or restarted. It is preferred to withhold digoxin for the first 12 to 24 hours after surgery because the myocardium is extremely sensitive to its effects. However, if it is required, a loading dose of 1 mg within a 24-hour period is most often ordered, with the initial dose being 0.5 mg intravenously. In situations in which the ventricular response is affecting the CO, a more rapidly acting drug such as verapamil or a beta-blocker may be used to control the rate.
   b. Perform synchronized cardioversion. If cardioversion is used, it is usually attempted before digitalization, because digoxin predisposes the myocardium to ventricular tachycardia and fibrillation. Cardioversion is usually attempted with 25 to 100 watt-seconds.
   c. Perform carotid sinus massage.
   d. Institute atrial overdrive pacing. Atrial pacing at a rate of 300 to 500 beats/minute for a few seconds may break the re-entry dysrhythmia mechanism and return the patient to normal sinus rhythm.[248]

(4) Junctional rhythms or heart blocks. Longstanding hypertension, left main coronary disease, and preoperative use of digitalis are predisposing factors associated with developing new fascicular conduction blocks.[238] First- and second-degree atrioventricular heart blocks are usually well tolerated and therefore not treated. However, therapy for third-degree atrioventricular heart block consists of the following measures:
   a. Initiate cardiac pacing, specifically ventricular or atrioventricular pacing. Owing to its atrial kick, atrioventricular sequential pacing is preferred because it provides a greater increase in CO. However, ventricular demand pacing may be adequate in patients who require a pacemaker at the time of discharge because third-degree atrioventricular block generally is resolved within 2 months after surgery.[7]

(continued)

NURSING CARE PLAN SUMMARY   Postoperative Period   Continued

Patient Outcome	*Nursing Orders*

(5) Premature ventricular contractions (PVCs). Premature ventricular contractions are commonly occurring dysrhythmias after surgery and are treated in the following manner:

    a. Maintain optimum serum potassium levels. Serum potassium levels should be maintained at levels greater than 4.0 to 4.5 mEq. Intravenous potassium replacement can be achieved by administration of 15 mEq of potassium chloride in 50 cc of solution infused intravenously over a 60 minute period. Constant monitoring of the ECG during potassium infusion is essential.

    b. Administer pharmacologic drugs such as lidocaine, procainamide, and bretylium.

    c. Initiate pacing to overdrive the PVCs. Either atrial, atrioventricular, or ventricular pacing can accomplish this effect.

(6) Ventricular tachycardia. Sustained ventricular tachycardia with hemodynamic deterioration requires immediate attention. Therapy includes the following measures:

    a. Administer a precordial thump. (Some physicians prefer that a precordial thump not be attempted in these patients in the immediate postoperative period because it may cause a sternal dehiscence.)

    b. Administer a bolus of lidocaine.

    c. Perform synchronized cardioversion with 50 to 360 joules in patients with ventricular tachycardia with a pulse but with falling blood pressure (see Chap. 14).

    d. Perform unsynchronized cardioversion for pulseless ventricular tachycardia at 200 to 300 to 360 joules (see Chap. 14 and Appendix I).

    e. If ventricular tachycardia persists or ventricular fibrillation ensues, external cardiac massage may be instituted to sustain these patients. This technique is usually quickly replaced by internal massage once the chest cavity is reopened.

(7) Ventricular fibrillation. Therapy consists of the following measures:

    a. Administer a precordial thump (see (6) (a)).

    b. Immediate defibrillation (see Chap. 14). During an open chest resuscitation procedure, internal defibrillation is initially performed using 25 to 40 watt-seconds and increasing the energy level per the physician's order.

B. Monitor, assess, and record any predisposing factors that contribute to dysrhythmias.

(1) Observe the patient's electrolyte results, especially for the presence of hypokalemia. Signs and symptoms of hypokalemia in addition to a serum level of less than 4.0 to 4.5 mEq include the following:

    a. Prolongation of the QT interval on the ECG

    b. T-wave inversion on the ECG

    c. ST-segment depression on the ECG

    d. Urinary pH below 5 due to excessive excretion of hydrogen ions

    e. Restlessness and irritability

(2) Monitor the patient's arterial blood gas levels and acid-base status to identify hypoxemic or acidotic/alkalotic states.

(3) Observe the chest x-ray for placement of the pulmonary artery catheter.

(4) Monitor and assist in maintaining filling pressures at optimum levels to avoid hypotension and hypertension and their potential dysrhythmogenic effects.

(5) Sedate and medicate the patient appropriately to reduce anxiety and minimize shallow breathing from splinting, which can lead to hypoxemia.

(continued)

NURSING CARE PLAN SUMMARY   *Postoperative Period*   *Continued*

Patient Outcome	*Nursing Orders*
	C. Monitor, assess, and record dysrhythmias in the following manner: (1) Monitor the ECG continuously. (2) Assess and record the heart rate and rhythm every 15 minutes from admission until the patient is stable and thereafter every 30 to 60 minutes. (3) Assess the patient's hemodynamic, cerebral, renal, and peripheral vascular responses to dysrhythmias. D. Notify the physician of dysrhythmia development. E. Institute therapies per the physician's orders or unit policy for dysrhythmia control. F. Assess and document the patient's response to therapies.

NURSING DIAGNOSIS

5. *Decreased cardiac output related to inappropriate volume status (exchanging pattern)*

Patient Outcomes	*Nursing Orders*
1. The patient will exhibit signs of adequate CO and volume status as evidenced by adequate CO/CI, adequate filling pressures, normotension, and absence of physical signs and symptoms of hypovolemia.	1. Causes of inadequate circulating volume or hypovolemia include inadequate volume replacement after or in conjunction with rewarming or vasodilator and diuretic therapy, hemorrhage from an active bleeding or oozing vessel in the chest, or hemorrhage from coagulopathies associated with cardiopulmonary bypass or medications. A. The hypovolemia associated with rewarming or vasodilator and diuretic therapy is the most common form of inadequate circulating volume. In this form, the patient develops a relative hypovolemia as the venous capacitance vessels dilate. Therapy centers on direct volume replacement and mobilizing fluids from the interstitial or third space. There may be a variable degree of fluid in the interstitial space depending on the particular effects the patient experienced from cardiopulmonary bypass. Bypass can alter vascular wall permeability somewhat, causing a capillary leak. Prolonged bypass times, particularly in a compromised patient, may significantly increase capillary permeability. Normally, compensatory mechanisms will return capillary permeability to normal levels. However, during the early postoperative period, these compensatory mechanisms may not be particularly helpful. Owing to the stress of surgery and the consequent release of antidiuretic hormones, aldosterone, and endogenous catecholamines, the body tends to sequester and retain fluid and maintain a state of vasoconstriction. These mechanisms may not fully deactivate until the third or fourth postoperative day. When they deactivate, the patient may experience a massive non–pharmacologic-induced diuresis or night sweats as the body attempts to shed this excess fluid. B. The type of volume replacement appropriate for these patients may vary. Crystalloid replacement may be well suited for the patient who has a minimal capillary leak as evidenced by minimal amounts of peripheral edema. Colloidal replacement may be more appropriate in patients with moderate amounts of peripheral edema. The therapeutic goal in this situation would be to retrieve the edematous fluid back into the intravascular space by increasing the plasma colloid osmotic pressure with colloid solutions. In severely edematous patients, replacement fluid of either kind may have a tendency to leak into the interstitium and increase the problem. Volume replacement in this situation is usually not aggressive, and the type of solution is determined by the patient's response. C. Another cause of hypovolemia, hemorrhage, occurs in approximately 5% of patients undergoing cardiac surgery.[57] Factors responsible for hemorrhage

(continued)

NURSING CARE PLAN SUMMARY *Postoperative Period* *Continued*

Patient Outcomes	*Nursing Orders*
	include medications, prolonged operative times, clotting abnormalities, and technical factors. Hemorrhage associated with medications centers on their ability to alter the normal clotting mechanism. Drugs that alter platelet adhesiveness and which are commonly ingested by cardiac patients include aspirin, dipyridamole, and clofibrate. Additionally, agents that have antiplatelet activity include indomethacin, papaverine, phenylbutazone, and sulfinpyrazone, to name a few. Sodium warfarin (Coumadin) should be stopped 4 to 7 days preoperatively. If its antithrombotic effects are absolutely essential, it can be replaced with heparin, which can be quickly reversed with protamine should bleeding become a problem. If immediate surgery is required in a patient receiving Coumadin, vitamin K or fresh frozen plasma can be administered to limit bleeding.

D. Prolonged exposure to cardiopulmonary bypass can alter blood component integrity, and additionally, in the severely compromised patient, an intravascular coagulopathy can develop. In all the preceding situations, evaluation of the coagulation system is essential, and platelet counts, prothrombin times (PT), and partial thromboplastin times (PTT) are obtained for this purpose. Prothrombin times evaluate factors I, II, V, VII, and X, whereas PTT evaluate factors V, VIII, IX, X, XI, and XII. Depending on the results, replacement components can include fresh frozen plasma, platelet concentrate, cryoprecipitate, antihemophiliac factor concentrate, and factor II, VII, and IX concentrates.

E. Hemorrhage may also develop due to *heparin rebound*. Although heparin is reversed in the operating room with protamine, this effect may be only a transient one. After admission to the recovery area, there may be a reappearance of circulating heparin in the blood. This can be caused by a slow release of heparin from adipose tissue or from rewarmed peripheral tissues and a dissociation of the heparin-protamine complex or by the administration of blood products such as fresh frozen plasma, which can render any remaining unneutralized heparin more effective.[215,250] Heparin rebound can be monitored by obtaining activated clotting times (ACT) and treated by giving the patient additional doses of protamine or desmopressin.

F. Technical factors causing hemorrhage and, thus, hypovolemia occur as a result of inadequate hemostasis or rupture of suture lines. Rupture is most often associated with inadequate control of postoperative hypertension. In addition, patients undergoing reoperation are at high risk because their normal dissection planes may be altered by adhesions from previous surgical procedures. In this situation, significant hemorrhage may occur from numerous small areas. Volume replacement for these situations is most appropriately accomplished with autologous blood, whole blood, or packed cells.

G. Monitor, assess, and record the following signs and symptoms of hypovolemia:

(1) Decreased CO/CI (CO less than 5 L/minute and CI less than 2.7 L/minute/m^2)

(2) Inadequate filling pressures. Normal filling pressures in postoperative patients reside in the upper portion of their normal ranges. Parameters less than this are generally indicators of hypovolemia.

(3) Fluctuations in the baseline of the RAP tracing with inspiration and expiration

(4) Hypotension: MAP less than 60 mm Hg. The arterial wave configuration in a hypovolemic state is characterized by a slow upstroke, a prolonged peak, and a dicrotic notch that is less than one third of the height of the curve (Fig. 26-9B, D).

(5) Tachycardia (Heart rate greater than 110 beats/minute)

(6) Urine output less than 0.5 to 1.0 cc/kg/hour

(7) Specific gravity greater than 1.020. The normal specific gravity is 1.015 to 1.020.

(continued)

NURSING CARE PLAN SUMMARY *Postoperative Period* *Continued*

Patient Outcomes	*Nursing Orders*
	(8) Weak, thready pulses
	(9) Dry mucous membranes
	(10) Decreased level of consciousness
	(11) Prolonged peripheral filling time
	(12) Poor skin turgor

2. The patient will not demonstrate signs or symptoms of hypervolemia.

    2. Causes of hypervolemia include overaggressive volume replacement, inadequate diuresis after cardiopulmonary bypass, and the development of a relative hypervolemia that ensues when there is a loss of myocardial contractility and the patient develops congestive heart failure.

    A. Monitor, assess, and record the following signs and symptoms of hypervolemia:

        (1) Decreased CO/CI (CO less than 5 L/minute and CI less than 2.7 L/minute/m^2)

        (2) Elevated filling pressures

        (3) Presence of *v* waves on the atrial pressure wave patterns. These waves develop when the ventricle is dilated with volume. This dilatation prevents the cusps of the mitral and tricuspid valves from touching each other during closing. Because of this, regurgitant flow can occur back into the atrium during ventricular systole. This regurgitant atrial flow creates exaggerated *v* waves on the respective atrial tracings. Once the dilatation resolves, these waves disappear.

        (4) Hypotension (MAP less than 60 mm Hg)

        (5) Tachycardia

        (6) Bounding pulses not easily obliterated with pressure

        (7) Peripheral edema

        (8) Weight gain greater than 0.5 kg/day

        (9) Pulmonary crackles

        (10) Engorgement of peripheral veins

3. If signs or symptoms of volume status alterations are observed, the patient will respond to the appropriate therapy.

    3. Implement the following strategies according to either the physician's orders or standing unit policies to assist in controlling the volume status:

    A. Identify therapies and pharmacologic and volume agents commonly used to control volume status as outlined in Box 26-3.

    B. Administer the agents outlined in Box 26-3 per physician's orders or routines of the unit. During administration of these agents and during periods of hypovolemia and hypervolemia, the nurse should perform the following:

        (1) Monitor the MAP and heart rate constantly and record every 15 minutes. Observe particularly for signs of myocardial ischemia.

        (2) Monitor filling pressures constantly. Left atrial pressure, PAS, and PAD pressures can be constantly monitored, because these lines are not used for volume replacement. Their values should be documented every 15 minutes during periods of aggressive fluid replacement.

        If the RAP line is not used for volume replacement, it should also be monitored constantly and recorded as above. If it is used as a volume replacement line, atrial pressures should be obtained and recorded every 30 minutes or after infusion of every 100 to 200 cc of volume.

        Pulmonary capillary wedge pressure should be determined per the physician's orders, but usually is obtained no more frequently than every hour.

        (3) Obtain CO/CI as needed.

        (4) Assess and correlate filling pressure values. The nurse should be aware that filling pressures from the right and left sides of the heart need to be assessed concurrently. If the RAP and LAP are both elevated, the patient is relatively or absolutely hypervolemic. Treatment includes the use of vasodilators (to reduce afterload) or diuretics with vasopressors if the patient is hypotensive. If both the RAP and LAP are low, the patient is relatively or absolutely hypovolemic and should be treated with fluids to increase the preload. If the RAP is normal and the LAP is elevated, the patient has left ventricular failure. Treatment includes the

(continued)

NURSING CARE PLAN SUMMARY *Postoperative Period Continued*

Patient Outcomes	*Nursing Orders*

use of positive inotropic drugs, diuretics, and vasodilators. If the RAP is elevated and the LAP is normal or low, the patient has right ventricular dysfunction and is treated with vasodilators, which will alter pulmonary vascular resistance, and positive inotropic agents.

BOX 26-3. Therapies Commonly Used to Control Volume Status

1. Prescribed fluid totals. Fluids are generally restricted to 1500 to 2500 cc/day because of the effects of antidiuretic hormone and aldosterone, which have been released by the stress of surgery. Solutions low in saline or 5% dextrose solutions are preferred for daily fluid maintenance.

2. Administration of diuretic agents. Mannitol, bumetanide, furosemide, and ethacrynic acid are commonly used diuretics for the cardiac patient. Mannitol, an osmotic diuretic, is usually given as the patient is removed from cardiopulmonary bypass. This initiates a diuresis that may be significant for the first 1 or 2 hours after surgery. After this, furosemide or bumetanide is heavily used owing to its rapid response and short-term action. In situations refractory to furosemide, bumetanide or ethacrynic acid may be given.

3. Crystalloid solutions. Ringer's lactate is a commonly used volume replacement solution and is frequently used in hypovolemic states due to normal vasodilatation.

4. Colloidal agents. Albumin in a 5% (Albumisol) or a 25% (25% albumin) saline solution can be administered. After major surgical procedures, albumin shifts from the plasma into the interstitial spaces. Administration of exogenous albumin assists in maintaining normal plasma colloidal osmotic pressure and therefore can assist in retrieving volume from the interstitial space. Hetastrach (Hespan), which is a synthetic colloid that provides direct volume and mobilizes interstitial fluid, also can be used.[117,133]

5. Autologous blood. Retrieval and reinfusion of the patient's own blood (see section on blood conservation, p. 449) can be performed both intraoperatively and postoperatively. Intraoperatively, as the patient is placed on cardiopulmonary bypass, 1 to 2 U of blood may be removed through the venous oxygenator line and replaced with crystalloid solution. This creates a hemodilution that is allowed to proceed to levels at which the hematocrit ranges from 23% to 25%. This removed blood is saved or is spun down to its packed-cell equivalent for reinfusion when needed. Intraoperatively, blood is retrieved from the surgical field by way of a sterile suction system and is also spun down, washed, and saved for later transfusion. As the

patient is weaned from bypass, all the volume in the cardiopulmonary bypass circuit may not be able to be reinfused into the patient. This "pump" blood is bagged and accompanies the patient to the critical care area, where it is reinfused when needed. Because the pump blood contains heparin, administration of this pump blood is accompanied by concurrent administration of protamine. The last technique for autologous blood retrieval is via the chest tube drainage system. Chest tubes are attached to a sterile system, which includes a sterile bag or a cardiotomy reservoir in which shed blood is collected. The nurse allows the blood to collect in the system and uses it for retransfusion when necessary to maintain filling pressures at ordered parameters. With this system, blood should be reinfused within a 1- to 2-hour period after it drains. Autotransfusion generally is not performed after 12 hours postoperatively. These methods of autologous blood reinfusion are well suited for both hemorrhage situations or hypovolemic states from vasodilatation.

6. Packed red cells. Infusion of packed cells is usually reserved for situations in which replacement of cell mass is required.

7. Whole blood. Use of whole blood is most often reserved for situations of hemorrhage. If hemorrhage is due to coagulopathies, whole blood less than 24 hours old is sought.

8. Fresh frozen plasma. Fresh frozen plasma is used to treat hemorrhage situations in which coagulation factors are sought. Fresh frozen plasma contains all coagulation factors but does not contain platelets.

9. Platelet concentrates. If thrombocytopenia is thought to contribute to the hemorrhage, then platelet concentrates are given.

10. Cryoprecipitate. In coagulation disorders in which fibrinogen is needed, cryoprecipitate is used. Cryoprecipitate also provides factors I and VIII.

11. Antihemophiline factor concentrate. This concentrate is used in rare situations in which lack of factor VIII is suspected as the cause of bleeding.

12. Factor II, VII, and IX concentrates. These concentrates are administered when coagulopathies are determined to be associated with inadequate amounts of factors II, VII, and IX. They also serve as a source of factor X.

(continued)

NURSING CARE PLAN SUMMARY   *Postoperative Period*   *Continued*

Patient Outcomes	*Nursing Orders*
	(5) Monitor and assess physical signs and symptoms of hypovolemia and hypervolemia.
	(6) Monitor and assess electrolyte, hematologic, and coagulation laboratory results.
	(7) Carefully ensure that all solutions are appropriately labeled, verified, and recorded.
	(8) Observe for development of adverse reactions, particularly with the infusion of blood and blood products.
	(9) Accurately record the patient responses to therapy.
	C. Monitor the patient's output and input as follows:
	(1) Observe chest tube drainage constantly. Rupture of major anastomoses will produce immediate filling of the chest tubes and collection systems and rapid deterioration of the patient's hemodynamic status. In this circumstance, immediate opening of the chest in the critical care area is essential to prevent death.
	(2) Measure and record the amount and quality of chest tube drainage every 30 minutes during periods of active bleeding and thereafter every 1 to 2 hours.
	(3) Observe urinary output constantly. Massive diuresis after diuretic administration can produce 1 to 2 L of urine in a few hours.
	(4) Measure and record the amount and quality of urine every 15 to 30 minutes during massive diuresis and then hourly once diuresis slows.
	(5) Assess for massive oozing from incisions and chest tubes and intravascular catheter insertion sites. Document the presence of oozing, site, and relative amount.
	(6) Measure and record the amount and quality of nasogastric tube drainage every 1 to 2 hours if greater than 50 cc/hour. Otherwise, measure and record every 8 hours.
	(7) Notify the physician if chest tube drainage exceeds 100 cc/hour, urine output exceeds 200 cc/hour, nasogastric drainage exceeds 500 cc in 8 hours, and massive oozing is present from incisions or insertion sites.
	(8) Calculating and recording fluid intake should be an ongoing process and should be performed after infusion of every 100 to 200 cc of volume.

NURSING DIAGNOSIS

6. *Actual or high risk for impaired gas exchange related to anesthesia and sedation, volume overloading, hemothorax/pneumothorax, or noncardiac permeability edema (exchanging pattern)*

Patient Outcome	*Nursing Orders*
1. The patient will exhibit signs of adequate gas exchange as evidenced by adequate respiratory rate and rhythm, adequate color, adequate arterial blood gases, normal breath sounds, absence of hemothorax or pneumothorax, and return to preoperative neurologic status.	1. Identify and describe the mechanisms or factors that contribute to impaired gas exchange after cardiac surgery. Factors responsible include effects of anesthesia and sedation, volume overloading, and the presence of a hemothorax or a pneumothorax. All these are usually self-limiting or easily resolved. The major effects of anesthesia and sedation wear off within the first few hours after surgery. In the case of volume overloading, the use of diuretics will gradually assist in resolving this problem. If a hemothorax or pneumothorax exists in the presence of chest tubes, then negative pressure can be applied to the chest tube system. If this fails, another chest tube may be required.
	The incidence of "bypass lung" or noncardiac permeability edema has greatly diminished in the past few years owing to the decrease in anesthesia, surgical, and cardiopulmonary bypass time needed to accomplish the surgery.

(continued)

NURSING CARE PLAN SUMMARY *Postoperative Period* Continued

Patient Outcome	*Nursing Orders*
	Additionally, a decreasing amount of blood transfused in these patients, particularly as a result of using autotransfused blood, has also significantly contributed to the decrease in this form of pulmonary edema, as has the use of modern oxygenators, hemodilution, and better arterial filters.

A. Monitor, assess, and record the following signs and symptoms of inadequate gas exchange:

   (1) Inadequate rate, rhythm, depth of respiration, color, and level of consciousness

   (2) Inadequate arterial blood gases

   (3) Presence of abnormal breath sounds. If breath sounds are not audible on the left side when the endotracheal tube is in place, it can be assumed that the tube has slipped into the right bronchus. In this situation, the endotracheal tube should be repositioned.

   (4) Abnormal chest x-ray. The chest x-ray should be observed for correct placement of the endotracheal, nasogastric, and chest tubes as well as placement of intravascular lines. Additionally, inspection for effusions or a pneumothorax should be performed.

B. Implement strategies according to either the physician's orders or standing unit policies to maintain or achieve adequate gas exchange.

   (1) Institute procedures or routines that should be performed in the immediate postoperative period:

     a. Keep the endotracheal tube and tubing secured and adequately supported.

     b. Use an oral airway to prevent the patient from clamping down on the endotracheal tube.

     c. Identify and correct any sudden abnormal functioning of the ventilator. The ventilator should provide adequate minute volume, oxygenation, and humidification of inspired gases.

     d. Use deep sterile tracheal suctioning as needed. Recently, Stone and colleagues have demonstrated that suctioning postoperative cardiac surgery patients can lead to significant rises in MAP. Constant monitoring for this phenomenon is essential to avoid these increases, which could place undue pressure on suture lines and result in hemorrhage.[224]

     e. Reposition the patient frequently. Repositioning the patient in the immediate postoperative period has been associated with a decrease in postoperative temperature elevation and length of stay in the critical care area as well as improvement in oxygenation.[45]

     f. Provide information and care to reduce the patient's anxiety and fear (see Chap. 8, Anxiety).

     g. Frequently remind the patient that the ventilator has taken over the work of breathing, but only temporarily.

     h. Provide the patient with a method of communication such as finger writing (see Chap. 8, Impaired Verbal Communication).

     i. Remind the patient frequently to practice the relaxation techniques learned in the preoperative period.

     j. If the patient is on controlled ventilation, assess whether the patient is out of phase with the ventilator and supply reassurance or sedation.

C. Institute procedures or routines that should be performed in the weaning period:

   (1) Assess the adequacy of the patient's arterial blood gases, chest x-ray, breath sounds, neuromuscular functioning, level of consciousness, and hemodynamic stability. If these are stable, weaning may be initiated.

   (2) Discontinue administering agents that depress respiration.

   (3) Explain the weaning process to the patient. Most often the controlled ventilation is discontinued and the patient is placed on or switched to

(continued)

NURSING CARE PLAN SUMMARY   Postoperative Period   Continued

Patient Outcome	Nursing Orders
	the intermittent mandatory ventilation (IMV) mode. In this mode, the ventilator's respiratory rate is decreased slowly, thereby requiring patients to increase their spontaneous respirations in order to maintain adequate minute volumes. As patients begin to generate an adequate respiratory rate, IMV is discontinued and patients are switched to continuous positive airway pressure (CPAP). On CPAP, patients maintain their own respiratory rate while the ventilator provides the positive pressure to the airway that normally is supplied by the glottis when the patient is not intubated. The use of positive pressure in this fashion prevents the development of microatelectasis and increases the functional residual capacity of the lung. Positive pressure in this situation is usually maintained at levels of 5 cm H_2O.

    (4) Continue to assess arterial blood gases during the weaning procedure.

    (5) Remind patients to practice their relaxation technique during weaning.

    (6) Observe the physiologic and psychologic responses to weaning.

    (7) Measure maximal inspiratory force and forced vital capacity. Maximal inspiratory force should be less than or equal to -28 cm H_2O, and forced vital capacity should be greater than 15 cc/kg before extubation.[106]

    (8) Assist with extubation.

  D. Institute procedures or routines that should be performed in the period immediately after extubation:

    (1) Observe for signs of laryngeal edema or spasm.

    (2) Administer a high-humidity mixture of air and oxygen. Most frequently patients will receive oxygen via nasal cannula for the next 24 hours and then oxygen therapy is discontinued. Rebreathing, nonrebreathing, and mask CPAP treatments may be necessary in some patients to maintain adequate oxygenation.

    (3) Assist the patient with coughing and deep breathing and use of incentive spirometry every 1 to 2 hours.

    (4) Perform chest physiotherapy and tracheal suctioning as needed.

    (5) Encourage the patient to engage in progressive activities and relaxation techniques.

    (6) Provide the patient with pain medication as necessary to avoid splinting and ineffective coughing. Recent use of patient-controlled analgesia in this group of patients has been found to be as safe as nurse-administered therapy and allows the patient more control over the pain.[52]

    (7) Continue to assess the respiratory status.

NURSING DIAGNOSIS

7. *Actual or high risk for impaired neurologic function related to transient neurologic defects, postcardiotomy delirium syndrome, alteration in sleep/rest cycles, or permanent neurologic defects (exchanging pattern)*

Patient Outcome	Nursing Orders
1. The patient will exhibit signs and symptoms of adequate neurologic status as evidenced by normal pupillary response; orientation to person, place, time, and situation; absence of motor and cognitive dysfunction; stable	1. Identify and describe mechanisms or factors that contribute to the development of neurologic dysfunction. Neurologic dysfunctions are generally of two types: transient deficits, which persist for hours or days, and permanent deficits. The *transient deficits* range from slowness to arouse the patient from anesthesia to confusion, memory loss, and delirium. This can occur in up to a quarter of patients undergoing operation, with the elderly being most affected.[17,170,232] This

(continued)

NURSING CARE PLAN SUMMARY Postoperative Period *Continued*

Patient Outcome	*Nursing Orders*
emotional state; and return to preoperative neurologic status.	syndrome is different from the *postcardiotomy delirium syndrome* (PCD), which usually occurs on the second to fifth postoperative day after a period characterized by normal arousal and orientation. Symptoms of PCD range from mild confusion to frank psychosis. Postcardiotomy delirium syndrome is self-limiting and resolves within a few days. Risk factors for PCD include sleep deprivation, prolonged intensive care residence times, advanced age, severe preoperative illness, and a history of preoperative psychiatric illness.[9,123,126,198,213] *Permanent deficits* involving cognition and motor and sensory functioning are attributed to embolic phenomenon or low-flow states.[85] Emboli can arise from intracardiac thrombi, calcified valve fragments, plaque dislodgment from the aorta, or air emboli from the bypass circuit or invasive lines.

A. Monitor, assess, and record the following signs and symptoms of neurologic impairment:
  (1) Abnormal pupillary response: Dilated, fixed, and nonreactive pupils involving one or both eyes.
  (2) Failure to arouse from anesthesia.
  (3) Presence of seizures.
  (4) Absence of motor function: As patients arouse from anesthesia, they should begin to move all four extremities. Absence of motor function may involve all or one extremity. Facial paralysis may not be identified until after extubation.
  (5) Absence of cognitive function: As patients continue to respond, they should be able to move their extremities to command. Strength of hand grasps can be assessed at this time and should be weak but equal. Final assessment of cognitive and communication functions cannot be performed completely until after extubation, when the patient's verbal responses can be evaluated.

B. Implement the following strategies to assist in maintaining or improving neurologic impairment:
  (1) Continue neurologic checks as needed.
  (2) Maintain MAP and CO at prescribed levels.
  (3) Provide frequent orientation to person, place, time, and situation.
  (4) Modify or limit extraneous environmental stimuli in the following manner:
    a. If possible, place patient in a separate room that has a window, a large clock, and a calendar.
    b. Limit the amount of monitoring equipment in the patient's room.
    c. Eliminate monotonous sounds such as the beep of the cardiac monitor.
  (5) Provide the patient with periods of uninterrupted sleep.
  (6) Provide sufficient and flexible visiting hours.
  (7) Attempt to normalize the environment and routines as much as possible. Encourage early ambulation and performance of self-care activities. Provide a radio, television, magazines, etc.
  (8) Attempt to reduce the patient's anxiety (see Chap. 8, Anxiety).

NURSING DIAGNOSIS

8. *Actual or high risk for impaired renal function related to inadequate renal perfusion, hemolysis, blood transfusion reactions, or renal emboli (exchanging pattern)*

Patient Outcome	*Nursing Orders*
1. The patient will exhibit signs and symptoms of adequate renal function as	1. Identify and describe the mechanisms or factors that contribute to the impairment of renal function in the cardiac surgical patient. Categories of

(continued)

NURSING CARE PLAN SUMMARY   *Postoperative Period*   *Continued*

Patient Outcome	Nursing Orders

Patient Outcome

evidenced by adequate amount and quality of urinary output, absence of fluid volume imbalances, absence of electrolyte abnormalities, and return to preoperative renal status.

Nursing Orders

postoperative renal complications include prerenal and acute renal failure. Prerenal failure develops in states of inadequate renal perfusion, which can occur from loss of myocardial contractile function or from conditions of hypovolemia. Correction of these entities will resolve the renal dysfunction. However, if they are allowed to continue, acute renal failure will ensue as renal parenchymal tissue is destroyed.

Other factors that can lead to acute renal failure include hemolysis, blood transfusion reactions, and renal emboli. Hemolysis of red cells is induced by excessive trauma that develops during bypass or with the constant use of operative field suctioning. The fragmented red cells liberate free hemoglobin, and free hemoglobin casts develop that have the ability to obstruct renal tubules. Transfusion reactions with their agglutination and release of hemoglobin also serve to obstruct the tubules. In both these instances, mannitol and sodium bicarbonate are used to neutralize the acidic environment and assist in clearance of the tubules.

Renal emboli may originate from intracardiac chambers, calcified valves, or plaque from the aortic wall. The consequent acute renal failure that develops from these processes can be either an oliguric or a nonoliguric failure. Oliguric failure is characterized by a urinary output of less than 500 cc/day. In this situation, the patient will most often exhibit signs of volume overload. Nonoliguric failure is characterized by the appearance of a hypovolemic patient whose urinary output exceeds 3 to 4 L a day.

A. Monitor, assess, and record the following signs and symptoms of renal dysfunction:
   (1) Elevated serum creatinine
   (2) Elevated blood urea nitrogen (BUN)
   (3) BUN: creatinine ratio greater than 10:1
   (4) Abnormal amount and quality of urinary output. In oliguric failure, urinary output is less than 0.5 cc/kg/hour. This urine is typically dark amber in appearance and may demonstrate the presence of particulate material. In nonoliguric failure, the urine is pale in color and exceeds 200 to 300 cc/hour.
   (5) Abnormal specific gravity. Normal specific gravity is 1.015 to 1.020. The specific gravity of urine may be low owing to overhydration, diuretics, or the inability of the kidneys to filter waste products. The specific gravity may be high owing to a decreased urinary output, dehydration, or the presence of fragmented red cells or of large molecular substances, such as glucose or proteins, in the urine.
   (6) Presence of physical signs and symptoms associated with hypovolemia and hypervolemia
   (7) Confusion and lethargy
B. Implement the following strategies to assist with the maintenance or recovery of renal function:
   (1) Assist in correcting the underlying cause of the renal dysfunction, if possible. In the case of inadequate renal perfusion, increasing the cardiac output or the intravascular volume may be beneficial.
   (2) Assist in maintaining adequate fluid volume status during the period of renal dysfunction.
   (3) Measure the patient's fluid intake and output. This should include the volume infused via pressurized intravascular lines. Intake and output should be calculated every hour in acute unstable situations, particularly in nonoliguric renal failure, to avoid the development of significant hypovolemia. If the patient is oliguric, the Foley catheter should be discontinued and daily catheterizations should be performed. This decreases the risk of infection.
   (4) Weigh the patient daily.

(continued)

NURSING CARE PLAN SUMMARY Postoperative Period   *Continued*

Patient Outcome	Nursing Orders
	(5) Observe electrolyte profiles. Observe for signs and symptoms of electrolyte imbalances and assist in administering corrective therapies. (6) Administer diuretics as ordered. (7) Order a low-sodium, low-potassium diet as directed. (8) Assist with isolated dialysis or continuous arteriovenous hemofiltration dialysis (CAVHD) procedures as necessary.

NURSING DIAGNOSIS

9. *Actual or high risk for impaired gastrointestinal function related to gastric distention, stress ulceration, mesenteric or splenic infarction, and pancreatitis and hyperbilirubinemia (exchanging pattern)*

Patient Outcome	Nursing Orders
1. The patient will exhibit signs and symptoms of adequate gastrointestinal function as evidenced by presence of normal bowel sounds, absence of gastric distention, and absence of symptoms of gastrointestinal bleeding or pancreatitis or hyperbilirubinemia.	1. Identify and describe mechanisms or factors that contribute to impairment of gastrointestinal function in the postoperative cardiac surgical patient. Common causes of gastrointestinal complications include gastric distention, stress ulceration (especially gastroduodenal), mesenteric or splenic infarction from inadequate cardiac output or embolism, and pancreatitis and hyperbilirubinemia. Gastric distention develops when the patient swallows air. This distention can cause pulmonary complications (due to the pressure it places on the diaphragm) and cardiac complications (such as dysrhythmias and inadequate venous return and cardiac output) as a result of the pressure it exerts on the vena cava. Stress ulceration can develop as a result of the stress of surgery, respiratory failure, sepsis, peritonitis, renal failure, and hypotension. Embolization from intracardiac structures, aortic wall processes, faulty intra-aortic balloon placement, and air embolization can cause mesenteric or ischemic infarction.[5,100] Lastly, pancreatitis most frequently develops in patients with multisystem failure, whereas multiple valve replacements, higher transfusion requirements, and cardiopulmonary bypass duration are associated with hyperbilirubinemia.

A. Monitor, assess, and record the following signs and symptoms of gastrointestinal impairment:
   (1) Presence of gastric air bubble. This can be identified on the chest x-ray as a significant bubble below the diaphragm. Percussion of the left upper quadrant will reveal an extensive tympanic percussion note. The abdomen is distended, and, if awake, the patient may complain of nausea and vomiting.
   (2) Distended, rigid abdomen
   (3) Presence of abdominal pain
   (4) Red or coffee-colored gastric secretions
   (5) Black or tarry stools
   (6) Fall in hematocrit unexplained by other causes of hemorrhage
   (7) Absence of bowel sounds
   (8) Gastric pH less than 3.5
   (9) Elevation in bilirubin
B. Implement the following strategies to alleviate or minimize gastrointestinal impairment:[100]
   (1) Assist in maintaining adequate gastrointestinal perfusion.
   (2) Ensure correct placement of the nasogastric tube and functioning of drainage and suction system. Nasogastric tubes can be placed on intermittent low suction or attached to gravity drainage.
   (3) Assist in maintaining the gastric pH at levels higher than 3.5 by administering antacids or other agents according to physician's order or per unit protocols.

(continued)

NURSING CARE PLAN SUMMARY *Postoperative Period* Continued

Patient Outcome	Nursing Orders
	(4) Hematest nasogastric drainage, stools, and vomitus for occult blood. (5) Identify pharmacologic drugs that potentiate ulceration, and monitor closely for this complication during their administration. (6) Attempt to minimize or eliminate psychologic stress.

NURSING DIAGNOSIS

10. *Actual or high risk for altered peripheral perfusion related to thromboembolic processes (exchanging pattern)*

Patient Outcome

1. The patient will exhibit signs of adequate peripheral circulation as evidenced by adequate peripheral pulses, adequate peripheral temperature, absence of edema, absence of engorged peripheral vessels, absence of pain in extremities, and normal peripheral motor function.

Nursing Orders

1. Identify and describe the mechanisms or factors that contribute to impairment of peripheral circulation. Problems of the peripheral circulation include both venous and arterial thrombus formation and embolism development. Venous thromboembolism can develop as a result of venous stasis from inactivity and immobilization and coagulation abnormalities occurring in the postoperative period. Arterial processes, although affected by postoperative coagulation abnormalities, are more often associated with embolic events from intravascular devices such as the intra-aortic balloon or other vascular catheters.
   A. Monitor, assess, and record the following signs and symptoms of inadequate peripheral circulation:
      (1) Absence or diminished peripheral pulses
      (2) Alterations in skin temperature. The extremities may be warm with a venous thrombosis and cold with an arterial embolism.
      (3) Alterations in peripheral skin color. Cyanosis will develop with venous obstructions, and pale extremities will develop with arterial obstruction.
      (4) Edema
      (5) Engorgement of superficial vessels or increases in vascular markings. These develop in situations of deep venous thrombosis when the venous blood is shunted to and engorges the peripheral vessels.
      (6) Pain. Patients will complain of excruciating pain with arterial thrombosis. Pain with venous thrombosis may be absent or negligible. A positive Homan's sign may be present.
      (7) Loss of motor function. Motor function will be absent distal to the site of an arterial embolism. Motor activity is not altered with venous processes.
   B. Implement the following strategies to alleviate or minimize inadequate peripheral circulation:
      (1) Assess peripheral perfusion frequently in the postoperative period, particularly after catheter manipulation or removal. After removal of a radial arterial line, an Allen test should be performed on the ulnar and radial arteries. The peripheral pulses should be monitored scrupulously after insertion or removal of the intra-aortic balloon.
      (2) Perform active and passive exercises.
      (3) Encourage early ambulation and progressive activities.
      (4) Apply antiembolism stockings for the patient.
      (5) Administer anticoagulant drugs as ordered.

(continued)

NURSING CARE PLAN SUMMARY *Postoperative Period*   *Continued*

NURSING DIAGNOSIS

11. *Actual or high risk for infection related to invasive lines, surgical incisions, immunologic derangements, or inadequate preoperative nutritional status (exchanging pattern)*

Patient Outcome	Nursing Orders

Patient Outcome

1. The patient will not develop infection as evidenced by lack of swelling, redness, drainage, or tenderness at insertion or incision sites; absence of temperature elevation; normal white blood cell count; negative cultures; clear, yellow urine; and normal sputum production and stable sternum

Nursing Orders

1. Identify and describe factors that contribute to the development of infection in the patient after cardiac surgery. Major factors that predispose the patient to the development of infection include multiple invasive lines, numerous surgical incisions, alteration in immunologic capabilities of various blood components by cardiopulmonary bypass, and inadequate preoperative nutritional status such as is seen in patients with cardiac cachexia. Patients undergoing prosthetic valve replacement are at high risk for the development of early or late prosthetic valve endocarditis (see Chap. 28).

   Mediastinitis or sternal wound infections are the most devastating of the incisional problems. They develop in 1% to 5% of patients undergoing sternotomy, with mortality ranging from 10% to 71%.[160,178] Sternal involvement can range from superficial wound infections to massive mediastinal infections involving the sternum, mediastinal area, and myocardium and its adjacent structures. Noninfectious mediastinal wound problems include drainage of serosanguineous fluid, unstable sternums, and sternal dehiscence due to inadequate wire closure or poor nutritional status. Management of infectious complications should be aggressive and includes antibiotic administration and wide surgical debridement with subsequent continuous irrigation with antibiotic or povidone-iodine or construction of grafts from major muscles such as the pectoralis major, rectus abdominus, latissimus dorsi, and omental to assist in closing the sternal cavity.[47,111,203,206] Split-thickness skin grafts also may be necessary. Management of noninfectious sternal wound complications centers largely on observation.

   Because symptoms of sternal wound complications can occur as late as a month after surgery, it is necessary to instruct the patient to report any signs or symptoms that may herald a problem, such as drainage, tenderness, or temperature elevation.

   A. Monitor, assess, and record the following signs and symptoms of infection:
      (1) Fever
      (2) Chills
      (3) Diaphoresis
      (4) Altered levels of consciousness
      (5) Warm peripheral skin temperature
      (6) Alterations in calculated SVR. Peripheral vasodilatation can occur in septic shock states. This vasodilatation will cause the calculated SVR to fall below normal levels.
      (7) Redness, induration, swelling, tenderness, and drainage from incision and vascular insertion sites
      (8) Sternal instability. This is assessed by placing the thumb and forefinger on opposite sides of the sternal incision or the palm over the sternal incision and asking the patient to cough. A palpable clicking or grating sensation indicates sternal instability. Sternal instability does not always indicate the presence of an infectious process, but it can be associated with a mediastinitis.
      (9) Mediastinal crunch. This is an audible sound heard over the sternum that is indicative of free air under the sternum.[225]
      (10) Cloudy, foul-smelling urine
      (11) Dysuria
      (12) Increased sputum production or alterations in sputum characteristics
      (13) Alterations in the chest x-ray, particularly the presence of patchy opacifications
      (14) Elevation in white blood cell counts or positive culture results

(continued)

NURSING CARE PLAN SUMMARY   *Postoperative Period*   Continued

Patient Outcome	*Nursing Orders*
	B. Implement the following strategies to prevent, minimize, or alleviate infectious complications: (1) Maintain aseptic technique when working with invasive devices. (2) Ensure that invasive devices are securely anchored with sutures or tape to prevent movement in and out of the insertion site, which serves as a mechanism for inoculation of bacteria into the blood stream. (3) Change sterile dressings on incisions and catheter-insertion sites every 24 hours using aseptic technique. Incisional dressings are removed once drainage subsides. (4) Change tubing to intravascular catheters every 48 hours. (5) Seal all stopcocks on intravascular tubing with sterile caps. (6) Record on care plan the time and date of the catheter insertion and the type and size of the catheter. Arrange for catheter changes according to hospital policy. (7) Record time and date of last tubing change either on dressing or on intravascular tubing. (8) Maintain a closed system for chest tube drainage. (9) Maintain a closed system for urinary drainage. Perform catheter care and perineal care per unit routine, and remove catheters as soon as possible after surgery. (10) Maintain sterile technique for tracheal suctioning. (11) Obtain the patient's temperature every 4 hours. (12) Administer antipyretic drugs for temperature elevations. Use cooling devices as necessary. (13) Administer antibiotics per unit routine.

NURSING DIAGNOSIS

12. *Actual or high risk for development of a postpericardiotomy syndrome related to trauma or residual blood in the pericardial sac (exchanging pattern)*

Patient Outcome	*Nursing Orders*
1. The patient will remain free from developing a postpericardiotomy syndrome as evidenced by absence of verbal and nonverbal indicators of pain or discomfort, absence of a temperature elevation, absence of a pericardial friction rub, normal white blood cell counts, absence of dysrhythmias and ECG changes, absence of effusions.	1. Identify and describe factors that contribute to the development of postpericardiotomy syndrome. Postpericardiotomy syndrome can occur days to weeks after cardiac surgery and is characterized by pericarditis, fever, pericardial and pleural pain, a friction rub, dysrhythmias, and elevation of the white blood cell count. Additionally, pericardial and pleural effusions may be present.[208] Although the exact etiology has not been determined, a common factor in this syndrome seems to be trauma or presence of residual blood in the pericardial sac. This syndrome can effect 10% to 40% of patients after cardiac surgery. Most cases are mild and generally self-limiting and therefore require no treatment. If treatment is necessary, it usually consists of administering anti-inflammatory drugs such as salicylates or nonsteroidal anti-inflammatory agents and providing the patient with rest. Occasionally, corticosteroids may be used. The development of cardiac tamponade is a major concern in these patients. A. Monitor, assess, and record the following signs and symptoms of postpericardiotomy syndrome: (1) Pain. The pain associated with postpericardiotomy syndrome is best characterized as stabbing and sharp, aggravated by inspiration or swallowing, and minimized by sitting up or leaning forward. (2) Temperature elevation (3) Elevated white blood cell counts (4) Presence of pericardial friction rub (5) Dysrhythmias (6) Alterations in ST-T wave configurations (7) Pericardial or pleural effusions

(continued)

NURSING CARE PLAN SUMMARY *Postoperative Period* *Continued*

Patient Outcome	Nursing Orders
	B. Implement the following strategies to prevent, minimize, or alleviate the inflammatory process:

B. Implement the following strategies to prevent, minimize, or alleviate the inflammatory process:
   (1) Maintain patency of the chest tubes to assure adequate evacuation of blood from the chest cavity.
   (2) Assist the patient in describing the pain or discomfort in order to differentiate it from other causes of postoperative discomfort such as incisional pain, angina pectoris, or chronic pain syndrome associated with internal mammary artery grafting.[153]
   (3) Provide a therapeutic balance between normal rehabilitative activity (*i.e.*, ambulation) and required rest periods.
   (4) Provide for adequate pain or discomfort relief via relaxation techniques or prescribed analgesics.
   (5) Provide the patient with sufficient information concerning postpericardiotomy syndrome to minimize or alleviate fear and anxiety.
   (6) Administer anti-inflammatory agents as ordered by the physician.

NURSING DIAGNOSIS

13. *Knowledge deficit related to the immediate rehabilitation period (knowing pattern)*

Patient Outcome

1. Before discharge, the patient will demonstrate an adequate knowledge concerning the rehabilitation period as evidenced by the ability to describe the surgical procedure and the underlying disease process, describe activity goals and restrictions, describe medications, describe dietary restrictions, describe methods for risk-factor modification, demonstrate adequate ability to perform physical care procedures, and list resource personnel and methods to contact them.

Nursing Orders

1. Develop an individualized discharge teaching plan for the patient and family.[116] Recent studies[188,220] have reported that major concerns expressed by patients in the early postoperative period (up to 8 months) included the persistance of incisional pain, the need for another bypass procedure, the return of angina, dependency on their spouses, death, and that better health in the future was their primary hope. In order to best prepare the patient and family to deal with these issues, discharge planning needs to begin immediately after surgery and should include the following general areas:
   A. Disease process
      (1) Review with patients the surgical procedure and provide them with a diagram depicting the graft or valve placement.
      (2) Describe the rationale for the procedure.
      (3) Identify general areas of risk-factor modification.
      (4) If valve surgery was performed, explain precautions to use to prevent endocarditis (see Chap. 28).
   B. Activities
      (1) Demonstrate the general activities involved with physical care (*i.e.*, incisional care and coughing and deep breathing).
      (2) Describe the signs and symptoms of infection and cardiac failure, which the patient should report to the physician.
      (3) Discuss exercise and activity goals and restrictions. Identify specific activities in relation to return to work, sexual expression, driving a car, lifting, etc.
      (4) Discuss the emotional lability that may occur after discharge. Discuss the potential for role alteration within the family unit after the surgical procedure.
   C. Medications
      (1) Describe discharge medications. Indicate their names, dosages, actions, indications, and side effects. Ensure that patients are discharged with prescriptions or have a 1- or 2-day supply of medication, particularly if they have a considerable distance to travel to go home.
   D. Diet
      (1) Describe rationale for dietary restrictions. Ensure that the patient meets with the dietitian for a detailed discussion of dietary components.

(continued)

NURSING CARE PLAN SUMMARY *Postoperative Period* *Continued*

Patient Outcome	*Nursing Orders*
	E. Return visits
	(1) Ensure that patients have secured a return visit appointment or are aware of the need to establish one with their physician.
	F. Resources
	(1) Supply patients with a list of resource names and their hospital phone numbers. The list should include the names of the primary nurse, social worker, dietitian, and physical therapist.

---

preoperative and postoperative nursing diagnoses, patient outcomes, and plan for the patient undergoing cardiac surgery.

INTERVENTION AND EVALUATION

The nursing diagnoses, formulated for preoperative and post-operative cardiac surgery patients, guide the development of the patient outcomes and nursing orders. Bedside nursing interventions are directed by the prioritized nursing orders, and the effects of the interventions are evaluated by the actual patient outcomes.

SUMMARY

To provide quality care to the cardiac surgical patient, the nurse needs a thorough knowledge of the pathophysiology, surgical indications, operative procedures, and complications. An interdisciplinary team approach is essential in coordinating the various phases of the patient's hospitalization. Nurses have the opportunity to demonstrate their expertise and skills in helping patients achieve optimum health postoperatively.

DIRECTIONS FOR FUTURE RESEARCH

1. Can relaxation techniques be useful in weaning the patient from the ventilator?
2. What nursing interventions are most useful in preventing shivering when rewarming the patient postoperatively?
3. What psychologic and physiologic variables are the best predictors for the development of postcardiotomy delirium syndrome, and what specific preoperative or postoperative nursing interventions can be designed to treat or prevent this syndrome?
4. What are the effects of nursing interventions on the incidence of postoperative bleeding?

REFERENCES

1. Abshagen, U. Organic Nitrates. In U. Abshagen (Ed.), *Clinical Pharmacology of Antianginal Drugs* (vol. 76). New York: Springer-Verlag, 1985:287–364.
2. Acinapura, A. J., Rose, D. M., Jacobwitz, I. J., *et al.* Internal mammary artery bypass grafting: Influence on recurrent angina and survival in 2,100 patients. *Ann. Thorac. Surg.* 48:186, 1989.
3. Alderman, E. L., Brown, C. R., Sanders, G. R., *et al.* Survival following bypass graft surgery. *Cleve. Clin. Q.* 45:157, 1978.
4. Alkasab, S., Al-Fagih, M. R., Shahid, M., *et al.* Valve surgery in acute rheumatic heart disease. *Chest* 94:830, 1988.
5. Aranha, G. V., Pickleman, J., Pifarri, R., *et al.* The reasons for gastrointestinal consultation after cardiac surgery. *Am. Surg.* 50:301, 1984.
6. Aris, A., Padro, J., Camara, M. L., *et al.* Clinical and hemodynamic results of cardiac valve replacement with the monostruct Bjork-Shiley prosthesis. *J. Thorac. Cardiovasc. Surg.* 95:423, 1988.
7. Baerman, J. M., Kirsh, M. M., de Buitleir, M., *et al.* Natural history and determinants of conduction defects following coronary artery bypass surgery. *Ann. Thorac. Surg.* 44:150, 1987.
8. Banasik, J. L., Bruya, M. A., and Steadman, R. E. Effect of position on arterial oxygenation in postoperative coronary revascularization patients. *Heart Lung* 16:652, 1987.
9. Barash, P. G. Cardiopulmonary bypass and postoperative neurologic dysfunction. *Am. Heart J.* 99:675, 1980.
10. Barash, P. G. Catheter-induced pulmonary artery perforation: Mechanisms, management and modifications. *J. Thorac. Cardiovasc. Surg.* 82:5, 1981.
11. Barcelona, M., Patague, L., Bunoy, M., *et al.* Cardiac output determination by the thermodilution method: Comparison of ice-temperature injectate contained in prefilled syringes or a closed injectate delivery system. *Heart Lung* 14:232, 1985.
12. Barlow, J. B., and Popcock, W. A. The mitral valve prolapse engima: Two decades later. *Mod. Concepts Cardiovasc. Dis.* 53:13, 1984.
13. Baumann, F. G. Vein contraction and smooth muscle cell extensions as causes of endothelial damage during graft preparation. *Ann. Surg.* 194:199, 1981.
14. Beall, A. C. Late results with cardiac valve replacement: Reduction of thromboembolic complications of mitral valve replacement. *J. Cardiovasc. Surg.* 13:261, 1972.
15. BHAT Study Group. A randomized trial of propranolol in patients with acute myocardial infarction. II. Mortality results. *J. Am. Med. Assoc.* 247:1207, 1982.
16. Blackburn, G. Nutritional support in cardiac cachexia. *J. Thorac. Cardiovasc. Surg.* 73:489, 1977.
17. Bojar, R. M., Najafi, H., DeLaria, G. A., *et al.* Neurological complications of coronary revascularization. *Ann. Thorac. Surg.* 36:427, 1983.
18. Bolooki, H. IABP for Myocardial Infarctions. In H. Bolooki (Ed.), *Clinical Application of Intra-Aortic Balloon.* Mount Kisco, NY: Futura, 1984.
19. Bolooki, H. IABP for Cardiogenic Shock. In H. Balooki (Ed.), *Clinical Application of Intra-Aortic Balloon.* Mount Kisco, NY: Futura, 1984.

20. Bolooki, H. Emergency cardiac procedures in patients in cardiogenic shock due to complications of coronary artery disease. *Circulation* (suppl. I)79:1989.

21. Borkon, A. M., Soule, L. M., Baughman, K. L., *et al.* Aortic valve selection in the elderly patient. *Ann. Thorac. Surg.* 46:270, 1988.

22. Braunwald, E. Valvular Heart Disease. In E. Braunwald (Ed.), *Heart Disease.* Philadelphia: W. B. Saunders, 1980.

23. Brenowitz, J. B., Johnson, D., Kayser, K. L., *et al.* Coronary artery bypass grafting for the third time or more: Results of 150 consecutive cases. *Circulation* (suppl. I)78:I–167, 1988.

24. Brower, R. W., Fioretto, P., Simmons, P., *et al.* Surgical versus non-surgical management of patients soon after acute myocardial infarction. *Br. Heart J.* 54:460, 1985.

25. Burckhardt, D., Striebel, D., Vogt, S., *et al.* Heart valve replacement with St. Jude medical valve prosthesis: Long-term experience in 743 patients in Switzerland. *Circulation* (suppl. I)78:I–18, 1988.

26. Buxton, M. J. Cost effectiveness of coronary grafting. *Curr. Opin. Cardiol.* 1:868, 1986.

27. Califf, R. M., Harrell, F. E., Lee, K. L., *et al.* Changing efficacy of coronary revascularization. *Circulation* (suppl. I)78:I–185, 1988.

28. Camm, J., Ward, D. E., Spurrell, R. A. J., *et al.* Cryothermal mapping and cryoablation in the treatment of refractory cardiac arrhythmias. *Circulation* 62:67, 1980.

29. Carpentier, A., Chauvand, S., and Fabiani, J. N. Reconstructive surgery of mitral valve incompetence—ten-year appraisal. *J. Thorac. Cardiovasc. Surg.* 79:338, 1980.

30. Cason, C. L., Lambert, C. W., Holland, C. L., *et al.* Effects of backrest elevation and position on pulmonary artery pressures. *Cardiovasc. Nurs.* 26:1, 1990.

31. Caspi, Y., Safadi, T., Ammar, R., *et al.* The significance of bundle branch block in the immediate postoperative electrocardiograms of patients undergoing coronary artery bypass. *J. Thorac. Cardiovasc. Surg.* 93:442, 1987.

32. CASS Principal Investigators, *et al.* Myocardial infarction and mortality in the coronary artery surgery study (CASS) randomized trial. *N. Engl. J. Med.* 310:750, 1984.

33. CASS Study Group. CASS principle investigators and their associates. Coronary Artery Surgery Study (CASS): A randomized trial of coronary artery bypass surgery. Survival data. *Circulation* 68:939, 1983.

34. Casson, W. R., Jones, R. M., and Parsons, R. S. Nifedipine and cardiopulmonary bypass. *Anaesthesia* 39:1197, 1984.

35. Chaitman, B. R., Davis, K. B., Dodge, H. T., *et al.* Should airline pilots be eligible to resume flight status after coronary artery bypass surgery? A CASS registry study. *J. Am. Coll. Cardiol.* 8:1318, 1986.

36. Chaux, A., Gray, R. J., Matloff, J. M., *et al.* An appreciation of the new St. Jude valvular prosthesis. *J. Thorac. Cardiovasc. Surg.* 81:202, 1981.

37. Chavez, A. M., Cosgrove, D. M., Lytle, B. W., *et al.* Applicability of mitral valvuloplasty techniques in a North American population. *Am. J. Cardiol.* 62:253, 1988.

38. Chesbro, J. H., Clements, I. P., Fuster, V., *et al.* A platelet-inhibitor drug trial in coronary artery bypass operations: Benefits of preoperative dipyridamole and aspirin therapy in early postoperative vein graft patency. *N. Engl. J. Med.* 307:73, 1982.

39. Chesbro, J. H., Fuster, V., Elveback, L. R., *et al.* Effect of dipyridamole and aspirin on late vein graft patency after coronary bypass operation. *N. Engl. J. Med.* 310:209, 1984.

40. Cheung, J. Y., Bonventre, J. V., Males, C. D., *et al.* Calcium and ischemic injury. *N. Engl. J. Med.* 314:1670, 1986.

41. Chiariello, M. Comparison between the effect of nitroprusside and nitroglycerin on ischemic injury during acute myocardial infarction. *Circulation* 54:766, 1976.

42. Christakis, G. T., Fremes, S. E., Weisel, R. D., *et al.* Reducing the risk of urgent revascularization for unstable angina: A randomized clinical trial. *J. Vasc. Surg.* 3:764, 1986.

43. Christakis, G. T., Fremes, S. E., Weisel, R. D., *et al.* Diltiazem cardioplegia: A balance of risk and benefit. *J. Thorac. Cardiovasc. Surg.* 91:647, 1986.

44. Christakis, G. T., Ivanov, J., Weisel, R. D., *et al.* The changing pattern of coronary artery bypass surgery. *Circulation* (suppl I)80:I–151, 1989.

45. Chulay, M. A. Effect of postoperative immobilization after coronary artery bypass surgery. *Crit. Care Med.* 3:176, 1982.

46. Chulay, M. A., and Miller, T. Effects of backrest elevation on pulmonary artery and pulmonary capillary wedge pressures in patients after cardiac surgery. *Heart Lung* 13:138, 1984.

47. Clancy, C. A., Wey, J. M., and Guinn, G. A. The effect of patients' perceptions on return to work after coronary artery bypass surgery. *Heart Lung* 13:173, 1984.

48. Cohen, M., Silverman, N. A., Goldfaden, D. M., *et al.* Reconstruction of infected median sternotomy wounds. *Arch. Surg.* 122:323, 1987.

49. Conaham, R. J. Complications of Cardiac Surgery. In J. A. Kaplan (Ed.), *Cardiac Anesthesia* (2nd ed.). New York: Grune & Stratton, 1987.

50. Connors, J. P., and Avioli, L. V. An update on cardiac surgery. *Heart Lung* 10:323, 1981.

51. Conti, C. R., Hutter, A., Rosati, R., *et al.* Unstable angina: A national cooperative study comparing medical and surgical therapy. *Cardiovasc. Clin.* 8:167, 1977.

52. Cosgrove, D. M., Loop, F. D., Lytle, B. W., *et al.* Primary myocardial revascularization: Trends in surgical mortality. *J. Thorac. Cardiovasc. Surg.* 88:673, 1984.

53. Cosgrove, D. M. Valve reconstruction versus valve replacement. *Cardiac Surgery: State of the Art Reviews* 1:143, 1987.

54. Coyle, J. P., Steele, J., Cutrone, F., *et al.* Patient controlled analgesia after cardiac surgery. *Anesth. Analg.* 70:S–71, 1990.

55. Crawford, F. A., Kratz, J. M., Sade, R. M., *et al.* Aortic and mitral valve replacement with the St. Jude's Medical prosthesis. *Ann. Surg.* 199:753, 1984.

56. Cukingnam, R. A., Carey, J. S., Wittig, J. H., *et al.* Influence of complete coronary revascularization on relief of angina. *J. Thorac. Cardiovasc. Surg.* 79:188, 1980.

57. Culliford, A. T. Postoperative Care. In D. C. Sabiston (Ed.), *Gibbon's Surgery of the Chest* (4th ed.). Philadelphia: W. B. Saunders, 1983.

58. Daily, E. K. *Techniques in Bedside Hemodynamic Monitoring* (3rd ed.). St. Louis: Mosby-Year Book, 1988.

59. Darovic, G. O. *Hemodynamic Monitoring: Invasive and Noninvasive Clinical Applications.* Philadelphia: W. B. Saunders, 1987.

60. Davidson, D. M. Long-term results of coronary artery bypass surgery for unstable angina: Incidence of mortality, myocardial infarction and angina resumption. *Clin. Cardiol.* 3:297, 1980.

61. DeBusk, R. F., Kraemer, H. C., and Nash, E. Stepwise risk stratification soon after myocardial infarction. *Am. J. Cardiol.* 52:1161, 1983.

62. Dion, R., Verhelst, R., Rousseau, M., *et al.* Sequential mammary grafting. *J. Thorac. Cardiovasc. Surg.* 98:80, 1989.

63. Doering, L., and Dracup, K. Comparison of cardiac output in supine lateral positions. *Nurs. Res.* 37:114, 1988.

64. Dorros, G., Lewin, R. F., and Daley, P. Coronary artery bypass surgery in patients over age 70 years: Report from the Milwaukee Cardiovascular Data Registry. *Clin. Cardiol.* 10:377, 1987.

65. Drop, L. J. Ionized calcium, the heart and hemodynamic function. *Anesth. Analg.* 64:432, 1985.

66. Edmunds, L., and Stephenson, L. Cardiopulmonary Bypass for Open Heart Surgery. In W. Glenn (Ed.). *Thoracic and Cardiovascular Surgery.* Norwalk, CN: Appleton-Century-Crofts, 1983.

67. Effler, D. B., Groves, K., Suarex, E. L., *et al.* Direct coronary artery surgery with endarterectomy and patch graft reconstruction. *J. Thorac. Cardiovasc. Surg.* 53:93, 1967.

68. Ehrlich, I. B. Patient selection and preoperative evaluation. *Heart Lung* 4:373, 1975.

69. Engeleman, R. M., Hadji-Rousou, I., Breyer, R. H., *et al.* Rebound

vasospasm after coronary revascularization in association with calcium antagonist withdrawal. *Ann. Thorac. Surg.* 36:469, 1984.

70. Engler, R. L. Is there a role for surgery in acute myocardial infarction? *Cardiovasc. Clin.* 8:213, 1977.

71. Epstein, S. E., Kent, K. M., Goldstein, R. E., *et al.* Reduction of ischemic injury by nitroglycerin during acute myocardial infarction. *N. Engl. J. Med.* 292:29, 1975.

72. Epstein, S. E., Palmeri, S. T., and Patterson, R. E. Evaluation of patients after acute myocardial infarction: Indications for cardiac catheterization and surgical intervention. *N. Engl. J. Med.* 307: 1487, 1982.

73. European Coronary Surgery Study Group. Long-term results of a prospective randomized study of coronary artery bypass surgery with stable angina pectoris. *Lancet* 2:1173, 1983.

74. Favalaro, R. G. Double internal mammary artery implants: Operative technique. *J. Thorac. Cardiovasc. Surg.* 55:457, 1968.

75. Favalaro, R. G. Saphenous vein graft in the surgical treatment of coronary artery disease: Operative technique. *J. Thorac. Cardiovasc. Surg.* 58:178, 1969.

76. Favalaro, R. G., Effler, D. B., and Cheanvechai, C. Acute coronary insufficiency (impending myocardial infarction and myocardial infarction): Surgical treatment by the saphenous vein graft technique. *Am. J. Cardiol.* 28:598, 1971.

77. Fisher, L. D., Kennedy, J. W., Davis, K. B., *et al.* Association of sex, physical size and operative mortality after coronary bypass in Coronary Artery Surgery Study (CASS) *J. Thorac. Cardiovasc. Surg.* 84:334, 1982.

78. Foex, P. Beta-blockade in anesthesia. *J. Clin. Hosp. Pharm.* 8: 183, 1983.

79. Forrester, J. S. Medical therapy of acute myocardial infarction by application of hemodynamic subsets. *N. Engl. J. Med.* 292: 1356, 1975.

80. Fox, M. H., Gruchow, H. W., and Barboriak, J. J. Risk factors among patients undergoing repeat aortic-coronary bypass procedure. *J. Thorac. Cardiovasc. Surg.* 93:56, 1987.

81. Fremes, S. E. Effects of postoperative hypertension and its treatment. *J. Thorac. Cardiovasc. Surg.* 86:47, 1983.

82. Fuller, J. A., Adams, G. G., and Buxton, B. Atrial fibrillation after coronary artery bypass grafting. Is it a disorder of the elderly. *J. Thorac. Cardiovasc. Surg.* 97:821, 1989.

83. Furlan, A. J., and Breuer, A. C. Central nervous system complications of open heart surgery. *Curr. Concepts Cerebrovasc. Dis.* 19:7, 1984.

84. Gardner, P. E., and Laurent-Bopp, D. Continuous SvO$_2$ Monitoring: Clinical application in critical care nursing. *Prog. Cardiovasc. Nurs.* 2:9, 1987.

85. Gardner, T. J., Stuart, R. S., Greene, P. S., *et al.* The risk of coronary bypass surgery for patients with postinfarction angina. *Circulation* (suppl. I)79:I–79, 1989.

86. Garrett, H. E., Dennis, E. W., and DeBakey, M. E. Aortocoronary bypass with saphenous vein graft: Seven year follow-up. *J.A.M.A.* 223:792, 1973.

87. Gerrity, R. G., Loop, F. D., Golding, L. A. R., *et al.* Arterial response to laser operation for removal of atherosclerotic plaques. *J. Thorac. Cardiovasc. Surg.* 85:409, 1983.

88. Gersh, B. J. Results of coronary artery bypass surgery conclusions from the Coronary Artery Surgery Study. *Curr. Opin. Cardiol.* 1: 870, 1986.

89. Gershan, J. A. Effect of positive end-expiratory pressure on pulmonary capillary wedge pressure. *Heart Lung* 12:143, 1983.

90. Gershlick, A. H., Lyons, J. P., Wright, J. E. C., *et al.* Long term clinical outcome of coronary surgery and assessment of the benefit obtained with postoperative aspirin and dypyridamole. *Br. Heart J.* 60:111, 1988.

91. Goe, M. R. Creatine kinase enzyme determination. *Prog. Cardiovasc. Nurs.* 2:44, 1987.

92. Goenen, M., Oneglio, P., Baele, P., *et al.* Amrinone in the management of low cardiac output after open-heart surgery. *Am. J. Cardiol.* 56:33B, 1985.

93. Goldstein, R. E. Intraoperative coronary collateral function in patients with coronary occlusion diseases: Nitroglycerin responsiveness and angiographic correlation. *Circulation* 49:298, 1974.

94. Goodman, L. The Use of Antibiotics in Cardiac and Thoracic Surgery. In D. C. Sabiston (Ed.), *Gibbon's Surgery of the Chest* (4th ed.). Philadelphia: W. B. Saunders, 1983.

95. Grose, B. L. Effects of mechanical ventilation and position upon pulmonary wedge pressure measurements. *Am. Rev. Respir. Dis.* 33:71, 1982.

96. Guiraudon, G., Fontaine, G., Frank, R., *et al.* Encircling endocardial ventriculotomy: A new surgical treatment for life-threatening ventricular tachycardias resistant to medical treatment following myocardial infarction. *Ann. Thorac. Surg.* 26:438, 1978.

97. Gutmann, M. C., Knapp, D. N., Pollock, M. L., *et al.* Coronary artery bypass patients and work status. *Circulation* 66:33, 1982.

98. Guzzetta, C. E. Can Critically Ill Patient Be Taught? In D. Bille (Ed.), *Practical Approaches to Patient Teaching.* Boston: Little, Brown, 1981.

99. Hamilton, W. M., Hammermeister, K. E., DeRouen, T. A., *et al.* Effect of coronary artery bypass grafting on subsequent hospitalization. *Am. J. Cardiol.* 51:353, 1983.

100. Hanks, J. B., Curtis, S. E., Hanks, B. B., *et al.* Gastrointestinal complications after cardiopulmonary bypass. *Surgery* 92:394, 1982.

101. Hansen, D. E., Cahill, P. D., Derby, G. C., *et al.* Relative contributions of the anterior and posterior mitral chordae tendineae to canine global left ventricular systolic function. *J. Thorac. Cardiovasc. Surg.* 93:45, 1987.

102. Harken, A. H., Horowitz, L. N., Josephson, M. E., *et al.* Comparison of standard aneurysmectomy and aneurysmectomy with directed endocardial resection for the treatment of recurrent sustained ventricular tachycardia. *J. Thorac. Cardiovasc. Surg.* 80: 527, 1980.

103. Harken, D. E., Soroff, H. S., Taylor, W. J., *et al.* Partial and complete prostheses in aortic insufficiency. *J. Thorac. Cardiovasc. Surg.* 40:744, 1960.

104. Harrison, D. C. Coronary bypass: The first 10 years. *Hosp. Pract.:* 49, June, 1981.

105. Heikkila, H., Jalonen, J., Laaksonen, V., *et al.* Metroprolol medication and coronary artery bypass grafting operation. *ACTA Anaesthesiol. Scand.* 28:677, 1984.

106. Hilberman, M., Kamm, R., Lancy, M., *et al.* An analysis of potential physiological predictors of respiratory adequacy following cardiac surgery. *J. Thorac. Cardiovasc. Surg.* 71:711, 1976.

107. Hultgren, H. N., Takaro, T., Detre, K., *et al.* Veterans Administration cooperative study of surgical treatment of stable angina: Preliminary results. *Cardiovasc. Clin.* 8:119, 1977.

108. ISIS Collaborative Group. Vascular mortality after early IV beta blockade in myocardial infarction. *Circulation* (suppl. 3)72:III–224, 1985.

109. Isom, O. W., and Spencer, F. C. The current status of bypass grafting for coronary artery disease. *South. Med. J.* 68:897, 1975.

110. IVAC Corporation. Titrator Module—Model 10K Closed Loop System for Sodium Nitroprusside Delivery [product information]. San Diego, CA: IVAC Corporation, 1989.

111. Jeevanandam, V., Smith, C. R., Rose, E. A., *et al.* Single-stage management of sternal wound infections. *J. Thorac. Cardiovasc. Surg.* 99:256, 1990.

112. Johnson, J. E. Effects of structuring patients' expectations on their reactions to threatening events. *Nurs. Res.* 21:499, 1972.

113. Johnson, W., Flemma, R. J., and Lepley, D. Extended treatment of severe coronary artery disease: A surgical approach. *Ann. Surg.* 170:460, 1969.

114. Jones, E. L., Craver, J. M., Guyton, R. A., *et al.* Trends in the treatment of severe coronary artery disease today: Selective use of PTCA and bypass surgery. *Ann. Surg.* 197:728, 1983.

115. Jones, R. H., Floyd, R. D., Austin, E. H., *et al.* The role of radionuclide angiocardiography in the preoperative prediction of pain relief and prolonged survival following coronary artery bypass grafting. *Ann. Surg.* 197:743, 1983.

116. Josephson, M. E., Horowitz, L. N., Spielman, S. R., et al. Comparison of endocardial catheter mapping with intraoperative mapping of ventricular tachycardia. Circulation 61:396, 1980.

117. Karanko, M. S., Klossner, J. A., and Laaksonen, V. O. Restoration of volume by crystalloid versus colloid after coronary artery bypass: hemodynamics, lung water, oxygenation and outcome. Crit. Care Med. 15:559, 1987.

118. Kay, J. H. Emergency operation for complications of myocardial infarction. Heart Lung 11:40, 1982.

119. Keating, D., Bolyard, K., Eichler, K., et al. Effect of sidelying positions on pulmonary artery pressures. Heart Lung 15:605, 1986.

120. Keck, S. Cardiac tamponade: An initial study of a preditive tool. Heart Lung 12:505, 1983.

121. Kennedy, J. W., Kaiser, G. C., Fisher, L. D., et al. Multivariant discriminary analysis of the clinical and angiographic predictors of operative mortality from the collaborative study in coronary artery surgery (CASS) J. Thorac. Cardiovasc. Surg. 80:876, 1980.

122. Kent, K. M., Borer, J. S., and Green, M. V. Effects of coronary-artery bypass on global and regional left ventricular function during exercise. N. Engl. J. Med. 298:1434, 1978.

123. Kimball, C. P. Psychologic response to the experience of open heart surgery. Am. J. Psychol. 126:96, 1969.

124. King, S. B., and Hurst, J. W. The Relief of Angina Pectoris by Coronary Bypass Surgery. In J. W. Hurst (Ed.), The Heart: Update II. New York: McGraw-Hill, 1980.

125. Kirklin, J. W. Cardiopulmonary Bypass for Cardiac Surgery. In D. C. Sabiston (Ed.), Gibbon's Surgery of the Chest (4th ed.). Philadelphia: W. B. Saunders, 1983.

126. Kolkka, R., and Hilberman, M. Neurologic dysfunction following cardiac operation with low flow, low-pressure cardiopulmonary bypass. J. Thorac. Cardiovasc. Surg. 79:432, 1980.

127. Kornfield, D. S., Heller, S. S., Frank, K. A., et al. Psychological and behavioral responses after coronary artery bypass surgery. Circulation 66:III–24, 1982.

128. Kouchoukos, N. T., Lell, W. A., and Rogers, W. J. Combined aortic valve replacement and myocardial revascularization. Ann. Surg. 197:721, 1983.

129. Krause, K. R., Hutter, A. M., Jr., and DeSanctis, R. W. Acute coronary insufficiency: Cause and follow-up. Arch. Intern. Med. 129:808, 1972.

130. Larach, D. R., Hensley, F. A., Pae, L. R., et al. A randomized study of diltiazem withdrawal prior to coronary artery bypass surgery. Anesthesiology 63:A23, 1985.

131. Laulive, J. L. Pulmonary artery pressures and position change in the critically ill adult. Dimens. Crit. Care Nurs. 1:28, 1982.

132. Lewis, H. D., Davis, J. W., Archibald, G. D., et al. Protective effects of aspirin against acute myocardial infarction and death in men with unstable angina: Results of a Veterans Administration cooperative study. N. Engl. J. Med. 309:396, 1983.

133. Ley, S. J., Miller, K., Skov, P., et al. Crystalloid versus colloid fluid therapy after cardiac surgery. Heart Lung, 19:31, 1990.

134. Liddle, H. V., Jensen, R., and Clayton, P. D. The rehabilitation of coronary surgical patients. Ann. Thorac. Surg. 34:374, 1982.

135. Litwak, R., Giannelli, S. Open Intracardiac Operations Employing Extracorporeal Circulation. In R. Litwak and E. Jurado (Eds.). Care of the Cardiac Surgical Patient. Norwalk, CT: Appleton-Century-Crofts, 1982.

136. Logue, B., Bone, D., Kaplan, J. The diagnoses and management of mechanical defects due to myocardial infarction. Cardiovasc. Rev. Rep. 1:446, 1980.

137. Loop, F. D. An 11-year evolution of coronary arterial surgery (1967–1978). Ann. Surg. 190:444, 1979.

138. Loop, F. D., Lytle, B. W., Gill, C., et al. Trends in selection and results of coronary artery reoperations. Ann. Thorac. Surg. 36:380, 1983.

139. Loop, F. D. Progress in surgical treatment of coronary atherosclerosis. Part 1. Chest 84:611, 1983.

140. Loop, F. D. Progress in surgical treatment of coronary atherosclerosis. Part 2. Chest 84:740, 1983.

141. Loop, F. D. Recent reports on long-term results after coronary artery bypass grafting. Curr. Opin. Cardiol. 1:884, 1986.

142. Lopes, M. G., Spivack, A. P., and Harrison, D. C. Prognosis of noninfarction coronary care patients. Am. J. Cardiol. 31:144, 1973.

143. Lorente, P., Gourgon, R., Beaufils, P., et al. Multivariant statistical evaluation of intraaortic counterpulsation in pump failure complicating acute myocardial infarction. Am. J. Cardiol. 46:124, 1980.

144. Luepker, R. V. What can be concluded from the three randomised coronary artery bypass surgery trials? Curr. Opin. Cardiol. 1:876, 1986.

145. Lytle, B. W., Kramer, J. R., Golding, L. A. R., et al. Young adults with coronary atherosclerosis: 10-year results of surgical myocardial revascularization. J. Am. Coll. Cardiol. 4:445, 1984.

146. Lytle, B. W., Loop, F. D., Cosgrove, D. M., et al. Long-term (5 to 12 years) serial studies of internal mammary artery and saphenous vein coronary bypass grafts. J. Thorac. Cardiovasc. Surg. 89:248, 1985.

147. Lytle, B. W., Loop, F. D., Cosgrove, D. M., et al. Bilateral internal mammary artery grafting: early and late clinical results for 1000 cases (1971–1985) [abstract]. Tenth World Congr. Cardiol. 81:459, 1986.

148. Lytle, B. W., Loop, F. D., Cosgrove, D. M., et al. Fifteen hundred coronary reoperations: Result and determinants of early and late survival. J. Thorac. Cardiovasc. Surg. 93:847, 1987.

149. Lytle, B. W. Long-term results of coronary bypass surgery. Is the internal mammary artery graft superior? Postgrad. Med. 83:66, 1988.

150. Lytle, B. W., and Loop, F. D. Coronary reoperations. Surg. Clin. North Am. 68:559, 1988.

151. Lytle, B. W., Cosgrove, D. M., Ratliff, N. B., et al. Coronary artery bypass grafting with the right gastroepiploic artery. J. Thorac. Cardiovasc. Surg. 97:826, 1989.

152. Lytle, B. W., Cosgrove, D. M., Taylor, P. C., et al. Primary isolated aortic valve replacement: Early and late results. J. Thorac. Cardiovasc. Surg. 97:675, 1989.

153. Mailes, A., Chan, J., Basinski, A., et al. Chest wall pain after aortocoronary bypass surgery using internal mammary artery graft: A new pain syndrome? Heart Lung 18:553, 1989.

154. Martin, J. L., Unterecker, W. J., Harken, A. H., et al. Aneurysmectomy and endocardial resection of ventricular tachycardia: Favorable hemodynamic and antiarrhythmic results in patients with global left ventricular dysfunction. Am. Heart J. 103:960, 1982.

155. Matsuki, O., Robles, A., Gibbs, S., et al. Long-term performance of 555 aortic homografts in the aortic position. Ann. Thorac. Surg. 46:187, 1988.

156. McCollum, C. H., Garcia-Rinaldi, R., Graham, J. M., et al. Myocardial revascularization prior to subsequent major surgery in patients with coronary artery disease. Surgery 81:302, 1977.

157. Miccolo, M. L., and Spagna, P. M. Late strut fracture and disc embolization in a 27-mm Bjork-Shiley mitral valve prosthesis. Am. Heart J. 110:898, 1985.

158. Michelson, E. L., Morganroth, J., and MacVaugh, J. Postoperative arrhythmias after coronary artery and cardiac valvular surgery detected by long-term electrocardiographic monitoring. Am. Heart J. 97:442, 1979.

159. Mickleborough, L. L., Harris, L., Downar, E., et al. A new intraoperative approach for endocardial mapping of ventricular tachycardia. J. Thorac. Cardiovasc. Surg. 95:271, 1988.

160. Miedzenski, L. J., and Keren, G. Serious infections complications of open-heart surgery. Can. J. Surg. 30:103, 1987.

161. Milano, A. D., Bortoslotti, U., Mazzucco, A., et al. Performance of the Hancock porcine bioprosthesis following aortic valve replacement: Considerations based on a 15-year experience. Ann. Thorac. Surg. 46:216, 1988.

162. Miller, D. C. Discriminant analysis of the changing risks of coronary artery operations. J. Thorac. Cardiovasc. Surg. 5:197, 1983.

163. Miller, D. C., Stinson, E. B., Oyer, P. E., *et al.* Discriminant analysis of the changing risks of coronary artery operations: 1971–1979. *J. Thorac. Cardiovasc. Surg.* 85:197, 1983.

164. Miller, D. W., Bruce, R. A., and Dodge, H. T. Physiologic improvement following coronary artery bypass surgery. *Circulation* 57:832, 1978.

165. Miller, D. W., Tobis, F. M., Ivey, T. D., *et al.* Risks of coronary arteriography and bypass surgery in patients with left main coronary artery stenosis. *Chest* 79:387, 1981.

166. Miller, P., Wikoff, R., McMahon, M., *et al.* Marital functioning after cardiac surgery. *Heart Lung* 19:55, 1990.

167. Mills, N. L., and Ochsner, J. L. Concepts of coronary bypass surgery. *Postgrad. Med.* 57:97, 1975.

168. Mirhoseini, M., Shelgikar, S., and Cayton, M. M. New concepts in revascularization of the myocardium. *Ann. Thorac. Surg.* 45:415, 1988.

169. Mock, M. B., Ringqvist, I., Fisher, L. D., *et al.* Survival of medically treated patients in the Coronary Artery Surgery Study (CASS) registry. *Circulation* 66:562, 1982.

170. Mohr, J. P. Neurologic Complications of Cardiac Valvular Disease and Cardiac Surgery, Including Systemic Hypotension. In P. J. Vinken (Ed.), *Handbook of Clinical Neurology.* Amsterdam: Elsevier North Holland, 1979.

171. Montague, N. T., Kouchoukos, N. T., Wilson, T. A. S., *et al.* Morbidity and mortality of coronary artery bypass grafting in patients 70 years of age and older. *Ann. Thorac. Surg.* 39:552, 1985.

172. Multicenter Postinfarction Research Group. Risk stratification and survival after myocardial infarction. *N. Engl. J. Med.* 309:331, 1983.

173. Mundth, E. D., and Austen, W. G. Surgical measures for coronary heart disease. Part I. *N. Engl. J. Med.* 293:13, 1975.

174. Mundth, E. D., and Austen, W. G. Surgical measures for coronary heart disease. Part III. *N. Engl. J. Med.* 293:124, 1975.

175. Murphy, M. L., Hultgren, H. N., and Detre, K. Treatment of chronic stable angina: A preliminary report of survival data of the randomized Veterans Administration Cooperative Study. *N. Engl. J. Med.* 297:622, 1977.

176. Norheim, C. Family needs of patients having coronary artery bypass graft surgery during the intraoperative period. *Heart Lung* 18:622, 1989.

177. Norwegian Multicenter Study Group. Timolol induced reduction in mortality and reinfarction in patients surviving acute myocardial infarction. *N. Engl. J. Med.* 304:801, 1981.

178. Ottino, G., DePaules, R., Pansini, S., *et al.* Major sternal wound infection after open-heart surgery: A multivariant analysis of risk factors in 2,579 consecutive operative procedures. *Ann. Thorac. Surg.* 44:173, 1987.

179. Pasque, M. K., and Weshsler, A. S. Metabolic intervention to affect myocardial recovery following ischemia. *Ann. Surg.* 200:1, 1984.

180. Penckofer, S., and Holm, K. Hopes and fears after coronary artery bypass surgery. *Prog. Cardiovasc. Nurs.* 2:139, 1987.

181. Pfisteres, M., Jockers, G., Regenass, S., *et al.* Trial of low-dose aspirin plus dipyridamole versus anticoagulants for prevention of aortocoronary vein graft occlusion. *Lancet* 8:1, 1989.

182. Phillips, R., and Skov, P. Rewarming and cardiac surgery: A review. *Heart Lung* 17:511, 1988.

183. Pierpont, G. L., Kruse, M., Ewald, S., *et al.* Practical problems in assessing risk of coronary artery bypass grafting. *J. Thorac. Cardiovasc. Surg.* 89:673, 1985.

184. Pierson, M. G., and Funk, M. Technology versus clinical evaluation for fluid management decisions in CABG patients. *Image* 21:192, 1989.

185. Rackley, C. E., Edwards, J. E., Wallace, R. B., *et al.* Aortic Valve Disease. In J. W. Hurst (Ed.), *The Heart* (6th ed.). New York: McGraw Hill, 1986.

186. Rackley, C. E., Edwards, J. E., and Karp, R. B. Mitral Valve Disease. In J. W. Hurst (Ed.), *The Heart* (6th ed.). New York: McGraw Hill, 1986.

187. Rahimtoola, S. H., Nunley, D., Grunkemeier, G., *et al.* Ten-year survival after coronary bypass surgery for unstable angina. *N. Engl. J. Med.* 308:676, 1983.

188. Rahimtoola, S. H. Coronary bypass surgery for unstable angina. *Circulation* 69:842, 1984.

189. Reddy, P. S. Cardiac tamponade: Hemodynamic observations in man. *Circulation* 58:265, 1978.

190. Reed, J. M., and Dargie, H. J. Risk stratification after myocardial infarction with and without coronary artery bypass grafting. *Eur. Heart J.* (suppl. G)9:691, 1988.

191. Reitz, B. A. Uses of Hypothermia in Cardiovascular Surgery. In A. K. Ream (Ed.), *Acute Cardiovascular Management: Anesthesia and Intensive Care.* Philadelphia: J. B. Lippincott, 1982.

192. Resnekov, L., Chediak, J., Hirsh, J., *et al.* Antithrombotic agents in coronary artery disease. ACCP-NHLBI, National Conference on Antithrombotic Therapy. *Chest* 89:54S, 1986.

193. Roberts, A. J., Sanders, J. H., Moran, J. H., *et al.* The efficacy of medical stabilization prior to myocardial revascularization in early refractory postinfarction angina. *Ann. Surg.* 197:91, 1983.

194. Robinson, W. A., Smith, R. F., and Stevens, T. W. Preinfarction syndrome: Evaluation and treatment. *Circulation* (suppl. 2)46:212, 1972.

195. Rocchiccioli, C., Chastre, J., Lecompte, Y., *et al.* Prosthetic valve endocarditis. The case for prompt surgical management. *J. Thorac. Cardiovasc. Surg.* 92:784, 1986.

196. Rosenkrantz, E. R., Okamota, F., Buckbery, G. D., *et al.* Safety of prolonged aortic clamping with blood cardioplegia. III. Aspartate enrichment of glutamate-blood cardioplegia in energy-depleted hearts after ischemic and reperfusion injury. *J. Thorac. Cardiovasc. Surg.* 91:428, 1986.

197. Rutan, P. M., Rountree, W. D., Myers, K. K., *et al.* Initial experience with the HEMOPUMP. *Crit. Care Nurs. Clin. North Am.* 1:527, 1989.

198. Sadler, P. D. Incidence, degree, and duration of postcardiotomy delirium. *Heart Lung* 10:1084, 1981.

199. Sawyer, P. N., Kaplitt, M., Sobel, S., *et al.* Experimental and clinical experience with coronary gas endarterectomy. *Arch. Surg.* 95:736, 1967.

200. Schaff, H. V., Gersh, B. J., Fisher, L. D., *et al.* Detrimental effect of perioperative myocardial infarction on late survival after coronary artery bypass. *J. Thorac. Cardiovasc. Surg.* 88:972, 1984.

201. Scheidegger, D., Drop, L. J., and Schellenberg, J. C. Role of the systemic vasculature in the hemodynamic response to changes in plasma ionized calcium. *Arch. Surg.* 115:206, 1980.

202. Schmidt, C. R., Frank, L. P., and Forsythe, S. B. Continuous SvO_2 measurement and oxygen transport patterns in cardiac surgery patients. *Crit. Care Med.* 12:523, 1984.

203. Scully, H. E., Leclerc, Y., Martin, R. D., *et al.* Comparison between antibiotic irrigation and mobilization of pectoral muscle flaps in treatment of deep sternal infections. *J. Thorac. Cardiovasc. Surg.* 90:523, 1985.

204. Seides, S. F., Borer, J. S., Kent, K. M., *et al.* Long-term anatomic fate of coronary-artery bypass grafts and functional status of patients five years after operation. *N. Engl. J. Med.* 298:1214, 1978.

205. Seifert, P. C. Protection of the myocardium during cardiac surgery. *Heart Lung* 12:135, 1983.

206. Sequin, J. R., and Loisance, D. Y. Omental transposition for closure of median sternotomy following severe mediastinal and vascular infection. *Chest* 88:5, 1985.

207. Sewell, W. H. Results of 122 mammary pedicle implantations for angina pectoris. *Ann. Thorac. Surg.* 2:17, 1966.

208. Shank, J. Postpericardiotomy syndrome. II. Nursing implications. *Cardiovasc. Nurs.* 19:15, 1983.

209. Shellock, F. G., and Riedeinger, M. S. Reproducibility and accuracy of using room-temperature vs. ice-temperature injectate

for thermodilution cardiac output determinations. *Heart Lung* 12:175, 1983.

210. Shelton, M. E., Forman, M. B., Virmani, R., *et al.* A comparison of morphologic and angiographic findings in long-term internal mammary artery and saphenous vein bypass grafts. *J. Am. Coll. Cardiol.* 11:297, 1988.

211. Silverman, K. H., and Grossman, W. Angina pectoris: Natural history and strategies for evaluation and management. *N. Engl. J. Med.* 1712:310, 1984.

212. Sladen, R. N. Management of the Adult Cardiac Patient in the Intensive Care Unit. In A. K. Ream, (Ed.), *Acute Cardiovascular Management: Anesthesia and Intensive Care.* Philadelphia: J. B. Lippincott, 1982.

213. Slogoff, S., Girges, K. Z., and Keats, A. S. Etiologic factors in neuropsychiatric complications associated with cardiopulmonary bypass. *Anesth. Analg.* 61:903, 1982.

214. Smith, T. W. Digitalis: Mechanisms of action and clinical use. *N. Engl. J. Med.* 318:358, 1988.

215. Soloway, H. B., and Christiansen, T. W. Heparin anticoagulation during cardiopulmonary bypass in an antithrombin III deficit patient: Implications relevant to the etiology of heparin rebound. *Am. J. Clin. Pathol.* 73:723, 1980.

216. Sones, F. M., Jr., and Shirey, E. K. Cine coronary arteriography. *Mod. Concepts Cardiovasc. Dis.* 31:735, 1962.

217. Spencer, F. C. Bypass grafting for preinfarction angina. *Circulation* 45:1314, 1972.

218. Spencer, F. C. Surgical Management of Coronary Artery Disease. In D. C. Sabiston, (Ed.), *Gibbon's Surgery of the Chest* (4th ed.). Philadelphia: W. B. Saunders, 1983.

219. Stanford, J. L. Who profits from coronary artery bypass surgery? *Am. J. Nurs.* 82:1068, 1982.

220. Stanton, B., Jenkins, D., Savageau, J., *et al.* Preceived adequacy of patient education and fears and adjustments after cardiac surgery. *Heart Lung* 13:525, 1984.

221. Starr, A., and Edwards, M. L. Mitral replacement: Clinical experience with a ball valve prosthesis. *Ann. Surg.* 154:726, 1961.

222. Stein, P. D., Collins, J. J., and Kantrowitz, A. Antithrombotic therapy in mechanical and biological prosthetic heart valves and saphenous vein bypass grafts. ACCP-NHLBI National Conference on Antithrombotic Therapy. *Chest* 89:465, 1986.

223. Still, J. E., Nugent, M., Moyer, T. P., *et al.* Influence of propranolol plasma levels on hemodynamics during coronary artery bypass surgery. *Anesthesiology* 60:455, 1984.

224. Stone, K. S., Vorst, E. C., Lanham, B., *et al.* Effects of lung hyperinflation on mean arterial pressure and post suctioning hypoxemia. *Heart Lung* 18:377, 1989.

225. Stradtman, J. C., and Ballenger, M. J. Nursing implications in sternal and mediastinal infections after open heart surgery. *Focus Crit. Care* 16:178, 1989.

226. Suma, H., Fukumoto, H., and Takeuchi, A. Coronary artery bypass grafting by utilizing in situ right gastroepiploic artery: Basic study and clinical application. *Ann. Thorac. Surg.* 44:394, 1987.

227. Suma, H., Takeuchi, A., and Hirota, Y. Myocardial revascularization with combined arterial grafts utilizing the internal mammary and the gastroepiploic arteries. *Ann. Thorac. Surg.* 47:712, 1989.

228. Takaro, T., Hultgren, N. H., Detre, K. M., *et al.* The Veterans Administration Cooperative Study of stable angina: Current status. *Circulation* 65:60, 1982.

229. Teoh, K. H., Christakes, G. T., Weisel, R. D., *et al.* Accelerated myocardial metabolic recovery with terminal warm blood cardioplegia. *J. Thorac. Cardiovasc. Surg.* 91:888, 1986.

230. Teoh, K. H., Mickle, D., Weiset, R. D., *et al.* Improving myocardial metabolic and functional recovery after cardioplegic arrest. *J. Thorac. Cardiovasc. Surg.* 95:788, 1988.

231. Thomas, C. S., Alford, W. C., Burrus, G. R., *et al.* Urgent operation for acquired ventricular septal defects. *Ann. Surg.* 195:706, 1982.

232. Townes, B. D., Bashein, G., Hornbein, T. F., *et al.* Neurobehavioral outcomes in cardiac operations. *J. Thorac. Cardiovasc. Surg.* 98:774, 1989.

233. Varnauskas, E. Twelve-year follow-up of survival in the randomized European Coronary Surgery Study. *N. Engl. J. Med.* 319:332, 1988.

234. Vennix, C. V., Nelson, D. H., and Pierpont, G. L. Thermodilution cardiac output in critically ill patients: Comparison of room-temperature and iced ejectate. *Heart Lung* 13:574, 1984.

235. Veterans Administration Coronary Artery Bypass Cooperative Study Group. Eleven-year survival in the Veterans Administration randomised trial of coronary bypass surgery for stable angina. The Veterans Administration Coronary Artery Bypass Surgery Cooperative Study Group. *N. Engl. J. Med.* 311:1333, 1984.

236. Vineberg, A. M. Development of an anastomosis between the coronary vessels and a transplant internal mammary artery. *Can. Med. Assoc. J.* 55:117, 1946.

237. Weschsler, A. S., and Junod, F. L. Coronary bypass grafting in patients with chronic congestive heart failure. *Circulation* (suppl. I)79:I–92, 1989.

238. Wexelman, W., Lichstein, E., Cunningham, J. N., *et al.* Etiology and clinical significance of new fascicular conduction defects following coronary bypass surgery. *Am. Heart J.* 111:923, 1986.

239. Wheatley, D. J. Coronary artery bypass graft surgery: Late survival and follow-up. *Eur. Heart J.* 9:107, 1988.

240. Whitman, G. R. Comparison of maximal temperature elevations following reversal of hypothermia with four rewarming techniques. *Circulation* 64:II–4, 1981.

241. Whitman, G. R. Comparison of cardiac output measurements in 20-degree supine and 20-degree right and left lateral recumbent positions. *Heart Lung* 11:256, 1982.

242. Whitman, G. R. Bedside Hemodynamic Monitoring. In P. T. Horvath, (Ed.), *Care of the Adult Cardiac Surgery Patient.* New York: John Wiley & Sons, 1984.

243. Whitman, G. R. Prosthetic cardiac valves. *Prog. Cardiovasc. Nurs.* 2:116, 1987.

244. Williams, D. B., Ivey, T. D., Bailey, W. W., *et al.* Post infarction angina: Results of early revascularization. *J. Am. Coll. Cardiol.* 2:859, 1983.

245. Windsor, T. Phlebostatic axis and phlebostatic level. Reference levels for venous pressure in man. *Proc. Soc. Exp. Biol. Med.* 58:165, 1945.

246. Woods, S. Effect of backrest position on pulmonary artery pressure in critically ill patients. *Cardiovasc. Nurs.* 18:19, 1982.

247. Wright, G. J., Pifarre, R., Sullivan, H. J., *et al.* Multivarient discriminant analysis of risk factors for operative mortality following isolated coronary artery bypass graft. Loyola University Medical Center Experience, 1970–1984. *Chest* 91:394, 1987.

248. Wulff, K. S. Use of temporary epicardial electrodes for atrial pacing and monitoring. *Cardiovasc. Nurs.* 18:1, 1982.

249. Xiaodong, Z., Jiaqiang, G., Yingchun, C., *et al.* Ten-year experience with pericardial xenograft valves. *J. Thorac. Cardiovasc. Surg.* 95:572, 1988.

250. Young, J. A. Coagulation abnormalities with cardiopulmonary bypass. In J. R. Utley, (Ed.), *Pathophysiology and Techniques of Cardiopulmonary Bypass.* Baltimore: Williams & Williams, 1982.

27

Acute Pericarditis

Linda M. Sulzbach   *Barbara Montgomery Dossey*

CREATING AN INTUITION LOG

Intuition is your knowledge of the truth as it comes to you, or a heightened sense of awareness and a sense of attaining the whole. Intuition comes to you as flashes of insight when you have not relied on the usual logical conscious process of reasoning. Keep a small notebook with you, and any time you sense a vague impression or feeling or hear your quiet, inner voice saying something insightful, record it.

Recognizing intuition is a skill that can be developed (see Chapt. 7). As you learn to validate your new skill, you become more comfortable acting on your intuitive insights in many day-to-day decisions. You will find that over time your entries are nonverbal descriptions in which you use words such as ''feel'' and ''knew.'' The following exerpt from an intuition log is an example:

> While driving along today I started thinking about my dear friend, Elizabeth. So funny, I've been so busy I haven't seen or talked to her in months. Called her, and she said that she had been thinking about me that same morning. She's under a lot of stress, and we talked for 30 minutes. Back at my desk, I had a sense that the big red book above my head might fall from the shelf. I looked up and it looked fine. Went back to my desk work. I heard nothing. A few minutes later, jack-hammering from the construction on the floor above my desk shook the walls, and that book—and the only book—fell from the shelf. I caught it and had a great laugh! I just reached up and caught it with both hands—like in slow motion. Interesting experience. I rehearsed that event before it happened.

Keeping an intuition log and answering your questions concerning the information gathered from intuitions can strengthen your intuitive skills. Answer such questions as how the intuition appears, and what you were doing right before the intuition. This log is similar to dream logs (see p. 789) and can be modified to fit both dreams and intuitions.

LEARNING OBJECTIVES

After reading this chapter, the nurse should be able to do the following:

1. State the pathophysiology of acute pericarditis.
2. List the symptoms of acute pericarditis.
3. State the serious complications of acute pericarditis.
4. Recognize the danger signals of pericardial effusion and cardiac tamponade.
5. Perform critical care nursing assessment and management of the patient with acute pericarditis, pericardial effusion, and cardiac tamponade.

CASE STUDY

Mr. H.B., age 38, was hospitalized with complaints of fever, severe shortness of breath, cough, and chest pain. His patient profile and social history described him as a 5 foot 10 inch, 175-lb Mexican-American farm worker from Laredo, Texas. His wife, age 36, was also a farm worker.

Mr. B. was visiting relatives in Dallas when he became ill. He was taken to the city-county hospital, where he was hospitalized. His present and past medical histories were obtained with the help of Mr. B.'s sister; Mr. B. did not speak English.

Mr. B.'s sister said that Mr. B. had complained of recurrent chills and fever. At first, Mr. B. was reluctant to cooperate in giving his history because he had been sick for more than a month without seeking medical help. Despite his illness, he took his vacation as planned because he felt that "getting away from work will make me feel better."

Through his sister, Mr. B. gave the following information. He had had a perforated gastric ulcer 3 years earlier that required an emergency gastrectomy. One year later, his epigastric distress recurred. At that time, an upper gastrointestinal series revealed no new findings.

History of Mr. B.'s Present Illness

Four weeks before his present hospitalization, Mr. B. developed a nonproductive cough and a recurrent fever accompanied by nocturnal chills and drenching sweats. He had pain in the right lateral and substernal chest, as well as aching pain in many muscles and joints. He also described gnawing epigastric pain and right upper quadrant fullness, but, he said, they were unlike the distress he had had with his gastric ulcer. He had had gradually increasing exertional dyspnea and orthopnea during the week before his admission. He had no history of cardiac murmur, jaundice, rheumatic fever, or tuberculosis. He was taking no medications, and he had no known allergies.

Mr. B. was an orphan; he knew nothing of his family history. His wife and children, ages 12, 13, 15, and 16, were well. He and his family were Catholic. He smoked a pack of cigarettes each day, and he drank about six beers a day.

The physical examination showed Mr. B. to be a well-developed, well-nourished, middle-aged man who was anxious, short of breath, and in pain. His temperature when he was admitted was 103°F; his pulse, 120; his respiration, 28; and his blood pressure, 120/70 mm Hg. During quiet respirations, he had a pulsus paradoxus of 10 mm Hg. His neck was supple. His cervical veins were distended to the angle of the mandible at 35° of elevation. He had no palpable lymph nodes in his cervical and axillary regions. Diminished breath sounds and dullness to percussion were heard over the lower third of the right lung posteriorly. The point of maximum cardiac impulse was not palpable, the left border of cardiac dullness was 1 cm beyond the midclavicular line in the fifth intercostal space, and a grade 2/6 systolic murmur was audible at the apex. He had a loud to-and-fro pericardial friction rub, which was heard best at the lower left sternal border. The edge of his liver was felt 8 cm below the right costal margin, and it was moderately tender. His extremities were normal, without clubbing or edema. The initial diagnostic studies revealed that Mr. B.'s hematocrit was 31%, his white cell count was 7400, and his differential count was normal. Blood cultures were done. A thoracentesis yielded 350 ml of serous fluid containing 175 red cells and 1250 white cells/mm³ composed of 75% lymphocytes, 16% monocytes, and 9% neutrophils; the protein content was 4 g/dl. A cytologic examination was negative for tumor cells, and a pathologic examination revealed sheets of histiocytes with inflammatory cells. Examination of Mr. B.'s sputum revealed acid-fast bacilli. His urine was normal. The results of the tests of his renal and hepatic function were all normal.

An electrocardiogram (ECG) showed sinus tachycardia; the QRS voltage was low, and the T waves were inverted in leads 2, 3, and V_1 through V_5. The chest radiograph showed a large cardiopericardial silhouette, with diminished pulsations on fluoroscopic examination. A small right pleural effusion was present. A patchy, streaky infiltrate extended from the right hilum to the apex of the right lung. No hilar lymphadenopathy was present.

Clinical Diagnosis

On admission, Mr. B. had a febrile illness. The clinical diagnosis of tuberculous pericarditis was suggested by the recurrent fever, anemia, chills, drenching sweats, and associated radiographic findings, including apical lung infiltrates and pleural effusion.

The lack of pulsations and the large cardiac silhouette shown by fluoroscopic examination were thought to be due to a pericardial effusion. Mr. B.'s dyspnea, friction rub, elevated venous pressure, and ECG findings were consistent with the diagnosis of tuberculous peri-

carditis. The murmur was considered functional in origin and associated with the anemia. The high cervical venous pressure and the hepatomegaly were due to the pericardial disease, which impaired venous return and thereby produced the elevation of the central venous pressure.

Mr. B. was admitted to the critical care unit, and isolation precautions were instituted. Close observation of him was necessary because of pericardial effusion and possible cardiac tamponade. Appropriate antituberculosis chemotherapy was begun.

Late on the afternoon of his admission, Mr. B., who was resting in bed, felt short of breath. He called for help; when the nurse arrived, she found him in acute distress. She called for the immediate help of another critical care nurse and had an emergency call placed to the physician. Her immediate assessment showed a blood pressure of 70/50 mm Hg, a pulsus paradoxus of 20 mm Hg, faint heart sounds, a respiratory rate of 32, and a radial pulse of 150. Mr. B.'s neck veins were fully distended on inspiration, but decreased on expiration. The nurse placed Mr. B. in a semi-Fowler's position and prepared him for an emergency pericardiocentesis. She administered intravenous morphine sulfate and started an intravenous infusion as ordered.

When the physician arrived, he performed a pericardiocentesis immediately after he examined the patient. The pericardiocentesis yielded 575 ml of straw-colored fluid. Mr. B.'s condition improved immediately. By the end of the day, he was sitting beside his bed.

Mr. B.'s cardiac tamponade, which was due to a slow accumulation of fluid without early symptoms, was manifested by dyspnea and other characteristic signs that were recognized quickly.

Mr. B. was discharged 14 days after his admission. He and his family were given detailed information about his medication and diet.

REFLECTIONS

Mr. B. had been ill with recurrent chills and fever for a month before he was taken to the hospital. To the nurses caring for him, the delay was significant. Mr. B. seemed to them a stoic person who accepted illness as an unavoidable part of life. Mr. B. did not seek medical help for each trivial illness, as his history showed.

It began to seem to the nurses that Mr. B.'s pattern of not seeking medical care was not a matter of his denying that he was sick (as some of the nurses had postulated). Rather, Mr. B. seemed to be living according to a particular conviction about sickness and health. His conviction was an expression of his culture. Because health care was expensive, Mr. B. treated it as a luxury. He felt that people should be seriously ill before they asked for treatment.

At a weekly team conference, the nurses spoke of the significant mind-body aspects of Mr. B.'s illness, but those aspects were not seen as psychological in the usual sense. The nurses asked, "How did Mr. B.'s endurance of his illness for a month contribute to its seriousness and complications? How do one's convictions affect the outcome of one's illnesses? How is illness related to one's cultural milieu?"

The nurses realized that illness and beliefs about illness were intimately related. If Mr. B. had gone to a physician early in the course of his illness, he might not have developed pericardial infection and tamponade.

The effect of the relationship that exists between a patient's mind and his body on his illness became more evident to the staff after the team conference. Mr. B.'s illness became a more interesting event than a simple case of disseminated tuberculosis. His problems were seen as a complex of phenomena transcending the usual definition of disease as a simple "body" process.

Mr. B. presented a challenge to the nursing staff both because of his acute illness as well as his inability to speak English. The language problem was solved by first making a list of the Spanish-speaking nurses in the hospital, what days and shifts they worked, and what times they could visit Mr. B. and his family, and then arranging the visits. When they visited and during the emergency procedure, the Spanish-speaking nurses explained the procedures to Mr. B. and elicited questions from him.

During Mr. B.'s hospitalization, his wife was educated about tuberculosis and was tested to see if she also had tuberculosis. She was found to have an active case of tuberculosis, and she was placed under the care of a physician. The family was given information about the county health department in their hometown, about the need for follow-up medical care, and about nutrition and self-care.

Although the nurses had taken care of patients with acute pericarditis many times, their experience with Mr. B. illustrated the need to be prepared for the complications of the disease. The nurses learned that they must always watch carefully for signs of developing tamponade. During Mr. B.'s cardiac tamponade, they were made aware of the need for adequate preparation to assist with a pericardiocentesis in order to save a patient's life in an emergency.

NORMAL PHYSIOLOGY OF THE PERICARDIUM

The space surrounding the heart is called the *pericardial cavity.* The dynamics in the pleural cavity are essentially the same as those in the pericardial cavity. The pressure within the pleural and the pericardial cavities is negative during inspiration. During expiration and during filling of the heart, the pericardial pressure often rises intermittently to a positive value.[11] This phenomenon forces excess fluid into the lymphatic channels of the mediastinum.

The visceral pericardium is a serous membrane that is separated by a small amount of fluid from a fibrous sac, the parietal pericardium (Fig. 27–1). Normally, the pericardial sac contains less than 50 ml of fluid.

The pericardium has several important functions. It holds the heart in a fixed position and minimizes friction between the heart and the surrounding structures.[11] It prevents sudden dilatation of the cardiac chambers during hypervolemia and exercise. It helps facilitate atrial filling during ventricular systole as the result of development of negative intrapericardial pressure during ejection. The pericardium also probably retards the spread of infections from the pleural cavity and lungs to the heart.[11,18] In some situations, however, the pericardium can be removed, and its absence does not lead to clinical disease.

ETIOLOGY AND PRECIPITATING FACTORS OF ACUTE PERICARDITIS

Acute pericarditis is an inflammation of the pericardium. Pain is the most important symptom of acute pericarditis, and a pericardial friction rub is the most important physical finding.

The classification of pericarditis according to causes is as follows: noninfectious pericarditis, infectious pericarditis, pericarditis related to hypersensitivity or autoimmunity, and drugs (Table 27–1).[3]

The causes of noninfectious pericarditis include myocardial infarction, uremia, neoplasia of benign or malignant origin,

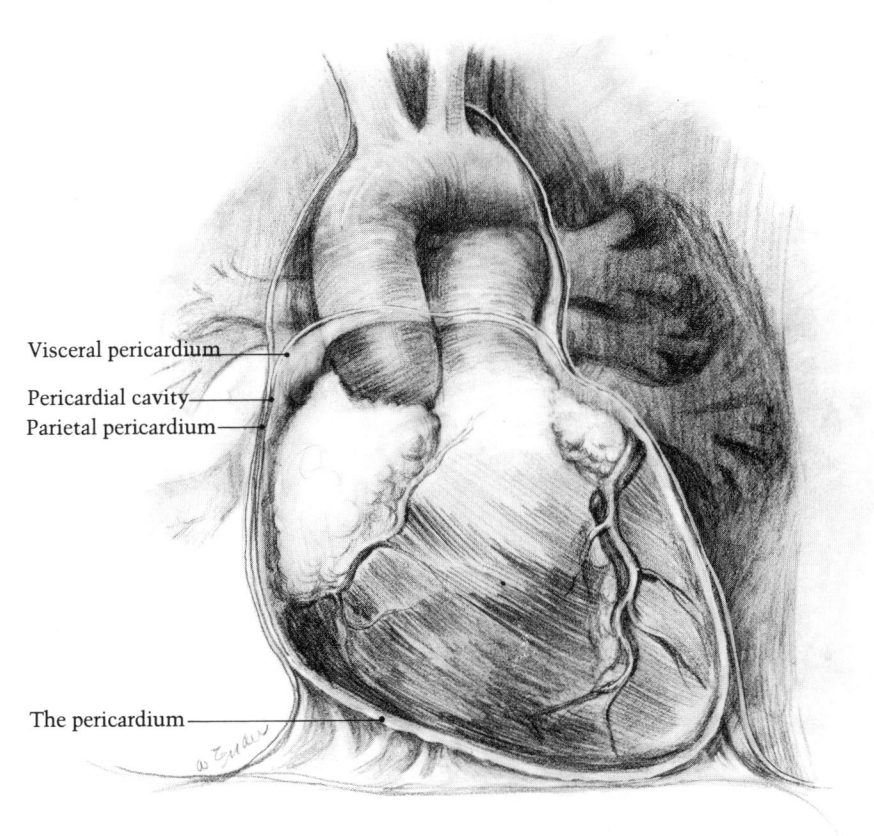

Visceral pericardium
Pericardial cavity
Parietal pericardium

The pericardium

Figure 27–1

A heart with a normal pericardium.

trauma, myxedema, irradiation, acute idiopathic causes, aortic aneurysm with leakage into the pericardial sac, and severe chronic anemia. The causes of infectious pericarditis are bacterial, viral, tuberculous, rickettsia, fungal, and mycotic infections.[5,11] Pericarditis related to hypersensitivity or autoimmunity can be caused by postcardiac injury, such as postpericardiotomy, Dressler's syndrome, rheumatic fever, and collagen vascular diseases, such as systemic lupus erythematosus. Drugs that can cause pericarditis are anticoagulants such as heparin and warfarin, cromdyn sodium, dantrolene, hydralazine, methysergide, and procainamide.

PSYCHOPATHOPHYSIOLOGY OF ACUTE PERICARDITIS

The pathophysiologic changes that occur in acute pericarditis include inflammation of the pericardium, the membranous sac that envelops the heart. A variety of inflammatory processes may involve the pericardium as secondary complications of acute pericarditis. Infection from bacteria, viruses, or other organisms usually occurs by way of the blood stream; however, an infection from a nearby organ may also extend to the pericardium. Noninfectious pericardial inflammation may occur secondary to acute myocardial infarction, uremia, and collagen-vascular (autoimmune) disorders.

The nurse should focus on the patient's perceptions of this illness. It is important for the patient's family or significant others to also be included in explanations of pericarditis and its course. Family perceptions of the patient's illness are also important information for the nurse to recognize. Anxious families can only compound an already stressful situation.

NURSING PROCESS

ASSESSMENT

Astute nursing assessment can detect the diagnosis of acute pericarditis. Pericarditis can mimic other diseases. Understanding the disease process as well as knowing the signs and symptoms can lead to early diagnosis and intervention. If left untreated, the illness could be fatal.

Pain

In the initial assessment and observations, the nurse should focus on the symptoms of the patient's illness. Patients are almost always anxious with pain. Pain, the dominant symptom in most forms of acute pericarditis, is often aggravated by coughing, swallowing, inspiration, and rotation of the trunk. Most of the pain of acute pericarditis is caused by inflammation of the adjoining diaphragmatic pleura (Fig. 27–2). It has been shown that only the lower portion of the external surface of the parietal pericardium is pain-sensitive.[3,14] The pain may be felt either in the precordium or in one or both shoulders. It is characteristically aggravated by recumbency, and it is eased by sitting upright and leaning forward. Patients frequently complain of dyspnea, which results from compression of the bronchi or the parenchyma of the lung by the distended pericardium. Patients may also have pleuritic pain if the surrounding pleura becomes secondarily inflamed. The dyspnea and pleuritic pain can frighten patients, and they need constant reassurance that the discomfort is temporary.

Pericardial Friction Rub

Probably the most important physical sign of acute pericarditis is the pericardial friction rub. The pericardial friction rub is heard most frequently during forced expiration while the patient leans forward or rests on the hands and knees (Mohammed's sign).[7] The friction rub is often evanescent and may vary in intensity from hour to hour and day to day.[11,18,21] It is best heard with the diaphragm of the stethoscope held firmly over the left third and fourth interspaces close to the sternum. If it cannot be heard in one position, the patient's position should be changed and the examination repeated. It may have up to three components, occurring with atrial systole, ventricular systole, or ventricular diastole. When all three sounds are present, the rub is triphasic.[18] It has been described as a to-and-fro leathery sound. One study of 50 consecutive, prospectively studied patients with pericardial friction rubs showed that 24% of the rubs were of the to-and-fro type and of several biphasic patterns, 18% were monophasic, and 58% were triphasic.[21] The pericardial sound is thought to be due to the roughening of the two serous membranes by fibrin deposits. With the accumulation of fluid in the pericardial sac, the friction rub may disappear. The nurse must be aware that pericardial fluid can accumulate slowly in amounts up to 100 ml to 150 ml without producing noticeable symptoms. If pericarditis is due to a bacterial infection, the fluid is likely to be purulent. If the effusion is due to a viral infection, the fluid is usually serous.

Pericardial Effusion

The rapid accumulation of fluid over a short period of time is especially ominous and may result in cardiac tamponade. With the rapid accumulation of fluid, the heart sounds become faint,

Table 27–1
Etiology of Pericarditis

NONINFECTIOUS	INFECTIOUS	HYPERSENSITIVITY	DRUGS
Anemia	Bacterial	Collagen vascular disease, such as lupus	Anticoagulants (heparin and warfarin)
Aortic dissection	Fungal		
Idiopathic	Mycotic	Dressler's syndrome	Cromdyn sodium
Irradiation	Parasitic	After cardiac surgery	Dantrolene
Myocardial infarction	Rickettsial	Rheumatic fever	Hydralazine
Myxedema	Tuberculous	Scleroderma	Methysergide
Neoplasia	Viral		Procainamide
Uremia and dialysis-related			
Trauma			

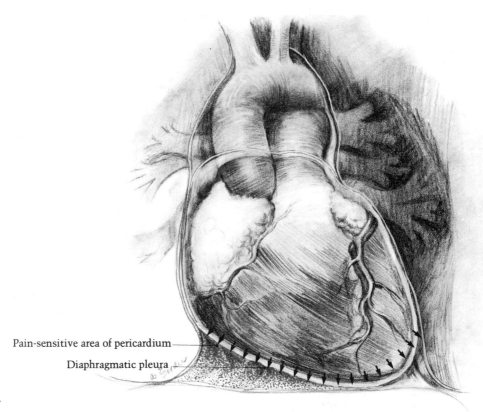

Pain-sensitive area of pericardium

Diaphragmatic pleura

Figure 27-2
Pain-sensitive area of the pericardium.

the friction rub may or may not disappear, and the apical impulse may vanish. If the effusion is large, one may find Ewart's sign. The compression of the lung by a large effusion may cause tubular breath sounds and area of dullness at the left scapular angle.

Clinical signs suggesting pericardial effusion are tachypnea and diminished heart sounds due to distention of the pericardial sac; hypotension and tachycardia resulting from reduced cardiac output; Kussmaul's sign, indicating impaired right-sided cardiac filling (Kussmaul's sign is increased neck vein distention on inspiration; normally, neck vein distention disappears on inspiration); and pulsus paradoxus resulting from an accumulation of pericardial fluid and increasing venous pressure.

Pulsus Paradoxus

Pulsus paradoxus is an exaggeration of the normal variation in systolic blood pressure that is usually associated with inspiration. The normal variation of systolic blood pressure during inspiration is 3 mm Hg to 10 mm Hg in the healthy person. It is thought that the normal variation in blood pressure that accompanies respiration results from the pooling of blood during inspiration in the pulmonary vasculature because of lung expansion and increased negative intrathoracic pressure.[7] Pulmonary vascular pooling normally occurs during inspiration, with a resultant decrease in blood return to the left side of the heart, causing decreased left ventricular output. The fall in systolic blood pressure is exaggerated when venous return to the heart is impaired for any reason.[7,8,16,18] There are other hypotheses to explain the exaggerated blood pressure response to inspiration that occurs in pericardial tamponade.

The presence of pulsus paradoxus, however, does not always mean the presence of pericardial disease. Pulsus paradoxus

may also be present in chronic obstructive pulmonary disease, heart failure, or any physiologic condition that augments a variation in the left-sided heart filling pressure.[2,12,13,19]

Pulsus paradoxus may be measured by using cuff sphygmomanometry or an arterial line wave.

Cuff Sphygmomanometry

When using a cuff sphygmomanometer to measure pulsus paradoxus, explain to the patient that a special type of blood pressure reading will be taken, and that it may take longer than usual. A quiet environment is important to hear the changes in the Korotkoff sounds, and proper functioning of the cuff sphygmomanometer is essential. Ensure that when the manometer is at maximal pressure, the mercury does not drift down.[23]

Assess the patient's ability to tolerate lying supine. This position will augment the pulsus paradoxus. If the patient has severe paradoxus, however, he may not tolerate this position and may require a semi-Fowlers or upright position to breathe. Auscultate the patient's normal systolic blood pressure on expiration and then inflate the pressure cuff to about 4 mm Hg to 8 mm Hg above the patient's systolic blood pressure on expiration. Deflate the pressure cuff slowly, at a rate of approximately 1 mm Hg to 2 mm Hg/respiratory cycle.[23]

Listen for the first Korotkoff sound, which will occur on expiration. Note the pressure at which the first sound is heard. The Korotkoff sound disappears with each inspiration and reappears on expiration. As the blood pressure cuff is slowly deflated, the Korotkoff sounds will ultimately be heard during both inspiration and expiration. Note the pressure when the Korotkoff sounds are heard during both inspiration and expiration. Subtract the pressure at which the Korotkoff sound is heard during both inspiration and expiration from the max-

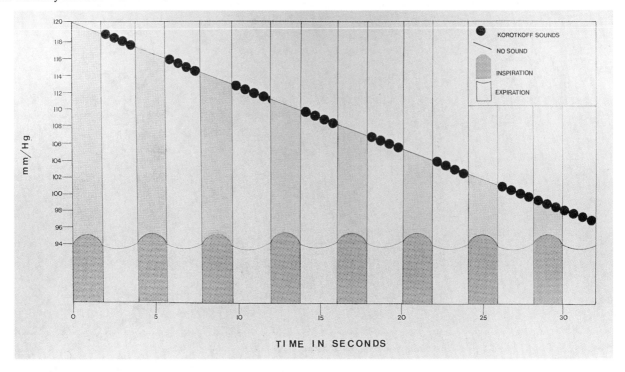

Figure 27–3

Visual representation of the Korotkoff sounds of pulsus paradoxus measured by cuff sphygmomanometry. Systolic blood pressure during the first Korotkoff sound is heard at 119 mm Hg. On inspiration, the Korotkoff sound disappears. It reappears again during expiration. The difference in pressure between when the first Korotkoff sound is heard and where it was heard during both inspiration and expiration is pulsus paradoxus. Subtracting 102 mm Hg from 119 mm Hg gives a pulsus paradoxus value of 17 mm Hg. (Sulzbach, L. M. Measurement of pulsus paradoxus. *Focus Crit. Care* 16:142, 1989; with permission.)

imal pressure (heard during expiration). The difference in pressure is the pulsus paradoxus.[23] Figure 27–3 shows the pulsus paradoxus using cuff sphygmomanometry.

A Doppler stethoscope may be used to amplify the Korotkoff sound. When using the Doppler stethoscope, the Korotkoff sound will slowly increase on inspiration, but the measurement of the paradoxic pulse of pulsus paradoxus is made when the sounds (during inspiration and expiration) are equal in intensity.

Arterial Line Wave

Normal respiratory variation is displayed with an arterial line wave recording, making it possible to measure pulsus paradoxus visually.

Place the arterial line on full scale. Zero and calibrate the transducer to atmospheric pressure. Record the arterial line trace and note the patient's respirations. Subtract the maximal systolic pressure during inspiration from the systolic pressure during expiration. The difference in the pressure is the pulsus paradoxus.[23] Figure 27–4 displays an arterial line wave with a pulsus paradoxus of 36 mm Hg.

Cardiac Tamponade

The major clinical manifestations of cardiac tamponade are a fall in cardiac output and systemic venous congestion. Both

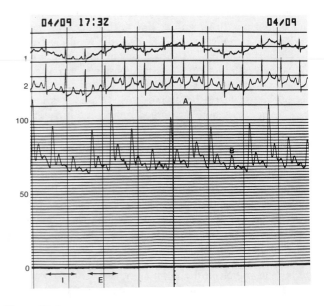

Figure 27–4

Standard electrocardiographic leads 1 and 2 with an arterial line wave simultaneously below. The arterial wave is scaled 0 mm Hg to 100 mm Hg. Peak systolic pressure during expiration (E) is 112 mm Hg (A). Systolic pressure during inspiration (I) is 76 mm Hg (B). Subtracting 76 mm Hg at B from 112 mm Hg at A gives a pulsus paradoxus value of 36 mm Hg. (Sulzbach, L. M. Measurement of pulsus paradoxus. *Focus Crit. Care* 16:142, 1989; with permission.)

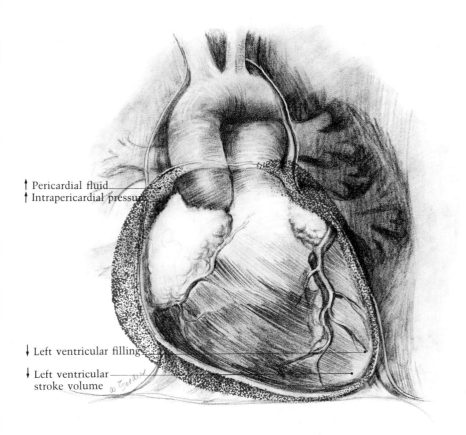

Figure 27-5

Pericardial effusion and cardiac tamponade. The following hemodynamic effects may result after pericardial effusion: accumulation of pericardial fluid resulting in intrapericardial pressure, elevation of right atrial pressure, elevation of left ventricular end diastolic pressure, reduction in left ventricular end-diastolic volume and cardiac output, and elevated venous pressure.

↑ Pericardial fluid
↑ Intrapericardial pressure

↓ Left ventricular filling

↓ Left ventricular stroke volume

phenomena are caused by obstruction of the inflow of blood to the heart (Fig. 27–5).[5] When tamponade develops slowly, the patient's condition resembles that seen in right-sided congestive heart failure. The patient has tachycardia, dyspnea, orthopnea, edema, hepatic engorgement, and a positive hepatojugular reflex. When severe tamponade develops, such as in cardiac trauma, faint heart sounds, electrical alternans, and arterial hypotension occur. When a patient has acute cardiac trauma after direct cardiac trauma from gunshot or stab wounds, his condition is critical (see Chap. 22).

Diagnostic Tests

Electrocardiogram

The ECG is observed closely to distinguish the changes of acute pericarditis from those of acute myocardial infarction (Fig. 27–6) (Table 27–2). Electrocardiographic changes of acute pericarditis evolve through four stages. These changes can occur a few hours or days after the onset of pericardial pain. Stage 1 electrocardiographic changes are present at the time of onset of chest pain, and are virtually diagnostic of acute pericarditis. Stage 1 consists of ST-segment elevation that, unlike the ST-segment elevation in acute myocardial infarction, is concave upward and is usually present in all leads except a V_r and V_1 (Fig. 27–7). The T waves are usually upright in the leads with ST-segment elevation.[22,24] In some cases PR segment is depressed.[20,21]

Stage 2 occurs several days later. The ST segments return to baseline, along with T-wave flattening. The PR segment may become depressed. The T-wave inversion occurs after the ST segment returns to the baseline, whereas T waves in

myocardial infarction often become inverted before ST segment returns to baseline.[11,18,22]

Stage 3 is characterized by T-wave inversion. T-wave inversion is generally present in most leads and is not associated with the loss of R-wave voltage or the appearance of Q wave, either of which may appear in myocardial infarction.[11,22]

Stage 4 consists of normalization of the ECG, which may occur weeks or months later. However, T-wave inversion may persist for several months or be permanent.[11,18,22]

The QRS complex with pericardial effusion may reveal a low QRS voltage (Fig. 27–8). Electrical alternans (Fig. 27–9), the alternation of the QRS complex amplitude from beat to beat, is usually found only when a large pericardial effusion is present. It is thought to be produced from an exaggerated swinging of the heart in a pericardial sac filled with fluid.[9,22]

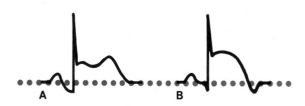

Figure 27-6

(*A*) Represents the electrocardiographic changes of acute pericarditis. The PR interval is depressed, and the ST segment is elevated with a concave curvature. (*B*) Represents the electrocardiographic changes of acute myocardial infarction. Q wave is present, and ST segment elevation is a convex curvature with T-wave inversion.

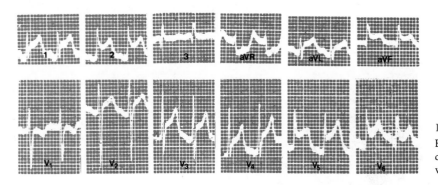

Figure 27-7

Electrocardiogram of a patient with acute pericarditis. The ST segment shows a characteristic elevation in leads 1, 2, V_1, V_3, and V_6.

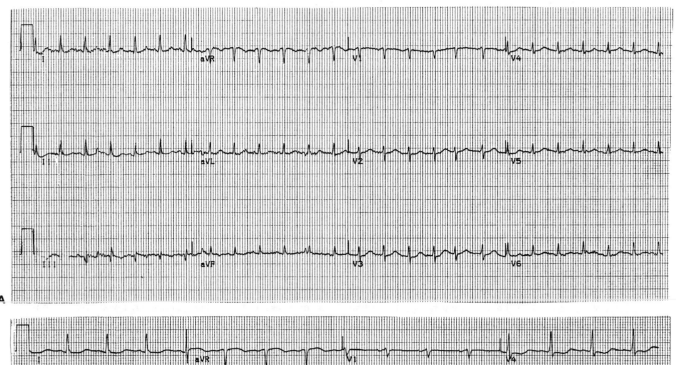

A

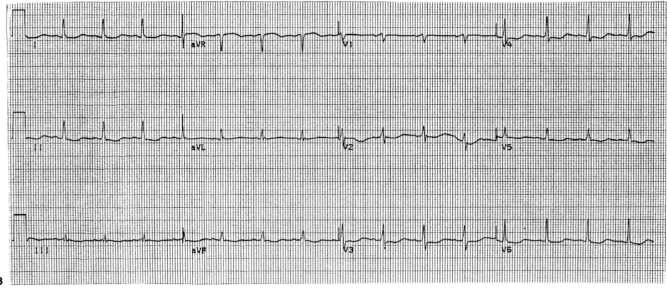

B

Figure 27-8

(A) Patient with pericardial effusion presents with low QRS voltage. (B) Same patient following pericardiocentesis. The QRS voltage is increased.

Table 27–2
Electrocardiographic Changes With a Myocardial Infarction and Acute Pericarditis

ELECTROCARDIOGRAM	MYOCARDIAL INFARCTION	ACUTE PERICARDITIS
PR interval	Normal	Depression
Q wave	Present	Absence
QRS	Various changes	Pulsus alternans
ST segment	Depression or elevation	Elevation with an upwardly concave appearance in limb leads and anterior precordial leads
T wave	Negative with elevated ST segment	Flat and inverted
Voltage	Normal	Low

Sinus tachycardia is the most common dysrhythmia to occur in the setting of pericarditis. Paroxysmal supraventricular tachycardia, atrial flutter, and atrial fibrillation may also occur.[22]

Chest Radiograph

The chest radiograph is usually normal in limited acute pericarditis. However, when a significant pericardial effusion is present, with at least 250 ml of fluid, the cardiac silhouette is usually enlarged and may have a globular shape.[1,4,11] The chest radiograph may be helpful in establishing the specific etiology of pericarditis, such as pulmonary parenchymal lesion or enlarged hilar lymph nodes. It is also helpful in supporting the diagnosis of pericardial effusion when there is a rapid increase in the size of the cardiac silhouette and the presence of clear lung fields (Fig. 27–10A and B).

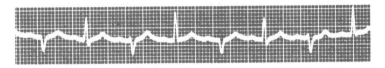

Figure 27–9
Partial electrocardiogram of a patient with pericardial effusion and tamponade. The V$_3$ lead shows "total electrical alternans," with an every-other-beat variation in the amplitude of P, QRS, and T waves.

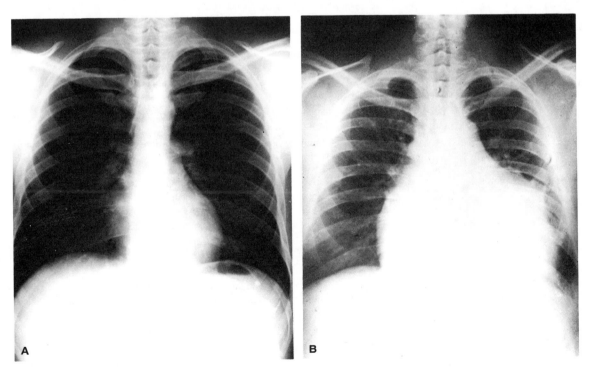

Figure 27–10
(A) Normal chest radiograph. (B) Chest radiograph of a patient with a large pericardial effusion that resulted in pericardial tamponade.

Echocardiography

Echocardiography is a noninvasive method of outlining the borders of the cardiac chambers by directing sound waves across the heart and recording the reflections of the waves (echoes) off solid structures in their path.[3,5,17] Pericardial fluid appears as a relatively echo-free space between the posterior left ventricular wall or anterior right ventricular wall and the parietal pericardium.[1,11,22]

The echocardiogram is the simplest and most effective test for demonstrating pericardial effusion, location, and quantity.[10,25] Two-dimensional echocardiography permits assessment of the extent of the effusion and the quantity of fluid.[1] It has replaced carbon dioxide injection as a diagnostic technique.

Cardiac Catheterization and Angiography

Catheterization of the right side of the heart may support the diagnosis of pericardial effusion. As the catheter traverses the right atrium, its tip is pushed against the inner wall of the atrium; an abnormal widening of the distance between the catheter tip and the radiolucent lung (normally represented by the very thin atrial wall) suggests pericardial effusion. Contrast material injected into the atrium can give a better idea of the increase in thickness of the pericardial shadow. In the presence of pericardial constriction by effusion, pressure recordings from the right ventricle show an abnormally rapid fall in pressure during diastole due to the impairment of filling.[5,11] Hemodynamic measurements show an equalization of pressure in the right atrial, left atrial, and ventricular diastolic pressures.

Laboratory Studies

Blood studies often show minor elevations in the leukocyte count and an increased erythrocyte sedimentation rate in infectious pericarditis. The results will depend on the etiologic agent causing the acute pericarditis. Cardiac enzyme levels may be normal or increased. The increase in creatine kinase-MB is usually small[1] and results from myocardial inflammation from surrounding infection.

NURSING DIAGNOSES, PATIENT OUTCOMES, AND PLAN

The preceding material on anatomy, physiology, nursing assessment, and diagnostic tests guides the nurse in establishing nursing diagnoses, patient outcomes, and plan for the patient with acute pericarditis.

NURSING CARE PLAN SUMMARY Patient with Acute Pericarditis

NURSING DIAGNOSIS

1. *Acute pain/discomfort related to pericardial inflammation (feeling pattern)*

Patient Outcomes	Nursing Orders

1. The patient will be pain-free.	1. Administer analgesics as ordered to relieve the pain. Document response to all medications, frequency of pain occurrence, pain description, pain relief:
	  A. Give salicylates and nonsteroidal anti-inflammatory agents as ordered to reduce fever and inflammation.
	  B. For rapid pain relief, give steroids as ordered to control the symptoms of pericarditis and to reduce the inflammatory process.

2. The patient will demonstrate resolution of pericardial friction rub.	2. Administer analgesic salicylates, nonsteroid anti-inflammatory agents, and steroids to relieve acute pericarditis when the cause is an infectious or immunologic one (*e.g.,* tuberculosis, rheumatic fever, or a fungus).
	  A. Assure the patient that the pain of pericarditis is temporary and will decrease when therapy, or other specific therapy is given.
	  B. Observe the patient for signs and symptoms of pain, and determine what activity or position precipitates or alleviates pain. The pain may be
	    (1) Increased by breathing
	    (2) Increased by coughing, swallowing, rotation of the trunk, and changes in the flexion, extension, or rotation of the spine (including the neck)
	    (3) Increased by lying on the back
	    (4) Decreased by sitting up or leaning forward.
	    (5) Take vital signs every 2 hours or as necessary.
	  C. Listen with the stethoscope for increasing or decreasing intensity of the

(continued)

NURSING CARE PLAN SUMMARY *Patient with Acute Pericarditis*   *Continued*

Patient Outcomes	Nursing Orders
	friction rub. The friction rub is often evanescent, with a leathery sound, and may have up to three components. Assess friction rub for the following: (1) Location (2) Quality (3) Continuous or intermittent (4) Number of cardiac components (5) Be aware of persistent clinical symptoms: 　a. Pain in the precordial area (mild to sharp or severe) 　b. Dyspnea 　c. Fevers, chills, and sweating (more significant if salicylates have not been given to reduce the patient's fever)
3. The characteristic ECG changes with pericarditis will resolve.	3. Observe ECG for persistent ST-segment and T-wave changes and dysrhythmias. Distinguish changes of acute pericarditis from those of acute myocardial infarction. A. Assess for presence of dysrhythmias. B. Assess for changes in QRS voltage or appearance of electrical alternans. C. Place rhythm strips of changes on patient's chart. D. Notify physician of any changes. E. Be alert to impending complications of pericardial effusion or cardiac tamponade.

NURSING DIAGNOSIS

2. *Anxiety (mild, moderate, or severe) related to lack of knowledge of disease process or to chest-wall pain (feeling pattern)*

Patient Outcome	Nursing Orders
1. The patient will show a decrease in anxiety.	1. Explain the usual course of pericarditis. 2. Explain all procedures to patient to decrease anxiety. 3. Teach the patient the use of relaxation imagery and music exercises to decrease pain and anxiety.

NURSING DIAGNOSIS

3. *Decreased cardiac output related to fluid in pericardial sac from pericardial effusion or high risk for cardiac tamponade related to pericardial effusion (exchanging pattern)*

Patient Outcomes	Nursing Orders
1. The patient will show resolution or absence of effusion or tamponade.	1. Be alert to the possibility of cardiac tamponade and do the following: A. If cardiac tamponade is suspected, check for Kussmaul's sign (distention of the neck veins on inspiration; normally, the veins collapse on inspiration). B. Check for pulsus paradoxus. (If it is greater than 10 mm Hg, pericardial tamponade should be suspected; 10 mm Hg or less is normal.) C. If pericardial effusion develops rapidly, watch for signs of a decreased cardiac output. D. Watch for changes in the ECG (electrical alternans, tachycardia, or a decrease in QRS complex voltage). E. Watch for a decrease in heart sounds, hypotension, and orthopnea. F. Have emergency equipment at hand.

(continued)

NURSING CARE PLAN SUMMARY   Patient with Acute Pericarditis   Continued

Patient Outcomes	Nursing Orders
2. If pericardial effusion is present, the patient will be prepared for special tests to determine the presence and amount of pericardial fluid.	2. Give oral corticosteroids as ordered for rapid resolution of pericardial effusion.
3. If cardiac tamponade is present, the patient will receive emergency treatment.	3. Be prepared for rapid infusion of saline solution or blood intravenously in order to make the venous pressure greater than the pericardial pressure in cases of cardiac tamponade (medical treatment).

NURSING DIAGNOSIS

4. *High risk for noncompliance related to inadequate knowledge about illness and future care (choosing pattern)*

Patient Outcome	Nursing Orders

The patient will verbalize knowledge of pericarditis and methods of prophylactic care.	1. Teach the patient the following knowledge base:
	  A. Heart function
	  B. Definition of pericarditis
	  C. Signs and symptoms of pericarditis
	  D. Pathophysiologic changes
	  E. Medications—action, dosage, time, side effects
	  F. Reasons to avoid exposure to upper respiratory infection and when to report signs and symptoms of cold, cough, or sore throat
	2. Teach about activity patterns during recovery and after discharge.
	3. Explain when to contact physician for help.
	4. Assess for motivation for a healthier state.
	5. Teach when to return for follow-up appointments and laboratory tests.
	6. Explain where to obtain Medic-Alert bracelet and importance of wearing bracelet if discharged on steroids.

IMPLEMENTATION AND EVALUATION
Clinical Course

Patients who present with acute pericarditis are almost always hospitalized for at least a few days to distinguish it from other problems that can cause acute chest pain. These conditions are acute myocardial infarction, acute pulmonary embolism, pleurisy without associated pericarditis, dissecting aortic aneurysm, mediastinal emphysema, spontaneous pneumothorax, or mediastinitis from esophageal rupture.[15]

The usual clinical course of acute pericarditis is self-limiting, short-term, and can last from 2 to 6 weeks. This refers to patients who have pericarditis related to acute myocardial infarction, Dressler's syndrome, or postpericardiotomy syndrome, pericarditis that is idiopathic, viral, traumatic, or drug-induced. Pericarditis related to idiopathic, viral, and connective-tissue etiologies may recur once or more over a 6-month to 12-month period. If left untreated, there is a higher morbidity and mortality in patients who have pericarditis related to tuberculous, fungal, or bacterial infections; neoplasms; uremia; or chest-wall trauma. Neoplastic pericarditis has a poor prognosis, even with appropriate treatment.[6] Bacterial pericarditis is an acute emergency with a 100% mortality if not treated early.

The nurse should continue to stay abreast of all tests and treatments of the underlying disease in the course of the illness in order to facilitate management and identify areas of knowledge the patient will need in order to understand the acute illness and future care. As nurses implement all nursing orders under Nursing Diagnoses 1 through 4, they should ascertain continually that the patient outcomes are being accomplished. Documentation should reflect whether the specific outcomes are being met. They should be stated in measurable terms. Teaching and learning evaluation are essential for the recovery of patients with pericarditis.

SUMMARY

Acute pericarditis is painful, and the pain often is aggravated by coughing, swallowing, breathing, and lying supine. Dyspnea also occurs frequently. The diagnosis of acute pericarditis is confirmed by the patient's clinical history and physical examination; a pericardial friction rub is a significant finding. Specific diagnostic procedures that help confirm the diagnosis are the ECG, the echocardiogram, cardiac catheterization and angiography, and laboratory studies.

Patients whose conditions have been diagnosed as acute pericarditis must be observed closely so that any complications of the illness can be detected as soon as they occur. If the complications of the illness are not detected, pericardial effusion and cardiac tamponade can cause death in a short time.

DIRECTIONS FOR FUTURE RESEARCH

Patients as well as family members are anxious about the many episodes of pain that occur in the setting of acute pericarditis. It is mandatory that nurses research specific modalities in order to help increase the knowledge base about effective nursing interventions to decrease the anxiety and fear these acutely ill patients experience.

Research questions that nurses may consider for improving care of patients with acute pericarditis follow:

1. What nursing interventions are most effective in relieving the anxiety of patients with acute pericarditis?
2. How can nurses use the families and significant others of patients with acute pericarditis to reduce the patient's stress?

REFERENCES

1. Brandenburg, R. O., and McGoon, D. C. The Pericardium. In R. O. Brandenburg (ed.), *Cardiology Fundamentals and Practice.* Chicago: Year Book Medical Publishers, 1987.
2. Callahan, M. Acute traumatic cardiac tamponade: Diagnosis and treatment. *J.A.C.E.P.* 7:306, 1978.
3. Chiaramida, S. A., Goldman, M. A., and Zema, M. J. Echocardiographic identification of intrapericardial fibrous strands in acute pericarditis with pericardial effusion. *Chest* 77:85, 1980.
4. Goldberger, E. Acute Cardiac Tamponade. In E. Goldberger (ed.), *Treatment of Cardiac Emergencies.* St. Louis: C. V. Mosby, 1982.
5. Goldberger, E. Acute Pericarditis. In E. Goldberger (ed.), *Textbook of Clinical Cardiology.* St. Louis: C. V. Mosby, 1982.
6. Hancock, E. W. ECG casebook: The case of the young woman with acute chest pain. *Hosp. Pract.* 17:33, 1982.
7. Henkind S., Benis A., and Teicholz L. The paradox of pulsus paradoxus. *Am. Heart J.* 114:198, 1987.
8. Himes V. Traumatic cardiac tamponade. *J.E.N.* 6(14a):28, 1980.
9. Holloway, J. D., Garcia, W., and Espinoza, L. R. Cardiac tamponade in a healthy young woman. *Hosp. Pract.* 22:128, 1987.
10. Horowitz, M. S., Schultz, C. S., Stinson, E. B., et al. Sensitivity and specificity of echocardiographic diagnosis of pericardial effusion. *Circulation* 50:239, 1974.
11. Lorell, B., and Braunwald, E. Pericardial Disease. In E. Braunwald (ed.), *Heart Disease: A Textbook of Cardiovascular Medicine.* Philadelphia: W. B. Saunders, 1988.
12. Markovchick, V., Evans, T., and Haftel, A. Traumatic acute pericardial tamponade. *J.A.C.E.P.* 6:562, 1977.
13. McGregor M. Pulsus paradoxus. *N. Engl. J. Med.* 301:480, 1979.
14. Murtash, J. Acute chest pain: A diagnostic approach. *Aust. Fam. Physician* 10:247, 1981.
15. Olson, H. G., Lyons, K. P., and Aronow, W. S. Technetium-99m stannous pyrophosphate myocardial scintigrams in pericardial disease. *Am. Heart J.* 99:459, 1980.
16. Pursley P. Acute cardiac tamponade. *Am. J. Nurs.* 83:1414, 1983.
17. Sawaya, J. I., Mujais, S. K., and Armenian, H. K. Early diagnosis of pericarditis in acute myocardial infarction. *Am. Heart J.* 100:144, 1980.
18. Shabetai, R. Diseases of the Pericardium. In J. W. Hurst and R. B. Logue (eds.), *The Heart Arteries and Vein* (6th ed.). New York: McGraw-Hill, 1986.
19. Shoemaker, W. Early diagnosis and management of pericardial tamponade. *Hosp. Med.* 17:7, 1978.
20. Spodick, D. H. Diagnostic electrocardiographic sequences in acute pericarditis: Significance of PR segment and PR vector changes. *Circulation* 48:575, 1973.
21. Spodick, D. H. Pericardial rub: Prospective multiple observer investigation of pericardial friction rub in 100 patients. *Am. J. Cardiol.* 35:357, 1975.
22. Sternbach, G. L. Pericarditis. *Ann. Emerg. Med.* 17:214, 1988.
23. Sulzbach, L. M. Measurement of pulsus paradoxus. *Focus Crit. Care* 16:142, 1989.
24. Surawicz, B., and Lasseter, K. C. Electrocardiogram in pericarditis. *Am. J. Cardiol.* 26:671, 1970.
25. Vignolo, P. A., Pohost, G. M., Curfrued, G. D., et al. Correlation of echocardiographic and clinical findings in patients with pericardial effusion. *Arch. Intern. Med.* 136:979, 1976.

28

Infective Endocarditis

Cathie E. Guzzetta

NONINTELLECTUAL APPROACHES TO BODY-MIND-SPIRIT

To believe in many of the "new therapies" (*e.g.*, biofeedback, relaxation techniques, meditation) is to be affected by them. The critical care nurse cannot merely say, "I believe," and leave the issue at that. To truly believe is to understand, and to understand is to experience personal change.

The emphasis is on *experience*, not *belief*.

Body-mind-spirit concepts are not "head trips." They are, first and last, *experiential*, not *intellectual*. They begin and end with feeling, not belief.

The personal experience of the nonintellectual approaches to body-mind-spirit considerations is possible. A word of caution is necessary, however. When one participates in the exercises with definite goals and results in mind, one may destroy the effectiveness and meaning of the experiences. As Watts* said, just as one cannot smell smelling, one cannot experience experiencing. It is the smell and the experience that are real, not the representational ideas of them. Similarly, when we try too hard to understand "what it's like" to experience a transcendent state, we may find that the experience eludes us. Abstractions are barriers to direct experience.

LEARNING OBJECTIVES

After reading this chapter, the nurse should be able to do the following:

1. Write a paragraph discussing the causes of subacute and acute endocarditis.
2. Compare and contrast the differences in the pathophysiologic mechanisms of subacute and acute endocarditis.
3. List the major clinical manifestations and complications of subacute and acute endocarditis.
4. Discuss the common laboratory and diagnostic findings for a patient with infective endocarditis.
5. Outline the nursing diagnoses, patient outcomes, nursing orders, and evaluation for a patient with infective endocarditis.

CASE STUDY
Hospital Admission

Mr. S.P., a 50-year-old man, was admitted to the coronary care unit with the chief complaint of new-onset, retrosternal chest pain. The

* Watts, A., *The Way of Zen*. New York: Vintage Books, 1957.

pain began the evening before his admission, it lasted for 15 to 20 minutes, and it was associated with nausea and shortness of breath. The patient complained of chills, fatigue, headache, and a poor appetite. He said that those symptoms began 2 weeks ago, and he called them "flu-like" symptoms.

Mr. P. had had rheumatic fever as a child, and he subsequently developed a murmur of mitral regurgitation. One month before admission, he had had an abscessed tooth extracted. He had not had antimicrobial prophylaxis before or after the extraction.

Mr. P. was a well-developed, 5 feet 10 inch, 165-lb man who was highly anxious during the admission interview. He talked constantly during his admission assessment, jumping from one topic to another without any purposeful intent. His temporal and jaw muscles were tensed.

Mr. P. denied any history of hypertension, smoking, high cholesterol, diabetes mellitus, family history of premature heart or vascular disease, or peripheral vascular disease such as claudication.

On examination, the patient's temperature was 100.4°F orally, his apical pulse was 110 beats/minute, his respirations were 16/minute, and the blood pressure was 126/80 mm Hg. The patient was pale, and his skin was warm and dry with normal tissue turgor. The patient's motor and sensory functions and reflexes were normal. Bilateral conjunctival petechiae were noted, and a 3-mm pale spot with a surrounding hemorrhagic zone (Roth spot) was seen in the right fundus at 2:00. The patient had poor oral hygiene. Bilateral rhonchi that cleared with coughing were heard. A left ventricular heave was palpated at the fifth left intercostal space, midclavicular line (MCL). The apical pulse was regular with a normal first and second heart sound. A third heart sound was heard at the apex. No fourth heart sound or rubs were heard. A grade 3/6 holosystolic heart murmur was heard at the lower left sternal border with radiation to the left axilla. The patient had normal bilateral arterial pulses. Splinter hemorrhages were noted on the distal third of the nails of the index and middle fingers of the right hand. No edema, clubbing, pain, swelling, or inflammation of the joints was noted. The initial electrocardiogram (ECG) suggested that Mr. P. had mild left ventricular hypertrophy and anteroseptal ischemia. The posteroanterior and lateral chest radiographs suggested slight cardiomegaly. Laboratory studies were done, including aerobic and anaerobic blood cultures.

Second Day

By the end of Mr. P.'s second day, his temperature had risen to 101°F. His stress level continued to be high. The critical care nurses noted that Mr. P. had a new splinter hemorrhage on the ring finger of his left hand and two new conjunctival petechiae in his left eye. There was no change in the intensity or quality of his heart murmur. There were no clinical manifestations of chest pain, dyspnea or palpitations.

Based on Mr. P.'s clinical history and assessment, the presumptive diagnosis of infective endocarditis was made by his primary physician. Mr. P. was given intravenous penicillin and intramuscular streptomycin.

The primary care nurse was concerned about Mr. P.'s stress level, and she had a conference with his attending physician, wife, and daughters.

Third Day

The next day, Mr. P.'s blood cultures were found to be positive for *Streptococcus viridans,* and the diagnosis of *Streptococcus viridans* endocarditis was made and entered in the nursing care plan.

The significant laboratory findings were anemia (manifested by a low red blood cell count, a low hemoglobin and hematocrit), an elevated erythrocyte sedimentation rate, a positive rheumatoid factor, and urine 2+ for protein with broad, coarsely granular casts and white and red blood cells. The cardiac enzyme levels were normal.

Discharge

Before Mr. P.'s discharge, the primary care nurse held sessions with the patient and his wife and daughters to discuss home intravenous therapy, prophylactic care, and the prevention of complications (see pp. 527 and 531).

REFLECTIONS

Patients who are admitted to critical care units often demonstrate high levels of psychophysiologic stress. Such patients have both primary physical and psychologic needs. Teaching during this initial crisis period has an important psychophysiologic impact and therapeutic benefits.

What we teach and how we teach are based on the Cartesian view of the human being—the idea that the individual is divided into two parts, body and mind, and that these two parts are separate and not connected in any meaningful way. Both nursing and medicine have gradually adopted the primary assumption that essentially it is the body that becomes sick; the mind may be secondarily involved but only in rare circumstances is it a causative factor in illness. Thus, our therapies, procedures, drugs, and surgery are body-oriented. Treatment for infective endocar-

ditis, for example, involves antimicrobial agents for the infection, antipyretic drugs for fever, and valve replacement for diseased valves that produce major complications, including emboli, heart failure, and valve-ring abscesses. Our teaching logically focuses on these areas. As a result, we administer body-oriented therapies, and we teach patients about the rationale, actions, and side-effects of such therapies. We do very little, however, to deal with the anxiety and fear that impacts on the illness and its outcome.

Holistic nurses clearly recognize that although body ailments may be eradicated with body-oriented therapies, patients' psychologic responses to the disease may impair their ability to return to full function and may actually interfere with the healing process. Body therapies and teaching related to those therapies are not enough.

In a holistic approach to patient care, the mind and body are seen as operating on a continuum. Disease is much more than a body process; it involves the whole person. The interconnections of mind and body, moreover, are reflected in reciprocal changes in emotions and physiology. Such interconnections may operate at the conscious or unconsciousness level. Thus, if we are able to educate the mind, we must be able to educate the body. Our challenge is to help patients understand that body and mind are connected and that mind therapies, used in conjunction with traditional medical therapies, can intensify the healing process.

Incorporating relaxation techniques, music therapy, imagery, and biofeedback into practice provide the nurse with the interventions needed to care for the whole patient. Such self-regulation techniques enlarge the nurse's options for effective therapy and can produce results as real as those produced by traditional body therapies.

Holistic self-regulation therapies are used to treat the anxiety, stress, and pain inherent to acute body illnesses. They are used to establish a sense of balance and control in one's emotions that, in turn, directly affects the physiologic processes. These therapies are used to appeal to the right brain.

To understand how self-regulation therapies work, an understanding of left-brain and right-brain functioning is necessary. In 1981, Dr. R. Sperry won the Nobel Prize in Medicine and Physics for his work on the hemispheric functioning of the brain.[84-86] This work revealed that we have two brains, or two central hemispheres that do not function in the same way. These two minds are different in terms of their goals and content and ways of processing information. The corpus callosum, a bundle of 200 million nerve fibers, provides for the hemispheric communication and the transmission of learning and memory between the two sides of the brain. The left brain is the rational, analytic, logical, linear, sequential, verbal, and problem-solving side of the brain. The right brain, in contrast, is the global, holistic, intuitive, nonlinear, nonverbal, melodic side of our brain.

It is likely that the right brain predominates during times of stress and crisis. In such situations, individuals primarily process information from the right hemisphere. All nurses have observed this situation. Nurses have seen, for example, families who are unable to cope with the acute hospitalization of a critically ill loved one and who are unable to function in the situation. These individuals express familiar expressions such as "I don't know what to do! My brain is not working! I can't think!" Such expressions are insightful. These individuals are telling us that they literally "can't think," which is entirely correct: They can't think from the rational, analytic left side of their brain because they are primarily processing information from the right hemisphere. The crisis has caused them to shift from the normal everyday left-brain mode of thinking to the right brain.

Extend this idea to patient teaching. Consider teaching a patient with infective endocarditis about antimicrobial therapy. We instruct the patient about how the antibiotics work, why they are needed, how long they are used, and what adverse reactions are associated with such therapy. This is left-brain teaching aimed at stimulating the left hemisphere, but our patient is in right hemispheric thinking. Hemispheric conflict results. At best, we are only half teaching. Is it any surprise that when we evaluate the outcomes of our teaching in critical care, we find that the patient understands or remembers very little of what has been taught!

In our critical care units, we need to initiate right-brain teaching. Self-regulation modalities provide patients with the intuitive experiences to stimulate the right brain and help patients make bodymind connections. Patients are extremely receptive to these therapies because they are in concert with their emotional needs as well as their current method of processing information. Such therapies relay the message that the patient's psychologic response to illness is as important in achieving therapeutic outcomes as their physical response.

In our units, we also need to implement whole-brain teaching. Because of Diagnosis-Related Groups, nurses are faced with developing creative ways to provide discharge teaching during progressively shorter in-hospital patient stays. Right-brain and left-brain learning techniques might be combined to achieve effective teaching and produce whole-brain learning.

Patients could be taught head-to-toe relaxation, for example, on the first day of their hospitalization. When patients are in a relaxed state with lowered anxiety levels, guided imagery techniques progressively could be added. The nurse might suggest that an intravenous access would soon be started. To facilitate a successful venipuncture, patients might be guided in visualizing relaxed, wide-open tubes (veins) in the periphery. Patients could be prompted to image the powerful antibiotic molecules rushing to the source of infection, rendering the bacteria weak and helpless. The 4-week to 6-week length of therapy can be discussed as an essential factor in rendering the bacteria defenseless. Patients then can be guided to visualize the progressive valvular healing that occurs with each week of therapy.

Such whole-brain teaching sessions could be developed for all other traditional content that is generally taught to patients with infective endocarditis. In doing so, patients are assisted in learning techniques that help them cope with the psychologic reactions to the illness and in learning the necessary information about the illness. The results of whole-brain teaching permit hemispheric integration to occur. The results also might revolutionize what we do and how we teach.

DEFINITION

Endocarditis is an infection of the endocardium or inner lining of the heart. It involves primarily the heart valves but also may affect the endocardium of the heart or the intima of the great vessels or both. Endocarditis is no longer termed *bacterial* endocarditis because, in addition to bacteria, other organisms, such as fungi and rickettsia, are known to be causative factors. The term *infective* endocarditis is preferred.[12,56] Even more descriptive is to use the name of the particular microorganism followed by the term endocarditis (*e.g., Streptococcus viridans* endocarditis).[38]

Before the days of antimicrobial therapy, infective endocarditis was classified according to the length of the patient's survival, and it was therefore divided into subacute endocarditis and acute endocarditis. Nearly everyone who had either form of endocarditis eventually died from it. The person with subacute endocarditis followed a chronic course and usually died in 6 to 8 months.[12] The patient with acute endocarditis, on the other hand, suffered a sudden, life-threatening episode and usually died in the first 6 weeks.

Currently, infective endocarditis is classified according to the virulence of the infecting organism. Organisms of low virulence that infect abnormal heart valves produce a more prolonged or "subacute" illness in the normal host. In the compromised host, immune-suppressed, or immune-incompetent patient, a more "acute" course would be expected. People with subacute endocarditis usually do not show signs of toxemia, and cardiac damage is seen only as a late complication. In contrast, acute endocarditis generally results from infection with a more pathogenic or virulent organism. Normal heart valves are often involved, and patients show early clinical manifestations of cardiac damage, septic embolism, and toxemia.[12,38]

INFECTIVE ENDOCARDITIS: SUBACUTE

Etiology

The organism that causes most cases of subacute endocarditis is *Streptococcus viridans,* a bacterium found in the oral cavity.[12,32,60] *Streptococcus viridans* is an alpha-hemolytic organism of low virulence that becomes opportunistically engrafted on abnormal heart valves. Other causative organisms include a nonhemolytic *Streptococcus* strain (gamma streptococcus) and microaerophilic strains, commonly found in the mouth and intestinal, female genital, and respiratory tracts. *Streptococcus faecalis* (enterococcus), a more virulent strain, is found in the gastrointestinal and genitourinary tracts. The alpha-hemolytic and nonhemolytic streptococci cause more than 90% of the cases of subacute infective endocarditis. The remaining 8% to 10% of the organisms causing the disease are of low virulence. About 1% of the patients have a mixed infection.

Pathogenesis

Streptococcus viridans is a selective bacterium that generally causes only the heart to become infected. Four mechanisms explain the selectivity and localization of the subacute infection: pre-existing valvular damage or other cardiac defects that cause a unique hemodynamic situation, the development of sterile platelet-fibrin thrombi, the presence of a bacteremia, and a high titer of agglutinating antibodies for the infecting organism.[27,93,94] These factors are discussed in the following sections.

Valvular Damage or Other Cardiac Defects

The first mechanism involves pre-existing valvular damage or other cardiac defects produced by rheumatic, congenital, or degenerative heart disease. Mitral or aortic valve abnormalities (including mitral valve prolapse, mitral stenosis, bicuspid aortic valves) are the most common deformities. Others include small intraventricular septal defects, coarctation of the aorta, tetralogy of Fallot, patent ductus arteriosus, pulmonic stenosis, and hypertrophic cardiomyopathies.[12] Prosthetic heart valves are also susceptible to infection.[30,32,46,60,91]

Valvular damage or other cardiac defects can produce a hemodynamic situation that allows organisms to settle out of the blood stream and localize around the irregularities of the valve.[12] The reason for this localization is not clearly understood, although a hydrodynamic theory developed by Rodbard helps to explain it (Fig. 28–1).[76] According to Rodbard's theory, the presence of valvular deformities creates a situation in which there is rapid blood flow, a narrowed valvular orifice, and a high-pressure gradient between two cardiac chambers. In mitral insufficiency, for example, the high left ventricular pressure observed during systole when the mitral valve is closed generates a high-velocity regurgitant jet from the left ventricle to the lower pressure of the left atrium.[76] The regurgitant jet produces a reduction in the lateral pressure on the atrial side of the valve, causing particulate matter to be deposited in the area because of a vortex-shedding effect, an increase in the local bacterial count during bacteremia, and a reduction in the endothelial nutrition. As a result, the atrium becomes highly susceptible to endocardial vegetation. Similar hemodynamic principles relevant to the localization of bacteria may apply also to other cardiac defects.[76,93]

Sterile Platelet-Fibrin Thrombi

The second mechanism responsible for the localization of the subacute infection is the development of sterile platelet-fibrin thrombi.[93] The endothelial surface is traumatized as a result of turbulence and the Venturi effect produced by various cardiac defects. As a result of the trauma, sterile platelet-fibrin thrombi form on the injured heart leaflets. The sterile thrombi are foci for infection if appropriate bacteria are introduced into the blood stream.

Bacteremia

The third mechanism necessary for localization of the infection is the entry of the infecting organism into the body to produce bacteremia (fungemia or rickettsemia). In most cases, organisms entering the body are either of such low virulence or are few enough that they fail to implant on normal heart valves. Although transient bacteremia occurs frequently in normal people, it rarely produces valvular infection. People with valvular damage or other cardiac defects, however, are susceptible to those organisms because of the presence of sterile platelet-fibrin thrombi.[4] Such thrombi are avascular and easily contaminated, allowing the microorganism to seed and proliferate.[12] In addition, some infecting organisms produce a polysaccharide coat that permits the organism to adhere more easily to the damaged valvular surface. Likewise, fibronectin, a glycoprotein in the plasma found on traumatized valvular tissue, is also a factor that promotes the adherence of organisms.[55,81]

Circulating Antibodies

The fourth major mechanism responsible for the localization and production of subacute endocarditis is the development of a high titer of agglutinating antibodies for the infecting organism. The platelet-covered valvular lesions probably provide a favorable surface for the organism. Also, circulating antibodies permit large numbers of bacteria to adhere to the platelet-fibrin thrombi. By clumping the organisms, circulating antibodies enhance the localization and multiplication of the infection.[43,93,95]

Pathology

The endocardial valvular lesions (called *vegetations*) develop slowly. They contain an inner mass of necrotic collagen and elastin, with platelets, fibrin, neutrophils, lymphocytes, red blood cells, and bacteria. Their middle layer is composed primarily of bacteria. Their outer layer is composed of fibrin and bacteria. The superficial irregular lesions are easily torn away.

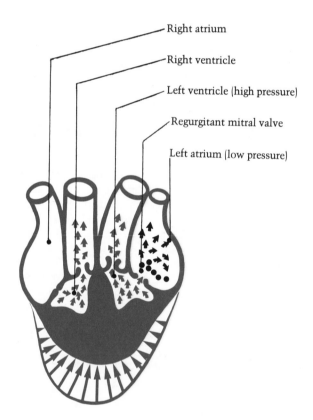

Right atrium

Right ventricle

Left ventricle (high pressure)

Regurgitant mitral valve

Left atrium (low pressure)

Figure 28–1

Hydrodynamic theory explaining the localization of lesions in subacute infective endocarditis. In the presence of mitral insufficiency, a regurgitant jet from the left ventricle to the left atrium during systole creates a reduction in the lateral pressure on the atrial side of the valve. The regurgitant flow causes a collection of particulate matter, an increase in local bacteria, and a reduction in nutrition in that area.

The mitral valve lesions are usually located on the atrial side with growth that can extend into the atrial wall (producing a ring abscess), but they can also involve the chordae tendineae on the ventricular side. Aortic lesions generally are found on the ventricular side of the valve, although they may develop on either side of the leaflet. The aortic and mitral valves are the most common sites of endocardial infection.

The infective process in subacute endocarditis can cause thinning or destruction of the valve, producing valvular incompetence (regurgitation) that leads to myocardial dysfunction and cardiac failure. In some instances, valvular thinning may also produce valvular aneurysms, which may rupture or perforate. Erosive complications, producing significant hemodynamic abnormalities, may result from the involvement of the chordae tendineae, papillary muscle, or conduction system.[93] Calcification, scarring, and deformities of the valve are common during the healing process, which may take as long as 2 or 3 months.[12]

INFECTIVE ENDOCARDITIS: ACUTE

Etiology

Typically, acute endocarditis is produced by a highly virulent organism that localizes on normal heart valves and produces rapid and extensive cardiac damage. The primary infection site is generally remote from the heart.

Staphylococcus aureus causes most cases of the acute infections.[58] Other organisms are *Diplococcus, Streptococcus pyogenes, Neisseria gonorrhoeae, Neisseria meningitidis, Escherichia coli, Proteus, Klebsiella, Pseudomonas, Salmonella, Hemophilus, Serratia, Listeria, Bacteroides, Candida,* and *Aspergillus.*[12,20,36,47]

Pathogenesis

It appears that the only mechanism responsible for the pathogenesis of acute endocarditis is the presence of bacteremia produced by a highly virulent organism. Fifty to 60% of the acute infections involve normal heart valves.[7,93] The aortic valve is the one most commonly affected. Right-sided heart valves are more frequently involved in the acute form of the disease, particularly in the parenteral drug abuser.

Pathology

The vegetations in acute endocarditis develop rapidly; they appear to be larger and softer than those in subacute endocarditis. They also tend to be more hemorrhagic, with significant inflammatory changes, granulation tissue, and polymorphonuclear infiltration. As a result, there is a greater tendency for larger vegetations to break away, leaving ulcerated lesions on the valve leaflets. The inflammatory process may spread into underlying tissue, causing destruction of the papillary muscle, chordae tendineae, and conduction system.[93]

MARANTIC ENDOCARDITIS

Marantic endocarditis (known also as degenerative nonbacterial thrombotic endocarditis, degenerative verrucous endocarditis, terminal endocarditis, and endocarditis simplex) is a *nonbacterial* form of endocarditis. It is characterized by the development of sterile thrombi on cardiac valves. Should the patient develop a bacteremia, the sterile platelet-fibrin thrombi can become the focus for infection and infective endocarditis can develop. Although marantic endocarditis is generally seen in patients with terminal malignant tumors or disease,[72] it may be associated with a variety of disorders, such as acute pneumonia, pulmonary embolism, glomerulonephritis, peritonitis, and other acute illnesses.[94]

Previously scarred heart valves appear to be more susceptible to marantic endocarditis than are normal valves. The precipitating factor, however, is related to a blood-clotting derangement, a chronic form of disseminated intravascular coagulation that is a part of certain underlying diseases.[72] Chronic disseminated intravascular coagulation is characterized by thrombotic and embolic manifestations. The lesions of marantic endocarditis are important because they can cause peripheral arterial embolism that results in infarction of the brain, kidney, spleen, or myocardium. Although anticoagulation therapy may be useful in preventing recurrent embolic complications, there is no definitive therapy.

Burn patients with indwelling pulmonary artery or central venous catheters are at high risk for developing right-sided nonbacterial thrombotic or infective endocarditis, because such catheters can induce trauma in the cardiac chambers.[66] Because burn-injured patients are in a hypercoagulable state with hyperdynamic cardiac functioning, such indwelling catheters can produce endocardial and endothelial injury that favors the development of nonbacterial thrombotic vegetations.[26] It is suggested that careful consideration be given to using such catheters in these and in other critically ill patients in order to prevent iatrogenic endocarditis.[80]

LIBMAN-SACKS ENDOCARDITIS

Systemic lupus erythematosus, the most common collagen disease, characteristically produces injury to the vascular system. Libman-Sacks endocarditis is a nonbacterial manifestation of systemic lupus erythematosus, occurring late in 50% of the cases. The myocardium and pericardium may also be affected, producing cardiac conduction disturbances, pericarditis, pericardial effusion, and tamponade.

NURSING PROCESS

ASSESS RISK FACTORS

A complete nursing assessment is carried out to evaluate the patient's nine human response patterns. When endocarditis is suspected, it is essential to identify high-risk patients and associated portals of entry for the infecting organism. High-risk patients include those with a history of congenital or rheumatic heart disease. Any patient who previously has had endocarditis or those with nonbacterial thrombotic endocarditis are at high risk for developing infective endocarditis.[67,72] Patients with idiopathic hypertrophic subaortic stenosis,[67] mitral valve prolapse with a precordial systolic murmur of mitral regurgitation,[19,24,35,57,67] or other acquired valvular diseases are also at risk. All of the high-risk patients are particularly susceptible to endocarditis if they do not receive prophylactic antibiotics when surgical or dental procedures are performed that involve mucosal surfaces or contaminated tissue that may cause a transient bacteremia.

Patients with surgically constructed systemic-pulmonary shunts and those who have undergone cardiac valve replacement are particularly at risk for developing endocarditis.[1,30,71,91] Infection of a prosthetic valve can occur at any time—during or after surgery or after discharge from the hospital. The major complication of prosthetic valve endocarditis is prosthetic valve detachment, which may lead to paravalvular regurgitation and generally to cardiac failure.[32] The overall mortality associated with prosthetic valve endocarditis is over 50%.[40]

Prosthetic valve endocarditis is divided into early and late categories.[20,32,35,48,53,73] *Early prosthetic valve endocarditis* occurs 2 months or less postoperatively and tends to be a serious problem.[25] It may be associated intraoperatively with contamination of prosthetic valves and patches, silk sutures, the cardiopulmonary bypass machines, operating room equipment, and intravenous solutions and blood products. Postoperatively, the patient is also exposed to many sources of infection, such as pacemakers; intravenous, arterial, and indwelling urinary catheters; endotracheal tubes; ventilatory equipment; postoperative wounds; and bacteremia during the convalescent period.[12,30,53,56,79,83,91] The common infective organism in these patients is usually one of the highly virulent organisms, such as *Staphylococcus aureus, Staphylococcus epidermis*, gram-negative bacilli, or fungi.

Frequently, endocarditis that develops in the early postoperative period is not recognized because of the administration of prolonged prophylactic antibiotic therapy. It is recommended that antibiotic prophylaxis for prosthetic valve surgery be directed toward staphylococci and be of short duration. The antibiotics should be started immediately before the surgery and continued no longer than 2 days postoperatively to reduce the occurrence of resistant microorganisms.[1] If a patient develops chills, marked toxemia, and a fever more than 3 days postoperatively, endocarditis should be suspected.

If the infection develops on a prosthetic valve, it is extremely difficult to eradicate. Microorganisms may be seeded before the prosthetic valve completely endothelializes, permitting them to become deeply embedded in the tissue and making treatment with antibiotics difficult.[29,32] Thus, patients with early prosthetic valve endocarditis frequently are advised to undergo a second prosthetic valve replacement.[20,29,32,35]

Late prosthetic valve endocarditis is suspected when the patient develops chills, fever, leukocytosis, or a new murmur more than 2 months after surgery and after the prothesis has had time to endothelialize.[55] It is usually caused by *Streptococcus viridans*. Although such patients are at risk for developing embolic complications or heart failure, the mortality associated with late prosthetic valve endocarditis is not as high as for those patients in the early category.[40,55] It is recommended, however, that patients with heart failure undergo reoperation.[32,35,48,73]

Other high risk patients include those who are immunologically suppressed because of cancer, hepatitis, diabetes mellitus, severe burns, systemic lupus erythematosus, or rheumatoid arthritis, or those who are receiving prolonged antibiotic, cytotoxic, or steroid medications or radiation.[20,32,35] Patients who are parenteral drug abusers are highly susceptible to endocarditis[20,21,27,32,35] secondary to the use of contaminated equipment and skin sites.[37] In such patients, right-sided endocarditis is common and frequently caused by *Staphylococcus aureus*, gram-negative bacilli, or fungi.[27,32,35,58]

When assessing high-risk patients, the nurse also must carefully investigate possible portals of entry. Because *Streptococcus* is normally present in the oral cavity, dental disease or procedures can produce a transient bacteremia that can cause endocarditis.[32,41] Thus, any recent history of dental work that has caused gingival bleeding, such as routine professional cleaning, or work that has produced trauma to the gingivae should be determined. The patient should be assessed for poor oral hygiene, including dental and periodontal disease, or poorly fitting dentures.

In patients with pre-existing cardiac abnormalities, infective endocarditis also can be associated with the development of skin abnormalities (*e.g.*, rashes, lesions, lacerations, trauma, or abscesses). Infections of the skin, respiratory, genitourinary, or gastrointestinal tracts, or central nervous system have been linked to the development of endocarditis. When exposed to surgical or invasive procedures of the ears, nose, and throat, or upper respiratory, genitourinary, or gastrointestinal tract, patients with pre-existing cardiac abnormalities are at high risk for infective endocarditis.[1,12,30,46,56,91,93]

Patients with prosthetic heart valves and those with surgically constructed systemic-pulmonary shunts are particularly at high risk for developing infective endocarditis if they do not receive prophylactic antibiotics even for low-risk procedures (*e.g.*, barium enemas, uncomplicated vaginal deliveries, uterine dilatation and curettage, cesarean section, therapeutic abortion, sterilization procedures, and "in-and-out" bladder catheterizations).[1]

Cases of acute endocarditis have been reported in patients with infected peripheral venous, pulmonary artery, and central venous lines, and indwelling transvenous cardiac pacemakers (usually from wound contamination at the time of surgery).[1,7,12,14,20,21,27,32,34–36,40,50,58,67,89,90,91] Patients with arteriovenous shunts or fistulas used for hemodialysis also are susceptible to developing endocarditis.[7,23,35,91] There is no evidence that patients undergoing coronary artery bypass graft surgery are at risk unless other cardiac abnormalities are also present.[1] Likewise, patients undergoing cardiac catheterization and angiography are not considered at risk, because aseptic techniques are involved.[1]

ASSESS CLINICAL MANIFESTATIONS

The clinical signs and symptoms of endocarditis are outlined in Table 28–1. They include those related to a reaction to the infection, cardiac involvement, embolism, and immunologic disorders.[30] These four factors are discussed in the following sections.

Reaction to Infection

Most patients infected with a low-virulent organism (*e.g.*, *Streptococcus viridans*) manifest subacute endocarditis by a persistent low-grade fever (99°F to 102°F).[12] Although bacteria are continuously released from the vegetations and could produce other sites of infections, the immune and cellular defenses generally protect the rest of the body against the organisms involved in the subacute infection. A high-grade fever (103°F to 104°F), recurrent chills, diaphoresis, and prostration are common reactions to the acute illness. Patients also tend to complain of a variety of nonspecific signs and symptoms, such as malaise, fatigue, back pain, headache, weight loss, and anorexia.[27,32,35]

Table 28–1
Clinical Findings in Infective Endocarditis

Reactions to infection
    Low-grade fever
    Chills, diaphoresis
    Cough
    Anorexia, weight loss
    Muscle aching
    Malaise, fatigue
Cardiac manifestations
    New murmur
    Change in the quality or intensity of an old murmur
    Congestive heart failure
    Myocardial ischemia or infarction
    Pericardial friction rub, pericarditis, cardiac tamponade
    Clubbing of the fingers
Embolic manifestations
    Confusion, weakness
    Psychotic behavior   *Central nervous system*
    Visual field defects   Cerebrovascular accident
    Hemiplegia, hemiparesis   Mycotic cerebral aneurysm or rupture
    Aphasia, dysphasia   Transient ischemic attacks
    Convulsions
    Coma

Substernal chest pain with radiation to arms, neck,   *Cardiovascular system*
    shoulder and associated with sweating,   Myocardial ischemia
    nausea, vomiting, and shortness of breath   Myocardial infarction
Sudden onset of abdominal pain with radiation to   *Gastrointestinal system*
    left axilla, shoulder, or precordium and   Splenic infarction
    associated with elevated temperature, chills,   Mesenteric infarction
    vomiting, leukocytosis, and toxemia
Flank pain with radiation to groin associated with   *Genitourinary system*
    hematuria and azotemia   Renal infarction
Immunologic derangements producing hypersensitivity reactions
    Petechiae
    Splinter hemorrhages
    Osler's nodes
    Janeway's lesions
    Roth's spots
    Arthralgia
    Arthritis
    Focal glomerulitis, acute or chronic glomerulonephritis
    Mycotic aneurysm
Laboratory and diagnostic findings
    Positive blood culture
    Anemia
    Elevated erythrocyte sedimentation rate
    Normal or slightly elevated white blood count
    Thrombocytopenia
    Positive rheumatoid factor (IgM anti-IgG antibodies)
    Elevated IgG and IgM levels
    Low serum complement levels
    Hematuria
    Albuminuria

Cardiac Involvement

Often patients suffering from subacute endocarditis have some form of cardiac involvement (see Table 28–1). About 85% to 95% of patients have heart murmurs.[12,32,35] With the rapid destruction of the valve in acute endocarditis, new murmurs may be produced or striking changes in the intensity or quality of an old murmur may occur owing to valve perforation or to functional hemodynamic changes.[20] Although endocarditis usually produces regurgitant murmurs, vegetations rarely are large enough to cause stenosis of the valve and stenotic murmurs.

Congestive heart failure is probably the most common complication of both acute and subacute endocarditis. It is also the most common cause of death. It is produced by perforation, erosion, or rupture of the valves or other associated structures.[32,43] The development of heart failure in a patient who has endocarditis carries a grave prognosis. The mortality is high despite effective antimicrobial therapy; thus, surgical intervention for such patients is advocated.[32,35]

A variety of other destructive hemodynamic changes occur as a result of friable lesions associated with infective endocarditis. Extension of the infection from the valve through the myocardial wall may lead to the formation of a fistula, abscess,

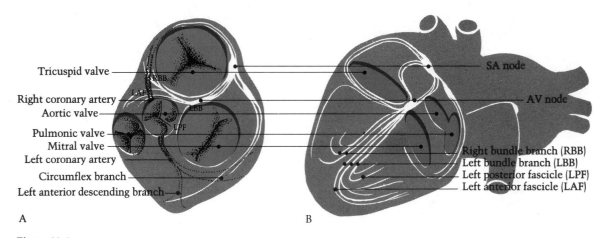

Figure 28–2

Anatomic relationships among heart valves, conduction system, and coronary arteries. (*A*) Idealized superior view of a coronal section of the heart without the atria and the great vessels. (*B*) Idealized anterior view of a sagittal section of the heart.

ventricular septal defect, or a conduction or rhythm disturbance (Fig. 28–2), pericarditis, and external rupture leading to cardiac tamponade. Myocardial ischemia or infarction may be caused by obstructive lesions around the coronary ostia or by coronary embolism.[12]

Clubbed fingers may be seen in the late stages of endocarditis. Clubbing is diagnosed by a spongy feeling over the skin proximal to the nail bed. In some instances, there is flushing and pulsation of the ends of the fingers. The proximal nail bed becomes convex and rises above the plane of the finger (Fig. 28–3). With successful antibiotic therapy, the nail beds may return to their original shape.

Embolism

Arterial embolism is a common complication of endocarditis (Fig. 28–4).[72] The friable vegetations, which are released continuously from the site of infection, produce changes in the arterioles.

Embolism and occlusion of major arterial vessels are also serious problems that occur often. Fungal infections characteristically produce fragments large enough to block major vessels. Occasionally, large embolic fragments detach to produce occlusion and infarctions in the kidney, spleen, brain, or heart (see Table 28–1). Pulmonary embolism and septic pulmonary infarction may develop in patients with right-sided endocarditis. Although embolic complications occur frequently in the early stage of the illness, embolization may continue for weeks, even after the institution of successful antimicrobial therapy.[35,39]

Immunologic Derangements

Immunologic derangements are also observed in infective endocarditis. Agglutinating, complement-fixing, and opsonizing antibodies specific for the infecting organism are commonly found.[5] A high titer of IgM anti-IgG antibodies (the rheumatoid factor), which inhibit the phagocytic action of the polymor-

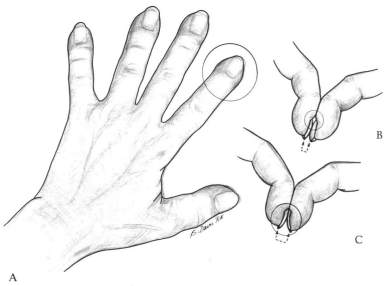

Figure 28–3

Clubbing of the fingers.[11] (*A*) The proximal nail beds are convex and rise above the flat plane of the finger. (*B*) Normal finger contour when placing the nail beds and dorsal surfaces of the terminal phalanges together, creating an aperture or diamond-shaped "window" at the nail-bed bases. (*C*) Clubbing of the fingers showing obliteration of the window and "beaking" or a wide distal angle between the ends of the nail bed extending more than halfway up the fingernail. Normally, this distal angle does not extend more than halfway. (Guzzetta, C. E. The Person with Infective Endocarditis. In C. E. Guzzetta, and B. M. Dossey, *Cardiovascular Nursing: Bodymind Tapestry.* St. Louis, C. V. Mosby, 1984; with permission.)

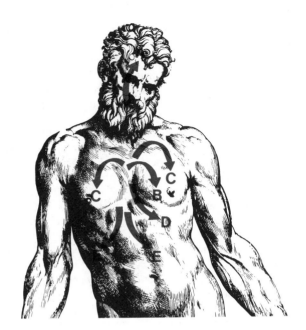

Figure 28–4

Common sites of arterial embolization in infective endocarditis. (*A*) Brain. (*B*) Heart. (*C*) Lungs. (*D*) Spleen. (*E*) Kidneys.

phonuclear leukocytes, is observed in up to 50% of all patients with infective endocarditis.[15,39,61,67,94] The high titer of IgM anti-IgG antibodies typically falls to low levels several weeks after effective antimicrobial therapy. A hypergammaglobulinemia is also frequently observed and is caused by stimulation of the humoral immune system, depression of the cellular immune system, or both.[15,70]

Circulating immune complexes (cryoglobulins) are often found in patients with infective endocarditis.[61] Circulating immune complexes produce a hypersensitivity reaction manifested as an allergic vasculitis (see Table 28–1). The arthralgia and arthritis associated with the disease are due to this allergic vasculitis. The classic peripheral manifestations of endocarditis, including petechiae, splinter hemorrhages, Osler's nodes, Janeway's lesions, and Roth's spots, are now also considered to be the result of the allergic vasculitis involving the arterioles rather than a result of embolic phenomena, as was formerly believed.[8,15,39,70,94]

Petechiae are commonly observed in the mucous membranes, conjunctiva (Fig. 28–5A), neck, wrist, and ankles. The petechiae are 1 mm to 2 mm in diameter, flat, red, nontender, and have white or gray centers. They appear in groups and fade away in a few days. Petechiae are not specifically diagnostic for endocarditis and can be observed in other types of patients, such as those undergoing cardiopulmonary bypass, who develop conjunctival petechiae from lipid microembolization.[35]

Splinter hemorrhages (linear subungual hemorrhages) are frequently seen early in infective endocarditis (Fig. 28–5B). They are black, longitudinal streaks generally found on the distal third of the nail beds. The hemorrhages are not specific for endocarditis, however. Frequently, they occur with trauma, age, hemodialysis, peritoneal dialysis, or mitral stenosis.[35,39]

Osler's nodes are a major manifestation of endocarditis (Fig. 28–5C). They are cutaneous nodules that vary in size from 1

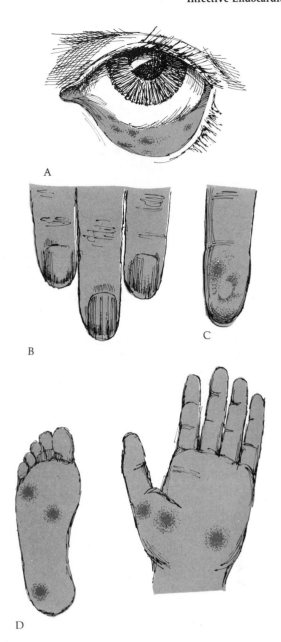

Figure 28–5

Findings in endocarditis. (*A*) Conjunctival petechiae. (*B*) Splinter hemorrhages. (*C*) Osler's nodes. (*D*) Janeway's lesions.

mm to 10 mm. They are reddish, *tender* lesions with a white center, and classically, they are located on the pads of the distal fingers or toes, sides of the fingers, palms, or thighs. They occur in 10% to 20% of patients with infective endocarditis.

Janeway's lesions are occasionally seen in subacute endocarditis (Fig. 28–5D). They are *nontender*, hemorrhagic, and erythematous lesions found on the palms, soles, arms, and legs. They are 1 mm to 5 mm in diameter, and they are accentuated when the extremity is elevated.

On funduscopic examination, *Roth's spots* are seen occasionally. They are boat-shaped retinal hemorrhages 3 mm to 10 mm in diameter, often have a pale or a white center, and are located near the optic nerve disk. They also occur in such diseases as leukemia, septicemia, thrombotic thrombocytopenia, and anemia.[35]

A number of musculoskeletal complaints, such as arthralgias, arthritis, myalgias, and severe lower back pain, occur in patients with infective endocarditis due to a localized immune response.[32,35,39,45] Splenomegaly may be observed, probably due to a continuous antigenic stimulation.[35,39]

Focal embolic glomerulitis and acute or chronic glomerulonephritis, previously thought to be the result of small emboli, are now also believed to be due to an allergic vasculitis.[35,39,70,94] The lesions may be associated with hematuria, acute renal failure, and uremia. The early administration of effective antimicrobial therapy is often helpful in reversing the pathologic changes associated with such complications.[8,70]

Mycotic aneurysm associated with both immunologic abnormalities and embolism is a rare but serious complication of subacute endocarditis.[32,35] It occurs even less commonly in acute endocarditis, especially when the infecting organism is *Staphyloccus aureus*. Injury from deposition of immune complexes in the arterial wall may, in combination with microembolism, produce inflammation, necrosis, thinning, and dilation of the artery. Mycotic aneurysms may rupture months or years after the subacute illness. Depending on their location, many mycotic aneurysms are potentially lethal. For example, rupture of a cerebral artery mycotic aneurysm can result in intracranial hemorrhage and death.[35,39]

LABORATORY AND DIAGNOSTIC FINDINGS

The most important laboratory finding in the diagnosis of infective endocarditis is a positive blood culture for the infective organism (see Nursing Diagnosis 1). Serial blood cultures are drawn to demonstrate a sustained rather than transient bacteremia. Because bacteria are continuously released into the circulation from the endocardial vegetations, blood cultures will remain positive during serial drawings.[61] Serial cultures are also done to prevent false-negative or false-positive interpretations. The organism causing the infective endocarditis will generally appear in all cultures, whereas a contaminant will usually appear in only one.[67]

Antimicrobial therapy should not be instituted until an adequate number of blood cultures have been obtained. Approximately 15% to 20% of patients have negative blood cultures, even though they show clinical and pathologic evidence of endocarditis.[32,69,74] Blood cultures may be negative because the culture techniques used are inappropriate for low levels of bacteria or for unusual organisms.[44] Probably the most common cause of negative blood cultures, however, is the early administration of antibiotics that suppress bacteremia when the culture samples are taken.[69]

A normochromic, normocytic anemia occurs in 60% to 70% of patients with endocarditis. Increased erythrocyte sedimentation rates are frequently observed.[32,67] Leukocyte counts are usually elevated. A thrombotic thrombocytopenic purpura-type syndrome has been reported in endocarditis patients. The syndrome is associated with a high titer of circulating immune complexes, a low serum complement level, and a low platelet count.[35,39]

Conduction abnormalities may occur in endocarditis because the noncoronary cusp and the right cusp of the aortic valve lie in close proximity to the conduction system (Fig. 28-2A and B).[75] A prolonged PR interval, a new left bundle branch block, or a new right bundle branch block may indicate extension of the infection from the aortic valve into the conduction system. The mitral annulus, however, lies close to the atrioventricular node and to the bundle of His. Extension of the infection from the mitral valve to the atrioventricular node and bundle of His may cause junctional dysrhythmias and first-, second-, or third-degree atrioventricular heart block. Ventricular dysrhythmias are observed occasionally when myocardial infarction, abscess, or myocarditis is associated with endocarditis.[32]

Cardiac catheterization is sometimes used to evaluate the extent of infection and to evaluate whether the patient may be a candidate for surgery. Visualization of large valvular vegetations can be done by transthoracic or transesophageal two-dimensional echocardiography.[7,61,63] Doppler echocardiography can be used to quantitate and confirm valvular lesions. Other laboratory findings are described in Table 28-1.[12,93]

NURSING DIAGNOSES, PATIENT OUTCOMES, AND PLAN

The preceding material on etiology, pathogenesis, nursing assessment, and diagnostic tests guides the nurse in establishing nursing diagnoses, patient outcomes, and the plan for the patient with infective endocarditis.

NURSING CARE PLAN SUMMARY *Patient With Infective Endocarditis*

NURSING DIAGNOSIS

1. Cardiac valve infection (name valve) related to (include name of organism) (exchanging pattern)

Patient Outcomes	Nursing Orders
1. The infecting organism will be identified from blood culture studies. The patient	1. Related to blood culture studies, do the following: A. Explain the procedure to the patient.

(continued)

NURSING CARE PLAN SUMMARY   *Patient With Infective Endocarditis*   *Continued*

Patient Outcomes	Nursing Orders

Patient Outcomes

will not experience any complications from the procedure.[38] The patient will verbalize the following:

A. Why blood culture studies are needed

B. A general description of the procedure, the frequency, and the amount of blood drawn

2. The patient will practice relaxation techniques and will not demonstrate a high level of anxiety during the procedure.

3. The patient will not experience any complications, such as infection, redness, swelling, bleeding, or discomfort, around the venipuncture site.

4. The patient will verbalize the following:

A. The rationale, frequency, and duration of the antimicrobial therapy

B. A general description of the therapy

C. Any discomfort, leaking, or pain around the venipuncture site

5. The patient will demonstrate symptomatic improvement from the antimicrobial therapy.

A. The patient's temperature will return to normal in 4 to 5 days.

B. The patient's appetite will improve.

C. The patient's blood cultures will become negative in 1 week.

D. The patient's circulating immune complexes and erythrocyte sedimentation rate will decline during the course of therapy.

E. The patient's rheumatoid factor will disappear.

F. The patient's complaints of malaise, fatigue, and headaches will decrease.

Nursing Orders

(1) Serial blood cultures are drawn to demonstrate a sustained rather than transient bacteremia. Three to six samples are drawn.

(2) Blood cultures are drawn so that the appropriate effective drug therapy can be selected.

(3) The amount of blood drawn during each venipuncture is generally not more than 1 tablespoon.

B. Assess patient's reaction to explanation of the procedure.

C. Supervise the drawing of blood samples for culturing *before* antimicrobial therapy is administered.

(1) Clean the patient's skin and the rubber diaphragm on top of the culture tubes with a solution of 2% iodine in 70% alcohol. After at least a 30-second drying time, remove iodine with a 70% isopropyl alcohol solution before doing the venipuncture. Strict aseptic technique is essential to prevent contamination of the blood cultures.

(2) In the less acutely ill patient, draw five or six blood samples for culturing over 24 to 48 hours.[35] In acutely ill patients with a spiking temperature and heart failure, draw three to five blood samples at 5- to 10-minute intervals. Each sample should be taken from a different venous site.

(3) Label the blood culture tubes.

(4) Incubate each sample under both anaerobic and aerobic conditions.

2. Teach patient some type of relaxation technique (see Chap. 3) that can be practiced during venipuncture sticks. Guide the patient with imagery during relaxation, suggesting the patient visualize relaxed, wide-open vessels (tubes) in the extremities. Explain that when the patient is anxious, peripheral constriction occurs. Explain that dilated veins are easier to stick than constricted ones and that relaxation techniques are useful in dilating peripheral vessels, warming the extremities, and reducing anxiety, fear, and a feeling of loss of control.[38] Assess the patient's reaction and level of relaxation during the procedure.

3. Check the venipuncture site for any signs or symptoms of complications, and instruct the patient to report any swelling, redness, bleeding, or discomfort around the venipuncture site.

4. Explain to the patient the rationale, frequency, and need for a 28-day (or longer) course of continuous intravenous antimicrobial therapy. Describe the general procedure, and explain that the patient should report any adverse effects.

5. Administer antimicrobial therapy and assess the patient's response.

A. Determine whether the patient has a history of allergic reactions to antimicrobial medication.

B. When the infecting organism is identified, write its name on the patient's care plan.

C. Administer the antimicrobial therapy as ordered by the physician immediately after all blood culture samples have been drawn. Antimicrobials are used to kill the organism, sterilize the vegetations, reduce symptoms, and prevent a relapse. For the patient with acute endocarditis, there must be no delay in giving antimicrobial therapy beyond the brief period of time required to do the blood cultures.

The type of medication chosen should have a narrow spectrum, the fewest possible adverse effects, and a bactericidal action.[16,67] High serum concentrations of the medication are needed because the avascular vegetations contain millions of organisms. The medication is given intravenously rather than orally to ensure absorption and compliance.[27]

(1) Treatment of streptococcal infections. Penicillin inhibits the synthesis of

(continued)

NURSING CARE PLAN SUMMARY   *Patient With Infective Endocarditis*   *Continued*

Patient Outcomes	*Nursing Orders*

G. The patient's renal disease will be reversed.
H. The patient's clubbing will disappear.
	the bacterial cell wall, making it more susceptible to lysis. Patients with *Streptococcus viridans* endocarditis are treated with 10 to 20 million U of parenteral penicillin daily given either as a continuous intravenous infusion or in six equally divided doses.[10] Such therapy is generally continued for 4 to 6 weeks.
	   In addition to penicillin, an aminoglycoside is given during the first 2 weeks of therapy.[10] Aminoglycosides enter the bacterial cell wall to produce changes within the bacterium that impair their survival. Streptomycin, 7.5 mg/kg (not to exceed 500 mg), is given intramuscularly every 12 hours. Alternatively, gentamicin, 1 mg/kg (not to exceed 80 mg), may be given intramuscularly or intravenously every 8 hours. When combined with aminoglycosides, penicillin has a higher potency and thus a greater bactericidal effect against certain organisms. Combination therapy with penicillin and an aminoglycoside is recommended for 6 weeks in patients whose infection involves prosthetic valves. Recently, high bacteriologic cure rates have been reported when combination penicillin and aminoglycoside therapy is given over a shorter (2-week) course for patients with uncomplicated *Streptococcus viridans* endocarditis.[10]
	   (2) Treatment of staphylococcal infections. Most strains of *Staphylococcus aureus* are resistant to penicillin because they produce penicillinase, an enzyme that inactivates penicillin. Penicillins that are structurally resistent to penicillinase (*i.e.*, penicillinase-resistant penicillins), such as the semisynthetic penicillins, nafcillin or oxacillin, are given in doses of 2 g intravenously every 4 hours for 4 to 6 weeks for patients with *Staphylococcus aureus* endocarditis. Gentamicin may be an optional addition to therapy, usually administered for 3 to 5 days.[10]
	   (3) Other infecting organisms. Gram-negative organisms are treated with specific antimicrobial therapy based on culture-proven sensitivity of the infecting organism to the antibiotic. Fungal infections are treated with amphotericin B. For patients who are allergic to penicillin, vancomycin can be used.[16,27,67]
	D. Assess the patient's therapeutic response to antimicrobial therapy.[38]
	   (1) Normal temperature
	   (2) Improved appetite
	   (3) Negative blood culture studies
	   (4) Declining circulating immune complexes and erythrocyte sedimentation levels
	   (5) Disappearance of rheumatoid factor
	   (6) Decreased complaints of malaise, fatigue, backache, and headache
	   (7) Reversal of renal disease
	   (8) Disappearance of clubbing
	E. Assess the patient carefully for clinical manifestations that may persist or develop despite effective antimicrobial therapy, such as heart murmurs, heart failure, rhythm or conduction disturbances, embolic manifestations, and hypersensitivity reactions such as petechiae.

6. The patient will not experience any complications from the antimicrobial therapy.
   A. No rash, diarrhea, urticaria, anaphylactic reactions, or other adverse effects will be present.
   B. The patient will verbalize any symptoms related to adverse effects.
	6. Be alert to any allergic reactions to penicillin or other antimicrobial drugs. The nurse should observe for the following:
	A. Allergic reactions such as mild skin rashes, hives, urticaria, fever, diarrhea, and anaphylactic shock (profound circulatory failure). If the patient has an allergic reaction, the nurse should assess the patient and consult with the physician before giving the next dose. Treatment for anaphylactic shock includes administering intravenous epinephrine (0.5 mg of a 1:10,000 solution). The dose should be repeated every 5 to 15 minutes until the patient responds. Other possible treatments that may be necessary include airway maintenance, cardiopulmonary resuscitation, use of a tourniquet above the injection site to delay absorption, and the intravenous administration of fluids, aminophylline, or hydrocortisone.

(continued)

NURSING CARE PLAN SUMMARY   *Patient With Infective Endocarditis*   *Continued*

Patient Outcomes	*Nursing Orders*
	B. The adverse effects of streptomycin include ototoxic complications such as possible irreversible damage to the eighth cranial nerve, which causes dizziness, lack of balance, and hearing loss. The adverse effects of gentamicin include nephrotoxic complications such as reduced renal function, with resulting blood urea nitrogen and creatinine elevations or oliguria.[10]
7. The patient will be assessed and prepared for home intravenous therapy.	7. Assess whether the patient is a candidate for home intravenous therapy. According to Diagnosis-Related Groups, a patient with infective endocarditis is allowed an inpatient stay of 18.4 days.[81] Because patients may need continuous intravenous therapy for 4 to 6 weeks, the need to administer intravenous therapy in the home has become an increasingly popular concept.[18,22,51,87]

A. A multidisciplinary team is involved that consists of a nurse, physician, and pharmacist who develop and implement a standardized patient teaching program. There is coordinated follow-up by a certified home health care agency as well as physician follow-up after discharge, and a means of monitoring and evaluating the effectiveness of and response to therapy.[22]

B. Evaluate potential candidates. Appropriate candidates should be given the choice of accepting or rejecting the program based on the teaching they receive. The degree of emotional stability, willingness to comply, family support systems, history of substance abuse, and motivation are important factors to assess. The patient will also need adequate manual dexterity to maneuver the equipment and perform the procedures. The home environment must be assessed and be conducive to meeting the patient's physical care needs. The availability of a responsible support person is highly desirable but not essential if the patient is able to manage the therapy effectively.[22]

(1) Appropriate candidates include those who have no need for additional hospitalization except for their intravenous therapy and who demonstrate clinical evidence that they are responding to the therapy without complications.[22] Patients should also have at least 7 days of remaining intravenous therapy for the program to be cost-effective.

C. Before discharge, assess the patient's knowledge, readiness, and ability to perform all phases of the treatment.[22]

(1) Teaching is necessary regarding the techniques of self-administered intravenous antibiotics. Whenever possible, premixed antibiotic solutions are used.

(2) Patients are frequently sent home with either a heparin lock or Hickman catheter.

(3) Patients need to be able to discuss thoroughly the potential complications, emergency measures, laboratory testing procedures, physician appointments after discharge, and physician/nurse availability for problem solving and questions.

D. After discharge, a nurse visits the patient in the home for the first antibiotic administration to ensure continuity of care and to provide reinforcement and emotional support.

(1) Additional visits are determined by the patient situation and the need to assess compliance, response to therapy, and to replace heparin locks. Heparin locks are changed every 48 to 72 hours by home care nurses[87] or by an intravenous nurse team when the patient returns to the hospital.[51] Insurance coverage is available for home intravenous therapy from most insurance companies.[22]

The results of home intravenous therapy are dramatic. In one study of 12 patients receiving intravenous therapy at home, a total savings of $109,767 (mean of $9,114/patient) was realized, and the length of hospital stay was reduced by a total of 260 days.[22] Home intravenous therapy allows patients to become active participants in their own care and gain tangible control of their therapy. Patients contract for self-care responsibility and learn the necessary techniques involved. They are

(continued)

NURSING CARE PLAN SUMMARY   *Patient With Infective Endocarditis*   Continued

Patient Outcomes	*Nursing Orders*
	able to return home and resume a more normal life-style. The psychologic experience of being in control and returning to an environment that is preferred clearly could augment physiologic recovery. These programs have demonstrated a safe, effective, and economical alternative to in-hospital intravenous therapy. Nurses have the ability to develop and coordinate such programs. We encourage nurses to accept this challenge.

NURSING DIAGNOSIS

2. *Decreased cardiac output related to complications of infected heart valve (name valve) (exchanging pattern)*

Patient Outcomes

1. The patient will not experience any hemodynamic complications associated with the infected valve, such as decreased cardiac output manifested by anxiety, restlessness, loss of feeling of well-being, hypotension, tachycardia, decreased urinary output, elevated blood urea nitrogen level, cyanosis, cold and clammy skin, change in mentation, or change in the quality and intensity of the heart murmur; no major recurrent arterial emboli; and no persistent infection or infection refractory to antimicrobial therapy.

2. If complications of infective endocarditis arise or if the patient is at high risk for hemodynamic deterioration, the patient will be evaluated as a candidate for cardiac valve surgery.

Nursing Orders

1. Assess the patient frequently to determine the severity of the illness and identify clinical manifestations related to the following:
   A. The infection (temperature, blood cultures, and laboratory studies; see Table 28–1).
   B. Cardiac involvement (heart rate, regularity, rhythm, blood pressure, respiration, and heart murmur [if any]). Listen for new or changing murmur, and note when it occurs in the cardiac cycle (*i.e.,* is it systolic or diastolic?) and its pitch, intensity, duration, and radiation. Be alert for new organic murmurs due to rupture of a valve or torn chordae tendineae, fever, anemia, or hypermetabolism.
   C. Cardiac complications include the following:
      (1) Signs and symptoms of congestive heart failure as a complication of perforation, erosion, or rupture of the valve
      (2) Pericarditis or a pericardial friction rub
      (3) Clubbing of the proximal nail beds
      (4) A conduction disturbance, such as a prolonged PR interval, new left bundle branch block, or new right bundle branch block, or first-, second-, or third-degree atrioventricular heart block
      (5) Atrial fibrillation or flutter, or junctional or ventricular dysrhythmias
   D. Arterial embolism to the central nervous, cardiovascular, gastrointestinal, or genitourinary system (see Table 28–1).
   E. Immunologic derangements producing hypersensitivity reactions (see Table 28–1).

2. Continue to assess any changes in the patient's reaction to infection, cardiac manifestations, microembolic manifestations, or hypersensitivity reactions. If the patient experiences major complications from endocarditis or falls into the high-risk category, then evaluation for cardiac valve replacement is considered.[92] Prosthetic valve replacement is recommended for high-risk endocarditis patients because of the destructive and erosive complications that can lead to intractable congestive heart failure. The most important factor in determining if patients are candidates for surgery is their hemodynamic status.[20,96,97] Survival of high-risk patients is improved if surgery is done at the first signs of cardiac failure rather than waiting until cardiac function is severely impaired.[2,59,67,88] If the patient is severely ill, valve replacement may be done during the active stage of infection and may be undertaken after only one preoperative dose of antimicrobial medication is given.[52] Antimicrobial therapy is continued after surgery.
   A. Carefully assess other high-risk patients. Those patients who are at high risk for intractable heart failure include patients with the following: aortic valve endocarditis,[35,58,59,71] mitral valve endocarditis,[9,31] *Staphylococcus aureus* endocarditis,[58,69,73] gram-negative bacilli endocarditis, fungal endocarditis,

(continued)

NURSING CARE PLAN SUMMARY   *Patient With Infective Endocarditis*   Continued

Patient Outcomes	*Nursing Orders*
	prosthetic valve endocarditis, recurrent arterial emboli, persistent infection, and severe hemodynamic deterioration.[9,52,59,68]
	B. Report any signs of cardiac decompensation, persistent infection, or major embolic phenomenon immediately to the physician. Prepare the patient for preoperative testing and cardiac valve replacement surgery (see Chap. 26). Cardiac valve replacement is done to eradicate the infection, to eliminate the source of emboli, and to treat heart failure that is refractory to medical therapy.[27,30,38,68] The surgery involves excising the infected tissue, unroofing any abscesses, and correcting the valvular lesion by replacing it with a prosthetic valve.[52,62]
	C. Assess less severely ill patients who might be candidates for valve reconstruction, repair, or vegetectomy.
	(1) Although tricuspid valve endocarditis (commonly a disease of intravenous drug abusers) is caused by a highly virulent organism, it frequently responds well to antibiotic therapy and is associated with a good prognosis.[17] About one quarter of the cases, however, require surgical intervention.[17] Recent reports have suggested that patients with right-sided endocarditis who fail medical therapy but who have localized infection can successfully undergo valve reconstruction or reparative approaches, such as valvuloplasty, because of the low right-sided intracardiac pressures and the three-leaflet configuration of right-sided heart valves.[99,100]
	(2) Vegetectomy or local excision of the vegetation with leaflet repair has also been reported for patients with well-circumscribed vegetations with little or no valve damage.[28,42]
	D. Reinforce and clarify the physician's explanation for surgery.
	E. Assess the patient's and family's reaction and stress levels with regard to the impending surgery.
	F. Assist the patient in practicing relaxation exercises and imagery before and after the surgery.

NURSING DIAGNOSIS

3. *High risk for complications of infection or phlebitis related to intravenous therapy (exchanging pattern)*

Patient Outcomes	*Nursing Orders*
1. The patient will not experience any complications related to intravenous therapy, such as thrombophlebitis, cellulitis, or occult intravenous site infection, as manifested by erythematous skin over an indurated or tender vein, or pus, inflammation, induration, swelling, heat, or bleeding near the insertion site or over the vein.	1. Implement the following nursing care measures to reduce the risk of complications from intravenous therapy:[33,54,82]
	A. Specially trained intravenous teams are recommended to insert, maintain, and replace intravenous needles or cannulas to reduce the risk of infection.
	B. Examine all bags and bottles for precipitates or turbidity. Examine bottles for cracks, and check that bottles have a vacuum when opened. Bags should be gently squeezed for leaks.
	C. Wash hands and maintain strict aseptic technique while preparing for and giving intravenous therapy.
	D. Prepare the patient's skin for venipuncture by shaving any hair and using tincture of iodine (a solution of 2% iodine in 70% alcohol). After at least a 30-second drying time, wash off the iodine solution with 70% isopropyl alcohol. Apply the solutions with friction, working from the center to the periphery.
	E. Use "scalp vein" or stainless steel needles when possible in an attempt to reduce the incidence of catheter-related infection and phlebitis.
	F. Upper extremities are preferred for catheter placement.

(continued)

NURSING CARE PLAN SUMMARY *Patient With Infective Endocarditis* *Continued*

Patient Outcomes	*Nursing Orders*
	G. Tape the needle or cannula securely to avoid to-and-fro motion, which could transport bacteria into the insertion site.
	H. Apply a topical polyantibiotic ointment and a sterile dressing. The dressing, not the tape, should cover the wound.
	I. Write the needle or cannula size, date, time, and site of venipuncture on the dressing and in the patient's chart or care plan.
	J. Use infusion pumps for administering a continuous 24-hour antimicrobial intravenous solution.
	K. Although intravenous terminal membrane filters do not reduce infections related to intravenous therapy, they have been recommended to block particulate matter and prevent a variety of noninfectious complications of intravenous therapy.[82]
	L. Single-use (single-dose) containers (vials) should be used for admixtures whenever possible.[82] If the patient complains of discomfort associated with the antibiotic infusion, reassure the patient and further dilute the medication or administer the solution a little more slowly.
	M. Refrigerate any admixed intravenous fluids until used. Use solutions as soon as possible after opening.
	N. Label all intravenous solutions after opening with the patient's name and date of opening. Add a supplementary label naming any admixtures, the dose, the date and time it was mixed, the expiration date, and the name of the person who mixed the solution. Disinfect injection port before adding medications.
	O. Maintain an accurate intravenous therapy fluid record on the patient's chart (include time, date, when each solutions was started and discontinued, the type of fluid, amount of additive, rate of administration, and amount of medication and fluid received).
	P. Replace all intravenous solutions every 24 hours.
	Q. Replace the intravenous tubing, extension sets, and administration sets every 24 hours and when the intravenous solution is changed. All tubing and solutions should be changed when the catheter is replaced. All tubings should be changed after the administration of blood, blood products, or lipid emulsion. Label the new tubing with the time and date.
	R. Palpate the insertion site through the intact dressing every 24 hours. (The use of transparent dressings may be useful so that the site can be both palpated and inspected every 24 hours without removing the dressing.)[54] If the patient has unexplained fever, pain, or tenderness, remove the dressing and inspect the site for signs and symptoms of phlebitis or infection. If the catheter insertion was traumatic, the nurse should record that fact on the notes and observe the insertion site even more carefully using the protocol just described.
	S. Replace all needles or plastic cannulas every 48 to 72 hours. Alternate sites, if possible.
	T. If peripheral needles or cannulas remain in place for prolonged periods, inspect the intravenous site, cleanse the site with iodine and alcohol, and change the sterile dressing at 48 to 72 hours. The time and date of the dressing change should be written on the dressing. Thereafter, inspect the site and reapply antibiotic ointment and a new sterile dressing every 24 hours.
	U. Avoid flushing or irrigating the intravenous line.
	V. Blood samples should not be withdrawn through the intravenous tubing except in emergencies or when the cannula and tubing will be discontinued immediately.
	W. At the first sign of infection or phlebitis, insert a new needle or catheter and remove the old one. Assess the patient carefully for potential catheter-related complications, such as systemic infection, fever, and septicemia, and document and report this information.

(continued)

NURSING CARE PLAN SUMMARY   *Patient With Infective Endocarditis*   *Continued*

Patient Outcomes	Nursing Orders
	X. If infection is suspected and associated with a plastic catheter, do the following: (1) Discontinue the intravenous solution. (2) Remove the catheter by thoroughly cleansing the venipuncture site with alcohol and allowing the alcohol to dry before aseptically removing the catheter from the vein without allowing it to touch the skin. Clip off the tip of the catheter with a sterile scissors, place it in a blood culture tube, and send it to the laboratory for analysis. Report the findings to the physician. Purulent drainage around the venipuncture site should be gram stained and cultured. Y. If contamination of the intravenous solution is suspected, discontinue the solution, culture the fluid, save the bottle, and notify local health officials, the Center for Disease Control in Atlanta, GA, and the Food and Drug Administration.
2. The patient will participate in range-of-motion exercise.	2. Assist the patient in passive and active range-of-motion exercises of the involved extremity every 2 hours.
3. If complications of the intravenous therapy arise, the patient will respond to the appropriate therapy.	3. If intravenous complications arise, institute therapy appropriate for the problem (warm soaks, heating pads, elevation of the extremity, administration of antipyretics, analgesics, or appropriate antimicrobial medications).[33,49,65]

NURSING DIAGNOSIS

4. *Anxiety related to diagnostic testing, acute illness, and prolonged treatment (feeling pattern)*[38]

Patient Outcome	Nursing Orders
1. The patient will demonstrate reduced anxiety levels, as demonstrated by the following: A. The patient will verbalize questions, concerns, and stressors. B. The patient will participate in and practice relaxation, imagery, or music therapy for 20 minutes twice a day (see Chap. 3, p. 34). C. The patient will demonstrate reduction in levels of stress from baseline data (see Chap. 3, pp. 34–36). (1) Lowering of heart rate (2) Raising of finger temperatures (3) Verbal reports of greater feelings of calmness and relaxation and reduced feelings of isolation and helplessness	1. See Chapter 3, page 34).

NURSING DIAGNOSIS

5. *High risk for noncompliance to medical regimen related to inadequate knowledge of illness and future prophylactic care (choosing pattern)*[38,98]

Patient Outcome	Nursing Orders
1. Patients will verbalize knowledge of endocarditis, the medical regimen, and	1. Teach the patient (and family) about endocarditis.[1,37,46,98] The teaching should include information related to the following:

(continued)

NURSING CARE PLAN SUMMARY *Patient With Infective Endocarditis* Continued

Patient Outcome	Nursing Orders
methods of prophylactic care. Patients will do the following: A. Discuss the normal function of the heart, valves, and circulation. B. Define endocarditis, identify which valve is involved, and why they are susceptible to the illness. C. Describe the valvular changes that occur with endocarditis and the susceptibility to reinfection. D. Describe the signs and symptoms of endocarditis. E. Demonstrate how to take their own oral temperature, and state the need for taking and recording temperatures daily after discharge for 1 month. F. List the possible portals of entry for a potential reinfecting organism. G. Demonstrate techniques of good oral hygiene, and discuss avoidance of devices that cause gum trauma. H. State the need for regular dental checkups. I. Discuss the need for prophylactic antibiotics before and after dental or surgical manipulations or procedures.	A. The normal functioning of the heart, the heart valves (use heart models and drawings), and circulation B. A definition of endocarditis, which valve is involved, and why the patient is susceptible to it. (Susceptible patients are those who have a history of endocarditis, rheumatic, congenital, or degenerative heart disease that has produced valvular deformities, other cardiac defects, or those with prosthetic heart valves.) C. The pathophysiologic changes associated with endocarditis and the patient's susceptibility to reinfection D. The signs and symptoms of endocarditis, such as chills, fever, sweating, fatigue, weight loss, and anorexia, and the necessity of contacting a physician at the first sign of fever or reinfection E. Directions about taking and recording one's own temperature daily for 1 month F. The portals of entry for the infecting organism (see Assessment, p. 520). (1) Sites of dental problems (2) Skin lesions (3) Infections (4) Sites of surgical procedures (5) Sites of invasive tests or manipulations G. Good oral hygiene, which consists of brushing the teeth twice a day with a soft-bristled toothbrush, using a firm, gentle motion, and avoiding trauma to the gums. The patient should also be told not to use a Water-Pik, dental floss, toothpicks, or any other devices that might cause the gums to bleed. Flossing the teeth can promote good oral hygiene and healthy gums; therefore, this precaution remains somewhat controversial.[38,46] H. The importance of regular dental examinations (even for patients who wear dentures) I. The need for antimicrobial prophylactic care before procedures listed in 1F above. Patients must understand that antibiotics are given shortly before, not several days before, the procedure. Many procedures require that antibiotics also be given after the procedure. It is important to note that the prophylactic regimen for rheumatic fever is different from that for preventing endocarditis.[1] Thus, for patients on antibiotics to prevent recurrences of acute rheumatic fever, additional antibiotics are necessary when undergoing surgery or other high-risk procedures. Despite the widely publicized guidelines distributed by the American Heart Association regarding recommendations for prophylaxis against endocarditis, recent studies have documented low compliance to these guidelines by both physicians and dentists.[13,29,64,77,78] Inconsistencies have been reported regarding the selection, dosage, and timing of the appropriate antibiotics by dentists caring for patients at high risk for developing endocarditis.[64,77,78] Physician compliance regarding antibiotic prophylaxis (as recommended by the American Heart Association) for patients with prosthetic valves who are undergoing high-risk diagnostic or operative procedures was only 30% in one study.[13] These studies suggest a lack of knowledge or understanding by the physician, dentist, and patient regarding the need for antibiotic prophylaxis and the danger of bacteremia associated with certain procedures. Undoubtedly, the impracticality of administering the prophylactic antibiotic intravenously in the physician's or dentist's office or the need to hospitalize patients for parenteral antibiotics for procedures

(continued)

NURSING CARE PLAN SUMMARY   *Patient With Infective Endocarditis*   *Continued*

Patient Outcomes	*Nursing Orders*
	that are generally done on an outpatient basis has been an important factor influencing the compliance rate.[6,29] An advisory committee of the American Heart Association is currently formulating new guidelines for the prevention of endocarditis that are likely to recommend the use of oral prophylactic antibiotics.
	(1) Patients must understand that it is their responsibility to inform their physician and dentist about their history of valvular heart disease or endocarditis. Patients should be encouraged to be assertive about asking the physician or dentist their plans for antimicrobial prophylaxis before and after invasive procedures and whether such a regimen is in compliance with the American Heart Association guidelines. The patient should be given and be able to discuss the information published by the American Heart Association in *Prevention of Endocarditis*.[1] This booklet discusses what groups of people are susceptible to endocarditis, lists the dental and medical procedures and instrumentations that are associated with the development of bacteremia, and suggests dosages for prophylactic antimicrobial therapy.
J. For women of childbearing age who are at high risk for developing endocarditis: Discuss antibiotic prophylaxis during labor, delivery, cesarean section, or therapeutic abortion.	J. For high-risk patients of childbearing age, the risk of infection during childbirth. Pregnant women who are at high risk for developing endocarditis should be told about the need for antimicrobial prophylaxis during labor, delivery, cesarean section, or therapeutic abortion.
K. For patients who are intravenous drug abusers: Discuss the high incidence of recurrent endocarditis, and express the need to enroll in a drug rehabilitation program.	K. For patients who are intravenous drug abusers, the high incidence of recurrent endocarditis.[3] The issue of drug abuse must be dealt with, and every effort must be made to help the patient understand the multiple dangers of drug addiction, including recurrent endocarditis. Every attempt must be made to have patients enroll in a drug rehabilitation program.
L. Describe their inpatient and outpatient activity schedules, and state reasons for no strenuous work, competitive sports, or activities for 1 month after discharge.	L. Restricted activities (no strenuous activities or competitive sports for 1 month to help the healing process). Provide the patient with a written inpatient and outpatient progressive activity schedule (a modified acute myocardial infarction activity program can be used).
M. Discuss stress reduction and relaxation techniques. Emphasize the potentially improved healing process and why these techniques should be practiced at home after discharge.	M. Stress reduction and relaxation techniques, which may enhance the healing process and should be continued at home
N. Explain and successfully demonstrate techniques of home intravenous therapy (see p. 527).	N. Techniques related to home intravenous therapy (see p. 527)
O. State where and when to return for blood tests.	O. The necessity of returning for follow-up blood culture studies every 2 weeks for 6 weeks after the completion of antimicrobial therapy
P. State the names and telephone numbers of their primary care nurse and cardiologist or clinic.	P. The name and phone number of the attending cardiologist or clinic and the primary care nurse. Encourage the patient to call with questions or problems.

IMPLEMENTATION AND EVALUATION

Implementation of care involves carrying out the nursing and medical orders, including blood culture studies to identify the infecting organism; administration of antimicrobial therapy for a long enough time to bring about sterilization of the vegetations; assessment and prevention of severe hemodynamic deteriorization; prevention of iatrogenic complications; and teaching the patient and family about the illness.[4,19]

The effectiveness of patient care is determined by evaluating each of the patient outcomes as previously described. Although the primary management of endocarditis involves the use of antibiotic therapy, prosthetic valve replacement is used to treat patients in whom antimicrobial therapy fails to eradicate the disease or in whom lethal complications develop. For such patients who do not meet the expected patient outcomes, a new patient care plan must be developed to reflect the patient's current status, and the patient outcomes must be revised. After surgery, these patients require education regarding both a cardiovascular rehabilitation and an endocarditis prophylaxis program. All patients should be assisted and encouraged to continue their relaxation exercises during hospitalization and after discharge.

SUMMARY

The critical care nurse must understand the etiology, pathophysiology, diagnosis, and treatment of infective endocarditis. A thorough understanding of the illness enables the nurse to play an important role in the assessment and management of patients with infective endocarditis as well as in its prevention.

DIRECTIONS FOR FUTURE RESEARCH

Research questions that nurses may consider for improving care of infective endocarditis patients are the following:

1. What are the effects of daily practicing music therapy on level of anxiety, length of hospitalization, and complication rate of infective endocarditis patients?
2. What is the most effective home intravenous therapy program that can be implemented to permit infective endocarditis patients to be discharged from the hospital earlier and continue intravenous therapy at home?
3. What is the difference in the intravenous complication rate between patients who receive intravenous therapy in the hospital versus those who receive it at home?
4. What are effective teaching methods to enhance understanding of and compliance with treatments used for patients with infective endocarditis?

REFERENCES

1. American Heart Association. *Prevention of Bacterial Endocarditis.* Dallas: National Center of the American Heart Association, 1985.
2. Aslamaci, S., Dimitri, W. R., and Williams, B. T. Operative considerations in active native valve infective endocarditis. *J. Cardiovasc. Surg.* 30:328, 1989.
3. Baddour, L. M. Twelve-year review of recurrent native-valve infective endocarditis: A disease of the modern antibiotic era. *Rev. Infect. Dis.* 10:1163, 1988.
4. Barry, J., and Gump, D. W. Endocarditis: An overview. *Heart Lung* 11:138, 1982.
5. Bayer, A. S., and Theofilopoulos, A. N. Immunopathogenetic aspects of infective endocarditis. *Chest* 97:204, 1990.
6. Bayer, A. S. New concepts in the pathogenesis and modalities of the chemoprophylaxis of native valve endocarditis. *Chest* 96:893, 1989.
7. Bayer, A. S. Staphylococcal bacteremia: Distinguishing endocarditis. *Am. Fam. Physician* 19:147, 1979.
8. Bayer, A. S., Theofilopoulos, A. N., Eisenberg, R., *et al.* Circulating immune complexes in infective endocarditis. *N. Engl. J. Med.* 295:1500, 1976.
9. Becker, R. M., Frishman, W., and Frater, R. W. M. Surgery for mitral valve endocarditis. *Chest* 75:314, 1979.
10. Bisno, A. L., Dismukes, W. E., Durack, D. T., *et al.* Antimicrobial treatment of infective endocarditis due to viridans streptococci, enterococci, and staphylococci. *J.A.M.A.* 261:1471, 1989.
11. Blumsohn, D. Clubbing of the fingers, with special reference to Schamroth's diagnostic method. *Heart Lung* 10:1069, 1981.
12. Bornstein, D. L. Bacterial Endocarditis. In H. L. Conn and O. Horwitz (eds.), *Cardiac and Vascular Diseases.* Philadelphia: Lea & Febiger, 1971.
13. Brooks, R. G., Notariom, F., and McCabe, R. E. Hospital survey of antimicrobial prophylaxis to prevent endocarditis in patients with prosthetic heart valves. *Am. J. Med.* 84:617, 1988.
14. Bryan, C. S., *et al.* Endocarditis related to transvenous pacemakers: Syndromes and surgical implications. *J. Thorac. Cardiovasc. Surg.* 75:758, 1978.
15. Cabane, J., *et al.* Fate of circulating immune complexes in infective endocarditis. *Am. J. Med.* 66:277, 1979.
16. Cassey, J. I., and Miller, M. H. Infective endocarditis: II. Current therapy. *Am. Heart J.* 96:263, 1978.
17. Chan, P. I., Ogilby, J. D., and Segal, B. Tricuspid valve endocarditis. *Am. Heart J.* 117:1140, 1989.
18. Christopherson, D. J., and Sivarajan Froelicher, E. S. Infective Endocarditis. In S. L. Underhill, S. L. Woods, E. S. Sivarajan Froelicher, *et al.* (eds.), *Cardiac Nursing* (2nd ed.). Philadelphia: J. B. Lippincott, 1989.
19. Clemens, J. D. *et al.* A controlled evaluation of the risk of bacterial endocarditis in persons with mitral valve prolapse. *N. Engl. J. Med.* 307:776, 1982.
20. Cohen, P. S., Maguire, J. H., and Weinstein, L. Infective endocarditis caused by gram-negative bacteria: A review of the literature, 1945–1977. *Prog. Cardiovasc. Dis.* 22:205, 1980.
21. Cohle, S. D., Graham, M. A., Sperry, K. L., *et al.* Unexpected death as a result of infective endocarditis. *J. Forensic Sci.* 34:1374, 1989.
22. Corby, D., Schad, R. F., and Fudge, J. P. Intravenous antibiotic therapy: Hospital to home. *Nurs. Manag.* 17:52, 1986.
23. Crespo, J. Dialysis-related infections. *Heart Lung* 11:111, 1982.
24. Danchin, N., Voiriot, P., Briancon, S., *et al.* Mitral valve prolapse as a risk factor for infective endocarditis. *Lancet* 1:743, 1989.
25. Downham, W. H., and Rhoades, E. R. Endocarditis associated with porcine valve xenografts. *Arch. Intern. Med.* 139:1350, 1979.
26. Ehrie, M., *et al.* Endocarditis with the indwelling balloon-tipped pulmonary artery catheter in burn patients. *J. Trauma* 18:664, 1978.
27. Everett, E. D. Infective endocarditis. *Mo. Med.* 75:167, 1978.
28. Evora, P. R., Brasil, J. C., Elias, M. L., *et al.* Surgical excision of the vegetation as treatment of tricuspid valve endocarditis. *Cardiology* 75:287, 1988.
29. Finkelmeier, B. A., Hartz, R. S., Fisher, E. B., *et al.* Implications of prosthetic valve implantation: An 8-year follow-up of patients with porcine bioprostheses. *Heart Lung* 18:565, 1989.
30. Finland, M. Current problems in infective endocarditis. *Mod. Concepts Cardiovasc. Dis.* 16:53, 1972.
31. Fowler, N. O., and Van Der Bel-Kahn, J. M. Indications for surgical replacement of the mitral valve. *Am. J. Cardiol.* 44:148, 1979.
32. Garvey, G. J., and Neu, H. C. Infective endocarditis: An evolving disease. *Medicine* 57:105, 1978.
33. Goldmann, D. A., Maki, D. G., Rhame, F. S., *et al.* Guidelines for infection control in intravenous therapy. *Ann. Intern. Med.* 79:848, 1973.
34. Greene, J. F., Fitzwater, J. E., and Clemmer, T. P. Septic endocarditis and indwelling pulmonary artery catheters. *J.A.M.A.* 233:891, 1975.
35. Gregoratos, G., and Karliner, J. S. Infective endocarditis: Diagnosis and management. *Med. Clin. North Am.* 63:173, 1979.
36. Grehl, T. M., Cohn, L. H., and Angell, W. W. Management of *Candida* endocarditis. *J. Thorac. Cardiovasc. Surg.* 63:118, 1972.
37. Guzman, L. Nursing management of the parenteral drug abuser with infective endocarditis. *Heart Lung* 10:289, 1981.
38. Guzzetta, C. E. The Person with Infective Endocarditis. In C. E.

Guzzetta and B. M. Dossey, *Cardiovascular Nursing: Bodymind Tapestry.* St. Louis: C. V. Mosby, 1984.

39. Heffner, J. E. Extracardiac manifestations of bacterial endocarditis. *West. J. Med.* 131:85, 1979.

40. Heimberger, T. S., and Duma, R. J. Infections of prosthetic heart valves and cardiac pacemakers. *Infect. Dis. Clin. North Am.* 3: 221, 1989.

41. Hollanders, G., DeScheerder, I., De Buyzere, M., et al. A six years' review of 53 cases of infective endocarditis: Clinical, microbiological, and therapeutical features. *Acta. Cardiol.* 43:121, 1988.

42. Hughes, C. F., and Noble, N. Vegetectomy: An alternative surgical treatment for infective endocarditis of the atrioventricular valves in drug addicts. *J. Thorac. Cardiovasc. Surg.* 95:857, 1988.

43. Hutter, A. M., and Moellering, R. C. Assessment of the patient with suspected endocarditis. *J.A.M.A.* 235:1603, 1976.

44. Infective endocarditis with negative blood cultures [editorial]. *Br. Med. J.* 2:4, 1979.

45. Irvin, R. G., and Sade, R. M. Endocarditis and musculoskeletal manifestations. *Ann. Intern. Med.* 88:578, 1978.

46. Kaplan, E. L., Anthony, B. F., Bisno, A. L., et al. Prevention of bacterial endocarditis (American Heart Association Committee Report). *Circulation* 56:139A, 1977.

47. Kaplan, E. L., et al. A collaborative study of infective endocarditis in the 1970s. *Circulation* 59:327, 1979.

48. Karchmer, A. W., et al. Late prosthetic valve endocarditis: Clinical features influencing therapy. *Am. J. Med.* 64:200, 1978.

49. Kaye, W. Catheter- and infusion-related sepsis: The nature of the problem and its prevention. *Heart Lung* 11:221, 1982.

50. Khoo, D. E., Zebro, T. J., and English, T. A. Bacterial endocarditis in a transplanted heart. *Pathol. Res. Pract.* 185:445, 1989.

51. Kind, A. C., et al. Intravenous antibiotic therapy at home. *Arch. Intern. Med.* 139:413, 1979.

52. Kinsley, R. H., Colsen, P. R., and Bakst, A. Emergency valve replacement for primary infective endocarditis. *S. Afr. Med. J.* 53:86, 1978.

53. Kluge, R. M. Infections of prosthetic cardiac valves and arterial grafts. *Heart Lung* 11:146, 1982.

54. Lenox, A. C. IV therapy: Reducing the risk of infection. *Nurs. '90* March:60, 1990.

55. Marrie, T. J. Infective endocarditis: A serious and changing disease. *Crit. Care Nurs.* 7:31, 1987.

56. Maschak, B. J. Patient education and prevention of endocarditis. *Nurs. Clin. North Am.* 11:319, 1976.

57. Mathewson, M. A. Prolapsed mitral valve syndrome. *Am. J. Nurs.* 80:1431, 1980.

58. May, J. M., et al. S. aureus endocarditis: A review and plea for early surgery. *Virol. Med.* 106:829, 1979.

59. McAnulty, J. H., and Rahimtoola, S. H. Surgery for infective endocarditis. *J.A.M.A.* 242:77, 1979.

60. McNeill, K. M., Strong, J. E., and Lockwood, W. R. Bacterial endocarditis: An analysis of factors affecting long-term survival. *Am. Heart J.* 95:448, 1978.

61. Miller, M. H., and Casey, J. I. Infective endocarditis: New diagnostic techniques. *Am. Heart J.* 96:123, 1978.

62. Mills, S. A. Surgical management of infective endocarditis. *Ann. Surg.* 195:367, 1982.

63. Mintz, G. S., et al. Survival of patients with aortic valve endocarditis: The prognostic implications of the echocardiogram. *Arch. Intern. Med.* 139:862, 1979.

64. Nelson, C. L., and Van Blaricum, C. S. Physician and dentist compliance with American Heart Association guidelines for prevention of bacterial endocarditis. *J. Am. Dent. Assoc.* 118:169, 1989.

65. Oakley, C. Use of antibiotics. *Br. Med. J.* 2:489, 1978.

66. Pace, N. L., and Horton, W. L. Indwelling pulmonary catheters: The relationship to aseptic thrombotic endocardial vegetations. *J.A.M.A.* 233:893, 1975.

67. Pankey, G. A. The prevention and treatment of bacterial endocarditis. *Am. Heart J.* 98:102, 1979.

68. Parrott, J. C., Hill, J. D., Kerth, W. J., et al. The surgical management of bacterial endocarditis: A review. *Ann. Surg.* 183:289, 1976.

69. Pesanti, E. L., and Smith, J. M. Infective endocarditis with negative blood cultures. *Am. J. Med.* 66:43, 1979.

70. Phair, J. P., and Clarke, J. Immunology of infective endocarditis. *Prog. Cardiovasc. Dis.* 22:137, 1979.

71. Rapaport, E. The changing roles of surgery in the management of infective endocarditis [editorial]. *Circulation* 58:598, 1978.

72. Reagan, T. J. Cerebral ischemia in nonbacterial thrombotic endocarditis. *Curr. Concepts Cerebrovasc. Dis.* 10:13, 1975.

73. Richardson, J. V., et al. Treatment of infective endocarditis: A 10-year comparative analysis. *Circulation* 58:589, 1978.

74. Roberts, K. B., and Sidlak, M. J. Satellite streptococci: A major cause of "negative" blood cultures in bacterial endocarditis. *J.A.M.A.* 241:2293, 1979.

75. Roberts, N. K., Child, J. S., and Cabeen, W. R. Infective endocarditis and the cardiac conducting system. *West. J. Med.* 129: 254, 1978.

76. Rodbard, S. Blood velocity and endocarditis. *Circulation* 27:18, 1963.

77. Sadowsky, D., and Kunzel, C. Usual and customary practice versus the recommendations of experts: Clinician noncompliance in the prevention of bacterial endocarditis. *J. Am. Dent. Assoc.* 118:175, 1989.

78. Sadowsky, D., and Kunzel, C. Recommendations for prevention of bacterial endocarditis: Compliance by dental general practitioners. *Circulation* 77:1316, 1988.

79. Sande, M. A., Johnson, W. D., Hook, E. W., et al. Sustained bacteremia in patients with prosthetic cardiac valves. *N. Engl. J. Med.* 286:1067, 1972.

80. Sasaki, T. M., et al. The relationship of central venous and pulmonary artery catheter position to acute right-sided endocarditis in severe thermal injury. *J. Trauma* 19:740, 1979.

81. Scrima, D. A. Infective endocarditis: Nursing considerations. *Crit. Care Nurs.* 7:47, 1987.

82. Simmons, B. P. CDC guidelines for the prevention and control of nosocomial infections: Guideline for prevention of intravascular infections. *Am. J. Infect. Control* 11:183, 1983.

83. Spaccavento, L. J., and Hawley, H. B. Infections associated with intraarterial lines. *Heart Lung* 11:118, 1982.

84. Sperry, R. Lateral Specialization of Cerebral Function in the Surgically Separated Hemispheres. In F. McGuigan (ed.), *The Psychology of Thinking.* New York: Academic Press, 1973.

85. Sperry, R. Interhemispheric Relationships: The Neocortical Commissures: Syndromes of Hemisphere Disconnection. In P. Vinken (ed.), *Handbook of Clinical Neurology.* Amsterdam: North Holland Publishing Co., 1969.

86. Sperry, R. Hemispheric disconnection and unity in conscious awareness. *Am. Psychol.* 23:723, 1968.

87. Stiver, H. G., et al. Intravenous antibiotic therapy at home. *Ann. Intern. Med.* 89:690, 1978.

88. Stulz, P., Pfisterer, M., Jenzer, J. R., et al. Emergency valve replacement for active infective endocarditis. *J. Cardiovasc. Surg.* 30:20, 1989.

89. Terpenning, M. S., Buggy, B. P., and Kauffman, C. A. Hospital acquired infective endocarditis. *Arch. Intern. Med.* 148:1601, 1988.

90. Ward, C., Naik, D. R., and Johnstone, M. C. Tricuspid endocarditis complicating pacemaker implantation demonstrated by echocardiography. *Br. J. Radiol.* 52:501, 1979.

91. Watanakunakorn, C. Infective endocarditis as a result of medical progress. *Am. J. Med.* 64:917, 1978.

92. Weinstein, L. Modern infective endocarditis. *J.A.M.A.* 233:260, 1975.

93. Weinstein, L., and Schlesinger, J. J. Pathoanatomic, pathophysiologic and clinical correlations in endocarditis. Part I. *N. Engl. J. Med.* 291:832, 1974.

94. Weinstein, L., and Schlesinger, J. J. Pathoanatomic, pathophysiologic and clinical correlations in endocarditis. Part II. *N. Engl. J. Med.* 291:1122, 1974.

95. Williams, R. C. Subacute bacterial endocarditis as an immune disease. *Hosp. Pract.* 6:111, 1971.

96. Wilson, W. R., *et al.* Valve replacement in patients with active infective endocarditis. *Circulation* 58:585, 1978.

97. Wilson, W. R., *et al.* Cardiac valve replacement in congestive heart failure due to infective endocarditis. *Mayo Clin. Proc.* 54: 223, 1979.

98. Wingate, S. Rehabilitation of the patent with valvular heart disease. *J. Cardiovasc. Nurs.* 1:52, 1987.

99. Yee, E. S., and Khonsari, S. Right-sided infective endocarditis: Valvuloplasty, valvectomy or replacement. *J. Cardiovasc. Surg.* 30:744, 1989.

100. Yee, E. S., and Ullyot, D. J. Reparative approach for right-sided endocarditis. Operative consideration and results of valvuloplasty. *J. Thorac. Cardiovasc. Surg.* 96:133, 1988.

VI

The Critically Ill Adult With Neurologic and Neurosurgical Problems

RECOGNIZING YOUR HEALING JOURNEY

As you become more aware of where you are on your personal healing journey, you are better able to assist yourself or others with peace in living and dying. As you recognize and honor your spirit, a sense of healing awareness emerges. This makes you more aware of being authentic, that is, of being consistent, in each lived moment, with what you believe to be true. Authenticity allows for harmony in your actions, behaviors, thoughts, and feelings. When you participate from your spiritual nature and healing awareness, consciously or unconsciously, the experience is translated and evoked in yourself and others. Living from authenticity, you are in a better position to act with intention and clear purpose and to have the freedom to create choices and rituals that can empower your life. You must be willing to explore and acknowledge your inner wisdom as a first step on your journey toward wholeness.

Answer or begin a process of answer the following questions:

- What is caring?
- How do people show caring?
- What is showing care?
- How do you care for yourself?
- What is goodness to you?
- How do people show goodness?
- Why do you think it is so hard to see goodness?
- What is forgiveness?
- Can you forgive yourself and others?

29

Neurologic Assessment

Cornelia Vanderstaay Kenner

TAKING CARE OF YOURSELF

Being a critical care nurse is intense, requires attention, and can be draining. To be present for yourself or another, you must honor your personal needs or you will be a physical and emotional wreck. What are the current circumstances in your life? Accept them. Release control of things over which you have no control. Honor yourself each day. You might daily practice quality quiet time with relaxation, imagery, music, meditation, or prayer, which assist in the process of letting go. Create an exercise program, take long, hot baths or showers, eat nutritious foods, eliminate excess caffeine or junk food, and ask other people for help if needed. Tell yourself over and over what a good job you are doing. Repeat it until you believe it.

Caring for yourself each day requires simple things. When waking up in the morning and before getting out of bed, ask yourself "The part of me that is most in need of healing right now is . . ." and "The things that I can do to bring about my healing are. . . ." The answers are usually simple, such as "I need to take a morning break and a lunch break, have a massage or take a walk, or ask a friend to meet me for lunch." Repeat this as often as necessary during the day. This increases your awareness of your human spirit. By honoring yourself, you allow fear, depression, aloneness, suffering, feelings of discouragement, crisis, or tragic moments to be released so that being with yourself or another is quality time.

LEARNING OBJECTIVES

After reading this chapter, the nurse should be able to do the following:

1. List the tests for the functioning of the cranial nerves and reflexes, cerebellum, motor system, and sensory system.
2. Develop an assessment tool for the neurologic examination of the eyes to be used for examining both conscious and unconscious patients.
3. Write a paragraph describing the major points in the assessment of consciousness.
4. Compare and contrast the possible respiratory patterns exhibited by the patient.
5. List the assessment findings in common pathophysiologic conditions.
6. Differentiate decorticate from decerebrate posture.
7. Develop nursing orders for the patient for whom the neurologist or neurosurgeon has ordered diagnostic studies.
8. Compare and contrast the interviewing techniques used for two types of patients admitted to the critical care unit: the patient with ascending paralysis and the patient with head injuries.

9. Monitor the physiologic parameters that are relevant to patients with neurological dysfunction.

HISTORY

The *chief complaint* is a precise statement of the patient's subjective problem. The details may have to be elicited from others if the patient has a mental impairment.

History of the Present Illness

The history of the present illness consists of an in-depth description of the problems of greatest concern. The patient's own evaluation should include strengths, deficiencies, what he or she thinks is happening, and what has helped the situation.

Past Medical History

The past medical history may be divided into perinatal, childhood, and adult history. Notation is made about any history of head trauma, meningitis, poliomyelitis, encephalitis, tuberculosis, otitis media, mastoiditis, venereal disease, viral infections, heavy alcohol consumption, and use of anticoagulants.

Family History

Many conditions have a familial incidence (*e.g.*, migraine headaches, diabetes, epilepsy, tremor, spinocerebellar degenerations, hereditary spastic paralysis, Huntington's chorea, and familial periodic paralysis). Symptoms and signs rather than names of diseases are elicited, because many illnesses may not have been diagnosed. Notation is also made about any history of psychiatric illness.

Review of Systems

In the review of systems and psychiatric problems, a quick determination is made of other problems. Patients are asked general questions, and if they answer in the affirmative, specific information is elicited.

- Central nervous system: Headache, syncope, seizures, vertigo, amaurosis (loss of vision), diplopia, paralysis, paresis, muscle weakness, tremor, ataxia, dysesthesia, fainting, drowsiness, insomnia, speech, memory, concentration, disorientation
- Eyes: Vision, scotomata, ptosis, reading difficulties, blinking
- Ears: Tinnitus, loss of hearing
- Nose, throat, and sinuses: Hoarseness
- Cardiorespiratory system: Tightness in the chest, palpitations
- Gastrointestinal system: Abnormalities of smell, taste, chewing, swallowing
- Urinary tract: Impairment of sphincter control, polyuria
- Reproductive system: Impotence, menstrual disturbances
- Musculoskeletal system: Motor disturbances of the face, trunk, extremities; sensory disturbances of the face, trunk, extremities; muscle weakness, muscle wasting, rigidity; problems in walking, or sitting
- Psychiatric: Hallucinations, hyperventilation, nervousness, depression, insomnia, nightmares, memory loss

Activities of Daily Living, Personal and Social History

To assemble a profile of the patient, a complete nursing history must be obtained. The history should include information about the patient's education, life-style, drug and alcohol intake, exposure to toxins, recent travels, and employment. It should be determined whether the patient finds his work interesting and enjoyable or stressful. If possible, the patient's relationship with his spouse and other family members as well as feelings, attitudes, goals, and frustrations should be assessed.

EXAMINATION

The neurologic examination is divided into broad areas for testing integrated functions: level of consciousness, mentation, respiratory pattern, cranial nerves, motor system, sensory system, coordination, and reflexes. This approach is the traditional one used to describe the neurologic examination. It is used throughout the chapter and is included in Figure 29–1. The general outline is as follows:

- Consciousness: Arousing
- Mentation: Thinking, remembering, feeling, use of language
- Motor: Seeing, eating, expressing, speaking, moving
- Sensory: Smelling, hearing, tasting, feeling (pain, touch, temperature, point discrimination)

For complete assessment, refer to the Critical Care Response Pattern Assessment Tool, Figure 5–2, page 59.

Consciousness

Consciousness or arousing is assessed with regard to level of consciousness and content of consciousness. Level of consciousness is principally controlled by the reticular-activating system in the brain stem. This system is analogous to an "off-on" switch with regard to consciousness, and it is subtentorial in location. The content of consciousness is controlled by the cerebral hemispheres, which are above the cerebellar tentorium.

To compare the patient's level of consciousness at one examination period with the level of consciousness at another period, it is best to describe the behavior of the patient, including information about spontaneous activity and responsiveness. Even if the nurse does not totally understand the significance of the findings, an accurate description is needed to make serial determinations and identify trends in the patient's status. Critically ill people often lose their orientation first to time, then to place, then to persons, but the exceptions are many.

The Glasgow Coma Scale is extremely helpful in assessing and monitoring the level of consciousness. It is simple, accurate, objective, reliable, and easy to use. Although several other coma scores are under investigation to increase the accuracy of trend determination, the Glasgow score (Table 29–1) is the standard.[11]

The following is a general description of the classic states of consciousness.[14] A precise delineation of each state is difficult, and most descriptions are subjective. For this reason, in clinical practice it is recommended that nurses use the Glasgow Coma Scale or one of its derivatives.

- The *alert, wakeful state* is characterized by much spontaneous activity and prompt, appropriate response to command.
- *Lethargy* is a state of drowsiness characterized by some spontaneous activity.
- *Obtundation* is a state of extreme drowsiness characterized by little spontaneous activity. The obtunded patient responds sluggishly and inconsistently to strong voice commands.
- *Stupor* is a state of extreme drowsiness characterized by a complete lack of spontaneous motor activity. The stuporous patient is aroused only by strong stimuli. Responses tend to be stereotyped and simplified.
- *Deep coma* is a state in which the patient cannot be aroused. It is not always easy to determine whether or not a person is in coma. An accurate description of the person's behavior is imperative.

It is important to determine whether the cause of the altered level of consciousness is structural or metabolic-toxic, the direction the disease process is taking, and what part of the brain might be the most affected.

Mentation
1. Thinking _____
2. Remembering _____
3. Feeling _____
4. Language _____

Motor
1. Seeing: O.D. _____
   O.S. _____
   Confrontation fields _____
   Palpebral fissures _____
   Ptosis _____ Exophthalmos _____
   Eye movements _____
   _____

   Eye opening
   Spontaneously _____ To speech _____
   To pain _____ None _____
   Pupils
   Size L _____ R _____ Shape _____
   Direct reaction to light
   L _____ R _____
   Consensual R to L _____
   L to R _____
   Reaction to near vision
   L _____ R _____
2. Eating _____
3. Expressing _____
4. Speaking _____
   Verbal: Appropriate _____ Confused _____
   Inappropriate _____
   Incomprehensible sounds _____
   No response _____
5. Moving
   a. Tone _____
   b. Strength _____
   c. Coordination: R   L
      Finger-nose   _____
      Finger-finger   _____
      Heel-shin   _____
      Posture holding   _____
      Rapid alternating
         movements   _____
      Rebound   _____
      Past-pointing   _____
      Equilibrium   _____
      Gait   _____
      Romberg   _____

d. Posture _____
   Purposeful: Obeys _____ Localized _____
   Semipurposeful _____ Flexion _____
   Extension _____ Flaccid _____
e. Involuntary movements
   (type and rate)

f. Reflexes: R   L
   Biceps   _____
   Brachioradialis _____
   Triceps   _____
   Patellar   _____
   Achilles   _____
   Plantar   _____

Sensory
1. Smelling _____
2. Blinking _____
3. Hearing _____
4. Tasting _____
5. Feeling _____

Figure 29–1

Sample of a neurologic assessment sheet.

Mentation

If an impairment in the content of consciousness is present, it must first be determined whether the cause is functional or organic. Bizarre thoughts and behavior with intact intellectual functioning point to a functional cause.[6] The markedly depressed patient, however, may demonstrate problems with tests of mental status that mimic the signs of an organic disorder. If it is determined that the patient has a true organic encephalopathy, it must be determined whether it is generalized or represents focal hemispheric dysfunction.

The person's alertness, ability to cooperate, educational level, and handedness are evaluated first. The person's general facial expression, level of consciousness, mood, and behavior are assessed. Next, the person's general intellectual level is determined (based on the person's occupational history, activities, vocabulary, grammar, and knowledge of the subjects discussed) to help the examiner structure the questions and evaluate the patient's responses.

The mental status examination tests the patient's immediate recall, recent or short-term memory, remote memory, interpretation and use of previously gained knowledge, and behavior.[4,7] The test of the patient's immediate recall evaluates his attention span. Short-term memory is evidenced by the ability to recall information about dates, time, or current political happenings, and to learn information, such as the plot of a short story, and to tell the story in several minutes. Remote

Table 29–1
Glasgow Coma Scale*

SCALE	SCORE	EXPLANATION
Eye Opening		
1. No eye opening	1	No eye opening. If the patient cannot open his eyes due to bandaging or swelling, the letter *E* is recorded after the total score. The nurse determines the minimum stimulus to cause opening of one or both eyes.
2. To pain	2	Eye opening only to pain. A noxious stimulus is used. It may be the same stimulus used to determine the best motor response.
3. To speech	3	Eye opening only to speech. The nurse may call the patient by name or may command the patient to open his or her eyes.
4. Spontaneous	4	Spontaneous eye opening.
Best Verbal Response		
0. Intubated	0	
1. Mute	1	Mute—no verbal response. No sound or vocalization is made even after stimulation with a noxious stimulus.
2. Incomprehensible sounds	2	The sounds made are not comprehensible. The patient makes groans or moans that are not discernible as words.
3. Inappropriate words	3	The patient is not able to use words appropriately. He can speak words, but can make no intelligible sentences. He often utters curses or disorganized ramblings but cannot enter into conversation.
4. Confused conversation	4	The patient can form sentences and group words, but his manner is confused. He is not fully oriented.
5. Oriented	5	The patient is appropriate and oriented to time, place, and person and can carry on a conversation.
Best Motor Response		
1. Flaccid	1	The patient demonstrates no motor response. Arms and legs are lax and weak. The nurse must be sure that the stimulus is noxious, and there is no spinal cord injury.
2. Extensor response	2	The patient exhibits decerebrate rigidity. Legs and arms are extended and in internal rotation. The wrists are flexed, and the patient makes a fist. The patient assumes this position in response to a noxious stimulus. If there is a question between the upper and lower extremities, the position of the upper extremities is used.
3. Flexor response	3	Upon stimulation, the patient flexes the upper extremities, but the lower extremities remain in extension. The wrist is flexed, and the patient makes a fist. The patient exhibits decorticate rigidity.
4. Semipurposeful	4	The patient has a generalized flexion withdrawal to pain. The patient briskly flexes either or both arms or may grimace or frown. There is no manual and purposeful attempt to stop the stimulus.
5. Localizes to pain	5	The patient withdraws from the pain or tries to locate and stop the stimulus. The patient does not follow commands but tends to move the arms toward the stimulus. The stimulus should be maximal, and the site used should be changed.
6. Obeys commands	6	The patient can follow commands. The patient will raise a certain number of fingers, hold up an arm, or release a grip.

* The basis of the scale is the patient's response to the examiner's specific requests. For each of the three parameters on the scale—eye opening, best verbal response, and best motor response—the patient function is graded and scored. The three parameters are summed for the overall score. The highest score possible is 15.

memory is evaluated by the patient's ability to remember information about childhood or young adult life.

The ability to interpret and use previously gained knowledge is evaluated by a series of tests. Abstract thinking may be tested by the patient's ability to point out similarities between objects. Second, a slightly more difficult test involves proverb interpretation. An even more difficult test involves problem solving, which requires the person to think through a problem and arrive at a solution.

Behavior is assessed by subjectively evaluating the person's affect and judgment. Essentially, *affect* is the person's emotional status, and such factors as happiness, sadness, and irritability are noted. Also, patients are asked to evaluate themselves with regard to their own feeling state and their perspective on the illness. The patient's judgment is assessed by the appropriateness of behavior; often judgment is difficult to assess on the first interview. The family is frequently asked for their assessment of the patient's behavior.

Respiratory Patterns

Identification of respiratory patterns helps to identify the lesion site and to anticipate patient problems. Respiratory abnormalities may be listed as posthyperventilation apnea, Cheyne-Stokes breathing, and central neurogenic hyperventilation (Fig. 29–2). It is important to recognize that a change from one pattern to another may herald a change in the patient's condition that allows little time for reversal.

Posthyperventilation apnea is a transient cessation of breathing after hyperventilation. Usually, hyperventilation causes a lowered partial pressure of arterial carbon dioxide and removes the major stimulus to the inspiratory stimulus

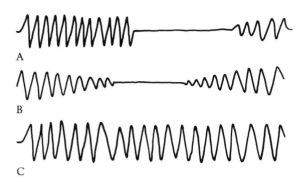

Figure 29-2
Abnormal respiratory patterns. (*A*) Posthyperventilation apnea. (*B*) Cheyne-Stokes respiration. (*C*) Central neurogenic hyperventilation.

in the medulla. A normal person would continue to breathe, because control areas in the cerebral cortex have priority over respiratory medullary control. However, if the patient has a bilateral impairment of cerebral functioning, the control is removed and posthyperventilation apnea may be exhibited.

Cheyne-Stokes breathing is a waxing and waning respiratory pattern. The respiration starts with apnea, increases to a maximum (crescendo), and then decreases to apnea (decrescendo). It is characterized by intermittent periods of hyperventilation followed by gradually decreasing breathing and then periodic apnea followed by gradually increasing breathing. In Cheyne-Stokes breathing, an increased ventilatory response to arterial carbon dioxide levels exists in the medulla, resulting in hyperventilation which, together with the loss of cortical influence on respiration, results in posthyperventilation apnea. Cheyne-Stokes breathing is usually seen in patients with bilateral deep lesions of the cerebral hemispheres and basal ganglia that damage the internal capsule.[16] Patients with increased intracranial pressure also often exhibit this pattern of breathing.

Central neurogenic hyperventilation is sustained, regular, deep, rapid breathing. It results from a lowered threshold to respiratory stimulation and leads to decreased arterial carbon dioxide tension and respiratory alkalosis. The syndrome normally is caused by lesions involving the tegmentum of the lower midbrain or upper pons.

Other types of abnormal respirations (apneustic breathing and ataxic respirations) that have been described in the literature do not correlate well with the site of damage.

Cranial Nerves

Olfactory Nerve

The *first cranial nerve*, the olfactory nerve, serves the sense of smell. Loss of smell (anosmia) may be unilateral or bilateral. The most common causes of anosmia are upper respiratory illness, fracture of the cribriform plate, and tumor of the olfactory groove or frontal lobe. Although the test is frequently not included in the examination, it is included if anosmia, trauma, visual problems, intellectual deterioration, or other neurologic problems are present. Defects in the olfactory bulb and tract or in the olfactory receptors in the nasal mucosa may interfere with smell. Familiar and mild odors, such as those of coffee, tea, vanilla, or peppermint, are used in testing,

and volatile, irritating substances, such as ammonia or vinegar, are avoided. The ability to distinguish between odors is more important than the ability to identify odors exactly.

Optic Nerve

The *second cranial nerve*, the optic nerve, is tested by direct examination with regard to visual acuity, visual fields, and pupillary response. On fundoscopic examination, the head of the optic nerve can be viewed directly. The examiner notes the color, size, and shape of the optic disk; presence of physiologic cup; distinctness of the edges of the optic disc; size, shape, and configuration of vessels; and presence of exudate, hemorrhage, or pigment. Pallor indicates chronic changes. Visual acuity may be tested by the use of a standardized chart, such as the Snellen chart, or the patient may be asked to read various sizes of print. If the patient usually wears glasses, they should be worn for the test. Visual fields may be roughly tested by the confrontation test. Gross hemianopic field defects or scotomas may be detected by the examination, and a more accurate determination may be performed with a perimeter or tangent screen.[16] All quadrants must be tested separately and carefully. The particular areas impaired are often diagnostic. Pupillary response is considered in the discussion that follows.

Oculomotor, Trochlear, and Abducens Nerves

The oculomotor nerve (*third cranial nerve*), trochlear nerve (*fourth cranial nerve*) and abducens nerve (*sixth cranial nerve*) are usually tested together, because they supply the muscles that rotate the eyeball. The observer looks for strabismus, nystagmus, ptosis, and exophthalmos. The size of each pupil and, in particular, the size relative to the other are noted.[5,6,13] The size is determined by the balance between the sympathetic and parasympathetic fibers. Next, the patient's direct light and consensual responses are evaluated.[3] The examiner should note whether the pupil is dilated or constricted and whether the abnormality is unilateral or bilateral. The response to light is tested by shining a focused bright light onto one pupil and then onto the other. Both pupils normally constrict when light is focused on one eye. The eye that receives the direct light shows the direct light response, and the other eye shows the consensual response. Accommodation and convergence are tested simultaneously (the ophthalmic signs most commonly assessed are shown in Table 29–2). The patient focuses on a distant object, such as a penlight, and continues to look at it as it is brought to the nose. The patient's eyes should begin to look at the penlight in a cross-eyed, or convergent, manner. At the same time, the pupils constrict, showing the accommodation response. Ocular movements are observed to note any defects in conjugate movements or nystagmus. Individual eye movements are tested by covering one eye and observing movement in all axes.

A lesion affecting the oculomotor nerve changes the pupillary reflexes and eye movements.[10] An expanding mass in one portion of the cerebral hemisphere may cause the uncal gyrus to herniate through the opening of the tentorium. As the uncus is pushed downward, the oculomotor nerve is compressed against the tentorium. The pupil is maximally dilated and unreactive. If the compression continues, ptosis ensues and the eye deviates laterally as oculomotor function is lost.

Table 29–2
Pupillary Reflexes Commonly Assessed

REFLEX	STIMULUS	CLINICAL SIGN	PATHWAY
Accommodation			
Pupillary phase	Far-to-near focusing	Pupil constricts	Optic nerve, visual cortex, Edinger Westphal nucleus, oculomotor nerve, ciliary ganglion, iris circular muscle
Convergence phase		Eyes converge	Visual cortex, oculomotor nucleus, oculomotor nerve, medial and lateral recti
Refractive phase		Ciliary muscle constricts, lens thickens	Visual cortex, oculomotor nerve, Edinger Westphal nucleus, ciliary ganglion, ciliary muscle
Light	Response to increased light/brightness	Pupil constricts	Optic nerve, pretectal area Edinger Westphal nucleus, oculomotor nerve, ciliary ganglion, iris circular muscle
Ciliospinal	Pinch skin on neck	Pupil dilates	Pain afferents, cervical sympathetics fibers, cervical ganglion, dilator muscle of iris
Nystagmus	Displace cristae	Fast and slow eye movements	Vestibular nerve and nucleus, oculomotor nucleus, extraoculomotor muscle

Observation of the direct light and consensual responses helps the examiner to pinpoint the problem to the optic or oculomotor nerve. The retina and the optic nerve form the afferent limb of the light reflex and carry sensory stimuli toward the brain. The oculomotor nerve, the efferent limb of the light reflex, carries motor stimuli away from the brain. If the optic nerve is injured, the pupil is dilated and the direct light response is lost. Because the consensual response, or motor pathway, remains intact, the pupil constricts when light is shown in the other eye. If the oculomotor nerve is impaired, both the direct light and consensual responses are absent in that eye.

Significant intracranial disease is not always present when an abnormality in pupillary size, reactivity, and symmetry is noted. Approximately 5% of the normal population has a difference in size greater than 1 mm, and about one fifth of all people have a smaller variation.

It is of particular importance to observe the pupillary reflexes and eye movements of the patient with impaired consciousness. Formerly, the presence of the ciliospinal reflex—dilatation of an ipsilateral pupil secondary to noxious stimuli at the neck—was thought to reflect the structural integrity of the brain stem, but it is now thought to reflect only the integrity of the cervical spinal cord and the peripheral sympathetic fibers to the eye.[14] The following observations should be made with regard to each eye: resting position, spontaneous motion, and the oculocephalic and oculovestibular reflexes. First, each eye is observed in the resting position, noting conjugate or disconjugate positioning. This applies whether the eyes are in midposition or deviated in any direction. The direction of any deviation is particularly important. Notation is made of the eye(s) involved and whether the deviation is conjugate or disconjugate. A skew position is present when one eye is up and the other down (disconjugate vertical position) (Fig. 29–3).

The normal resting position of the eyes is midposition. A forced lateral conjugate gaze results from lesions of the frontal lobe or pons. A unilateral destructive lesion in the frontal lobe produces a forced lateral conjugate gaze toward the side of the lesion. A unilateral irritative lesion in the frontal lobe and a unilateral destructive lesion in the pons produce a forced lateral conjugate gaze away from the side of the lesion. A lesion of the third cranial nerve causes the eye to deviate outward, alterations in pupillary size and reflexes, and ptosis.

Skewing of the eyes is produced by brain-stem lesions. Skewing cannot be used to further localize the lesion within the brain stem.

Next, the presence of any spontaneous movement of the eyes is noted. A normal finding is no spontaneous movement or conjugate or disconjugate roving of the eyes (similar to that seen in a normal sleeping person). The four major types of abnormal spontaneous eye movements are shown in Figure 29–4. They must be differentiated from the normal roving, conjugate, or disconjugate eye movements. Retraction nystagmus is a conjugate irregular jerking movement that seems to pull both globes into the orbits. It results from simultaneous contraction of all the eye muscles. There is rapid retraction of the globes, followed by a slow return to normal position. It occurs with lesions in the midbrain tegmentum. Ocular bobbing consists of quick downward conjugate eye movements, followed by a slow return to neutral position; it occurs with lesions of the lower pons. Convergence nystagmus is a slow, drifting, divergent movement of each eye followed by a quick compensatory jerk of convergence. It sometimes is associated with retraction nystagmus, and it occurs with lesions of the midbrain. The fourth type of abnormal spontaneous eye movement is occasional jerking of only one eye in any direction; it occurs with large lesions of the pons.

Additional tests can be performed by the physician to determine the integrity of the oculocephalic and oculovestibular reflexes. These tests evaluate the integrity of the extraocular muscles and the vestibular system.

The test of the oculocephalic reflex (the doll's head maneuver) consists of rapidly and carefully turning the patient's head to one side or the other and up and down and noting how the patient's eyes follow the head movements. In the normal, awake person, the eyes will follow the head unless the gaze is fixed. The test is performed by rotating the head first to one side and then to the other; recordings consist of conjugate

Figure 29–3
Skew position.

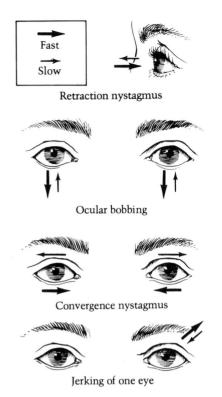

Figure 29-4

Four major types of eye movements.

deviation (normal), disconjugate or asymmetric eye movement (abnormal), and no movement of either eye (absent). Normally, in the unconscious patient, the eyes do not move with the head. Thus, movement lags, and what is seen on rotating the head to one side is an apparent deviation of the eyes to the opposite side, followed by a slow return to midposition. Abnormalities consist of the eyes moving with the head or not deviating in certain directions—up, down, in, or out. The test must not be performed if any question concerning integrity of the spinal cord exists.

There are many reasons for an abnormal oculocephalic reflex. A large lesion in the brain stem will limit all eye movements, and the person's eyes will move with the head in all directions. A lesion in the cerebral cortex above the level of the nucleus of the third cranial nerve will cause the eyes to deviate to one side. The eyes will come to, but not cross, the midline. If the person has a unilateral lesion in the medial longitudinal fasciculus, the eye ipsilateral to the lesion will be unable to deviate toward the midline, and the opposite eye will deviate laterally. The condition is known as *internuclear ophthalmoplegia*, and the disconjugate lateral position is either unilateral or bilateral. If the person has a lesion in the midbrain pretectal area, the eyes cannot move upward conjugately.

If full range of eye movements cannot be elicited with the oculocephalic reflex, the oculovestibular reflex (cold calorics) is tested. The test employs similar reflex mechanisms as does the oculocephalic reflex, but it uses stronger stimulation. After checking for an intact tympanic membrane, approximately 10 ml to 20 ml of cold water or a puff of cold air is injected into the patient's external auditory canal while the patient is in an elevated position (30°). In the comatose patient, the test will usually elicit prolonged conjugate deviation to the same side

if the oculovestibular pathways are intact. For example, in patients with brain-stem injuries and tonic eye deviation, cold water irrigation to the opposite ear does not produce an effect.

Trigeminal Nerve

The *fifth cranial nerve*, the trigeminal nerve, has both motor and sensory functions. In a test of the motor portion of the trigeminal nerve, the patient clenches his teeth, and the examiner palpates the volume and firmness of the muscles. The patient then opens the mouth against resistance. While the patient's mouth is open, any deviation of the mandible to the weak side is more apparent. In a test of the sensory portion of the trigeminal nerve, pain is evaluated with a pin, and light touch is evaluated by passing a piece of cotton over the patient's face and anterior half of scalp. Temperature may also be tested, if indicated. Sensation on each side of the face is compared in each of the three divisions of the trigeminal nerve (ophthalmic, maxillary, and mandibular) (Fig. 29–5). Last, the corneal reflex is tested. A hair or piece of cotton so fine that it is invisible to the person is used. The patient's cornea is approached from the side and touched lightly with the hair or cotton. A normal reaction is a rapid forceful contraction of the eyelid. A contralateral blink is also common. If the patient has no reaction, he is asked whether anything was felt. (Care is taken not to touch the eyelashes or conjunctiva, because the response to such a touch would also be a forceful blink.)

Facial Nerve

The *seventh cranial nerve* is the facial nerve. In tests of the facial nerve, expression, symmetry, and mobility during

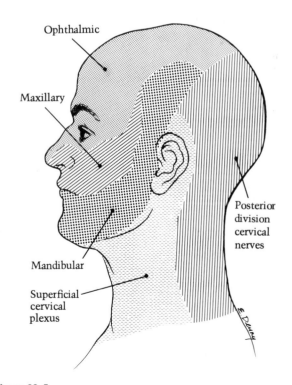

Figure 29-5

Ophthalmic, maxillary, and mandibular divisions of the trigeminal nerve.

speaking, smiling, and laughing are assessed. The patient performs all the voluntary movements that can be done with the face. The patient frowns or scowls, wrinkles the forehead, closes the eyelids (the examiner attempts to forcibly open the patient's eyes), opens the mouth, retracts the mouth, blows out the cheeks, puckers the lips, shows the teeth, whistles, and screws up the nose. Careful observation is made of any asymmetry of the nasolabial folds and of eye blinking. If a paralysis is noted on one side of the facial musculature, taste (which may be lost on the affected side) is tested on the anterior two thirds of the tongue with small quantities of sweet (sugar), salty (saline), bitter (quinine), and sour (lemon or vinegar) substances. The person is asked to identify each substance without putting the tongue back into the mouth.

Auditory Nerve

The *eighth cranial nerve*, the auditory nerve, is tested with regard to its cochlear and vestibular portions. The cochlear portion is tested with regard to the ability to hear the spoken voice, a whisper, or a watch ticking. The patient repeats a sentence whispered from across the room, occluding each ear in turn. If further assessment is needed, the Rinne test and the Weber test may be performed. The Rinne test determines air conduction. The vibrating tuning fork is placed on the mastoid process until sound is no longer heard, and it is moved in front of the patient's ear. Usually air conduction is greater than bone conduction. In the Weber test, a vibrating tuning fork is placed on a patient's forehead, and the patient states where he hears sound. Normally, sound is heard equally well in both ears. In nerve deafness, sound is not heard in the diseased ear, even with occlusion. If further testing is needed, an audiometer is used. Next, the vestibular portion is tested in three ways. First, the past-pointing test is performed by having the patient bring the index finger of an outstretched arm down on the examiner's finger. The patient does this vertically and horizontally with the eyes opened and then with the eyes closed. In vestibular disease, the finger past-points to one side or the other consistently. Then the patient is tested for nystagmus. The patient is told to look to one side. In true nystagmus, there is a sustained movement with two components: a fast jerk to the side of the deviation and a slow jerk back to the midline. The nystagmus may be horizontal or vertical or rotary. The third test consists of stimulation of the semicircular canal by injection of cold water or a puff of cold air into the normal ear canal with the patient sitting (if possible).

Glossopharyngeal Nerve

The *ninth cranial nerve*, the glossopharyngeal nerve, is normally tested when the vagus nerve is tested. Its chief function is sensory; its motor function involves a minor muscle of the pharynx.

Vagus Nerve

The *tenth cranial nerve* is the vagus nerve. The pharynx and larynx are assessed by noting swallowing and elevation of the uvula. While the patient says "Ah," the pharynx is observed. Normally, the soft palate and uvula are pulled up in the midline. If the vagus nerve is weak, the affected side droops and the healthy side elevates. If the paralysis is bilateral, there is no palatal movement. The gag reflex is tested by touching the soft palate. Its absence is most significant if it is unilateral.

The character, sound, and volume of the patient's voice and pulse and respirations are also noted. The nerve may be indirectly assessed by laryngoscopy.

Spinal Accessory Nerve

The *eleventh cranial nerve* is the spinal accessory nerve. The innervation of the trapezius muscle is tested by asking the patient to shrug his shoulders against resistance. Then the opposite sternocleidomastoid muscle is tested by asking the patient to rotate his head against a resistance applied to the side of the chin. In the test of both sternocleidomastoid muscles, the patient flexes the head forward against a resistance applied under the chin.

Hypoglossal Nerve

The *twelfth cranial nerve*, the hypoglossal nerve, is the motor nerve to the tongue. In the test of this nerve, the person protrudes the tongue and the observer looks for atrophy, involuntary movements, or fasciculations. A paralysis of the muscles on the left will produce a protrusion to the left. Strength is tested by having the person push his tongue against each cheek or by pushing against a tongue blade.

Motor System

The fourth major part of the physical examination is assessment of the motor system. The examination includes determination of muscle bulk, tone, posture, strength, symmetry, and presence of abnormal muscle movements. Both sides are compared. Any lateralizing signs are documented and reported. The presence of such signs suggests a structural nonmetabolic lesion.

If the functional approach is selected, integrated abilities assessed are seeing, eating, expressing, speaking, and moving. Cranial nerve observations are combined with those of the motor system.

Any hypertrophy or atrophy of muscles should be noted. To check any suspected asymmetry, a tape measure is used to measure corresponding muscles at corresponding places on the limbs. Muscle tone is evaluated by passive range-of-motion exercises and active movement, noting any involuntary resistance, spasticity, flaccidity, or rigidity. Muscle strength is tested by having the patient push against resistance. Any abnormal movements, such as swift, jerking motions or slow, irregular movements, twistings, tics, tremors, or choreiform movements are noted. The results may be graded as follows: 0 = no movement, 1 = flicker of movement, 2 = movement with gravity eliminated, 3 = movement against gravity, 4 = mild impairment of power, and 5 = normal power.

The hands and arms are assessed by having the patient squeeze two of the examiner's fingers. The strength of the hand is estimated by the force the examiner must exert to withdraw his or her fingers. Next, the patient clenches a fist and fixes the wrist, and the examiner tries to overcome the dorsiflexion. The procedure is repeated to test for abduction of fingers and apposition of thumbs. Next, the patient flexes and extends an arm against resistance. Last, arm abduction at the shoulders is tested. Assessment of the trunk may be done by having the patient rise from a lying to a sitting position. The lower extremities may be tested in several ways. First, the patient flexes and extends the legs against resistance. One leg is elevated at a time and held for 10 to 20 seconds. The power of leg extension at the knee and at the hip is evaluated. Then dorsiflexion is tested by having the patient push the partially flexed foot against the examiner's hand. Plantar flexion is tested by having the patient push down against the examiner's hand.

Subtle weakness due to an upper motor neuron (or "pyramidal") lesion may be evidenced by a downward drift in one of the patient's outstretched arms while the eyes are closed. With pyramidal lesions, muscles that abduct and extend the joints in the upper extremities are weaker than their antagonists. In patients with vascular disease, a positive drift may be an early clue to rebleeding. The clot formed acts as a pyramidal tract lesion and thus produces the drift. In the lower extremities, the flexors of the hips and knees and the dorsiflexors of the feet are the weaker. Testing can be performed manually by having the patient exert maximum pressure against the examiner's resistance.

If the patient is unconscious, the motor system is assessed by observation of the resting posture, spontaneous movement, any asymmetry of position, and abnormal movement. With regard to localizing the lesion, posture, muscle tone, and the position of each limb are important for the nurse to observe. Posture may be decerebrate, decorticate, or hemiplegic (Fig. 29–6). Certain patients may consistently assume the first two postures, but mainly these postures are assumed in response to pain stimulation.

The patient with decerebrate posture (extensor response) exhibits extension, internal rotation, and wrist flexion in the upper extremities and extension, internal rotation, and plantar flexion in the lower extremities. Such a patient's jaw may be clenched and the neck hyperextended. The patient with decorticate posture (flexor response) exhibits adduction of the shoulders, pronation and flexion of the elbows and wrists, and extension, internal rotation, and plantar flexion of the lower extremities. Although the responses are often bilateral, a patient may be decerebrate or decorticate on one side only. He may be decerebrate on one side and decorticate on the other. On one side, responses may be purposeful, whereas on the other side they may be semipurposeful.

In hemiplegia, the affected side and the normal side are not symmetric. Initially, the affected extremities show an outward rotation and decreased muscle tone. A hemiplegic extremity lifted off the bed and allowed to fall drops abruptly, much like a dead weight. An extremity with normal muscle tone falls to the bed in a smooth motion. Later (the time varies), there is spasticity and resistance to passive movement. The upper extremity exhibits adduction of the shoulder and pronation with flexion of the elbow and wrist. The lower extremity exhibits extension, internal rotation, and plantar flexion.

Sensory Assessment

There are three aspects of the sensory examination: qualitative, to determine what elements of sensation are affected; quantitative, to determine the degree of impaired sensation; and regional, to determine the exact distribution of sensory impairment or loss. If the functional approach is used, parameters assessed include smelling, hearing, tasting, and feeling (pain, touch, and temperature discrimination). Sensory findings are combined with those from the cranial nerve assessment to determine functional ability.

In testing for light touch, the skin surface is stroked with the tip of a finger, a wisp of cotton, or a camel's hair brush. Care is taken to avoid tickling. Pain sense is tested by asking the patient to distinguish the sharp from the dull end of a pin in a side-to-side comparison. Temperature is tested by having the patient differentiate test tubes filled with hot water from those filled with ice.

Deep sensation assesses the posterior columns and pain. In vibration testing, a tuning fork (C128) is placed over elbows, wrists, ankles, shins, and other bony prominences. The patient is asked to identify sensation and then to determine when sensation ceases. When testing position sense, many joints of the body are evaluated. Most commonly, the big toe is tested. When testing for deep pain, muscle pain is assessed by pressing on a muscle (usually the trapezius muscle) to the point of pain. The standard stimulus is pressure applied to the nail bed. Moderate supraorbital pressure gets mixed responses and is contraindicated in patients with facial fractures. Tendon pain sense is tested by pressing on a tendon (usually the Achilles tendon). The tendon is compressed between the knuckle of the thumb and the tip of the index finger. Testicular pain sense is tested by squeezing the testicle gently between the thumb and finger.

Tests of stereognosis evaluate the patient's ability to recognize objects placed in the hand. Familiar objects, such as a coin, key, or knife, are used. The patient closes his eyes, the object is placed in the hand, and the patient attempts to identify the object. In a test of graphesthesia, numbers or letters are traced on the patient's skin with a blunt object, and the patient tries to identify what has been drawn. In a test of two-point discrimination, the patient indicates whether he feels one point or two points pressed over various parts of the body with the use of a calibrated compass. (The shortest normal

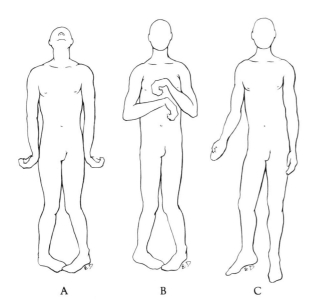

Figure 29–6

Abnormal posturing. (*A*) Decerebrate position. (*B*) Decorticate position. (*C*) Position in early hemiplegia.

distances are fingertips, 0.3 cm to 0.6 cm.) In a test of topognosis (tactile localization), the patient closes his eyes and the examiner touches a spot on the patient's body. The patient points to the spot. Corresponding areas of both sides of the body are tested. Normally, the patient is more accurate with regard to tests on the fingers and hands than with regard to tests on the arms.

Assessment of Coordination

The cerebellum functions primarily in balance and coordination. Incoordination is usually seen in attempted cooperative muscle movement; it results from involvement of the cerebellum or the nerve systems associated with the cerebellum. Most commonly, the movement is jerking and inaccurate.

Movement in the upper extremities is assessed by several tests. In the finger-to-nose test, the patient brings the tip of the index finger to the tip of the nose, first with the eyes open and then closed, first slowly and then rapidly. The test is considered positive if the movement to the nose is irregular or if the tip of the nose is missed consistently. In the finger-to-finger test, the same sequence is used, but the examiner's finger is substituted for the patient's nose. In assessment of rapid alternating movements of the fingers, the patient is asked to flex and extend the fingers rapidly or to tap a table rapidly with the fingers extended. In the patting test, the patient rapidly pats his leg on the examiner's hand. Amplitude and rhythm are noted. In supination and pronation of the forearm, continuous rapid alternations using the elbows as a fulcrum are tested. A positive finding is the inability to perform the test quickly and smoothly (adiadokokinesia).

The same type of tests are used in the lower extremities. In the heel-to-knee test, the patient places one heel on the opposite knee and then slides the foot down the shin. The test is positive when the person has difficulty placing or holding the heel on the knee or cannot keep the heel firmly on the leg as the heel is moved downward. In the patting test, the patient pats the foot quickly on the floor. In the figure-of-eight test,

the patient draws an 8 in the air with the big toe. In the toe-finger test, the supine patient touches the examiner's finger with his or her big toe. Then the examiner moves the finger to a new position approximately 6 to 18 inches away, and the patient follows the finger with his toe.

Tests for gait and station to assess truncal coordination and dorsal column function are usually not performed in the critical care unit. If the patient is mobile, his gait can be assessed when he moves from the bed to the chair.

Reflexes

Reflexes are specific muscular responses to stimuli (Table 29–3). They are usually evaluated along with the cranial nerves with regard to functions served. The reflexes tend to be increased in upper motor neuron disease and decreased in lower motor neuron disease. The examiner uses the lightest percussion needed on the appropriate part to elicit a reflex. Stronger taps can be used to assess maximum reflex output.

Superficial Reflexes

Two superficial reflexes are commonly evaluated: the abdominal reflex and the cremasteric reflex. The abdominal reflex is composed of abdominal muscle movements in all four quadrants. With the patient lying supine and the abdominal muscles relaxed, the skin of each quadrant is stroked with a pin, key, brush, or blunt end of an orangewood stick; the movement is from the periphery toward the umbilicus or in the shape of a diamond. A normal response consists of movement of the abdominal muscles and a pull of the umbilicus toward the quadrant that was stroked. (The response is difficult to elicit in patients who are overweight.) The cremasteric reflex is elicited by stroking the inner aspect of a man's thigh. The normal response is contraction of the scrotum on that side. Absence of an abdominal or cremasteric reflex may indicate a spinal cord lesion.

Table 29–3
Commonly Assessed Reflexes

REFLEX	STIMULUS	RESPONSE	LEVEL	PERIPHERAL NERVE
Tendon				
Biceps	Biceps tendon	Flexion of the elbow	Cervical 5–6	Musculocutaneous
Triceps	Triceps tendon	Extension of elbow	Cervical 6–7	Radial
Radial	Styloid process of the radius	Flexion of the elbow	Cervical 5–6	Radial
Knee	Quadriceps tendon	Extension of the knee	Lumbar 2–4	Femoral
Ankle	Calcaneus tendon	Plantar flexion of the ankle	Sacral 1–2	Sciatic
Superficial				
Plantar	The skin of outer border of sole of foot	Plantar flexion of toes with dorsiflexion of foot at ankle	Sacral 1	Lateral plantar nerve of posterior tibial
Cremasteric	Inner surface of thigh	Elevation of ipsilateral testicle	Lumbar 1, sacral 2–3	Ilioinguinal and obturator
Abdominal	Skin on upper or lower abdomen	Contraction of ipsilateral abdominal muscles	Thoracic nerve 7–12	Anterior cutaneous branches of thoracic nerves
Oppenheim's	Firm, moving pressure on skin of tibia	Same as Babinski, or extensor plantar reflex	Lumber 4–5	Saphenous

Deep Tendon Reflexes

The common deep tendon reflexes elicited are the biceps, triceps, radial, Achilles, and patellar reflexes. The biceps reflex tests the intactness of the innervation of C5-6. The patient flexes the elbow while the examiner presses his thumb against the patient's biceps tendon in the antecubital space. The examiner's thumb is hit with the percussion hammer to produce a quick sharp contraction of the biceps tendon. The result is flexion of the arm.

The radial reflex also indicates the intactness of C5-6. With the patient's forearm midway between pronation and supination, the lower third of the radius is tapped. The result is flexion of the forearm on the arm with slight pronation and, usually, flexion of the fingers and hand. If there is a lesion at the fifth cervical segment, the radial response consists of flexion of the hand and fingers but not of the forearm.

The triceps reflex tests the intactness of C6-7. The tendon is put under slight tension by placing the forearm on a horizontal plane in front of the chest or by holding the upper arm straight out from the body and allowing the lower arm to dangle loosely. In the supine patient, the arm is drawn across the chest and the forearm is slightly flexed. Directly striking the triceps tendon with the percussion hammer produces extension of the arm.

The patellar (knee) reflex tests the intactness of L2-4. The patient is sitting with knees hanging loosely over the side of the bed. In the supine position, several test methods are possible: flex the patient's knees over the examiner's arm and have the heels resting lightly on the bed; place a pillow under the knees; or cross the legs. The reflex is elicited by striking the tendon immediately below the patella. The normal response is contraction of the quadriceps muscle and extension of the knee, much like a kick. If the response is difficult to elicit, it can be strengthened by having the patient lock the fingers of both hands and pull as hard as possible in opposing directions.

The Achilles tendon (ankle) reflex tests the intactness of L5-S2, particularly S1. The patient relaxes his foot and lies prone, kneels on a chair, or lies supine with the legs flexed and the hip rotated outward. Gentle pressure is applied to the ball of the foot, and the Achilles tendon is tapped with the percussion hammer. The normal response is plantar flexion of the foot. If a response is not forthcoming, a distractor should be used (*i.e.*, ask the patient to bite and pull his hooked fingers apart just before tapping). In this way, the patient's mind will be distracted from the test, and the natural response can be elicited.

Abnormal Reflexes

The plantar reflex is elicited by stroking the sole of the foot with a blunt object from the heel up the lateral margin of the foot to the ball of the foot and then across the ball to the base of the big toe. The normal response is flexion of the toes. The abnormal (Babinski) response consists of extension (dorsiflexion) of the big toe, flexion of the small toes, spreading of the small toes, and flexion of the leg. A Babinski response suggests an upper motor neuron lesion.

Chaddock's sign is elicited by stroking the lateral aspect of the dorsum of the foot and the external malleolus. The abnormal response is extension of the big toe. Oppenheim's sign is elicited by stroking the medial aspect of the tibia in a firm downward motion. The abnormal response is extension of the big toe. Gordon's sign is elicited by firm compression of the calf. The abnormal sign is extension of the big toe. Ankle clonus is elicited with the foot relaxed and the knee flexed. The foot is quickly pushed with a moderate force in a dorsal direction and held in that position. The abnormal response is a persistent clonic contraction of the posterior muscles of the leg.

Several similar abnormal flexion reflexes may be seen in the upper extremity. These finger reflexes are common in the healthy person, and they do not have the importance of an abnormal plantar response. Hoffman's sign is indicative of increased reflex activity. With the patient's wrist and fingers relaxed, the wrist is held in horizontal pronation. Two techniques are common: light snapping of the nail of the middle finger or flexing of the distal phalanx of the middle finger over one of the examiner's fingers and quickly releasing the phalanx. The abnormal response is flexion of the fingers and thumb. The response increases nonspecifically with generalized hyperreflexia. If it is increased unilaterally, an upper motor neuron lesion may be present. Trömner's sign is elicited by tapping the patient's middle or index finger on the palmar surface. The abnormal response is flexion of all five fingers. The grasp reflex is elicited by placing something in the patient's hand. The abnormal response is a strong grasp.

Three additional reflexes are commonly noted. The snout reflex is elicited by tapping the mandible or maxilla. The abnormal response is a rooting movement; it is indicative of cerebral dysfunction. The sucking reflex is elicited by oral stimuli. The abnormal response is sucking or pursing of the lips; it is indicative of cerebral dysfunction and is classified as a severely abnormal snout response. The jaw reflex is elicited by tapping the partially open, relaxed mandible downward at the tip of the lower jaw. The abnormal response is a very brisk upward movement of the jaw.

Recording

The response elicited after testing the reflex is graded and recorded from 0 to 4+: 0 = absent, tr = trace, 1+ = hypoactive, 2+ = normal, 3+ = hyperactive, and 4+ = sustained clonus.

Several different methods may be used for recording the results of testing the reflexes. If the data base does not include a printed method, the examiner may select the method preferred. Three different examples commonly accepted for recording the reflexes are shown in Figure 29–7.

DIAGNOSTIC STUDIES

What diagnostic studies the neurologist or neurosurgeon chooses depends on the individual patient's pathophysiology. The studies most commonly ordered are skull and spinal films, lumbar puncture, angiography, brain scanning, electroencephalography, and computed axial tomography.

Skull films are ordered as a screening procedure. In patients with trauma, the skull fracture may be outlined or a foreign body may be visualized. If the pineal gland is calcified, a shift in its position may indicate the side of the intracranial mass. Cervical, dorsal, or lumbosacral spinal films are ordered whenever a disease process in the particular area is suspected.

(1)

	Bi	Tri	F	K	A	Plantar	Abdomen	Snout	Grasp	Jaw	Suck
R											
L											

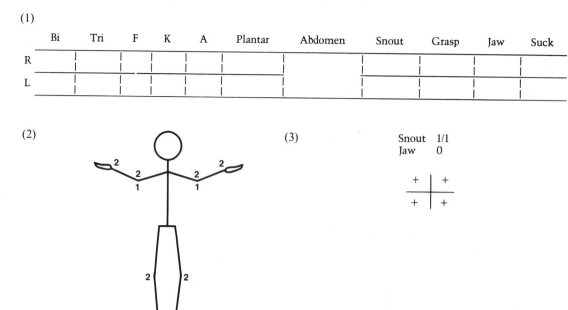

(2)

(3)

Snout 1/1
Jaw 0

$$\frac{+\ \ |\ \ +}{+\ \ |\ \ +}$$

Figure 29–7
Three different examples of recording test results for reflexes.

The lumbar puncture is particularly valuable in patients with suspected subarachnoid hemorrhage or meningitis. It is sometimes deferred when the patient has increased intracranial pressure because of the possibility of uncal or cerebellar herniation. Normally, the spinal fluid pressure varies from 70 mm H_2O to 200 mm H_2O. Pressures over 200 mm H_2O are considered elevated, and they result from tumors, abscesses, cysts, subdural hematoma, infection, cerebral hemorrhage or thrombosis, subarachnoid hemorrhage, hydrocephalus, and pseudotumor cerebri. Under normal circumstances, the cerebrospinal fluid is colorless and has a low blood cell count. A white blood cell count of more than six cells, and any red blood cells are considered abnormal. The normal protein content is 15 mg to 45 mg/100 ml. Protein electrophoretic rather than colloidal gold reaction studies may be ordered to evaluate the patient for inflammatory disease, such as multiple sclerosis. The glucose content is 50 mg to 75 mg/100 ml, and it is normally 20 mg/100 ml less than that found in the blood.

Cerebral angiography is one of the most useful neurodiagnostic techniques available for the assessment of structural abnormalities, abnormal positioning of blood vessels, and alterations in flow patterns. Catheterization of the carotid, brachial, or femoral arteries enables the contrast material to be injected directly into the carotid or vertebral arteries or indirectly into the brachial vessels or aortic arch. The cerebrovascular system is outlined clearly. Serial evaluation in the lateral and anteroposterior planes is then possible as the contrast material progresses through the arteries, capillaries, and veins. The films are read by the neurologist or neurosurgeon and radiologist for size and placement, changes in the position of vessels, abnormal proliferation of vessels, and direction and velocity of blood flow. Angiography has replaced air studies in most situations, but it is still considered an invasive procedure, because a catheter is threaded through vital arteries.

The possibility exists that blood supply to a vital organ may be disrupted or that the procedure could cause a stroke or myocardial infarction. Allergic reactions to the contrast material are also possible. The complications vary from minor to life-threatening.

Electroencephalography is used in the diagnosis of seizure disorders, focal and generalized encephalopathies, and brain death. The electrical activity of the brain is amplified, transmitted, and recorded by means of electrodes applied to the scalp. The waveform tracings are analyzed and interpreted according to the frequency, amplitude, form, and distribution of the wave activity.

Evoked potentials provide sensitive, quantitative extensions of the clinical examination and are particularly useful for patients with tumors, stroke, multiple sclerosis, and trauma. The brain's response to an external stimulus is seen as an electrical manifestation, an evoked potential. Three evoked potential tests are particularly useful: pattern-shift visual, brain stem auditory, and short-latency somatosensory. The tests are used to demonstrate abnormal sensory system function when it cannot be determined by history and physical examination, to define the anatomy of the particular manifestation of the disease process, to identify as yet unsuspected lesions, and to monitor nerve pathways that cannot be determined clinically. Primarily numerical data are produced, although there is a certain amount of waveform interpretation and measurement. Computer-signal averaging is the technique used to extract the evoked potential from background activity. One or more potentials or electric waves are seen after a repeated stimulus. Clinical interpretation primarily uses the presence or absence of these waves, the time from stimulus to wave peak, and the time measured between peaks.

Radioisotope brain scanning is used to identify abnormal areas of isotope concentration and to help in the diagnosis of abscesses, cerebral infarctions, subdural hematomas, and especially neoplasms. Brain scanning relies on the phenomenon of the blood-brain barrier, where the brain's blood vessels have a natural filter that keeps out noxious agents circulating in the blood. The barrier allows only the substances needed for brain functioning to pass. When pathology is present, the natural filter breaks down. Circulating radiopharmaceuticals leave the vessels in the diseased areas and enter the brain substance. Today, relatively few scans are performed, because computed tomography (CT) has largely supplanted other diagnostic studies.

Imaging technology with the CT scan has revolutionized diagnosis because the accuracy is so great. Computer memories and microcircuits store and process the information needed. Vast quantities of information are necessary to produce a single image. Coupled with radiographic techniques, the image produced is a *tomograph*, the depiction of a single cross-sectional plane. The CT scan is rapid and noninvasive, and it localizes lesions accurately and allows for the assessment of multiple lesions.[2] The scanner sweeps a narrow, highly focused beam of x-ray across the section of the head to be imaged. Sensitive sodium iodide crystal detectors record the amount of x-ray absorbed by the body as the beam circles 360°. Any changes in absorption in different tissues, even though minute, are stored and processed in the computer. The computer then displays the image on the cathode ray tube of the viewing unit (much like a television screen), from which Polaroid pictures can be taken. The image is produced by hundreds of thousands of calculations performed in only seconds. The resulting cross-sectional image of the head distinguishes structures and surrounding space in three dimensions and appears as a front-to-back slice of the head. The scanners are so sensitive to even small changes in x-ray absorption that differences in the gray and white matter can be identified. Injection of a contrast material can enhance visualization of vascular structures or abnormalities present. If the blood-brain barrier has been disturbed, the contrast material will leak out and the blood vessels in the affected area will be visualized on a subsequent CT scan.[16] In some institutions, curare is given to reduce erratic movements during the scan.

Magnetic resonance imaging (nuclear magnetic resonance or NMR imaging) is the newest noninvasive procedure available. Two advantages are paramount: It is completely safe, and it images tissues high in water and fat content that cannot be seen with other techniques. Thus, magnetic resonance imaging can show the soft bone marrow, whereas x-rays can show only the hard bone. The basic technique has been used since the 1940s in chemistry and has become the most important structural tool available to the organic chemist. On imaging, only nuclei are seen, and only one type of nucleus at a time is seen (*e.g.*, ^1H or ^{13}C nuclei). Magnetic resonance imaging uses the hydrogen atoms of water molecules in brain tissue. When the brain is exposed to a high-frequency magnetic field, the hydrogen nuclei interact with the radiation and change energy levels. The net result is the absorption of electromagnetic radiation that gives rise to the signal evaluated. The magnetic resonance imaging system is a cylindric, hollow superconducting magnet with a magnetic density as high as 0.35 Testa, more than 7000 times greater than the natural magnetic field of the earth. When the patient lies within the hollow core of the magnet, the hydrogen atoms in his body orient themselves to the magnetic field. Then, as a response to high-frequency radio waves, the hydrogen nuclei resonate and change energy levels. The precise frequency that changes the energy level of a particular nucleus is the *resonance frequency* of that nucleus. Each nucleus reacts according to its molecular environment. Nuclei with the same environment react in the same way and increase the amplitude of the response. In a way, the hydrogen nuclei are just like tuning forks hit at just the right pitch, they respond to the radio signals with their own characteristic wave broadcast, or in other words, their own *magnetic resonance*. A computer then analyzes the data from all the resonating atoms and creates a cross-sectional image.

At the present time, magnetic resonance imaging can be used to measure fluid flow, localize hemorrhage, and identify or map areas of cerebral edema and tumors. It is contraindicated in patients with pacemakers and metal aneurysm clips, and in patients with epilepsy.

MONITORING

Monitoring, reassessment, and evaluation are an ongoing process (Table 29–4). Only by reassessment and monitoring are trends in the patient's condition noted. Data should be gathered to help the physician make a medical diagnosis regarding the pathologic process or the location and nature of the lesion, and to formulate the nursing diagnoses regarding human responses to health problems and aspects of daily living—abilities, disabilities, and potential abilities. The same techniques and similar data are used, but the purposes differ. The physician needs to interpret information for the medical diagnosis. The nurse needs to interpret information for the nursing diagnosis. Both work together to help one another in the gathering as well as the interpretive aspects of the process. No domain exclusively belongs to one discipline. The essence of teamwork and joint practice is mutual respect and collaboration. For example, while asking the patient to lift his or her gown so that the heartbeat can be heard, the nurse observes the patient's movements and coordination. If the patient is not able to follow commands or has no coordination in movements, the nurse knows that assistance will be needed in the activities of daily living. The findings must also be documented and communicated to the physician to aid in his or her interpretation.

Table 29–4
Monitoring Parameters

Level of consciousness
Clinical assessment:
    Coma score, pupillary signs, motor function, pulse, respiration
Temperature
Arterial blood pressure
Hourly urine output
Intracranial pressure
Cerebral perfusion pressure
Swan-Ganz pressures:
    Central venous pressure, pulmonary artery systolic and diastolic pressure, pulmonary capillary wedge pressure
Laboratory studies:
    Electrolytes, blood urea nitrogen, glucose, creatinine
Complete blood count
Coagulation studies:
    Prothrombin time, partial thromboplastin time, platelets

The initial assessment should be performed as soon as possible after the patient's arrival in the critical care unit. A baseline for later comparison is established. The times of the next assessment(s) or check(s) depend on the patient's condition and may be every 15 minutes or every 1 to 2 hours. The time is dependent on anticipation of clinical changes. Although sleep is a priority for all critically ill patients, the nurse needs to be sure assessments are performed if needed. A sleeping patient may be an unconscious patient. The common practice is for the physician to write an order for time frequency of vital signs or "neuro check" (vital signs, level of consciousness, pupillary signs, and motor signs). This practice is in contra-

distinction to all points made about dependence on the patient's condition. A much more natural practice is for the nurse and physician to plan the patient's care and for the nurse to make the periodic assessments as the patient's condition requires. The person on site at the bedside is much more capable of noting alterations and titrating therapy.

Flow sheets (Fig. 29–8) have been developed in most units and are instrumental in organizing and recording data needed repeatedly at different time periods to monitor the patient's condition. Recording is concise and consistent. Usually the flow sheet remains at the patient's bedside so that the health team members may evaluate the data collected. Flow sheets

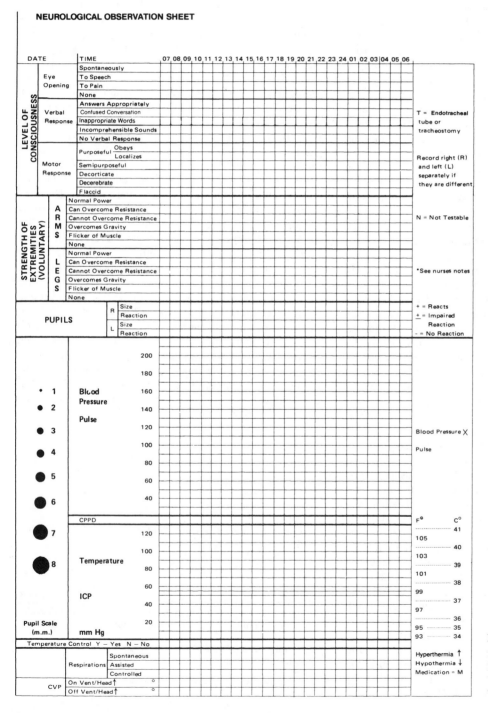

Figure 29-8

Sample flow sheet. (Courtesy of Sarah Moody, R.N., Department of Nursing, Dallas County Hospital District, Dallas, Texas.)

contain the parameters representative of the patient's condition and are used to serially monitor the patient's condition in order to identify trends.

The neurologic assessment need not take a lot of time. A great deal of information can be gathered in a few minutes by organizing the approach.

Monitoring Intracranial Pressure

Detailed clinical observation is still the forte of assessment and management, but the development of the technique to measure intracranial pressure (ICP) directly aids in diagnosing, prognosing, managing, and monitoring the patient's condition. Direct measurement of ICP is now an established technique.

Although nothing can be done to salvage brain tissue destroyed initially with the primary problem, much can be done to prevent the secondary phenomena that adversely affect potentially viable tissue. In particular, monitoring and subsequent control of ICP elevations likely have a beneficial effect on the ultimate survival and quality of life of patients with intracranial hypertension. Monitoring of ICP is a useful adjunct in both operative and nonoperative patients. Although an invasive procedure, it is the most accurate available. Many patients undergoing craniotomy develop elevations of ICP in the postoperative period. Intracranial pressure monitoring identifies these patients and facilitates decision making regarding lowering these elevations. In postoperative patients with nontraumatic lesions, such as tumors, such monitoring can bring impending problems to the nurse's attention.

Measurement

Monitoring systems are based on simple principles. Initially, a type of energy (pressure or electric activity) must be evaluated. Some means is then developed to transmit and perhaps convert this energy so that it can be measured. Intracranial pressure monitoring equipment consists of a transducer, a sensor (a movable diaphragm, a balloon, a solid-state probe, or a fluid column), and a recording device. It is particularly important that the system does not become even partly blocked, because the pressure recording will be damaged or lost. Although the ideal monitoring system is not yet available, the following characteristics should be considered: simplicity, noninvasiveness, ability to remain in place for long periods of time, ability to remain relatively infection-free, and ability to remain accurate under a wide variety of clinical conditions.

The ICP can be monitored in several places: ventricles, subarachnoid space, epidural space, and subdural space. Ventricular catheterization involves the insertion of a catheter into the frontal horn of a lateral cerebral ventricle through a small burr hole; it permits pressure monitoring, cerebrospinal fluid sampling and draining, ventriculography, and the administration of drugs (Fig. 29–9). The potential for infection is reduced if the catheter does not remain in place longer than 3 days.[18] Infection, the risk factor most consistently associated with ICP monitoring, is directly related to duration of monitoring.[12] Additional factors related to the development of infection are age and diagnosis of the patient being monitored, the consistency of maintaining a closed system, the insertion, environment, technique, and the type of ICP monitoring device used. In trauma, cannulation of a small, swollen, and possibly shifted ventricle poses technical difficulties. The procedure is particularly useful for monitoring during surgery, because problems with ventilation or positioning can be quickly identified and assessed. Postoperatively, the catheter is useful for ventricular draining, detection of a hematoma, monitoring the patency of a shunt, and identification of intracranial hypertension. Ventriculostomies can also be performed in the critical care unit by the neurosurgeon. Tubing and transducers are set up by the nurse using sterile techniques. Patients are usually placed on prophylactic antibiotic coverage. Tubing is changed every 48 hours. Dressings should be totally occlusive and changed only if they become soiled or nonocclusive.

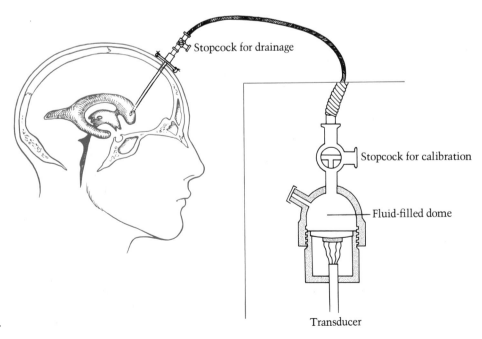

Figure 29–9
Ventricular catheterization.

Stopcock for drainage

Stopcock for calibration

Fluid-filled dome

Transducer

Mainly because of problems with infection and with accurate stabilization of the ventricular catheter, the subarachnoid, epidural, and subdural techniques have been developed. The subarachnoid technique using the Richmond screw (bolt) is perhaps the most popular. In this technique, the ICP is monitored by means of a sensor and transducer, and the output of the transducer is displayed on an oscilloscope or on a digital pressure-reading device. The tip of a hollow screw rests in the subarachnoid space so that pressure recordings are obtained intermittently or continuously. The device is easy to insert at the bedside and is accurate. The proximal end of the screw consists of a Luer-Lock and a hexagonal collar for insertion. The distal thread fits a 1¼-inch twist drill hole made through a 1-cm incision. The screw is connected to a stopcock assembly through a saline-filled extension tube. Then the transducer is opened to the subarachnoid space and a calibrated ICP reading is taken. Isovolumetric measurements can be made because of the use of the transducer. Periodic flushing is required or the readings become damped and inaccurate, because brain tends to herniate up into the screw. Intravenous normal saline is used for flushing, because bacteriostatic saline may cause seizures. Infections must be considered if the screw remains in place longer than 3 days.

With epidural monitoring, the nervous system is not exposed to the risk of contamination because the dura is left intact. After a burr hole is drilled, the dura is gently stripped from the inner table, and a pressure sensor is placed. Because the dura remains intact, the sensors can remain in place for 10 to 14 days as long as the readings are reliable.

The subdural space can be monitored with a pediatric feeding tube inserted through the dura by way of a small burr hole. If the ICP is greatly elevated, the brain is tight, and insertion will damage neural tissue. This system works for 4 to 5 days and rarely requires flushing.

Evaluation of Measurement of Intracranial Pressure

With regard to outcome criteria, the ICP levels are not as significant as the clinical signs of severe cerebral and brain-stem dysfunction. The ICP levels are of value in patients with diffuse brain damage; the higher the patient's ICP on admission, the greater is the risk of his developing recurrent or persistent hypertension. In patients with purposeful motor responses, persistent ICP elevation is associated with a poor outcome.

In trauma, patient outcome is determined ultimately by the degree and distribution of injury. Increased ICP reflects a potentially severe injury. However, a normal ICP does not guarantee a favorable outcome.

Intraventricular pressures between 0 mm Hg and 10 mm Hg are generally regarded as normal. There is no agreement about whether 10 mm Hg, 15 mm Hg, or 20 mm Hg is the mean-level threshold for intracranial hypertension. The indication for treating increased ICP generally is a sustained increase to over 30 mm Hg or any increase that is associated with neurologic deterioration. Unless arterial blood gas alterations or head and body position changes are determined to be the cause of the increase, the treatment usually consists of further hyperventilation by increasing the tidal volume, using closed drainage, or administering intravenous mannitol intermittently or continuously.

The ICP trend along with sequential neurologic and radiologic examinations must be evaluated in the overall context of the patient's systematic assessment.[8] The following example compares normal ICP and increased ICP.

	Normal ICP (mm Hg)	Increased ICP (mm Hg)
Systolic blood pressure	120	90
Diastolic blood pressure	60	30
Mean arterial pressure	80	50
ICP	8	40
Cerebral perfusion pressure	72	10

Cerebral perfusion pressure (mean arterial pressure − ICP) should be maintained at levels greater than 60 mm Hg for adequate perfusion.

Pressure waves (or fluctuations in the ICP) are spontaneous transient waves produced by systemic problems, such as alterations in the arterial blood gases with hypercapnia. *Plateau* (alpha or A) waves usually arise from an elevated ICP baseline and are probably caused by changes in cerebral blood volumes and cerebral vasomotor paralysis. They are rapid, spontaneous increases in pressure followed by rapid decreases and may be accompanied by a temporary or permanent increase in neurologic deficit. If no change in neurologic function is observed with the wave, measures should be taken immediately to reduce ICP and prevent deterioration. The plateau waves are more likely to occur when ICP is already elevated; they may increase to 50 mm Hg to 115 mm Hg and usually last 5 to 20 minutes. The ICP then precipitously falls to the original level. Probably because of the increased use of prophylactic measures (*e.g.*, controlled hyperventilation and ventricular drainage), plateau waves are not observed as frequently as they were previously.

As pressure increases, blood circulation is eventually slowed and systemic blood pressure must be raised to maintain intracranial perfusion. The pulse slows, and the pulse pressure widens. The respirations are usually slow and deep. Breathing becomes irregular as the patient's condition worsens. The blood supply to the brain is finally cut off, and the respirations cease (Fig. 29–10). However, although a rising systolic pressure, a widening pulse pressure, and a slow, bounding pulse are important indicators of increasing ICP, they do not necessarily correlate with the actual measurements of increased ICP. The only way to assess the ICP accurately is to measure it directly. It has even been shown that there is no absolute correlation between CT scan findings and levels of ICP.[2]

BRAIN DEATH

Termination of extraordinary life support and determination of death are questions that plague everyone in critical care. Medical, technical, clinical, and emotional responses occur.[11] Particularly in the brain-dead patient from whom organ retrieval and transplantation are possible, the question of diagnosis of cessation of total brain function assumes vast importance. Kidney, skin, eye, and bone transplants are common, and even pancreas, liver, lung, and heart procedures are being refined.

A consistent legal definition of brain death is not possible, because only about 25 states have a legal definition.[9] Although

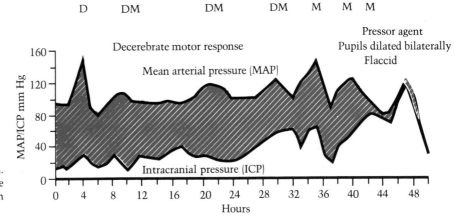

Figure 29-10

Progression of intracranial hypertension. Despite treatment with ventricular drainage (D) and mannitol (M), cerebral perfusion decreased and the patient died.

the Harvard criteria are now used in many units, other criteria are being proposed. The model statute that is being suggested for adoption follows:

An individual who has sustained either (1) irreversible cessation of circulatory and respiratory functions or (2) irreversible cessation of all functions of the entire brain, including the brainstem, is dead. A determination of death must be made in accordance with acceptable medical standards.

Partly as an outgrowth of problems with determination of brain death and partly because of public questions concerning ethical considerations, the hospital-based ethics committee was started. Such committees are being formed in most large teaching hospitals and will probably become commonplace in all hospitals where critical patients are present. There are four general functions: prognosis, counseling, policy making, and review. A great deal of variation exists in how these committees are formed and how many functions are undertaken. More evaluations will have to be made to determine the appropriate functioning of these committees and to decide whether the concept of an ethical committee has long-term viability.

SUMMARY

Techniques of neurologic assessment are important for the critical care nurse to master. The basis of assessment and monitoring is to determine a baseline for future comparisons, to assess the patient's ability for self-care, and to identify trends to determine if the patient is getting better or worse.

REFERENCES

1. Ad Hoc Committee of Harvard Medical School. A definition of irreversible coma. *J.A.M.A.* 205(6):35, 1968.
2. Auer, L., Oberbuer, R., and Titthart, H. Relevance of CAT Scan for the Level of ICP in Patients with Severe Head Injury. In K. Schulman (ed.), *Intracranial Pressure IV*. Berlin: Springer-Verlag, 1980.
3. Bates, B. Guide to Physical Examination. Philadelphia: J. B. Lippincott, 1987.
4. Bickerstaff, E. R. Neurological Examination in Clinical Practice. Oxford: Blackwell, 1973.
5. Bires, B. Head trauma: Nursing implications from prehospital through emergency department. *Crit. Care Nurs. Q.* 10:1, 1987.
6. Brown, S. L. Practical points in the assessment and care of the patient having a carotid endarterectomy. *J. Postanesth. Nurs.* 11:41, 1987.
7. Chusid, J. G. Correlative Neuroanatomy and Functional Neurology. Los Altos, CA: Lange, 1984.
8. Core Curriculum for Neuroscience Nursing. Chicago: American Association for Neuroscience Nursing, 1984.
9. Davis, K. M., and Lemke, D. M. Brain death: Nursing roles and responsibilities. *J. Neurosci. Nurs.* 17:114, 1985.
10. Fisher, C. M. Some neuro-opthalmological observations. *J. Neurol. Neurosurg. Psychiatry* 39:383, 1967.
11. Hickey, J. V. The Clinical Practice of Neurological and Neurosurgical Nursing (2nd ed.). Philadelphia: J. B. Lippincott, 1986.
12. Hickman, K. M., Mayer, B. L., and Muwaswes, M. Intracranial pressure monitoring: Review of risk factors associated with infection. *Heart Lung* 19:84–92, 1990.
13. Nikas, D. L. Critical aspects of head trauma. *Crit. Care Nurs. Q.* 10:19, 1987.
14. Plum, F., and Posner, J. G. The Diagnosis of Stupor and Coma. Philadelphia: F. A. Davis, 1972.
15. Rauman, P. T., Reddy, P. R., and Sarasvaniv, R. Orbiculris oculi reflex and facial muscle electromyelography: Pre- and post-surgical evaluation of posterior fossa lesions. *J. Neurosurg.* 44:550, 1976.
16. Roper, A. H., Griswald, K., McKenna, D., et al. Computer-assisted neurological assessment in the neurologic intensive care unit. *Heart Lung* 10:54, 1981.
17. Sabin, T. D. The differential diagnosis of coma. *N. Engl. J. Med.* 290:1062, 1974.
18. Smith, K. A. Head trauma: Comparison of infection rates for different methods of intracranial pressure monitoring. *J. Neurosci. Nurs.* 19:310, 1987.

30

Head Injuries

Susan Kay Mitchell   *Rowena R. Yates*
Cornelia Vanderstaay Kenner

MUSIC AS MEDICINE

Tommy was a 3-year-old patient with neurotrauma who had been placed in a pentobarbital coma secondary to increasing intracranial pressure. Although the penobarbital dose was at high levels, Tommy also required morphine and pavulon. Any stimulation increased his heart rate, blood pressure, and intracranial pressure. His mother talking near his bed, monitoring alarms, or any noises would cause abrupt changes in his vital signs.

I wanted to see if music therapy would decrease his vital signs to normal levels consistently. I played soft music and lullabies at all times. He still required his pentobarbital, but I was able to decrease the frequency of his morphine and pavulon. Since that time, I have used music therapy with children and adults. It has been a helpful nursing intervention to promote sleep, decrease anxiety, provide a focus for patients exposed to the stimulation of an intensive care unit, and encourage relaxation.

Pam Davis, RN, BSN, RNC, CCRN
Special Care Unit
Maine Medical Center
Portland, Maine

LEARNING OBJECTIVES

After reading this chapter, the nurse should be able to do the following:

1. Describe the mechanism of head injury.
2. Differentiate among the types of head injury.
3. Compare and contrast uncal herniation and central herniation.
4. Compare and contrast the patient with increased intracranial pressure with the patient in shock.
5. Perform the initial assessment of a patient who has a head injury.
6. Monitor the physiologic parameters that are relevant to patients with head injuries.
7. Observe and protect the patient who is having a seizure.

CASE STUDY

At a construction site where he was working, R. A., an 18-year-old man, fell down eight steps and struck his head. He was extremely difficult to arouse. The emergency medical technicians who came to

help Mr. A. summoned the helicopter evacuation service, which quickly transferred him to the nearest trauma center.

Mr. A.'s health before the accident had been excellent. On arrival to the trauma center, his blood pressure was 118/62 mm Hg, his pulse was 104 beats/minute and regular, and his respirations were 22 and of regular rate and depth. A general physical examination revealed no gross abnormalities. His Glasgow Coma Scale rating was 14; his eyes opened spontaneously, his conversation was confused, and he obeyed commands with his right upper and lower extremities. Mr. A. was drowsy and displayed minimal spontaneous activity, his responses to verbal commands were sluggish, his pupils were 4 mm in diameter, they were equal, and they reacted briskly to light. His ciliospinal and corneal reflexes were intact. He had spontaneous ocular movement with full lateral range. A fundoscopic examination revealed no hemorrhages and no papilledema. He exhibited a flaccid left hemiplegia with no reflexes and a diminished sensitivity to painful stimuli. His arterial blood gas measurements were pH, 7.4; PaO_2, 90 mm Hg; $PaCO_2$, 40 mm Hg; and delta base, 0. Complete blood count and serum electrolyte results were within normal limits, and his skull, cervical spine, and chest radiographs were unremarkable.

Forty-five minutes later, Mr. A.'s level of consciousness had decreased, he had become extremely drowsy, and he displayed no spontaneous motor activity. He could be aroused only by noxious stimuli, and his responses tended to be stereotyped and simplified. His Glas-

557

gow Coma Scale rating was 12. His eyes opened on command, he responded with inappropriate words, and he obeyed commands with his right upper and lower extremities. His eye examination revealed the following: His right pupil was 6 mm in diameter, and it reacted sluggishly to light; on testing of his oculocephalic reflex, his right eye did not move entirely in the medial direction; his left pupil was 4 mm in diameter, and it reacted briskly to light. Thirty minutes later, a computed tomographic (CT) scan was done that revealed a right-sided subdural hematoma; Mr. A. exhibited flexion posturing on his left side. His respirations were 30 and regular and very deep. His right pupil was 8 mm in diameter, and it was fixed and dilated. He was immediately taken to the operating room for surgical evacuation of the subdural hematoma.

After surgery, Mr. A. was returned to the neurosurgical intensive care unit with an intracranial pressure monitor in place. On his first and second postoperative days, his level of consciousness increased consistently. He obeyed commands and displayed semipurposeful spontaneous movements. His family, who were devoted to him, voiced their optimism. His primary care nurse asked the family liaison nurse and chaplain to support the family however possible. The nurses, who were never without hope, encouraged the family in every positive occurrence. At the same time, they reinforced to the family that this period remained a critical one in Mr. A's care and that the final outcome remained unknown. On the third postoperative day, Mr. A.'s level of consciousness decreased, and he exhibited semipurposeful movements only with deep pain stimulus. His intracranial pressure increased from 20 mm Hg to 25 mm Hg; it was controlled with mannitol and mechanical hyperventilation. On Mr. A.'s fourth postoperative day, his intracranial pressure rose to 40 mm Hg, and it could not be controlled with mannitol and hyperventilation. A CT scan at this time revealed diffuse cerebral swelling without evidence of hematoma. On the fifth postoperative day, Mr. A. exhibited systolic hypertension and bradycardia. His pupils became fixed and dilated, and he had no corneal or oculocephalic reflexes. On sternal pain stimulation, his arms and legs assumed extension posturing. On the sixth postoperative day, Mr. A. exhibited hypotension, tachycardia, and total flaccidity of all extremities. He suffered a full cardiopulmonary arrest that was not responsive to aggressive resuscitative measures.

REFLECTIONS

Often, the brain-injured patient is in a state of unconsciousness, functioning on a subcortical level, seemingly unaware of his surroundings. But is he? Do stimuli somehow reach him even on a subconscious level? For years, nurses have been cautioned to talk to the patient, to give heed to what is said at the bedside, and always to be cognizant that the patient may hear. How often it has been said that "hearing is the last to go." What of the other senses? Changes in the patient's environment have been shown to have an effect on intracranial pressure.[10,24] It is not known for sure whether the changes are coincidental or whether there really might be some fundamental effect on the patient. There is much to be studied; there is much to be learned.

It is well accepted in the neuroscience nursing literature that many movements the patient makes will increase the intracranial pressure and should be avoided, but only a few references say what can decrease intracranial pressure. Assuredly, in many instances reduction of intracranial pressure would be of benefit to the patient. Because most patients with severe head injury have been shown to be functioning with low scores on the Glasgow Coma Scale, traditional approaches that affect cortical functioning do not show a lot of promise. Techniques such as the creative

use of sound and touch are potentially fruitful therapy and are only beginning to be adopted in nursing practice. One innovative researcher[41] looked at the effect of purposeful touch on intracranial pressure (ICP). This study revealed a significant decrease in ICP when smooth, circular motion was applied to the patient's cheek. However, no significant decrease in ICP was seen with stroking of the patient's hand.

Other research studies have examined the effects of both conversation and family presence on a patient's ICP.[12] One study indicated that family presence had a positive effect on ICP either significantly or nonsignificantly in the majority of the patients observed. Another study revealed that there could be a significant decrease in ICP when conversation unrelated to the patient took place within the patient's hearing. However, the available literature on the effects of conversation on ICP is contradictory as well as inconclusive.[15]

What implications these discoveries have for the art as well as the science of nursing! For a minute, let your mind expand. Consider potential ramifications of these studies. If purposeful touch would prove to be beneficial, would therapeutic touch be even more beneficial? If coincidental family presence has a positive effect on ICP, would planned presence be of even greater benefit? If conversation can serve to lower a patient's ICP, how much more could therapeutic conversation help? Up until this time, therapeutic touch, conversation, and family presence as treatments for increased ICP have not withstood the test of scientific inquiry. Perhaps with more study and a different perspective, the trend will change, and a firm basis for these interventions will be identified. Perhaps researchers will learn how to study the effects of these interventions. It is possible that the correct tools and protocols have not yet been identified.

As care is provided at the bedside, why not incorporate purposeful touch and therapeutic conversation into nursing practice? Think carefully about what is being done, and carefully observe the patient's response. Make assessments only after analyzing all the available data. Perhaps in this way, salient research questions can be identified and systematically investigated. Nursing is a doing profession. Touch and vocal interaction are a part of a doing art. It is time to bring these techniques out into the open, use them, study them, and find out if they really have a beneficial role in nursing practice.

ETIOLOGY AND INCIDENCE

Head injuries are caused by automobile accidents, gunshot wounds, stabbings, diving accidents, and falls or blows to the head—to name only a few causes. Most head injuries are caused by automobile accidents. In such accidents, the chances for serious head injury are great because the speed is often high and the riders' heads are not supported.[28] The head is injured in more than two thirds of all automobile accidents, and injury to the brain is the single most common cause of death in victims of automobile accidents. Hyperextension, hyperflexion, and lateral flexion injuries constitute over 50% of head injuries resulting from automobile accidents involving two or more vehicles. Hyperflexion injuries result from head-on collisions, whereas hyperextension injuries result from rear-end collisions. Lateral flexion injuries result from a lateral impact. Hyperflexion and lateral flexion injuries are more serious than hyperextension injuries. The incidence of associated spinal cord injury with severe head injury is approximately 5%. If the head injury has caused the death of the patient, the incidence increases 20%.

Central nervous system trauma accounts for 50% of the total of accidental deaths and follows heart disease, neoplasm, and cerebrovascular disease as the leading causes of death.[24] Much of this trauma is actually preventable, and significant advances are being made in the area of prevention and in promoting public awareness.

Brain and spinal cord injuries may occur simultaneously, at the time of the accident or at any time up to several months later. Important factors that influence the severity of injury are force, duration, location, and type of injury; associated injuries; age; prior health status; and emergency treatment.

The incidence of spinal cord injury in the United States is estimated to be 30 to 35 persons in 1 million, with 8,000 to 10,000 new cases annually. About 50% result from motor-vehicle accidents, 15% from falls, 15% from sports injuries, and 15% from gunshot wounds. In the category of sports-related injuries, an average of 10% is sustained by diving accidents in which the mean age of the victim is 22 years.[34]

Injuries to the spinal cord are caused by several types of trauma. Penetrating injury caused by a stab wound, bullet, or other high-speed missile may result in direct damage to the spinal cord. In motor-vehicle and motorcycle accidents, the head and spinal cord can move in any direction. Injuries caused by diving into shallow water are usually hyperextension injuries. Blows to the occiput and then to the vertex account for many compression fractures. A whiplash injury or a direct blow to the forehead results in sudden hyperextension. The areas of the body able to have the most movement experience an even greater motion, which then becomes abnormal. When a force is applied to a body, the force continues until the ligaments and bones are involved. This is true of the C4 and C6 areas (and of the T11 to L2 area), which are the most mobile. The type of spinal cord injury that occurs in association with head injury is usually of the cervical spine.

PATHOPHYSIOLOGY

Head injuries may be open (compound) or closed. They may be mild, moderate, severe, or lethal. In open head injuries, there is "communication" between the outside environment and the intracranial vault. Compound fractures of the skull, caused by both blunt and penetrating trauma, are open head injuries. They may result in different degrees of cerebral dysfunction. In open head injuries, the skull's contents have been exposed to the environment. Surgical debridement for cleansing and hemostasis is mandatory. Certain types of compound and penetrating injuries may be considered nonoperable under specific circumstances. Vigorous surgical management may not be indicated when vital signs show periods of apnea and bradycardia, when unconsciousness is profound, when pupils are fixed and dilated, and when reflexes are absent.

Immediate surgical intervention is usually not necessary in patients with a cerebrospinal fluid leak (rhinorrhea or otorrhea), because spontaneous closure is the usual course. If meningitis does occur, the infection is usually due to *Diplococcus pneumoniae*, or occasionally *Staphylococcus aureus*, and is responsive to methicillin and chloramphenicol. Prophylactic

antibiotics may be ordered in the presence of a cerebrospinal fluid leak.

In closed head injuries, there is no communication with the environment, although a simple fracture may be present. In mild head injuries, retrograde amnesia may be present, but the loss of consciousness is brief. In moderate head injuries, unconsciousness is longer (hours to days) and is associated with abnormal neurologic signs. In severe head injuries, unconsciousness is even longer and is commonly associated with a larger number of abnormal neurologic signs. Death is inevitable in lethal injuries.

Formerly the terms *concussion, contusion,* and *laceration* were commonly used to categorize injuries. These terms are explained here, although the terminology now used is *mild head injury, moderate head injury,* and *severe head injury*. In a concussion, the most common kind of head injury, the injury is less severe and the loss of consciousness is brief. Dizziness, loss of memory, and headache are of short duration. A contusion is much more serious; bruising and many small hemorrhages may be present, as may true laceration (tearing). There may be extensive permanent injury. On early evaluation, contusion is often clinically indistinguishable from laceration, but the difference can be seen on the CT scan. The term *contusion* is really very descriptive, because contusions are the most obvious sign of brain injury when the brain is examined with the naked eye.[21] In situations in which the head is accelerated after a blow or when the moving head undergoes sudden deceleration, contusions occur most frequently on the undersurfaces of the frontal lobes and around the poles of the temporal lobes. Contusions may be more severe on one side but are usually present bilaterally.

MECHANISM

There are many theories regarding the causes of cerebral injury. The factors mentioned include the transmission of waves of force, skull deformation, skull vibration, formation of a pressure gradient in the cranial cavity, brain displacement, brain rotation, and transient brain cavitation. No one theory has been generally accepted. Essentially, injuries to the head are caused by a force that is either focal or general, or both. All three types of force are serious, but the nursing observations and expectations are slightly different for each one. The types of force may be conceptualized by considering the difference between a moving object that strikes a stationary head and a moving head that strikes a stationary object. The former example involves a focal injury (coup contusion), and the latter example usually involves a generalized injury, a much more profound injury.

When the force is focal, the type of injury sustained depends on the local area involved and the extent of the injury. Symptoms will likely arise from the area injured, and observations for dysfunction would depend on what that area is. For example, a blow to the head by a blackjack is likely to cause a depressed skull fracture. Deformation and depression occur because the object has relatively low velocity.

Several problems may result from a generalized force. First, the energy either dissipates into a fracture or is directly transmitted to the brain with resultant damage as the force is absorbed and the direction of force changes. Second, particularly during acceleration and deceleration, the brain strikes the skull and the dura and may even strike the inner skull surface on the opposite side. Linear stresses can cause bruising of the brain on the side opposite the impact (the contrecoup effect). Third, generalized force is particularly dangerous if the direction of the blow is tangential and rotation occurs. For example, the brain may strike the sphenoid ridges or falx, or the brain stem may be compressed by rotation of the cerebrum. Vectoral force can be aimed at deep centers. For example, at the time of injury, the person may be traumatized to the point where no or only minimal linear skull fractures are observed on the radiograph, and the remaining energy is transmitted to the brain substance itself. If the force is caused by the head striking the ground, the injury is usually on the opposite side of the brain, a contrecoup contusion with the coup contusion being smaller or even absent.

On postmortem examination, many patients are found to have a laceration of the corpus callosum that results from its being compressed against the falx. A lacerated corpus collosum has been found by CT scan to usually occur with a lethal head injury.[3]

Movement and Forces That Produce Injury

The mechanism of head injury depends on the mass and velocity of the type of injury. The brain is well protected by the scalp, the skull, and the cerebrospinal fluid. At the time of impact, several things may occur. As the scalp moves across the skull, bleeding or a hematoma may result. The skull then may be fractured or may bend internally. The brain may be bruised locally. Also, gas bubbles (microcavitation) may be formed locally in the cerebral hemisphere and disrupt neural tissue. In turn, white matter may be lacerated. A significant problem may result from the movement of the brain across the many rough areas on the inside of the "bony box." The brain can move front to back or back to front so that the orbital surfaces are raked across the medial floor of the frontal fossa and the frontal lobes are contused (usually) or lacerated (occasionally). In particular, the temporal lobe is in a precarious position. The anterior part of the temporal lobe, which is bordered by the sphenoid bone, may become contused and edematous. Commonly, movement causes resonance cavitation, which is followed by movement in the temporal fossa and across the frontal fossa. Shearing forces result; they may be great enough to cause death. Significantly, the shearing force may cause injury at the spinal medullary junction, because the brain is attached at the base of the skull and must rock back and forth. The rotary motion produces a vector of force toward deep midline structures. It probably is the cause of unconsciousness. In some instances, the motion is so intense that the brain stem strikes the tentorium and thus causes primary brain stem injury. Pressure waves follow the impact. They can injure the brain by compression and tension. Thus injury can occur anywhere and can be of any severity. The injury is then compounded by hypoxia and swelling, and the injured brain is far more susceptible to a second insult of any type.

INCREASED INTRACRANIAL PRESSURE

One of the consequences of head injury is an increase in the ICP. Increased ICP is a result of swelling or hemorrhage. The term *swelling* is preferred to the term *edema* because the probable mechanism is massive dilatation of blood vessels after injury and not edema, as seen with tumors. (Cerebral edema produces a volumetric enlargement of the brain, an increase in tissue water content, and is one cause of swelling.) Damage to the cerebral cells and their functioning is caused by the increased size or volume of the brain and by the intrinsic and extrinsic pressure. The fluid in the intracranial compartments (intracellular, cerebrospinal fluid, and intravascular compartments) is contained in a bony box that cannot expand.

According to the modified Monro-Kellie hypothesis, the skull is a rigid compartment filled to capacity with essentially noncompressible contents. The volume of these contents, brain matter, intravascular blood supply, and cerebrospinal fluid, is nearly constant. If any one of these three components increases in volume, one of the other components has to decrease in volume to prevent the ICP from rising. For example, increases in blood or fluid will result in increases in volume. Therefore, increased ICP can result from those factors influencing the volume of these components, such as hypoventilation, alterations in arterial carbon dioxide levels, and decreased cerebral venous return. In effect, hypoventilation produces increased carbon dioxide levels that produce vasodilatation that results in increased ICP.

When prolonged high levels of increased ICP are associated with an intracranial hematoma, the expected patient outcome is poor. Poor outcome is defined as a severe disability, vegetative state, or death. Intracranial pressure levels of 0 mm Hg to 20 mm Hg are associated with a 27% poor outcome, 20 mm Hg to 40 mm Hg are associated with a 46% poor outcome, 40 mm Hg to 60 mm Hg are associated with a 76% poor outcome, and ICP levels greater than 60 mm Hg are associated with a 100% poor outcome.[21]

Compensatory Mechanisms

Compensatory mechanisms are brought into play by the body in an effort to ensure adequate blood supply to the brain. In the presence of increased ICP, Cushing's reflex (increased blood pressure and decreased pulse, and respiratory abnormality) is activated in an attempt to decrease the amount of blood in the head without decreasing the perfusion of brain tissue.

Cerebral perfusion pressure = mean arterial pressure − ICP

It is thought that compression of or interference with a small region in the medulla is critical for the production of arterial hypertension. If increased ICP is diffuse, or if there are no pressure gradients along the craniospinal axis, the pressor response does not occur until the ICP equals or exceeds the diastolic blood pressure.[7] In contrast, a mass lesion that causes compression or distortion of the brain stem may produce a pressor response at relatively low levels of ICP. This increase in blood pressure is due to peripheral vasoconstriction from increased sympathetic activity and to increased cardiac output. Such compensatory mechanisms are not active with excessively increased levels of ICP; the patient exhibits a decreased blood pressure and increased or decreased and irregular pulse and respirations shortly before death.

When the contents of the fluid compartments continue to expand and thereby increase pressure, shifts occur within the parenchyma of the brain. The shifts depend also on the rate of expansion. A rapid expansion of a small mass causes a larger increase in ICP and the degree of brain malfunctioning than does a slow expansion of a much larger mass, because the brain is able to accommodate a slowly growing mass without as much loss of functioning. Eventually, vascular problems or obstruction of the spinal fluid circulation becomes so great that compensation is no longer possible.

Pressure Transmission

Pressure is transmitted evenly and quickly to all intracranial compartments as long as there is fluid connection among the compartments (Pascal's law). In the event of obstruction, pressures in the various compartments are very different.

The intracranial space contains displaceable fluid (cerebrospinal fluid and blood) that can be expressed into the extracranial vascular system. A certain amount of cerebral or intracranial expansion is possible, because cerebrospinal fluid is approximately 10% of the intracranial volume,[19] and blood is approximately 2% to 11% of the intracranial volume. The entire normal ventricular system accounts for 35 ml, and part of this amount may be displaced (Fig. 30–1). In order to accommodate an enlarging mass, the fluid is displaced, and the intracranial pressure does not change as long as the volume displaced equals the volume added. However, the volume of fluid that can be displaced is limited. If the mass continues to expand, the ICP increases monotonically (i.e., increments in the mass produce an ever-increasing rise in the ICP) (Fig. 30–2). At the point when almost all the fluid has been displaced, an additional small increase in the mass produces a very large increase in the ICP.

Swelling develops gradually in the first hours after injury; the maximum development is usually reached in 36 to 48 hours. If the swelling reaches the point that the ICP equals the arterial blood pressure, circulation through the brain ceases and death results.

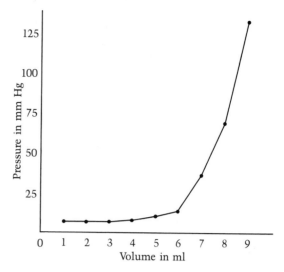

Figure 30–2

Volume and pressure relationship. The volume of fluid that can be displaced is limited, and if the volume continues to expand, the intracranial pressure elevates at an increasingly rapid rate.

Brain Edema

Hydrostatic and oncotic pressures in plasma and tissues are responsible for the movement of water across the capillary membrane in the brain, just as in the peripheral circulation. However, the movement of water and solutes across the epithelium in brain capillaries is lower than in the rest of the body's circulation. This phenomenon is largely attributable to the special properties of the blood-brain barrier. Several different mechanisms may produce the three types of edema: vasogenic, cytotoxic, or interstitial.[9]

Vasogenic edema, the most common form, which is usually produced by mechanical trauma, is characterized by an increased permeability of the capillary endothelial cells. Because of the dysfunction in the blood-brain barrier, osmotically active proteins move from the intravascular compartment into the interstitial extracellular space. The osmotic pressure in the tissues therefore increases, and more fluid is attracted into the interstitial extracellular space. If vasogenic edema is accompanied by venous engorgement, there may be severe brain swelling. Although not fully understood, cerebral white matter is known to be susceptible to vasogenic edema. This susceptibility may be related to the fact that capillary density and blood flow are normally lower in white matter than in cortical and subcortical gray matter.

Cytotoxic edema is the result of defective osmoregulation, cerebral ischemia, and intracellular fluid accumulation. It is characteristically seen after cardiac arrest with hypoxemia and in water intoxication. The fluid is composed of sodium and intracellular water and results from the failure of the adenosine triphosphate–dependent sodium pump. The neurons, glia, and endothelial cells swell, reducing the extracellular fluid space in the brain and significantly decreasing the size of the capillary lumen (mainly because of the swelling of the endothelial cells).

Interstitial edema is the result of an increase in the sodium and water content of the periventricular white matter. It is characteristically seen in obstructive hydrocephalus. Cerebrospinal fluid moves across the ventricular walls, but the peri-

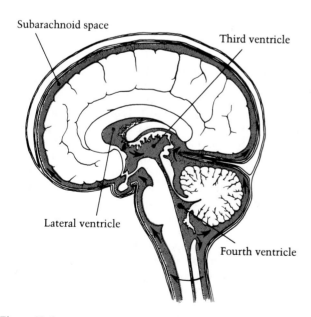

Figure 30–1

Ventricular system showing cerebrospinal fluid circulation from lateral ventricles to subarachnoid space.

ventricular white matter decreases in size rather than increases. As the hydrostatic pressure within the white matter increases, the myelin lipids decrease rapidly, resulting in the decrease in periventricular white matter rather than in the anticipated increase.

AUTOREGULATION

The brain has the unique capability to autoregulate; therefore, of particular significance are the impairments in pressure and metabolic autoregulation. *Pressure autoregulation* is a change in the diameter of blood vessels in the brain produced by a change in transmural pressure across the walls of the autoregulatory vessels so as to maintain a constant blood flow during a change in perfusion pressure.[17] Normally, cerebral blood flow is kept constant because of arterial constriction and dilatation, and it is only partly dependent on the systemic arterial blood pressure and body posture. After trauma, the autoregulatory capacity to change caliber and flow rate is impaired, producing swelling and dilation of intracranial vessels under the influence of the systemic blood pressure.

Because vasoconstriction would decrease cerebral blood flow, the explanations offered for the phenomena include Cushing's reflex. In the presence of increased ICP, when there is a threat to the blood supply to the brain, increases in sympathetic vasoconstriction elevate the blood pressure (increased ICP → medullary vasomotor center ischemia → vasomotor inhibitory fibers are sensitive to the hypoxia resulting from ischemia, whereas the sympathetic fibers are not → vasoconstriction → increased blood pressure). Once the systemic blood pressure rises in response to increasing ICP, the hydrostatic pressure in the arterial side of the cerebral circulation also rises, and the amount of hydrostatic edema increases.

Even more important in the person with a closed head injury is the compensatory change in blood flow to meet the altered metabolic demands of the tissue. Here the premise concerns chemical regulation dependent on local oxygen requirements and carbon dioxide production. The hydrogen ion concentration in the extravascular space is the key determinant of the diameter of the vessel. As more hydrogen ions are produced locally and diffuse to the vessels, the vessels dilate and increase the cerebral blood flow. Also, increased carbon dioxide levels decrease the extracellular pH and cause vasodilation and increased cerebral blood flow.

Cerebral Blood Flow

Although cerebral blood flow is an important consideration, assessment of brain functioning as well as brain damage in humans and experimental animals cannot be determined accurately by measuring the cerebral blood flow.[13] In injured people with severe neurological dysfunction and depressed brain metabolism, cerebral blood flow may be normal. The converse can also be true (*i.e.*, the brain may be able to function normally with a decreased cerebral blood flow as long as the decrease in metabolism is proportional to the decrease in cerebral blood flow). The hypothermic patient exemplifies that concept in that decreased temperature decreases metabolism, which in turn decreases cerebral blood flow.

Research studies on cerebral blood flow must be evaluated carefully. Most studies do not truly simulate the pathophysiology of head injury. Actually, questions remain as to whether clinical head injury has ever been simulated by an existing investigational model.[6] Usually the model includes rapid infusion of fluid into the subarachnoid space, resulting in a diffuse increase in the ICP. The clinical situation can be quite different in the case of the intracranial expansion of a supratentorial mass, which causes fluid obstruction and a difference in pressure gradients; hence, information about pressure from the subarachnoid space is not sufficient to evaluate the complex situation (*e.g.*, knowledge of local tissue pressures is needed to establish a relationship between pressure and flow).

In the clinical situation, it is difficult to measure cerebral blood flow and certainly difficult to measure it as part of a research protocol. Changes in cerebral perfusion pressure and cerebral blood flow are often temporary and last only a very short period of time. It is hard to document the occurrence at that moment in time.[21]

Cerebral blood flow is a function of the diameter of the cerebrovascular bed, blood viscosity, pressure, vascular bed resistance, and cerebral perfusion pressure. In the usual case, the brain receives 50 ml of blood/100 g of brain tissue each minute (15% of the cardiac output). Because of autoregulation, cerebral blood flow remains relatively constant even with a wide variance in cerebral perfusion pressure. After head injury, the situation is different. Autoregulation is compromised severely or even lost, so that blood flow becomes pressure-dependent. Therefore, any decrease in cerebral perfusion pressure may result in a decrease in cerebral blood flow.

HEMORRHAGE

An early potential complication after traumatic head injury is acute bleeding from an epidural (extradural), acute subdural, or intracerebral hemorrhage. Acute bleeding can cause unconsciousness, increasing abnormal neurologic signs that indicate rostrocaudal deterioration, or herniation and death. These are signs of true surgical emergencies. A decrease in the level of consciousness after head trauma is assumed to be caused by a hemorrhage. Further emergency neurodiagnostic tests may be indicated.

An epidural hematoma (Fig. 30–3) may be caused by arterial or venous bleeding in the frontal or temporal regions (very rarely in the posterior fossa). Most epidural hematomas are over the cerebral convexity, are usually related to the temporal lobe, and result from a laceration of the middle meningeal artery caused by a skull fracture.[23] The recovery rate for patients diagnosed and treated early is extremely good. Only a minority of individuals undergo the classic progression of symptoms—from unconsciousness to a conscious lucid interval and back to unconsciousness—but the nurse must always ask about the sequence when obtaining historic data. Although the clinical sequence apparent to the observer varies, the most common progression is as follows[22,26]: As the hematoma expands, the brain is first pushed away from the skull, then it is compressed, and then herniation occurs. The signs and symptoms are headache, possibly followed by a subtle change in behavior, a decreased level of consciousness, and then a change in the ipsilateral pupil signs followed by contralateral motor paralysis. When the eye on the side of the hematoma is tested, first the pupil constricts, then it reacts more slowly, and then it becomes fixed and dilated. Paralysis of the extraocular muscle follows quickly. The same sequence occurs in the contralateral pupil. If both pupils are fixed and dilated for

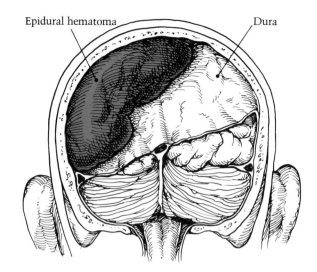

Figure 30–3

Epidural hematoma. Usually the bleeding is arterial in origin. The epidural hematoma tends to have a concave, localized formation because the dura is firmly affixed to the skull.

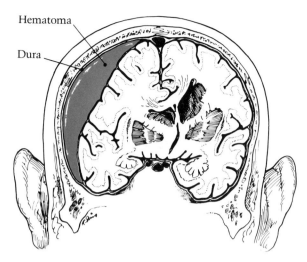

Figure 30–4

Subdural hematoma. Usually the bleeding is venous in origin. The subdural hematoma tends to have a convex, diffuse formation, because the brain is not as firmly affixed to the dura as the dura is to the skull. The bleeding may encircle the hemisphere and have an elliptic, convex appearance.

more than 30 minutes, it is highly unlikely that the person will survive.

Acute subdural hematoma (Fig. 30–4) may be unilateral or bilateral, as well as arterial or venous in origin. Arterial bleeding, although uncommon, is usually caused by a tear in the brain; the patient has a decreased level of consciousness and may demonstrate a focal neurologic deficit. Venous bleeding commonly occurs from tearing of the veins that go from the brain to the dural sinuses. The mortality can be extremely high if the hematoma develops suddenly so that the brain is unable to withstand rapid compression. The shearing force that produces the intracranial shifting and vascular tears also produces dramatic intracerebral shearing forces. It is these intracerebral forces that are probably so destructive. The expanding lesion compresses the midline structures to one side. The patient's death occurs in the same sequence: hemorrhage, compression, edema, and herniation. The pupil signs are ipsilateral, and the motor findings are contralateral. In adults under the age of 30, the survival rate is 50%. For those 30 to 50 years old, the survival rate is 20%. For those over the age of 50, the survival rate is extremely low.

Traumatic intracerebral hematoma in salvageable patients is less common than subdural hematoma but more common than epidural hematoma; often it mimics or accompanies one or both. The most common site is the temporal lobe. The occipital and frontal lobes are also common sites. Usually the hemorrhage is the result of acute contusion of the blood vessels in the brain. The symptoms are a decreased level of consciousness and a progressive focal neurologic deficit.

Computed tomographic scanning is commonly used (before surgery if time permits) to help localize the lesion. Arteriography is now done less frequently.

HERNIATION

Severe head trauma with symptoms of an expanding supratentorial mass resulting in herniation is a true surgical emergency. Unless treatment is instituted rapidly, the pressure and

vascular injuries associated with herniation produce death by deterioration in a rostrocaudal progression. Accurate observations and recording are imperative to help determine whether the person is getting better or getting worse. Once the masses enlarge so that the skull is not large enough to hold its contents, the cerebral structures shift and compress other areas. These areas then swell and shift. A shift may occur from one side of the brain to another or from the supratentorial compartment to the posterior fossa through the tentorial notch (the large semioval opening in the center of the tentorium). Displacement from the posterior fossa into the spinal canal produces tonsilar herniation through the foramen magnum. Compression of the medulla leads to respiratory arrest and death.

Tentorial herniation may occur by either of two processes: uncal herniation or central herniation. In rapidly expanding hematomas, it is usually uncal. The process of herniation is well described by Plum and Posner.[26]

Transfalcian Herniation

In transfalcian or cingulate herniation, cerebral ischemia and edema are increased by the compression of blood vessels (the anterior cerebral arteries) and tissues. The falx is a fold of dura mater that separates the two cerebral hemispheres and extends down into the interhemispheric fissure. Once the force produced by the enlarging mass is great enough, the hemisphere herniates under the falx. Also, ischemia in the distribution of the anterior cerebral artery can lead to paralysis of one or both legs.

Uncal Herniation

Uncal herniation (Fig. 30–5) occurs after a temporal mass has shifted the inner basal edge of the uncus and hippocampal gyrus over the lateral edge of the tentorium. Crowding at the tentorial notch compresses the midbrain and oculomotor nerve

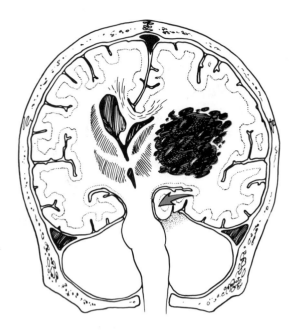

Figure 30–5
Uncal herniation.

against the opposite edge. Classically, the uncus herniates over the free edge, pushes the posterior cerebral artery down, and compresses the oculomotor nerve. The temporal lobe then herniates into the notch. As the posterior cerebral artery is occluded, ischemia of the occipital lobe increases, and infarction results. The aqueduct is compressed, and spinal fluid circulation is blocked. The brain stem is damaged by ischemia and hemorrhage.[26]

The signs of herniation may be described as those seen early and late. According to Plum and Posner,[26] a significant exception to the norm may occur in that the first observable sign is not a decreased level of consciousness but a sluggishly reactive pupil. Clinically, however, this is not a consistent finding, and a decreased level of consciousness often precedes a change in the pupil. In any event, the patient may arrive at the hospital with a subtle eye sign, such as a unilaterally dilated pupil. Also, the classical signs of increased blood pressure and slowed pulse may not occur unless the posterior fossa is involved. A progressive sequence of pupillary, respiratory, and motor signs is seen. Deterioration proceeds quickly once the signs of midbrain dysfunction occur.[27,37]

The criteria used for evaluation are described in Chapter 29 (Neurologic Assessment). The evaluative criteria for early herniation are the following:

1. Level of consciousness: Near wakefulness to coma
2. Respirations: Eupnea
3. Eyes:
    A. Pupil size: Unequal, unilateral dilation (6 mm in diameter)
    B. Pupil reaction: Dilated pupil, sluggish reaction, opposite pupil reacts
    C. Ciliospinal reflex: Intact
    D. Eye movements: Unimpaired
    E. Oculocephalic reflex: Unimpaired
    F. Oculovestibular reflex: Unimpaired (the dilated pupil may not turn toward a cold stimulus)

4. Motor signs: No change
5. Pain: Purposeful

The signs of late uncal herniation are those of midbrain dysfunction. They are the following:

1. Level of consciousness: Stuporous or comatose
2. Respirations: Cheyne-Stokes or central neurogenic hyperventilation
3. Eyes:
    A. Pupil size: Unequal, unilaterally dilated (8 mm in diameter)
    B. Pupil reaction: Direct response absent in dilated pupil, present in other pupil
    C. Ciliospinal reflex: Intact but difficult to test in a fully blown pupil
    D. Eye movements: Oculomotor paralysis
    E. Oculocephalic reflex: Irregular
    F. Oculovestibular reflex: Sluggish
4. Motor signs: Frequently ipsilateral hemiplegia and contralateral flexion or extension posturing
5. Pain: Bilateral extensor plantar response, extension posturing

The signs of deterioration continue, and the signs of midbrain damage appear and progress caudally. The damage is due to secondary ischemia and necrosis. The patient's chances of full recovery are extremely poor. The portion of the midbrain compressed by the uncus is the cerebral peduncle.[35] Because that area is the carrier of motor fibers to the spinal cord, communication between the cerebrum and the midbrain is interrupted. Brain stem reflexes appear.

The signs of midbrain and upper pons damage are the following:

1. Level of consciousness: Stuporous or comatose
2. Respirations: Sustained central neurogenic hyperventilation
3. Eyes:
    A. Pupil size: Irregularly at midposition (4 mm to 6 mm in diameter)
    B. Pupil reactivity: Fixed bilaterally
    C. Ciliospinal reflex: May disappear
    D. Eye movements: Paralysis
    E. Oculocephalic reflex: Absent or impaired (when the reflex is elicited, eye movements are dysconjugate and the medially moving eye does not move as far as the laterally moving eye)
    F. Oculovestibular reflex: Impaired
4. Motor: Resting position or bilateral extension posturing
5. Pain: Bilateral extension posturing

Without therapy, damage due to ischemia and necrosis continues down the brain stem. The following signs of the lower pons and upper medullary dysfunction appear:

1. Level of consciousness: Comatose
2. Respirations: Shallow, rapid eupnea (20 to 40 breaths), and apneustic
3. Eyes:
    A. Pupil size: Midposition
    B. Pupil reactivity: Fixed
    C. Ciliospinal reflex: Unobtainable

D. Eye movements: Unobtainable
E. Oculocephalic reflex: Unobtainable
F. Oculovestibular reflex: Unobtainable
4. Motor signs: Flaccid, bilateral extensor plantar response
5. Pain: Occasional flexion or perhaps response in lower extremity

Before death, the patient passes through a state exhibiting signs of medullary dysfunction. Respirations are slow, ataxic, and interrupted by deep sighs or gasps. Blood pressure drops, and the pulse may be fast or slow.

Central Herniation

After head injury, the patient may also herniate centrally (transtentorial). The diencephalon, the midbrain, the pons, and then the medulla are affected in an orderly progression. Preceding the sequence might have been a lateral shift and cingulate herniation that resulted in increased ischemia and edema from the compression of the cerebral artery and vein.

Downward pressure from the cerebral hemispheres then compresses the diencephalon and even the midbrain through the tentorial notch. Several brain stem changes occur (they are the same as those in uncal herniation): compression of the posterior cerebral artery, spinal fluid circulation blockage, brain-stem ischemia, and then continued destruction. The early signs are different from those in uncal herniation, but after the midbrain and upper pons stage, they are the same.

One of the most reliable early signs of central herniation is a decrease in the level of consciousness. Other early signs are as follows:

1. Level of consciousness: Obtunded–stuporous–comatose
2. Respirations: Cheyne-Stokes with deep sighs or yawns
3. Eyes:
   A. Pupil size: Small (1 mm to 3 mm in diameter)
   B. Pupil reaction: Brisk but hard to see
   C. Ciliospinal reflex: Intact
   D. Eye movements: Conjugate or roving and slightly divergent
   E. Oculocephalic reflex:
      (1) If the eyes are conjugate at rest, they do not move when the head turns.
      (2) There is only a slight alteration from the resting eye movement.
      (3) Vertical movement may be impaired.
   F. Oculovestibular reflex: Movement of eyes toward a cold stimulus
4. Motor signs:
   A. If hemiplegia is present, it may worsen. The other side may develop paratonic resistance (that includes the whole body). There is bilateral plantar extension.
   B. Later, grasp reflexes are present.
5. Pain:
   A. The nonhemiplegic side may respond appropriately to pain.
   B. In the hemiplegic limb, flexion posturing appears, particularly in response to pain.
   C. Occasionally, the hemiplegic side responds to pain with extension posturing, and the opposite side (ipsilateral to the mass) responds to pain with flexion posturing.

ASSOCIATED SPINAL CORD INJURY

A patient with head trauma may have spinal cord injury associated with intracranial head injury, or spinal cord injury may be seen as a separate entity. The clinical findings in spinal cord injury are presented in the following sections.

The syndrome of swelling, hemorrhage, and transection occurs in cord injuries, but actual evaluation of spinal trauma is difficult, because there is no way to determine the amount of damage. It has been known for many years that a weight of greater than 600 g/cm^2 dropped on an animal's spine renders the animal permanently paralyzed. When the weight is less than 400 g/cm^2, the animal will recover from paralysis. It was learned much later that when a stainless steel wire was passed between the ligaments above and below the injury, the wire raised the weight needed to cause permanent paralysis from 600 g to 800 g/cm^2. In other words, eliminating mobilization produced a decreased incidence of paralysis.

Nervous tissue withstands compression poorly, and the more rapid the compression, the poorer the tolerance. Even though the cord compression is transient, with sufficient force the result is total disruption of the cord. If the cord were viewed approximately 30 minutes after impact, a small number of petechial hemorrhages in the central gray matter would be seen. Two hours later, the hemorrhages would be larger in number and the expanding hematoma would compress the cord and extend up and down the cord for several segments. The result within 24 hours is dissolution of the central cord, edema within the surrounding white matter, and necrosis of the cord. The pathophysiologic processes after trauma are the same within the brain and spinal cord, but the results differ because of anatomic variations.

Mechanisms of Spinal Trauma

The most vulnerable part of the spine is the cervical area. The head is mobile, relatively heavy, and supported poorly—by rather weak muscles, so any head injury may well damage the spine. The mechanisms of spinal trauma must be analyzed to afford understanding of the clinical and pathologic findings; the injuries are defined by the movement of the head in relationship to the spine: axial loading, flexion, and hyperextension (Fig. 30–6).

In an axial loading injury, the force is upward and downward with no posterior or lateral bending of the neck. Commonly, a burst fracture of the vertebral body or a disc extrusion results. A typical axial loading injury is one that occurs in an automobile accident in which the person is thrown up against the roof and strikes the vertex of his head. The classic presentation is fracture of the first cervical vertebra (Jefferson's fracture), in which the head is impacted from above and the ring at the first cervical vertebra bursts. It is unusual to have associated cord injury, because the cervical space is relatively large at this site and the fracture site is not greatly displaced.

In a flexion injury, the head is bent forward on the cervical spine. Flexion, both with and without rotation, produces a more complex injury. The person may have a residual compression fracture with more destruction anteriorly, posterior points of spinal dislocation, and a disc herniated posteriorly against the cord. If rotation accompanies the flexion, there may be more compression of one side of the body than the other. At the time of the flexion injury, one vertebral body

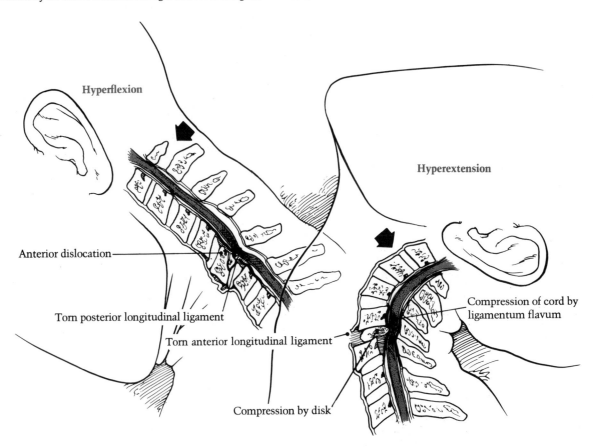

Figure 30–6
Mechanism of spinal injury.

moves forward and the cord is essentially totally compressed. Not a lot of force is required to produce a flexion injury. Characteristically, the type of spinal cord injury produced is complete paralysis with no functional segment of any kind below the transection. A typical flexion injury can occur to a football player who "spears" another player during a tackle.

When spinal flexion of the cervical spine occurs with disc extrusion (it occurs rarely), the anterior cervical spine syndrome is produced. Paralysis of all four limbs occurs, with loss of pain and temperature sense, but with preservation of position sense and light touch, because the posterior columns remain intact. Many surgeons consider the syndrome an indication for surgical decompression.

In a hyperextension injury, the cord is angulated acutely as the head is bent back sharply. If the direction of the force is significantly downward, varying degrees of compression of the vertebral bodies result. The wedging force may crush one of the adjacent vertebrae, and bony fragments may be driven posteriorly into the spinal canal. Depending on the direction and intensity of the force, there may also be a fracture of the pedicles or laminae. The fracture may be further complicated by forward dislocation of the upper vertebra on the lower if the posterior longitudinal ligament or the articular ligaments are torn. Hyperextension injuries caused by forces applied to the anterior skull or face result in a stretched anterior longitudinal ligament. If the force is sufficient to carry the upper vertebra backward, the vertebral body above the break may separate from the one below, leaving the disc intact but stripping the posterior longitudinal ligament from the vertebra be-

low. The spinal cord is carried backward with the vertebra above and may be contused against the lamina of the vertebra below. The alignment of the vertebra about the break depends on the type of injury and on how the patient is handled after the injury.

People who have spinal cord injuries often also have a narrow spinal canal and their spinal cord is essentially squeezed. The central cervical cord syndrome may result. Characteristically, the spinal cord lesion is incomplete; the arms, especially the hands, are more involved than are the legs. The loss of sensory function varies. A common injury occurs when the person falls and strikes his head, extending it backward; the hallmark is a bruise on the forehead.

Severity of Spinal Trauma

Cervical spine fractures do not necessarily cause a neurologic deficit. The more severe and extensive the fracture, the more likely the person is to have a neurologic deficit. Likewise, the greater the amount of subluxation, the more likely the person is to have a neurologic deficit. In patients who have congenitally narrow spinal canals with or without spinal spondylosis, spinal cord injury and a neurologic deficit may be present, even in the absence of fracture or subluxation. Relatively small degrees of subluxation in a narrowed area may cause severe and irreversible damage.

Fracture dislocations characterized by bony displacement in which the interarticular joints have been subluxed and the pedicles broken do not usually cause spinal cord compression.

The presence of subluxations may be attributed to the facts that the spinal cord takes up a considerably smaller cross-sectional area than does its surrounding vertebral canal and that as the fracture separates, the canal may widen and take more room.

Thoracolumbar fractures are much less of a problem for the following reasons: the cord becomes smaller as it approaches the end in the conus medullarus, and so the amount of free space is much larger; the conus is more likely than the higher, more proximal areas of the spinal cord to recover; and peripheral nerves are involved in the lumbar area.

The severity of the spinal injury varies according to the degree of pathology produced. The cord can look normal at surgery, but the patient can have no function. There may be a simple contusion (bruising), laceration (tearing), or compression due to fracture dislocation and subluxation. If the cord has been contused, swelling occurs within the tough, inelastic pia with subsequent partial or complete interruption of conduction. Anatomical transection is exceedingly rare. The swelling increases for 48 hours and gradually subsides in a week.

Spinal cord compression abolishes all functions below the segment compressed. Ischemia to a cord segment that lasts for an hour produces irreversible infarctions, mainly in the gray matter. If the onset of the cord compression is slow, the deficit is seen first in the pyramidal tract and posterior columns. The deficit is manifested by loss of motor function and joint position; loss of pin sensation from spinothalamic dysfunction is temporally the last modality to be affected in spinal cord compression. Neurosurgical decompression can sometimes halt and even reverse the process.

Studies suggest that mechanical trauma severe enough to produce paralysis initiates a process in the spinal cord tissues that destroys the spinal cord parenchyma in 24 to 48 hours.[34] A biphasic phenomenon in blood flow to regions of the cord has been described in which perfusion to the center of the spinal cord is severely decreased, whereas perfusion to the surrounding white matter is severely increased. Thus, vessels and tissues that are unable to survive profound hypoxia become necrotic.[33] The microvasculature is the most trauma-sensitive tissue in the cord. Early metabolic changes are similar to those described in other organ systems, with alteration of sodium-potassium ATPase and elevation of calcium.

Spinal Shock

Spinal shock occurs with acute physiologic or anatomic spinal cord transection; it results in sympathetic collapse, paralysis, anesthesia, areflexia, and the loss of sphincter function below the level of the lesion. Spinal shock may last up to 6 weeks; it ends when the reflexes are regained. At that point, the reflexes are generally hyperactive or spastic. The shock state appears to be due to loss of facilitation from descending tracts, inhibition of spinal segments, and degeneration of the axons. Corticospinal and reticulospinal stimuli no longer reach either the part of the trunk that is below the lesion or the extremities. The patient does not lose consciousness, but he displays a flaccid paralysis accompanied by a loss of sensation and reflexes in the involved parts. Vasomotor control is lost in the periphery, because the reflex pathways in the spinal cord are cut. Blood then pools in the extremities. Both pulse and blood pressure are decreased.

In complete lesions of the spinal cord, neurologic deficits below the level of the lesion include complete flaccid paralysis, total loss of sensation, loss of sweating below the level of the lesion, and paralysis of the bowel and bladder. The duration of spinal shock depends on the extent of injury to the spinal cord. If the cord is completely transected, spinal shock may last several weeks. After that period, the tendon reflexes become hyperactive, with marked clonus. Retention of urine is common when reflex activity returns because the sphincter recovers before the detrusor muscle. The leg muscles particularly show varying degrees of spasticity, mainly the extensors. Damage is considered to be functionally complete and permanent if the patient has an immediate motor and sensory paralysis that lasts for 24 hours. However, because reflexes below the injury are not operant in the presence of spinal shock, a complete lesion is not considered permanent until the return of the bulbocavernosus perineal reflex.

In incomplete spinal cord lesions, the period of spinal shock is shorter. The deep and superficial reflexes return in days or weeks. Sensation gradually returns. Motor function may return in varying degrees, and depending on the severity of the injury, it may be asymmetric.

NURSING PROCESS

ASSESSMENT

The outcome of severe head injury is determined primarily by the severity of the initial injury, and it is modified by the subsequent assessment and management of the neurosurgical team. Initially, whether at the scene of the accident or in the emergency room, the patient must be assessed for any life-threatening condition. He may have an obstructed airway, an open chest injury, or a severe hemorrhage. The level of consciousness may be decreased. A sign of neurologic dysfunction, such as a dilated pupil or unconsciousness, also indicates an emergency. In a closed head injury, once the pupil dilates, herniation will soon follow (unless the patient has had a direct injury to the eye or a direct brain-stem injury). The cause of unconsciousness must be ascertained (*e.g.,* hypoxia, shock, drug or alcohol ingestion, hypoglycemia, or head injury). The cause is not always easy to determine, and the condition may have a number of causes. Often a patient is brought into the emergency room after having been drinking and then involved in an automobile accident. If the patient exhibits decreasing levels of consciousness, it is difficult to determine to what degree the condition is caused by alcohol and to what degree it is caused by the head injury.

The thrust of observation has changed in the assessment of head-injured patients. The advent of the CT scanner has meant that problems can be identified and treated before any deterioration is seen in the patient. Previously, monitoring of the level of consciousness meant that the team would watch for any deterioration in the patient's condition, any deterioration would be justly noted, and treatment would be instituted to prevent further deterioration. Today, the goal is to avoid any deterioration. Recognition of the circumstances that might lead to problems and CT scanning to identify problems are considered the proper protocol.[21]

History

The patient's medical history is very important. The first details to be gathered are those of the accident. What happened in the accident? What caused it? What happened afterward? All the circumstances surrounding the accident may be vitally important. What was the person's state of consciousness before, during, and after the accident? (For example, was the person unconscious and then conscious?) Did the patient hit his head? Did the patient have convulsions? Does the past history point to any significant pre-existing problems?

Baseline Examination

The initial examination is the emergency examination (ABCD—the basic approach of cardiopulmonary resuscitation). The patient's respirations should be easy, even, and near a normal rate. If respirations are deep, irregular, or slow, the team should be alert to the possibility of head injury. The patient's pulse should be regular and normal to fast. Hemorrhagic shock is not caused by intracranial bleeding, because the amount of cerebral bleeding is not sufficient to cause the signs and symptoms of shock; it indicates another problem. Only rarely (and usually only in children) is hemorrhagic shock due to a scalp laceration. Most patients with head injuries who are in shock also have a thoracoabdominal injury or a fractured pelvis.

A spinal fracture must always be considered. Examination of the head may reveal significant bleeding or an open skull fracture. Drainage from the nose or ear may be bloody. A bruise over the mastoid area (Battle's sign) should alert the team to a possible basilar skull fracture. Palpation must be done gently, because further neurologic damage can be caused by pressure on skull fragments.

The initial neurologic examination is used as a baseline.[36] Changes in the patient's level of consciousness are determined. The patient's respiratory pattern must be assessed and followed; it may be normal. The abnormal patterns are Cheyne-Stokes, central neurogenic hyperventilation, apneustic, or ataxic respirations. Central neurogenic hyperventilation is not common and must often be differentiated from a similar pattern, one that is produced by a chest injury. This pattern is often not neurologic but a response to a ventilatory problem. It must be monitored closely, because overbreathing lowers the $PaCO_2$ (respiratory alkalosis) and reflexly results in cerebral vasoconstriction (decreased cerebral blood flow). Although hyperventilation with the $PaCO_2$ maintained at 20 mm Hg to 30 mm Hg is the treatment of choice for increased ICP, arterial tension levels below 20 mm Hg are dangerous.

Examination of the eyes consists of noting pupillary size and reactivity, the ciliospinal reflex, eye movements, and the oculocephalic and oculovestibular reflexes. The position of the eyes at rest is noted. Any abnormalities, such as forced gaze, ocular bobbing, skew deviations, or nystagmus, are documented. The pupillary signs are of utmost importance. Widely dilated pupils produced by third cranial nerve compression are an ominous sign and indicate impending brain-stem injury or oculomotor nerve compression by a herniating temporal lobe. This unilateral expanding mass is usually ipsilateral to the abnormal pupil. Funduscopic examination performed by the physician helps to assess hemorrhages and pre-existing disease, as well as to establish a baseline (papilledema is not usually apparent for 36 to 72 hours). Eye signs give valuable information about the person's status. A rule of thumb is this: If there is a difference in eye signs and motor signs, rely on the eye signs.

Motor signs help the staff to focus on the neurological problems (Fig. 30–7). After noting the movements of the face and extremities, appraise the reflexes. In addition, cranial nerve functioning must be evaluated, and any focal problem must be thoroughly assessed. Failure of a patient to respond to pinprick raises the possibility of associated spinal cord injury.

In the event of increased ICP, serial determinations must be done to monitor the patient. Ninety to 95% of patients with closed head injuries do not require an intracranial procedure. The initial accurate neurologic examination is only the first in a succession of examinations. The trend in the patient's condition is most important. The patient's level of consciousness is the best clinical sign of his neurologic status. The Glasgow coma score is used as the standard for serial assessments. Complete, concise, accurate, and descriptive standard terminology must be used in evaluating changes.

Emergency laboratory measurements commonly used are baseline blood tests (complete blood count, typing and crossmatching, blood sugar, blood urea nitrogen, and serum electrolyte tests) and urine tests (for sugar, acetone, protein, and formed elements). Arterial blood gas levels must be determined and monitored.

Spinal Cord Injury

The main symptom of spinal fracture is local pain that may radiate into the arms, thorax, abdomen, or legs. If the patient is in pain, he should not be moved until after examination by

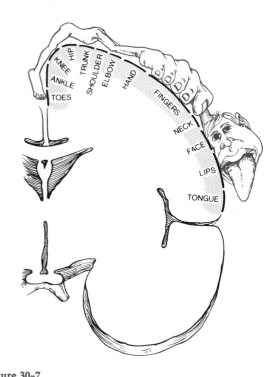

Figure 30–7

Precentral gyrus with localization of motor functions in the cortex. Localized findings on clinical examination help pinpoint the area of the brain affected.

the medical team. With the patient supine, the examiner should slip his hand underneath the patient and palpate the spine for displacement, crepitus, and abnormal mobility. Other examinations are done as indicated, and the appropriate radiographs are then ordered by the physician.

Assessment of spinal cord damage entails examination for motor and sensory abnormalities, changes in reflexes, and autonomic alterations. Initially, the patient is observed for diaphragmatic breathing, flexion of the forearms across the chest, and a decreased blood pressure without other signs of shock. Injury to the cord is suspected when patients with altered levels of consciousness do not move their limbs, but grimace, open their eyes to pain, or make sounds. Spinal cord functioning is assessed by noting the patient's ability to move the extremities, his ability to respond to a pinprick on the hands and feet, his response to reflex stimulation, and the tone of the rectal sphincter. On rectal examination, if the patient feels the finger palpate or if the patient contracts the perineal muscles voluntarily, the lesion is incomplete. It is not enough to have the patient move his extremities; each muscle group should be assessed (deltoid, biceps, triceps, finger flexor, finger extensors, finger spreader, hip flexors, knee flexors, dorsiflexion, and plantar flexion). The patient may suffer from modification in spinal function (Table 30–1). Muscle weakness may indicate cord damage. In the patient who has an altered level of consciousness, the presence of spinal cord injury is determined by a reduced or absent motor response to a deep pain stimulus. For example, facial grimaces may be noted when stimuli are applied above the clavicle, but not when they are applied below the clavicle. A complete spinal cord injury is associated with no voluntary movements or sensation on or below the level of cord trauma.

The key signs of damage to the various levels of the spinal cord are as follows:

1. C2-to-C3 vertebral level:
   A. Respiratory paralysis (the outcome is probably death)
   B. Flaccid paralysis
   C. Areflexia (the patient who has complete areflexia that lasts longer than 24 hours has almost no chance of recovery)
   D. Loss of sensation below the level of the mandible
2. C5-to-C6 vertebral level:
   A. Diaphragmatic breathing
   B. Paralysis of the intercostal and abdominal muscles

C. Quadriplegia (shoulder girdle functioning and a minimal amount of deltoid, pectoral, and biceps functioning may remain, but motor power is essentially lost below the shoulder level)
   D. Anesthesia below the clavicle and anesthesia of the ulnar half of the arms
   E. Areflexia, with the possible exception of the biceps reflex
   F. Fecal and urinary retention
   G. Priapism
3. T12-to-L1 vertebral level:
   A. Paraplegia
   B. Anesthesia in the legs
   C. Areflexia in the legs (the upper abdominal reflexes may be present)
   D. Fecal and urinary retention
   E. Priapism
4. L1-to-L5 vertebral level:
   A. Flaccid paralysis to partial flaccid paralysis
   B. Abdominal and cremasteric reflexes present
   C. Ankle and plantar reflexes absent

The *functional level* is the level of the lowest nerve root that demonstrates muscle function. Muscle strength is graded on a scale of 0 to 4; grade 4 refers to good muscle strength manifested by complete motion against gravity and some resistance. Muscle innervations below the level of the injury are either paralyzed or weaker. The level of injury is determined by noting the lowest level of innervation that is functioning. In cervical spinal injury, the key muscles to determine particular functional levels are as follows:

C4 functional level: Neck and upper trapezius
C5 functional level: Weak deltoids and biceps
C6 functional level: Strong deltoids and biceps, wrist extensors
C7 functional level: Wrist flexors, pronators, and weak triceps
C8 functional level: Finger flexors

The results of the assessment of spinal cord injury should be recorded in three ways:

1. At the fracture level, which is determined by radiograph.
2. At the neurologic level, or the lowest dermatome where there is impaired or intact sensation or where there is some degree of muscle function.
3. At the functional level (*i.e.*, at the level of the lowest key

Table 30–1
Spinal Cord Lesions

SYNDROME	MECHANISM OF INJURY	FUNCTION LOSS
Anterior cord	Flexion injuries	Weakness or paralysis with loss of pain and temperature sense (maintained are light touch, vibratory sensation, and joint position sense)
Posterior cord (rare)	Hyperextension injuries	Decrease in touch and proprioception
Central cord	Hyperextension injuries	Greater loss of motor function and sensation in upper extremities than in lower extremities
Brown-Sequard (incomplete forms also occur)	Stab and gunshot wounds	Ipsilateral weakness or paralysis with loss of position sense, light touch, and vibration; contralateral loss of pain and temperature sensation modalities

muscle in which there is a "good" grade). This applies only to complete injuries.

Diagnostic Studies

Skull and chest radiographs, radioactive brain scans, cerebral angiograms, echoencephalograms, electroencephalograms, CT scans, magnetic resonance imaging (MRI), or monitoring of ICP (p. 575 and Fig. 30-10) may be done.

For head injuries, skull radiographs and cervical spinal radiographs are ordered. The radiographic examination is specific, and it is dictated by the findings. For example, with patients who are unconscious or who are suspected of having a cervical injury, the physician orders initial lateral radiographs that include C7 and T1. (Taking anteroposterior radiographs requires lifting or moving the patient, a dangerous undertaking unless the personnel are appropriately trained.) After the lateral radiographs, the neurosurgeon may order other films. Radiographs of the skull are helpful if the pineal gland is calcified, because a shift from its midline position signifies that a mass is present. However, the pineal gland is usually not calcified until after the age of 40, and most patients with head injury are younger than 40 years of age. Also, a depressed skull fracture (or fractures) that transverses the arterial vessel grooves in the skull (the middle meningeal artery), a foreign body, or air in the skull (resulting from a tear in the coverings of the brain) may be demonstrated on radiographs. In the event of additional trauma, a radiographic evaluation of the appropriate area is made.

Cerebral angiography, a very useful tool, is a specific neurodiagnostic technique. If time permits, the procedure is often used for accurate location of the problem. Although angiography has been superseded largely by CT scanning, it will certainly provide useful diagnostic information when CT scanning is not possible. It is especially useful in distinguishing extracerebral hematomas from intracerebral mass lesions.

Electroencephalography is used only under rare circumstances, and its primary value for comatose patients remains the evaluation of the coma.

Brain stem auditory-evoked responses offer some aid in determining the extent of brain stem damage and response to treatment. Brain stem auditory-evoked responses provide information about the structural and functional integrity of the brain stem auditory pathway and are a sensory-evoked potential occurring very quickly after stimulation. The origin of the wave is known, and the peak latencies are highly reliable. Abnormalities are useful in localizing damage within the brain stem.

Computed tomographic scanning for head-injured patients is the most valuable and reliable diagnostic tool available. In CT scanning, the entire brain is routinely visualized. An antilog picture is obtained by the emission of x-rays through the head to a densitometer. (Sodium iodide crystal detectors receive the x-rays after passage through the patient's head. A further crystal detector measures the intensity of the x-ray source, and the readings taken can be used to calculate the absorption by the material along the x-ray path.) The scanner is moved in small increments, and the process is repeated again and again. The readings are stored on a magnetic disc file for processing at the end of a scanning run. The result is a digital computer printout of the x-ray densities of tissues that gives a picture of the part of the body through which the x-ray beam was passed. Anything that is in the way of the beam, such as blood (iron) or bone (calcium), alters the densities. Various lesions can be identified as a function of their densities, nature, and appearance (Fig. 30–8). Now commonly used in emergencies—and considered by many to be the procedure of choice—a CT scan series can be completed in a short time and with minimal radiation exposure. Also, the patient may be monitored before and after therapy, and the densities can be measured to determine the effectiveness of the treatment

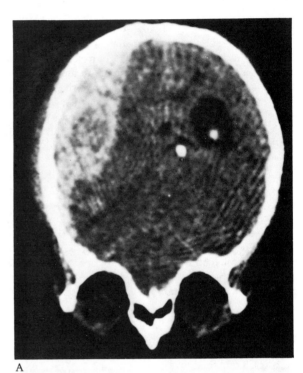

A

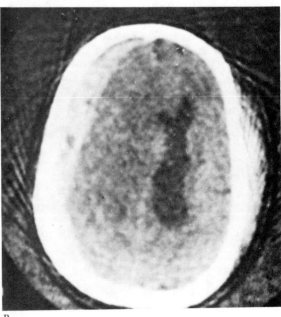

B

Figure 30–8

Computed tomography scans. (*A*) Epidural hematoma. (*B*) Subdural hematoma.

and to visualize any new lesions. Both intracerebral and extracerebral hematomas in all skull compartments can be identified. Delayed complications, such as late hematomas and hydrocephalus, can also be identified.

The newest noninvasive diagnostic procedure is MRI (see Chap. 29, p. 551).

NURSING DIAGNOSES, PATIENT OUTCOMES, AND PLAN

The preceding material on anatomy, physiology, nursing assessment, and diagnostic tests guides the nurse in establishing nursing diagnoses, patient outcomes, and plan for the patient with head injuries.

NURSING CARE PLAN SUMMARY Patient with Head Injury

NURSING DIAGNOSIS

1. Altered cerebral perfusion related to closed head injury (exchanging pattern)

Patient Outcomes	Nursing Orders
1. The patient should demonstrate stable vital signs. Intracranial swelling should be reduced.	**Emergency Department/Critical Care Unit**

Emergency Department/Critical Care Unit

1. Initially assess the patient for any type of life-threatening trauma, such as an obstructed airway or a hemorrhage. Perform oral or nasotracheal intubation as needed. Assess the patient's cardiopulmonary status. Consider the possibility of a spinal injury.[8]
   A. If there is respiratory abnormality or Cushing's triad, notify the physician. If the symptoms of shock are present and persist, the cause is probably a hemorrhage.
   B. Maintain the arterial oxygen tension at greater than 80 mm Hg.
   C. Monitor the vital signs, and note the pupillary responses.
   D. Assess the chest and abdomen.
   E. Look for fractures, especially of the pelvis, because fractures are the most common cause of shock.
   F. Ascertain the level of consciousness. Use the Glasgow coma score.

   (1) The Glasgow Coma Scale has three assessment parameters: Eye opening, best verbal response, and best motor response. The patient who is completely awake will score 15. The patient who scores 10 or less usually needs to be intubated and hyperventilated. The following values are assigned to the assessment parameters:

   Eye opening:

Do not open at all	1
Open after pain stimulation	2
Open on command	3
Open spontaneously	4

   Best verbal response:

Intubated	0
Mute	1
Incomprehensible sounds	2
Inappropriate words	3
Conversation confused	4
Appropriate and oriented	5

   Best motor response:

Flaccid	1
Extensor	2
Flexor	3
Semipurposeful	4
Localized to pain	5
Obedient to command	6

   (2) Take into account the patient's ability to cooperate, awareness of environment, response to questions, and the following:

(continued)

NURSING CARE PLAN SUMMARY *Patient with Head Injury* *Continued*

Patient Outcomes	*Nursing Orders*

Nursing Orders

    a. Depth of consciousness can be judged by the patient's reactions to external stimuli on various levels.

    b. The patient may be completely unconscious and not respond to external or internal stimuli. Urinary retention is common. Corneal reflexes, the swallowing reflex, or some of the tendon reflexes may be present, but they are usually absent in deep coma, which indicates severe damage to the brain stem. No meaningful response is made to questions. The bladder empties reflexly when distended.

  (3) A patient can respond to stimuli by painful, purposeful movements (*e.g.*, grimacing or hand movements to push away the examiner's hand). Purposeful movements are considered defensive. Non-purposeful movements (*e.g.*, a thrust toward the stimulus or some aberrant behavior) are considered defenseless.

  (4) Level of consciousness can be evaluated by describing the patient's behavior, including spontaneous activity and responses. The patient's orientation must be determined. The patient may be disoriented with regard to time, place, or person. Thoughts may be suddenly interrupted by inappropriate statements or behavior. In addition to the Glasgow coma score, the following classification is helpful:

    a. Mild confusion. The patient is capable of coherent conversation, and his behavior is appropriate.

    b. Moderate confusion. The patient is out of touch with the environment, but on some insistence, he may respond to simple questions (*e.g.*, about his age or where he lives).

    c. Severe confusion. The patient is out of touch with the environment, but able to follow simple and repeated commands (*e.g.*, "Open your eyes," or "Stick out your tongue").

G. Assess the patient's respiratory rate, depth, and pattern. Using the following guidelines, assess pupillary size and reactivity and eye movements:

  (1) Pupils: Size, position, reactivity, and consensual response

  (2) Eye movements: Spontaneous movements and doll's-eye response

  (3) Mild injury: Pupils equal, react to light, conjugate gaze, resistant to forced opening

  (4) More serious injury: Absent or deviant reactivity, fixed gaze with dilation, lack of response

H. Assess the patient's skeletal responses. The nurse should compare the strength in the patient's right side to the strength in his left side and the strength in his arms to the strength in the legs. The following comparison should also be made on both sides of the body:

  (1) Arms: Patient's ability to hold the arms at a right angle to the body (watch for pronator drift)

  (2) Legs: Patient's ability to hold the legs 10° off the bed and ability to dorsiflex the feet against the pressure of the nurse's hands

  (3) Reflexes

  (4) Pain response

  (5) The nurse should observe any failure of a body part to move, focal or generalized seizures, responses to verbal or noxious stimuli, extensor spasms, or lateralization of neurologic signs (mainly evident in facial grimacing, movements of the extremities, absent deep tendon reflexes or superficial abdominal reflex, and a Babinski response).

I. Check the patient's vital signs—temperature, pulse, respiration, blood pressure—every hour (more often if indicated).

J. Obtain baseline laboratory data. Any clear nasal drainage should be tested for glucose.

K. Place a Salem pump nasogastric tube for acute gastric distention. Insertion is contraindicated in patients with gunshot wounds to the head if the

(continued)

NURSING CARE PLAN SUMMARY Patient with Head Injury Continued

Patient Outcomes	Nursing Orders
	nasopharynx or the tissues surrounding it have been removed by the blast or if there is any danger of disrupting a hematoma at the base of the neck. Antacids, anticholinergics, or antihistamines are given as ordered. L. Be aware that a lumbar puncture is usually not done, because it provides little useful information and is potentially disastrous. M. Ascertain that the patient has had a cervical spine series with negative results before a CT scan is done, because positioning the patient for the CT scan requires considerable manipulation. N. Before a CT scan of an agitated patient is done, administer intravenous diazepam if ordered, to minimize artifact movement.

2. The patient should be free of any further injury during this emergent phase.	2. Assume that the patient has a cervical or other type of spinal fracture and treat accordingly.
	
	A. Determine the serial values and assess any trends.
	
	B. Look for open head wounds; bloody drainage from the ears, nose, or posterior pharyngeal wall; or blood in the middle ear with an intact eardrum.
	
	C. Obtain the relevant information about the patient and the accident. Find out about the patient's state of consciousness before, during, and after the accident (especially note any period of unconsciousness); the circumstances surrounding the accident (clues to the amount of force transmitted to the brain and the severity of the injury are often given in a description of the accident); the treatment rendered; and any history of pre-existing disease (*e.g.*, cardiovascular or cerebrovascular disease, diabetes, chronic alcoholism, or epilepsy, and any medicine the patient has been taking (*e.g.*, an anticoagulant). While obtaining these data, the nurse should also assess the patient's use of language, memory, orientation, and clarity of speech.
	
	D. Using the following guidelines, assess pupillary size and reactivity and eye movements:
	  (1) Pupils: Size, position, reactivity, and consensual response
	  (2) Eye movements: Spontaneous movements and doll's eye response
	  (3) Mild injury: Pupils equal, react to light, conjugate gaze, resistant to forced opening
	  (4) More serious injury: Absent or deviant reactivity, fixed gaze with dilatation, lack of response
	
	E. Assess the patient's skeletal responses. Compare the strength in the patient's right side to the strength in the left side and the strength in the arms to the strength in the legs. The following comparison should also be made on both sides of the body:
	  (1) Arms: Patient's ability to hold the arms at a right angle to the body (watch for drift)
	  (2) Legs: Patient's ability to hold the legs 10° off the bed and dorsiflex the feet against the pressure of the nurse's hands
	  (3) Reflexes
	  (4) Pain response
	  (5) Failure of a body part to move, focal or generalized seizures, responses to verbal or noxious stimuli, decerebrate spasms, or lateralization of neurologic signs (mainly evident in facial grimacing, movements of the extremities, absent deep tendon reflexes or superficial abdominal reflex, and Babinski response)

3. The patient should be free of the complications of seizures.	3. Take the patient's seizure history. Avoid circumstances that might precipitate seizures (*e.g.*, stress, interference with normal sleeping patterns, irregular eating, fever, hypoxia, and electrolyte disturbance).
	
	A. If a seizure occurs, screen the patient, remove the bed clothes, and stand at the foot of the bed to observe closely while another health team member maintains safety precautions. Note and record the following:
	  (1) Level of consciousness before, during, and after the seizure
	  (2) Presence or absence of an aura

(continued)

NURSING CARE PLAN SUMMARY *Patient with Head Injury* *Continued*

Patient Outcomes	*Nursing Orders*
	(3) Progression and involvement of activity
	(4) Deviation of head and eyes
	(5) Length of the tonic and clonic phases
	(6) Respiratory changes
	(7) Pupillary reactions during and after the seizure
	(8) Incontinence
	(9) Tongue biting
	(10) Ability to handle salivation
	(11) Muscle weakness
	(12) Duration of seizure
	(13) Character and duration of status after the seizure and the presence of paralysis or dysphasia

B. During convulsion, observe all safety precautions.
   (1) If possible, before the tonic phase, place a soft object (*e.g.*, a padded tongue blade, napkin, or oral airway) between the patient's teeth. (Once the jaws are clenched, do not attempt to place anything between the teeth.)
   (2) Loosen any tight clothing.
   (3) If at all possible, guide the patient's movements.
   (4) Protect the patient's head and the rest of the body; do not try to stop movement.
   (5) Move with the patient's body to help protect the patient.
   (6) Remain in the patient's room.
C. Anticipate that the physician will order medication such as intravenous phenytoin sodium. Monitor vital signs carefully, and place the patient on a cardiac monitor. Diphenylhydantoin infusion should be monitored carefully, because ventricular dysrhythmias may occur with rapid administration.
D. Administer medication ordered by the physician. Depending on the assessment, the physician may not order any medication after the first seizure (but perhaps sodium phenobarbital or another medication). If the seizures continue, sodium amobarbital, paraldehyde, phenobarbital, diazepam, or thiopental sodium may be ordered.
E. Take the patient's temperature rectally only.
F. Keep an oral airway and suctioning equipment at the patient's bedside.
G. Perform mouth care while the patient is taking diphenylhydantoin.
H. Pad the headboard and side rails; keep side rails up, unless the nurse is in direct attendance.
I. Keep the bed height at the lowest level.
J. Observe the patient carefully, particularly during the night.
K. Plan patient education and family education.

NURSING DIAGNOSIS

2. *Impaired gas exchange related to altered respiratory drive and cerebral dysfunction (exchanging pattern)*

Patient Outcomes	*Nursing Orders*
1. The patient should maintain pulmonary stability.	1. Draw arterial blood gas samples as ordered and send them for analysis.
	A. Notify the physician of any decrease in PaO_2 or pH or any increase in $PaCO_2$. Arterial carbon dioxide levels above 42 mm Hg or arterial oxygen levels below 50 mm Hg may produce vasodilation and a sustained increase in the ICP.
	B. If respiratory distress is noted, notify the physician. Observe closely, and do not leave the patient unattended.

(continued)

NURSING CARE PLAN SUMMARY   *Patient with Head Injury   Continued*

Patient Outcomes	Nursing Orders
	C. Prepare the patient for endotracheal intubation if PaO_2 decreases to 70 mm Hg. D. Monitor vital capacity, blood gases, and respiratory effort to assess respiratory status. Maintain pulmonary hygiene and suctioning as indicated by the arterial blood gas measurements and the chest examination. Encourage inspiration. Give the patient 100% oxygen for 1 to 2 minutes before and after suctioning, and limit the suctioning to 15 seconds.
2. The patient should maintain adequate arterial oxygenation.	2. Assess and maintain the patency of the upper airway. A. Give 40% oxygen through a mask as ordered. B. Observe and record the pattern of respirations. C. Persistent hypocarbia ($PaCO_2$ < 30 mm Hg) and increased respiratory rate (>25/minute) are associated with a poor prognosis. D. Have equipment for suctioning and endotracheal intubation at the patient's bedside. E. If hyperventilation measures and a paralyzing drug are ordered, monitor the ICP closely. F. Turn the patient onto the side, and change sides every hour.

NURSING DIAGNOSIS

3. *High risk for altered cerebral function related to head injury (exchanging pattern)*

Patient Outcomes	Nursing Orders

1. The patient should be free of the symptoms of increased cerebral swelling in order to sustain neural cell metabolism.	1. Observe the patient for changes in levels of responsiveness, restlessness, and bilateral motor response, as well as for changes in pupils and respirations. Any changes should be reported to the physician immediately.[9] Serial assessments will identify trends (see Fig. 30–9, p. 580 for examples).
	A. Every hour, observe for, report, and record the following:
	  (1) Pupillary changes (in size, equality, position, direct response, and consensual response)
	  (2) Respiratory irregularity (a decreased rate, an increased rate, or periods of apnea). One of the most important changes in respiration is from normal respirations to Cheyne-Strokes respirations of central neurogenic hyperventilation, which indicates actual or impending central herniation.
	  (3) Motor changes (movement and pain on the right side compared with movement and pain on the left side)
	  (4) Vomiting or incontinence
	  (5) Increased blood pressure with widened pulse pressure. When the mean arterial pressure is 60 mm Hg to 170 mm Hg, the cerebral blood flow remains within normal limits. However, arterial pressures below 90 mm Hg that are associated with an increased ICP and that peak to 60 mm Hg to 90 mm Hg may produce a low perfusion pressure and cerebral hypoxia.
	  (6) Cerebral perfusion pressure. Abnormal cerebral function is associated with pressures below 50 mm Hg.
	  (7) Pulse less than 60 or greater than 100
	  (8) A moderately elevated temperature.
	B. Administer intravenous mannitol as ordered.
	C. Administer intravenous furosemide as ordered.

2. The patient will attain intracranial pressure within normal limits.	2. Assess and record the patient's level of consciousness every 15 minutes. Do not confuse progressive restlessness and agitation with an improvement in the level of consciousness; these signs may indicate increased ICP. A. For serial determination, use the Glasgow coma score for patients who do not have lateralizing signs.

(continued)

NURSING CARE PLAN SUMMARY   *Patient with Head Injury*   *Continued*

Patient Outcomes	*Nursing Orders*

B. Maintain controlled hyperventilation and induced hypocarbia by keeping the arterial carbon dioxide levels at about 25 mm Hg. Adjust the minute ventilation. The arterial carbon dioxide tension level should not be allowed to drop below 20 mm Hg, because further arterial constriction may result in tissue hypoxia and acidosis.

C. Use ventricular drainage via a closed system to vent and remove cerebrospinal fluid so that the ICP is kept below 25 mm Hg as the ICP may rise rapidly. The nurse should remember that just as the addition of a 1-ml to 2-ml aliquot of cerebrospinal fluid to the total brain volume can at times increase the ICP exponentially (see Fig. 30–2), so the removal of 1 ml to 2 ml can make a vast difference.

D. Elevate the head of the bed 30° to 45°. Maintain the patient's neck in a neutral position using pillows wrapped in sheets. To prevent jugular vein compression, the patient's head should not be allowed to rest on a pillow.

E. Keep the patient's temperature below 38°C (101°F).

F. Administer intravenous furosemide as ordered. Normally 40 mg is the initial dose, and the repeat dose is 20 mg.

G. Administer intravenous mannitol as ordered. Normally, 0.18 g to 2.5 g/kg (in a 20% solution) is administered as a bolus over 2 to 30 minutes.

H. Monitor the ICP. Intracranial pressure of 4 mm Hg to 10 mm Hg with an upper limit of 15 mm Hg are considered normal; ICPs of 15 mm Hg to 30 mm Hg are considered to be moderately elevated; and ICPs of 30 mm Hg to 40 mm Hg are considered to be elevated (see Fig. 30–10, p. 581 for example).

I. Measure the ICP at least hourly concurrent with the neurologic vital signs. Research substantiates that the ICP recorded hourly by nursing staff is a reasonable estimate of the patient's mean ICP for the entire hour as measured continuously and averaged by a computer for the same 60-minute period. The nurse should do the following:
   (1) Use the monitoring system prescribed by the physician and follow the protocol established by the institution's intensive care unit.
   (2) Notify the physician of ICP greater than 20 mm Hg that persists in the absence of stimulation.
   (3) Drain cerebrospinal fluid as ordered. Record ICP before drainage, length of time (in seconds) drain is open, and ICP following drainage.
   (4) Maintain a sterile, occlusive dressing over the monitor insertion site. Change the dressing only if it becomes soiled or nonocclusive in order to decrease incidence of infection.

3. The patient should attain maximal neurologic functioning.

3. Check the vital signs every 15 minutes. If they are stable for 2 hours, check them every 30 minutes for 2 hours, and then every 60 minutes. Although there is not a definite correlation between vital signs and progressive increases in the ICP, in many instances there is a certain relationship. Because the classic changes are late ones, clinical monitoring must cover all the parameters.

A. Avoid sedation.

B. Monitor the patient for headaches (they occur rarely). A headache that is severe and is associated with agitation indicates an epidural hematoma. Because opiates (*e.g.,* morphine) mask neurologic signs, they are not used. Administer dexamethasone sodium phosphate as ordered. Normally 4 mg to 10 mg is given intravenously as the initial dose; then 4 mg to 6 mg is given every 4 to 6 hours for 5 to 10 days. Dexamethasone is never discontinued abruptly. The patient is weaned off in decreasing doses.

4. The patient should be free from further complications.

4. Observe all safety precautions. The patient is particularly susceptible to a second insult. Report blood pressures of less than 100 and pulse rates of greater than 100.

A. Administer an anticholinergic, antacid, or cimetidine as ordered to prevent gastrointestinal bleeding. If otorrhea or rhinorrhea occurs, notify the physician and lightly place a sterile cotton pad over the patient's ears or

(continued)

NURSING CARE PLAN SUMMARY *Patient with Head Injury*   *Continued*

Patient Outcomes	Nursing Orders
	drip pad under his nose. Tell him not to blow his nose or sneeze. Use a commercially prepared pH-sensitive tape to determine whether glucose is present.

Nursing Orders continued:

B. If bleeding starts from the ear or the nose, notify the physician and collect some blood in a test tube and on a tissue. The presence of cerebrospinal fluid is indicated by nonclotting blood and by blood with a ring about it. If the patient becomes combative, pad the side rails, put mittens on the patient, and assess the need for a chest restraint.

C. Determine the cause of any restless behavior. Have an oral airway and suctioning equipment in the patient's room.

D. Protect the patient's eyes from corneal irritation.
   (1) Inspect the eyes with a flashlight.
   (2) Apply methycellulose drops every 1 to 2 hours or a bland ophthalmic ointment at least as often as pupillary function is evaluated but not less than every 4 hours. Tape should be applied horizontally to the eyes, ensuring complete closure with apposition of the upper and lower lid margins. Taping of the eyelid is preferred over patching and should continue for as long as the patient has incomplete eyelid closure.
   (3) Report any corneal drying, irritation, or ulceration to the physician.

E. Observe patients for bulging eyes or red vessels in the sclera. Ask them whether they hear a humming or roaring noise in their head.

F. Observe for signs of the postconcussion syndrome.

G. If patients develop a cranial nerve deficit, observe them carefully. A patient with a cranial nerve deficit is particularly prone to residual injuries.

H. Observe the patient for endocrine abnormalities.

NURSING DIAGNOSIS

4. Altered fluid and electrolyte balance related to closed head injury (exchanging pattern)

Patient Outcome	Nursing Orders
The patient should maintain fluid and electrolyte balance.	1. Administer intravenous fluid. 2. Record fluid intake. Weigh the patient daily. 3. Place a Foley catheter if indicated. 4. Measure and record the hourly and daily urinary output. 5. Obtain baseline data about the urinary output and report any change in the amount or appearance of the urine. 6. Monitor the patient's serum and urine electrolyte levels every 8 hours. 7. Administer potassium as ordered. 8. Check the hematocrit and the blood urea nitrogen levels daily. 9. Observe the patient for symptoms of hyponatremia. 10. If urine output is greater than 250 ml/hour for 2 hours in a row or greater than 6000 ml/day, alert the physician.

NURSING DIAGNOSIS

5. Altered nutrition: less than body requirements related to catabolic response to injury (exchanging pattern)

Patient Outcome	Nursing Orders
The patient should attain a positive caloric balance.	1. Administer intravenous fluids as ordered. 2. Initiate oral feedings (or nasogastric feedings) after return of bowel sounds, as ordered.

(continued)

NURSING CARE PLAN SUMMARY Patient with Head Injury   Continued

Patient Outcome	*Nursing Orders*
	3. If the patient is obtunded, nasogastric feedings will probably be withheld because of the danger of aspiration; continuous feedings via a Dobhoff tube, gastrostomy tube, or a similar technique may be ordered. 4. See Nursing Diagnosis: Altered Nutrition, page 682.

NURSING DIAGNOSIS

6. *Altered thought processes related to cerebral dysfunction (knowing pattern)*

Patient Outcome	*Nursing Orders*
The patient will become less confused and will be reoriented to reality.	1. Assess reasons for confusion: Head injury, fear, bizarre behavior, physical status (vital signs, neurological status, blood urea nitrogen, fluid and electrolyte status). 2. Make contact with the patient: 　A. Speak clearly, slowly, and distinctly. 　B. Use eye-to-eye contact. 　C. Use gentle touch. 　D. Provide comfort. 　E. Do not startle. 3. Establish rapport. 4. Explain surroundings. 5. Assess patient's need of safety measures. 　A. Bedrails that extend to foot of bed in upright position 　B. Bed in lowest position 　C. Room in close proximity to nurse's station 　D. Observe closely; keep intercom on 　E. Continual presence of family member 　F. Vest restraints (attached to bed, not side rails)

NURSING DIAGNOSIS

7. *Sensory/perceptual alterations related to closed head injury (perceiving pattern)*

Patient Outcome	*Nursing Orders*
The patient should regain contact with the outside world and demonstrate an awareness of the immediate environment.	See Nursing Diagnosis: Sensory/Perceptual Alteration, page 114.

NURSING DIAGNOSIS

8. *High risk for ineffective thermoregulation related to altered hypothalamic processes (exchanging pattern)*

Patient Outcome	*Nursing Orders*
The patient should maintain a normal temperature range or mild hypothermia (32°C to 36°C; 90°F to 97°F) or moderate hypothermia (27°C to 31°C; 81°F to 89°F).	1. Take the patient's temperature every 2 hours with a tympanic membrane, esophageal, or rectal sensor. 2. Administer aspirin or Tylenol every 4 hours as ordered. 3. When the temperature is elevated, bathe the patient with tepid water sponges rather than alcohol sponges.

(continued)

NURSING CARE PLAN SUMMARY   *Patient with Head Injury*   *Continued*

Patient Outcome	Nursing Orders
	4. Make sure fluid intake is at least 3000 ml/day as ordered.
	5. Keep the room temperature at 20°C (68°F). Keep the amount of bed clothes at a minimum.
	6. Put a hypothermia blanket on the patient's bed before arrival in the critical care unit.
	7. Determine the mechanism of cooling to be ordered and make preparations for its institution: Surface cooling, blood-stream cooling, barbiturate hypothermia, or medications.
	8. Use a cooling blanket when the patient's temperature elevates as ordered.

NURSING DIAGNOSIS

9. Anxiety (patient and family's) related to the threat of further neurologic damage (feeling pattern)

Patient Outcome	Nursing Orders
The patient and family will demonstrate decreased anxiety.	See Nursing Diagnoses: Anxiety, page 111.

NURSING DIAGNOSIS

10. High risk for further injury related to traumatic fracture of the cervical vertebra and cervical traction (exchanging pattern)

Patient Outcome	Nursing Orders

The patient should not have further cord damage.	1. Maintain a patent airway.
	  A. Avoid moving the neck. Treat the unconscious patient as if he or she had a cervical injury.
	  B. Insert an airway.
	  C. Prepare the patient for endotracheal intubation or tracheostomy if he or she needs ventilatory assistance. Airway management has the highest priority.
	  D. Determine baseline information against which later estimates of the extent of injury can be compared.
	  E. Maintain the patients' $PaCO_2$ level at 20 mm Hg to 30 mm Hg.
	  F. Monitor the patients' respiratory status. Assess pre-existing pulmonary problems, determine if there is diaphragmatic breathing and if intercostals are functioning, auscultate breath sounds frequently, and assess tidal volume and vital capacity every 2 hours.
	  G. Determine the serial values, and assess the trends.
	  H. Monitor the vital signs and pupillary responses.
	  I. Place a urethral catheter.
	  J. Place a nasogastric catheter unless there is a gunshot wound to the head.
	  K. Administer tetanus prophylaxis as ordered.
	  L. Know that analgesics and sedatives are to be avoided.
	  M. Assess the presence or absence of movement and sensation (pain and touch). Report any progression of neurologic deficit.
	  N. Categorize muscle strength as strong, weak, or absent.
	  O. Compare the left and right sides and the arms and legs. Assess and record any differences.
	  P. Categorize the reflexes as normal, increased, decreased, or absent.

(continued)

NURSING CARE PLAN SUMMARY   *Patient with Head Injury*   Continued

Patient Outcome	*Nursing Orders*
	Q. Communicate specifics concerning radiographs ordered by the physician.
	R. Use aseptic technique in cleansing the lacerations.
	S. Maintain the immobilization of a fracture or dislocation (whether or not the patients have a neurologic deficit), using skeletal traction if ordered.
	T. Monitor the patients for spinal shock. Check them for decreased blood pressure, paralysis, and bladder and bowel distention. Elevate lower extremities or place Ace wraps or antiembolic stockings.
	U. Be prepared to plan and implement nursing care for any of the following: Role disturbance, ineffective airway clearance, alterations in bowel elimination/constipation, anticipatory grieving/acute grief reaction, impaired physical mobility, self-care deficit, potential impairment of skin integrity, alteration in patterns of urinary elimination, and lack of knowledge of the family.

IMPLEMENTATION AND EVALUATION

A significant percentage of all patients admitted with head injuries also have systemic injuries, so their treatment must include management of both their head injuries and their systemic injuries. Adequate perfusion of the injured brain is needed to minimize morbidity and to increase the patient's chances of surviving. If the mean arterial pressure declines or if the ICP rises, the cerebral perfusion pressure falls. Thus,

the mean arterial pressure must be maintained at normotensive levels in patients who have multiple injuries. The morbidity and mortality of patients with head injuries who are hypotensive on admission are two to three times higher than the morbidity and mortality of patients with head injuries who are not hypotensive on admission. All possible measures must be taken to prevent increased ICP as a result of intracranial hematomas or swollen brain tissue.

Because initially it is not possible to determine clinically

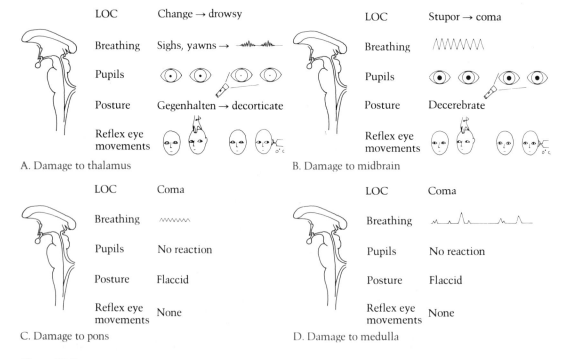

Figure 30-9

Progression of central herniation. Serial assessments will identify trends. The nurse may observe signs, beginning with diencephalic compression and progressing to lower brain stem involvement.

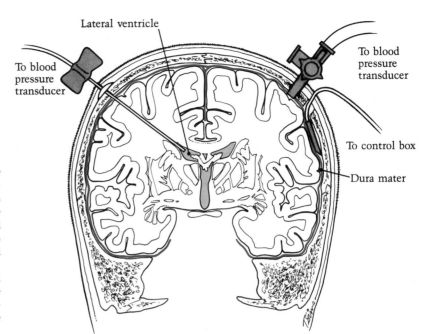

Lateral ventricle

To blood
pressure
transducer

To blood
pressure
transducer

To control box

Dura mater

Figure 30-10

Measurement techniques for intracranial pressure monitoring. On the left is shown a method for intraventricular catheterization. The catheter is placed in the uninjured side, and, if possible, the left side is avoided. On the top, the subarachnoid method is pictured. Here, a plastic stopcock is passed through the skull into the subarachnoid space. On the right, the epidural method is shown. The transducer is placed between the skull and dura through a burr hole. The transducer in the illustration is enlarged for clarity; the actual transducer is much smaller—approximately 1 cm wide by 2 mm thick.

whether a patient with a severe head injury has an increased ICP, it is assumed so. The neurosurgical resuscitation measures are described in the following paragraphs.

Intubation is often performed, and hyperventilation measures are taken so that the patient does not become hypoxic or hypercarbic. Hypercarbia is a potent cerebral vasodilator, and when the intracranial blood vessels are dilated, the ICP can increase significantly. Conversely, with hypocarbia induced by hyperventilation, cerebral vasoconstriction will occur with a rapid decrease in the ICP. Hyperventilation decreases the cerebral metabolic use of oxygen. Thus, intubation and hyperventilation are used to maintain the patient's arterial carbon dioxide levels at about 25 mm Hg.

To decrease brain water and thus brain volume in patients suspected of having increased ICP, 500 ml of a 20% mannitol solution is given intravenously for 30 minutes. Intracranial pressure decreases rapidly, and a patient who has a dilated pupil frequently has constriction of that pupil as the brain is dehydrated and the ICP returns to more normal levels. Mannitol is contraindicated in a patient who is hypotensive on admission, because the intravascular volume must be maintained.

Efforts are made to keep the ICP levels below 15 mm Hg. Often mannitol must be infused in 25-g to 50-g boluses every 4 to 6 hours as indicated. Because mannitol can cause renal failure when serum osmolality is elevated significantly (usually to levels above 340 mOsm to 350 mOsm), the serum sodium levels and the indices of renal function have to be monitored. Mannitol is customarily not administered to any patient whose serum sodium level is greater than 155 mEq/L. Also, cerebrospinal fluid may be drained to decrease the ICP.

The patient is best positioned with the neck in a neutral position and the head of the bed elevated 30° to 45°. The jugular venous pressure and, in turn, the ICP are reduced.

Control of temperature is important, because the patient often is thermolabile because he or she has a brain stem injury, blood in the subarachnoid space, increased heat production with extension posturing, or a central nervous system infection.

Hyperthermia greatly increases the cerebral edema and thus the ICP, and it increases the cerebral metabolism at a time when the tissue viability is borderline. Control of hyperthermia should be instituted whenever the temperature rises to 38°C (101°F) or greater. If hyperthermia control is not instituted until the temperature has reached higher levels, the hyperthermia is much more difficult to control. The use of aspirin or acetaminophen (Tylenol) in appropriate doses and a hypothermia blanket is effective. Hyperthermic patients usually have their temperatures lowered to normothermic (not hypothermic) levels. Injections of intramuscular thorazine (10 mg) may be ordered to help to lower an elevated temperature. Thorazine, an alpha-adrenergic blocking drug, causes peripheral vasodilation, which helps dissipate heat and prevents or reduces the shivering sometimes seen. (The shivering tends to retard the lowering of body temperature.)

Patients with severe extensor spasms accompanied by a significantly increased ICP may be helped by the administration of muscle relaxants. Intravenous morphine or drugs that exert a blocking effect at the myoneural junction (*e.g.*, pancuronium bromide) are the drugs of choice.

The administration of steroids to patients with severe head injuries is still being studied. The potential benefit of steroids is associated with stabilization of the endothelial and glial membranes and, thus, reduction of edema formation. Although much research must still be conducted, the benefits of steroid use in treating both traumatic and ischemic cerebral edema are inconclusive. Neither high-dose nor low-dose corticosteroids have been scientifically proved to be effective in head-injured patients. Owing to the potentially harmful side-effects of steroid therapy, one should always exercise discretion in their use. However, corticosteroids are still the treatment of choice for edema resulting from space-occupying lesions of the brain, including neoplasms.[11]

Barbiturate coma is a fairly widely accepted therapy to control the brain's metabolic activity and enhance cerebrovascular microcirculation. The brain is protected and preserved through the postinjury phase by reducing the metabolic needs. Increased ICP is rapidly reduced, and cerebral perfusion is maintained. The goal is maintenance of brain activity close to the level of an isoelectric electroencephalogram. If used, physiologic monitoring is mandatory because of the potential cardiopulmonary complications. Because the patient is deeply anesthetized, intubation and mechanical ventilation are necessary. Different medications can be used. As one example, sodium phenobarbital, 150 mg to 500 mg daily, can be administered. However, owing to the high mortality rate associated with barbiturate coma in adults, this type of therapy is a "last-ditch" effort when all else fails to lower ICP.

Complications

The nurse must carefully observe the patient for any complications. Through collaboration with other health team members, many complications can be prevented and, at the least, minimized.

Pulmonary Problems

Pulmonary problems occur often, and they are frequently lethal. Monitoring of arterial blood gas levels and of the other pulmonary parameters is important. Decreased consciousness brings the threat of hypoxemia, hypercapnia, and a secondary insult to the brain. Aspiration is always possible.

Alterations in respiratory function may be caused by cerebral or pulmonary injury. Loss of the sighing mechanism leads to microatelectasis (secondary to a decrease in pulmonary surfactant). Patients so affected tend to breathe at the same tidal volume, and atelectasis results in nonventilated portions of the lung that continue to be perfused so that ventilation-perfusion abnormalities arise. The venous admixture results in right-to-left shunts, systemic hypoxemia, and an increased $PaCO_2$. A problem that can compound the situation is a rapid reduction in $PaCO_2$, because the cerebral vessel will constrict and decreased amounts of oxygen will be available.

Another cause of alterations in respiratory function is that neurogenic stimuli open pulmonary arteriovenous shunts that bypass the alveoli. In animals, after a head injury, prophylaxis with various sympatholytic antiepinephrine and general anesthetics (but not isoproterenol or atropine) prevents pulmonary complications and thus suggests a neuroendocrine influence on pulmonary surfactant and compliance. Also, increased ICP and brain compression, although uncommon, may cause acute pulmonary edema. The cause has not been identified, but it may be pulmonary vein constriction or left-heart failure. The two most critical periods are the admission period and the first 2 postoperative days. As a rule of thumb, a decrease in PaO_2 to below 70 mm Hg is an indication for endotracheal intubation.

Fluid and Electrolyte Problems

Fluid and electrolyte problems are potential complications.[1] Usually only maintenance fluids are required, and the patient is kept dry. With the breakdown of the blood-brain barrier at the capillary endothelial level, edema fluid passes into the brain parenchyma. Excess intravenous fluid enhances edema formation, negates the effects of mannitol, and produces increases in the ICP. If the 24-hour urinary output and the laboratory values (serum electrolytes, blood urea nitrogen, and creatinine levels, and the hematocrit) are normal, 1500 to 2000 ml of fluid is usually administered (Ringer's lactate solution or half-normal saline solution). Patients who have a fever, third-space loss, or excessive movement require increased fluids. The use of dehydrating drugs to control cerebral swelling has not been well defined. Although a rebound effect may occur after administration of hyperosmotic agents, the immediate situation must be considered a critical event. The use of hyperosmotic agents is based on the idea that if the osmolarity of the blood is increased to a higher level than that of the tissues, fluid will move out of the brain tissue into the blood and subsequently be excreted in the urine. However, some of the hypertonic agent enters the brain parenchyma. As blood is cleared of the hypertonic agent, the hypertonic agent that has entered the brain cells causes the cells to be hypertonic relative to the brain. The result is that fluid moves into the cells, producing cellular swelling (i.e., rebound swelling). Agents such as mannitol or glycerol are used, and they are supplemented with furosemide.

The hypothalamus and the posterior pituitary may be damaged, causing a decreased secretion of antidiuretic hormone and resulting in diabetes insipidus. The urinary output is quite high, even several liters per hour, and the specific gravity and osmolar concentration are low. Diabetes insipidus is diagnosed by the physician when the urine cannot be concentrated to greater than 1.005 and the 24-hour urinary output is more than 4000 ml. Because the water loss is great, hypernatremia is a threat.

Because polyuria may result from many conditions (i.e., sodium loss, adrenal insufficiency, water diuresis, fluid overload, osmotic diuresis, or elevated blood glucose levels), a dehydration test is often done. The patient is not permitted fluids during the night, and blood and urine specimens are obtained from 3 A.M. to 6 A.M. The patient with antidiuretic hormone insufficiency exhibits a low urine osmolality and is evaluated as follows: If he or she is alert and thirsty and has mild polyuria, he or she can probably maintain fluid balance by drinking. If he or she is alert but the urinary output is greater than 250 ml/hour or if the patient is not alert and is not thirsty, aqueous pitressin (2 U to 5 U subcutaneously) is usually ordered.[32] Fluid replacement matches urinary output, and 700 ml to 1000 ml additional replacement is given for insensible water loss. The fluids are replaced with a 5% dextrose in water solution (1000 ml/24 hours) given with Ringer's lactate solution, because the urine is low in electrolytes. Fluid balance and electrolyte levels must be assessed serially.

On the other hand, antidiuretic hormone secretion may be inappropriately increased, resulting in water retention and dilutional hypovolemia. The mechanisms involved are an increased glomerular filtration rate, volume expansion, suppression of renin-angiotensin-aldosterone secretion, and decreased distal tubular sodium reabsorption, all of which result in increased sodium excretion. Clinically, the patient has renal sodium excretion associated with hypovolemia, normal thyroid-renal-adrenal functioning, a lack of peripheral edema, a lack of the signs of volume depletion, and an increased urine osmolarity that is inconsistent with the plasma hypotonicity. If the serum sodium levels are below 120 mEq/L, the patient may exhibit the cerebral signs of irritability, confusion, lethargy, or even psychosis. If the serum sodium levels are below 110 mEq/liter, the patient may have convulsions. Therapy usually is water restriction or administration of 500 ml of normal saline daily. If convulsions occur or if severe hyponatremia is present, the therapy usually is the administration of a 3% to 5% hypertonic saline solution and mannitol or furosemide for free-water clearance. If the condition becomes chronic, the physician may order demeclocycline to inhibit antidiuretic action at the renal tubular site.

Gastric Bleeding

Cushing's ulcers are probably caused by marked hypersecretion of gastric acid.[5] In patients with severe head injuries resulting in coma and (particularly) decerebrate rigidity, the degree of gastric hyperacidity correlates roughly with the amount of gastric bleeding, approximating the levels attained in the Zollinger-Ellison syndrome.[40] The hypothesis that the hyperacidity is the result of direct stimulation of the vagal nuclei by increased ICP has been supported by the fact that the routine administration of parenteral anticholinergics blocked and reduced gastric acid secretion and essentially prevented the syndrome.[21,22] Also, with the advent of prophylactic antacid therapy and cimetidine therapy, bleeding rarely occurs. It is considered almost a complication of the past.

Epilepsy

Secondary epilepsy refers to structurally induced seizure that has a known cause. These seizures result from cerebral scarring due to head injury, cerebrovascular accident, infection, degenerative central nervous system disease, or recurrent childhood febrile seizures. Traumatic head injury is one of the main causes of secondary epilepsy. Approximately 10% of patients who have an acute head injury may have seizures, probably because of bleeding, edema, and neuronal death. The incidence of posttraumatic seizures has been reported to range from 5% to 50%, depending on the severity of the underlying injury or disease, whether or not unconsciousness was present, and whether or not the dura was penetrated.[43]

Seizures are classified as partial or generalized. *Partial seizures* refer to those seizures initially involving only one hemisphere. Simple partial seizures usually involve only one hemisphere and are not accompanied by a loss of consciousness or responsiveness. Complex partial seizures always involve both hemispheres and result in a loss of consciousness. Generalized seizures are those whose first electroencephalogram and clinical changes indicate involvement of both cerebral hemispheres. Partial seizures have evidence of a local onset but not a discreet focus, whereas generalized seizures do not exhibit a local onset. The term *aura* has been used in the past to describe a warning sign of an impending seizure. However, due to the fact that consciousness is maintained and only a small portion of the brain is involved, the aura is now thought to be a simple partial seizure. Because simple partial seizures may progress to complex partial seizures or generalized tonic-clonic seizures that result in unconsciousness, the aura may in fact be a warning sign of impending complex partial seizures.[43]

The first rule of treatment with any person experiencing seizure activity is to maintain a patient airway and protect the person from injury. The next rule is to treat the underlying disease, which may reduce the frequency of seizures. Once the underlying disease is treated, the goal of treatment is to bring the seizures under control. This goal is accomplished primarily through anticonvulsant drug therapy. Sixty to 80% of persons with epilepsy can obtain good seizure control with proper drug management.[43]

Bacterial Meningitis

Although bacterial meningitis can be a primary disease of the central nervous system, it is also a possible complication related to neurosurgical procedures, diagnostic procedures such as lumbar punctures, ICP monitoring, trauma, and ear/sinus or systemic infections. Bacterial meningitis affects the pia mater, arachnoid space, and cerebrospinal fluid. Owing to the circulatory properties of the cerebrospinal fluid, the infection can spread throughout the entire subarachnoid space and affect the ventricles of the brain. The accumulation of exudate may spread into the cranial and spinal nerves as well as obstruct the normal flow of cerebrospinal fluid, resulting in the development of hydrocephalus. Secondary encephalitis and neuronal degeneration may occur if the brain's surface adjacent to the meninges becomes involved.

Signs and symptoms of bacterial meningitis include fever, severe headache, nuchal rigidity, generalized seizures, alteration in the level of consciousness, and positive Kernig's (inability to completely extend the legs) and Brudzinski's (forward flexion of the head causing hip and knee flexion response) signs. Because the signs and symptoms of meningitis are usually the same as those of the primary insult, (*i.e.*, head injury, subarachnoid hemorrhage, arteriovenous malformation, ischemic insult), a definitive diagnosis must be made by examining the cerebrospinal fluid. Diagnostic findings usually include increased spinal fluid pressure, increased protein levels, increased leukocyte count, decreased glucose content, and a positive Gram stain and culture.

Treatment for bacterial meningitis includes temperature control as well as administration of systemic or intrathecal antibiotics depending on the causative organism. The resolution of the inflammatory process and degree of recovery depend largely on the stage at which the infection is controlled and how it has further impacted the initial insult. If bacterial meningitis persists, the chance of further cerebral damage increases. In the patient who is already neurologically compromised, this complication can significantly impact the ultimate recovery.

A carotid cavernous sinus fistula, which is an abnormal communication between the carotid artery and the cavernous sinus, may develop as a result of head trauma. Blunt trauma is the most common cause of this complication. Pulsating exophthalmos, bruit (the most common initial symptom), chemosis, headache, papilledema, opthalmoplegias, and visual loss are the major presenting symptoms of a carotid cavernous sinus fistula. Carotid cavernous fistulas are rarely life-threatening, and 4% to 12% close spontaneously.[20] Treatment of these fistulas is indicated for impending blindness, intolerable bruit, or unacceptable cosmetic appearance. The goal of treatment is to occlude the fistula while still preserving blood flow in the carotid artery.[20]

Other possible problems, particularly for the unconscious patient, are pulmonary complications, thrombi, pulmonary embolism, decubitus ulcer, and urinary tract infections.

Many problems occur after the initial danger is past. The Glasgow outcome score may be used for assessment. With it, the patient is classified as having made a good recovery, being moderately disabled, being severely disabled, being vegetative, or as dead.[13] Personality changes may occur. Sexual dysfunction (*e.g.*, impotence) and dysmenorrhea occur often. It is hypothesized that these problems are secondary to energy forces directed toward deep midline structures, such as the hypothalamus.[7] Focal neurologic deficits are dependent on the site of the injury and on the nerve involvement. Intelligence can be decreased, depending on the severity of the injury. For example, it is not unusual that an engineer resumes his working life as a draftsman.

Often postconcussion syndrome occurs for up to 2 years, and even for the rest of the patient's life. It is characterized by the loss of memory, dizziness, headaches, decreased concentration, and insomnia.

SUMMARY

Accurate assessment and management by the neurologic team are essential in aiding patient recovery from head trauma. Because nurses are at the bedside, they are responsible for monitoring patients and quickly managing critical situations. Although the initial extent of injury cannot be altered, prolonged elevations of ICP and cardiopulmonary complications can be prevented. It is hoped that such interventions will prevent patient death and improve the patient's quality of life.

DIRECTIONS FOR FUTURE RESEARCH

Past research efforts have been geared primarily toward pathophysiology and treatment regimens. Great advances have been made. Current research efforts can now be targeted at clinical care delivery. The long-term effects of head injury have many implications for nursing. Several nursing units in different locales can join forces and select one question toward which to direct their efforts. Sometimes there is not enough information to answer a question, so more fundamental questions must be answered first. Examples of important questions follow:[18]

1. What factors are associated with attracting and keeping nurses in neurosurgical nursing?
2. How can nurses involve families to help reduce patient stress?
3. How do families react to increased technology?
4. What clinical parameters can be used to assess and monitor anxiety and pain?
5. What techniques are most helpful to assess and relieve pain?
6. How is ICP affected by patient position changes?
7. How is increased ICP affected by verbal and environmental stimuli?
8. Does touch have a place in the care of the head-injured patient?

REFERENCES

1. Balestrieri, F. J., Chernow, B., and Cainey, T. G. Post-craniotomy diabetes insipidus: Who's at risk? *Crit. Care Med.* 10:108, 1982.
2. Cohen, C. B. Interdisciplinary consultation on the care of the critically ill and dying: The role of one hospital ethics committee. *Crit. Care Med.* 10:776, 1982.
3. Cooper, P. R., Maravilla, K., Moody, S., *et al.* Serial computerized
4. tomographic scanning and the prognosis of severe head injury. *Neurosurgery* 1(5):566, 1979.
4. Cowley, R. A., and Trump, B. J. *Pathophysiology of shock, anoxia, and ischemia.* Baltimore: Williams & Wilkins, 1981.
5. Cushing, H. Peptic ulcers and the interbrain. *Surg. Gynecol. Obstet.* 55:1, 1932.
6. Dempsey, K. J., and Kindt, G. W. Experimental augmentation of critical blood flow by mannitol in epidural intracranial masses. *J. Trauma* 22:449, 1982.
7. Ensin, J. Nutritional assessment of a severely injured multi-trauma patient. *J. Neurosurg. Nurs.* 14(5):262, 1982.
8. Fisher, C. M. Some neuro-ophthalmological observations. *J. Neurol. Neurosurg. Psychiatry* 30:283, 1967.
9. Fishman, R. A. Brain edema. *N. Engl. J. Med.* 293:706, 1975.
10. Hall, J. W. III. Auditory evoked responses in acute severe head injury. *J. Neurosurg. Nurs.* 14(5):225, 1982.
11. Harper, J. Use of steroids in cerebral edema: Therapeutic implications. *Heart Lung.* 17(1):70, 1988.
12. Hendrickson, S. Intracranial pressure changes and family presence. *J. Neurosci. Nurs.* 19(1):14, 1987.
13. Jennett, B. Assessment of outcome after severe brain damage. *Lancet* 1:480, 1975.
14. Jennett, B., Miller, J. D., and Broakman, R. Epilepsy after non-missile depressed skull fracture. *J. Neurosurg.* 41:208, 1974.
15. Johnson, S., Omery, A., and Nikas, D. Effects of conversation on intracranial pressure in comatose patients. *Heart Lung* 18(1):56, 1989.
16. Kuhl, D. E., Alevi, A., Hoffman, E. J., *et al.* Local cerebral blood volume in head injured patients: Determination by emission computed tomography of Tc^{99m}-labeled red cells. *J. Neurosurg.* 52:309, 1980.
17. Langfitt, T. W. Cerebral circulation and metabolism. *J. Neurosurg.* 40:461, 1974.
18. Lewandowslci, L. A., and Kositsky, A. M. Research priorities for critical care nursing. *Heart Lung* 12:35, 1983.
19. Lundberg, N. Clinical Indications for Measurement of ICP. In M. Brock and H. Dietz (eds.), *Intracranial Pressure: Experimental and Clinical Aspects.* New York: Springer-Verlag, 1972.
20. Martin, E., and Hummelgard, A. Detachable balloon occlusion of carotid-cavernous sinus fistula. *J. Neurosci. Nurs.* 19(3):132, 1987.
21. Mendelow, A. D., and Teasdale, G. M. Pathophysiology of head injuries. *Br. J. Surg.* 70:641, 1983.
22. Miller, J. D., Becker, D. P., Ward, J. D., *et al.* Significance of intracranial hypertension in severe head injury. *J. Neurosurg.* 47:503, 1977.
23. Miller, J. D., and Becker, D. P. Secondary insults to the injured brain. *J. R. Coll. Surg. Edinb.* 27:292, 1982.
24. Mitchell, P. H., and Mauss, W. K. Relationship of patient-nurse activity to intracranial pressure variations: A pilot study. *Nurs. Res.* 27:4, 1978.
25. Prendergase, V. Bacterial meningitis update. *J. Neurosci. Nurs.* 19(2):95, 1987.
26. Plum, F., and Posner, J. *The Diagnosis of Stupor and Coma.* Philadelphia: F. A. Davis, 1983.
27. Rimel, R. W. Emergency management of the patient with central nervous system trauma. *J. Neurosurg. Nurs.* 10:185, 1978.
28. Rottenberg, D. A., and Posner, J. B. Intracranial Pressure Control. In J. E. Cottrell and H. Turndoff (eds.), *Anesthesia and Neurosurgery.* St. Louis: C. V. Mosby, 1980.
29. Rudy, E. Magnetic resonance imaging: New horizon in diagnostic techniques. *J. Neurosurg. Nurs.* 17(6):331, 1985.
30. Sabin, T. D. The differential diagnosis of coma. *N. Engl. J. Med.* 290:1062, 1974.
31. Shatsky, S., Evans, D., Miller, F., *et al.* High-speed angiography of experimental head injury. *J. Neurosurg.* 41:523, 1974.
32. Shucart, W. A., and Jackson, I. Management of diabetes insipidus in neurosurgical patients. *J. Neurosurg.* 44:65, 1976.

33. Shulman, K., Marmorov, A., Miller, J. D., *et al. Intracranial Pressure IV*. New York: Springer-Verlag, 1980.

34. Sitz, W. V. Blunt Force Injury. In W. V. Spitz and R. S. Fisher (eds.), *Medicolegal Investigation of Death*. Springfield, IL: Charles C. Thomas, 1980.

35. Spielman, G. Coma: A clinical review. *Heart Lung* 10:700, 1981.

36. Teasdale, G. Assessment of coma and impaired consciousness: A practical scale. *Lancet* 2:81, 1974.

37. Teres, D., Brown, R. B., and Lemeshow, S. Predicting mortality of intensive unit patients: The importance of coma. *Crit. Care Med.* 10:86, 1982.

38. Turner, H., Anderson, R. L., and Ward, J. D., *et al.* Comparison of nurse and computer recording of ICP in head injured patients. *J. Neurosci. Nurs.* 20(4):236, 1988.

39. Vries, J., Becher, D., and Young, H. A subarachnoid screw for monitoring intracranial pressure. *J. Neurosurg.* 39:416, 1973.

40. Walleck, C. Primary nursing: Providing continuity of care to the neurosurgical patient. *J. Neurosurg. Nurs.* 11:21, 1979.

41. Walleck, C. The Effect of Purposeful Touch on Intracranial Pressure. *In Proceedings of the Tenth Annual National Teaching Institute*. Newport Beach, CA: American Association of Critical Care Nurses, 1983.

42. Watts, C., and Clark, K. Gastric acidity in the comatose patient. *J. Neurosurg.* 30:107, 1969.

43. Wierenga, M. Disorders of Cerebral Function. In Porth (ed.), *Pathophysiology*. Philadelphia: J. B. Lippincott, 1986.

44. Wincek, J., and Ruttem, M. Exposure keratitis in comatose children. *J. Neurosci. Nurs.* 21(4):241, 1989.

31

Cerebrovascular Disease

Susan Kay Mitchell   *Rowena R. Yates*

BUILDING MIND MAPS AND CLUSTERING
An excellent tool to begin a flow of visions of healing and a free association of ideas and thoughts is called "mind mapping" or "clustering." Whenever you feel stuck with your ideas or problem-solving steps, make a mind map and see how many possibilities and new patterns come up. You can cluster ideas on a piece of typing paper. However, it makes a marvelous visual impact when you are working on a piece of paper that is 14 inches × 17 inches or larger. The bigger piece of paper helps you play with ideas.

Here is how to begin. Let yourself sit quietly and become focused within. Let a central word or theme come to you and write it in the center of your paper and draw a circle around it. This theme word may be a name, symptoms that might be present, a short statement about a problem, an image, a metaphor, or a symbol.

As associated words arise, you can write them around the central word, circle them, and connect them to the center or each other with appropriate lines.

Remember that this activity should be like a brain-storming session; nothing should be censored, and no idea should be ignored. Within a few minutes, your web-like grouping of key words will begin to point to relationships and possibilities of which you were probably unaware. This shifting from a nebulous, indeterminate form to a focus on patterns and relationships is called an "inner shift" and is a state that occurs during any creative act. From seemingly disconnected random words and thoughts, there suddenly emerges a direction, a clarity of purpose that may lead you out of the dark and into a solution.

You will know when the clustering project is complete because it just feels that way. Step back from it and enjoy the visual and felt pleasure of your free flow of ideas.

LEARNING OBJECTIVES

After reading this chapter the nurse should be able to do the following:

1. Describe normal cerebral vasculature, identifying the major vessels and the area of the brain each supplies.
2. List the major causes of cerebrovascular disease and the major signs and symptoms of each.
3. Describe the different signs and symptoms particular to ruptured cerebral aneurysm, hypertensive intracerebral hemorrhage, ruptured arteriovenous malformation, and thrombotic versus embolic insult.
4. List the major complications associated with hemorrhagic cerebrovascular insult.
5. List the major complications associated with ischemic cerebrovascular insult.
6. Describe the major medical and surgical management for cerebrovascular disease.
7. List the correct nursing actions to institute when caring for a patient with cerebrovascular disease.
8. Identify and initiate correct nursing actions for specific complications of cerebrovascular disease.

CASE STUDY

Mrs. W., a 52-year-old housewife, suddenly collapsed at breakfast after having a generalized seizure. Her husband and daughter responded quickly and called the paramedics, who promptly transported her to an outlying community hospital. On arrival to the hospital's emergency department, Mrs. W. was lethargic and mute. She had a disconjugate gaze to the right and right hemiparesis. Mr. W. stated that his wife had complained of a slight headache over the past few days, but that it had not been severe or associated with nausea and vomiting.

The patient profile described Mrs. W. as a thin woman (5 feet 7 inches, 120 pounds). She occasionally took over-the-counter medications for sinus difficulties. She had a 40 pack/year history of cigarette smoking and occasionally drank alcohol. She slept 7 to 8 hours a night and rarely awakened. Her dietary pattern consisted of three meals a day with occasional snacks in the afternoon. Mrs. W.'s past medical history was significant only for a hemorrhoidectomy 7 years before this admission. She had no known history of heart disease, diabetes mellitus, or cerebrovascular disease.

The physical examination revealed eye opening to speech but with no response to verbal commands. Mrs. W. would localize briskly with her left extremities to painful stimuli, and the right extremities would flicker to same. There were positive Babinski's reflexes bilaterally. Pupils were equal and round and reacted briskly to light. The rest of the physical examination was unremarkable. An emergency computed axial tomographic scan (CT scan) with contrast dye was obtained that showed generalized subarachnoid hemorrhage (SAH) involving most of the cisterns of the brain with normal-sized ventricles. Mrs. W. was admitted to the intensive care unit (ICU) and scheduled for an arteriogram and an electroencephalogram the following day. She was intubated due to her decreased level of consciousness and inability to maintain an adequate airway and was placed on medical management consisting of dexamethasone, phenytoin sodium, and aminocaproic acid. A four-vessel angiogram was performed that revealed two large saccular aneurysms, each measuring 2 cm, that arose from the internal carotid artery with no other abnormalities of the cerebral vessels. The electroencephalogram was normal, with no seizure activity or focal abnormalities shown.

Mrs. W.'s status improved with resulting extubation and continued ICU care. At this time, she was verbalizing but not oriented, using abusive language at times.

Seven days after her admission, a repeat CT scan was obtained with and without contrast dye. These CT scans showed an increase in ventricular size with subarachnoid blood still present. Right frontal edema was present and was noted to be more prominent than in the previous scan, suggesting the possibility of a second hemorrhage since admission. Due to the location and size of the aneurysms, Mrs. W. was referred to a large county teaching hospital whose surgeons had the needed expertise.

Eight days after the initial hemorrhage, Mrs. W. was admitted to the neurosurgical ICU to be monitored for further rebleeding and vasospasm until surgery was performed. A central line was placed to monitor fluid status, and an arterial line was placed to monitor blood pressure. At this time, Mrs. W. was oriented to person, place, and time with continued use of abusive language at times. The family was reassured that this abusive language was a result of her disease, as were such physical changes as her sleepiness and weakness. Mrs. W. obeyed commands bilaterally, with the right side weaker than the left in response. Pupils were equal and round and reacted to light. Vital signs and neurologic signs were stable. The aminocaproic acid infusion was discontinued, but the patient remained on dexamethasone and phenytoin sodium, and magnesium hydroxide was added to the regimen.

On day 10 after her initial SAH, Mrs. W. was taken to surgery, where a left internal carotid artery aneurysm and an ophthalmic artery aneurysm were identified and clipped. An intraoperative arteriogram documented a patent left internal carotid artery. Mrs. W. returned to the neurosurgical ICU, intubated. Her neurologic examination at this time revealed spontaneous eye opening, pupils equal and reactive, with left extremities localizing and right extremities semipurposeful to painful stimuli. Her vital signs were stable, with a blood pressure of 130/60, a heart rate of 60, and respirations of 20.

Late in the afternoon of postoperative day 1, Mrs. W. became progressively less responsive. Her pupils were noted to be equal but nonreactive to light. Despite induced hyperventilation and diuresis with mannitol, the right pupil became dilated and both extremities extended to painful stimulus. An emergency CT scan was performed that revealed left hemispheric and right frontal ischemia with a left-to-right shift of the midline. At this time, ventricular catheter placement was attempted but unsuccessful owing to massive swelling and small ventricles. A subarachnoid screw was placed to monitor the intracranial

pressure (ICP), which measured 0 mm Hg to 5 mm Hg initially. Owing to the patient's rapid deterioration and unresponsiveness to other measures, barbiturate coma was induced using thiopenthal sodium. The goal of the barbiturate coma was to decrease the metabolic needs of the brain and to help prevent further ischemia. A dopamine drip was begun simultaneously to keep the systolic blood pressure above 100 mm Hg. The central line remained in place to monitor fluid status, because the surgeons opted not to place a Swan-Ganz catheter. The patient's status remained unchanged in barbiturate coma until postoperative day 3, when she developed diabetes insipidus, as documented by a urine output of 800 cc/hour for 2 consecutive hours, serum osmolality of 320 (nl 290), and urine osmolality of 120 (nl 650 to 1200) with a urine specific gravity of 1.002 (nl 1.005 to 1.021). The diabetes insipidus was treated with intravenous fluids to replace urine output and aqueous vasopressin to control fluid and electrolyte loss. The ICP readings continued to be less than 20 mm Hg, but Mrs. W.'s pupils continued to dilate until both were fixed at 8 mm. Thiopenthal was stopped at this time, and supportive care consisting of ventilator support, intravenous fluids, and dopamine to maintain systolic blood pressure above 90 were continued because of the gravity of her condition.

On postoperative day 7, the thiopenthal levels were zero and Mrs. W.'s neurologic status was re-evaluated. At this time, she was flaccid to painful stimuli in all four extremities. She had negative doll's eyes as well as negative corneal, cough, and gag reflexes. Pupils remained fixed at 8 mm. Because she had no brain function, documented by absence of cranial nerve function, no spontaneous respiratory drive, and inability to maintain systemic pressure without drug support, the surgeons pronounced her brain-dead and opted to remove cardiovascular support. The surgeons talked with the family and discussed with them the negative prognosis. The family, who had been by the bedside as much as was possible, expressed interest in the possibility of organ donation. They were told that because of the high doses of cardiovascular drugs and the prolonged periods of time in which her blood pressure was below 60 systolic, this was not an option. The family was allowed to remain at the bedside as much as possible. The dopamine was slowly weaned, and the patient's blood pressure fell to zero, resulting in cardiovascular collapse and death.

REFLECTIONS

Patients who experience a severe cerebrovascular insult are suddenly placed in a situation in which they are unable to communicate with others. However, although unable to respond verbally, they need outside stimuli to help them relate to their surroundings. There are many ways of stimulating these patients in an effort to keep them aware of their environment. One way to accomplish this goal is to work with the family or significant others in setting up a program that involves the use of the patient's favorite music, family photographs, and favorite objects to stimulate the patient and help increase his awareness. The music is taped and then played for 15 to 30 minutes six to eight times a day using a tape recorder placed near the patient; earphones are used if possible. In addition, the family is encouraged to ask relatives, close friends, and significant groups to send taped messages instead of cards. In this manner, the patient can hear voices that are familiar in the hope of stimulating the patient's memory and awareness of his surroundings. This action is based on the generally accepted theory that hearing is one of the last senses to leave and the first to return. The family is encouraged to talk to the patient, showing photographs and pointing out objects that have been placed nearby. The family is asked to tell the patient what is happening within the family unit and who has come to see him in the hospital. In this way, the family is able to support and relate to the patient and help in recovery.

The professional staff also plays an important role in promoting awareness in the patient who is neurologically impaired. It is important to incorporate constant reassurance into the plan of care through touch and tone of voice. Reorienting the patient to date, time, place, circumstance, and person if necessary is an integral part of the recovery process. Last, but not least, reassurance and reorientation should be accompanied by an explanation of all treatments and procedures involving the patient. Because it is not known how much the patient is actually cognizant of, it should be assumed by the professional caregivers and family members that the patient hears what is said to him and is aware of what is done to him.

ANATOMY AND PHYSIOLOGY

In order to understand the neurologic manifestations of cerebrovascular disease one must first have an adequate understanding of the normal vascular anatomy of the central nervous system and the major factors regulating cerebral blood flow.

Cerebral Vasculature

The brain is supplied by two pairs of arteries: the two internal carotid arteries and the two vertebral arteries (Figs. 31–1 and 31–2). The internal carotid artery (ICA) supplies blood to the vascular tree of the anterior two thirds of the brain and constitutes the anterior circulation of the brain. The vertebral basilar system supplies the posterior third of the brain, as well

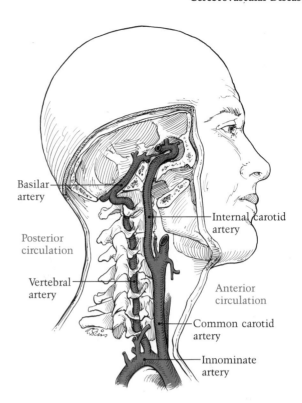

Figure 31–2
Lateral view of the origins of the anterior and posterior circulation.

as the brain stem and cerebellum, and constitutes the posterior circulation.

The internal carotid arteries originate from two different vessels, although both vessels arise from the aorta. The left common carotid artery originates directly from the aorta, and the right common carotid artery arises from the innominate artery, which originates from the aorta. The common carotids branch to form the external and internal carotid arteries. The internal carotid artery enters the cranial vault through the foramen lacerum. Most of the cerebral hemispheres, excluding the occipitals, the basal ganglia, and the upper two thirds of the diencephalon, are supplied by the internal carotid arteries and their branches. The cerebral branches of each carotid artery include the posterior communicating artery, the anterior cerebral artery, and the middle cerebral artery.

The vertebral arteries originate from the subclavian arteries and enter the skull through the foramen magnum, ventrolateral to the spinal cord. In general, blood is supplied to the brain stem from the bulb to the lower third of the diencephalon (thalamus and hypothalamus), the cerebellum, and the occipital region of the cerebral hemispheres. The vertebral arteries unite to form the basilar artery.

The branches of the vertebrobasilar system and the internal carotid arteries are joined by the posterior communicating artery on each side to form an anastomotic circle of Willis on the base of the brain. The two anterior cerebral arteries, whose longest sides are connected by the one anterior communicating artery, essentially connect the two internal carotids (Figs. 31–3 and 31–4).

The cerebral veins, excluding the sinuses, have even thinner walls than the arteries in proportion to their size and lack of muscle layer. The veins and sinuses have no valves; therefore,

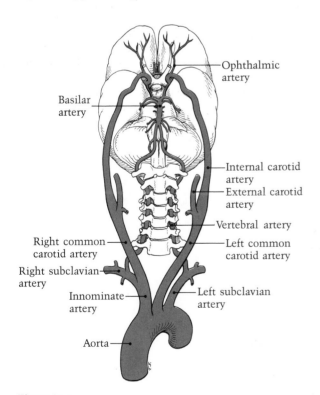

Figure 31–1
Origins of the anterior and posterior circulation.

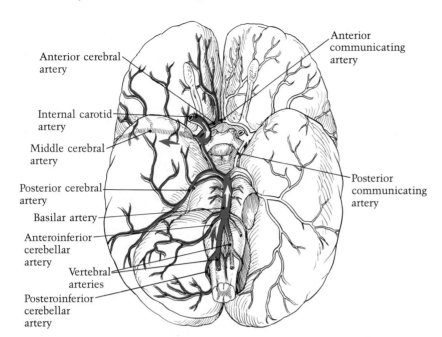

Anterior cerebral artery

Anterior communicating artery

Internal carotid artery

Middle cerebral artery

Posterior cerebral artery

Posterior communicating artery

Basilar artery

Anteroinferior cerebellar artery

Vertebral arteries

Posteroinferior cerebellar artery

Figure 31–3
The circulation of the circle of Willis.

cerebral drainage is dependent on the head position. The venous return does not retrace the course of corresponding arteries but follows a pattern of its own. The veins of the convexity of the brain drain principally into the superior longitudinal sinuses. The cavernous sinus collects venous drainage from the inferior surface, whereas the inferior longitudinal sinuses collect venous drainage from the medial surface. There are also other less important sinuses that collect the venous return. The dural sinuses are large venous chambers lying between the two layers of the dura. The veins empty into the dural sinuses, which in turn empty into the jugular veins for the return of the blood to the heart.

Cerebral Blood Flow

Functionally, the anterior circulation and the posterior circulation usually remain separate. The circle of Willis may be thought of as a protective mechanism by which blood is shunted to compensate for alterations in cerebral blood flow or pressure. However, collateral circulation through the circle of Willis depends on the patency of its components. The vessels of the circle, particularly the communicating arteries, are frequently anomalous. In greater than 25% of the population, the functional efficiency of the circle of Willis is compromised congenitally so that communication between the anterior and posterior circulation is poor. Nevertheless, in favorable instances, the circle does permit an adequate blood supply to reach all parts of the brain, even after ligation of one or more of the four supplying vessels has occurred.

Functional and useful collateral blood supply in the cerebrovasculature comes from large vessels at the base of the brain or occasionally from small branches on the surface. Other major sources of collateral blood supply, besides the external carotid to the eye, are the anterior, middle, and posterior cerebral anastomoses on the surface of the brain and the posterior and anterior inferior cerebellar arteries on the cerebellar

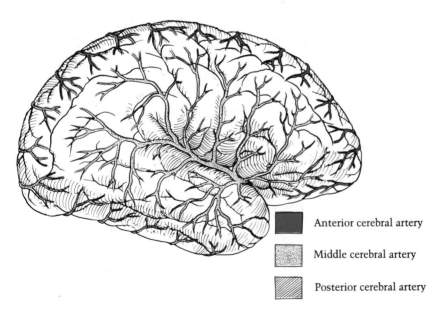

Anterior cerebral artery

Middle cerebral artery

Posterior cerebral artery

Figure 31–4
Cerebrovascular distribution.

surface, through which blood may bypass a vertebral artery occlusion. Most of the time, the anastomotic connections between the cortical branches of the major vessels are ineffective in preventing infarction.

Autoregulation

Although the brain accounts for only 2% of total body weight, it receives almost 15% of the cardiac output and uses almost 20% of the oxygen consumed by the body.[53] This substantial need for both blood and oxygen requires an intact and functioning cerebrovascular system. In the normal person, the brain maintains blood flow to meet these demands by automatically regulating the diameters of the arteries and arterioles, thus maintaining a very constant level of flow despite any changes in the systemic needs of the body. This mechanism is known as *perfusion autoregulation.* To maintain normal blood flow to the brain, the cerebral blood flow is dependent on a pressure gradient known as cerebral perfusion pressure (CPP). This gradient is calculated by taking the mean systemic arterial pressure (MAP) minus the ICP to give a pressure that is measured in millimeters of mercury. The normal range for CPP is 50 mm Hg to 100 mm Hg. In this range, an adequate blood supply to the brain will be provided. If the CPP should drop below 30 mm Hg, it is considered to be incompatible with life and results in neuron hypoxia and cell death. Normally, MAP is greater than the ICP; however, when the MAP equals the ICP, the CPP becomes zero and cerebral blood flow will terminate. This effect can occur with damage to the brain resulting in increased ICP. Other factors that affect cerebral blood flow are hypercapnia, hypoxia, blood viscosity, and temperature changes. For an in-depth discussion of cerebral blood flow, autoregulation, and increased ICP, see Chapter 30.

ETIOLOGY

At least 5% of the population may harbor ruptured and unruptured cerebral aneurysms. They are most prevalent in the 35-year to 60-year age group and are rarely seen in children, especially during the first decade of life. However, peripheral fusiform aneurysms and giant aneurysms occur with greater frequency in children than in adults. More women than men have aneurysms after the age of 40, especially on the internal carotid artery, although the reason remains unknown. Middle cerebral artery aneurysms are slightly more common in women, but men predominate below the age of 40 years. Anterior communicating artery aneurysms are more common in men. Multiple aneurysms occur in 15% to 30% of patients, and a few families in which more than one member has an aneurysm have been reported. In some of these families, the occurrence was suggestive of autosomal dominant inheritance, an inherited weakness of the vessel wall that may predispose these individuals to aneurysm formation.

By definition, *hypertensive hemorrhages* usually occur in patients with hypertension who are experiencing blood pressures grossly elevated in the range of 200/100 mm Hg. Age distribution extends from the third to the ninth decade, with the great majority occurring between 40 and 70 years of age. Sex distribution has varied from report to report and is generally insignificant.

With *arteriovenous malformations,* hemorrhage is the most frequent initial symptom. Fifty percent bleed before the age of 30 years, and 72% have bled by the age of 40 years. The possibility of bleeding does not appear to be directly related to size, site, age, or sex.

Factors predisposing a person *to ischemic cerebrovascular disease* all involve some compromise of the vascular system. These factors include aging, hypertension, atherosclerosis, cardiac disease (especially valvular or coronary artery disease and dysrhythmias such as atrial fibrillation), peripheral vascular disease, vasospasm of cerebral arteries, diabetes mellitus, polycythemia, clotting abnormalities, obesity, hyperlipidemia, smoking, history of oral contraceptive use, and compression of vertebral arteries when the head is turned.

Embolic insults are most often the result of heart disease. A thrombus within the heart breaks into fragments and is carried to the brain. Patients with atrial flutter are five times more likely to experience embolic stroke than those without flutter. Other less common causes of embolic infarction are fat- or tumor-cell emboli, septic emboli, exudate from subacute bacterial endocarditis, or emboli precipitated during cardiac or vascular surgery.

PATHOPHYSIOLOGY

Hemorrhagic Disease

The most common causes of hemorrhagic insult are ruptured cerebral aneurysm, hypertensive intracerebral hemorrhage, and ruptured arteriovenous malformation.

Ruptured Cerebral Aneurysms

A cerebral aneurysm is a round, saccular dilatation of the arterial wall that develops as a result of weakness of the wall. Most aneurysms are referred to as *saccular aneurysms,* and they have a stem and a neck (Figs. 31–5, 31–6, and 31–7). Many people refer to saccular aneurysms as *berry aneurysms.* *Fusiform aneurysms* appear as a puckering or ballooning of the blood vessel without a neck. *Giant aneurysms* have been defined as aneurysms larger than 2.5 cm in diameter.

The cause of aneurysms is uncertain, although many theories have been proposed. One explanation suggests that aneurysms are due to congenital defects in the media of the cerebral arteries. The wall of the aneurysm is thin and usually composed of intimal and subintimal connective tissue without any muscle or elastic tissue in the sac itself. Other theories propose that aneurysms represent vestigial remains of the embryonic circulatory system or result from arteriosclerotic changes in the blood vessels. These theories are still speculative, and research continues in an attempt to uncover an accurate explanation for the presence of cerebral aneurysms.

Trauma may result in the formation of a cerebral aneurysm. The wall of an artery may be weakened at the fracture line of a basilar skull fracture or by a careening missile such as a bullet. With each pulsation, the damaged arterial wall expands until clinical symptoms or bleeding occurs.

Eighty-five percent of all aneurysms develop on the anterior portion of the circle of Willis, arising from the internal carotid artery, the anterior and posterior communicating arteries, the middle cerebral artery, or the anterior cerebral artery. The most frequent site of occurrence is the juncture of the posterior communicating artery and the internal carotid artery (see Fig. 31–3). Fifteen percent arise within the vertebrobasilar system.

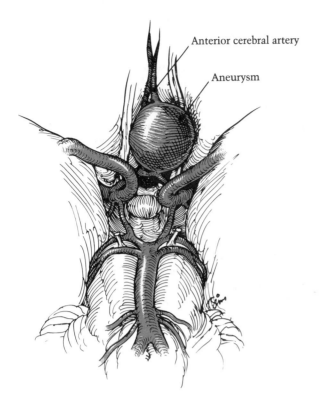

Anterior cerebral artery

Aneurysm

Figure 31-5
Saccular aneurysm arising from the anterior communicating artery.

Most aneurysms occur at the point of bifurcation of arterial vessels, because a potential weakness exists when two arteries form a junction. Occasionally, fusiform aneurysms occur at sites other than arterial forks and are usually found in the posterior circulation on a severely atherosclerotic artery.

Hemorrhage from the bleeding aneurysm may occur into the subarachnoid space, into the cerebral substance, or into both areas. Bleeding into the subarachnoid space is referred to as *subarachnoid hemorrhage* (SAH). Bleeding into the cerebral substance results in an *intracerebral hematoma*.

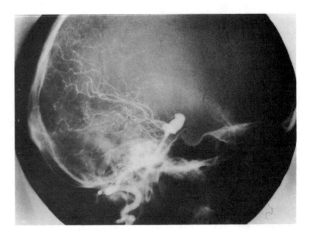

Figure 31-7
Lateral view of an aneurysm depicted on angiography.

Vasospasm

Cerebral vasospasm, prolonged contraction of a blood vessel, is the most serious complication for patients with SAH after aneurysm rupture. It most frequently occurs 7 to 10 days after the initial SAH and can have devastating consequences for the patient's prognosis. Vasospasm alters cerebral blood flow and cerebral circulation by producing a focal constriction along one or more of the cerebral arteries or within the branches of the circle of Willis. The diagnosis and severity of vasospasm may be demonstrated by angiography and the patient's clinical symptoms (Figs. 31–8 and 31–9). The degree of alteration in cerebral circulation will be manifested by focal or diffuse neurologic changes. Regional blood flow alterations will result in focal neurologic deficits, such as hemiplegia or aphasia. Alterations in general or diffuse blood flow will be manifested in the patient's level of consciousness.

The underlying mechanism of vasospasm has not been determined, although there are several theories. The most widely accepted theory is that certain vasoconstrictive agents (serotonin, prostaglandins, and catecholamines) are released from

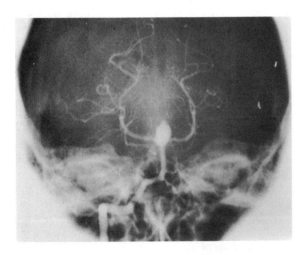

Figure 31-6
Anteroposterior view of an aneurysm depicted on angiography.

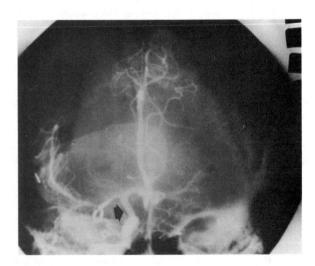

Figure 31-8
Angiogram of clipped middle cerebral artery aneurysm depicting normal cerebral blood flow.

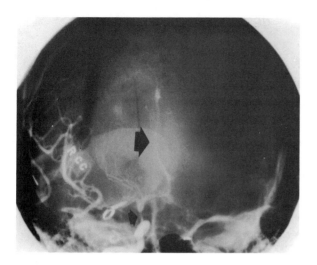

Figure 31-9

Same as Figure 31–8 of clipped middle cerebral artery aneurysm depicting vasospasm (*small arrow*) and decreased blood flow distally (*large arrow*).

the breakdown of blood products in the subarachnoid space, producing a reflex spasm in the cerebral arteries.

Vasospasm was originally thought to be a biphasic event, with the initial episode occurring immediately after rupture of the aneurysm in an attempt to control bleeding. However, current research indicates that a sudden increase in ICP, not arterial constriction, causes a tamponade effect that reduces cerebral blood flow and promotes the formation of a platelet plug to inhibit bleeding. The second phase of this event occurs 4 to 14 days after rupture of the aneurysm and is now considered true vasospasm. This episode is considered to be due to the spasm of arteries adjacent to the site of aneurysmal hemorrhage.[19] Vasospasm that occurs during this phase produces clinical symptoms and threatens the patient's neurologic recovery. There appears to be a direct correlation between the amount of blood in the subarachnoid space as evidenced by CT scan and the incidence and severity of vasospasm.[35]

When chronic vasospasm persists, a series of severely threatening events occurs. One of these is the disturbance in or loss of autoregulation. Its loss causes cerebral blood flow to follow mean arterial blood pressure. Fluctuations in blood pressure may rapidly lead to cerebral ischemia and infarction as cerebral circulation is further compromised. Cerebral acidosis ensues, which alters cerebral microcirculation. This alteration produces vasogenic edema and intracranial hypertension, which raise ICP. If the process continues, the patient usually succumbs to the syndrome with areas of massive infarction and ischemia. The mortality rate from vasospasm after SAH may be as high as 25%.[42] Therefore, much of the preoperative and postoperative treatment of patients who have had a SAH secondary to a ruptured aneurysm is directed toward combating vasospasm. A method of preventing vasospasm from occurring would be the ideal treatment for these patients; however, such a method does not exist at the present time. Drug studies are being conducted currently to determine the effectiveness of calcium-channel blockers such as nimodipine and nicardipine in treating vasospasm. These studies are based on the theory that smooth muscle contraction is a calcium-dependent phenomenon.[19]

A recent development in predicting the onset of vasospasm is transcranial Doppler ultrasound. The lumen of the cerebral vessel will narrow, resulting in an increase in the velocity of blood flow in an attempt to deliver an adequate volume of blood to the cerebral tissues. This technique is still under investigation, but studies show its promise in identifying spasm of certain cerebral vessels.[19]

Rebleeding

Another major cause of morbidity and mortality after SAH is rebleeding. Traditionally, it was thought that the peak time of rebleeding is at the end of the first week after aneurysm rupture. However, data from the Cooperative Aneurysm Study[25] suggest that rebleeding may be maximal within the first 24 hours after SAH and that there is no late peak of rebleeding at the end of the first and the beginning of the second week after the insult.

Some institutions continue to use aminocaproic acid to prevent rebleeding from cerebral aneurysms. However, because inhibiting clot breakdown may actually promote vasospasm,[35] the use of antifibrinolytics is controversial, and the only proven effective preventive measure for rebleeding is surgical intervention.

Hydrocephalus

A third complication after a SAH is hydrocephalus. It results from blockage or malabsorption of cerebrospinal fluid from the ventricles of the brain. Diagnosis is usually confirmed by CT scan, which reveals increased ventricular size with darkened areas due to decreased absorption of cerebrospinal fluid. Treatment of hydrocephalus may consist of temporary manual drainage by ventriculostomy or lumbar drain. Permanent treatment consists of insertion of a ventriculoperitoneal shunt.

Hypertensive Hemorrhages

Hypertension causes continued pressure on the cerebral artery, which results in rupture of the vessel and bleeding into the brain tissue (Fig. 31–10). Initially, bleeding does not occur into the subarachnoid space; however, as the clot enlarges from

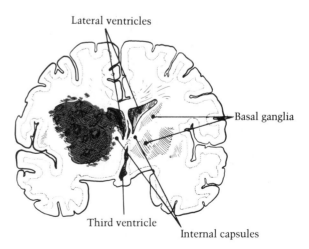

Figure 31-10

Hemorrhagic insult with bleeding into lateral ventricle.

continued bleeding, there is seepage into the ventricular system in approximately 90% of patients. Normally, a clot would form at the rupture site and seal off the vessel; however, with the blood pressure so high, the force behind the clot is too great to allow the ruptured vessel to be sealed. The clot displaces and compresses the adjacent cerebral tissue, resulting in increased ICP. A major bleeding episode can cause midline displacement, brain stem herniation, and death.

Ruptured Arteriovenous Malformation

An arteriovenous malformation (AVM) is composed of a tangled array of dilated vessels that forms an abnormal communication network between the arterial and venous systems (Figs. 31–11, 31–12, and 31–13). The arterial blood is shunted directly into the venous system without the usual connecting capillary network. The venous vessels of the AVM form huge, dilated, pulsating channels that carry away the oxygenated arterial blood. If only one vein is responsible for drainage of the malformation, the vessels can develop into a huge aneurysmal sac. Arteriovenous malformations usually become symptomatic between the ages of 10 and 30 years.

ISCHEMIC DISEASE

Ischemic insults are usually classified according to their etiologic basis and are identified as thrombotic or embolic.

Thrombotic Insults

Thrombotic insults are the most common type of cerebral ischemic injury. It is associated with atherosclerosis, which causes the artery lumen to narrow. The most common site for atheromatous plaque build-up in the extracranial arteries is the bifurcation where the common carotid artery divides into its external and internal branches. The origin of the vertebral arteries is also a common site. In the intracranial arterial system, the most common site of atherosclerosis is the middle cerebral artery. More than half of all strokes resulting in hemispheric symptoms are probably the direct result of atherosclerosis in the internal carotid artery. Plaque formation begins

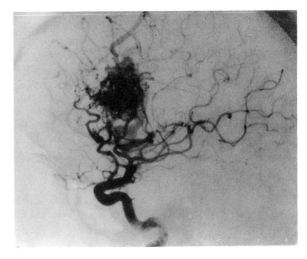

Figure 31–12
Lateral view of an average-sized arteriovenous malformation depicted on angiography.

with the accumulation of fat under the intimal lining of the arterial wall, especially at bifurcations, which is then covered with fibrous tissue. As the plaque enlarges, it reduces blood flow and may eventually cause occlusion. Complete occlusion may take hours to occur. Sixty percent of all complete occlusions occur during sleep.

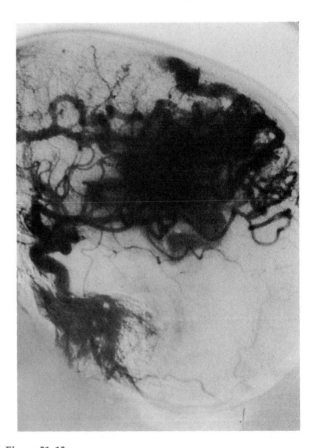

Figure 31–13
Lateral view of a massive arteriovenous malformation depicted on angiography.

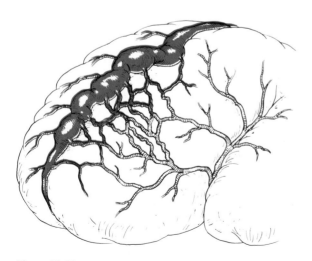

Figure 31–11
Cortical presentation of an arteriovenous malformation.

An ulcerated plaque forms when growth of the lesion disrupts the intimal lining, exposing the rough surface of media. Debris or platelet thrombi may lodge and embolize on the roughened surface, causing either an ischemic attack or a completed stroke. Antiplatelet drugs such as aspirin or dipyridamole help prevent thrombi from forming.

Embolic Insults

Embolic infarcts develop rapidly within seconds to minutes with no warning signs. Emboli arising from the heart most often enter the cerebral circulation by way of the carotid arteries. Large emboli can plug the internal carotid artery, resulting in severe hemiplegia. Smaller emboli are more common and may obstruct a branch of the middle cerebral artery, resulting in monoplegia or aphasia.

As an embolus passes through a vessel, it may produce temporary dysfunction. A large embolus may lodge in an area for a few hours, fragment into pieces, and move. When the obstruction breaks down, symptoms will probably be reversed. These small fragments will eventually obstruct a smaller vessel, causing symptoms of neurologic deficit appropriate to that area of the brain.

If the underlying cause of the embolic infarct is not treated aggressively, many patients will have subsequent episodes of stroke.

NURSING PROCESS

ASSESSMENT

The outcome of the patient who has cerebrovascular disease is determined primarily by the severity of the initial insult. However, subsequent assessment and management by the health care team may help improve the final outcome. It is of great importance to obtain a complete history from the patient or family and to establish a thorough baseline examination. This assessment will form a solid foundation on which to evaluate changes in neurologic condition as well as highlight systems that are compromised by other disease processes, such as chronic obstructive lung disease, diabetes mellitus, and cardiovascular and thyroid disease.

Initially, the patient will be assessed for an adequate airway and stable vital signs. Then a thorough neurologic examination should be performed (see Chap. 29). The patient's level of consciousness and respiratory pattern must be assessed and followed. An examination of the eyes consists of noting pupillary size and reactivity and extraocular eye movements. Motor signs will reveal the extent and area of the neurologic dysfunction. Contralateral paresis or plegia of the extremities due to the motor neurons decussating in the brain stem–spinal cord region will be seen (Fig. 31–14). Facial movement and cranial nerve function must also be evaluated for deficits.

Psychologic Aspects

Psychologic aspects are an important part of the initial assessment, because the information will assist understanding of the patient as a whole person in a complex unit of interpersonal relationships. In all types of cerebrovascular disease, the patient and family will experience a drastic disruption of life-style. During the patient's hospitalization, the family must

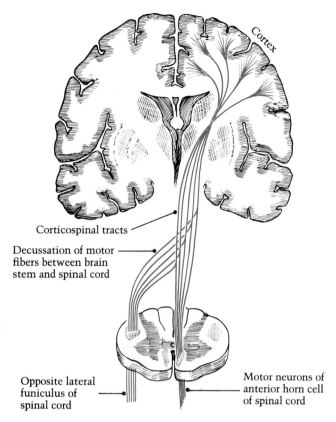

Figure 31–14
Motor neuron pathways.

make adjustments to the temporary loss of their family member. They may also feel a degree of frustration as the patient transfers some of his dependency onto the nursing staff.

During this time, patients experience much frustration over their difficulty or inability to perform their usual activities of daily living. They must depend on others to assist with or do for them activities that in the past they took for granted. It is up to the nurse to set realistic goals for rehabilitation, a process that begins on the first day of hospitalization. The patient and family must be given the opportunity to discuss their feelings of anxiety, fear, and anger about the patient's hospitalization and possible surgery.

The relationship between the nurse in the critical care unit and the patient is a special one. The patient's recovery depends on the nurse in more ways than one, and the nurse is also in a position to assist the family through a very difficult period. At times it will be necessary for the nurse to aid the family in accepting the impending death of their loved one. The nurse must be aware of the patient's prognosis as well as what has been communicated to the family by other members of the health care team in order to be as realistic as possible and to keep from offering them any false hope. The main role of the nurse in interacting with the family during this time is to support them and allow them to work through the grieving process.

Specific Conditions
Cerebral Aneurysms

Clinical signs and symptoms arising from a cerebral aneurysm may be divided into two categories: before rupture or leak and after rupture or leak. *Rupture* means that there is a forcible tearing apart or a major break in the aneurysmal sac. The term *leaking* is used to mean a weeping or sweating of blood from a very thin aneurysmal sac without actual rupture.

Before Rupture or Leak.   Many patients are completely asymptomatic until the time of bleeding, whereas other patients may complain of generalized headaches with subsequent lethargy, neck pain, and localization of headache. Warning signs or symptoms are noted in about 48% to 60% of patients. In women, the incidence of these warning signs is higher than in men, but declines rapidly with advancing age.

Okawara[37] classified these signs and symptoms into three categories: those due to expansion of the aneurysm and adjacent artery (visual-field defects, extraocular muscle palsy, eye pain, face pain, and localized head pain); those due to minor rupture (generalized headache, nausea, neck and back pain, lethargy, and photophobia); and those due to an ischemic lesion, vascular spasm, occlusion, or embolism (motor or sensory impairment, visual hallucinations, loss of balance, dizziness, and so on). The most frequent warning symptoms in all patients are headache and dizziness, both nonspecific.

After Rupture or Leak.   At the time of bleeding, the patient experiences a violent headache that is commonly described as "explosive" in nature. Other signs and symptoms include a decreased level of consciousness, deficit of the cranial nerves (especially the oculomotor), visual disturbances, deficit of the voluntary muscles resulting in hemiparesis or hemiplegia, and possible vomiting. All these signs and symptoms are related to increased ICP. If the blood from the bleeding aneurysm has come into contact with the meninges, as in SAH, symptoms include stiff neck, positive Kernig's and Brudzinski's signs, neck pain, photophobia, blurred vision, irritability and restlessness, and possible elevation in temperature. The presence and severity of symptoms depend on the amount, location, and extent of the bleeding.

Classification of Subarachnoid Hemorrhage.   Subarachnoid hemorrhages are classified according to the extent of the neurologic deficit exhibited by the patient. The extent of the neurologic deficit coincides with the severity of the hemorrhage and helps predict the ultimate patient outcome. Grades I and II are considered "good" grade hemorrhages and have the highest percentage of favorable patient outcome. Grade III

subarachnoid hemorrhages are considered borderline, and their outcome is more difficult to predict. Grade IV/V hemorrhages usually indicate an outcome of severe neurologic impairment or death. The two most commonly used grading systems for SAH are described in Table 31–1.

Hypertensive Hemorrhages

The symptoms experienced by patients with hypertensive hemorrhagic insults include some or all of the following: severe headache, nuchal rigidity, vomiting, focal seizures, and hemiplegia.

Arteriovenous Malformations

There are three major assessment parameters involved in the diagnosis of AVM: headache, bruit, and seizure. Headache is a common complaint of patients with AVM, but it is also common in many other avascular conditions. A bruit is auscultated in 2% to 10% of these patients. The possibility of auscultating one depends on the size and location of the AVM and the thickness of the skull; a bruit is more likely to be heard in a child because the skull is thinner. Seizures are also an important indication of AVM; they may initially be partial but often become generalized.

Other presenting symptoms of AVM include transient episodes of syncope, fainting, dizziness, motor weakness, sensory deficits or tingling, aphasia, dysarthria, visual deficits (usually hemianopsia), and mental confusion. Some patients may develop dementia or intellectual impairment as a result of chronic ischemia of the frontal lobes.

Ischemic Insults

Signs associated with thrombosis or embolism in the branches fed by the internal carotid artery are usually *hemispheric*. Inadequate perfusion of the brain's right lobes due to problems in the right internal carotid artery results in sensory-motor deficits on the body's left side. Upper extremity signs occur more commonly than lower extremity signs because the upper extremities are controlled by the opposite branches of the middle cerebral artery. The middle cerebral artery has the potential for adequate collateral circulation. The lower extremities are controlled by the opposite branches of the anterior cerebral

Table 31–1
Patient Symptomatology in Subarachnoid Hemorrhage

CLASSIFICATION	GRADE	DESCRIPTION
Hunt-Hess	1	Asymptomatic, minor headache, mild meningeal signs
	2	Normal consciousness level, headache, meningeal signs, possible cranial nerve palsy
	3	Depressed consciousness level, mild neurologic deficit
	4	Depressed consciousness level, moderate to severe neurologic deficit
	5	Deep coma—brain-stem reflexes
Botterell	1	Normal consciousness level, possible meningeal signs
	2	Depressed consciousness level, neurologic deficit
	3	Depressed consciousness level, hemispheric neurologic deficit, possible intracranial hematoma
	4	Depressed consciousness level, major neurologic deficit with intracranial hematoma

(Samson D. S., *et al.* A Comparison of the Results of "Early" vs. "Late" Aneurysm Surgery in the Good Grade Patient. In R. H. Wilkins (ed). *Cerebral Spasm*. Baltimore: Williams & Wilkins, 1980; with permission.)

artery. Occlusion of this artery can produce dementia, confusion, or coma, contralateral hemiplegia, and cortical sensory loss. The one exception to the contralateral principle is the eye. Eye symptoms occur on the same, or ipsilateral, side.

The posterior cerebral artery perfuses the midbrain and feeds the posterior temporal and occipital lobes. Decreased blood flow in one of these branches may result in visual loss, contralateral flaccid hemiparesis, loss of deep sensation, burning pain, and ataxia or tremors.

Symptoms from vertebrobasilar branches are not easily evaluated. These nonhemispheric events are usually caused by decreased cerebral perfusion from stenosis or occlusion rather than embolization. Generalized nonhemispheric symptoms consist of syncope, "drop attacks," visual changes, unsteady gait, vertigo, and headaches.

Ischemic insults may be further classified according to developmental process into transient ischemic attack, reversible ischemic neurologic deficit, stroke in evolution, or completed stroke.

Transient Ischemic Attack. The symptoms of transient ischemic attack (TIA) come on suddenly and usually last from a few seconds to minutes, but not longer than 24 hours. Transient ischemic attacks are reversible; they repeat themselves and usually affect the same part of the body (because the same cerebral vessel is involved each time). Transient ischemic attacks may occur days to months apart. They do not usually cause loss of consciousness, and they may subside spontaneously or progress to a completed stroke. The probability of a completed stroke following a TIA is 25% to 35%. It is the number-one factor in predicting completed stroke.

Reversible Ischemic Neurologic Deficit. Reversible ischemic neurologic deficits present similarly to TIAs, but their symptoms last for a few days to a week. The patient also has a complete or nearly complete recovery.

Stroke in Evolution. Strokes in evolution must be seen to be diagnosed; therefore, they are seldom seen because the deficit has usually become fixed by the time of the initial examination. These patients experience a progressive neurologic deficit, and the principal indicator of its progression is usually hemiparesis.

Completed Stroke. Completed stroke represents a neurologic deficit that is stable over a period of weeks. The clinical consequences of ischemia are complete; infarction (irreversible brain cell damage or cell death) has followed. Varying degrees of functional recovery through retraining other parts of the brain to take over may come about over weeks to months. Although the patient can regain many former capabilities, completed stroke rarely allows total recovery.

Diagnostic Tests

Various tests and procedures are used to differentiate between hemorrhagic and ischemic injury. Baseline laboratory work should be obtained, including cerebrospinal fluid values, electrolytes, blood counts, and clotting studies, to monitor changes and to aid in managing any fluid and electrolyte imbalances that may occur related to the initial insult and its medical or surgical management.

Noninvasive Procedures

Computed Axial Tomography. The CT scanner utilizes an x-ray beam in conjunction with a computer to provide extremely accurate images of thin cross sections of the brain and skull. The CT scan will demonstrate areas of subdural and epidural hematoma, intracerebral hematoma, abscesses, cysts, infarctions, contusions, hydrocephalus, edema, and tumors. The CT scan using contrast dye will identify aneurysms and AVMs.

Brain Scan. During the brain scan, a small amount of radioisotope is administered to the patient to measure tissue uptake of the isotope. The brain scan can identify only the presence of a space-occupying intracranial lesion; it cannot differentiate between types of lesions. The CT scan has all but replaced this test in recent years.

Nuclear Magnetic Resonance. Refer to Chapter 29, page 551, for details.

Blood Flow Studies. To evaluate total or regional cerebral blood flow to determine areas of normal, increased, or decreased blood supply, cerebral blood flow studies are performed. Various methods of introducing a radioactive tracer into the patient are used, including inhalation or intravenous administration. The tracer immediately saturates the cerebral tissue. The tracer removal rate from the cerebral tissue will be proportioned to the rate of blood flow. A tracer detector placed over the head will record the radioactivity of the tracer and will determine the regional tracer clearance. This calculation will indicate regional blood flow rates. The average value is 50 ml/100 g of cerebral tissue per minute of observation.

Blood flow studies aid in evaluating areas of ischemia and infarct, the presence and degree of vasospasm and edema, and the differential diagnosis between communicating and noncommunicating hydrocephalus. Another use for blood flow studies is to determine the pathogenesis and possible treatment of dementia.

Invasive Procedures

Lumbar Puncture. The lumbar puncture is used to ascertain the presence of blood in the cerebrospinal fluid. In addition, the cerebral fluid pressure may be measured to check for elevation. Analysis of the cerebrospinal fluid in a person who has had an SAH usually demonstrates an increased blood cell count and a glucose level that is normal or slightly decreased. Lumbar punctures should be performed only when there is no question of the ICP being elevated, because herniation may result.

Cerebral Arteriogram. An arteriogram of cerebral vessels is the most valuable tool in identifying vascular abnormalities. Angiography can provide a multitude of information. It can identify cerebral aneurysms, their size and number, the configuration of the neck of the aneurysm, evidence of surrounding spasm, relation to the surrounding arteries, and a possible association with other malformations (arteriovenous angiomas or tumors). Angiography can also provide an assessment of the permeability of the circle of Willis and visualize patency, narrowing or stenosis, thrombosis, and occlusions of vessels.

Approximately 2% of the population will develop some complications after angiography, and one source quotes the figure as high as 10%.[22] The following complications are those most commonly seen:

- Hematoma formation at the catheter insertion site
- Sensitivity to iodine resulting in allergic rash, bronchospasm, and cardiovascular or respiratory failure
- Further damage to an already diseased renal system due to delayed excretion of the contrast medium
- Development or aggravation of central nervous system signs (Hemiplegia or dysphasia present before the study may temporarily increase. Fragments set free as emboli from needling through an atheromatous plaque may enter the cerebral circulation. Reflex spasm in cerebral vessels or occlusion of the carotid artery may result from injection into the carotid sheath or subintimal lining. Systemic arterial hypotension induced by anesthesia or by the injection of contrast medium may aggravate spasm. If there is already occlusion of the opposite carotid artery or of either of the vertebral arteries, any of the accidents may result in an inadequate cerebral blood supply.)

- Patients already critically compressed may suffer increased ICP due to the action of the contrast medium or saline injected between films on abnormal vessels with an altered blood-brain barrier
- Seizures may occur on injection of the contrast medium
- Nausea may occur after the first contrast injection and rarely after subsequent ones
- Syncope can occur from the needle being in the carotid sinus
- Occlusion of the femoral artery may result
- Carotid aneurysms and carotid-jugular (arteriovenous) fistulas are rare late developments. The risk of complications developing, the quality of films produced, and the amount of discomfort suffered by the patient under local anesthesia depend largely on the skill of the operator and team.[22]

NURSING DIAGNOSES, PATIENT OUTCOMES, AND PLAN

The preceding material on anatomy, physiology, nursing assessment, and diagnostic tests guides the nurse in establishing nursing diagnoses, patient outcomes, and plan for the patient with cerebrovascular disease.

NURSING CARE PLAN SUMMARY   *Patient With Cerebrovascular Disease*

NURSING DIAGNOSIS

1. High risk for further injury related to rebleeding and additional episodes of cerebrovascular disease (exchanging pattern)

Patient Outcome	Nursing Orders

The patient should experience absence or resolution of rebleeding hemorrhagic or ischemic insult.	1. Establish neurologic baseline and vital signs on admission.
	  A. Monitor neurologic status and vital signs as ordered and as needed, especially for changes in the following:
	    (1) Level of consciousness
	    (2) Motor and sensory functioning
	    (3) Behavior or personality
	    (4) Pupil equality, size, and reaction; extraocular movements; ptosis
	    (5) Visual abilities, including acuity, diplopia, nystagmus, and photophobia
	    (6) Presence and extent of headache, nausea or vomiting, and nuchal rigidity
	    (7) Communication abilities
	    (8) Cranial nerve functioning
	    (9) Presence or worsening of pronator drift. Check every 4 hours, and notify physician as indicated.
	  B. Follow the unit policy and orders regarding the minimization of external stimuli. These may include the following:
	    (1) A single, quiet, dark room
	    (2) Absolute bed rest
	    (3) Feeding, turning, and bathing of the patient
	    (4) Limitation of visitors to the immediate family; a certain number for a limited time period
	    (5) Minimization of patient's verbalization
	    (6) The head of the bed elevated at the degree specified (usually 15° to 30°)

(continued)

NURSING CARE PLAN SUMMARY   Patient With Cerebrovascular Disease   Continued

Patient Outcome	*Nursing Orders*
	(7) Side rails in the up position
	(8) No smoking by the patient or in the patient's room
	(9) Restriction or no use of the telephone, television, or radio
	(10) Restriction of coffee or tea and very hot or cold foods
	(11) No rectal temperatures or treatments
	C. Notify the physician immediately of any change in neurologic status or vital signs.

NURSING DIAGNOSIS

2. *High risk for altered cerebral function (ICP) related to physiologic changes, such as cerebral edema from vasospasm, ischemic infarct, rebleeding, hematoma formation, and hydrocephalus (exchanging pattern)*

Patient Outcome	*Nursing Orders*
The patient will demonstrate an absence or resolution of increased ICP.	1. Monitor neurologic signs every hour (or more frequently), and notify the physician of changes (see Nursing Diagnosis 1 for specifics).
	A. Monitor vital signs for widened pulse pressure and decreased heart rate (Cushing's response), and notify the physician if present.
	B. Monitor respirations for changes in pattern and effectiveness of gas exchange.
	C. Monitor the temperature for an increase; treat as ordered with hypothermia and antipyretics to keep the temperature lower than 38.5°C rectally.
	D. Maintain strict bed rest, keeping the head of the bed elevated 30° with proper head alignment to promote venous return.
	E. Monitor ICP by the intracranial device as placed by the physician. If there is a ventriculostomy, vent to keep the ICP less than 20 mm Hg as ordered by the physician.
	F. Administer medications as ordered. Monitor serum electrolytes and urine output with the administration of intravenous diuretics.
	G. Avoid maneuvers that increase ICP (*i.e.,* prolonged suctioning, Valsalva maneuver, straining, and coughing).

NURSING DIAGNOSIS

3. *High risk for or presence of impaired physical mobility related to cerebral insult and alterations in life-style (moving pattern)*

Patient Outcome	*Nursing Orders*
The patient will achieve maximum physical mobility, will be free of the complications of immobility, will achieve maximal neurologic functioning, and will become independent in activities of daily living within his capabilities.	1. Encourage patient to participate as able and do the following:
	A. Assess for the degree of physical deficit, and evaluate limitations in the activities of daily living. Initiate referrals for physical and occupational therapy as necessary.
	B. Allow the patient to participate in the activities of daily living as much as allowed by the physician, and assist as needed.
	C. Turn the patient on bed rest at least every 2 hours, inspect pressure points, give skin care with lotion, and position in correct body alignment with pillows.
	D. Ensure that the patient has some type of pressure mattress (*i.e.,* alternating air mattress, egg-crate mattress, or sheep skin on bed).

(continued)

NURSING CARE PLAN SUMMARY *Patient With Cerebrovascular Disease*   *Continued*

Patient Outcome	*Nursing Orders*
	E. Perform the passive range-of-motion exercises at least every 8 hours and as needed.
	F. Promote the maximum respiratory function (see Nursing Diagnosis 4).
	G. Place antiembolism stockings on the patient's legs and assess for signs of venous thrombosis. The stockings should be thigh-high.
	H. Prevent problems of bowel and bladder elimination.

NURSING DIAGNOSIS

4. *Impaired gas exchange related to decreased level of consciousness and/or immobility (exchanging pattern)*

Patient Outcome	*Nursing Orders*
The patient will maintain an adequate gas exchange and airway clearance and will not develop pulmonary complications.	1. Monitor gas exchange.
	A. Maintain the patent airway by using mechanical devices as needed. Insert an oral airway as indicated.
	B. Check the ventilator settings with the physician's order, and check that alarms are functioning.
	C. Assess pulmonary secretions for amount, consistency, and odor.
	D. Turn the patient every 2 hours, and suction every 1 to 2 hours and as needed.
	E. Ensure that respiratory treatments and chest radiographs are done as ordered. Avoid the head-down position in all patients and the head-flat position in patients with uncontrollable ICP.
	F. Auscultate breath sounds before and after suctioning and treatments to document their effectiveness.
	G. Observe and report signs of hypoxia (restlessness, airway obstruction, and cyanosis).
	H. Assess skin color, nail beds, and mucous membranes for cyanosis.
	I. Assess for the presence and strength of gag, cough, and swallow reflexes.
	J. Encourage all cooperative patients to cough and deep breathe unless contraindicated by the physician's orders.
	K. Provide for additional oxygen and humidification as indicated and ordered by the physician.
	L. Assist with intubation as necessary.
	M. Give mouth care every shift and every 4 to 6 hours in intubated patients to prevent drying of mucous membranes.
	N. Keep intubated patients restrained to prevent accidental extubation.
	O. Administer medications as ordered to ensure the patient's compliance with mechanical ventilation.

NURSING DIAGNOSIS

5. *High risk for altered fluid and electrolyte balance related to cerebrovascular insults (exchanging pattern)*

Patient Outcome	*Nursing Orders*
The patient should maintain fluid and electrolyte balance within normal limits.	1. Administer intravenous fluids as ordered (D5W is not a fluid of choice because it contributes to brain swelling).
	2. Keep accurate intake records of intravenous lines, tube feedings, and fluids by mouth every 1 to 2 hours until the fluid status is stable.

(continued)

NURSING CARE PLAN SUMMARY   *Patient With Cerebrovascular Disease*   *Continued*

Patient Outcome	*Nursing Orders*
	3. Keep accurate output records of urine, gastric drainage, and other losses that can be measured.
	4. Weigh the patient daily.
	5. Monitor for signs of dehydration and overhydration at least every 8 hours.
	6. Monitor serum and urine electrolytes and osmolality every 8 to 12 hours.
	7. Measure urine specific gravity every 4 to 8 hours if ordered.
	8. Check hemoglobin and hematocrit daily for hemoconcentration or dilution.
	9. Monitor for insensible losses, including respiratory, excessive diaphoresis, emesis, and diarrhea.
	10. Administer medications as ordered to correct electrolytes.
	11. If the patient is receiving steroids, monitor urine glucose and acetone levels at least every 6 hours or as ordered.
	12. If the urine output is greater than 200 cc for 2 consecutive hours or less than 30 cc for 2 consecutive hours, notify the physician.
	13. Notify the physician of any fluid or electrolyte imbalances.

NURSING DIAGNOSIS

6. *High risk for gastrointestinal bleeding related to stress or steroid administration (exchanging pattern)*

Patient Outcome	*Nursing Orders*
The patient should have no or a resolution of gastric ulceration or bleeding.	1. Establish if bleeding is present.
	A. Monitor the hemoglobin and hematocrit for changes indicative of bleeding.
	B. Check for occult blood from nasogastric aspirate and stool every shift on all unresponsive patients and those on steroids.
	C. Check gastric pH every 2 to 4 hours on patients with nasogastric tubes, and keep the pH greater than 5.0 with antacids.
	D. Administer antacids along with steroids to help minimize gastric acidity.
	E. Monitor for signs of gastrointestinal bleeding, including abdominal tenderness, distention, hypotension, and sudden tachycardia.
	F. Notify the physician of any occult or frank blood from nasogastric aspirate or stool.

NURSING DIAGNOSIS

7. *High risk for impaired neurologic function (seizures) related to increased ICP (exchanging pattern)*

Patient Outcome	*Nursing Orders*
The patient should have no or control of seizures and be free of injury to self after seizures.	1. Provide care to avoid seizures.
	A. Avoid precipitating factors, such as fever, hypoxia, water intoxication, and electrolyte imbalances.
	B. Institute seizure precautions if indicated, such as padded side rails that are up at all times, bed in lowest position, padded tongue blade and oral airway at bedside, and emergency equipment and medications readily available.
	C. Administer anticonvulsive medications as ordered, and monitor their levels in the blood.

(continued)

NURSING CARE PLAN SUMMARY   *Patient With Cerebrovascular Disease*   *Continued*

Patient Outcome	*Nursing Orders*
	D. If a seizure occurs, monitor and record its activity and notify the physician. E. Take all temperatures rectally until seizures are controlled and the patient is seizure-free for at least 5 to 6 days.

NURSING DIAGNOSIS

8. *High risk for systemic infection related to invasive procedures or meningitis (exchanging pattern)*

Patient Outcome	*Nursing Orders*
The patient will be free of infection during the course of the illness.	1. Assess for signs of infection A. Monitor temperature every 4 hours and as needed by any elevation. B. Obtain blood, sputum, urine, and cerebrospinal fluid cultures as ordered. C. Evaluate intravenous sites every 4 to 8 hours for signs of redness, tenderness, and phlebitis. Discontinue intravenous lines and start new sites as indicated. D. Observe the patient for sources of infection, including pulmonary and urinary. E. Monitor white blood cell counts for elevation (may be falsely high if the patient is on steroids). F. Ensure strict sterile technique for such procedures as catheterization, endotracheal tube/tracheostomy tube suctioning, and dressing changes on central lines and on arterial lines. G. Ensure strict sterile technique when assisting with such procedures as ventriculostomy placement, Swan-Ganz and central line placement, and other invasive line insertions. H. Administer antibiotics as ordered.

NURSING DIAGNOSIS

9. *Altered nutrition: less than body requirements related to catabolic response to injury (exchanging pattern)*

Patient Outcome	*Nursing Orders*
The patient will attain a positive caloric balance and will maintain a baseline weight.	1. Initiate nutritional support as soon as the patient's condition is stable and fluid limitations are no longer in effect. A. Initiate oral feeding (tube feedings if the patient is not awake) as soon as possible. B. Assess for tolerance to tube feedings by checking for residuals, and hold feedings if greater than 150 cc of aspirate is obtained. C. Keep the head of the bed elevated and turn feedings off (if on continuous feeding infusion) for any procedure that requires the head of the bed to be lowered to prevent aspiration. D. If the patient does not tolerate oral or tube feedings, notify the physician and assist the physician with central line placement for parenteral feedings. E. Monitor for constipation or diarrhea after feedings have been initiated. F. Supplement the diet with high-calorie foods if the patient's appetite is poor. G. Ask the family or patient for a list of food likes and dislikes to help stimulate appetite. H. Encourage the family to bring in favorite foods once or twice a week.

(continued)

NURSING CARE PLAN SUMMARY   Patient With Cerebrovascular Disease   Continued

NURSING DIAGNOSIS

10. *Ineffective patient or family coping related to deficit and possible alterations in life-style (choosing pattern)*

Patient Outcome	*Nursing Orders*
The patient or family will verbalize acceptance of the situation at this time, as well as realistic expectations of the patient's ability to function independently.	See Nursing Diagnosis: Ineffective Patient Coping and Ineffective Family Coping, page 112.

IMPLEMENTATION AND EVALUATION

The course of a patient suffering from cerebrovascular disease is highly variable. It is important that the team members collaborate and have a unified approach to the patient's care. The physician as well as other members of the health team must know what the nursing plan of care is for each patient. It will be the responsibility of the nursing staff to coordinate the patient information (medical and surgical intervention, laboratory results, and procedure outcomes) and communicate the plan of care. Continual evaluation and reassessment of patients for complications or changes in their condition should also be performed. This evaluation and reassessment will be reflected by updates in the nursing orders and documentation in the patient record. In order to achieve maximum rehabilitation, patient and family teaching should also be incorporated and evaluated on a continuing basis.

Medical and Surgical Implementation

Therapy for all types of cerebrovascular disease consists of multisystem stabilization and support. The appropriate amounts of fluid, electrolytes, and nutrients must be administered to the patient, and proper elimination of body wastes must be maintained. Adequate care must be provided for the skin and lungs, and fever must be controlled. Medications are administered for headache, restlessness, hypertension or hypotension, and seizure control. Control of ICP will also be of major importance.

Hemorrhagic Disease

Cerebral Aneurysms

The preferred treatment for a cerebral aneurysm is surgical intervention to prevent additional hemorrhage and death. The surgeon clips the aneurysm with a special clip, wraps the aneurysm with fine muslin gauze, or glues it; the decision is made on the basis of the size, location, and shape of the aneurysm. There is continued controversy as to the optimal time for surgery. Some surgeons recommend a wait of 1 to 2 weeks after the bleed to allow the patient's neurologic status to improve and cerebral edema and vasospasm to be controlled.

However, this creates a complex situation, for it is within the first 2 weeks that the chances are greatest for both rebleeding and vasospasm to occur; the medical treatment for these two complications is diametrically opposed. To decrease the chances of rebleeding, medical care consists of keeping the blood pressure in the lower end of normal by sedation, fluid restrictions, and special drips, such as sodium nitroprusside or nitroglycerin. Antifibrolytic therapy is also used in some institutions. Aminocaproic acid (Amicar) delays the lysis of the clot present in and around the aneurysmal sac. Although some studies involving the use of aminocaproic acid (Amicar) have been encouraging (because it retards clot lysis), other studies show that the incidence of vasospasm is greatly increased. If during the time before surgery vasospasm should occur, the treatment is that of hypertension and hypervolemia by special drips, such as dopamine, and large volumes of intravenous fluids and volume expanders, such as fresh frozen plasma, albumin, or plasmanate. Because of the difficulty in treating vasospasm and minimizing the chances of rebleeding concurrently, many surgeons now operate as soon as possible in SAH grades I to III. In this manner, vasospasm can be treated effectively without the danger of rebleeding. Antiinflammatory corticosteroids will also be used both preoperatively and postoperatively to treat cerebral edema. The drug most often used is dexamethasone, because it does not pose the problem of fluid retention characteristic of other steroids. Postoperative management consists of blood pressure control, fluid and electrolyte balance, and administration of medications to decrease swelling, prevent seizures, and control blood pressure if needed. If surgery is not performed, the chance of rebleeding after the sixth month after the initial bleed is 3%/year. However, about 50% of patients who survive the initial bleed will rebleed by the end of the fourth week, with mortality being extremely high. Thus, surgery should always be the first choice of treatment when dealing with a ruptured cerebral aneurysm.

Intracranial Hemorrhage

For patients who have hypertensive intracerebral hemorrhage, medical management consists of controlling their hypertension with appropriate medications, such as hydralazine, clonidine, and methyldopa, and special drips, such as nitroprusside (Table 31–2) to bring the blood pressure within acceptable limits as determined by the physician. This will aid in decreasing the chances of rehemorrhage due to sustained elevation in systemic and cerebral blood pressure. If the hematoma is of considerable size or is causing massive edema and compression of surrounding viable tissue, surgery may be performed to evacuate the clot and relieve pressure within the cranium. Postoperative care consists of maintaining the blood pressure within set parameters, which decreases the chances of recurrent hematoma formation. Maximal return of neurologic functioning will depend on the amount of infarction and resulting impairment caused by the initial clot. If the infarct is on the patient's dominant cerebral hemisphere and affects the speech centers, expressive or receptive aphagias of varying degrees of severity will be seen (Fig. 31–15). Deficits of the extremities may range from a slight hemiparesis to a total hemiplegia. Additional deficits include memory loss and perceptual disorders.

Arteriovenous Malformation

Arteriovenous malformations are also most effectively managed by surgical excision at the present time. This consists of resection of the AVM mass with clipping or cauterizing of all arterial and venous feeders. The entire AVM mass must be resected, or there is no benefit from surgery because the remaining AVM may still bleed. Depending on the size and location of the AVM, the neurologic deficit after surgery can be minimal or it can consist of total loss of motor movement on one side as well as aphasias, visual loss, and intellectual impairment. If surgery is not an option, the chance of successive bleeds with increasing impairment and possible death is around 3%/year.

Sterotactic radiosurgery, the closed-skull destruction of a precisely defined intracranial target by ionizing beams of radiation, is the newest technique for treating AVMs.[29] So far, the patient population undergoing radiosurgery with the gamma knife has consisted of those with lesions considered inoperable or those with residual lesions after attempted surgical resection. Use of the gamma knife in neurosurgery shows great promise, because no surgical mortality or significant morbidity has been associated with it, and patients can be discharged from the hospital within 18 hours after radiosurgery.[29]

Although gamma knife stereotactic radiosurgery is a safe, effective, and cost-effective alternative to conventional neurosurgery by craniotomy in a select patient population, the number of patients and the size of AVMs that can be treated effectively by this process are currently unknown.[29]

The rehabilitation period for patients with hemorrhagic disease will depend on the extent of damage done by the insult and the individual patient. It will range from minimal to extensive, and may last for years if neurologic impairment is extensive.

Ischemic Disease

The medical prophylactic treatment in patients with TIA and reversible ischemic neurologic deficit may consist of the administration of anticoagulants or antiplatelet therapy. Anticoagulants will prevent the fibrin formation at the end of the hemostatic process. Antiplatelet therapy will prevent the initial platelet adhesion, the release of platelet constituents, the synthesis of the prostaglandin endoperoxides, and the platelet aggregation.

In transient cerebral ischemia due to cerebral embolism from the heart with persistent source of embolism (*i.e.*, atrial fibrillation and mitral stenosis, especially combined with rheumatic heart disease or cardiomyopathy), long-term anticoagulant treatment is indicated, as in patients with an artificial heart prosthesis or hypertension.

In most cases of cerebrovascular accident, recovery occurs in the first 6 months after the insult. Complications include visual deficits, aphasia, dysphagia, loss of memory, poor comprehension ability, and various perceptual disorders.

Much attention is now being paid to the development of stroke units within the hospital setting for the specific purpose of caring for patients with ischemic cerebrovascular disease; however, the value of such units is still in question.[7] Most studies do suggest that not only do patient and family benefit from units specialized for the care of ischemic stroke patients, but that diagnosis is probably also enhanced because of the concentration of professional expertise. In addition to improved patient care and subsequent reduction in the need for long-term hospitalization and its associate costs, stroke units can also benefit the health care team by serving as a focal area for continuing education concerning cerebrovascular disease.[7]

Carotid Endarterectomy

The role of carotid endarterectomy in patients experiencing definite hemispheric symptoms (TIAs and reversible ischemic neurologic deficits) is to prevent embolization and distal occlusion by removing the atheromatous plaque. Its role in patients with stroke in evolution and early completed stroke is controversial. It sometimes worsens the stroke by causing a hemorrhagic infarction.

The aim of carotid endarterectomy in patients experiencing vertebral circulatory symptoms is to augment clinically deficient anterior cerebral circulation (the collateral support of the vertebral system) by increasing flow from a stenotic internal carotid.

During a carotid endarterectomy, a vertical incision is made in the carotid artery and the plaque build-up is removed. It is important not to be deceived by the small neck dressing, because the potential for several complications is present postoperatively.

The major problem in the early postoperative period after carotid endarterectomy is the instability of blood pressure, which usually appears before the operation is completed or in the recovery room and is manifested by hypotension or hypertension. Almost half of all patients undergoing carotid endarterectomy develop an abnormal increase or decrease in blood pressure that rarely leads to permanent sequelae with treatment. It is possible that this circulatory instability results from impairment of carotid sinus reflexes. The intimate anatomic relationship between the carotid sinus and the carotid occlusive lesions makes this a reasonable possibility. Left uncontrolled, the extremes of hypotension or hypertension may precipitate a stroke.

Another complication of carotid artery surgery is loss of carotid body function. A loss of carotid body function results in a loss of the normal ventilatory and circulatory responses to hypoxia. This loss, whether temporary or permanent, is a potentially serious hazard. Instead of the normal response, in

Table 31-2
Nitroprusside Dosage Chart*

CAL FACTOR (3.33/kg)	WT. (kg)	5 cc/hr	10 cc/hr	15 cc/hr	20 cc/hr	25 cc/hr	30 cc/hr	35 cc/hr	40 cc/hr	45 cc/hr	50 cc/hr	55 cc/hr	60 cc/hr	65 cc/hr	70 cc/hr	75 cc/hr	80 cc/hr	85 cc/hr	90 cc/hr	95 cc/hr	100 cc/hr	105 cc/hr	110 cc/hr	115 cc/hr
0.074	45	0.37	0.74	1.11	1.48	1.85	2.22	2.59	2.96	3.33	3.70	4.07	4.44	4.81	5.18	5.55	5.92	6.29	6.66	7.03	7.40	7.77	8.14	8.51
0.066	50	0.33	0.66	0.99	1.32	1.65	1.98	2.31	2.64	2.97	3.30	3.63	3.96	4.29	4.62	4.95	5.28	5.61	5.94	6.27	6.60	6.93	7.26	7.59
0.061	55	0.31	0.61	0.92	1.22	1.53	1.83	2.14	2.44	2.75	3.05	3.36	3.66	3.97	4.27	4.58	4.88	5.19	5.49	5.80	6.10	6.41	6.71	7.02
0.056	60	0.28	0.56	0.84	1.12	1.40	1.68	1.96	2.24	2.52	2.80	3.08	3.36	3.64	3.92	4.20	4.48	4.76	5.04	5.32	5.60	5.88	6.16	6.44
0.051	65	0.26	0.51	0.77	1.02	1.28	1.53	1.79	2.04	2.30	2.55	2.81	3.06	3.32	3.57	3.83	4.08	4.34	4.59	4.85	5.10	5.36	5.61	5.87
0.048	70	0.24	0.48	0.72	0.96	1.20	1.44	1.68	1.92	2.16	2.40	2.64	2.88	3.12	3.36	3.60	3.84	4.08	4.32	4.56	4.80	5.04	5.28	5.52
0.044	75	0.22	0.44	0.66	0.88	1.10	1.32	1.54	1.76	1.98	2.20	2.42	2.64	2.86	3.08	3.30	3.52	3.74	3.96	4.18	4.40	4.62	4.84	5.06
0.042	80	0.21	0.42	0.63	0.84	1.05	1.26	1.47	1.68	1.89	2.10	2.31	2.52	2.73	2.94	3.15	3.36	3.57	3.78	3.99	4.20	4.41	4.62	4.83
0.039	85	0.20	0.39	0.59	0.78	0.98	1.17	1.37	1.56	1.76	1.95	2.15	2.34	2.54	2.73	2.93	3.12	3.32	3.51	3.71	3.90	4.10	4.29	4.49
0.037	90	0.19	0.37	0.56	0.74	0.93	1.11	1.30	1.48	1.67	1.85	2.03	2.22	2.41	2.59	2.78	2.96	3.15	3.33	3.52	3.70	3.89	4.07	4.26
0.035	95	0.18	0.35	0.53	0.70	0.88	1.05	1.23	1.40	1.58	1.75	1.93	2.10	2.28	2.45	2.63	2.80	2.98	3.15	3.33	3.50	3.68	3.85	4.03
0.033	100	0.17	0.33	0.50	0.66	0.83	0.99	1.16	1.32	1.49	1.65	1.82	1.98	2.15	2.31	2.48	2.64	2.81	2.97	3.14	3.30	3.47	3.63	3.80
0.032	105	0.16	0.32	0.48	0.64	0.80	0.96	1.12	1.28	1.44	1.60	1.76	1.92	2.08	2.24	2.40	2.56	2.72	2.88	3.04	3.20	3.36	3.52	3.68
0.030	110	0.15	0.30	0.45	0.60	0.75	0.90	1.05	1.20	1.35	1.50	1.65	1.80	1.95	2.10	2.25	2.40	2.55	2.70	2.85	3.00	3.15	3.30	3.45
0.029	115	0.15	0.29	0.44	0.58	0.73	0.87	1.02	1.16	1.31	1.45	1.60	1.74	1.89	2.03	2.18	2.32	2.47	2.61	2.76	2.90	3.05	3.19	3.34
0.028	120	0.14	0.28	0.42	0.56	0.70	0.84	0.98	1.12	1.26	1.40	1.54	1.68	1.82	1.96	2.10	2.24	2.38	2.52	2.66	2.80	2.94	3.08	3.22
0.027	125	0.14	0.27	0.41	0.54	0.68	0.81	0.95	1.08	1.22	1.35	1.49	1.62	1.76	1.89	2.03	2.16	2.30	2.43	2.57	2.70	2.84	2.97	3.11
0.026	130	0.13	0.26	0.39	0.52	0.65	0.78	0.91	1.04	1.17	1.30	1.43	1.56	1.69	1.82	1.95	2.08	2.21	2.34	2.47	2.60	2.73	2.86	2.99
0.025	135	0.13	0.25	0.38	0.50	0.63	0.75	0.88	1.00	1.13	1.25	1.38	1.50	1.63	1.75	1.88	2.00	2.13	2.25	2.38	2.50	2.63	2.75	2.88
0.024	140	0.12	0.24	0.36	0.48	0.60	0.72	0.84	0.96	1.08	1.20	1.32	1.44	1.56	1.68	1.80	1.92	2.04	2.16	2.28	2.40	2.52	2.64	2.76
0.023	145	0.12	0.23	0.35	0.46	0.58	0.69	0.81	0.92	1.04	1.15	1.27	1.38	1.50	1.61	1.73	1.84	1.96	2.07	2.19	2.30	2.42	2.53	2.65
0.022	150	0.11	0.22	0.33	0.44	0.55	0.66	0.77	0.88	0.99	1.10	1.21	1.32	1.43	1.54	1.65	1.76	1.87	1.98	2.09	2.20	2.31	2.42	2.53
0.021	155	0.11	0.21	0.32	0.42	0.53	0.63	0.74	0.84	0.95	1.05	1.16	1.26	1.37	1.47	1.58	1.68	1.79	1.89	2.00	2.10	2.21	2.31	2.42
0.020	160	0.10	0.20	0.30	0.40	0.50	0.60	0.70	0.80	0.90	1.00	1.10	1.20	1.30	1.40	1.50	1.60	1.70	1.80	1.90	2.00	2.10	2.20	2.30

* This dosage chart was developed using the standard concentration of 50 mg of nitroprusside in 250 cc of 5% dextrose in water (D5W). Its author suggests keeping a copy at the patient's bedside to enable easy calculation with every subsequent dose adjustment.

To calculate dose, first find cal factor (3.33/kg). Multiply cal factor times cubic centimeters on intravenous pump. Dose is in micrograms per kilogram per minute. Example: If a patient weighs 70 kg and is receiving nitroprusside at 60 cc/hr, the dose is 2.88 µg/kg/hr.

(Morris, L. Dosage calculation charts. Crit. Care Nurse 9 (5):92, 1989.)

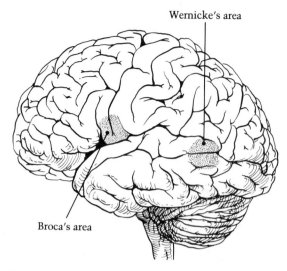

Wernicke's area

Broca's area

Figure 31–15
Speech centers of the cerebral hemispheres.

which ventilation and blood pressure increase with hypoxia, ventilation and blood pressure decrease. Avoidance of situations that provoke hypoxemia will prevent sudden deaths from hypoxic respiratory or circulatory failure.

A less common complication of carotid endarterectomy is acute respiratory insufficiency. The symptoms vary according to the patient's state of consciousness. The patient may show signs of hypoxemia (confusion, restlessness, and uncooperativeness). Respirations may be labored, and wheezing or stridor may be heard. The trachea may be deviated to one side.

The most common cause of acute postoperative respiratory insufficiency is distortion or compression of the trachea by a hematoma at the wound site. Drainage of an incisional hematoma in the neck should be done in the operating room, except in an emergency, when immediate drainage may be a life-saving procedure. Drainage may be necessary before an endotracheal tube can be passed.

Vocal cord paralysis is a rare complication after carotid endarterectomy. It is caused by retraction and trauma to the vagus nerve and usually does not become manifest until the first or second postoperative day. This complication usually requires only symptomatic treatment. Respiratory insufficiency occurs only when additional factors, such as laryngeal edema or polyps, are present.

Cerebral Artery Bypass Surgery

The purpose of the extracranial-intracranial (EC-IC) arterial bypass is to augment collateral circulation to a symptomatic or potentially symptomatic ischemic area of cerebral circulation. Although approximately 3000 of these operations are performed annually in the United States,[49] the indications and effectiveness of the operation remain controversial.

Extracranial-intracranial arterial bypass involves the surgical construction of an end-to-side anastomosis between a branch of the external carotid circulation and a cortical branch of the symptomatic internal carotid circulation. The donor artery is most frequently one or both branches of the superficial temporal artery, which is palpated at the temple. The recipient artery is the middle cerebral artery.

In some patients thought to require bypass surgery, the external carotid branches are unavailable or quite small. Under these circumstances, a free vein graft harvested from the arm or leg can be anastomosed proximally to the external carotid artery or one of its branches and distally to a cortical branch of the middle cerebral artery.

The International Cooperative Study of Extraranial/Intracranial Arterial Anastomosis was completed and analyzed in 1985. The results of this study revealed that anastomosis of the superficial temporal artery to the middle cerebral artery did not reduce the rate of subsequent events of stroke and stroke-related death among patients with symptomatic atherosclerotic disease of the internal carotid and middle cerebral arteries. Both fatal and nonfatal stroke occurred more frequently and earlier in patients assigned to the surgery group.[49]

Patients undergoing this surgery should take aspirin for the rest of their lives. Aspirin is an antiplatelet-aggregating agent that assists in the prevention of formation of tiny clots at the areas of anastomoses.

SUMMARY

Cerebrovascular disease poses a tremendous threat to the health and well-being of far too many individuals. The lasting neurologic deficits can be devastating and even fatal.

The uncomplicated course of many hemorrhagic insults will keep a patient hospitalized for a minimum of 10 days, during which time the disease process is diagnosed, evaluated, and treated. These patients usually resume their activities of daily living with no limitations to their life-style. A course complicated by vasospasm, rebleeding, or infection may prolong the hospital stay for weeks and even months.

Many ischemic insults and some hemorrhagic insults result in an extensive rehabilitation process. The rehabilitation processes may last as long as 2 years.

The needs of the family are great during this time, especially when the patient undergoes an extensive rehabilitation process. The nursing plan of care must incorporate the needs of the patient and the needs of the family to ensure optimal recovery for the patient who has cerebrovascular disease.

DIRECTIONS FOR FUTURE RESEARCH

Increasingly, nursing is becoming a profession requiring specialization. It is readily apparent that generalized nursing research is unable to cover all areas of nursing to the degree to which they deserve to be covered. Therefore, it is necessary for each nursing specialty to assume the responsibility of generating research that deals with problems particular to its individual focus. The following questions are examples of the need for research in the area of cerebrovascular disease and its nursing implications:

1. What are the effects on increased ICP of changes in patient position?
2. What are effective nursing interventions to minimize anxiety and helplessness in patients with impaired communication?
3. What is the effect of early initiation of nursing measures (*e.g.*, passive and active range-of-motion exercises, positioning, sleep/rest periods) on the rehabilitation of patients with a cerebrovascular insult?
4. What are the specific advantages of "stroke units" for patients who experience cerebrovascular insult?

5. What positive effects do unlimited visiting hours in the critical care unit have on patient outcome?
6. How do changes in patient condition relate to periods of hypotension, and what is their effect on the neurologic manifestations of cerebral vasospasm?

REFERENCES

1. Adams, H. P. Current status of antifibrolytic therapy for treatment of patients with aneurysmal subarachnoid hemorrhage. *Stroke:* 13:256, 1982.
2. Allwood, A., and Lundy, C. Cerebral artery bypass surgery. *Am. J. Nurs.* July:1284, 1980.
3. Bader, D. Micro-surgical treatment of intracranial aneurysms. *J. Neurosurg. Nurs.* 11:221, 1979.
4. Baum, P. Carotid endarterectomy: One strike against stroke. *Nursing '83* March:50, 1983.
5. Bock, J. Stroke: A review. *Can. Nurse* May:47, 1980.
6. Burt, M. Perceptual deficits in hemiplegia. *Am. J. Nurs.* 70:1026, 1970.
7. Clark, S., A neurovascular unit as an adjunct to therapy. *BNI Q.* 3(2):37, 1987.
8. Dignan, M., Howard, G., Toole, J. F., *et al.* Evaluation of the North Carolina stroke care program. *Stroke* 17(93):382, 1986.
9. Doolittle, N. Arteriovenous malformations: The physiology, symptomatology and nursing care. *J. Neurosurg. Nurs.* 11:221, 1979.
10. Easton, J. D., and Sherman, D. G. Management of cerebral embolism of cardiac origin. *Stroke* 2:433, 1980.
11. Eliasson, S. G., and Prensby, A. L. *Neurological Pathophysiology.* New York: Oxford University Press, 1978.
12. Feldman, J., and Schultz, M. Rehabilitation after stroke. *Nurs. Dig.* Summer:63, 1976.
13. Flynn, E. Cerebral vasospasm following intracranial aneurysm rupture: A protocol for detection. *J. Neurosci. Nurs.* 21(96):343, 1989.
14. Gray, R. Caring for patients with cerebral aneurysms. *A.O.R.N. J.* 37:631, 1983.
15. Grotta, J. Current medical and surgical therapy for cerebrovascular disease. *N. Engl. J. Med.* 317(24):1505, 1987.
16. Go, G. K., Van Dyk, P., Luden, L., *et al.* Interpretation of nuclear magnetic resonance tomograms of the brain. *J. Neurosurg.* 59 (4): 1983.
17. Hickey, J. *The Clinical Practice of Neurological and Neurosurgical Nursing* (2nd ed.) Philadelphia: J. B. Lippincott, 1986.
18. Hopkins, M., Valberg, B., and Robinson, L., A report on the EC/IC bypass study. *J. Neurosci. Nurs.* 18(4):211, 1986.
19. Hummel, S. Cerebral vasospasm: Current concepts of pathogenesis and treatment. *J. Neurosci. Nurs.* 21(4):216, 1989.
20. Jacobansky, A. Stroke. *Am. J. Nurs.* 72:1260, 1972.
21. Jan, M., Buchheit, F., and Tremoulet, M. Therapeutic trial of intravenous nimodipine in patients with established cerebral vasospasm after rupture of intracranial aneurysms. *Neurosurgery* 23(2):154, 1988.
22. Jennet, B. *An Introduction to Neurosurgery.* Chicago: Year Book Medical Publishers, 1977.
23. Johanson, B., Wells, S., and Hofmeister, D. *Standards for Critical Care.* St. Louis: C. V. Mosby, 1988.
24. Kappert, A. New noninvasive methods of investigating cerebrovascular insufficiency. *Triangle* 21:1, 1982.
25. Kassel, N. F., and Torner, J. C. Aneurysmal rebleeding: A preliminary report from the Cooperative Aneurysm Study. *Neurosurgery* 13:479, 1983.
26. Lee, K. Aneurysm precautions: A physiologic basis for minimizing rebleed. *Heart Lung* 9(2):336, 1980.
27. Little, J., Moufarrif, H., and Furlan, A., Early carotid endarterectomy after cerebral infarction. *Neurosurgery* 24(3):334, 1989.
28. Loftus, C., Biller, J., Godersky, J. C., *et al.* Carotid endarterectomy in symptomatic elderly patients. *Neurosurgery* 22(4):676, 1988.
29. Lunsford, L., Flickinger, J., Lindner, G., *et al.* Stereotactic radiosurgery of the brain using the first United States 210 Cobalt-60 source gamma knife. *Neurosurgery* 24(2):151, 1989.
30. MacDonald, E. Aneurysmal subarachnoid hemorrhage. *J. Neurosci. Nurs.* 21(5):313, 1989.
31. Mee, E., Dorrance, D., Lowe, D., *et al.* Controlled study of nimodipine in aneurysm patients treated early after subarachnoid hemorrhage. *Neurosurgery* 22(3):484, 1988.
32. Meyer, J. S., *et al.* (eds.). *Cerebral Vascular Disease 4.* Hachinski, V. Extracranial/Intracranial Bypass Surgery: Technique or Therapy. Amsterdam: Excerpta Medica, 1983.
33. Miller, E., and Williams, S. Alteration in cerebral perfusion: Clinical concept or nursing diagnosis. *J. Neurosci. Nurs.* 19(4):183, 1987.
34. Millikan, C. Stroke intensive care units: Objectives and results. *Stroke* 10(3):235, 1979.
35. Mitchell, S., and Yates, R., Cerebral vasospasm: Theoretical causes, medical management, and nursing implications. *J. Neurosci. Nurs.* 18(6):315, 1986.
36. Newell, D., Grady, S., Scrotta, P., *et al.* Evaluation of brain death using transcranial Doppler. *Neurosurgery* 24(4):509, 1989.
37. Okawara, S. H. Warning signs prior to rupture of an intracranial aneurysm. *J. Neurosurg.* 38:575, 1973.
38. Olsson, J. E. Recent Advances in the Treatment of Cerebrovascular Diseases. *Acta Scandinavica* 26 (Suppl. 78):77–78.
39. Peck, S. Calcium blocking agents for treatment of cerebral vasospasm. *J. Neurosurg. Nurs.* 15:123, 1983.
40. Pia, H. W., *et al.* (eds.): *Cerebral Aneurysms: Advances in Diagnosis and Therapy.* New York: Springer-Verlag, 1977.
41. Rudy, E. Magnetic resonance imaging: New horizon in diagnostic techniques. *J. Neurosurg. Nurs.* 17(6):331, 1985.
42. Sahs, A. L., *et al. Intracranial Aneurysms and SAH: A Cooperative Study.* Philadelphia: J. B. Lippincott, 1969.
43. Samson, D. S., and Boone, S. Extracranial-intracranial (EC-IC) arterial bypass: Past performance and current concepts. *Neurosurgery* 3(1):79–86, 1978.
44. Sasaki, T., Kassell, N. F., Colohan, A. R. T., *et al.* Cerebral Vasospasm Following Subarachnoid Hemorrhage. In McDowell, F. H., and Caplan, L. R. (eds.), *Cerebrovascular Survey Report.* The National Institute of Neurological and Communicative Disorders and Stroke, 1985.
45. Seiler, R., Reulen, H. J., Huber, P., *et al.* Outcome of aneurysmal subarachnoid hemorrhage in a hospital population: A prospective study including early operation, intravenous nimodipine, and transcranial Doppler ultrasound. *Neurosurgery* 23(5):598, 1988.
46. Sekhar, L. N., and Heros, R. C. Origin, growth and rupture of saccular aneurysms: A review. *Neurosurgery* 8:248, 1981.
47. Sekhar, L., Wechsler, L. R., Yonas, H., *et al.* Value of transcranial Doppler examination in the diagnosis of cerebral vasospasm after subarachnoid hemorrhage. *Neurosurgery* 22(5):813, 1988.
48. Solomon, R., Fink, M., and Lennihan, L. Early aneurysm surgery and prophylactic hypervolemic hypertensive therapy for the treatment of aneurysmal subarachnoid hemorrhage. *Neurosurgery* 23(6):699, 1988.
49. Stewart-Amidei, C., and Penckofer, S. Quality of life following cerebral bypass surgery. *J. Neurosci. Nurs.* 20(1):50, 1988.
50. Samson, D. S., *et al.* A Comparison of the Results of "Early" vs. "Late" Aneurysm Surgery in the Good Grade Patient. In R. H. Wilkins (ed.), *Cerebral Arterial Spasm.* Baltimore: Williams & Wilkins, 1980.
51. Willis, D., and Harbit, M. A fatal attraction: Cocaine-related subarachnoid hemorrhage. *J. Neurosci. Nurs.* 21(3):171, 1989.
52. Wylie, E. J., and Ehrenfeld, W. K. *Extracranial Occlusive Cerebrovascular Disease: Diagnosis and Management.* Philadelphia: W. B. Saunders, 1970.
53. Youmans, J. (ed.). *Neurological Surgery: Physiology, Homeostasis and General Care* (Vol. 2). Philadelphia: W. B. Saunders, 1982.
54. Youmans, J. (ed.). *Neurological Surgery: Vascular Abnormalities* (Vol. 3). Philadelphia: W. B. Saunders, 1982.

VII

The Critically Ill Adult With Renal and Gastrointestinal Problems

THE NURSE'S WORLD VIEW

A *world view* is those set of beliefs each of us has about how the world operates, why things happen the way they do, and the rules they follow. We usually never give a thought to what our world view is, but it is a powerful, guiding force in all our lives. We cannot escape the effects of our world view. It begins to operate the very moment we begin our day. No one can *not* have a world view.

The moment we walk onto the unit, we put our world view in action. Do things happen by accident, or is there some purpose or meaning behind the events I'm dealing with (*e.g.,* this patient's heart attack, that patient's cancer, this child's birth defect)? Does this patient have any control over the illness, or is it only a function of the physiologic processes occurring in the body? Does choice exist in health and illness, or is the body entirely "on automatic"?

Our world view gives us answers to difficult questions like these. The more conscious we become of the assumptions we make about what our world view actually is, about "how things work," the more effective we will become in our interactions with others.

32

Abdominal and Renal Assessment

Miranda Toups   Barbara Montgomery Dossey

BLENDING THE BREATH AND THOUGHT

Can you remember the last time you said out loud "ahhhh" to release some tension and calm yourself? The simple release of the breath and the "ah" sound is an ancient way for you or your patients to release worries, fear, and pain, to evoke relaxation, and to die in peace.

For centuries, mystics have said that the breath connects consciousness to life. This practice of releasing the breath allows a space to emerge so that you or your patients can enfold all emotions, pains, and memories that emerge into conscious experience. Blending the breath and thought facilitates sensations of inner peace to be present.

The following steps will help you guide a patient in blending the breath and thoughts.* At first, the "ahhhh" sounds might be like an echoing of words, but staying with the sounds allows releasing of tension, fears, and pain. The following steps can help you guide the patient in a powerful process:

- Position yourself comfortably and close to the patient who is full of fear, in pain, or who is dying, and sit by his side for a short time or longer, if necessary. A session may last 5 to 10 minutes or can even last up to an hour or longer. Obtain whatever is necessary to maintain comfort for the person, such as pillows, a light blanket, and so forth. (For a longer session, ask if the family may wish to participate.)
- Suggest to the patient that watching the breath is an ancient method of calming the body and the mind. Let the person first begin noticing the rise and fall of his or her abdomen with each breath in and out.
- Sitting at the patient's midsection, focus on the rise and fall of his or her abdomen with each inhalation and each exhalation. With this focused intention, breathe in unison with the patient. At the top of the patient's exhalation, begin sounding softly and out loud the sound "ahhhh" matching the respiration of the patient.
- Simple, powerful phrases such as "peaceful heart" or "releasing into the breath" may be said occasionally. However, the fewer words spoken, the more powerful is the breath work.

LEARNING OBJECTIVES

After reading this chapter, the nurse should be able to do the following:

1. Perform a systematic abdominal assessment.
2. Perform a systematic renal assessment.
3. Establish nursing diagnoses after assessment.

* Modified from Boerstler, R. *Letting Go.* Watertown, MA: Associates in Thantology, 1982.

LOCATION OF THE ABDOMINAL ORGANS

To permit accurate description of the abdomen, it is divided anteriorly by imaginary lines into quadrants. A horizontal line passes through the umbilicus, and a vertical line extends from the xiphoid process to the symphysis pubis (Fig. 32–1).

The abdomen is sometimes divided into nine sections. Two imaginary horizontal parallel lines cross at the lower costal margin border and the anterior superior spine of the iliac bones. Two vertical lines drop from the midclavicular lines to the approximate borders of the abdominal muscle.

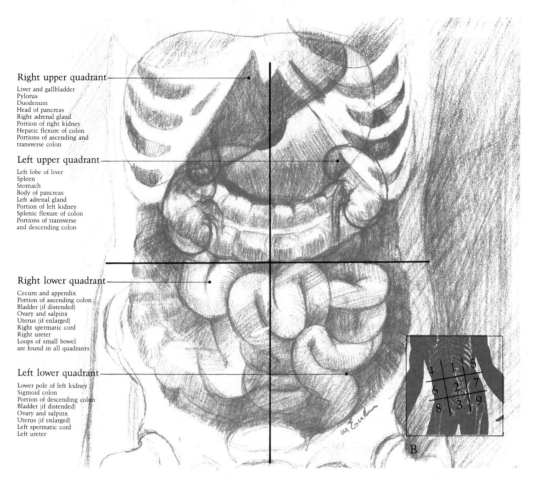

Right upper quadrant
Liver and gallbladder
Pylorus
Duodenum
Head of pancreas
Right adrenal gland
Portion of right kidney
Hepatic flexure of colon
Portions of ascending and
transverse colon

Left upper quadrant
Left lobe of liver
Spleen
Stomach
Body of pancreas
Left adrenal gland
Portion of left kidney
Splenic flexure of colon
Portions of transverse
and descending colon

Right lower quadrant
Cecum and appendix
Portion of ascending colon
Bladder (if distended)
Ovary and salpinx
Uterus (if enlarged)
Right spermatic cord
Right ureter
Loops of small bowel
are found in all quadrants

Left lower quadrant
Lower pole of left kidney
Sigmoid colon
Portion of descending colon
Bladder (if distended)
Ovary and salpinx
Uterus (if enlarged)
Left spermatic cord
Left ureter

Figure 32–1

(*A*) The four regions of the abdomen identified are the right upper quadrant, left upper quadrant, right lower quadrant, and left lower quadrant. (*B*) The nine areas of the abdomen are the (1) epigastric, (2) umbilical, (3) pubic, (4 and 5) right and left hypochondriac, (6 and 7) right and left lumbar, and (8 and 9) right and left inguinal areas.

Normally, the only areas that are palpable in the abdomen are the edge of the liver at the right costal margin, the lower pole of the right kidney (in a thin person), and the sigmoid colon in the left lower quadrant. The abdominal aorta is palpable in some people, especially women. If the patient's bladder is full, it may be palpable in the lower midline area.

The renal system comprises the kidneys, the ureters, the urinary bladder, and the external male genitalia. Except for the male genitalia, these organs are relatively inaccessible for palpation. Physical complaints and the medical history often provide the first clues to problems occurring in the abdomen or kidneys. Laboratory tests and special radiologic studies are necessary to confirm the diagnosis.

HISTORY OF PRESENT ILLNESS

Abdominal Complaints

The nurse must obtain the patient's history and assess for the four major gastrointestinal symptoms: pain, vomiting, abdominal distention, and alterations in bowel activity.[5] The correlation between pain and nausea is important. Pain can cause nausea and must be differentiated from nausea that originates from a problem in the gastrointestinal tract.

With regard to a patient's abdominal complaints, the nurse should ask the patient to describe the character, duration, frequency, location, and distribution of the discomfort in relation to food, drugs, activity, and defecation.[2] Abdominal pain is frequently the reason a person may seek medical advice. However, pain alone is not an early or common symptom of gastrointestinal disorders. The pain may be experienced as a general sensation throughout the abdomen or referred to a specific quadrant (see Fig. 32–1). Table 32–1 lists the common causes of abdominal pain.

The pain stimulus may be elicited by local traction, stretching, or palpation. Thus, patients may use local muscle guarding as a protective mechanism to protect pain-sensitive structures. Information about constipation, diarrhea, frequency of bowel movements, and the use of enemas and laxatives must be obtained.

The nurse should ask the patient about any problems with swallowing, nausea, and vomiting, as well as about the types of food and drinks (including alcoholic drinks) he consumes

Table 32–1
Causes of Abdominal Pain

CAUSES	LOCATION OF PAIN	FINDINGS
Appendicitis	Initially epigastric, umbilical, later localized in lower right quadrant	Fever, nausea, and vomiting, local iliac tenderness, anorexia
Acute gastritis	Epigastric	Nausea and vomiting
Acute pancreatitis	Epigastric	Vomiting, low-grade fever, tachycardia, hypotension, referred pain to midback or flank
Cholecystitis	Right epigastric, severe	Nausea and vomiting, especially after a heavy meal, referred pain to subscapular area or back
Colon obstruction	Lower abdomen	Frequent vomiting, increased distention, constipation
Dissecting abdominal aneurysm	Initially thoracic; later epigastric	Tachycardia, cyanosis, hypotension, loss of pulses below aneurysm, referred pain to back
Diverticulitis	Left iliac	Alternating diarrhea and constipation, abdominal tenderness, leukocytosis
Gastroenteritis	Initially epigastric; later lower bowel	Nausea and vomiting, cramping, diarrhea
Gastric ulcer	Left epigastric; gnawing or burning	Pain relieved by food
Intussusception	Epigastric	Sudden onset of pain, tachycardia, hypotension, shock, legs drawn up, sausage-shaped abdominal swelling, rectally passed mucus and blood, referred pain to back
Mesenteric thrombosis	Epigastric, severe, generalized, unrelenting	Nausea and vomiting, abdominal muscle spasms, cyanosis, tachycardia, shock
Small intestine obstruction	Epigastric	Repeated vomiting, abdominal distention
Perforated duodenal ulcer	Initially epigastric; later generalized	Abdominal rigidity, absent bowel sounds, tachycardia, hypotension, cyanosis, shock
Renal colic	Flank pain over affected kidney	Nausea and vomiting, costovertebral angle tenderness; referred pain to groin or testicle in man, bladder in woman
Ruptured ectopic pregnancy	Lower abdomen; sharp	Cramping and spotting, abdominal tenderness and rigidity, tachycardia, shallow and rapid breathing, shock, referred pain to shoulder.

and any changes in eating and drinking habits. Special attention should be given to complaints of weight loss.

Gastrointestinal Symptoms

Gastrointestinal symptoms frequently accompany genitourinary complaints. The right kidney lies in the right quadrant with the liver, gallbladder, duodenum, and hepatic flexure of the colon. The left kidney lies in the left quadrant with the stomach, spleen, pancreas, and splenic flexure of the colon. Because these organs have a common autonomic sensory innervation, a patient with renal disease may present with gastrointestinal symptoms.[3] Because the kidneys are surrounded by the peritoneum, inflammation of the kidneys frequently produces an irritation of the peritoneum. If it does, rebound tenderness and muscle rigidity mimicking peritonitis are present.

Most renal conditions are painless, because distention of the renal capsule progresses slowly. Renal pain is usually a constant, dull ache in the costovertebral angle. Table 32–2 lists common types of genitourinary symptoms of pain.[4]

Ureteral pain due to spasm of smooth muscle and hyperperistalsis can be observed, or the patient may tell about expelling a foreign object (a kidney stone). Patients may complain of severe back pain—intermittent pain radiating from the midback to the lower anterior abdomen. Women may complain of pain in the vulva, whereas men may complain of pain in the testicles and scrotum. Overdistention of the bladder can cause severe suprapubic pain. When the examiner feels a suprapubic bulge, an overdistended bladder due to acute urinary retention is suspected.

Prostate pain is rare. Usually men complain of a feeling of fullness or discomfort in the perineal or rectal area. Discomfort from cystitis and referred pain to the lumbosacral area are not uncommon. Pain in the testicles caused by trauma or infection is severe. Spermatic cord involvement usually causes referred lower abdominal pain. Infection involving the epididymis causes pain in the lower abdomen, groin, and, sometimes, the adjacent testicle. The pain can mimic that of a ureteral stone or appendicitis. Leg and back pain can be the result of more severe problems. The nurse should ask the patient about the quantity, quality, setting, and course of any renal pain.

Complaints of dysuria must be investigated. A burning sensation on urination usually indicates some kind of irritation.

Table 32–2
Common Causes of Genitourinary Symptoms of Pain

TYPES	CAUSES
Urethral pain	Spasm of smooth muscle; hyperperistalsis after passage of a kidney stone; back pain, intermittent or severe; men may complain of pain in testicles or scrotum; women may complain of pain in vulva
Suprapubic pain	Severe bladder distention because of urinary retention
Prostate pain	Inflammation and swelling of prostate; rare
Lumbosacral pain	Cystitis
Testicular pain	Trauma, infection, spermatic cord involvement; may also mimic pain of urethral stone

Spasm of the bladder and anal sphincter associated with pain and a desire to evacuate the bladder and bowel is referred to as *tenesmus*. Frequency of urination is usually a result of an inflamed mucosa, a decreased bladder capacity, or the loss of bladder elasticity. Nocturia (excessive urination that interrupts sleep) is common in obstructive conditions and renal diseases in which there is a loss of parenchymal concentrating power.

Patients may describe abnormalities that are characteristic of acute or chronic obstruction of the neck of the bladder or the prostate. Urinary hesitancy (a delay in initiating a urinary stream) or an increased physical effort in starting the flow of urine is the most common abnormality. Loss of force and caliber of the urinary stream is not the only phenomenon associated with increased muscular effort. Terminal dribbling refers to the urine continuing to drip despite muscular effort to stop it. Abrupt interruption of the urinary flow can occur, and it may often be accompanied by suprapubic pain.

The nurse should investigate any complaints of incontinence. With stress incontinence, a patient urinates involuntarily during physical exertion such as sneezing or laughing. With urgency incontinence, urination occurs involuntarily after the patient experiences an urge to void. With true incontinence, urination occurs periodically without warning. In patients with renal disease, complaints of itching, nausea, and vomiting, and changes in sensorium usually indicate advanced renal disease.

Nurses in the acute care setting must be aware of any abnormalities in the urine volume. The amount of urine voided, as well as the amount of fluids lost through drainage and through daily insensible loss, must be compared with the intake of fluids. Oliguria is present when a patient voids less than 400 mL/day. Anuria, the absence of urine, indicates a malfunction of the kidneys or a bilateral ureteral obstruction. Both phenomena are critically important and warrant immediate medical attention.

SYSTEMATIC ASSESSMENT OF THE ABDOMEN

The nursing assessment of the abdomen should proceed in a systematic manner from quadrant to quadrant and in the se-

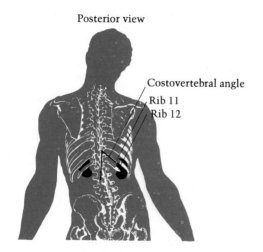

Posterior view

Costovertebral angle
Rib 11
Rib 12

Figure 32–2
Renal pain can be elicited in the area of the costovertebral angle formed by the vertebral column and the rib cage.

quence of inspection-auscultation-percussion-palpation. Auscultation is performed before percussion and palpation because percussion and palpation are apt to alter the frequency of bowel sounds.[2,9]

Inspection

While inspecting the patient's abdomen, the nurse can put the patient at ease by talking with the patient and making certain that the patient is as comfortable as possible. The nurse should always be aware of any facial expressions or body language that might indicate signs of anxiety or pain. The general inspection is best done from the patient's right side. It should include observation of the abdominal surface, striae, old or new scars, rashes, lesions, or dilated veins. Size, shape, contour, and symmetry should be noted. Any complaints of severe abdominal pain with distention must be investigated immediately. An altered abdominal contour may be due to abdominal masses, hernias, or distention from ascites. Table 32–3 helps the nurse determine whether there is intestinal obstruction present.

The nurse can instruct the patient to cough in order to elicit bulges or pain. Striae may be a result of pregnancy, obesity, ascites, or edema. Scars may be present from trauma, surgical procedures, or healed incision sites. Dilated veins may be due to obstruction of the vena cava or portal vein and circulation from the abdomen. Peristalsis can be observed by watching the abdomen. Sometimes it may be several minutes before peristalsis can be seen. Visible frequent peristalsis may result from pyloric or intestinal obstruction. Peristalsis usually is not visible except in thin people. Other normally visible abdominal pulsations may be from the aorta in the epigastric region.

Auscultation

Auscultation of the abdomen is performed in a systematic manner, with the nurse moving from quadrant to quadrant. The diaphragm of the stethoscope is kept in place long enough to determine the frequency, quality, and pitch of bowel sounds (Fig. 32–3). Most intestinal sounds originate in the small bowel; they are high-pitched and gurgling. The frequency of bowel sounds varies with meals. Absence of bowel sounds may indicate paralytic ileus, peritonitis, or severe hypokalemia. Increased high-pitched sounds at frequent intervals, referred to as *borborygmi*, are heard with increased peristalsis in early intestinal obstruction or complete obstruction.[6]

After listening to bowel sounds, the nurse should listen for bruits, which are vascular sounds. The nurse should listen in the midepigastrium for bruits that indicate stenosis of the renal arteries and in the iliac region for bruits that indicate stenosis of the iliofemoral artery. If splenic infarction or liver tumor is suspected, the nurse should listen over the spleen and liver for peritoneal friction rubs.

Percussion

Percussion is done to determine the degree of resonance, tympany, and dullness. Tympany usually is more dominant owing to presence of a small amount of swallowed air in the gastrointestinal tract. When a flat or dull sound is elicited, this occurs over a solid structure such as distended bladder, enlarged uterus, or abdominal masses. The patient should be

Table 32-3
Does the Patient Have Intestinal Obstruction?

ASSESSMENT	NURSING DIAGNOSES	PATIENT OUTCOMES	INTERVENTION
History			
Often follows history of previous surgeries; note time of last bowel movement	Acute pain related to abdominal abnormality	1. The patient will be pain-free. 2. The patient will be free of major complication of abdominal pain.	1. Place patient in a comfortable position. 2. Call physician. 3. Prepare to obtain abdominal radiographs and laboratory studies; insert intravenous line and nasogastric tube 4. Give pain medicine after radiographs so that the pain is not masked.
General Appearance			
Lies still; breathes quietly at first; as distention increases, respirations are short and shallow			
Chief Complaint			
Localized pain; cramps; any body movement increases pain; patient feels that having a bowel movement may relieve pain.			
Physical Examination			
Acute onset of pain; fever; rapid pulse; nausea and vomiting; hard, distended abdomen; borborygmus or no bowel sounds with complete obstruction			

observed at all times for any tenderness or pain. Percussion of the liver provides only a good estimate of liver size.[2,5] To percuss the liver, the nurse starts in the right midclavicular line below the umbilicus and percusses upward toward the liver (Fig. 32–4). The lower border of the liver can be found in the midclavicular line. Next the nurse percusses downward from lung resonance in the right midclavicular line until dullness is heard. The distance from the border of upper dullness and lower dullness indicates the height of the liver. Normal liver heights are 6 cm to 12 cm in the right midclavicular line and 4 cm to 8 cm in the midsternal line. Borders of liver dullness can be obscured by gas in the colon, by lung consolidation, or by right pleural effusion.

The stomach is percussed on the left side in the area of the left lower anterior rib cage (see Fig. 32–4). The nurse can hear the tympany of a gastric air bubble. If abdominal distention is obvious, and if the size of the gastric air bubble is increased, gastric dilatation is suspected.

The spleen is more difficult to percuss.[2] In the area of the left tenth rib posterior to the midaxillary line, a small oval area may be identified (Fig. 32–5). If it cannot be identified, the patient should take a deep breath, and the nurse should percuss in the lowest intercostal space in the left anterior axillary line. That area is usually tympanic.

Palpation

Both light palpation and deep palpation are done in the abdominal examination to give the nurse information about abdominal tenderness, muscular resistance, and masses. Begin palpation at the pubis and work upward to the costal regions.

As the nurse moves from one quadrant to the next, the entire hand is moved to avoid causing the patient an uncomfortable feeling or irritation to the abdominal skin surface. If the patient is sensitive to palpation and cannot relax, the nurse can have the patient place the patient's own hand on the abdomen under the nurse's hand. Then as the patient relaxes, his hand can be moved to the side. Light palpation helps to relax and reassure the patient. In a light, gentle, rotating motion, the nurse places fingertips together and palpates with the fingertips. Areas of tenderness, any masses, and organs are identified. A true danger sign is rebound tenderness (known as *Blumberg's sign*). Rebound tenderness is intense abdominal pain caused by rebounding of palpated tissue. It can be localized, as with abscesses, or generalized if an intra-abdominal organ has been perforated.[8] Deep palpation is usually needed to detect abdominal masses and organs. If masses are palpated, their shape, size, consistency, mobility, tenderness, and pulsation are determined and recorded. It is possible to distinguish an abdominal wall mass from an abdominal cavity mass. A mass in the wall remains palpable when the patient tightens the abdominal muscles, whereas a mass in the abdominal cavity is obscured when the patient tightens the abdominal muscles.

The liver is palpated by having the patient breathe with the abdominal muscles (Fig. 32–6). By placing the examining hand lateral to the rectus muscle, with the fingers pointing to the patient's head, the nurse should try to feel the liver as it comes down to meet the fingertips.

At the peak of inspiration, it may be necessary to release the pressure of the right hand and move up a little toward the costal margin. The edge of a normal liver is a firm, regular

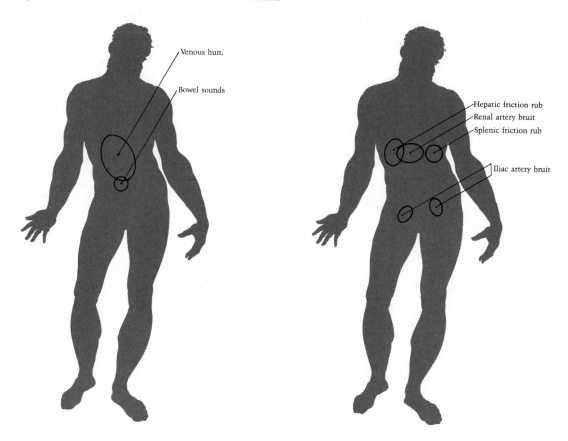

Figure 32–3

Abdominal auscuitation. (*A*) Bowel sounds are best heard over the area of the small circle. Listen for at least 1 to 2 minutes to determine whether they are present or absent. The venous hum may be heard over the area of the large circle. The venous hum is a systolic bruit heard sometimes over the patient with a cirrhotic liver; it is due to an increased flow through the portal and the systemic venous collaterals. (*B*) The systolic bruit heard in the epigastrium or anterior lumbar region may be a sign of renal artery stenosis. The systolic bruit heard over the iliac region may be a sign of stenosis of the iliofemoral artery. Peritoneal friction rubs can be heard over the spleen in splenic infarction and over the liver in liver tumor.

ridge with a smooth surface. If the liver is felt, its distance below the costal margin is recorded in centimeters. The liver may also be palpated by the hooking technique (see Fig. 32–6). The nurse should stand to the right of the patient and face the patient's feet. Next the nurse places both hands side by side on the patient's right abdomen below the border of liver dullness. As the nurse asks the patient to take a deep breath, the nurse presses in with her fingers and up toward the costal margin.

If palpable, the spleen is felt by palpation in the left upper quadrant. The nurse remains on the right side of the patient and reaches across the abdomen with both hands. The nurse's right hand is placed below the left costal margin. The left hand is placed around the patient and is used to press upward on the lower left rib cage for support. At this point, the right fingertips are pressed in toward the area of the spleen. An enlarged spleen is fragile, and it should be percussed or palpated gently only by an experienced nurse.

SYSTEMATIC ASSESSMENT OF THE RENAL SYSTEM

The examining techniques that are used for the renal system are inspection, palpation, percussion, and auscultation. (The

discussion of the ausculation of the abdomen lists some specifics that are appropriate to auscultation of the renal system.)

Inspection

With inspection, the nurse looks for any raised area that may indicate a kidney mass. The ureters are not accessible for direct assessment. The urinary bladder is inspected in the suprapubic area for any evidence of bulging. If urinary retention is present, the nurse can determine the level of the bladder by percussing and listening for a dull fluid sound. The outline of a distended bladder can be determined by palpation. The nurse will elicit pain if distention is present.

Palpation

The nurse palpates the kidneys by placing the fingertips of the upper hand at the costal margin in the midclavicular line and the lower hand posteriorly at the costovertebral angle (Fig. 32–7). At this point, the patient, who is supine, is instructed to take a deep breath. The nurse exerts firm upward pressure on the patient's right upper quadrant, with the upper hand exerting slightly more pressure above than below. The nurse may feel the right kidney. If the right kidney is palpable,

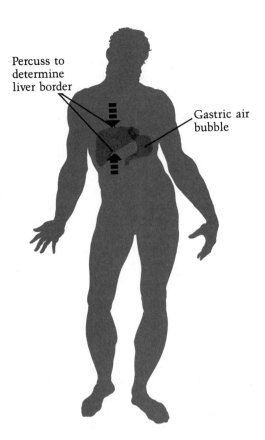

Percuss to
determine
liver border

Gastric air
bubble

Figure 32–4
Percussion of the liver. A gross estimate of the liver size can be made by identification of the borders of the liver. The *dark arrows* show percussion from the level of the umbilicus upward and from lung resonance downward until liver dullness is elicited. The normal heights are 6 cm to 12 cm in the right midclavicular line and 4 cm to 8 cm in the midsternal line. Percussion of the stomach. The tympany sound of the gastric air bubble is in the left lower anterior rib cage.

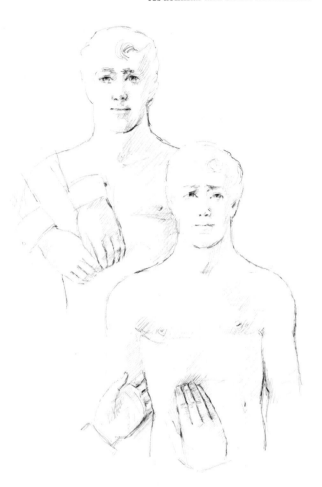

Figure 32–6
Two methods for palpation of the liver.

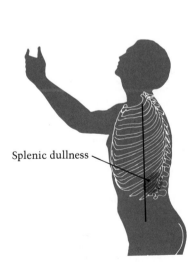

Splenic dullness

Figure 32–5
Percussion of the spleen. Splenic dullness can be elicited by percussion posterior to the left midaxillary line near the tenth rib.

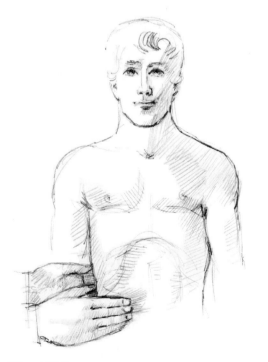

Figure 32–7
Palpation of the kidney.

the size, contour, and degree of tenderness should be recorded. The same maneuver is repeated for palpation of the left kidney. A normal left kidney is rarely palpable.

Percussion

While assessing the patient's back, the nurse should check for kidney tenderness by placing the palm of the left hand over each costovertebral angle and striking it with the ulnar surface of the right fist.

Auscultation

The nurse should auscultate in the costovertebral angles posteriorly and listen in the upper quadrants anteriorly for bruits. If bruits are present, they should be investigated further through diagnostic procedures.

ASSESSMENT OF THE RECTUM AND GENITALIA

Examination of the rectum is usually deferred in the critically ill patient or in the patient who had a coronary, stroke, or head injury. Rectal examination and rectal temperatures can cause a vasovagal effect and cause the patient's heart rate to slow down. If the examination is done, however, it is accomplished by the patient lying in the left lateral position. The patient's buttocks are spread apart by the hand of the nurse. The perianal and sacracoccygeal areas are inspected for lesions, inflammation, excoriation, external hemorrhoids, and masses. In order to palpate the anus, the nurse lubricates the index finger of the examining hand and inserts it into the patient's anal canal.

This may be done by the critical care nurse when impaction is suspected. When done, note anal sphincter tone, tenderness, and irregularities.

The nursing assessment of the male genitalia can be done during routine physical care. Inspection for discharges, lesions, engorged vessels, or structural abnormalities can be done while inserting a catheter or giving catheter care. The shaft of the penis is inspected for size, shape, skin color, edema, and

placement of the urethral meatus. A common condition in uncircumcised men is phemosis (restriction of the opening of the prepuce). If the man is uncircumcised, the foreskin should be retracted to inspect for any irritation. Palpation for masses can be done during routine perineal care.

Palpation for tenderness, nodules, or edema of the penis and scrotum can be done at the same time. The inguinal region is palpated for nodules or masses. Inguinal hernias are best felt with the patient in a standing position. This is rarely done in the critical care unit.

The female genitalia can also be examined during routine care. First, the mons pubis, labia majora, and perineum are inspected for swelling, inflammation, discharge, abnormal bleeding, growths, lesions, and scars. The labia minora, clitoris, urethral opening, and vaginal introitus are then inspected for the preceding abnormalities. If the situation warrants, internal inspection of the vagina is done with the use of a speculum by a specially trained nurse.

SPECIAL STUDIES

A complete assessment of the gastrointestinal and renal systems includes special studies. Table 32-4 lists the special studies done most frequently.

After a thorough history has been taken and a complete physical examination has been done by the physician, all the data are gathered and tests are ordered that can support or provide the medical diagnosis.[4,5]

The tests that are done frequently for gastrointestinal diagnosis are complete blood count, urinalysis, and examination of stool specimen. The stool specimen is examined by gross inspection. Stools are inspected for odor, amount of mucus, consistency, number, and color. Stool color is normally brown and may be altered. Red in stools indicates lower gastrointestinal bleeding. Tarry indicates upper gastrointestinal bleeding. Gray or tan indicates lack of bile or biliary obstruction. White indicates barium. Specific laboratory and microscopic studies are done when parasites are suspected. Specimens for parasites should be kept warm and sent directly to the laboratory for inspection.

Table 32-4

Studies Ordered to Confirm Specific Gastrointestinal and Renal Diagnosis

TESTS	DATA RESULTS
Radiographs: gastrointestinal	Visualizes stomach and intestinal tract
Barium enema	Visualizes colon
Fluoroscopic study	Shows shadows of all organs from esophagus to anus
Gastric drainage	Determines level of gastric acidity
Fiberoptic gastroscopic exam	Gastric biopsy and photographs of gastric lesions
Anoscopic, proctoscopic, and sigmoidoscopic exam	Visualizes directly colon mucosa
Urinalysis	Detects blood (hematuria), cloudiness (phosphate constitutes precipitated in alkaline medium), specific gravity, pH, and protein
Blood chemistries	Electrolyte studies, serum calcium, creatinine, blood urea nitrogen, phosphorus, total serum protein; other specific studies may be ordered depending on history and physical findings
Excretory urogram	Visualizes renal structures
Renal arteriography	Determines renal circulation, cysts, tumors, or other renal diseases
Renal biopsy	Determines specific cause of renal disease

Radiographic Examination of Gastrointestinal System

Radiographic examination of the patient includes a gastrointestinal series to visualize the stomach and intestinal tract. Barium enema examination reveals information about the colon; barium double-contrast enema examination examines the colonic mucosa.

Fluoroscopy

Fluoroscopic examination shows shadows of all the organs from the esophagus to the anus. Gastric contents obtained by Levine drainage may be examined for gastric acidity.[1] A fiberoptic gastroscope may be used for a biopsy study and photographs of any gastric lesions. Anoscopic, proctoscopic, and sigmoidoscopic examinations permit direct observation of the mucosa lining the colon.[4,7] Because of risks that are involved with these studies, the nurse must obtain the patient's signed consent for diagnostic procedures of the abdomen and renal system.

Urinalysis

Special studies that are done for patients with renal problems involve frequent urinalysis. Urine is inspected for evidence of blood (hematuria), for cloudiness (due to phosphate constituents precipitated in an alkaline medium), leukocytes (pyuria), feces (fecaluria), red blood cells, and casts. The specific gravity of urine is checked. A diseased kidney is unable to dilute or concentrate urine normally. Urine is excreted with solute concentration equivalent to that of plasma. The pH of urine is measured for alkalinity or acidity. Urine is usually acidic, and its acidity is affected by food intake. Consistently alkaline urine is abnormal; it can result from an alkaline-producing organism such as *Proteus*, which causes a urinary tract infection; alkalinity may also indicate that the kidneys are unable to acidify urine. Urine is examined for the presence of protein, most commonly albumin. The presence of protein in the urine usually indicates an abnormality.

Hematology and Blood Chemistries

Hematologic and electrolyte studies are done routinely. Other laboratory data that are significant in renal disease are the levels of serum calcium, creatinine, blood urea nitrogen, phosphorus, uric acid, and total protein.

Abnormalities in serum calcium levels may cause abnormalities in excretion. Because the urinary creatinine level is constant and is relative to a person's total body mass, determination of the creatinine level is a useful test to measure kidney function.[5] When renal function is reduced, the creatinine level is elevated. Urea, a byproduct of protein, is filtered by the glomerulus and reabsorbed in the renal tubule. The blood urea nitrogen level rises in conditions that reduce renal function, such as acute and chronic renal failure, chronic glomerulonephritis, chronic pyelonephritis, nephrosclerosis, and obstructive uropathy. In conditions characterized by decreased renal perfusion, such as shock or congestive heart failure, the blood urea nitrogen level may rise.

Elevated serum phosphate and serum uric acid levels are observed in renal insufficiency. When serum uric acid and the total-body pool of uric acid increases, deposition of uric acid may occur in the kidney and renal collecting system. Uric acid stones, which can disturb kidney function, are formed.

Total serum protein comprises albumin and globulin. Serum proteins have many functions, including normal clotting and distribution of water in the body due to their osmotic activity. When serum protein levels are reduced, the albumin fraction is most often affected by excessive loss from the kidney. Hypoalbuminemia is seen in the nephrotic syndrome.

Radiographic Examination and Special Studies of Renal System

If necessary, cystoscopic study is done for direct visualization of renal structures. Plain abdominal films are obtained when some abnormality of the urinary tract is suspected. Stones in the urinary tract can be identified when a patient has renal colic. Intravenous pyelograms, also referred to as *excretory urograms*, may be ordered with urinary tract abnormalities, such as hematuria, recurrent urinary tract infection, and pain of renal colic, as well as to investigate an abdominal mass or to evaluate hypertension. Renal arteriography is done to look specifically at the circulation of the kidneys and for any cysts, tumors, or other renal diseases. Other special techniques can be done as indicated to study structures adjacent to or related to the urinary tract.

In patients who require both abdominal and renal contrast films, the intravenous pyelogram and cholecystogram are done before the barium studies. When both barium enema studies and upper gastrointestinal tract studies are to be done, the barium enema study is done before the upper gastrointestinal tract study, because barium from that study may be retained in the colon for a long period and may thus delay the barium enema test.

Renal Biopsy

A renal biopsy study is sometimes necessary to make a diagnosis in a patient with known or suspected renal disease. It is most helpful in any renal disease when the disease process is distributed evenly throughout the kidney tissue, affecting the glomeruli specifically and causing hematuria and proteinuria. Some examples of these diseases are the nephrotic syndrome and any form of glomerulonephritis. Other disease processes in which renal biopsy study may be helpful are the collagen diseases, unexplained acute oliguric renal failure, and inflammatory and infectious diseases of the kidney, after healing in reversible conditions. The renal biopsy study may also assist in determining early stages of renal disease that are not explained by other diagnostic studies. A renal biopsy study should be done only by an experienced physician. A dangerous invasive procedure, it is performed only after comprehensive evaluation of the patient. The patient's signed consent must be obtained. The most common complications are bleeding and hematuria, and the nurse must understand what nursing care is to follow the procedure. Firm pressure is applied to the biopsy site immediately, followed by application of a pressure dressing. The patient must remain prone for 30 minutes and then flat for 1 hour; bed rest should follow for 24 hours. The patient's condition is assessed. The vital signs are taken, and any patient complaint must be investigated, especially with regard to pain at the biopsy site or to frequent or urgent urination.

SUMMARY

The abdominal and renal assessment must be approached in an organized and systematic manner in order to obtain clear and concise data. The nurse must have a knowledge of abdominal anatomy and physiology as well as an awareness of psychosocial issues that may be involved in problems of the abdominal and renal region.

REFERENCES

1. Becker, K. L., and Stevens, S. Performing in-depth abdominal assessment. *Nursing* 18:60, 1988.
2. Bates, B. A. *Guide to Physical Examination* (3rd ed.). Philadelphia: J. B. Lippincott, 1987.
3. Guyton, A. C. *Textbook of Medical Physiology* (7th ed.). Philadelphia: W. B. Saunders, 1986.
4. O'Connell, E. A. Assessing the bladder. *Nursing* 15:44, 1985.
5. Patras, A. C. Gastrointestinal assessment. *AORN* 40:726, 1984.
6. Smith, C. E. Assessing bowel sounds. *Nursing* 18:42, 1988.
7. Smith, C. E. Detecting acute abdominal distention: What to look for, what to do. *Nursing* 15:34, 1985.
8. Tollison, A. A. Danger signs: Rebound tenderness. *Nursing* 18:78, 1988.
9. Williams, P. *Gray's Anatomy* (36th ed.). Philadelphia: W. B. Saunders, 1980.

33

Acute Renal Failure

Barbara Giordano

BODYMIND THERAPIES AND RELIGION

Some persons who are deeply committed to a particular religious point of view are sometimes quite unsympathetic to certain mind-body therapies such as meditation or other forms of voluntary, intentional relaxation. Meditation in particular may be threatening, because the emptiness of mind that is promoted in many meditative traditions may seem to conflict with religious instruction always to hold Jesus, Christ, or God uppermost in consciousness. Making a void of the mind, some say, violates this teaching and sets the stage for the entry of negative or satanic forces.

In the early 1970s, Herbert Benson* at Harvard Medical School examined the physiologic effects of many types of inner quiet—Christian prayer, transcendental meditation, progressive relaxation, and autogenic therapy. They found that the physical changes produced in all these states were virtually identical. Oxygen consumption, carbon dioxide production, blood lactate levels, and many other indices were the same whether prayer, meditation, or the other two types of relaxation were employed.

Based on these findings, nurses should feel confident in recommending a variety of relaxation techniques to patients, because of the common physical responses to many of them. The specific technique can be chosen by the patient, in accord with his or her religious persuasion. From the point of view of the body, many techniques are effective. From the point of view of religion, the choice is individual, and should be honored and respected by the nurse, whatever it may prove to be, and whether it coincides with his or her personal religious views.

LEARNING OBJECTIVES

After reading this chapter, the nurse should be able to do the following:

1. Describe the anatomy and physiology of the normal kidney.
2. Identify the categories of acute renal failure.
3. Identify the clinical manifestations of acute renal failure.
4. Describe the major medical therapies for acute renal failure.
5. Describe the basic diagnostic urine tests.
6. List the methods of reducing hyperkalemia.
7. Describe the nursing care objectives for a patient who has acute renal failure.

CASE STUDY

Mr. T. S., 39 years of age, was admitted to the hospital emergency room with the chief complaint of fever, generalized muscle weakness,

* Benson, H. *The Relaxation Response*. New York: William Morrow, 1975.

malaise, and pain, tenderness, and swelling of both lower extremities. He was accompanied by his wife, who said that her husband started a physical training program, including working with weights and jogging, about a week ago.

His temperature was 102°F, his blood pressure was 100/80, his apical pulse was 128 and irregular, and his respirations were 32.

Mr. T. S. was 6 feet, 0 inches tall and weighed 205 pounds. He was a full-time writer and part-time professor in English at local university. He was married and the father of two children, ages 5 and 1. He smoked one pack of cigarettes per day, and drank two six-packs of beer per week. His hobbies included reading, photography, fishing, and mechanics.

Physical Examination

The patient was a tall, well-developed, dark-haired man lying on a stretcher in his jogging suit. His skin was covered with perspiration. The patient had thick brown curly hair distributed evenly over head.

His hearing was intact, and his ear canals were clear. Patient had history of sinusitis. His vision was 20/20 in each eye. Patient denied having diplopia, headaches, or spots before eyes. His pupils were equal, round, regular, and reacted to light and accomodation. Extraocular eye movement was intact. Conjunctiva were pale. Visual fields were normal by confrontation.

The patient's lips were dry, his tongue was coated, and his mucous membranes were dry. No saliva was present. Breath odor was present. Multiple fillings were visible. Tongue was at midline, uvula raised on phonation, and gag reflex was intact. Tonsils were not present. Patient complained of feeling "parched."

Patient had full range of motion in neck. Trachea was at midline. Thyroid was nonpalpable. There was no lymphadenopathy.

The patient's respirations were 32, and his breathing was shallow and purse-lipped. There was no costovertebral angle tenderness. Lungs were clear anteroposteriorly. There were no adventitious sounds.

The patient's blood pressure was 100/80, and his apical pulse was 120 and irregular. No heaves and thrills were present. PMI 5th ICS, MCL.

The abdomen was nontender and soft. Bowel sounds were heard in all four quadrants. Patient admits to no food intolerances. He denied any history of mononucleosis or hepatitis. Examination of the genitourinary system was deferred.

Femoral pulses were 2+; other pulses were nonpalpable. Nonpitting edema (4+) was present from midthigh to ankle. Patient could lift legs off stretcher, but did so with much difficulty and complained of pain. Patient admitted to increasing his jogging distance from 1 mile to 5 miles in 5 days' time. Today, despite the 100°F weather, he started to jog, jogging 5½ miles. His legs began to cramp, and he was unable to continue.

Laboratory Results

Sodium was 145 mEq/L; potassium, 5.8 mEq/L; chloride, 112 mEq/L; carbon dioxide, 12 mM/L; glucose, 75 mg/100 ml; blood urea nitrogen, 95 mg/100 ml; creatinine, 1.6 mg/100 ml; calcium, 7.3 mEq/L; phosphorus, 5.8 mg/100 ml; and uric acid, 17.2. All liver function tests were within normal limits. Complete blood count was within normal limits. Haptoglobin was normal. Creatine kinase level was 1575 U/L. Urine was dark yellow, almost brown. Specific gravity was 1.006, and pH was 5.0. Urine was glucose negative. Acetone was 4+, protein was 4+, and hemetest was positive. Red blood cell count was zero.

Summary of Findings

Mr. S. is a 39-year-old dehydrated man who had an essentially negative past medical history until he came to the emergency room today. A week ago, he changed from his sedentary habits and began an unsupervised physical training program.

Physical examination confirmed his complaints of pain in lower extremities. The laboratory results of dehydration hyperkalemia, hyperuricemia, hypocalcemia, hyperphosphatemia, elevated creatine kinase level, and hemetest-positive urine confirmed the diagnoses of dehydration and rhabdomyolysis, which were nontraumatic in origin.

Nursing Diagnosis

The nursing diagnoses were electrolyte abnormalities related to massive skeletal muscle destruction, and complications of physical training related to knowledge deficit about physical training program and relationship to stress on body.

Medical Diagnosis

The medical diagnosis was rhabdomyolysis that was nontraumatic in origin and dehydration.

Mr. S. was admitted to the intensive care unit for fluid therapy and observation. Over the next 24 hours, his urine output was 105 cc, his weight increased 2.0 kg, he became significantly fluid-overloaded, and his serum potassium rose to 7.2 mEq. Hemodialysis therapy was initiated through a subclavian catheter. Over the next 2 weeks, Mr.

S. received five more treatments, and on hospital day 15, his urine output was 400 cc. After not receiving hemodialysis for 2 more days, Mr. S.'s urine output increased to 1000 cc and his laboratory results did not indicate a need for additional hemodialysis.

Mr. S. was discharged 36 days after his admission, with his serum creatinine level elevated slightly at 2.8 mg/100 ml.

REFLECTIONS

Mr. S. began a diet and exercise program several times before this one, but he lost interest in continuing it after several days. This time he vowed it would be different. He would start and complete a program that would be his until he decided to stop. He was determined to become "lean and mean."

Before instituting his program, he researched the topic of physical fitness. The regimen he decided on was a compilation of bits and pieces from various authors' recommendations. As he embarked on his physical fitness regimen, he was accompanied by his ever-present friend, Mike, his 3-year-old Pug dog.

When Mr. S. was admitted to the hospital, he was very upset. He had never been sick, let alone a patient in a hospital. What would happen to him? What would happen to Mike? Would Mike become sick because they were running together? His admission to the intensive care unit was seen as a crisis. When hemodialysis became necessary, Mr. S. felt hopeless. His primary nurse identified two categories influencing his hopelessness—his internal and external resources. Part of the threat to his internal resources was the loss of a vital part of himself when his kidneys failed. He seemed to be making no progress. It was as if time was standing still. His days seemed to be marked by the days on the hemodialysis machine, the length of dialysis treatment, and the wait for a decision about when the next treatment run would occur. His feelings of desperation were intense. Specific nursing interventions were established to help Mr. S. tap into his internal resource of motivation. Although he spent a lot of time sleeping during the first few days in intensive care, the nurses were able to convince Mr. S. that his complication of acute renal failure could be reversed. It simply took time. This gave him hope and motivation. His primary nurse helped Mr. S. identify his strengths and focus on the simple accomplishment of daily tasks. She assured him that his having to relinquish his normal control of self-responsibility was temporary.

Mr. S. remained despondent. His wife began to take on her husband's despair as well. In an effort to motivate Mr. S. from his negative state, his primary and associate nurses decided that the significance of Mike in his life could not be overlooked. Mike must come to visit.

Familiar social contacts can lessen the painful, physiologically arousing feelings associated with uncertainty, loneliness, and isolation. The positive health effects of human–animal relationship and bonding have focused on the animal's ability to offer love and tactile reassurance without criticism, and it is this perpetual infantile, innocent dependency that becomes a source of stability.

Pets are constant. They always have the same gestures and enthusiasm, do not grow up, remain unaffected by human progress or failure, and are oblivious to their owner's status. Attentiveness, one of the most important psychologic benefits, can be scheduled on demand by the owner, in almost any quantity, without bargaining or begging.[5] Dogs are more attentive to their family members than vice versa. Having a pet is having someone to talk to that listens. Companion animals provide a socially acceptable outlet for women as well as men for touching. Talking to and touching animals resemble intimate dialogue. When petting an animal, a person's face relaxes, a smile becomes less forced, more relaxed, and open. The unambivalent nature of such an exchange of affection is different from the familiar interpersonal relationships that are frequently ambivalent and charged with negative emotions.

When the owner faces real adversity, the pet's affection takes on a new meaning. The pet's continuing affection is a sign that the essence of the person has not been changed.[1]

Both the nursing and medical directors agreed to have Mike visit once. Before he could enter the unit, the Infectious Disease Team was consulted to develop guidelines.

Mike did come to visit. When he saw his master, he became very animated—so animated that he almost wriggled from the arms of Mrs. S. The two friends visited and then napped together. Not only did Mr. S. become visibly more relaxed and energetic, but each member of the nursing staff found an excuse to visit and talk to both. Mike's one visit became an every-other-day event. Another group of people, the nurses, seemed to benefit from Mike's visits. A seemingly simplistic nursing intervention translated into communication, support, motivation, coping, and improved body image. The primary nurse's loving, honest, caring human guidance facilitated the patient's movements toward insight and balance. Nurses have many different types of therapeutic techniques at their disposal if they give themselves permission to take a risk and be creative.

ANATOMY AND PHYSIOLOGY OF THE KIDNEY

The kidneys are paired, somewhat flattened, bean-shaped structures that have indented medial borders. The indented borders, which are called *hila* (singular: *hilum*), are the entrance sites for the renal blood vessels and the renal pelvis. The kidneys lie in the retroperitoneal space, between the twelfth thoracic and the third lumbar vertebrae, behind the liver on the right side and behind the spleen on the left side. They are separated from the abdominal cavity anteriorly by layers of peritoneum; they are protected posteriorly by the lower thoracic wall. The kidney surface is a strong fibrous capsule that is covered by fat tissue.

Internal Structure of the Kidney

Internally, each kidney is composed of a cortex, a medulla, and a pelvis. The cortex, the outer layer of the kidney, contains the glomeruli and tubules.

The medulla is composed of 5 to 15 pyramids, conical arrangements of tubules that project into the minor and major calyces of the renal pelvis. The major calyces are contiguous with the minor calyces, which in turn contain the medullary pyramids. Each of the 5 to 15 pyramids is made up of parallel tubules that form larger collecting ducts that penetrate the

papilla (or apex) of the pyramid. Minor calyces form major calyces, which also vary in number from two to four. Major calyces form the renal pelvis, which becomes the ureter at a point called the *ureteropelvic junction.*

Once the urine reaches the renal pelvis, it leaves the kidney through the ureter to be passed to the urinary bladder. Each ureter extends downward within the retroperitoneal space to the bladder. Because the walls of the calyces, pelvis, and ureter contain smooth muscles that contract rhythmically, the urine is propelled along its course in peristaltic spurts.

Renal Blood Flow

The kidney is a highly vascular organ that normally provides little resistance to blood flow through it. Blood enters each kidney at the hilus through a large renal artery. Each artery then divides into five smaller segmental branches, the *interlobar arteries,* which ascend to the corticomedullary junction, where they terminate into the arcuate arteries. The vessels continue to nourish the kidneys by traversing the bases of the pyramids. *Interlobular arteries* branch off at right angles for the arcuate arteries, which continue to ascend through the cortex to the capsular surface of the kidney. The interlobular arteries form the afferent arteries.

The total renal blood flow is between 1000 and 1200 ml/minute, or about 20% to 25% of the resting cardiac output. About 90% of the renal blood flow nourishes the cortex,[8,9] and the remaining 10% goes through the medulla. The high cortical perfusion is probably related to the kidney's evolution as an organ of high filtering capacity and not to its need for oxygen. The relatively low medullary blood flow is crucial to the kidney's important function of concentrating urine and conserving water.

After nourishing the entire kidney from the inside to the outside, from the medulla to the cortex, the blood flow then becomes unique to the kidney. From the interlobar arteries to the interlobar veins, the renal circulatory system features two different capillary beds, or microcirculations, arranged serially and separated only by the efferent arteriole. Each of these microcirculations not only has a specialized role but is found in different regions of the kidney. The structural and vascular properties of each are uniquely suited to the specific exchange processes that occur at the capillary level, producing the final urine of required volume and composition.

The afferent arterioles give rise to the glomerular capillaries, which are specialized for filtration, the first step in the formation of urine. The narrower efferent arterioles are formed from the glomerular capillaries. These arterioles, carrying blood away from the glomerulus, divide into the cortical and medullary peritubular capillary networks. The peritubular capillaries are highly anastamotic and surround the short loop of Henle nephrons and collecting ducts found in the outer and midcortex. In the juxtamedullary region of the inner cortex, the peritubular capillaries penetrate deep into the medulla. The cortical peritubular capillary network is specialized for reabsorption of fluid, whereas the medullary network is specialized for the concentration and dilution of urine.

The vascular supply to the cortical nephrons is different from that to the juxtamedullary nephrons. In the cortical nephrons, the efferent arteriole immediately breaks up into numerous freely anastomosing networks of capillaries that surround the convolutions of the proximal and distal tubules and the cortical aspects of the ascending and descending thick limbs of the loops of Henle and collecting ducts. The capillary network of one glomerulus is so lush and dense that it is impossible to distinguish the capillary network of one glomerulus from that of another.

However, the vascular supply to the juxtamedullary nephrons is more complex than that to the cortical nephrons. The diameter of the efferent arteriole of these nephrons is equal to or larger than that of the afferent arteriole. Just as with the cortical nephrons, the efferent arteriole is devoid of muscular elements, although it gives off one or more side branches to envelop the cortical convolutions of the proximal and distal tubules. The unique feature of the juxtamedullary circulation is the countercurrent arrangement of the blood flow that follows the descending or "arterial" limb of the loop of Henle through the medulla and papilla, turns at the bend of the loop, and then traverses upward with the ascending or "venous" limb, which ultimately reassembles into a venule that then enters into an interlobular vein. This countercurrent arrangement of descending and ascending blood flow appears specialized to retain solutes in the medulla by establishing and maintaining a gradient of osmolar concentration between the cortex and the tip of the papilla.

In all the peritubular capillary networks, most of the basement membranes are in close apposition to those of the tubules. It is the physical closeness of the basement membranes to that of the endothelial lining that is responsible for the exchange of solutes.

The serial arrangement of the glomerular and peritubular capillary networks does not permit the blood flow from the interlobular arteries to be shunted directly into the peritubular capillary bed or into the venous drainage system. Thus, diseases producing inflammation and edema of the glomerular capillaries may have a profound effect on renal blood flow.

Renal blood flow remains remarkably constant under most normal physiologic conditions. The ability of the kidney to maintain this near constancy of renal perfusion, despite variations in arterial pressure between 80 mm Hg and 200 mm Hg, depends on alterations in arteriolar tone. Within a range of 30 mm Hg above or below normal systolic blood pressure, the arterioles respond by directly changing vascular tone so that glomerular filtration rate and renal blood flow are held nearly constant. This phenomenon, termed *autoregulation*, is largely a function of the renal cortical circulation. Because 80% to 90% of the total renal blood flow is distributed to the cortical zone, autoregulation becomes a matter of some consequence.

The Nephron

Each kidney is composed of approximately 1 million nephrons, the functional workhorses. Each is basically similar in structure and presumably grossly similar in function. Each nephron is composed of a renal corpuscle, where the plasma ultrafiltrate is formed, and a tubule, which reabsorbs many of the filtered substances and subsequently delivers the highly modified plasma ultrafiltrate known as *urine* to the renal pelvis. About 75% of the nephrons can be destroyed before the patient has problems, because the remaining nephrons compensate.

The main functions of the nephrons are to filter the plasma of the waste products of metabolism and to maintain fluid balance by the regulation of sodium, water, and pH. There

are two different types of nephrons—cortical and juxtamedullary. The cortical nephrons have a short, thin loop of Henle, whereas the juxtamedullary nephrons have a long loop of Henle that goes deep into the medulla of the kidney. Both types of nephrons have similar but not identical functions. The juxtamedullary nephrons have a greater ability to concentrate urine (see Countercurrent Mechanism).

Nephron Structure

Each nephron is composed of a glomerulus (Bowman's capsule and capillary tufts), a proximal tubule, a loop of Henle, a distal tubule, and a collecting duct system. Just as the nephron segments are arranged serially, anatomically, the function of each segment depends on the compositional changes of tubular fluid brought about by transport processes that occur in the more proximal portion of the nephron.

Glomerulus

The glomerulus is a hollow spherical bulb situated between the afferent and efferent arterioles. At the vascular pole, the afferent arteriole expands into a relatively wide chamber that branches into five to seven capillary loops. Each loop further subdivides into some 20 to 40 capillary loops. Numerous anastomoses join the loops within a given lobule. These loops then recombine to form the emergent efferent arteriole. At the urinary pole, the proximal tubule begins.

Glomerular Filtration

Glomerular filtration is the rate at which fluid flows from the glomerulus into Bowman's capsule. The process of filtration is governed by Starling forces, which predict that ultrafiltration ceases when the sum of the forces favoring filtration are offset by the net sum of the forces opposing filtration (Fig. 33–1).

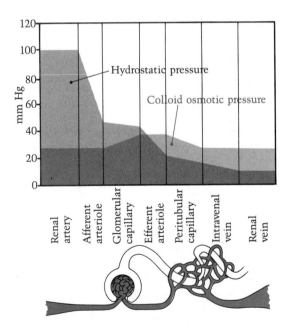

Figure 33–1

Starling forces in operation within the nephron.

Thus, fluid movement from the plasma to the interstitium is governed by the balance of hydrostatic and oncotic pressures of the glomerular capillary. The Starling forces are oriented to filter at the glomerulus, where the hydrostatic pressure exceeds the oncotic pressure. Pressure is higher inside the glomerulus than it is in Bowman's capsule, causing fluid to constantly pass into Bowman's capsule. The plasma ultrafiltrate in Bowman's capsule then enters the lumen of the proximal tubule.

The driving force behind filtration is the effective hydrostatic pressure generated not by the expenditure of energy from an active metabolic event, but by a physical one, the contraction of the heart. Thus, if something interrupts the normal functioning of the heart, interrupting the effective arterial blood volume, blood flow to the kidney is also interrupted. The kidney maintains constancy of the glomerular hydrostatic pressure by changes in afferent and efferent arteriolar tone in response to blood flow from the renal arteries through the capillary beds into the renal veins. Therefore, the arterioles not only control the hydrostatic pressure and blood flow, but they also control the filtration rate through the capillary.

Proximal Tubule

Like its parent glomerulus, this part of the nephron is entirely within the cortex. The tubule is joined to Bowman's capsule by a short connecting segment. It then coils extensively and twists about itself in the neighborhood of the glomerulus and then straightens out to penetrate into the deeper layers of the cortex and outer medulla.

The most important function of this part of the tubule is to reduce the volume of glomerular filtrate from the overwhelming 170 L/day to a more manageable 30 L to 40 L/day. The proximal tubule accomplishes this task by reabsorbing 60% to 70% of the salt and water in the glomerular filtrate. The brush border of the tubule increases the reabsorbing surface area tremendously and is also highly permeable to water.

Approximately 85% of all electrolytes are reabsorbed in the proximal tubule. Sixty to 70% of sodium is reabsorbed in the proximal tubule each day. All the filtered glucose is normally reabsorbed here and returned to the peritubular capillaries. Amino acids, urea, bicarbonate, phosphate, potassium, and calcium are reabsorbed here to varying degrees.

Loop of Henle

The loop of Henle is composed of the straight portion of the proximal tubule, a thin limb, and the straight portion of the distal tubule. In spite of the absence of gross morphologic differences, the functional properties of the descending segment differ from those of the ascending segment. The descending segment of the loop possesses no known acute transport systems. In the cortex, the interstitial fluid that surrounds the loop has an osmotic concentration close to that of the tubular fluid, so little reabsorption occurs in the thin limb of the cortical nephrons. In the medullary region, the environment of the thin limb of juxtamedullary nephrons is different. The concentrations of sodium, chloride, and urea in the medullary interstitial fluid increase from the corticomedullary junction to the tip of the papilla. Thus, as the thin limb descends into the medulla, the tubular fluid is exposed to an ever-increasing osmotic concentration. The interstitial fluid has

a progressively higher concentration of sodium and urea from cortex to papilla. The reabsorption of water in response to this gradient raises the osmotic concentration of the tubular fluid as it flows deeper into the medulla. As the fluid travels down the descending limb, the osmotic pressure created by the sodium and urea gradient causes water in the descending limb to move out into the interstitium. The remaining fluid enters the ascending limb, which is permeable to fluid. The ascending limb is impermeable to water but is able to reabsorb sodium chloride without water against a substantial concentration gradient. The reabsorption of sodium and chloride with little water raises the osmotic and salt concentrations of the medullary interstitium. This consequence is one of the important features of the countercurrent mechanisms.

Distal Tubule

As the ascending thick limb of the distal tubule returns to the cortex, it passes between the afferent and efferent arterioles of its glomerulus and continues as a distal convoluted segment. In the area where the distal tubule passes near its arterioles, the macula densa is formed (the macula densa is discussed later). The distal convoluted tubule joins directly with a collecting tubule in the cortex.

The distal tubule is where the final qualitative changes in ion and water excretion are made. In the absence of antidiuretic hormone (ADH), the entire tubule acts as a diluting segment. In the presence of ADH, 5% to 8% of the glomerular filtrate may be reabsorbed by the distal tubule.

Collecting Duct System

The collecting tubules are the site of the major qualitative changes in urinary concentration. They accomplish this task of maintaining water and ion homeostasis by varying the reabsorption of water, sodium, and potassium and the secretion of potassium and hydrogen.

Antidiuretic hormone controls the water permeability of the collecting tubule throughout its length. In the presence of this hormone, the membranes of the collecting duct become highly permeable to water. In the absence of ADH, the hypotonic fluid entering the collecting tubule may further dilute by active salt reabsorption.

Countercurrent Mechanism

The kidneys have a mechanism for concentrating urine called the *countercurrent mechanism*. This mechanism depends on the anatomic arrangement of the loops of Henle, of the juxtamedullary nephrons, and of the vasa recta loops, which supply blood to the medulla. The osmolality of the interstitial fluid in the outer medulla and papilla is hyperosmotic to arterial blood as the glomerular filtrate enters the proximal tubule; its normal osmolality is about 300 mOsm/L. Because the osmolality of the interstitial fluid of the medulla of the kidney becomes progressively greater deeper into the medulla, there is an increase from 300 mOsm/L in the cortex to 1200 mOsm/L at the pelvic tip of the medulla. The osmolality is about four times that of plasma. The increase is due to the sodium ions that are trapped in the medulla. As fluid returns through the ascending limb, there is a reversal in the osmolality. Fluid entering the distal tubule is hypotonic (100 mOsm/L) compared with the fluid in the proximal tubule (300 mOsm/L). .

It is theorized that as the small volume of fluids travels through the ascending limb, sodium chloride is actively pumped out of the tubular lumen. Because the ascending limb is impermeable to water, water does not follow the sodium chloride; therefore, the fluid becomes hypotonic relative to the fluid in the papilla. The osmolality is raised by the sodium ions that are pumped into the interstitium; they cause water to leave the water-permeable descending limb. Fluid that descends the loop becomes progressively more concentrated. Fluid that started out at 300 mOsm/L at the outer medullary junction increases to 1200 mOsm/L at the tip, only to fall to 100 mOsm as it leaves the ascending limb. From there, the ascending thick-limb urine passes to the distal convoluted tubules, where active sodium transport continues. Antidiuretic hormone from the pituitary controls the permeability of the distal tubule to water. Excretion of potassium occurs there. Although approximately 85% of water resorption has occurred as it passed from the proximal to the distal tubule, ADH increases water resorption in the distal tubule and collecting duct. Aldosterone aids in sodium resorption in the distal tubules. Cortisols, which are salt-regulating hormones, also help in sodium resorption and decrease potassium resorption at this point.

Distal tubule fluid then enters the collecting ducts in the medulla, where concentration and fine adjustments of sodium, chloride, potassium, and acid-base occur. At this point, aldosterone accelerates sodium resorption and is matched by passive chloride resorption; thus, potassium and hydrogen are exchanged.

Fluid in the collecting ducts is also exposed to the osmotic forces from the cortex to the medulla, as previously discussed. Water permeability in the collecting ducts, which is also controlled by ADH, causes water to move by osmosis into the medullary interstitium.

The collecting ducts filter the fluids, which are converted into urine, the end product of kidney function. Urine flows from the collecting tubules to the pelvis of the kidney. From there the urine goes through the ureters to the urinary bladder.

Regulatory Mechanisms

Because the blood flow through the kidneys and the glomerular filtration rate remain almost constant, it is logical to assume that the mechanics of autoregulation are intertwined with the regulation of the effective circulating blood volume. Although the mechanisms of the process of autoregulation are not clear, the available evidence suggests that the following factors are intimately tied together: baroreceptors, intrarenal vasoactive systems, and glomerulotubular feedback.

Baroreceptors

The body responds to variations in the effective circulating blood volume by appropriately varying vascular resistance, cardiac function, and renal sodium and water excretion. Subtle changes in the volume of the arterial compartment are sensed as changes in the systemic blood pressure by baroreceptors in the carotid sinuses and aortic arch and by an intrarenal baroreceptor.

As a result of the decreased volume and reduced activity of the stretch receptors, the activation of a variety of effector mechanisms occurs. Because ADH secretion varies inversely with left atrial pressure, one of the effective mechanisms activated is the release of ADH and the subsequent alteration in renal water excretion.

Renal function may be altered by a 10% loss in blood volume, a loss too small to alter the systemic blood pressure.[2] The afferent arteriole, acting as a baroreceptor, can directly alter renin release in response to a decreased arterial pressure. Additionally, changes in the rate of delivery of fluid to the macula densa through the distal tubule can also alter the rate of renin-angiotensin release. The juxtaglomerular apparatus is also a secondary receiver of information.

Renin

The juxtaglomerular apparatus, an important structure in the distal tubule, is a specialized part of the afferent arteriole. It contains specific granulated cells and the macula densa, a part of the distal tubule. In the macula densa, the distal tubular cells have a different morphology. The basement membrane outside the macula densa disappears, bringing the macula densa and the afferent arteriole into close contact. The close relationship between the distal tubule and the afferent arteriole appears to be the basis for the following feedback mechanism, which controls the blood flow through the afferent arteriole. When the blood pressure is low, the juxtaglomerular cells secrete renin, which converts angiotensin, a plasma protein produced by the liver, into angiotensin I. Angiotensin I is converted to angiotensin II by an enzyme found in pulmonary tissue. Angiotensin II, a vasoconstrictor, causes the systematic arterioles to constrict. It stimulates the adrenal cortex to secrete aldosterone. The aldosterone causes increased sodium resorption and, thus, increased extracellular fluid. As the sodium level rises, the macula densa slows the secretion of renin. The amount of angiotensin II in the body also reflects the amount of circulating renin. Thus, as renal blood flow is decreased, renin secretion increases. When renal blood flow increases, renin secretion is decreased.

Glomerulotubular Feedback

The term *glomerulotubular balance* describes a phenomenon in which the nephron itself is a feedback loop. Glomerulotubular feedback implies that an interrelationship exists between changes in the proximal tubular resorption of sodium and water and parallel increases or decreases in glomerular filtration rate. The net result of this relationship is to maintain a relatively constant percentage of reabsorbed sodium. The significance of each nephron maintaining a constant fraction of reabsorbed sodium is to preserve the extracellular fluid volume.

The mechanism by which proximal tubular sodium reabsorption varies with changes in the glomerular filtration rate so as to keep the proportion of filtered sodium reabsorbed relatively constant is not clearly understood. The results of experiments designed to determine the mechanism of glomerulotubular balance conclude that an increase in the single-nephron glomerular filtration rate in an intact nephron causes an increase in the tubular flow rate or a change in the chemical composition of tubular fluid past the macula densa cells. This change from the normal is sensed by the macula densa cells, and they, through unknown mechanisms, increase the synthesis and release of renin-angiotensin-aldosterone, causing a resultant decrease in glomerular filtration rate.[2] As a result of the feedback loop, it is suggested that whole-kidney glomerular filtration rate and, secondarily, renal blood flow are autoregulated.[2]

Intrarenal Vasoactive Systems

In addition to functioning as a filtering organ, the kidney also functions as an endocrine organ. As the primary receiver of information (with the afferent arteriole acting as its baroreceptor), the juxtaglomerular apparatus can directly alter the rate of the release of renin in response to changes in arterial pressure and the subsequent generation of angiotensin II. This hormone is a potent vasoconstrictor as well as being able to stimulate the release of aldosterone from the adrenal cortex.

Angiotensin II restores renal perfusion toward normal by increasing systemic blood pressure and, through aldosterone, by augmenting the effective circulating blood volume. Angiotensin II causes renal arteriolar constriction; therefore, it is believed to play a role in the regulation of intrarenal blood flow and glomerular filtration rate.[9] A negative-feedback loop occurs as angiotensin II, acting directly on the juxtaglomerular cells, and aldosterone, by its action to augment volume, decrease renin secretion.[9]

Aldosterone is an important factor in the body's response to a fall in extracellular fluid volume. The major factor controlling aldosterone secretion is the plasma concentration of angiotensin II, which in turn is controlled by the rate of renin secretion. Angiotensin II stimulates the zona glomerulosa of the adrenal cortex to produce aldosterone. Aldosterone acts on the distal tubule and collecting ducts to increase the reabsorption of sodium and hydrogen. The subsequent increase in salt and water reabsorption tends to increase extracellular fluid volume, which, acting through the renin system, exerts a negative-feedback influence on plasma angiotensin II concentration. As a result of the increased osmotic concentration in the extracellular fluid volume, ADH secretion is stimulated to produce a further increase in water reabsorption.

The secretion of aldosterone is not dependent only on the renin-angiotensin axis. Other factors influence aldosterone secretion. In addition to the plasma level of sodium, the secretion of aldosterone varies directly with plasma potassium. This effect is not mediated by renin-angiotensin, but rather acts directly on the zona glomerulosa.[9] Small increments in plasma potassium levels can induce a significant rise in aldosterone secretion. In addition to enhancing sodium reabsorption, aldosterone has the additional effect of promoting potassium secretion. The resultant increase in potassium excretion returns the plasma potassium toward normal and subsequently decreases aldosterone secretion.

The regulation of sodium balance and the maintenance of extracellular volume constancy are intimately related functions. Changes in sodium balance in general lead to corresponding changes in extracellular balance, and, conversely, changes in extracellular fluid volume exercise a feedback control over the rate of renal excretion of sodium. Extracellular fluid volume is regulated by a variety of receptors and overlapping effector mechanisms.

The osmotic changes in plasma result in the hypothalamic release of ADH from the posterior pituitary. Antidiuretic hormone acts primarily on the distal tubule cells and the collecting ducts. If the extracellular fluid is concentrated, ADH causes water to be resorbed and results in concentrated urine. If the extracellular fluid is diluted, ADH is not released, extracellular volume is decreased, and diluted urine results.

Renal Control of Water

Three basic processes are involved in the renal control of water: delivery of the filtrate to the ascending limb of the loop of Henle, separation of water from electrolytes in the ascending limb, and controlled resorption of water from the collecting duct under the influence of ADH.

Acid-Base Balance

Acids are formed continuously by the metabolic processes of the body. Each day, the healthy person eats food that contains proteins. The breakdown of the proteins produces hydrogen ions that contain sulfur and phosphorus, which form acids. Organic acids that are not metabolized by the body are also produced.

In order to maintain a normal acid-base balance, the lungs and kidneys constantly regulate the hydrogen ion concentration in the body fluids. The lungs act in minutes to eliminate carbonic acid. The kidneys can also directly excrete hydrogen ions. However, the correction of acid-base imbalances by the kidneys is a matter of hours or days, not minutes.

Maintenance of the acid-base balance implies the regulation of the hydrogen ion concentration in the body fluids. If the hydrogen ion concentration is great, the fluids are acidic; if the hydrogen ion concentration is low, the fluids are basic.

The mechanisms for maintaining the acid-base balance by the kidneys may be described as follows. Hydrogen ions are removed from the extracellular fluids when the hydrogen ion concentration becomes too great. Sodium and bicarbonate ions are removed when the hydrogen ion concentration becomes too low. For example, if the pH of extracellular fluid is alkaline, the urine pH also becomes alkaline owing to the loss of alkaline substances from the body fluids. If the pH of the extracellular fluid becomes acidic, the urine pH also becomes acidic owing to the loss of large amounts of acidic substances from the body fluids. In either situation, the pH is returned toward normal because of the loss of alkaline or acid substances.

Hydrogen ions are secreted continually into the tubular fluid by the distal tubule epithelium. Weak acids are formed when the hydrogen ions combine with the sodium salts contained in the tubular fluid and, thus, free the sodium ions bound in the salts. The sodium is then able to be resorbed through the tubular wall to return to the extracellular fluid. The hydrogen ion concentration is decreased by the loss of hydrogen ions from the extracellular fluid and sodium ion resorption. Thus, a net exchange of hydrogen for sodium ions occurs owing to the hydrogen ions' being excreted into the urine and the sodium ions' being resorbed. The process helps keep the fluid more basic and helps control the continuous formation of acid by the normal daily metabolic processes.

The hydrogen ion secretion into the distal tubules is determined by the carbon dioxide concentration in the extracellular fluid. An excess of carbon dioxide in the extracellular fluid is usually associated with increased carbonic acid and hydrogen ion concentrations, which indicate acidosis. When fluids are acidic, the hydrogen ion secretion is greater; thus, the kidneys attempt to eliminate the excess acid.

In alkalosis, alkaline substances combine with carbonic acid, forming bicarbonate salts; thus, the extracellular bicarbonate ion concentration is increased. As the bicarbonate ion concentration increases, the ions are excreted into the urine in the form of sodium bicarbonate. The excretion causes the loss of alkaline substances by the body, thus correcting the alkalosis.

CAUSATIVE AND PRECIPITATING FACTORS IN ACUTE RENAL FAILURE

Acute renal failure does not occur alone, but often is a multifactorial event in which a combination of concurrent or secondary etiologies may be involved (Table 33–1).

Surgery

The surgical patient, both intraoperatively and postoperatively, is exposed to a number of potential insults. Hypovolemia, hypotension, ischemia, sepsis, toxic pigments, and nephrotoxic agents are clinical events that might adversely affect the surgical patient. Even in the absence of these hazards, acute renal failure can occur.

General anesthesia almost always poses a threat to the kidney. Anesthesia alters the renal hemodynamics and water and electrolyte excretion and increases the level of circulating catecholamines, angiotensin, and ADH. The net result of this hormonal imbalance is the disturbance of renal autoregulation and a subsequent compromise in normal renal blood flow.

Several surgical subgroups appear to be at high risk for developing ARF; these include patients undergoing cardiopulmonary bypass, abdominal aortic surgery, or major biliary tree surgery, elderly persons undergoing lengthy or major surgery, patients with pre-existing renal disease who are undergoing surgery, and those with major trauma.

Patients undergoing cardiac surgery have a 30% risk of developing acute renal failure.[2] The risk factors associated with cardiac surgery that predispose the patient to develop postoperative acute renal failure include the increased age of the patient undergoing this type of surgery, the presence of underlying renal disease, operations involving the tricuspid valve, severe congestive heart failure, and the duration of the operation. However, the most consistent factor is the duration of "pump time." Other factors increasing the risk of acute renal failure include low urinary output or the use of large doses of vasopressors to maintain a systolic pressure of 80 mm Hg during surgery.

Another subgroup of surgical patients at risk to develop postoperative acute renal failure are patients undergoing biliary tree surgery. Patients with obstructive jaundice have up to a 35% incidence of developing acute renal failure as opposed to those without jaundice.[2] Biliary tree obstruction interferes not only with biliary emptying but also with the blood supply, thus providing an opportunity for the rapid growth of bacteria. Patients with acute cholecystitis have positive bile cultures in 70% of cases; when common duct obstruction is present, this incidence increases to 90%.[2] Compounding biliary tree obstruction may be volume depletion secondary to vomiting and decreased oral intake, the sensitization of the renal tubules by the conjugated bilirubin to the development of ischemic damage, renal tubular endothelial damage by bile salts, and the development of endotoxic shock associated with gram-negative sepsis.

Sepsis is the most common cause of acute renal failure among surgical patients. The now-frequent gram-negative bacilli that often colonize surgical wounds cause devastating infections. Sepsis not only alters renal hemodynamics but also impairs renal function through immunologic mechanisms. Trauma, postoperative, and critically ill patients are at risk to develop sepsis because they have both an altered immune response and a decreased resistance to infection. Thus, such patients are unable to mount effective immune responses to combat septic processes from developing. Because the degree

Table 33–1

Causes and Precipitating Factors of Acute Renal Failure

	CLINICAL SITUATION	
CAUSE	**Decrease in Extracellular Fluid**	**Normal Extracellular Fluid**
Surgery	Hemorrhage Fluid and electrolyte losses Obstetrical complications Cardiac surgery Biliary tree obstruction	Cardiogenic shock Renal artery clamping Sepsis: genitourinary, biliary tract Intravascular catheters Intravascular clotting
Trauma	Thoracoabdominal wounds Malnutrition Sepsis Traumatic rhabdomyolysis Crush injuries, burns, electric shock	
Pigment-induced nephropathy	Nontraumatic rhabdomyolysis: physical exertion/heat stroke, prolonged coma, carbon monoxide poisoning Hemoglobinuria: mismatched blood transfusions, hemolysis	
Nephrotoxic drugs	Allergic interstitial nephritis: penicillin, diuretics (furosemide, thiazides), allopurinol, anticonvulsants Obstructive nephropathy: intratubular precipitation of drug or intratubular obstruction Acute tubular necrosis: aminoglycosides	

of immune suppression is related to the magnitude of the stress, the more contributory factors, the more likely the patient is to develop an infection.

Trauma

Trauma may either directly, as in abdominal, or indirectly, as in circulatory or respiratory failure, affect organ function. Hypoxia, especially if associated with decreased tissue perfusion, is a common factor contributing to acute renal failure. The interrelationships between organ systems help to explain the hazards of both acute postoperative renal failure and multiple organ trauma. Because the decline of one system challenges the functioning of the other organ systems, patient survival depends on identifying how to interrupt the cascading effect compounding this particular clinical situation. The patient with trauma may lose as much as 30% of his total body weight in as little as 11 days. The associated malnutrition contributes to impaired wound healing, wound dehiscence, and wound infection.

Pigment-Induced Acute Renal Failure

Drugs and chemicals may produce hemoglobinuria and myoglobinuria, with myoglobin-induced acute renal failure being the most common form. Rhabdomyolysis and myoglobinuria can occur under a variety of traumatic or nontraumatic circumstances in which muscle is subjected to stress beyond its capacity to produce energy.

Trauma still accounts for most cases of acute renal failure, although nontraumatic rhabdomyolysis is occurring with increasing frequency, especially in the substance-abuse patient. Rhabdomyolysis, long known to occur in crush injuries, extensive burns, and muscle inflammation, also occurs in a variety of clinical settings in which blood flow and metabolism are disturbed by inadequate oxygenation or muscle energy production is increased.[8] Mechanisms responsible for rhabdomyolysis in the patient with prolonged coma from alcohol or drug overdose are multiple: prolonged immobilization in one position, hypotension, dehydration, chronic malnutrition, and acidosis.

The prognosis of acute renal failure in traumatic rhabdomyolysis is poor primarily because of the underlying disease processes. Nontraumatic rhabdomyolysis and its associated acute renal failure, however, have a good prognosis.

Drug-Induced Acute Renal Failure

Nephrotoxic drugs may be ingested, inhaled accidentally in a confined space, given therapeutically, or taken in a suicide attempt. It is estimated that drug nephrotoxicity may cause as many as 20% to 30% of the instances of acute renal failure in teaching hospitals.[2] Patients with pre-existing renal disease, advanced age, and multiple medical problems are most likely to develop renal toxicity. Additionally, certain aspects of renal anatomy and physiology account for the system's susceptibility to various toxins.

Aminoglycosides, used widely to treat life-threatening infections from gram-negative organisms, are a prime causative agent of this form of acute renal failure. All the drugs in this group of antibiotics have demonstrated nephrotoxicity. Within the group, however, a spectrum of nephrotoxicities is seen.

The least nephrotoxic is spectinomycin, the most nephrotoxic is neomycin, and gentamicin, tobramycin, and amikacin have intermediate toxicity.

Another group of antibiotics that is potentially nephrotoxic is the cephalosporins, although the incidence of acute renal failure from this group is declining. Cephalosporins, particularly cephalothin, used in combination with an aminoglycoside potentiate aminoglycoside toxicity. The observed renal toxicity with the use of the cephalosporins appears to be dose-related, with frequency increasing in patients receiving more than 8 g/day.

Classification of Acute Renal Failure

A classification of acute renal failure must be considered when evaluating the patient with an impairment in renal function. The ability to identify the causative or precipitating factor of acute renal failure permits the nurse to recognize treatable or preventable causes of diminished renal function, to use findings gleaned from the history and physical examination, and to make use of the results of laboratory and radiographic studies.

Acute renal failure exists in three forms: prerenal oliguria, intrinsic renal failure (intrarenal), and postrenal failure. Table 33–2 summarizes the categories of acute renal failure with clinical situations.

Prerenal

Acute prerenal oliguria refers to decreased renal perfusion secondary to either a decline in cardiac output or fluid and electrolyte deficits resulting in diminished circulating blood volume. In prerenal oliguria, renal parenchymal damage usually does not occur. The kidneys remain physiologically normal and maintain their ability to excrete nitrogenous wastes in an economically small amount of water. As a direct result of renal hypoperfusion and subsequent reduced glomerular filtration rate, azotemia and a decreased load of filtered sodium excretion occur. The physiologic response to hypovolemia or an ineffective circulating blood volume is to call into play the extrarenal defense mechanisms of autoregulation, baroreceptors, and osmotic receptors.

Because the abnormalities observed in prerenal oliguria are functional, prompt diagnosis is important; otherwise, prolonged hypoperfusion may result in the development of renal parenchymal damage or intrarenal failure. It is important to remember that the only difference between prerenal oliguria and intrarenal failure is the lack of parenchymal renal damage and the rapid reversibility of the former.

Intrarenal

The intrarenal causes of acute renal failure are a change in the interstitium, the site of resorption in the kidneys, and diseases that involve the nephron. When the cause is intrarenal, the kidneys are no longer able to excrete the nitrogen waste produced by protein metabolism. The tubules are damaged and cannot concentrate urine.

Postrenal

The postrenal causes of acute renal failure occur in 1% to 10% of patients with a sudden decrease or increase in the urine

Table 33–2
Major Categories of Acute Renal Failure

CATEGORIES	CLINICAL SITUATION
Prerenal	
Hypovolemia	Extracellular fluid volume loss, *e.g.*, from internal or external sources
	Burns
	Hepatorenal syndrome
Cardiovascular failure	Cardiogenic shock, dysthythmias
	Congestive heart failure
	Cardiac tamponade
Systemic arterial hypotension	Vascular pooling from sepsis or anaphylaxis
	Obstetrical complications
Venous thrombosis	Embolic phenomena resulting from myocardial infarction, ventricular aneurysm, atrial fibrillation, trauma, cholesterol or atheromatous clot after major surgery
Intrarenal	
Damage to basement membranes Interstitial diseases	Systemic lupus
	Allergic interstitial disease secondary to antibiotics, anesthesia and contrast agents, solvents, heavy metals
	Chemical dependency abuse
Miscellaneous	Eclampsia, thrombolic phenomenon from hemolytic uremic syndrome, idiopathic postpartum renal failure
Pigment nephropathy	Transfusion reactions, muscle damage from crush injuries or extensive exercising, heat stroke
Postrenal	
Extrarenal or intrarenal obstruction	Renal calculi, blood clots, neoplasms, ureteral edema, benign prostatic hypertrophy, extensive retroperitoneal disease
Bladder rupture	Trauma or surgical accident

output. An output that varies from day to day when the intakes are stable increases the suspicion that a bladder outlet obstruction is present. In postrenal states, the kidney functions properly, but the urine does not leave the bladder. The obstructions occur below the level of the collecting ducts, anywhere from the pelvis of the kidney to the external urethral orifice. The obstructions are either functional or anatomic. Functional obstructions can follow the use of drugs that interrupt the autonomic supply to the urinary passages or the bladder (*e.g.*, antihistamines and ganglionic blocking drugs). Anatomic obstructions may be caused by the encroachment of adjacent abdominal or pelvic organs on the bladder or by tumors, stones, or strictures.

Differential Diagnosis

The diagnosis of acute renal failure is primarily exclusion of causative factors. Tables 33–3 and 33–4 summarize the problem-solving process of establishing the diagnosis of acute renal failure. The following laboratory and radiographic investigations are done in patients suspected of having or known to have acute renal failure.

Laboratory Studies

Laboratory studies include determinations of the serum sodium, chloride, potassium, bicarbonate, creatinine, uric acid,

Table 33–3
Assessment Parameters of Patient With Acute Oliguria

Does true oliguria exist?	Total 24-hour urine output
	Daily weight
	Serial laboratory values
	Rule out outlet obstruction: ultrasound, intravenous pyelogram
	Rule out physiologic oliguria
	Rule out circulatory insufficiency
Does intrinsic renal failure exist?	
If intrinsic acute renal failure exists, is the cause hidden or apparent?	Medical history
	Clinical setting
	Input and output
	Physical examination: tachycardia; blood pressure, sitting and lying; decreased skin turgor; dry mucous membranes
	Urinary electrolytes
	Urine creatinine clearance
	Renal failure index

Table 33-4
Laboratory Differential Diagnosis of Acute Renal Failure

LABORATORY DETERMINATIONS	OPTIMUM RENAL FUNCTION	PRERENAL	RENAL	POSTRENAL
Plasma				
Creatinine	0.6–1.5 mg/100 ml			
Urea nitrogen				
Urea-creatinine ratio	10–15:1	>15:1	~10:1	~10:1
Urine				
Volume (ml/day)	500–2500	<500	Variable	<500
Specific gravity	1.010–1.015	>1.015	~1.010	~1.010
Osmolality (mOsm/kg H_2O)	400–600	>500 or >100 mOsm more than plasma	<350 or equal to plasma	<400
Sodium (mEq/L)	15–40	<10	>40	Usually >20, but <40
Potassium (mEq/L)	15–40	Variable	Variable	Variable
Urine-Plasma Concentration Ratios				
Osmolality	1.5:1–2:1	>1.5:1	<1.1:1	<1:1
Creatinine	1.2–1.7 g	>40	<20	24 hours
Urea	20	>10:1	<4:1	<8:1
FeN_a	7%	<1.0	>1.0	<1.0
Renal failure index	1%	<1.0	>1.0	<1.0

and blood urea nitrogen (BUN) levels and of the osmolality. If there is no extensive muscle damage, the serum creatinine level is less sensitive than the BUN level to prerenal and to other catabolic factors; therefore, it reflects renal function more closely.

Determinations of the hemoglobin, hematocrit, and the white blood cell count should be done, and a blood smear should be evaluated. Because it has become more widely known that disseminated intravascular coagulation can cause acute renal failure, coagulation studies are often done, depending on the clinical setting. The coagulation studies include determinations of the prothrombin time, clotting time, bleeding time, partial thromboplastin time, platelet count, and the fibrinogen level. If disseminated intravascular coagulation is detected, the early administration of heparin could prevent permanent renal damage.

Urinalysis

A few studies of the renal function and of the urine can show whether the renal function is normal or abnormal and, if it is abnormal, to what degree. If bladder outlet obstruction is suspected, an in-and-out bladder catheterization should be performed. Urine specimens should be obtained before the patient is given diuretics; only then are the sodium determinations reliable. The test results that are most helpful in the diagnosis of acute renal failure are a urine plasma osmolality ratio of 1:1, a urine urea nitrogen–blood urea nitrogen ratio of less than 10:1, and an elevated urinary sodium level (usually one that is higher than 20 to 30 mEq/L).

Creatinine Clearance

The creatinine clearance test measures renal excretory function. Creatinine, a byproduct of muscle metabolism, is excreted in the urine because of glomerular filtration. Therefore, it is in-dicative of the glomerular filtration rate. The creatinine clearance can be determined in the following manner:

U = urine creatinine (mg/100 ml)

V = urine volume (ml/min)

P = plasma creatinine concentration (mg/100 ml)

$$\text{Creatinine clearance} = \frac{UV}{P}$$

The normal serum values are about 0.6 mg to 1 mg/100 ml in women and 0.8 mg to 1.3 mg/100 ml in men. Throughout the day and from day to day, the plasma creatinine level varies little. Because the plasma creatinine concentration remains constant in persons with stable renal function, creatinine clearance can be determined by obtaining a 24-hour urine sample (or some other "timed" urine sample), determining the urine volume and the urine creatinine concentration, and obtaining a blood sample to determine the plasma creatinine concentration. To obtain accurate values, the urine sample must be a complete one.

When the kidneys are damaged by a disease, the creatinine clearance decreases and the serum creatinine concentration rises. In acute renal failure, the serum creatinine concentration is an adequate index of renal dysfunction. The urine creatinine clearance is often difficult to determine in a state of oliguria or anuria.

In some centers, two indices are being more frequently used. These are the fractional sodium excretion (*i.e.*, U/P Na/U/P creatinine $\times$ 100)—a comparison of the clearance of sodium to creatinine—and the renal failure index (*i.e.*, U Na/U/P creatinine $\times$ 100)—a modified version that assumes that plasma sodium concentration is equal in all patients and thus can be dropped from the equation.[3] A value of less than 1 for either index suggests that tubular function is intact and that prerenal acute oliguric failure may be reversible.

Electrocardiogram

An electrocardiogram (ECG) is obtained for baseline information and to assess the cardiac rhythm and any ectopy. During the phases of acute renal failure, the ECG can also serve as an immediate index of the serum potassium concentration.

Radiographs

The routine radiographic studies are a chest radiograph and a plain abdominal radiograph. The plain abdominal radiograph may be useful in determining the cause of acute renal failure. In acute renal failure, the kidneys are usually normal or may be enlarged. Radiologic evidence that the kidneys are small is a clue to chronic renal failure. Calcific densities indicate possible obstruction. In some patients, retrograde studies and ultrasound may be needed to gather further evidence of an obstruction.

Ultrasound

In general, ultrasonography has come to play an important role in the diagnosis of acute renal failure. Because ultrasound is basically morphologic and is independent of physiologic function, it can assess renal size, contour, and internal architecture. Thus, ultrasound can provide the clinician with the length of the kidney and can delineate any structural enlargement or obstructive uropathy to identify hydronephrosis and post–kidney transplant complications.

A major advantage of ultrasound is that it does not require the administration of contrast material. Another advantage is that the machine may be brought to the bedside and each kidney evaluated with the patient lying either prone or in a decubitus position. The diagnostic information from noninvasive ultrasound makes it an ideal for screening as well as for follow-up of treatment in many conditions.

Renal Biopsy

Rarely, a renal biopsy may be indicated for unexplained acute oliguric renal failure. The kidney biopsy is an invasive procedure, but it may be needed to arrive at a diagnosis and to manage the patient. It should be done only by the experienced physician, and some type of localization method should be used. A renal biopsy carries the risk of bleeding and hematuria. In some medical centers, ultrasonic guidance for renal biopsy is the method of choice.[3]

Pyelography

Valuable diagnostic information may be obtained by careful ureteral catheterization and retrograde dye injection or by the newer method of guided antegrade pyelography. The procedure demonstrates obstruction or stricture, the contour of an intraluminal mass, and it also allows the selective sampling of urine from each kidney.

It is important to remember that any procedure that might introduce infection may initiate pyelonephritis and subsequently increase intrarenal damage. If a ureteral catheter is left in place, sterile technique is essential. It is imperative that the closed drainage system not be broken for any reason. Frequent urine culture samples should be sent to identify pathogens and antibiotic sensitivities so that specific antibiotic treatment may be started early.

NURSING PROCESS

ASSESSMENT

The assessment phase of a patient suspected of having or of being at high risk for acute renal failure should include the history and physical examination. The history includes recent surgery, trauma, infections, or diseases involving the kidneys, diseases that are associated with low kidney perfusion, drug history, ingestion of toxins, recent hypersensitivity response, urination patterns, and cardiac or liver disease.

In the acute situation, the physical examination should include blood pressure and pulse, noting any significant changes, hypotensive state, or orthostatic changes. The change from normal in the patient's level of consciousness is assessed. The nurse must observe the urine output pattern, urine volumes, and specific gravity along with the patient's weight. Hydration states should be assessed along with pallor. With hypovolemia, tachycardia, tachypnea, decreased skin turgor, and any mucous membranes may be present. Blood pressure is usually low, with small pulse pressure, and there may be orthostatic hypotension. The temperature is usually not elevated. States of hypervolemia must also be assessed. With hypervolemia, the patient's pulse is rapid and may be bounding. Respirations are rapid, and symptoms of dyspnea may be observed. Moist rales can be heard with auscultation. Blood pressure can be normal to high. The patient's tongue may be moist, and the saliva may be excessive and frothy. Signs of pitting edema may be seen over bony prominences. The patient's skin may be moist, warm, and wrinkled from the pressure of linens or clothes. Hydration states should always be assessed along with electrolyte data.

Acute renal failure can occur in any clinical setting. Typically, a rapid decrease in renal function accompanied by progressive azotemia with or without oliguria is seen. In progressive azotemia, the BUN and creatinine levels become elevated over several days (about 20 mg to 30 mg/100 ml/day and 1 mg to 2 mg/100 ml/day, respectively). The BUN and creatinine levels rise as a result of a decrease in urea clearance by the kidney. The normal ratio of BUN to creatinine is 10 to 15:1, and the ratio of elevation is maintained in a stepwise fashion. Disproportionate elevations are observed closely in the differential diagnosis of acute renal failure. The progressive elevations of plasma BUN and creatinine levels over several days with or without oliguria are an indication of acute renal failure. Oliguria implies that the urinary output is less than 400 ml/day. Although the clinical course of acute renal failure can be dramatic, it is one of the few kinds of organ failure that is completely reversible.

NURSING DIAGNOSES, PATIENT OUTCOMES, AND PLAN

The preceding material on anatomy, physiology, nursing assessment, and diagnostic tests guides the nurse in establishing

NURSING CARE PLAN SUMMARY *Patient With Acute Renal Failure*

NURSING DIAGNOSIS

1. *Altered fluid and electrolyte balance related to renal dysfunction and massive muscle destruction (exchanging pattern)*

Patient Outcome	Nursing Orders
The patient will not develop complications as a result of abnormal serum levels.	1. Weigh patient once a day. 2. Observe for distended neck veins or dyspnea every hour. Listen to heart rate, rhythm, and the presence or absence of a gallop rhythm. 3. Measure central venous pressure every hour. 4. Keep an accurate record of input and output, and total every 8 hours. Total 24-hour intake should be restricted to 1500 cc. 5. Monitor heart rate, rhythm, and presence or absence of U wave. 6. Measure serum K potassium level every 8 hours. 7. Perform complete blood count daily. 8. Care of CVP catheter: Change dressing every 3 days. Keep dressing air-occlusive at all times. Send blood specimen and swab of skin around insertion site every 3 days. Change dressing using strict aseptic technique. Take temperature every 4 hours. 9. Assess arterial blood gases every 12 hours. 10. Measure serum creatinine levels every 24 hours.

NURSING DIAGNOSIS

2. *High risk for impaired gastrointestinal function related to uremic syndrome (exchanging pattern)*

Patient Outcome	Nursing Orders
Patient will not develop parotitis or a gastrointestinal bleed.	1. Exercise careful mouth care to prevent crusting and ulceration. 2. Have hard candies at bedside. 3. Use soft toothbrush. 4. Guaiac test all stool and vomitus. 5. Measure complete blood count and platelets every day. Obtain prothrombin and partial thromboplastin and clotting time twice a week or on nondialysis days. 6. Administer Zantac, 150 mg orally, every 12 hours. 7. Use electric razor when shaving.

NURSING DIAGNOSIS

3. *Altered nutrition: less than body requirements (anorexia) related to uremic syndrome (exchanging pattern)*

Patient Outcome	Nursing Orders
Patient will maintain normal weight or not exceed expected daily weight loss of 0.3 to 0.5 kg.	1. Explain to the patient and family the reason for a 300-g carbohydrate, 100-g protein, and 3-mEq potassium diet. 2. Ask dietitian to consult with patient to plan food preferences to be within dietary constraints. 3. Maintain 1500-cc fluid restriction. 4. Weigh patient daily. 5. Measure BUN and creatinine levels predialysis and on nondialysis days. 6. Assess and record level of consciousness in nurses notes.

(continued)

NURSING CARE PLAN SUMMARY *Patient With Acute Renal Failure* *Continued*

NURSING DIAGNOSIS

4. *Altered activities of daily living related to acute renal failure processes (moving pattern)*

Patient Outcomes	*Nursing Orders*

1. Patient or family will discuss situation and ask for help with methods of coping.	1. Explain usual course of acute renal failure.
	  A. Explain all procedures and treatments, and assess patient and family understanding.
	  B. Help patient and family express anxiety stressors and fears.
	  C. Maintain contact with patient in daily care to increase patient participation in recovery.

2. Patient or family will use relaxation techniques.	2. Teach patient and family to use relaxation techniques.

NURSING DIAGNOSIS

5. *High risk for noncompliance related to inadequate knowledge of acute illness (choosing pattern)*

Patient Outcome	*Nursing Orders*

The patient will verbalize knowledge of acute renal failure and follow-up care during the recovery phase of acute renal failure.	1. Teach the patient the following knowledge base:
	  A. Definition of acute renal failure
	  B. Pathophysiologic changes
	  C. Medications
	  D. Diet
	  E. Rest and progressive activity schedule. Encourage some daily exercise such as walking.
	2. Inform patient that it may be 6 to 12 weeks or longer (3 to 12 months) before kidney function returns to normal.
	3. Encourage activity within patient's limitations. He may return to work within 4 to 6 weeks after discharge or, if recovery is prolonged, within 3 to 12 months.
	4. Explain when to contact physician or clinic for follow-up care.
	5. Maintain contract with patient during recovery. Help patient set realistic goals.

---

nursing diagnoses, patient outcomes, and the plan for the patient with acute renal failure.

IMPLEMENTATION AND EVALUATION

The diverse etiologies of acute renal failure make the clinical course extremely variable. Acute renal failure may be either oliguric or nonoliguric. The incidence of acute nonoliguric renal failure is difficult to estimate, because often it goes unrecognized because the patient seems to have an adequate urine output.

Clinical Picture and Course of Acute Nonoliguric Renal Failure

Acute nonoliguric renal failure usually occurs as a complication of surgery, shock, trauma, nephrotoxic drugs, or infection. If it is diagnosed early, it can be managed easily and conservatively. It is usually not fatal.

Although oliguria is considered a cardinal feature of acute renal failure, nonoliguric acute renal failure was considered to be an uncommon clinical entity. Acute nonoliguric renal failure is now recognized not only for its prevalence, perhaps accounting for as many as 20% to 30% of all cases of acute renal failure but also for its more favorable natural history.[2,3]

The patient who has acute nonoliguric renal failure has progressive azotemia without oliguria. He usually voids from one to several liters of urine per day. Typically, such a patient has increasing azotemia for 10 to 12 days and a return toward normal for the next 10 to 12 days. During the peak period of azotemia, the patient's urine volumes also peak and then slowly return to normal. The electrolyte and BUN levels must be observed closely so that the physician can regulate the patient's electrolyte management according to daily urine output. Even when a patient's urine output is normal, fluid overload can still occur and precipitate pulmonary edema. Dialysis is often not required in acute nonoliguric renal failure. The complications of the condition are similar to those of acute oliguric renal failure, but electrolyte, fluid, and nutritional problems are more easily managed. Infection, overhydration, dehydration, and hyperkalemia are the most frequently occurring complications, and they are managed as they are in acute oliguric renal failure.

Clinical Picture and Course of Acute Oliguric Renal Failure

Initiating Phase

The important point of the initiating phase is prevention. This means recognizing the clinical situations that potentially may result in acute renal failure and identifying preventive measures. As a general rule for ensuring adequate extracellular volume, no uniform prophylactic measure is available for avoiding acute renal failure.

The customary therapy revolves around ensuring an adequate circulating blood volume by replacing any deficits and by using diuretics, either mannitol or furosemide. The mechanism or mechanisms by which diuretics are useful remain unclear. Regardless of how they work, their usefulness remains controversial. When administered early to a select group of patients, diuretics may favorably alter the course of acute renal failure.[3] However, the use of diuretics is not without hazards, because these drugs may precipitate acute renal failure in the patient with prerenal azotemia and marginally effective renal perfusion.

Mannitol, an osmotic diuretic, is believed to have a beneficial effect on the kidney itself and to prevent the development of renal insufficiency when administered before a high-risk situation begins. Mannitol has no known biologic or metabolic activity. It is readily filtered across the glomeruli into the tubular lumen, but it is not reabsorbed.

The main principle with the clinical use of mannitol is to administer the smallest continual or intermittent dose to maintain a urine volume of 50 ml to 100 ml/hour or more. The method of administration depends on the goal of treatment. However, mannitol is not without hazard. Its administration may result in an abrupt increase in plasma volume with precipitation of pulmonary edema or congestive heart failure, especially when urine flow rates remain low. However, if a brisk diuresis occurs, a much larger proportion of mannitol is excreted, and it is unlikely that a significant increase in plasma volume will occur.

Another group of medications that may be used in the initiating phase are the "loop" diuretics, furosemide or ethacrynic acid. Loop diuretics block tubular reabsorption of sodium and water, but they do not have the volume-expanding effects of mannitol. Therefore, loop diuretics are not likely to precipitate pulmonary edema or congestive heart failure. When effective, however, the loop diuretics are likely to induce more volume depletion than mannitol.

At the present time, furosemide is the most commonly used loop diuretic. When given intravenously, furosemide begins to act within minutes, and its effects last 2 to 3 hours. The majority of side-effects consist of fluid and electrolyte imbalances.

Maintenance Phase

Once the patient has established acute renal failure, therapy is directed toward problems that contribute to the morbidity and mortality of this phase. With the cessation of renal function, fluid and electrolyte balance, acid-base balance, endocrine and metabolic functions, and excretory functions must be assumed by medical personnel caring for the patient.

Fluid Balance. The major cardiovascular complications in acute renal failure are due to volume overload or electrolyte abnormalities; pulmonary edema, hypertension, and cardiac dysrhythmias can complicate medical management. Consequently, fluid management must be carefully monitored to prevent circulatory overload. Fluid management is based on the assessment of fluid status, by physical examination or hemodynamic monitoring, and by matching of input and output with consideration for insensible losses. Water ingestion is carefully recorded. Accurate daily weights are a must. Adult water need has been determined to average 400 ml/day. This amount will maintain serum sodium concentrations around 140 mEq/L. When the patient's sodium concentration rises above 140 mEq/L, his water intake should be increased to avoid excessive thirst. If the patient's serum sodium falls below 135 mEq/L, water should be reduced. Because of the increased catabolism, a stable daily weight may actually represent loss of lean body mass and thus indicate fluid retention. Patients can also develop hyponatremia because of the kidneys' inability to excrete free water to match free-water intake. Urine electrolytes should be measured and fluid replacement tailored to match salt and water excretion. Fluid intake may be restricted to the volume required to replace renal and extrarenal losses. Diuretics also may be used to attempt to treat volume overload; frequently, however, the response is either absent or inadequate. Continuous arteriovenous hemofiltration (CAVH) is a procedure that has become popular in critical care settings as an effective method of ultrafiltration. One indication for the use of CAVH is hypervolemia with or without renal failure in patients with acute pulmonary edema or congestive heart failure who are unresponsive to diuretic therapy. However, in the overall clinical picture, dialysis may be the only choice in treating the patient's fluid balance.

Potassium Balance. Hyperkalemia is the most feared metabolic complication of acute renal failure. Hyperkalemia occurs despite adherence to a potassium-restricted intake. The cessation of obligatory potassium excretion and the resulting uremia and acidosis of acute renal failure favor the accumulation of potassium in the extracellular compartment.

Because hyperkalemia has significant effects on the cardiac conduction system, the serial ECG results must be evaluated carefully; the plasma potassium levels do not always correlate with the ECG results. Dysrhythmias occur often. Probably they are most often caused by an electrolyte imbalance and a fluid overload, but they can be caused by hyperkalemia. Digitalis intoxication is also a cause of dysrhythmias in those patients with electrolyte imbalance. It has been suggested that hyperkalemia can be classified as minimal, moderate, or severe. Hyperkalemia can be treated by several different methods, depending on the degree of hyperkalemia. Potassium can be removed from the body by ion exchangers (*e.g.*, Kayexalate) in minimal hyperkalemic states. If Kayexalate is used, for every milliequivalent of potassium removed, 1 mEq of sodium is put in as the exchange. If a patient is in cardiac failure, the physician must be careful not to overload him or her with sodium. If the patient cannot take an oral medication, the cation exchange resin may be administered by a retention enema.

Kayexalate, which is given by mouth or in an enema, usually reduces an elevated serum potassium level by 1 or 2 mEq every 24 to 48 hours. If Kayexalate is given in an enema, the patient should retain the enema for 30 to 60 minutes so that the potassium can be removed. It is preferable to give Kayexalate by mouth because the oral route allows the resin to come in direct contact with more of the gastrointestinal tract and thus pick up more potassium. Sorbital may be given with Kayexalate to cause osmotic diarrhea and thus help excrete potassium and prevent constipation.

Kayexalate should not be given in fruit juices because the potassium in the fruit juices binds with the resin and so renders Kayexalate ineffective.

In moderate hyperkalemic states, potassium can be shifted from the extracellular to the intracellular fluid by the infusion of hypertonic glucose and insulin. This treatment can be effective within 30 minutes. If the patient is acidotic and not fluid-overloaded, sodium bicarbonate may be added to the infusion.

In severe hyperkalemia, the most effective treatment for cardiac intoxication is calcium infusion. Cardiac intoxication may be antagonized by raising the serum calcium concentration without altering the serum potassium concentration. This treatment has an effect in 5 minutes. Because the effect is of short duration, it should be followed by the intravenous administration of glucose and bicarbonate. Hyperkalemia increases the neuromuscular excitability by lowering the resting potential toward the threshold level, and hypercalcemia opposes this state by decreasing the threshold level. It is usually necessary to begin dialysis for patients who have moderate-to-severe hyperkalemia because the measures just discussed have only transient effects.

Sodium Balance.   Hyponatremia is a common event during the maintenance phase of acute renal failure, and it is usually due to a failure to consider endogenous water production and exogenous fluid administration in calculating fluid balance. Sodium intake should be limited to measured losses, which usually amount to about 20 mEq/day in the oliguric patient and more in the nonoliguric patient.

The most practical and readily available guide to sodium requirements in the patient revolves around daily weights. Sometimes it is useful to measure urinary sodium excretion as a guide to replacement therapy.

Acid-Base Balance.   In acute renal failure, metabolic acidosis is common and arises from the kidney's inability to excrete the normal acid load resulting from catabolism. Basal acid production is approximately 1 mEq/kg/day, but when there is increased catabolism or superimposed acid load, metabolic acidosis may be severe. Because protein restriction to minimize the azotemia usually decreases the acids of metabolism, unless the serum bicarbonate falls below 15 mEq/L, specific sodium bicarbonate replacement is not usually required. If acidosis is a clinical problem, bicarbonate replacement should be undertaken with caution in acute renal failure. In particular, bicarbonate replacement represents a considerable salt and water load to a patient who has an impaired ability to handle salt and water.

Endocrine Dysfunction: Calcium and Phosphate Metabolism. In mild renal failure, serum phosphate levels remain within normal range owing to a decrease in tubular reabsorption of phosphate mediated by parathyroid hormone. Aluminum-containing antacids may be used to bind phosphate in the gastrointestinal tract in order to avoid or treat hyperphosphatemia. However, at a glomerular filtration rate of less than 25 cc/min, the significant decrease in filtered phosphate produced hyperphosphatemia in spite of decrease in tubular reabsorption. At this level of glomerular filtration rate, the level of serum calcium decreases owing to a combination of physiologic events: decreases in vitamin D synthesis and abnormalities of parathyroid hormone action. Often phosphate control associated with mild hypocalcemia does not require therapy. Sometimes hypocalcemia can be severe, especially in the early stages of acute renal failure or rhabdomyolysis. Under these conditions, intravenous administration of calcium may be necessary. Should it be necessary to correct acidosis, it is important to remember that acidosis increases and alkalosis decreases the fraction of serum calcium that is in the ionized form. The significance of this is that rapid correction of systemic acidosis or the presence of alkalosis may precipitate acute manifestations of hypocalcemia, including tetany and convulsions.

Nutrition.   Proper dietary management in acute renal failure is aimed at minimizing protein catabolism, limiting the accumulation of nitrogenous wastes, nonvolatile acids, and potassium in the extracellular fluid, and preventing malnutrition so that healing is not delayed and resistance to infection is not decreased. The patient with acute renal failure is in a hypercatabolic state and as such requires a greater caloric intake and a protein diet of higher biologic value than the diet of the metabolically stable patient. Because acute renal failure is a physiologic stress, the patient's metabolic status is such that endogenous stores of carbohydrate, fat, and protein are all catabolized concurrently to provide energy for metabolic processes. The first principle of nutritional management is to supply enough carbohydrate to prevent protein breakdown. A minimum of 100 g of carbohydrate is administered first because it is protein-sparing and because the carbon fragments can be metabolically recycled to produce the nonessential amino acids. The second principle is to supply enough total calories and enough total protein to restore positive nitrogen balance. This is accomplished by supplying 1800 to 2500 calories/day and 20 to 25 g of protein/day.

When clinical circumstances preclude oral intake, the principles of proper dietary management are incorporated into the formulation of an appropriate regimen for parenteral nutrition. The specific composition of total parenteral nutrition in patients with acute renal failure must reflect their need for high energy requirements, insulin resistance, and negligible water and urea clearance.

Use of intralipid infusions also provides a source of nonprotein calories, and in catabolic patients with uremia who need greater quantities of energy, these emulsions can be used in lieu of glucose to avoid any potential problems resulting from glucose loading.

Metabolic parameters must be followed closely to ensure that fluid and electrolyte hemostasis are maintained adequately.[4] In order to accommodate the volume of hyperalimentation necessary to achieve fluid and electrolyte hemostasis, CAVH or dialysis may become necessary.

Hematologic Complications. Anemia is a complication that usually occurs during the first week of oliguria. It is caused by a mild increase in the erythrocyte destruction and a deficiency in the red blood cell production. Both erythropoiesis and red cell survival are diminished in acute renal failure. The predominant mechanism varies with the type and the acuteness of the renal disease. Blood replacement is usually not required. If it is required, it should be given in the form of packed red blood cells to avoid serious overexpansion of the plasma volume.

Bleeding abnormalities are common in uremia and have been a significant cause of morbidity and mortality. Prolonged bleeding time is the result of platelet dysfunction.[4] Infusion of cryoprecipitate and administration of DDAVP have been used in patients with uremia for temporary correction of the bleeding time in special situations.

Infection is one of the primary causes of death in patients with acute renal failure. The uremic state depresses cellular immunity and phagocyte function[4] and may well contribute to susceptibility to infection. The incidence of pulmonary, urinary tract, and wound infections are common, with a 51% to 89% incidence of septicemia.[4]

For the patient with acute renal failure who is in a critical care unit, it is imperative to avoid infection by diligent pulmonary hygiene, vigorous wound care, removal of bladder catheter, and refraining from using unnecessary venous and arterial catheters.

Excretory Dysfunction: Gastrointestinal Complications. Anorexia, nausea, vomiting, mucosal ulcerations, and gastrointestinal bleeding are the major gastrointestinal complications associated with acute renal failure. In the critically ill population, stress ulcers are common, and the bleeding tendency in uremia puts that patient at particular risk.

The approach to managing bleeding in the critically ill patient is the same as in any patient: prophylaxis with antacids or their antagonists. Should active bleeding occur, endoscopy is indicated.

Dialysis

Peritoneal Dialysis Versus Hemodialysis During Oliguria. Uncontrolled hyperkalemia, severe fluid overload, severe acidosis, and uremic symptoms are the chief indications for dialysis in acute renal failure.[2,4] When the BUN of the patient in acute renal failure exceeds 100 mg/dl, dialysis is usually seriously considered. A complicated clinical picture, in which early and severe manifestations of uremia can be expected, often leads to early and repeated dialysis before the overt signs and symptoms of uremia occur. Hemodialysis is usually highly preferable; it is a highly developed technology in centers where it is routinely used. The patient who requires dialysis must be assessed individually to determine whether he needs peritoneal dialysis or hemodialysis. Peritoneal dialysis may be the treatment of choice for the patient with acute renal failure in the absence of peritoneal pathology. It is contraindicated in the catabolic patient and is most useful in the noncatabolic patient who requires infrequent dialysis. Peritoneal dialysis

has the advantage that it can be done in virtually any hospital. The advantage of hemodialysis is that it can be done in a shorter period of time on patients who are not candidates for peritoneal dialysis and the same goals can be achieved.

Peritoneal Dialysis. Peritoneal dialysis involves a combination of three basic mechanisms: osmosis, diffusion, and filtration. Waste products are removed, and the fluid and electrolyte balance is re-established. The patient's peritoneum is used as the dialyzing membrane to replace the damaged kidneys via a closed drainage system (Fig. 33–2). The peritoneum approximates the surface area of the glomerular capillaries. In an acute situation in which dialysis might be life-threatening, peritoneal dialysis is time-consuming and inefficient. Technical problems are frequent, especially obstruction in the outflow and inflow of dialysate. In order to carry out peritoneal dialysis, the patient must be immobilized, which can predispose to pulmonary complications.

Two additional disadvantages of peritoneal dialysis are peritonitis (chemical versus bacterial) and protein and amino acid losses. It is impossible to avoid the loss of protein and amino acids during a course of peritoneal dialysis. Accumulated losses may be as great as 60 g of protein and 5 g to 10 g of amino acids during a 36- to 48-hour series of exchanges.

Hemodialysis avoids many of the problems described for peritoneal dialysis and is preferred if there is severe catabolism or if life-threatening hyperkalemia is present. However, hemodialysis requires special vascular access to an artery and a vein as well as greater technical support. Prompt access to the blood stream can be obtained through relatively simple percutaneous catheter placement into one of the subclavian or femoral veins may be performed at the bedside by an experienced physician. Such catheters may be left in place for two or three treatments, provided adequate attention is given to bleeding and infection at the insertion site.

The principles of peritoneal dialysis apply to hemodialysis as well. In hemodialysis, the semipermeable membrane is a

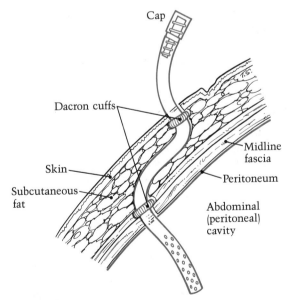

Figure 33–2
Placement of peritoneal catheter.

thin, porous plate of cellophane. Blood and dialysate are circulated on opposite sides of a semipermeable membrane that permits passage of low-molecular-weight substances, such as potassium and urea, but increasingly restricts the passage of high-molecular-weight substances, such as creatinine and uric acid. Because the dialysate is similar to the ultrafiltrate or the extracellular fluid, the appropriate adjustment of dialysate composition can either electively remove or add to the blood stream during hemodialysis. Therefore, hemodialysis has two major functions: solute removal and fluid removal.

Regardless of the technique selected for dialysis, many nephrologists believe that early prophylactic dialysis can potentially avoid much of the mortality and morbidity due to uremia, hyperkalemia, and severe acidosis. The role of early dialysis is controversial,[4] and the improvement in mortality probably rises according to the ability to provide support for severely catabolic patients and to prevent the occurrence of sepsis.

Continuous Arteriovenous Hemofiltration

Continuous arteriovenous hemofiltration is a recent advancement in the management of patients with multiple organ failure who have fluid and electrolyte disturbances and are hemodynamically unstable. This therapeutic technique is remarkably simple, because it avoids the use of an external blood pump and uses the patient's own blood pressure to deliver arterial blood to and through a biocompatible hemofilter. Systemic blood pressure is the driving force across the hemofilter to form an ultrafiltrate. The basic principles responsible for the efficiency of treatment are filtration, hydrostatic pressure, and convective solute removal. Within the hemofilter, an ultrafiltrate is produced by a transmembrane pressure gradient between hydrostatic pressure and the oncotic pressure. Initially, the pressure gradient favors formulation of a protein-free ultrafiltrate; as water is removed, the plasma protein concentration in the blood compartment rises gradually, and as the oncotic pressure equals the hydrostatic pressure, ultrafiltration ceases.[6] The ultrafiltrate drains by gravity through tubing into a collection bag. The height of the collection bag attached to the ultrafiltrate port creates a mild negative pressure in the blood chamber of the filter, further favoring ultrafiltration. Because blood cells and protein are returned through the venous access to the patient, the filter efficiently removes plasma, water, and dissolved solutes from the vascular space while retaining the cellular and protein constituents of the circulating blood.

Continuous arteriovenous hemofiltration is an extracorporeal system similar to that used in hemodialysis: Blood moves from the patient's arterial circulation through a filter and is returned to the patient's venous circulation. The filter consists of a semipermeable membrane that is composed of a bundle of fibers that are surrounded by a mesh covering and housed in a plastic cylindric filter. The surface area of the membrane is quite large and conductive to the passage of water and small solutes with a molecular weight of less than 50,000.[7] The CAVH membrane is extremely permeable, and large amounts of fluid can be removed with a relatively small pressure gradient. Arterial and venous tubing leave the filter at each end and attach to the patient's vascular access. The filter and tubing is primed with 40 ml of a special solution.

Internally, the filter is divided into blood and ultrafiltration compartments. Between the mesh covering and the plastic

filter is the ultrafiltration compartment. In the system, the patient's blood pressure acts as the pump that drives the blood through the blood compartment producing a filtrate. The amount of fluid that is removed is determined by the patient's blood pressure and the amount of volume overload present. Because there is the potential for rapid depletion of the vascular space, intravenous fluids must be administered to support the ultrafiltration rate and the integrity of the vascular space. Continuous arteriovenous hemofiltration has distinct advantages over hemodialysis, permitting large amounts of fluid removal slowly without associated osmolar changes. Therefore, the inappropriate autonomic function associated with rapid vascular compartment shift of hemodialysis does not occur with CAVH. The vascular response during CAVH acts to support cardiovascular stability. The main disadvantage of CAVH is its limited capacity to remove wastes and excess solute with minimal volume replacement.

Continuous arteriovenous hemofiltration does not change the osmolality of the extracellular fluid. The filtrate is free of protein and red blood cells and contains potassium, sodium, chloride, glucose, urea, and creatinine in amounts equal to concentrations present in the patient's plasma. Hence, CAVH does not effectively lower uremic toxins and potassium quickly in spite of the removal of significant quantities of plasma water. While the hemofilter removes the extracellular water and solutes, administering a predilutional filter replacement fluid enhances both the net urea clearance and ultrafiltration rate. The filter replacement fluid, a substitute for the ultrafiltrate that was removed, replaces all the plasma water constituents except for the unwanted uremic solutes. Thus, the filter replacement fluid used is a modified saline solution with added calcium and magnesium and either acetate or lactate as the major buffering anion.[6] Failure to replace the ultrafiltrate with an appropriate solution can cause hyperkalemia.

After the initial preparation of the filter and the institution of CAVH, the critical care nurse is responsible for maintaining the system and monitoring the patient. As with any procedure or treatment, safety and effectiveness depend on the nurse's keen assessment and her ability to identify complications. When complications do arise, the nurse must determine whether the problem is with the patient or with the equipment. In order to do so, the nurse must consider the CAVH common complications of bleeding, blood leak, decreases in ultrafiltration rate, and difficulty at the insertion site.

The nursing care of the patient requiring CAVH focuses on the following:

- Obtain baseline data: weight, vital signs, prothrombin time, partial thromboplastin time, arterial blood gas, complete blood count, creatinine concentration, and electrolyte levels.
- Keep accurate records of fluid losses and gains by monitoring intake and output, vital signs, and ultrafiltration rate hourly. Monitor clotting times every 6 hours. Maintain continuous heparin infusion to keep partial thromboplastin time 1.5 times normal. Monitor electrolytes and arterial blood gases every shift as indicated. Check complete blood count daily. Weigh patient daily.
- Assess the circuit for any mechanical problems. Observe the ultrafiltrate for clots or blood streaks every 2 hours. Test ultrafiltrate for blood with reagent strip every 4 hours. Keep Kelly clamp taped to the bed, and tape all connections. In order for the system to work efficiently, the arterial line

should be short, the tubing remain unobstructed, the hemo-filter kept below the level of the patient's heart, and the collecting system kept at least 18 inches below the filter. Obtain ultrafiltrate specimens to evaluate serum chemistries every 4 to 6 hours. Call physician if ultrafiltrate rate falls below 5 ml/min.

- Maintain aespsis of the system. Insertion sites must be assessed frequently for signs of bleeding or infection, and dressings should be changed daily.
- Prime filter and tubing according to manufacturer's recommendations, prepare replacement fluid and heparin infusion, connect the system using strict aseptic technique, administer initial heparin bolus, and then begin procedure by obtaining baseline ultrafiltration and blood flow rates.

Recovery Phase

The recovery phase is marked by a stepwise increase in urine volume, typically doubling each day. During the early diuretic phase, urine output may be high enough to be considered polyuric, because the patient may excrete more than 3 L/day.

Unless rigid fluid restriction is maintained, quantitative replacement will only perpetuate the obligatory salt and water losses. The patient should not be permitted a total oral intake of more than 3500 ml/day. The calculation of fluid intake is based on an amount equal to two thirds of the previous day's output.

Renal function may take up to 1 year to return to normal or to plateau at near-normal levels. Persistent abnormalities will exist in patients over 40.

SUMMARY

Acute renal failure is a condition in which renal excretory function is severely compromised. Acute renal failure may be due to hypovolemia, a decreased cardiac output, an altered peripheral resistance, and renal tubular degeneration from renal ischemia, toxic drugs, obstructions, or stricture. Acute renal failure has an abrupt onset and three clinical phases. The first phase is the initiating phase. The second is oliguria (a urine output of less than 400 ml/day), which usually lasts 10 to 14 days. The aim of treatment during the maintenance phase is to maintain the fluid and electrolyte balance and to avoid the complications of a negative nitrogen balance and fluid and electrolyte imbalances, which usually result in over-hydration, hyperkalemia, and infection. The third phase is the recovery phase. In this phase, the patient begins to show a progressive return of normal urine output. This phase lasts from 3 to 12 months. During the recovery phase, the patient must be educated about diet, medications, and follow-up medical care.

DIRECTIONS FOR FUTURE RESEARCH

Acute renal failure has an abrupt onset and is often a reversible condition. It is mandatory that critical care and hemodialysis nurses continue investigation in order to provide skillful management of the complex problems that can occur in this setting. Based on the research priorities for critical care nursing, research questions that may be considered are as follows:[5]

1. What methods for developing and implementing interdisciplinary teams in critical care are the most effective for reducing conflict and developing mutual support and respect?
2. What nursing interventions are effective in helping patients with acute renal failure maintain basic stress reduction?
3. What are the effects of different administration methods of nutritional alimentation on absorption, gastrointestinal mobility, patient comfort, and prevention of complications in the patient with acute renal failure?
4. Which nursing interventions are the most effective in creating a sense of independence and control in the patient with acute renal failure?
5. Which indicators most accurately reflect the nutritional status of the patient with acute renal failure?

REFERENCES

1. Beck, A., and Katcher, A. *Between Pets and People*. New York: G. P. Putnam's Sons, 1983.
2. Brenner, B. M., and Lazarus, J. M. *Acute Renal Failure* (2nd ed.). New York: Churchill Livingston, 1988.
3. Corwin, H. L., and Bonventre, J. V. Acute renal failure in the intensive care unit. Part 1. *Intensive Care Med.* 14:10, 1988.
4. Corwin, H. L., and Bonventre, J. V. Acute renal failure in the intensive care unit. Part 2. *Intensive Care Med.* 14:86, 1988.
5. Friedmann, E. Animal companions and one-year survival of patients after discharge from a coronary care unit. *Public Health Rep.* 95:307, 1980.
6. Golper, T. A. Continuous arteriovenous hemofiltration in acute renal failure. *Am. J. Kidney Dis.* 6:373, 1985.
7. Kiely, M. A. Continuous arteriovenous hemofiltration. *Crit. Care Nurse.* 49:39, 1984.
8. Kurokawa, K. Acute renal failure and rhabdomyolysis. *Kidney Int.* 23:888, 1983.
9. Rose, B. D. *Clinical Physiology of Acid-Base and Electrolyte Disorders.* New York: McGraw-Hill, 1989.

34

Gastrointestinal Disorders

James A. Fain

WHEN THINGS GO WRONG

Most of us want days filled with sunshine and flowers, with no upsetting moments to deal with. We spend much of our lives trying to achieve what we call "happiness," which we perceive as a state of continual, uninterrupted pleasure. Is this realistic? Is such a state possible? Is it even desirable?

In 1977 the Belgian physical chemist Ilya Prigogine was awarded a Nobel Prize for his theory of dissipative structures. The key idea is that orderliness in nature arises from chaos. Chaos is even necessary in many situations for the existence and origin of order. This means that order does not, and *cannot* exist on its own.*

Although developed in the physical sciences, Prigogine's idea has been applied to many other areas, including the domain of human experience. It says something important about the way we react when things go wrong. When chaos (*e.g.*, illness, poor health, financial setbacks), assails us this may be a blessing in disguise. Chaos in our lives may be setting the stage for a higher degree of order and happiness in our lives. Above all, it tells us we cannot have one without the other.

Nurses can draw on these ideas not only in interpreting their own experiences but in counseling patients as well. When a patient seems devastated, we can remind him of Prigogine's idea in terms he can understand (*e.g.*, "It is always darkest before the dawn," or "Every cloud has a silver lining"). These folksy expressions are not just empty consolations. They have the validation of modern science.

LEARNING OBJECTIVES

After reading this chapter, the nurse should be able to do the following:

1. Describe the structure and function of organs within the gastrointestinal tract.
2. List the common causes of upper gastrointestinal tract bleeding.
3. Describe the pathophysiology and pathogenesis of acute pancreatitis.
4. Identify the major signs and symptoms of acute pancreatitis.
5. Differentiate between acute and chronic pancreatitis.
6. Recognize abnormal laboratory and radiologic findings associated with pancreatitis.
7. Write appropriate nursing orders for a patient with pancreatitis.
8. Describe various treatment modalities associated with acute pancreatitis.

9. Identify major complications associated with acute pancreatitis.

CASE STUDY

Mr. P., age 58, was referred to the Medical Center for evaluation of chronic abdominal pain and weight loss. Mr. P. was 5 feet 10 inches tall and weighed 150 pounds. His temperature, obtained orally, on admission was 100°F, his resting pulse was 96, and his blood pressure was 126/76 mm Hg. He noted this onset of epigastric and left upper quadrant pain about 6 months earlier.

On physical examination, Mr. P. was underweight and appeared chronically ill. Abdominal examination revealed a well-healed laparotomy scar with no palpable masses. Rectal examination was normal, with stool being negative for occult blood. A complete blood count demonstrated a white blood cell count of 8200, a hemoglobin of 15.6, and a hematocrit of 45. Serum electrolytes, blood urea nitrogen, and creatinine concentrations were within normal limits. Fasting blood glucose was 152, and the 2-hour postprandial glucose level was 190. An upper gastrointestinal series was negative, with small bowel films revealing pancreatic calcification.

* Dossey L., Dissipative Structures. In *Space, Time and Medicine.* Boston: Shambhala, 1982: 82–97.

History of Past Illnesses

Eight years ago, Mr. P. was taken to the emergency room after vomiting bright red blood for 2 hours. The day before, he had vomited coffee-ground–colored material with some blood but was reluctant to come to the emergency room. Mr. P. had a nasogastric tube inserted that was irrigated with iced saline. After an endoscopy, Mr. P. was transferred to SICU. His diagnosis was upper gastrointestinal bleeding. On the third day after admission, Mr. P.'s condition began to stabilize. Two years later, Mr. P. had an oral cholecystogram that revealed cholelithiasis. At that time, Mr. P. underwent a cholecystectomy. The gallbladder contained six small, pigmented stones, and chronic inflammation was noted on histologic examination. The pancreas at that time was described as hard and nodular.

After the cholecystectomy, Mr. P. continued to experience frequent episodes (six to eight times a week) of epigastric pain. The pain, which was aching in nature, radiated to his back and was exacerbated by ingestion of large meals. Mr. P. gave a history of drinking three to four beers a day for 15 or so years. However, Mrs. P. revealed that he had actually been drinking six to eight beers a day for close to 20 years. Mr. P. smoked a pack of cigarettes each day.

At age 56, Mr. P. was admitted to the emergency room once again with a 2-day history of severe epigastric pain associated with nausea and vomiting and a low-grade fever. Based on his physical examination, laboratory results, and past history, a diagnosis of acute pancreatitis was made.

During the 6 months before admission for evaluation, Mr. P. had lost 15 to 18 pounds. On questioning him about his bowel habits, he reported his stools were greasy and left an "oily ring" in the toilet bowl. He denied the use of any medications except for an occasional aspirin. Review of his medical records revealed no history of polyuria, nocturia, hypercalcemia, hypertriglyceridemia, or abnormal liver tests.

REFLECTIONS

For Mr. P., the sight of vomiting bright red blood was a terrifying experience. In Mr. P.'s case, the event was rather sudden and unexpected. As for the cause of the bleeding, it was not readily apparent. In spite of not knowing the exact cause, fear and anxiety are two predictable responses that can occur when patients are severely bleeding. Mr. P. was no exception. Although it was obvious that immediate action needed to be taken to stabilize and manage Mr. P., it was essential not to lose sight of the need for emotional support for both him and his family.

Although fear and anxiety are predictable responses, critical care nurses must be aware that each individual's expression of fear and anxiety will be different depending on such factors as age, ethnic background, past experiences with similar situations, and usual coping patterns. Because of his joking with the staff about his experience of vomiting blood, Mr. P. could have been viewed by the nurses with disapproval. However, critical care nurses should be accepting and supportive when patients are thought to behave or respond inappropriately. Patients like Mr. P. are coping the best way they can and want to be assured that those caring for them are aware that they have anxieties that cannot be expressed. Thus, patients who appear to be calm and in control may be as frightened and unable to cope with their fears and anxieties as patients who overtly express their feelings. In order to deal with patients in these ever-changing and uncertain situations, nurses must foster personalization and communicate effectively.

The most important role critical care nurses can play in fostering personalization is to be open and talk to the patient while providing care. It means that nurses will meet and respond to the patient's face and eyes. It means that nurses will feel free to exchange thoughts, ideas, and feelings on a human level. It means that nurses will think about and feel what the patient is going through without turning away or without rushing.

Personalization begins as soon as the patient arrives in the critical care area. The attitude with which the patient is received will determine how he responds to those caring for him. Communicating with the patient involves conveying a warm, receptive attitude; meeting his eyes with concern; and offering a touch or gesture. Supportive measures in themselves are not always helpful or comforting; it is the way in which they are administered that makes a difference. Thus, the nurse's attitude can foster in the patient a feeling of personal uniqueness or a feeling of anonymity.

Mr. P.'s illness was unique to him. It was quite easy for him to magnify his fears and anxieties and distort the reality of the situation. The key to a personalized approach lies in the nurse's ability to create a supportive environment. Thus, the nurse must see Mr. P. as an individual who is trying to master his internal biologic crisis and cope with an unfamiliar environment. Once the nurse has achieved this perspective, Mr. P. will be viewed as a person, not an illness.

NORMAL PHYSIOLOGY OF THE GASTROINTESTINAL SYSTEM

The gastrointestinal tract can be thought of as a continuous tube running from the mouth to the colon. The gastrointestinal tract comprises the mouth, esophagus, stomach, small intestine, and large intestine. Each organ plays a vital role from the time food is eaten until it is digested and prepared for elimination. Muscular contractions in the wall of the gastrointestinal tract break down food physically, whereas secretions produced by various cells along the tract aid in the chemical breakdown of food.

A second group of organs, termed *accessory structures*, lie outside the gastrointestinal tract and produce or store secretions that likewise aid in the chemical breakdown of food. Such secretions are released in the gastrointestinal tract by way of ducts. These organs include salivary glands, liver, gallbladder, and pancreas.

The body is divided into various anatomic cavities. Organs of the gastrointestinal tract are located within the abdominopelvic cavity. This cavity is large and contains many organs. It is further divided into smaller areas called *quadrants* or *regions* (see Fig. 32–1, Chap. 32, p. 612).

Esophagus

The esophagus is a muscular, collapsible tube that lies behind the trachea and is about 23 cm to 25 cm (10 inches) long. It begins at the end of the laryngopharynx and terminates in the superior portion of the stomach. It neither produces digestive enzymes nor carries out the function of absorption. It secretes mucus and is responsible for transporting food to the stomach. Food is pushed through the esophagus by involuntary muscular movements called *peristalsis*. The passage of food (bolus) from the esophagus into the stomach is regulated by the lower esophageal sphincter (gastroesophageal).

The walls of organs from the esophagus to the large intestine have three distinct layers: mucosa, which is the innermost layer and lines the cavity or lumen of organs; submucosa, which is found just beneath the mucosa and consists primarily of connective tissue that contains blood vessels and nerve endings; and muscularis externa, which is the muscular layer commonly made up of smooth muscle cells.

Stomach

The stomach is a C-shaped enlargement of the gastrointestinal tract located directly under the diaphragm in the epigastric region that acts as a storage area for food as well as a site for food breakdown. It is divided into four sections: cardia, fundus, body, and pylorus. As food enters the stomach, secretions from gastric glands begin to reduce the bolus into a liquid called *chyme*. Most chemical digestion takes place in the plyoric region of the stomach through the action of an enzyme called *pepsin*. The convex lateral surface of the stomach is the greater curvature; its concave medial surface is the lesser curvature. After the food has been processed, it passes through the pyloric sphincter and enters the small intestine. This sphincter acts as a gatekeeper, controlling movement of food into the small intestines and preventing it from being overwhelmed (Fig. 34–1).

Small Intestine

Major portions of digestion and absorption occur in the small intestine, which extends from the pyloric sphincter to the ileocecal valve. It is divided into three divisions: the duodenum, which originates at the pyloric sphincter and curves around the head of the pancreas; the jejunum; and the ileum, which is the section that joins the large intestines at the ileocecal valve.

Large Intestine

The major functions of the large intestines are the completion of absorption and the formation and expulsion of feces from the body. It is divided into the cecum, appendix, colon, rectum, and anal canal. The saclike cecum is the first part of the large intestine. Attached to the cecum is a twisted, coiled tube called the *vermiform appendix*. The colon is divided into several regions. The ascending colon ascends on the right side of the abdominal cavity and makes a turn (right hepatic flexure) across the abdomen as the transverse colon. It curves again (left splenic flexure) and continues downward to the level of the iliac crest as the descending colon. The sigmoid colon begins at the iliac crest and terminates at about the third sacral vertebrae. The anal canal ends at the anus, which has an external voluntary sphincter and an internal involuntary sphincter (Fig. 34–2).

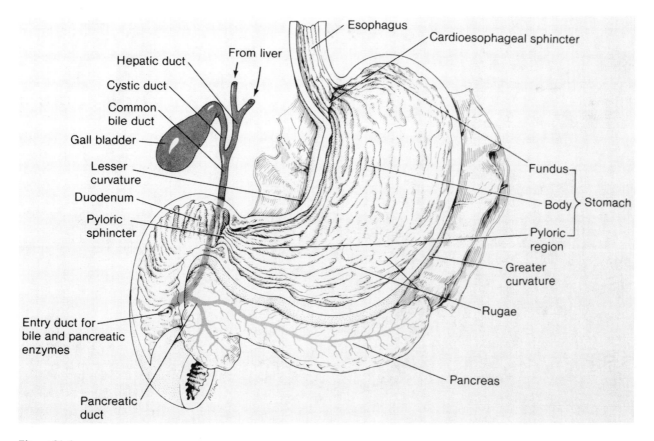

Figure 34–1

Anatomy of the stomach with hepatic, cystic, and pancreatic ducts.

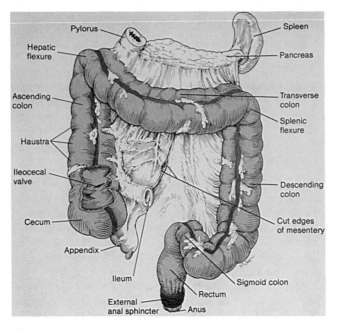

Figure 34–2
Anatomy of the large intestines.

Pancreas

The pancreas is a soft, oblong gland that extends across the abdomen and has both exocrine and endocrine functions. It lies behind the stomach and is divided into a head, body, and tail. The head of the pancreas is thicker and fills the C-shaped curve of the duodenum. The tail end reaches the spleen, whereas the middle portion, which extends horizontally, is the body. The pancreas is linked to the small intestines by two ducts. The large duct is called the *pancreatic duct* (duct of Wirsung). This duct unites with the common bile duct from the liver and gallbladder and enters the duodenum at the hepatopancreatic ampulla (ampulla of Vater). The smaller of the two ducts is the accessory duct (duct of Santorini), which originates from the duct of Wirsung and empties into the duodenum about 1 inch above the ampulla of Vater (Fig. 34–3).

Acini cells within the pancreas produce 1 to 2 quarts of pancreatic juice daily. It consists of water, sodium bicarbonate, electrolytes, and enzymes for digesting all three major food types (proteins, fats, and carbohydrates). Pancreatic juice is slightly alkaline (pH of 7.5 to 8.2), which stops the action of pepsin in the stomach and creates a proper environment for enzymes in the small intestines.[6,17] The enzymes in pancreatic juice include pancreatic amylase, a carbohydrate-digesting

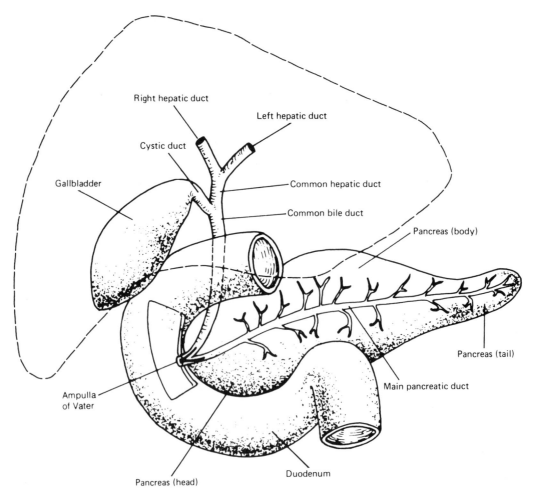

Figure 34–3
Anatomy of the pancreas.

enzyme; pancreatic lipase, which breaks down fats into glycerol; and proteolytic enzymes (trypsin, chymotrypsin, carboxypeptidase, ribonuclease, deoxyribonuclease), which break down proteins into essential amino acids.[6,10]

The exocrine pancreas protects itself from autodigestion in two ways. First, proteolytic enzymes do not become activated until they have been secreted into the intestines. The powerful splitting enzymes are secreted as inactive proenzymes. Trypsinogen is converted to the active enzyme trypsin by enterokinase, which is secreted by the duodenal mucosa. Trypsin converts chymotrypsinogen and other proenzymes into active enzymes (Fig. 34–4). Second, the same cells that secrete the proteolytic enzymes into the acini of the pancreas simultaneously secrete another substance called *trypsin inhibitor,* which prevents autodigestion. Trypsin inhibitor is stored in the cytoplasm of the glandular cells surrounding the enzyme granules and prevents activation of trypsin both inside the secretory cells and in the acini of the pancreas. Because trypsin activates the other pancreatic proteolytic enzymes, trypsin inhibitor also prevents the subsequent activation of other enzymes. If a duct becomes blocked or damaged, however, secretions are backed up and their concentration increases to the point that they overpower the trypsin inhibitor. This process activates trypsinogens and, subsequently, other proteolytic enzymes.[6]

The endocrine function of the pancreas focuses on the effects of two major hormones. Islets of Langerhans are distributed throughout the pancreas and are called *pancreatic islets.* The pancreatic islets are composed of three different types of cells: alpha, beta, and delta. Alpha cells secrete glucagon and increase blood glucose concentrations. Glucagon is sometimes referred to as a *gluconeogenic hormone* or a *hyperglycemic factor.* Beta cells are the major source of insulin and decrease blood glucose concentrations. Delta cells secrete a recently identified hormone called *somatostatin.* Somatostatin, can inhibit the secretion of glucagon and insulin, although its function is not fully understood. Its function is similar to that of growth hormone.[10]

Liver and Gallbladder

The liver is located under the diaphragm and occupies most of the right hypochondrial region of the abdomen. It is divided into left and right lobes that are separated by the falciform ligament. The liver has many metabolic and regulatory roles. Its digestive function is to produce bile, which leaves the liver by way of the hepatic duct and enters the duodenum through the common bile duct. Bile is not an enzyme; rather, it emulsifies fats by physically breaking apart large fat globules and producing smaller globules for the fat-digesting enzymes to work on. About 1 quart of bile, which consist of water, bile salts, cholesterol, lecithin, and bile pigments, is produced daily.

The gallbladder is embedded in the inferior surface of the liver. When digestion is not occurring, bile backs up the cystic duct and enters the gallbladder to be stored. In the gallbladder, bile is concentrated by the removal of water. Later, when fatty foods enter the duodenum, a hormonal stimulus causes the gallbladder to contract and release bile, making it available to the duodenum.

ETIOLOGIC AND PRECIPITATING FACTORS OF ACUTE PANCREATITIS

Acute pancreatitis is an inflammation of the pancreas that can occur at any age, but it is considered rare in children and young adults. In the later group, it has been associated with infections (particularly mumps), physical trauma, drugs, or heredity. The major etiologic factors associated with acute pancreatitis are biliary tract disease and sustained alcohol abuse.[1–3,5,8,14]

A common channel theory has been related to pancreatitis based on the fact that gallstones migrate to the lower end of the common bile duct and obstruct the outflow of biliary and pancreatic secretions. This allows bacteria from the inflamed biliary tract to reflux into the pancreatic duct.[1,2,8] Secondly, spasms of the pylorus and spincter of Oddi interfere with the outflow of pancreatic secretions.

Although the relationship between alcohol abuse and pancreatitis has been well documented, the pathogenesis of this relationship is uncertain. Alcohol ingestion may produce increased gastric acid production and secondary stimulation of pancreatic secretion. It may also induce duodenal stimulation and ampullary obstruction. If such is the case, pancreatic stimulation in the presence of an obstruction will result in inflammation and, thus, pancreatitis.[16]

The alcohol-related form is usually found in individuals less than 50 years of age, whereas the biliary disease form manifests itself in middle-aged and older adults. Approximately 80% of patients respond well to conservative medical treatment; the remaining 20% require intensive, aggressive therapy because of life-threatening complications.[15] Other factors associated with acute pancreatitis are listed in Table 34–1.

PATHOLOGY OF GASTROINTESTINAL DISORDERS

Gastritis

Gastritis is an inflammation of the gastric mucosa in the stomach that may be either acute or chronic. It is associated frequently with heavy alcohol intake or prolonged use of aspirin, anticoagulants, phenylbutazone, and steroids. It is manifested clinically by malaise, epigastric pain, and hematemesis. Diagnosis is made on the basis of a history and gastroscopy. Gastritis is one of the most common causes of upper gastrointestinal bleeding, although the bleeding is rarely massive. In most instances, the gastric mucosa is capable of repairing itself

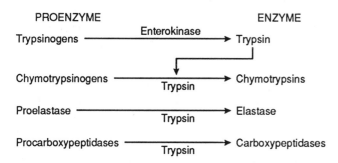

Figure 34–4
Activation of pancreatic proteolytic enzymes.

Table 34–1
Etiologic Factors in the Development of Acute Pancreatitis

Alcohol abuse
Biliary tract disease
    Gallstones
    Common bile duct (duodenal obstruction)
Gastric disease
    Peptic ulcers
Metabolic
    Hypercalcemia
    Hyperlipoproteinemia
    Drugs (*i.e.,* thiazides, sulfonamide derivatives)
Physical trauma
    Penetrating injuries
Postoperative gastrointestinal surgery
Infections
    Mumps
Hereditary

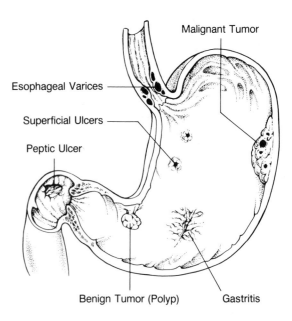

Figure 34–5
Common area of upper gastrointestinal tract bleeding.

after a bout of gastritis.[7,13] Other causes of upper gastrointestinal bleeding are listed in Table 34–2.

Peptic Ulcer

Peptic ulcers are a break in the continuity of the gastrointestinal tract that may involve the mucosa, submucosa, or muscular layers of the esophagus, stomach, duodenum, or (after gastroenterostomy) jejunum. A peptic ulcer is referred to frequently as a gastric, duodenal, or esophageal ulcer, depending on its location. Ulcerations develop as a result of an imbalance between the digesting power of acid secretions and the ability of the mucosa to resist this digestive action. The resistance can be decreased by factors such as inadequate blood supply, inadequate regeneration of tissue, and an inadequate quantity of mucus.

Gastric ulcers are more common in older age groups of both sexes and tend to occur in the lesser curvature of the stomach, near the pylorus. Peptic ulcers are more commonly found in the duodenum. Duodenal ulcers are more commonly found in young adults and in middle-aged men. Areas of upper gastrointestinal tract bleeding are shown in Figure 34–5. The duodenal ulcer is most often related to stress and life-style,

which leads to stereotyping the ulcer personality as a competitive, successful, nervous, compulsive executive in a position that demands high-powered decision-making and affords little opportunity for relaxation.

Acute Pancreatitis

Acute pancreatitis is a process of autodigestion caused by premature activation of proteolytic enzymes within the pancreas. Various mechanisms of enzyme activation have been postulated. They include reflux of duodenal contents, bile reflux, obstruction to the outflow of pancreatic juice, and lack of pancreatic secretory trypsin inhibitor (PSTI).[12]

NURSING PROCESS

ASSESSMENT
Patients With Gastrointestinal Bleeding

Vomiting of blood (hematemesis) and bloody or tarry stools (melena) are significant findings. Bleeding from the upper portion of the gastrointestinal tract (esophagus, stomach, duodenum) is manifested by hematemesis or passage of bloody, tarry stools. The vomited blood may be bright red or altered to resemble coffee grounds, the latter being caused by the action of gastric acid on hemoglobin to form acid hematin. As for melena, as little as 50 ml to 80 ml of ingested blood may produce a tarry stool. Blood within the stomach tends to stimulate peristaltic activity, which explains the presence of gross blood in the stool from bleeding in the upper tract. Gross blood from the rectum, in the absence of blood from nasogastric suctioning, places the site of bleeding in the lower gastrointestinal tract (jejunum, ileum, colon).

Abdominal findings may be minimal, although in upper gastrointestinal bleeds, tenderness can be found in the area of the duodenum, just above or to the right of the umbilical

Table 34–2
Causes of Upper Gastrointestinal Tract Bleeding

Common Causes

Gastritis
Peptic ulcer
Esophageal varices (usually associated with cirrhosis and portal hypertension)

Less Common Causes

Longstanding use of aspirin or other salicylates, anticoagulants, or steroids
Acute pancreatitis with duodenitis
Focal areas of gastritis in a hiatal hernia
Linear tears at the gastroesophageal junction (Mallory-Weiss syndrome)
Benign or malignant neoplasms of the stomach or duodenum
Congenial malformations of the stomach or duodenum (hemangioma, telangiectasia)
Stress ulcers associated with severe trauma or underlying disease (burns, central nervous system disorders)
Esophagitis

region (see Fig. 32–1). Nasogastric aspirate may contain whole blood or coffee-ground material. In the presence of normal gastric juice aspirate, some patients may be bleeding from a duodenal ulcer. In this instance, the plyoric ring may be closed to edema, thus preventing the regurgitation of contents into the stomach.

A patient history is of major importance. Most patients will give a history of peptic ulcer disease that has been identified by past gastrointestinal series; others report frequent use of medications (*i.e.*, salicylates, steroids, anticoagulants, anti-inflammatory agents, antacids).

Tachycardia, pallor, cold clammy skin, and low-value hematocrit are reliable indicators of hemodynamic compromise in acute bleeding.

Patients With Acute Pancreatitis

Initial clinical manifestations of acute pancreatitis can vary among patients and mimic those of myocardial or other gastrointestinal disease. The major symptoms associated with acute pancreatitis include pain, nausea and vomiting, low-grade fever, abdominal tenderness, fluid and electrolyte imbalance, and possible shock.

Pain

Abdominal pain is the first and most prominent symptom in acute pancreatitis.[5,8,17,18] It is located in the left upper quadrant, but it may be in the midepigastrium (see Fig. 32–1). It radiates to the back due to the retroperitoneal location of the pancreas and can be described as severe, steady, deep, and continuous. It is aggravated by eating large meals or after a drinking binge. The pain is usually not relieved after vomiting and may be accompanied by flushing or dyspnea. The pain is due to an inflamed pancreas, peritoneal irritation, and obstruction of the biliary tract.[8]

Nausea and Vomiting

Patients may present with nausea and vomiting and a low-grade fever. Abdominal tenderness to palpation with muscle guarding is common. Bowel sounds are often diminished but not absent. Mild abdominal distention develops in most patients and exhibits a characteristic fullness. Nausea and vomiting occur in approximately 80% of patients and may be aggravated by opiate analgesic medication. A fever suggests the development of an infection in the form of a possible pancreatic abscess or pneumonitis. The lungs are frequently involved, and crackles are present. Intravascular damage from circulating trypsin may cause areas of cyanosis or a greenish-yellow discoloration of the abdominal wall. In more severe cases, a bluish-brown discoloration of the flanks (Grey Turner's sign) or periumbilical area (Cullen's sign) is an uncommon symptom due to pancreatic bleeding into subcutaneous tissue.[5,8,17]

Diagnostic Tests and Studies

The diagnosis of acute pancreatitis is made by the presenting signs and symptoms as well as a history. Laboratory tests are used to help diagnosis, to evaluate the severity of disease, to monitor the course of an acute episode, and to guide appropriate treatment.

Acute pancreatitis should be suspected in patients who present with upper abdominal pain, elevated levels of serum pancreatic enzymes, and possible shock. A past history of repeated attacks diagnosed as biliary colic and a history of alcohol abuse provide valuable clues.

Laboratory Studies. Serum amylase levels are elevated in 95% of patients with acute pancreatitis (>500–2000 Somogyi units/100 ml). Levels tend to rise within 2 to 12 hours after the onset of symptoms and remain elevated for 3 to 5 days. Serum lipase levels tend to be elevated, but they remain elevated longer than serum amylase levels (>0.1–1.5 U/ml). Analysis of a 24-hour urine specimen for urine amylase demonstrates an increased excretion of amylase (>2–50 Wohlemuth units/ml for single specimen; >5000 Somogyi units/24-hour specimen). In some instances, enzyme levels may be elevated in patients who do not have pancreatitis. For example, conditions associated with renal insufficiency, cerebral trauma, intra-abdominal disease, and the administration of steroids, codeine, and opiates may cause false elevations in enzyme levels.[8] Although decisions should not be based solely on serum pancreatic enzyme levels, they are useful prognostic indicators.

Liver function tests such as SGOT, SGPT, LDH, and alkaline phosphate are elevated in about 50% of patients with acute pancreatitis. Alcoholism, liver disease, and common bile duct obstruction may also cause values to rise.

Serum calcium levels are decreased (hypocalcemia) in about 30% of patients with pancreatitis (<8.0 mg/100 ml). Levels decrease 2 to 3 days after onset of the disease and may persist for several weeks. Calcium levels below 8.0 mg/dl signify a poor prognostic sign. Serum potassium levels may also be decreased (<3.5–5.0 mEq/L) owing to nasogastric drainage or vomiting. Leukocytosis of 10,000 to 25,000 cells/mm^3 is present in about 80% of patients.

Transient or mild hypoglycemia is common during initial attacks of pancreatitis when excess glucagon is released from alpha cells or when there is damage to beta cells. Fasting hyperglycemia of greater than 200 mg/dl reflects pancreatic necrosis and can be a poor prognostic sign. A very small percentage of patients will go on to develop diabetes mellitus.

Radiologic Studies. Abdominal radiographs should be obtained in all patients with known or suspected pancreatitis. They indicate distended, gas-filled loops of intestine, suggesting a paralytic ileus. Such findings are not specific to pancreatitis, but they do point to the presence of an intra-abdominal or retroperitoneal process. It is likewise useful to rule out the presence of free intraperitoneal air caused by gastric and intestinal perforation. Diaphragmatic involvement and pulmonary complications (*i.e.*, pleural effusion, atelectasis) are recognized by chest radiographs.

Ultrasonography and Computed Tomography. Ultrasonography and computed tomography are used for the following reasons: to determine the presence of pancreatic disease, to assess the severity of pancreatitis and the development of local complications, and to evaluate the biliary tract for the presence of stones and dilatation. Ultrasonography can be performed at the bedside and does not involve the use of intravenous contrast medium. It is not specific, however, and has a limited role in diagnosing acute pancreatitis. It determines whether the gallstones are present and can visualize complications (*i.e.,* pseudocysts). Computed tomography scanning is the imaging method of choice for any pancreatic disease, especially in patients with suspected complications of acute pancreatitis. When intravenous contrast medium is given during the computed tomographic examination, enlargement of the pancreas as well as calcifications and dilatation of the bile ducts can be visualized. However, allergy to contrast medium or compromised

renal function precludes the use of such intravenous contrast material.

NURSING DIAGNOSES, PATIENT OUTCOMES, AND PLAN

The preceding material on anatomy, physiology, nursing assessment, and diagnostic tests guides the nurse in establishing nursing diagnoses, patient outcomes, and plan for the patient with gastrointestinal disorders.

NURSING CARE PLAN SUMMARY The Patient With Gastrointestinal Disorders

NURSING DIAGNOSIS

1. *Altered comfort related to pain from inflamed pancreas (feeling pattern)*

Patient Outcome	Nursing Orders
The patient will experience a reduction of pain to within a manageable or tolerable level.	1. Assess patient's pain with regard to the following: A. Onset B. Duration C. Type D. Intensity E. Location 2. Administer pain medication as ordered. Assess effectiveness. The drug of choice is meperidine (Demerol). Morphine is contraindicated because of its spasmodic effect on the sphincter of Oddi. 3. Allow the patient to express what makes the pain better and what makes it worse. 4. Reassure patient, and help relieve other sources of discomfort including fear and anxiety. Both fear and anxiety will increase release of pancreatic enzymes, producing more pain. 5. Assist the patient to assume positions of comfort.

NURSING DIAGNOSIS

2. *Fluid volume deficit related to vomiting, decreased fluid intake, fever, and diaphoresis (exchanging pattern)*

Patient Outcome	Nursing Orders

The patient will demonstrate normal fluid and electrolyte status.	1. Assess fluid and electrolyte status (*i.e.,* skin turgor, mucous membranes, urine output, vital signs).
	 A. Assess sources of fluid and electrolyte loss (*i.e.,* vomiting, diarrhea, nasogastric drainage, excessive diaphoresis).
	 B. Monitor for signs of shock (*i.e.,* note vital signs, hematocrit and hemoglobin levels).
	 C. Administer plasma, albumin, steroids, and blood as ordered.
	 D. Assess abdomen for ascites formation (*i.e.,* measure abdominal girth daily, weigh patient daily).
	 E. Assess for the following signs and symptoms of hypocalcemia:
	  (1) Increased neuromuscular irritability
	  (2) Decreased cardiac output
	  (3) Numbness or tingling of the fingers or toes
	  (4) Prolonged QT interval

(continued)

NURSING CARE PLAN SUMMARY   *The Patient With Gastrointestinal Disorders*   *Continued*

Patient Outcome	Nursing Orders
	(5) Palpitations (6) Carpopedal spasms after inflation of blood pressure cuff (hands folding in) (7) Positive Trousseau's sign (8) Laryngeal spasm and tetany (clinical emergency) F. When patient is in severe hypocalcemia, place him or her on seizure precautions. Make sure that padded side rails, an oral airway, and suction are available. G. Assess for the following signs and symptoms of hypokalemia: (1) Muscle weakness (2) Hyporeflexia (3) Abdominal distention (4) Electrocardiographic changes: flattened T waves, depressed ST segment (5) Apathy (6) Irritability H. Administer and monitor electrolyte replacements as needed.

NURSING DIAGNOSIS

3. *Ineffective breathing pattern related to abdominal pain with guarding and retroperitoneal inflammation (exchanging pattern)*

Patient Outcome	Nursing Orders
The patient will maintain normal respiratory rate and depth.	1. Assess respiratory status (*i.e.*, rate, pattern, breath sounds). A. Monitor for the following signs and symptoms of a pneumothorax: (1) Dyspnea (2) Hypotension (3) Tachycardia (4) Decreased breath sounds (5) Limited excursion on affected side (6) Restlessness B. Assist patient to turn and change position every 2 hours. C. Maintain semi-Fowler's position. This will help decrease pressure on the diaphragm and allow greater lung expansion. D. Instruct patients to take frequent and deep breaths. E. Assess for pain relief. F. Provide restful, quiet environment for patients. This will allow for the maximal amount of rest between nursing care activities. It is essential to decrease the metabolic rate, which in turn decreases the workload of the respiratory system and the use of oxygen by tissue. G. Perform chest physiotherapy every 4 to 6 hours. H. Encourage adequate hydration.

NURSING DIAGNOSIS

4. *Altered nutrition: less than body requirements related to inadequate dietary intake and impaired pancreatic secretions (exchanging pattern)*

Patient Outcome	Nursing Orders
The patient will have an improvement in nutritional status.	1. Assess patient's nutritional status based on medical history (*i.e.*, hepatic disease, alcohol abuse). A. Monitor albumin levels and symptoms of vitamin deficiencies. B. Provide hyperalimentation as nutritional adjunct. Monitor blood glucose levels closely. C. Give nutritional supplements as indicated. D. Provide high-carbohydrate, low-protein, low-fat diet when tolerated. E. Counsel patient to avoid excessive use of coffee, spicy foods, and alcohol.

IMPLEMENTATION AND EVALUATION

The major objectives in the implementation and evaluation of acute pancreatitis include relieving pain, decreasing pancreatic inflammation and secretions, controlling fluid and electrolyte imbalances, initiating nutritional support, and treating complications as they arise.

Pain

The pain associated with acute pancreatitis may be very severe and is a significant clinical problem. It is the result of edema and distention of the pancreatic capsule, obstruction of the biliary tree, and peritoneal irritation.[8] Meperidine (Demerol) is administered rather than morphine because of the spasms produced at the ampulla of Vater and the sphincter of Oddi.

Reduction in Pancreatic Secretions

It is important to reduce or suppress pancreatic enzymes in order to allow the pancreas to rest. This is accomplished by keeping the patient NPO and instituting nasogastric suction to reduce vomiting and abdominal distention. Nasogastric suction is maintained until abdominal pain and tenderness, fever, and leukocytosis have subsided. Hourly antacids or cimetidine (Tagamet) may be given when gastric contents reveal evidence of upper gastrointestinal bleeding. Once the nasogastric tube has been discontinued, the patient is kept NPO for a 24- to 48-hour period of observation before a low-fat diet is gradually introduced. If evidence of pancreatitis resumes when the patient begins eating, the diet is withdrawn. Anticholinergics, antispasmotics, and glucagon have also been recommended in order to decrease vagally mediated pancreatic secretions and reduce ampullary spasm.

Fluid and Electrolyte Replacement

Fluids are replaced rather aggressively because of the loss of electrolytes, blood, plasma, and extravascular fluids. Specifically, lactated Ringer's solution and sodium chloride are used frequently.[8] Hypovolemic shock can occur in about 60% of the patients with acute pancreatitis.[4] Plasma or plasma volume expanders such as dextran or albumin may be given. In many instances, a central venous catheter is inserted. In patients with associated cardiovascular disease, monitoring of pulmonary arterial pressures by means of a Swan-Ganz catheter may be essential to monitor fluid therapy.

As a result of prolonged hypovolemia or shock, the patient may develop acute tubular necrosis with renal insufficiency. Oliguria (<400 ml of urine/day) may develop; anuria is rare. Blood urea nitrogen and creatinine concentrations may rise steadily. Hyperkalemia and metabolic acidosis are the most feared metabolic complications.

Metabolic complications are seen frequently in patients with pancreatitis and include hypocalcemia and hypokalemia. Adequate replacement is needed. Hyperglycemia frequently occurs early in the course of pancreatitis. Mild hyperglycemia or glucosuria does not require treatment. Insulin therapy should be withheld unless the blood sugar level is greater than 300 mg/dl, because hypoglycemia can significantly increase mortality. If insulin is to be administered, blood sugar levels should be kept at 200 mg to 300 mg/dl to limit the possibility of hypoglycemia.[4]

Respiratory Monitoring and Support

Respiratory complications will vary from mild hypoxia to pulmonary edema. Severe insult to the respiratory system may lead to adult respiratory distress syndrome. Careful monitoring of the patient's respiratory status, including arterial blood gases and chest radiographs, leads to early recognition of problems. In patients who develop early hypoxemia, management consist of oxygen administration, respiratory physiotherapy, and close monitoring. In patients with severe respiratory failure, endotracheal intubation and positive end-expiratory pressure ventilation may be initiated.

Nutritional Support

Nutritional depletion in patients with acute pancreatitis is very common. In those with mild pancreatitis, feeding may resume in a few days. In patients with severe pancreatitis, oral feedings are not usually tolerated for prolonged periods of time. Hyperalimentation is begun with close monitoring of blood glucose levels.

Treatment of Local Complications

Pseudocysts are collections of fluid within or adjacent to the pancreas. Pseudocysts may be suspected if symptoms of pain, nausea, vomiting, fever, abdominal pain, or elevated amylase levels persist for 2 to 3 weeks after pancreatic injury. Ultrasonography and computed tomography have shown that pseudocysts occur in 25% of patients with acute pancreatitis and that about 85% resolve spontaneously within a few weeks of discovery. Those persisting for over 4 to 6 weeks are considered chronic and should undergo surgical drainage. Surgical intervention can be external or internal. The most common complication is spontaneous rupture, with drainage into the peritoneum (causing pancreatic ascites). Other complications are obstruction of organs (common bile duct, stomach) and hemorrhage from erosion into the gastrointestinal tract.[4,11,16]

Pancreatic Abscesses

Pancreatic abscesses may develop as a result of abdominal trauma or as a secondary infection within an acute pseudocyst. The incidence is directly related to the initial severity of the pancreatitis attack. Clinical symptoms include fever, chills, tachycardia, hypotension, leukocytosis, and, at times, a palpable mass. Drainage of abscesses may be accomplished surgically or by needle aspiration directed by computed tomography. Cultures of the drainage will establish or exclude the presence of bacterial infection. Most cultures yield species of *Escherichia coli, Enterococcus, Staphylococcus, Streptococcus faecalis, Proteus, Klebsiella*, and *Bacteroides*.[4,11,16] Treatment consists of surgical debridement followed by drainage and lavage of the infected area. Antibiotics are administered.

Pancreatic Ascites

Pancreatic ascites occurs most frequently in patients with chronic alcohol-induced pancreatitis. It is characterized by an increased abdominal girth and accompanied by abdominal pain and weight loss. Paracentesis reveals protein concentration of exudative fluid greater than 3.0 g/dl.[9]

Patients With Chronic Pancreatitis

Chronic pancreatitis is progressive destruction of the pancreas with fibrotic replacement of pancreatic tissue. The two major types of chronic pancreatitis are chronic obstructive pancreatitis and chronic calcifying pancreatitis. Chronic pancreatitis may follow acute pancreatitis, but it can occur in the absence of any history of an acute condition.[8,9]

Chronic obstructive pancreatitis is associated with inflammation of the sphincter of Oddi, which is associated with cholelithiasis. Other causes include cancer of the pancreas, ampulla of Vater, or duodenum that develops slowly and obstructs the pancreatic duct, thus producing signs of pancreatitis.[8]

Chronic calcifying pancreatitis is characterized by inflammation and sclerosis mainly in the head of the pancreas and around the pancreatic duct. Protein plugs form and eventually lead to ductal obstruction, acinar cell atrophy, fibrosis, and, in later stages, calcification, which forms calculi.[8,9]

Alcohol abuse is by far the most common cause of chronic pancreatitis and pancreatic exocrine insufficiency. Men with an average history of 10 years of chronic alcohol abuse are most often affected. Patients seek medical attention because of chronic abdominal pain and weight loss. As with acute pancreatitis, abdominal pain is a major problem. Attacks may become more frequent and are described as gnawing, heavy, or sometimes burning or cramplike. Other symptoms include constipation, mild jaundice with dark urine, steatorrhea, and diabetes. Steatorrhea may become severe, with foul, fatty stools. Abdominal tenderness is present, and pseudocysts are very common. Cysts and diabetes are sometimes considered complications, but due to their frequent occurrence, they may be considered late symptoms.

SUMMARY

Acute pancreatitis is an inflammation of the pancreas in which complications and mortality vary depending on cause and severity. In mild pancreatitis, mortality averages 3% and complications are infrequent. In severe pancreatitis, mortality and complications range from 30% to 60%. Among those patients whose first attack is related to the biliary tract, mortality is approximately 20%. For those whose etiology is alcohol-related, the mortality is less than 5%.[4]

Because severe pancreatitis and biliary-tract related pancreatitis have such a high mortality, early recognition of this gastrointestinal emergency is crucial. Critical care nurses must recognize pancreatitis as a multisystem disease and have a firm foundation of knowledge with respect to pathologies, associated etiologies, complications, and current therapy. Accurate assessment is vital to the survival and eventual recovery of the patient with pancreatitis.

DIRECTIONS FOR FUTURE RESEARCH

Research questions that critical care nurses may consider in the care of patients with pancreatitis are as follows:

1. What nonpharmacologic measures are most effective in relieving pain associated with pancreatitis?
2. What are the best nursing interventions in patients with altered nutrition: less than body requirements to help minimize nutritional depletion?
3. What nursing interventions are most effective in helping patients cope with the chronicity of alcohol-induced pancreatitis?

REFERENCES

1. Armstrong, C. P., and Taylor, T. V. Pancreatic-duct reflux and acute gallstone pancreatitis. *Ann. Surg.* 204:59, 1986.
2. Armstrong, C. P., Taylor, T. V., Jeacock, J., *et al.* The biliary tract in patients with acute gallstone pancreatitis. *Br. J. Surg.* 72:551, 1985.
3. Bank, S. Acute and Chronic Pancreatitis. In Dent T. L. (ed.), *Pancreatic Disease: Diagnosis and Therapy.* New York: Grune & Stratton, 1981:34, 421–429.
4. Barkin, J. S., and Garrido, J. Acute pancreatitis and its complications. *Postgrad. Med.* 79:241, 1986.
5. Brooks, F. P. *Diseases of the Exocrine Pancreas.* Philadelphia: W. B. Saunders, 1980.
6. Fain, J. A., and Amato-Vealey, E. Acute pancreatitis: A gastrointestinal emergency. *Crit. Care Nurs.* 8:47, 1988.
7. Geelhoed, G. W. Gastrointestinal bleeding. *Am. Fam. Physician* 29:115, 1984.
8. Given, B. A., and Simmons, S. J. *Gastroenterology in Clinical Nursing* (4th ed.). St. Louis: C. V. Mosby, 1984.
9. Greenberger, N. J. Chronic pancreatitis and exocrine insufficiency. *Hosp. Pract.* 20:33, 1985.
10. Guyton, A. C. *Textbook of Medical Physiology.* Philadelphia: W. B. Saunders, 1981:810–812, 966–967.
11. Jeffres, C. Complications of acute pancreatitis. *Crit. Care Nurs.* 9:38, 1989.
12. Kurfees, J. F. Acute pancreatitis: Pathology and pathogenesis. *Am. Fam. Physician* 23:156, 1981.
13. Levinson, M. J. Gastric stress ulcers. *Hosp. Pract.* 24:59, 1989.
14. Oria, A., Alvarez, J., Chippetta, L., *et al.* Risk factors for acute pancreatitis in patients with migrating gallstones. *Arch. Surg.* 124:1295, 1989.
15. Ranson, J. C. Risk factors in acute pancreatitis. *Hosp. Pract.* 20:69, 1985.
16. Sleisenger, M. H., and Fordstran, J. S. *Gastrointestinal Disease: Pathophysiology, Diagnosis, Management* (4th ed.), vols. 1 and 2. Philadelphia: W. B. Saunders, 1989.
17. Steinberg, W. B. Acute Pancreatitis. In G. L. Eastwood (ed.), *Core Textbook of Gastroenterology.* Philadelphia: J. B. Lippincott, 1984:233–252.
18. Warshaw, A. L. Pain in chronic pancreatitis. *Gastroenterology* 86:987, 1984.

VIII

The Critically Ill Adult With Metabolic Problems

THE DISEASE THAT "JUST WENT AWAY"

Every nurse and physician sees from time to time things that are difficult to believe—the cancer that disappeared without treatment, the person who was predicted to die but who did not, the case that breaks all the known rules. The old-fashioned term for these cases is *miracles*. Although the term is outmoded, nobody has a better word for these anomalous events.

No one likes to talk about these cases because they threaten our concepts about how disease "ought" to behave. These cases tell us that there are holes in our theories, that our knowledge is incomplete.

They also tell us something else: In any serious illness, there is at least the possibility that the unexpected can happen, that the miraculous may occur. This realization can be a hope and consolation for every one of our patients, no matter how grave the situation. This does not mean that we should hold out false hope or engage in dreamy optimism, and we should emphasize that these clinical twists are not the norm. However, it is just as wrong to strip our patients of hope by suggesting that everyone with "disease X" is dead at 5 years after diagnosis, for this simply is not true. Any and all diseases break the rules from time to time.

35

Metabolic Assessment

Loretta Forlaw   *Cornelia Vanderstaay Kenner*

ANCIENT WISDOM AND PSYCHOBIOLOGIC UNITY

It is interesting that science may be revealing what mystics of diverse cultures and ages have suggested all along. The idea of psychobiologic unity is as old as the history of ideas. However, we are only now coming to feel that we can legitimately adopt the psychobiologic view, because only recently has science begun to tell us that it is all right to do so.

Somewhere the mystics must be smiling, having held those beliefs about unity long before modern science was born.

There is a certain danger in a body-mind-spirit approach to illness and healing. When one reads reports, for example, of increased rates of healing and control of malignant dysrhythmias with biofeedback or meditation techniques, with or without the concomitant use of drugs, one is likely to become overly enthusiastic. One commonly feels exhilarated; after all, the idea of psychobiologic unity offers people a new way of seeing themselves. That new way may feel more "right," more "whole," than the old way.

Uncontrolled enthusiasm for the new ideas has been damaging to their development. As critical care nurses, we must continue to search for the data that demonstrate efficacious body-mind-spirit healing approaches.

LEARNING OBJECTIVES

After reading this chapter, the nurse should be able to do the following:

1. Locate tables with normal intakes and outputs of body fluids, electrolytes, and minerals and common nutrients.
2. List the common causes and clinical manifestations of each metabolic alteration.
3. Participate in the development of protocols or have access to protocols for medical and nursing treatment of each metabolic alteration.
4. Explain clinical manifestations and their causes to other personnel, the patient, or the family.

NUTRITIONAL DEFICIENCIES

The ravages of a critical illness quickly use up a patient's nutritional stores (see Chap. 36, p. 674). Additionally, many pa-

tients, especially elderly patients, arrive in the unit already malnourished.

Metabolic alterations may occur suddenly, at least as perceived by the patient or the family. It is important for the patient and family to receive information pertinent to the patient's expected physical (and often emotional) progress. The nurse should not assume that the patient or family does not need continual explanation about routine procedures just because they have experienced a specific situation in the past or have been experiencing the problem for an extended period during the present hospitalization. Emotional needs of the patient or family should be addressed and must be communicated to all personnel involved in the care. Clear, concise messages greatly help to reduce the anxiety associated with the patient's medical and nursing diagnoses. Opportunities for teaching frequently occur during care and should be used in addition to formalized teaching sessions.

Recommendations

The recommended daily allowance of protein for the patient without renal or liver failure is 0.8 g/kg of body weight/day.[9,11,14] Increases in protein delivery above 0.8 g/kg of body weight/day should be based on the patient's nitrogen-balance

Note: The opinions or assertions contained herein are the private views of the authors and are not to be construed as official or as reflecting the views of the Department of the Army or the Department of Defense.

data.[3] Twenty to 30% of the patient's calculated energy requirements is delivered as fat calories. At least 4% of the patient's estimated energy requirements must be delivered as fat calories to meet essential fatty acid requirements.[4]

Specific nursing diagnoses, patient outcomes, and nursing orders for alterations in nutritional metabolism follow.

NURSING CARE PLAN SUMMARY   Patient with Altered Metabolism

NURSING DIAGNOSIS

1. Altered nutrition: less than body requirements related to decreased intake or increased nutrient requirements (exchanging pattern)

Patient Outcome	Nursing Orders
The estimated nutrient needs of the patient will be met by enteral or parenteral nutrition.[16]	1. Assess the patient for the physical signs and symptoms of nutrient deficiency (see Chap. 36, p. 678). A. Monitor the patient's intake and output, urine glucose, and urine specific gravity. B. Monitor the patient's weight. C. Estimate the patient's fluid requirement. D. Estimate the patient's energy, protein, and fat requirements. The Harris-Benedict equation is used to calculate resting energy requirements (REE): $$REE \text{ (men)} = 66.47 + 13.7W + 5.0H - 6.76A$$ $$REE \text{ (women)} = 655.10 + 9.56W + 1.8H - 4.68A$$ where W = weight in kilograms, H = height in centimeters, and A = age in years.[1,10] Resting energy expenditure increases about 32% in patients with skeletal trauma. Bed rest increases REE about 20%, and usual activity (walking) increases REE about 30%.[6,7,14,19]

NURSING DIAGNOSIS

2. Altered metabolic processes related to inadequate nutrient intake or altered biochemical activity (exchanging pattern)

Patient Outcomes	Nursing Orders
1. The patient will not demonstrate signs or symptoms of hypoglycemia.	1. Assess the patient for clinical signs and symptoms of hypoglycemia (see Table 35–1). A. Assess the patient for altered laboratory values associated with hypoglycemia. (1) Decreased serum glucose levels (2) Increased serum insulin levels (3) Negative glucose values in urine B. Anticipate the following with hypoglycemia: (1) Obtaining serum glucose and serum insulin (2) Immediate delivery of glucose orally or 50% glucose intravenously (3) Continuous infusion of 10% dextrose until glucose levels stabilize (4) Cardiac monitoring if prolonged (5) Seizure precautions
2. The patient will not demonstrate signs or symptoms of hyperglycemia.	2. Assess the patient for clinical signs and symptoms of hyperglycemia (see Table 35–1). A. Assess the patient for altered laboratory values associated with hyperglycemia. (1) Elevated serum glucose (2) Elevated serum osmolality (3) Elevated or normal sodium (4) Normal or decreased potassium

(continued)

NURSING CARE PLAN SUMMARY   *Patient with Altered Metabolism*   Continued

Patient Outcomes	*Nursing Orders*
	B. Anticipate the following with hyperglycemia:
	(1) Obtaining serum glucose, osmolality, sodium, potassium, hematocrit
	(2) Administration of fluids to correct fluid loss
	(3) Administration of insulin to lower blood glucose
	(4) Correction of associated electrolyte abnormalities
	(5) Slow correction of hyperglycemia, essential to prevent cerebral edema
3. The patient will not demonstrate signs or symptoms of hyperosmolar nonketotic dehydration.	3. Assess the patient for clinical signs and symptoms of hyperosmolar nonketotic dehydration (see Table 35–1).
	A. Assess the patient for the following altered laboratory values associated with hyperosmolar nonketotic dehydration:
	(1) See Chapter 38.
	(2) Serum glucose greater than 600 mg/dl
	(3) Serum ketones may be positive
	(4) Serum potassium decreased
	(5) Serum sodium—pseudohyponatremia
	(6) Serum osmolality elevated
	(7) Hematocrit and hemoglobin elevated
	(8) Serum urea nitrogen elevated
	(9) Serum phosphorus decreased
	(10) Urine glucose values greater than 3$^+$
	B. Anticipate the following with hyperosmolar nonketotic dehydration:
	(1) Obtaining serum and urine tests
	(2) Fluid replacement
	(3) Insulin administration
	(4) Correction of associated electrolyte abnormalities
4. The patient will not demonstrate signs or symptoms of essential fatty acid deficiency.	4. Assess the patient for clinical signs and symptoms of essential fatty acid deficiency (see Table 35–1).
	A. Assess the patient for the following altered laboratory values associated with essential fatty acid deficiency:
	(1) Elevated serum triene-tetraene ratio
	(2) Elevated serum SGOT
	B. Anticipate the following with essential fatty acid deficiency:
	(1) Obtaining blood for laboratory evaluation
	(2) Delivery of fat emulsion solution to provide at least 4% of patient's calories as linoleic acid
5. The patient will not demonstrate signs or symptoms of excessive delivery of intravenous fat emulsion.	5. Assess the patient for the immediate and delayed signs and symptoms of excessive delivery of intravenous fat emulsion (see Table 35–1).
	A. Assess the patient for the following altered laboratory values associated with excessive delivery of intravenous fat emulsion:
	(1) Liver function tests elevated
	(2) Triglycerides elevated
	(3) Fingerstick hematocrit lipemic
	(4) Coagulopathies
	(5) Serum sodium—pseudohyponatremia
	B. Anticipate the following with excessive delivery of intravenous fat emulsion:
	(1) Obtaining blood for laboratory tests at time of excessive delivery and 6 hours after stopping fat emulsion
	(2) Potential bleeding in patients with clotting abnormalities
	(3) Slowing rate of fat emulsion
	(4) Do not administer fat emulsions at a rate greater than 2.5 g/kg/day to adult patients.

Table 35–1
Metabolic Alterations and Complications

TYPE OF METABOLISM	COMPLICATIONS	CLINICAL AND METABOLIC MANIFESTATIONS	ANTECEDENT CONDITIONS
Glucose	Hypoglycemia	Weakness Diaphoresis Hunger Nervousness Irritability Palpitations Tremors Headache Blurring or double vision Numbness of lips, tongue	Abrupt interruption of glucose infusion; excessive administration of insulin
	Hyperglycemia	Fatigue Thirst Polyuria Dry, hot, flushed skin	Excessive glucose administration; stress; glucocorticoids; inadequate endogenous or exogenous insulin; chromium deficiency
	Hyperosmolar nonketotic dehydration	Dry skin Dry mucous membranes Fever Polydipsia Osmotic diuresis Hypovolemia Somnolence Seizures Coma	Untreated hyperglycemia resulting in increased urine output with each molecule of glucose carrying two molecules of water
Protein	Prerenal azotemia	Symptoms of dehydration Elevated blood urea nitrogen Decreased urine output Increased urine specific gravity	Dehydration (possible hyperosmolar type); calorie nitrogen impairment
Fat	Essential fatty acid deficiency	Scaly dermatitis Poor wound healing Alopecia	Inadequate infusion of linoleic acid and/or arachidonic acid

	Essential fatty acid excess	Immediate signs:
		  Tachycardia
		  Tachypnea
		  Nausea, vomiting
		  Headache
		  Back pain
		  Dyspnea
		  Cyanosis
		  Histamine-like reaction
		  Fever and chills
		Delayed signs:
		  Low-grade fever
		  Headache
		  Hyperirritability
		  Lethargy
		  Abdominal pain
		  Nausea
			Excessive rate of delivery; inability of liver to metabolize fat emulsion

Water	Hypovolemia	Poor skin turgor Dry mucous membranes Decreased urine output Increased specific gravity Weight loss Increased pulse Lethargy, coma Convulsions Hypotension Tachycardia Abdominal distention Decreased or increased temperature Feeble to absent peripheral pulses Weight loss	Inadequate fluid replacement; hyperglycemia; excessive gastrointestinal losses; systematic infection; renal disease; intestinal obstruction; blood loss; burns; diuretics
	Hypervolemia	Confusion, apathy Facial edema Jugular vein distention Anorexia Nausea, vomiting	Excessive fluid replacement; postoperative antidiuretic hormone effect; renal disease; steroid therapy; excessive sodium; excessive sodium bicarbonate; congestive heart failure

(continued)

Table 35-1   (*Continued*)

TYPE OF METABOLISM	COMPLICATIONS	CLINICAL AND METABOLIC MANIFESTATIONS	ANTECEDENT CONDITIONS
Electrolyte	Hyponatremia	Dyspnea Orthopnea Dependent edema Anasarca Warm, moist skin Pallor Weight gain Rales Increased or decreased urine output Headache Muscle weakness Fatigue Apathy Postural hypotension Nausea, vomiting Abdominal cramps	Dilutional excessive urinary or gastrointestinal sodium losses
	Hypernatremia	Dry skin Dry mucous membranes Thirst Decreased urine output "Rubbery" tissue turgor Tachycardia Excitement Weight loss Hypotension	Dehydration; excessive infusion of sodium ion; high-protein feeding; diabetes insipidus; inability to perceive thirst
	Hypokalemia	Anorexia Nausea, vomiting Abdominal distention Paralytic ileus Muscle weakness Cardiac dysrhythmias	Anabolism; deficit of potassium in solution; excessive urinary or gastrointestinal losses; metabolic alkalosis; diuretics
	Hyperkalemia	Nausea, vomiting Diarrhea Muscle weakness Muscle irritability Oliguria, anuria Numbness, tingling Cardiac dysrhythmias	Excessive replacement of potassium; metabolic acidosis; renal failure; crushing injury; acute digitalis poisoning; mineralocorticoid deficiency
Mineral	Hypocalcemia	Numbness and tingling of nose, ears, fingertips, or toes Carpopedal spasm Muscle twitching Convulsions Tetany Positive Trousseau sign Positive Chvostek sign Nausea, vomiting Diarrhea Cardiac dysrhythmias	Insufficient calcium in solution; rapid correction of hypophosphatemia; vitamin D deficiency; increased urinary excretion; decreased parathyroid hormone; respiratory acidosis; acute pancreatitis; large amounts of citrated blood
	Hypercalcemia	Thirst Polyuria Anorexia Nausea, vomiting Lethargy Confusion Constipation Decreased deep tendon reflexes Psychoneurosis Bone pain Dehydration Cardiac dysrhythmias Weight loss Hypertension	Excessive calcium in solution; immobilization; excessive vitamin D intake; steroid therapy; multiple myeloma; carcinoma with bone metastasis; hyperparathyroidism
	Hypomagnesemia	Agitation Depression Confusion Convulsions	Insufficient magnesium in parenteral solution; excessive urinary and gastrointestinal losses; hypercalcemia; elevated aldosterone

(continued)

Table 35–1   (*Continued*)

TYPE OF METABOLISM	COMPLICATIONS	CLINICAL AND METABOLIC MANIFESTATIONS	ANTECEDENT CONDITIONS
		Paresthesias Tremor Ataxia Muscle cramps Tetany Tachycardia Hypotension Positive Chvostek sign	levels; chronic alcoholism; impaired gastrointestinal absorption
	Hypermagnesemia	Lethargy, coma Hypotension Loss of deep tendon reflexes Respiratory depression Cardiac dysrhythmia Tachycardia, bradycardia	Excessive infusion of magnesium-containing fluids; renal failure; severe dehydration
	Hypophosphatemia	Paresthesias Hyperventilation Lethargy coma Decreased erythrocyte 2,3-diphosphoglycerate	Anabolism, intracellular shift of phosphorus in response to concentrated glucose solution; inadequate phosphorus in total parenteral nutrition solutions; respiratory alkalosis; alcoholism; chronic use of phosphate-binding antacids
Acid-base	Metabolic acidosis	Hyperventilation Tachypnea Lethargy Lassitude Mental obtundation	Excessive metabolic acids; lactic acidosis; diabetic ketoacidosis; renal failure; hyperkalemia; starvation; hepatitis; anesthesia; excessive bicarbonate loss; diarrhea; hyperchloremia; fistula loss
	Metabolic alkalosis	Hypoventilation Cardiac dysrhythmias Hypotension Confusion Delirium Tetany Muscle weakness Paralysis Ileus Abdominal distention Muscle cramps Dysarthria	Decreased metabolic acids; nasogastric suction; vomiting; hypokalemia; excessive bicarbonate intake; excessive intake of sodium bicarbonate; potassium-free intravenous solutions; diuretics; excessive adrenocortical hormone therapy; low-sodium, low-potassium diet
	Respiratory acidosis	Hypoventilation Visual disturbances Headache Confusion Drowsiness Coma Ventricular fibrillation Yawning Flared nostril Tachycardia	Decreased ventilation and diffusion in the lungs with retention of carbon dioxide; abdominal surgery; chronic obstructive lung disease; lung infection; lung tumors; traumatic pneumothorax; central nervous system depression
	Respiratory alkalosis	Dizziness Hyperreflexia Muscle twitching Nausea and vomiting Convulsion Positive Chvostek sign	Increased ventilation of lungs with loss of carbon dioxide; mechanical ventilation; pregnancy; hysteria; elevated temperature; drug toxicity; encephalitis; pain; chronic alcoholism; impaired gastrointestinal absorption

(Modified from Forlaw, L. Parenteral nutrition in the critically ill child. *Crit. Care Q.* 3–4, 1980, 1–21, 1980; with permission.)

ALTERATIONS IN WATER, ELECTROLYTE, AND MINERAL METABOLISM

Alterations in water, electrolyte, and mineral metabolism are related intimately to one another.[13] Thus, physiologic changes often have concurrent effects. Most pathologic changes result from inadequate or excessive delivery or changes within the organism that alter the usual intake or output of water, electrolytes, and minerals.

The patient's daily intake of electrolytes, minerals, and trace elements is increased or decreased as indicated by serum and urinary levels.

Nursing interventions are common to the assessment of all metabolic alterations. The nurse should do the following:

- Assess the patient's mental, cardiovascular, pulmonary, gastrointestinal, renal, and integumentary status.
- Explain the signs and symptoms to the patient or family.

- Communicate with the physician and other staff members regarding improvement or worsening of the abnormality.
- Monitor the patient's intake and output (urinary, gastrointestinal, insensible losses) at least daily.
- Monitor the patient's weight at least daily.
- Monitor the patient's serum levels of glucose, potassium, chloride, urea nitrogen, carbon dioxide, phosphorus, calcium, magnesium, and triglycerides, and arterial blood gases.
- Monitor urine and gastrointestinal losses for potassium, sodium, chloride, glucose, ketones, and urea.

- Anticipate the influence of medications, especially diuretics, on serum and urinary levels.
- Investigate and correct precipitating factors.
- Provide education for patient, family, and other staff members.

Specific nursing diagnoses, patient outcomes, and nursing orders for alterations in water, electrolyte, and mineral metabolism follow.

NURSING CARE PLAN SUMMARY *Patient with Altered Metabolism* *Continued*

NURSING DIAGNOSIS

3. Actual fluid volume deficit related to inadequate delivery of fluid, patient's inability to report thirst, excessive fluid losses, or specific cause (exchanging pattern)

Patient Outcome	Nursing Orders

The patient will demonstrate normal fluid volume.	1. Assess the patient for clinical signs and symptoms of hypovolemia (see Table 35–1).
	  A. Assess the patient for altered laboratory and hemodynamic values associated with hypovolemia:
	    (1) Serum sodium value normal; decreased if hypovolemia is severe
	    (2) Serum glucose normal or elevated
	    (3) Hematocrit, hemoglobin, and red blood cells elevated
	    (4) Urinary specific gravity increased
	    (5) Urinary glucose 2+ to 4+ if hypovolemia is associated with elevated serum glucose
	    (6) Central venous pressure decreased
	    (7) Pulmonary capillary wedge pressure decreased
	    (8) Arterial pressure curve flattened
	    (9) Hypotension
	  B. Anticipate replacement of fluid deficits.

NURSING DIAGNOSIS

4. Actual fluid volume excess related to antidiuretic hormone effect, altered cardiovascular status/reserve, inadequate attention to total fluid delivery, and/or renal failure (exchanging pattern)

Patient Outcome	Nursing Orders

The patient will demonstrate normal fluid volume.	1. Assess the patient for clinical signs and symptoms of hypervolemia (see Table 35–1).
	  A. Assess the patient for altered hemodynamic or laboratory values associated with hypervolemia.
	    (1) Hematocrit decreased
	    (2) Hemoglobin decreased
	    (3) Red blood cells decreased
	    (4) Serum sodium normal; isotonic fluid excess
	    (5) Urinary sodium normal; isotonic fluid excess
	    (6) Central venous pressure increased
	    (7) Capillary wedge pressure increased
	    (8) Cardiac output increased

(continued)

NURSING CARE PLAN SUMMARY   *Patient with Altered Metabolism*   Continued

Patient Outcome	*Nursing Orders*
	B. Anticipate the following with hypervolemia: (1) Fluid restriction (2) Diuretic administration (3) Dialysis

NURSING DIAGNOSIS

5. *Altered electrolyte balance related to insufficient or excessive delivery of specific electrolyte or insufficient or excessive delivery of free water, renal failure, and specific etiology (exchanging pattern]*

Patient Outcomes	*Nursing Orders*

1. The patient will not demonstrate signs or symptoms of hyponatremia.	1. Assess the patient for clinical signs and symptoms of hyponatremia (water excess) (see Table 35–1).
	    A. Assess the patient for altered laboratory values associated with hyponatremia:
	        (1) Serum sodium decreased
	        (2) Serum osmolality decreased
	        (3) Serum urea nitrogen decreased
	        (4) Urinary output decreased
	        (5) Urinary osmolality equal to or greater than that of plasma
	        (6) Urinary sodium decreased
	    B. Assess the patient for clinical signs and symptoms of and alterations in laboratory values associated with pseudohyponatremia.
	        (1) If hyperglycemia is present, there may be a pseudohyponatremia. The hyperglycemic effect can be calculated by employing the excess of glucose over a normal of 100 mg/dl (*i.e.*, blood glucose mg/dl − 100 mg/dl) in the following formula:
	
	$$\frac{\text{Glucose excess}}{36} = \text{depression of sodium (mEq/L)}$$
	
	The actual serum sodium is the sum of the serum sodium plus the "depression" value calculated above.[2]
	        (2) If hyperlipemia or hyperproteinemia is present, there also may be a pseudohyponatremia. This should be suspected if the clinical signs of hyponatremia are not present. Lipid and protein falsely depress the serum sodium level by lowering the serum water concentration.
	    C. Anticipate the following with hyponatremia:
	        (1) Obtaining serum and urine samples for laboratory tests
	        (2) Fluid restriction and administration of diuretics if hyponatremia is due to excessive free water
	        (3) Administration of 5% sodium chloride with an intravenous pump if patient's serum sodium is less than 120 mEq/L
	        (4) Administration of insulin and/or decreased delivery of glucose solutions if associated with hyperglycemia
	        (5) Discontinuance of fat emulsions if associated with hyperlipemia
	        (6) Modification of delivery of protein solutions or dialysis if associated with hyperproteinemic states
	        (7) Slow correction to avoid complications of hypernatremia
	        (8) Seizure precautions if serum sodium is less than 110 mEq/L

2. The patient will not demonstrate signs or symptoms of hypernatremia.	2. Assess the patient for clinical signs and symptoms of hypernatremia (water deficit) (see Table 35–1). A. Assess the patient for altered laboratory values associated with hypernatremia.

(continued)

NURSING CARE PLAN SUMMARY   *Patient with Altered Metabolism*   *Continued*

Patient Outcomes	Nursing Orders

Nursing Orders

   (1) Serum sodium elevated
   (2) Serum osmolality elevated
   (3) Hemoglobin and hematocrit elevated
   (4) Serum plasma proteins elevated
   (5) Water deficit can be calculated by the following formula:

$$\frac{\text{Serum sodium (patient)} - \text{serum sodium (normal)}}{\text{serum sodium (normal)}} \times \text{body water}$$

B. Anticipate the following with hypernatremia:
   (1) Fluid replacement with 5% dextrose in water or 0.45% saline
   (2) Adding insulin if patient is diabetic, septic, or has received parenteral nutrition at an excessive rate
   (3) Slowed correction of excess to avoid cerebral edema
   (4) Seizure precautions

Patient Outcomes

3. The patient will not demonstrate signs or symptoms of hypokalemia.

Nursing Orders

3. Assess the patient for clinical signs and symptoms of hypokalemia (see Table 35–1).
A. Assess the patient for altered laboratory values or electrocardiographic changes associated with hypokalemia.
   (1) Serum potassium decreased
   (2) Serum chloride decreased
   (3) Flattening of T waves
   (4) ST-segment depression
   (5) Prominent U waves
B. Anticipate the following with hypokalemia:
   (1) Obtaining serum samples for laboratory tests
   (2) Parenteral replacement not exceeding 40 mEq/2-hour period; administering any potassium ordered over 20 mEq/hour with an infusion pump.[15]
   (3) Possibly decreasing glucose infusion rates (especially parenteral nutrition) during severe hypokalemia
   (4) Bicarbonate delivery may further decrease serum potassium levels
   (5) Cardiac monitoring
   (6) Digitalis effect possibly exaggerated

Patient Outcomes

4. The patient will not demonstrate signs or symptoms of hyperkalemia.

Nursing Orders

4. Assess the patient for clinical signs and symptoms of hyperkalemia (see Table 35–1).
A. Assess the patient for altered laboratory values or electrocardiographic changes associated with hyperkalemia.
   (1) Serum potassium elevated
   (2) Peaked T waves
   (3) Widening of the QRS complex
   (4) Absent or low P waves
   (5) Cardiac standstill or ventricular dysrhythmias
B. Anticipate the following with hyperkalemia:
   (1) Discontinuing exogenous sources of potassium, for example, drugs, stored blood
   (2) Obtaining the same concentration of plain glucose (*i.e.*, D25) and so on before discontinuing parenteral nutrition (glucose has been driving potassium into the cell; serum potassium level will increase if glucose concentration decreased too quickly)
   (3) Cation exchange resin (kayexalate—poor enema)
   (4) Sodium bicarbonate infusion
   (5) Calcium gluconate infusion
   (6) Glucose and insulin infusion
   (7) Dialysis

(continued)

NURSING CARE PLAN SUMMARY   *Patient with Altered Metabolism*   Continued

NURSING DIAGNOSIS

6. *Altered mineral balance related to excessive or inadequate delivery, renal failure, or specific etiology (exchanging pattern)*

Patient Outcomes	Nursing Orders

1. The patient will not demonstrate signs or symptoms of hypocalcemia.	1. Assess the patient for clinical signs and symptoms of hypocalcemia (see Table 35–1).
	 A. Assess the patient for altered laboratory values or electrocardiographic changes associated with hypocalcemia.
	   (1) Serum calcium decreased
	   (2) Serum magnesium normal to increased level
	   (3) Serum phosphorus low, normal, or high
	   (4) Prolonged QT interval
	 B. Anticipate the following with hypocalcemia:
	   (1) Intravenous calcium supplementation
	   (2) Oral calcium and vitamin D supplementation (hypoparathyroid hormone)
	   (3) Initiating seizure precautions
	   (4) Avoiding mixing calcium gluconate and sodium bicarbonate
	   (5) Emergency tracheostomy

2. The patient will not demonstrate signs or symptoms of hypercalcemia.	2. Assess the patient for clinical signs and symptoms of hypercalcemia (see Table 35–1).
	 A. Assess the patient for altered laboratory values or electrocardiographic changes associated with hypercalcemia.
	   (1) Serum calcium elevated
	   (2) Serum phosphorus low, normal, or high
	   (3) Shortened QT interval
	   (4) Heart blocks
	 B. Anticipate the following with hypercalcemia:
	   (1) Administration of isotonic saline, furosemide, mithramycin, and phosphate
	   (2) Cardiac monitoring
	   (3) Monitoring of digitalis levels

3. The patient will not demonstrate signs or symptoms of hypomagnesemia.	3. Assess the patient for clinical signs and symptoms of hypomagnesemia (see Table 35–1).
	 A. Assess the patient for altered laboratory values associated with hypomagnesemia.
	   (1) Serum magnesium decreased (but in some patients, *e.g.*, the burn patient, serum magnesium may be within a normal range even though total body magnesium is depleted.)[18]
	   (2) Increased outputs of gastrointestinal fluids[5]
	 B. Anticipate the following with hypomagnesemia:
	   (1) Administering magnesium supplements
	   (2) Seizure precautions

4. The patient will not demonstrate signs or symptoms of hypermagnesemia.	4. Assess patient for clinical signs and symptoms of hypermagnesemia (see Table 35–1).
	 A. Assess the patient for altered laboratory values or electrocardiographic changes associated with hypermagnesemia.
	   (1) Serum magnesium elevated
	   (2) Prolonged PR interval
	   (3) Prolonged QRS complex
	   (4) Elevated T wave
	   (5) Cardiac standstill
	 B. Anticipate the following with hypermagnesemia:
	   (1) Stopping administration of magnesium
	   (2) Administration of calcium gluconate

(continued)

NURSING CARE PLAN SUMMARY   Patient with Altered Metabolism   Continued

Patient Outcomes	*Nursing Orders*
	(3) Administration of additional intravenous fluids
	(4) Cardiac monitoring
	(5) Standby mechanical ventilation
5. The patient will not demonstrate signs or symptoms of hypophosphatemia.	5. Assess the patient for clinical signs and symptoms of hypophosphatemia (see Table 35–1).
	A. Assess the patient for altered laboratory values associated with hypophosphatemia.
	(1) Hemolytic anemia
	(2) Serum phosphorus decreased
	(3) Serum calcium decreased
	B. Anticipate the following with hypophosphatemia:
	(1) Stopping phosphate-binding antacids
	(2) Phosphorus supplementation
	(3) That rapid correction of hypophosphatemia may cause hypocalcemic tetany
	(4) That enteral and parenteral delivery of carbohydrate will decrease serum phosphate level

ALTERATIONS IN ACID-BASE BALANCE

Alterations in acid-base balance are of two basic types, as seen in Table 35–2: alkalosis, which results from increased arterial blood pH (decreased hydrogen in the blood); and acidosis, which results from decreased arterial blood pH (increased hydrogen in the blood).

Metabolic imbalances occur with derangement of the excretion or production of hydrogen or bicarbonate. Respiratory imbalances occur with derangement in carbon dioxide excretion. Mixed imbalances occur when two primary imbalances occur simultaneously or with inadequate compensation of a single imbalance. Mixed metabolic and respiratory disturbances usually neutralize pH changes. Actual bicarbonate, base excess, or the carbon dioxide content is used to evaluate compensatory mechanisms.

Acids and Bases

A substance that is dispersed in solution without undergoing any chemical change may or may not be dissociated. When the substance is dissociated, ions are dispersed in solution. Ions are molecules that have an excess or a deficit of electrons, and therefore have a net electrical charge. Ions with a positive charge are called cations, and ions with a negative charge are called anions. The hydrogen ion is a special cation with a positive charge and is called a proton. Proton donation or hydrogen ion donation is the concept involved in acidity. An acid is a substance that dissociates into component ions and donates a hydrogen ion or a proton to the solution. As the hydrogen ion is transferred to the solution, acidity is imparted to the solution. The strength of an acid is measured by the degree to which it dissociates. When an acid dissociates in solution, the base accepts the proton that is released. A base

is a hydrogen ion or proton acceptor. The most common base in the body is water. Each acid in the body dissociates into a hydrogen ion and its conjugate base. In general, a strong acid has a weak conjugate base, and a weak acid has a strong conjugate base. The strength of a base depends on its ability to extract protons from the dissociation (*i.e.*, the stronger the base, the stronger is the affinity for hydrogen ions).

Any discussion of acid-base balance must center around the hydrogen ion, for the level of the hydrogen ion controls the acidity of the solution. Although classification of acid-base balance is based on the changes in the extracellular fluid, those changes do not always parallel the condition found inside the cell. Actually, the changes might be in opposite directions.

Acidosis refers to any physiologic problem that tends to add acid to the extracellular fluid or to remove base from it. As the blood becomes more acid, the pH decreases. Because the hydrogen ion concentration is measured as the pH, as the hydrogen ion concentration increases, the pH decreases. The normal pH of arterial blood is 7.4. Compensation in the body may minimize or prevent any fall in pH of the blood, but if the pH is depressed significantly, the biochemical change is referred to as *acidosis*. A pH of less than 7.36 indicates an increase in the hydrogen ion concentration and thereby an increase in blood acidity. The opposite condition, a pH greater than 7.44, indicates a decrease in hydrogen ion concentration and is known as *alkalosis*.

$$\text{Acidosis} = \text{pH} < 7.36$$

$$\text{Alkalosis} = \text{pH} > 7.44$$

The Henderson-Hasselbalch Equation

Understanding the Henderson-Hasselbalch equation is the key to understanding acid-base balance. The equation is derived

Table 35–2
Differentiation Between Types of Acidosis and Alkalosis

	ACIDOSIS		ALKALOSIS	
	Metabolic	**Respiratory**	**Metabolic**	**Respiratory**
Antecedent Conditions	Lactic acidosis (inadequate circulation, drug induced, or prolonged fasting as in obesity) Ketoacidosis (diabetic ketoacidosis, starvation ketosis, or alcoholic ketoacidosis) Renal failure (primary tubular disease or azotemic renal failure) Poisoning (with or without increased anion gap)	Hypoventilation Chronic obstructive lung disease Depression of the respiratory center by cerebral disease or drugs Neuromuscular disorders Cardiopulmonary failure	Volume or chloride depletion (vomiting/gastric intubation with suctioning or diuretic therapy) Increased sodium bicarbonate administration Severe potassium depletion Hyperadrenocorticism	Brain-stem disease Overventilation with mechanical ventilator Hyperventilation, anxiety, pain Pulmonary embolism Secondary to hypoxia Hyperpyrexia Bacteremia Hepatic coma Salicylate poisoning
Clinical Findings	Highly variable and depend on severity and suddenness Minimal fatigue, anorexia, malaise, exertional dyspnea to stupor, coma	Headache Dyspnea Apprehension Obtunded ($PaCO_2$, 65 mm Hg to 75 mm Hg) Confusion, stupor, coma ($PaCO_2$, 90 mm Hg) Restless, pallor, sweating When significant amount present, patients are usually cyanotic with signs of pulmonary failure	When severe: apathy, confusion, slightly depressed respirations, only rarely tetany	Tingling, numbness, dizziness Restlessness, agitation Tetany Increased respiratory rate and depth
Laboratory Findings Arterial blood gases pH	↓ lowest pH compatible with life: 6.8 to 6.9	↓	↑	↑
HCO_3^-	↓	↑ in compensation	↑	↓ in compensation
$PaCO_2$	↓ in compensation about 1 mm Hg for each 1 mM/L reduction in bicarbonate	↑	↑ in compensation	↓
Electrolytes Potassium	↑	↑↓	↓	↓
Chloride	↑	↓	↓	↑ in compensation about equal to the decrease in bicarbonate

in the following way: As an acid (HB) dissociates into a proton (H^+) and a base (B^-), it does so in relation to an equilibrium constant (K):

$$\frac{[H^+][B^-]}{[HB]} = K$$

The brackets indicate that the concentrations of the various ions are being considered. Because the hydrogen ion concentration is primary, the equation can be rewritten as follows:

$$[H^+] = K\frac{[HB]}{[B^-]}$$

Because the hydrogen ion concentration is quite small, approximately in the range of 10^{-7} equivalents, this hydrogen

ion concentration is expressed as the negative logarithm, otherwise known as the pH. For example, a hydrogen ion concentration of 10^{-7} equivalents/L would be a pH of 7.00. Using log notation, the equation becomes the following:

$$\log [H^+] = \log K + \log \frac{[HB]}{[B^-]}$$

Using the pH notation or taking the negative log, the equation becomes the following:

$$-\log [H^+] = -\log K - \log \frac{[HB]}{[B^-]}$$

$$pH = pK + \log \frac{[B^-]}{[HB]}$$

The pH of a buffer solution is related to the constant, pK, plus the logarithm of the ratio of the base concentration divided by the weak acid concentration. A buffer consists of a weak or incompletely dissociated acid and its basic salt. The various body changes in the hydrogen ion concentration can best be explained in terms of one of the body's most important buffer systems, the bicarbonate-carbonic acid system. Here, excessive changes in the body's hydrogen ion concentration are prevented by maintenance of a ratio between the bicarbonate ion and carbonic acid. The ratio is 20 to 1 (*i.e.*, 20 parts bicarbonate to 1 part carbonic acid). The $PaCO_2$ is used to indicate carbonic acid. Carbonic acid may be calculated by multiplying the partial pressure of carbon dioxide, the $PaCO_2$, by the conversion factor of 0.03. Therefore, the $PaCO_2$ can be used in the Henderson-Hasselbalch equation in place of carbonic acid.

A modified version of the Henderson-Hasselbalch equation is usually used to calculate the ratio, because the pK is a constant. The equation then becomes the following:

$$pH = \frac{[B^-]}{[HB]} = \frac{base}{acid} = \frac{kidney\ function}{lung\ function}$$

$$= \frac{HCO_3^-}{H_2CO_3} = \frac{20}{1}$$

$$\updownarrow$$

$$PaCO_2 \times 0.03$$

The ratio expressed in the Henderson-Hasselbalch equation is fundamental to acid-base balance. When the ratio is changed, the pH will change. If the $PaCO_2$ increases, the denominator in the equation increases, and the pH decreases; therefore, the blood is more acid. The converse is also true. If the $PaCO_2$ decreases, the denominator becomes smaller and the pH increases; therefore, the blood is more alkaline. If the base or HCO_3^- increases, the numerator of the equation increases and the pH increases; therefore, the blood is more alkaline. If the amount of HCO_3^- decreases, less base is available to buffer and the pH decreases; therefore, the blood is more acid.

Changes in HCO_3^- are metabolic alterations—metabolic acidosis and metabolic alkalosis. Changes in $PaCO_2$ are respiratory alterations—respiratory acidosis and respiratory alkalosis. One must differentiate changes in pH as well as the metabolic versus respiratory component (Table 35–2). Mixed derangements do occur.

Metabolic Acidosis

All factors that alter the hydrogen ion concentration, other than changes in the $PaCO_2$, are metabolic or nonrespiratory in nature. As the bicarbonate level decreases significantly, the pH becomes more acidic. Metabolic acidosis is produced in the following ways:

- The hydrogen ion concentration may be directly increased by the endogenous addition of hydrogen ions. This is by far the most common mechanism, as in lactic acidosis. In the metabolism of glucose, if the cell is hypoxic, the Krebs cycle is blocked and lactic acid accumulates. It is the hydrogen ion of lactic acid that is usually responsible for the metabolic acidosis in surgical patients.

- The bicarbonate concentration may be decreased so that there is a surplus of hydrogen ions. For example, a biliary fistula with the resultant loss of large amounts of bicarbonate would produce a metabolic acidosis.

As the body attempts to compensate, respiration is stimulated, and the carbon dioxide level, like pH and bicarbonate concentration, will fall to values below normal. The compensatory respiration process stops short of normalizing pH at a point where the low pH is balanced by depression of the respiratory drive as a result of a decreased $PaCO_2$. The final acid-base status is one of primary metabolic acidosis and compensatory respiratory alkalosis.

Lactic acidosis may be due to a number of causes. Most often it is related to circulatory failure, as occurs in sepsis or shock. In such cases, lactic acid production is increased, because glycolysis is stimulated by tissue hypoxia. The acidosis may be severe, as in cardiopulmonary arrest, but usually is moderate, with the plasma lactate level less than 10 mg/dl.

Diabetic ketoacidosis is the most common cause of acute metabolic acidosis. The defect in carbohydrate use produces increases in the production of acetoacetic acid and beta-hydroxybutyric acid. These acids accumulate in the extracellular fluid in the place of bicarbonate.

Despite the body's attempt to compensate with hyperventilation and urinary acid excretion, blood pH is often reduced to extremely low levels. Ketoacidosis may also be associated with alcoholism and starvation. The typical alcoholic patient gives a history of a recent high alcohol intake, protracted vomiting, and lack of food intake. Ketone bodies and lactate accumulate in the plasma. With starvation, the use of fat as a body fuel results in a ketosis and a relatively mild acidosis.

Renal failure is the most common cause of chronic metabolic acidosis. The renal tubules are unable to excrete endogenous acids at a rate equal to that of their creation from intermediary metabolism. In some patients, this defect includes a deficiency in the renal absorption of bicarbonate, so that the acidosis is related not only to retention of acid but also to loss of alkali. When the tubular defect occurs in the absence of a significant reduction of the glomerular filtration rate, the reduction of bicarbonate is associated with an equivalent rise in plasma chloride, producing a hyperchloremic acidosis. The converse occurs when the glomerular filtration rate is very low and azotemia is present. Here, metabolic anions such as phosphates and sulfates are retained in the plasma. There is little rise in chloride concentration, and the condition is called *uremic acidosis*. The reduction in bicarbonate is balanced by a rise in anions.

With drug intoxication, the acidosis produced is greater than would be expected from the drug alone. Apparently, the drug or a breakdown product of the drug causes a metabolic block that results in excess production of endogenous organic acids. The unmeasured anions are increased.

Anion Gap

Calculation of the anion gap provides an index of acid-base status. Under normal circumstances, the total number of anions is counterbalanced by the same number of cations, so that equilibrium is maintained. The anions that can easily be measured are chloride and bicarbonate. The difference between the measured anions and cations is the anion gap. Normally, there is an anion gap of 12 mEq/L ± 2 mEq/L. An elevated anion gap implies that anions other than bicarbonate or chloride are present. This elevation in anion gap is synonymous with the presence of a metabolic acidosis. Clinically, the anion gap is calculated from serum electrolytes by the following formula:

$$Anion\ gap = Na^+ - (Cl^- + HCO_3^-)$$

Base Excess

In addition to the plasma bicarbonate, several other metabolic indices of base concentration are used to express acid-base balance (Table 35–3). There is no universal agreement about which test best measures metabolic acid-base derangements. The one test discussed in this section is base excess.

Base excess specifies the number of milliequivalents of acid or base needed to titrate 1 L of blood to pH 7.40 at 37°C while the $PaCO_2$ is held constant at 40 mm Hg. In other words, base excess quantitates the total amount of fixed acid or base present in the blood in excess of normal. The determination of base excess is widely used clinically. By convention, a *base deficit* is referred to as a negative base excess. In the body, base excess is independent of changes in the $PaCO_2$ and therefore is a measure of metabolic acid-base balance. For example, the normal base excess is zero. If 5 mEq of base, sodium hydroxide, were added to 1 L of blood, this blood would have a base excess of 5 mEq/L. The converse is true for acids. If 5 mEq/L of hydrochloric acid were added to 1 L of blood, there would be a negative base excess of 5 mEq/L.

The base excess concept is a derived binding index developed for its practical application. It consists of the bicarbonate concentration corrected for alterations in $PaCO_2$ plus the buffering capacity of hemoglobin, phosphates, and other blood proteins. After measurements of pH, $PaCO_2$, and hematocrit, the base excess is determined from nomogram calculations. As an index of deviation from the normal base concentrations, the base excess is expressed in milliequivalents per liter above or below the normal buffer base range and is changed only by nonvolatile acids.

Metabolic Alkalosis

Metabolic or nonrespiratory alkalosis is generally caused by either the addition of alkali to the body or the loss of fixed acids. Commonly, the body loses gastric secretions by vomiting or prolonged gastric suction. The result is a hypochloremic alkalosis. Because of the loss of hydrogen ions, the loss of hydrochloric acid produces an alkalosis. The chloride deficiency decreases the resorption of sodium from the renal tubules. Hydrogen and potassium then are exchanged for sodium in the distal tubules. It is this inappropriate loss of hydrogen ions that accounts for the paradoxic acid urine even in the presence of alkalosis. The loss of potassium is significant enough to cause a profound hypokalemia. As a matter of fact, hypokalemia alone will cause a corresponding metabolic alkalosis as seen with diarrhea, Cushing's disease, diuretic therapy, and steroid administration.

In metabolic alkalosis, the pH and HCO_3^- are elevated. As the pH increases, respiration is depressed. Retention of carbon dioxide then helps reduce the pH. Depression of respiration stops at the point where the independent effects of carbon dioxide and pH are equally balanced. The body changes in metabolic alkalosis are among the most complicated acid-base disturbances. As the bicarbonate concentration increases, extracellular potassium decreases. If alkalosis progresses beyond a pH of 7.55, the resultant hypokalemia is potentially fatal because of the possibility of cardiac arrest.

Respiratory Acidosis

In the normal patient, carbon dioxide excretion is determined by carbon dioxide production. An autoregulatory process, under chemoreceptor feedback control, occurs when the lungs are normal. For example, if carbon dioxide production is increased, ventilation immediately increases because of the increase in hydrogen ion concentration of the cerebrospinal fluid bathing the respiratory chemoreceptors. The increased ventilation continues until the $PaCO_2$ returns to normal. Because carbon dioxide is a volatile gas, its concentration is completely under the control of the respiratory system. Actually, the body cannot generate so much carbon dioxide that the arterial carbon dioxide level would be increased on a metabolic or nonrespiratory basis. Because carbon dioxide is the only major component of any buffer system that is under respiratory control, and because increased $PaCO_2$ would tend to elevate the hydrogen ion concentration, an increased $PaCO_2$ results in respiratory acidosis.

An acute rise in $PaCO_2$ above 44 mm Hg leads to an almost immediate rise in bicarbonate, owing to the buffering of carbonic acid by hemoglobin and other tissue buffers. This rise is minimal, about 0.8 mEq/L for each 10 mm Hg increase in $PaCO_2$, and has no real effect on the decreased pH. If the carbon dioxide retention continues for days, the plasma bicarbonate concentration will increase even more, because the renal excretion of acid increases and the renal threshold for bicarbonate simultaneously increases. With this renal compensation, the pH is closer to normal and the total increase in bicarbonate approximates 3 mEq/L for each 10 mm Hg rise in $PaCO_2$.

Respiratory Alkalosis

Respiratory alkalosis results from alveolar hyperventilation that reduces the alveolar carbon dioxide and, thus, the $PaCO_2$. In most patients, the hyperventilation is reflective of increased activity in the respiratory center. Although a mild respiratory alkalosis is generally harmless and requires no treatment, a severe alkalosis can be detrimental. The hemoglobin dissociation curve can be shifted to the left so that hemoglobin has a greater affinity for oxygen and decreased oxygen is available at the tissue level. Also, a decreased $PaCO_2$ results in con-

Table 35–3
Metabolic Parameters Indicative of Acid-Base Status

PARAMETER	NORMAL VALUE (mEq/L)
Base excess	0 ± 2
Bicarbonate	24 ± 2
Carbon dioxide combining power	25 ± 3
Carbon dioxide content	25 ± 2
Standard bicarbonate	23 ± 2
Whole buffer base	45 to 50

NURSING CARE PLAN SUMMARY   *Patient with Altered Metabolism*   Continued

NURSING DIAGNOSIS

7. *Altered acid-base balance related to excessive metabolic acids or renal failure (exchanging pattern)*
Note: *The remainder of the nursing diagnoses in this listing pertain to the acid-base balance discussion.*

Patient Outcome	Nursing Orders

The patient will not demonstrate signs or symptoms of metabolic acidosis.[12]	1. Assess the patient for clinical signs and symptoms of metabolic acidosis (see Table 35–1).
	   A. Assess the patient for altered laboratory values associated with metabolic acidosis.
	     (1) Serum potassium elevated
	     (2) Serum calcium elevated
	     (3) Serum chloride elevated
	     (4) Serum bicarbonate decreased
	     (5) Arterial blood pH decreased
	     (6) $PaCO_2$ normal or decreased
	   B. Anticipate the following with metabolic acidosis:
	     (1) Replacement of bicarbonate—60% to 100% of losses over 8 to 12 hours. The bicarbonate loss can be estimated by the following equation:
	
	 Deficit in bicarbonate (mEq)
	
	 $$= \text{normal } HCO_3^- \times \text{patient's } HCO_3^- \times \tfrac{1}{2} \text{ body weight (kg)}$$
	
	     (2) Correction of associated electrolyte abnormalities

NURSING DIAGNOSIS

8. *Altered acid-base balance related to hypokalemia, vomiting, a diuretic effect, or other specific etiology (exchanging pattern)*

Patient Outcome	Nursing Orders

The patient will not demonstrate signs or symptoms of metabolic alkalosis.	1. Assess the patient for clinical signs and symptoms of metabolic alkalosis (see Table 35–1).
	   A. Assess the patient for altered laboratory values associated with metabolic alkalosis.
	     (1) Arterial bicarbonate elevated
	     (2) Arterial pH increased
	     (3) $PaCO_2$ normal or elevated
	     (4) Serum chloride normal or decreased
	     (5) Serum potassium decreased
	     (6) Serum calcium decreased
	     (7) Urinary chloride elevated or decreased
	     (8) Gastrointestinal losses—chloride elevated
	   B. Anticipate the following with metabolic alkalosis:
	     (1) Replacement of chloride
	     (2) Replacement of potassium
	     (3) Saline infusion
	     (4) Mixed imbalances occurring frequently

(continued)

NURSING CARE PLAN SUMMARY *Patient with Altered Metabolism* *Continued*

NURSING DIAGNOSIS

9. *Altered acid-base balance related to retention of carbon dioxide (exchanging pattern)*

Patient Outcome	*Nursing Orders*

The patient will not demonstrate signs or symptoms of respiratory acidosis.	1. Assess the patient for clinical signs and symptoms of respiratory acidosis (see Table 35–1).
	    A. Assess the patient for altered laboratory values associated with respiratory acidosis.
	        (1) Serum potassium elevated
	        (2) Serum calcium elevated
	        (3) $PaCO_2$ elevated
	        (4) Arterial pH decreased
	        (5) Bicarbonate normal or elevated
	        (6) Ventricular fibrillation
	    B. Anticipate the following with respiratory acidosis:
	        (1) Identification of the precipitating factors
	        (2) Replacement of bicarbonate deficit
	        (3) Correction of electrolyte imbalance
	        (4) Not treating patient with compensated chronic obstructive pulmonary disease
	        (5) Aggressive pulmonary toilet
	        (6) That patient's sensorium may clear slowly because it takes longer for hydrogen ions to filter from the spinal fluid
	        (7) Careful administration of oxygen and the need to avoid carbon dioxide narcosis
	        (8) Seizure precautions

NURSING DIAGNOSIS

10. *Altered acid-base balance related to increased excretion of carbon dioxide (exchanging pattern)*

Patient Outcome	*Nursing Orders*

The patient will not demonstrate signs or symptoms of respiratory alkalosis.	1. Assess the patient for clinical signs and symptoms of respiratory alkalosis (see Table 35–1).
	    A. Assess the patient for altered laboratory values associated with respiratory alkalosis.
	        (1) Serum potassium decreased
	        (2) Serum calcium decreased
	        (3) $PaCO_2$ decreased
	        (4) Arterial pH elevated
	        (5) Arterial HCO_3^- normal or decreased
	    B. Anticipate the following with respiratory alkalosis:
	        (1) Use of methods to increase retention of carbon dioxide
	        (2) Correction of electrolyte imbalance
	        (3) Careful ventilator management of patient with chronic obstructive disease
	        (4) Administration of calcium gluconate
	        (5) Seizure precautions

striction of cerebral blood vessels and leads to hypokalemia with possible ventricular fibrillation.

As a compensatory mechanism in acute respiratory alkalosis with a $PaCO_2$ below 36 mm Hg, bicarbonate is reduced quickly by an adjustment in the equilibrium of the carbonic acid reaction. The kidneys compensate slowly, over hours or days, by excreting bicarbonate, so that a new relationship is established between bicarbonate and $PaCO_2$. Alkaline urine develops, and the serum potassium falls because it is exchanged with hydrogen in an effort to conserve hydrogen ions. The loss of bicarbonate in the urine results in a retention of chloride ion and a resultant increase in serum chloride proportional to the decrease in bicarbonate concentration.

Mixed Acid-Base Imbalance

A patient's acid-base status may be altered in one of the ways previously discussed, or in any combination. There are three ways in which abnormalities are seen:

1. The deviation from normal may be produced by one single physiologic process, either metabolic or respiratory in nature.
2. The metabolic or respiratory deviation from normal may be followed by a compensatory mechanism of the opposite system in the body's attempt to return to equilibrium.
3. The deviation from normal may be produced by multiple physiologic processes and the individual compensatory mechanisms.

The pH, HCO_3^- or base excess, and $PaCO_2$ must all be assessed in order to determine the primary derangement and the compensatory mechanism. For example, a patient with pH of 7.26, a $PaCO_2$ of 30 mm Hg, and a base excess of -15 mEq/L is acidotic. The base excess shows acidosis, and the $PaCO_2$ shows alkalosis. Because the pH is acid, the acidosis is primary and the alkalosis is compensatory. The decreased $PaCO_2$ helps to maintain the pH. The patient has metabolic acidosis and respiratory alkalosis. A systematic method of approaching blood gas analysis is described in Chapter 19.

IMPLEMENTATION AND EVALUATION

Table 35–1 identifies the common metabolic alterations and complications that the nurse should be able to identify. The nurse must be aware of the patient's response to planned therapeutic measures and alter nursing care as appropriate. Documentation of physical and emotional care and teaching activities should reflect whether specific outcomes are being met or the events that prevent achievement of any specific outcome. Teaching and evaluation are essential for the patient's immediate care needs, but they also address the potential for chronic problems related to metabolic alterations that can be prevented or minimized by the patient's self-care ability.

SUMMARY

Metabolic assessment is vital to the ongoing survival and eventual recovery of the critically ill patient. Alterations may occur in nutrition, water, electrolytes, minerals, or acid-base balance. Clinical signs and symptoms coupled with serum and urine values are important parameters. The nurse has the responsibility of identifying potential problems by making an accurate assessment and diagnosis and of alerting other members of the healthcare team about the patient's condition.

DIRECTIONS FOR FUTURE RESEARCH

A major research question that must be addressed by nursing is the re-evaluation of beginning to teach patients or families after their acute events but before their discharge from the critical care area to the ward. The current trend toward limiting hospital stays, which decreases available teaching time, makes consideration of this essential.

REFERENCES

1. Alpers, D. *Manual of Nutritional Therapy.* Boston: Little, Brown, 1983.
2. Burgess, A. *The Nurse's Guide to Fluid and Electrolyte Balance.* New York: McGraw-Hill, 1979.
3. Caldwell, M. D., and Kennedy-Caldwell, C. Normal nutrient requirements. *Surg. Clin. North Am.* 61:489, 1981.
4. Caldwell, M. D. Human Essential Fatty Acid Deficiency: A Review. In H. C. Meng and D. W. Wilmore (eds.), *Fat Emulsions in Parenteral Nutrition.* Chicago: American Medical Association, 1975: 24–28.
5. Dickerson, R. N., and Brown, R. O. Hypomagnesemia in hospitalized patients receiving nutritional support. *Heart Lung* 14:561, 1985.
6. Elwyn, D. H. Nutritional requirements of adult surgical patients. *Crit. Care Med.* 8:9, 1980.
7. Elwyn, D. H., Kinney, J. M., and Askanazi, J. Energy expenditure in surgical patients. *Surg. Clin. North Am.* 61:547, 1981.
8. Forlaw, L. Parenteral nutrition in the critically ill child. *Crit. Care Q.* 3–4:1, 1980.
9. Goodhart, R. S., and Shils, M. E. (eds.). *Modern Nutrition in Health and Disease* (6th ed.). Philadelphia: Lea & Febiger, 1980.
10. Harris, J. A., and Benedict, F. G. *A Biometric Study of Basal Metabolism in Man.* Publication No. 279, Washington: Carnegie Institute of Washington, 1919.
11. Hinson, L. R. Nutritional assessment and management of the hospitalized patient. *Crit. Care Nurs.* 5:53, 1985.
12. Janusek, L. W. Metabolic acidosis: Pathophysiology, signs, and symptoms. *Nursing, 90* 20:52, 1990.
13. Kennedy-Caldwell, C. Clinical triads: Water metabolism, the NPO patient, and parenteral nutrition. *Crit. Care Nurs.* 6:63, 1986.
14. Long, C. L., Schaffel, N., and Geiger, J. W. Metabolic response to injury and illness: Estimation of energy and protein needs from indirect calorimetry and nitrogen balance. *J.P.E.N.* 3:452, 1979.
15. Lunger, D. G. Potassium supplementation: How and why? *Focus Crit. Care* 15:56, 1988.
16. Moore, M. C., Guenter, P. G., and Bender, J. H. Nutrition-related nursing research. *Image J. Nurs. Sch.,* 18:18, 1986.
17. Valle, G. A., and Lemberg, L. Electrolyte imbalances in cardiovascular disease: The forgotten factor. *Heart Lung* 17:324, 1988.
18. Whang, R., Oei, T. O., Aikawa, J. K., *et al.* Predictors of clinical hypomagnesemia. *Arch. Intern. Med.* 144:1794, 1984.
19. Wilmore, D. W. *The Metabolic Management of the Critically Ill.* New York: Plenum Medical, 1980.

36

Altered Nutrition

Loretta Forlaw   *Cornelia Vanderstaay Kenner*

REWARDING YOURSELF

When was the last time you rewarded yourself? When was the last time you let yourself play regardless of how much work you needed to do? It is so easy to work, work, and work. However, it is very important to reward yourself in some small way each day. Keep in mind that rewards don't have to cost any money. The following list might spark some ideas about helping you bring more play into your life:

- Take a bubble bath and stay in 30 minutes longer than usual.
- Take a picnic in the country.
- Work on a hobby or project.
- Go to a free concert.
- Take a nap.
- Treat yourself to a massage, facial, or pedicure.
- Take time alone to just sit and think.
- Browse in a bookstore.
- Buy an item for a new craft.
- Take a continuing education course in something other than nursing.
- Cook a special meal.
- Go to a movie or rent a video.
- Spend time alone or with a friend.
- Take a half day off to do nothing.

LEARNING OBJECTIVES

After reading this chapter, the nurse should be able to do the following:

1. Compare and contrast starvation and the metabolic response to stress.
2. List the parameters involved in the nutritional assessment.
3. Provide alimentation for the critically ill patient orally, by tube, by peripheral vein, or by central vein.
4. Design a flow sheet by which to monitor the patient's weight or protein and calorie intake on a daily basis.
5. Identify salient questions in nursing research for the nutritionally depleted patient.

Note: The opinions or assertions contained herein are the private views of the authors and are not to be construed as official or as reflecting the views of the Department of the Army or the Department of Defense.

CASE STUDY

Mrs. H. is a 51-year-old real estate broker. On the date of her injury, Mrs. H. and her son had just closed their real estate office and gone for a late night supper at a nearby club. One of the patrons in the club pulled out a handgun and began to threaten the clientele. Mrs. H. was one of those shot. She sustained three wounds. The first bullet entered at the left anterolateral neck, injuring the left carotid artery and transversing to the right axillary area, causing bilateral hemopneumothoraces. The second bullet entered the abdomen at the right upper quadrant and exited at the right lateral back above the right iliac crest, causing injuries to the liver, small bowel, and colon. The third bullet entered the left lateral posterior buttock and was later palpable in the left posterior thigh.

In the emergency department, Mrs. H. had palpable pulses times four, right tracheal deviation, elevation of the left diaphragm, and mediastinal widening. Bilateral chest tubes were placed, and 2 U of uncrossmatched whole blood were administered. Mrs. H. was taken to the operating room for neck exploration, median sternotomy, thoracotomy, and exploratory laparotomy. Surgical procedures included repair of liver lacerations and small bowel injuries and a right transverse colostomy.

Mrs. H. was returned to the critical care unit in serious condition and placed on the mechanical ventilator. Mrs. H.'s postoperative course was complicated with a persistent infection that necessitated reexploration. The second procedure consisted of drainage of the pleural cavity with large argyl chest tubes, a tracheostomy for ventilatory support, and feeding jejunostomy. Internal tube feedings were initiated in the postoperative period through the jejunostomy catheter. Mrs. H.'s sepsis and pulmonary status improved, but she could not be weaned from the ventilator. A nutritional-metabolic assessment was done on the 22nd postoperative day and showed the following:

Clinical Measurements

Weight	81.4 kg
Height	152 cm
Triceps skinfold	21.0 cm
Total white blood cell count	13,050/cm^3
Lymphocytes	21%
Serum albumin	2.69/dl
Serum transferrin	105.6 mg/dl
Urine volume (24 hours)	1490 ml
Urine urea nitrogen	500 mg/dl
Urine creatinine	62 mg/dl
Serum creatinine	1.1 mg/dl
Positive skin tests	1
Intake last 24 hours:	
Dextrose 5% in water	900 ml
Magnacal, full strength	1800 ml
Indirect calorimetric measurements	
$\dot{V}O_2$	256 ml/min
$\dot{V}CO_2$	265 ml/min
Respiratory quotient	1.04

Derived Measurements

Percent ideal body weight	174%
Percent ideal triceps skinfold	95%
Calculated resting energy expenditure	1303 calories
Predicted resting energy expenditure	1468 calories
Total caloric intake	3780 calories
Total protein intake	126 g
Total nitrogen intake	20.2 g
Total urinary nitrogen	7.4 g
Nitrogen balance	9.8 g
Approximate calories needed per 24 hours	2280 to 2606 calories
Prognostic nutritional index	71.5%
Creatinine height index	108.9%

The nutritional assessment showed that Mrs. H. was receiving too many calories as a result of increased $\dot{V}CO_2$ and depressed pulmonary status. She was in positive nitrogen balance, as indicated by a positive creatinine height index and protein intake.

Mrs. H.'s caloric intake was reduced to the calculated amount needed, 2600 calories. Her pulmonary status improved. Four days later, indirect calorimetry showed a respiratory quotient of 0.82 with $\dot{V}CO_2$ of 164 ml/min and $\dot{V}O_2$ of 199 ml/min. She was successfully weaned from the ventilator.

REFLECTIONS

The nutritional requirements of patients are now recognized and addressed in most critical care settings. Little attention is given, however, to the nutritional needs of the family members of the critically ill patients. The crisis associated with responding to the patient's situation and the need for family members to make decisions for the impaired patient generally produce a stress response that results in anorexia and increased energy needs. Family members often relate their lack of appetite and inability to eat. In brief periods of 1 to 2 weeks, weight loss may be noticed by the family members themselves and the staff of the critical care unit.

The family members frequently exist on fast food because hospital cafeterias do not provide 24-hour services. Vending machine food is unappetizing, and often choices are limited or no food is available in the late evening. Families are reluctant to leave the critical care unit area, especially when the patient is severely ill, because it often seems to them that something happens each time they leave. The waiting room is often filled with empty coffee cups and partially completed fast foods. Microwave ovens are not common in waiting rooms, and tables may not be provided. Drink machines, when available, rarely contain juices or milkshakes.

Studies of normal volunteers have shown that a weight loss of 10% or greater can lead to apathy and irritability.[45] Modern technology has made it possible to support patients for extended periods of acute, nonstabilizing illness. Thus, families may be away from home with their normal routines and functioning under stressful conditions for weeks. Nutritional inadequacy, when coupled with sleep deprivation, may impact on the family member's ability to make decisions or provide support for the critically ill patient.

Nurses are in an optimal position to address these problems. A section can be included in the nursing care plan that directs the nurse to elicit information about the family's concerns, coping strategies, current eating and sleeping habits, and other pertinent information.

Common-sense measures could be implemented to address the potential effects of weight loss and its sequelae in family members. For example, can dietary services provide nutritious brown bag lunches for them for a reasonable fee? Can a refrigerator, microwave oven, and table be maintained in the waiting room? Is there a vending machine that stocks juices and milkshakes?

Evaluating and addressing ways that increase the health and quality of life of family members during the patient's time in the critical care unit should be of concern to the nursing staff and may enhance the family's ability to cope with the situation and provide support for the patient.

ETIOLOGY AND INCIDENCE

Many patients in critical care units suffer from hypermetabolism, anorexia, and malabsorption, resulting in protein and calorie undernutrition. Many, and probably most, become undernourished before hospitalization as a result of illness-related anorexia, a slightly smaller number become undernourished from the catabolic response to the stress of disease and infection, and still more from the ravages of trauma, surgery, nosocomial infections, and the semistarvation regimen of 5% dextrose in water administration. Table 36–1 lists the most common conditions associated with depletion of body-energy stores.

One study that reviewed patients awaiting heart valve replacement found that 40% had decreased lean body masses and suffered higher postoperative morbidity with a more prolonged stay in the hospital when compared with patients with normal lean body masses.[40] As many as 25% to 50% of patients hospitalized for 2 weeks or more suffer from protein and cal-

Table 36-1
Depletion of Energy Stores

Burns
Polytrauma
Fractures
Infections
High-risk or complicated major surgery
Fever
Endocrine diseases such as thyrotoxicosis
Hepatic insufficiency
Insidious protein loss such as gastrointestinal tract malignancy
Renal failure
Gastrointestinal fistula
Weight loss greater than 10% and inability to eat
Inability to eat 4 to 5 days postoperatively
Acute pancreatitis
Respiratory failure
Muscle wasting
Decubitus ulcers
Stress ulcers
Failure to heal wounds

orie undernutrition. Bistrian et al.[5,6] showed that 50% of the general surgical and 44% of the general medical patients at Boston City Hospital had undernutrition. Similarly, in an English study, 50% of surgical patients were nutritionally deficient 1 week postoperatively.[24] Undernutrition leads to increased hospital morbidity and mortality.[1,10]

PATHOPHYSIOLOGY

The normal person in a sedentary job uses 2000 calories each day. The average diet in the United States provides 70 g of protein, some 30 g to 35 g over the minimum requirement. The protein consumed has several uses in the body: formation and repair of lean tissue, visceral proteins, and immunocompetence systems.

After surgery, physical trauma, and sepsis, an inordinate amount of protein is lost from the body and can be measured in the urine as nitrogen. There is also a greater expenditure of energy (*e.g.*, after a surgical procedure such as a gastrectomy, the body's calorie requirements increase by 20% to 50%).

Undernourished patients have an increased susceptibility to develop complications such as decubitus ulcers or delayed wound healing. This tends to increase time in the critical care unit in the hospital and mortality.

Undernutrition and Stress

The body's response to stress reflects the effects of undernutrition and an altered metabolism. Although the mechanisms underlying the body's metabolic response have not been fully elucidated, many studies have identified significant alterations. Because of differences in people, site and severity of stress, treatment, and complications, the response varies. In all likelihood, alternate patterns of endocrine and metabolic response characterize different sequences.[32]

An imbalance between anabolism and catabolism is generally considered central to the problem.[14,16] Stress accentuates the use of body protein and increases gluconeogenesis for unknown reasons. Increases in nitrogen excretion tend to parallel increases in resting metabolic expenditure. Without nutritional supplements, people under stress lose weight to an

extent that is roughly proportional to the severity of the metabolic insult.

Moore[32] has described the metabolic response as having four phases: the *catabolic phase* (also called the *initial phase*, the *adrenergic-corticoid phase*, and the *negative nitrogen balance phase*); the *early anabolic phase* (also called the *turning point* and the *corticoid withdrawal phase*); the *anabolic phase*; and the *late anabolic*, or *convalescent*, phase.

The intensity of the changes in and the length of each phase vary considerably depending on the seriousness of the stressor. In the catabolic phase, the patient's energy requirements are increased, and the hormone levels (*e.g.*, the adrenergic and adrenal corticoid hormone levels) are elevated. The normal eating pattern is altered in most patients, and these patients must get their nourishment from their own bodies, exogenous alimentation, and the food they are able to eat.

The transition from the catabolic phase to the anabolic phase is called the *early anabolic phase*; it lasts for 1 to 2 days. The potassium balance becomes positive, and the nitrogen losses decrease.

In the anabolic phase, which lasts 2 to 5 weeks, the body is in positive nitrogen balance and body proteins are synthesized. The patient feels much better, begins to eat well, and gains weight.

In the late anabolic phase, the positive nitrogen balance becomes normal and the person returns to normal weight. The late anabolic phase lasts several months. Table 36–2 summarizes the metabolic responses during stressed and nonstressed starvation.

Table 36-2
Metabolic Responses During Starvation

WITHOUT STRESS	WITH STRESS
Brief Starvation	
Decreased metabolic rate	Decreased metabolic rate
Normal body temperature	Decreased body temperature
Decreased blood insulin levels	Decreased blood insulin levels
Increased blood glucagon levels	Increased catecholamine, glucagon, cortisol levels
Increased blood free fatty acids levels	Increased glucose levels
Increased urinary nitrogen excretion	Increased blood lactate levels
	Increased plasma free fatty acid levels
	Increased urinary nitrogen excretion
Prolonged Starvation	
Decreased metabolic rate	Increased metabolic rate— decreased rate
Decreased body temperature	Increased body temperature
Decreased blood insulin levels	Increased or normal insulin levels
Increased free fatty acid levels	Increased or normal catecholamine, glucagon, cortisol levels
Increased urinary nitrogen excretion	Increased or normal blood glucose levels
	Increased blood lactate levels
	Increased free fatty acid levels
	Increased urinary nitrogen excretion

(Forlaw, L. The critically ill patient: Nutritional implications. *Nurs. Clin. North Am.* 18:112, 1983; with permission.)

Starvation

The stress state is superimposed on the starvation state. During the first 2 days of food deprivation, body processes continue and the person still requires carbohydrates, proteins, fats, vitamins, and minerals. Calories are derived mainly from fat stores, because most of the small amounts of carbohydrate stored as glycogen in the liver and the muscles are quickly depleted the first day.[13]

The body's glucose requirements (about 150 g to 200 g/day) must be met by the formation of glucose (gluconeogenesis). The breakdown of tissue protein is the main source of the substrates, because glucose cannot be synthesized from fatty acids. The result is a breakdown of 50 g to 60 g of protein each day, resulting in a negative nitrogen balance of 8 g to 10 g.[20,21]

The body's protein is in a dynamic state; as such, it is not stored. Each molecule of protein has an essential purpose (*i.e.*, as part of an enzyme, an organ, a skeletal muscle, or an oncotic molecule). Thus, loss of protein means loss of function. The breakdown products of protein catabolism are excreted in the urine as urea and, to a smaller extent, as ammonia, creatinine, and uric acid. Thus, 10 g to 15 g of urinary nitrogen is usually measured in the 24-hour urine. The amount of urinary nitrogen is a good indicator of this process and accounts for most of the nitrogen loss. Although small amounts of nitrogen are lost in the urine and feces, these can be approximated in most patients (except those with diarrhea) and considered as a constant for all calculations.

Blood levels of glucose and insulin fall, and the blood levels of glucagon rise. Because insulin release is associated with a rapid reduction in the plasma levels of all amino acids by enhancing their deposition or reducing their release from muscle, decreased amounts of insulin produce the opposite effect. The release of glucagon from the alpha cells is stimulated by hypoglycemia and by the rise in the levels of plasma amino acids. It is associated with glycogenolysis, gluconeogenesis, muscle proteolysis, and the elevation of serum free fatty acids and triglycerides. A high insulin-to-glucagon ratio enhances synthesis and anabolism, and a low insulin-to-glucagon ratio enhances catabolism.

After about 48 hours, the body adapts to the starvation state by sparing protein, thus enhancing the chances of body survival. The total nitrogen loss is reduced to 3 g to 5 g/day. Although the mechanism of adaptation is not known, two changes seem to be important: the brain converts from glucose metabolism to ketone metabolism so that the body's glucose needs are reduced by 50%, or 100 g/day, and the low levels of alanine seem to limit the rate of gluconeogenesis. Most of the glucose is derived from glycerol, lactate, and pyruvate, and it is produced by the kidney as well as by the liver. The metabolic rate is reduced. Tissue fat supplies approximately 85% to 90% of the calories required; whole protein supplies 10% to 15%. An interesting side note is that obligatory water losses are decreased because nitrogen losses are decreased.

Hypermetabolism

In the changes that occur after stress, the patient is hypermetabolic. The greater the stress, the greater the catabolism. Protein is not spared. Gluconeogenesis is increased. Increases in the urinary excretion of potassium and nitrogen tend to parallel increases in the resting metabolic expenditure, but not necessarily in a cause-and-effect relationship.

Visceral and skeletal protein from all over the body is used in the catabolic response. The use of body protein as an energy source is an extremely significant phenomenon. Enzyme systems are disturbed. Use of liver protein itself from the time of the stress, coupled with therapy that produces hyperglycemia, may set the stage for deposition of fat in the liver and thus for liver failure. It is hypothesized that the catabolism of respiratory muscles as an energy source will decrease the size of the muscle mass and may limit respiration, thus setting the stage for pneumonia. Decreases in the albumin and immunoglobulin levels and in cellular immunity set the stage for infection.

Measurements of the oxygen consumption and the carbon dioxide production in surgical patients have shown that the increase in the resting metabolic expenditure approximates the increase in urinary nitrogen level.[20] In patients who have undergone uncomplicated surgical procedures, the preoperative and postoperative levels of urinary nitrogen showed no significant increases. In patients who had major fractures, the calorie expenditure increased toward 20% for 2 to 3 weeks. If major sepsis occurred in the postoperative clinical course, increases of 10% to 40% were measured. Fever superimposed on an underlying disorder raised the patient's calorie expenditure by more than the usually accepted value (a 7.2% increase for every Fahrenheit degree of increase in the body temperature). In general, the resting metabolic expenditure was elevated 20% to 50%.

The daily measurement of urinary excretion of urea nitrogen may be used to categorize patients according to severity of their stress and hypermetabolism (Table 36–3).[7–9] Patients who have a severe metabolic insult excrete more than 10 g of nitrogen daily for long periods, or they excrete higher levels of nitrogen daily for shorter periods. Corresponding problems of people who excrete more than 10 g of nitrogen daily also include hypermetabolism, metabolic disturbances, weight loss, and disturbances in the levels of electrolytes, vitamins, and trace minerals. Protein is depleted from the body in many other ways, including hemorrhage, plasma- or protein-containing fluid loss (as in a major soft tissue injury), and atrophy of bone and muscle from bed rest and other conditions of immobility.

The severity of the metabolic insult is also approximately proportional to the weight loss. For example, patients who have major fractures may lose 10% to 25% of their weight without nutritional therapy. The amount and rate of loss are accentuated if fever or sepsis is superimposed. The patient's actual weight is difficult to determine because weight is affected by the state of hydration (a large proportion of weight loss is a result of water loss).

The hypermetabolic response is at its extreme in the thermally injured patient. The metabolic rate is characterized by a rapid increase from its normal value to a peak rate and then a gradual decrease as the wound is closed. The peak rate is reached between the sixth and tenth postburn days. The amplitude of the response is proportional to the size of injury, with a maximum reached in burns involving 40% to 50% of the total body surface area. The body's oxygen consumption returns to normal when the wound is closed.[42]

Many authorities start nutritional supplementation early, and a 10% weight loss is commonly the maximum weight loss tol-

Table 36–3
Comparison of Degree of Stress Expressed as Urea Nitrogen Excretion and
Hypermetabolism Expressed as Oxygen Consumption

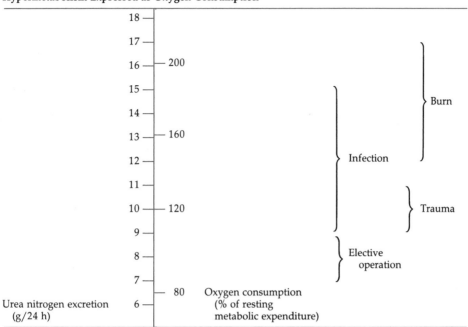

Metabolic Response

Sympathicoadrenal activity is rampant during the "fight-or-flight" response, resulting in an increased energy production, the release of glycogen and its conversion to glucose, an altered organ blood flow, an increased glucagon and a decreased insulin secretion, and gluconeogenesis. The cardiac output, heart rate, and systolic blood pressure rise. Because of capillary dilatation, the total peripheral resistance and the diastolic blood pressure decrease. The person feels anxious and is tachypneic. Intestinal peristalsis and pancreatic secretion cease. Renal blood flow decreases, as does the excretion of sodium, potassium, and chloride. In simple terms, the body has gathered all its forces and is operating at full speed in an effort to protect itself.

In another aspect of the nonspecific stress reaction, the release of corticosteroid by the adrenal cortex may be increased threefold. Glucose production increases because of the diminished release of insulin, the production of more glucose from amino acids, hepatic glycogenolysis, and the suppression of fat metabolism from carbohydrates. Protein synthesis is inhibited, and protein catabolism is enhanced. Also, the movement of water into the cell is retarded.

In trauma, the hyperglycemia is an expected response; the blood sugar returns to normal in a few hours in people who have only minor trauma. (Patients whose blood sugar levels become subnormal are probably close to death.) If the stress persists, the elevations persist. In most people, the blood glucose level is elevated for varying periods of time so that the substrate is ready for use. In others, excess glucose accumulates for a prolonged period and they demonstrate a diabetes-like syndrome (called the *diabetes of trauma* or *pseudodiabetes*).

erated before exogenous alimentation is started. A weight loss of 40% to 50% is invariably fatal, and amounts less than that result in malaise and impaired physical performance.

Insulin probably plays a central role in regulating the metabolic response.[43] The initiation and suppression of metabolic processes are regulated by the insulin-glucagon ratio. It is hypothesized that insulin reacts with the cell membrane to dispatch a second messenger inside the cell. Thus, insulin alters the metabolic response of the cell by the amount of second messenger dispatched. Muscle proteolysis is suppressed by the second messenger. In order to counteract whatever mechanism or factor produces the accelerated muscle catabolism, the insulin concentrations must increase.

CLINICAL IMPLICATIONS

Cardiovascular System

Reductions in cardiac mass and size associated with undernutrition decrease the ability of the cardiovascular system to meet the metabolic or mechanical demands that require increased myocardial work.[38] In the stressed, undernourished patient, the heart may be required to maintain constantly or intermittently, an accelerated response to compensate for decreased arterial oxygen content and increased oxygen uptake by the respiratory muscles, which reduces the quantity of oxygen available to other tissues.[38] Studies have demonstrated that the terminal event in individuals with prolonged dieting or anorexia nervosa is a cardiac dysrhythmia despite normal serum electrolyte levels.[38]

Early nutritional support minimizes weight loss and concomitant loss of cardiac mass and provides fuel for muscle work.

Pulmonary System

Undernutrition is associated with increased pulmonary infection. Pneumonia has been shown to occur more commonly in surgical patients with serum albumin levels less than 3.0 g/dl.[38]

Diaphragmatic muscle mass diminishes with weight loss. There is a significant effect on muscle strength and endurance.[26,38] Decreased vital capacity and lower peak inspiratory force are associated with malnutrition in patients without respiratory disease.[26,38] Maximal mid-expiratory flow rate and lung-diffusing capacity are decreased in malnourished patients with chronic pulmonary disease.[38]

Nutritional support has been shown to improve respiratory muscle function before complete repletion of lean body mass. This suggests that providing fuel reverses the deleterious effects of inadequate energy and mineral supplies associated with undernutrition.[26]

Renal System

Starvation has little effect on kidney mass, and microscopic changes are minimal.[38] Hypophosphatemia, which is common in malnourished patients, impairs the kidney's ability to excrete an acid load. The maximal concentrating ability of the kidney is decreased (660 mOsm versus 800 mOsm) with dehydration in the malnourished patient.[38] This effect may be related to a decreased urea concentration in the renal medulla.[38]

Maintaining normal serum phosphorus levels and providing a balanced total parenteral nutrition solution (potassium and sodium as chloride and acetate salts) decrease the workload of the kidney and enhance acid-base balance in the malnourished patient.

NURSING PROCESS

ASSESSMENT

Before undernutrition and stress can be treated, a nutritional assessment is in order. The results of this assessment then act as a baseline in serial monitoring and reassessment. Although many assessment parameters have been identified, accurate predictors of energy expenditure in undernourished critically ill patients are not available. At the present time, no single test is sufficient, and a metabolic profile of each patient must be determined. The following sections identify the components of assessment that are used (Table 36-4).

History

In relation to the dietary history, the patient should be asked the following questions:

- At what time does the patient eat?
- With whom does the patient eat?
- Are there any problems in eating or chewing (*e.g.*, poorly fitting dentures)?
- Has the patient recently noted any weight loss or gain?
- Does food smell or taste any different?
- Does the patient have any problems with nausea, vomiting, constipation, or diarrhea?
- What medications is the patient currently taking?
- What are the patient's favorite foods and beverages?
- What was ingested at the last meal? When was it?

Table 36-4
Parameters in Nutritional Assessment

Nutritional Status
Protein intake (in grams)
Caloric intake (in grams)
Nitrogen balance (derived, in grams)
Obligatory nitrogen loss (derived, in grams)
Net protein utilization (derived, in grams)
Basal energy expenditure (derived, in calories per 24 h)
Caloric intake (calories or derived as percent of basal energy expenditure)
Skin-test results (in mm and number of positive tests)

Anthropometrics
Height (in centimeters)
Weight (in kilograms)
Usual weight (in kilograms)
Sex
Ideal body weight (from standard tables, in kilograms)
Weight (derived, as percent of usual weight and as percent of ideal body weight)
Triceps skinfold (in millimeters and derived, as percent of standard)
Arm circumference (in centimeters)
Arm muscle circumference (derived, in cm and as percent of standard)

Laboratory Tests
Serum albumin (in g/dl)
Total iron-binding capacity (in μg/dl)
Serum transferrin (in mg/dl)
Lymphocytes (as percent)
White blood cell count (in number/mm^3)
Total lymphocyte count (derived)
24-hour urine urea nitrogen (in grams)
24-hour urine creatinine (in milligrams)
Creatinine-height index (derived, as percent of standard)

Clinical Signs

The nurse carefully assesses the status of protein, calorie, vitamin, and mineral intake. The status is reflected in the clinical physical signs of the patient:

Face	Seborrhea
Hair	Dull, dry, lacks luster, is easily removed or falls out easily, thin, sparse, transverse depigmentation (flag sign)
Eyes	Blepharitis, photophobia, cornea vascularization, dull and dry conjunctiva, mild yellow cast to sclera, fundal capillary microaneurysms
Lips	Cracks and sores around mouth, fissures
Mouth	Stomatitis
Tongue	Edema, glossitis, papillae, magenta tongue
Gums	Bleeding, swollen, peridontal problems
Teeth	Mottled
Neck	Enlarged thyroid or parotid glands
Skin	Pigmentation changes, dry and flaky, tight and drawn, pale, dermatitis, petechiae, hyperkeratosis
Nails	Brittle, spoon-shaped, lusterless, transverse ridging
Abdomen	Vomiting, diarrhea, enlarged, faulty liver, ascites

Neurosensory   Decreased position sense, vibratory sense, and reflexes; ataxia; weakness

Musculoskeletal   Dependent edema, wasted muscles (especially in temporal area, on dorsum of hand, or spinal area), flabby skin, tender calf muscles, and skeletal malformations such as tenderness

Anthropometric Measurements

Anthropometric measurements can be used with acutely ill and chronically ill patients. However, there remain some questions about the best way to use the measurements with critically ill patients. Chronically ill patients may be nutritionally depleted and admitted to the critical care unit in an acute episode. Previously healthy patients may be admitted to the critical care unit after an acute episode and quickly become nutritionally depleted. Figure 36–1 illustrates a sample nutritional assessment sheet on which to record anthropometric measurements and laboratory data.

The height and age are obtained directly from the patient. The weight record is graphed from those weights documented in the patient's record. A body weight below 90% of ideal body weight indicates depletion of body mass with protein and calorie undernutrition. Improvement in or maintenance of body weight can also be assessed by serial daily weights. However, weight loss is a difficult measurement to assess, because the loss may be masked by progressive edema. Body weight may be normal in the semistarved patient with protein and calorie depletion. Especially in patients who were obese before the stressful incident or illness, the lean body mass may be atrophic, although the adipose tissue is still enlarged.

Anthropometric measurements give a quantitative estimate of the triceps skinfold and midarm circumference. The triceps skinfold is estimated on three readings with calipers. The skin is measured at the back of the nondominant arm midway between the acromial process and the olecranon process of the ulna. Body fat or adipose stores are assessed by the triceps skinfold. The normal values are 12.5 mm for men and 16.5 mm for women. A reading of 3 mm or less is indicative of severely depleted fat stores. The measured values are often expressed as a percentage of the normal values, so that the caloric deficiency can be assessed as mild, moderate, or severe (mild being 90% to 51%, moderate being 50% to 30%, and severe being less than 30%).

The midarm circumference at the mid-upper arm is measured on the same site on the nondominant arm with a tape measure and acts as an indication of skeletal muscle mass or somatic protein. The normal values are 25.3 cm for men and 23.2 cm for women. The measured values are often expressed as a percentage of the normal values, so that protein deficiency can be assessed as mild, moderate, or severe (mild being 90% to 81%, moderate being 80% to 70%, and severe being less than 70%). In some hospitals, because lean muscle mass is really the desired parameter, the midarm circumference (MAC) is used to calculate the midarm muscle circumference (MAMC). The MAC is really a measurement of MAMC and fat stores.

Patient _____ Date _____ Age _____
Diagnosis _____ Height _____ cm Weight on Admission _____ kg

	Measurements	Normal	Patient	Less than Body Requirements			
				None	5–15%	16–30%	>30%
Somatic Protein and Fat Stores	Usual weight / Current weight	From standard tables					
	Triceps skinfold	Men 12.5 mm Women 16.5 mm					
	Midarm circumference	Men 25.3 cm Women 23.2 cm					
	Midarm muscle circumference	Men 21.4 cm Women 18.0 cm					
	Urinary creatinine	From standard tables					
	Creatinine-height index	Percent of standard					
Visceral Protein	Serum albumin Serum transferrin	≥3.5 gm/dl ≥150 mg/dl					
Cell-Mediated Immunity	Lymphocytes Skin tests	1500–3000/mm^3 >5 mm					

Figure 36–1

Nutrition assessment sheet.

To calculate skeletal muscle mass, the following formula is used:

$$MAMC \text{ (in cm)} = MAC \text{ (in cm)}$$
$$- [0.314 \times \text{triceps skinfold (in mm)}]$$

The normal values for the MAMC are 21.4 cm for men and 18.0 cm for women. Severe skeletal muscle wasting is indicated by a MAMC of less than 15 cm.

Diagnostic Tests

Diagnostic tests in the nutritional assessment usually include a combination of several of the following: complete blood count; white blood cell count and differential, with the lymphocyte count expressed as a percentage of the white blood cell count; total lymphocyte count; serum albumin, serum transferrin, or total iron-binding capacity; serum creatinine; serum alkaline phosphatase; a 24-hour urine specimen for urine urea nitrogen and creatinine; and skin tests.

The status of visceral protein is assessed by the hemoglobin, albumin, serum transferrin, and total iron-binding capacity. Serum albumin has been identified as an important indicator of undernutrition.[1] Edema results when serum albumin levels fall below 2.8 g/dl, provided there is no liver, cardiac, or venous disease. However, serum transferrin is a protein with a shorter half-life than albumin; therefore, during nutritional therapy, it reflects nutritional repletion more rapidly than albumin. Serum transferrin can be calculated from the total iron-binding capacity (TIBC) measurement by the following formula:

$$\text{Serum transferrin} = (0.8 \times \text{TIBC}) - 43$$

The hemoglobin and hematocrit values also assess nutritional iron status. Serum alkaline phosphatase is used as an indirect measurement of vitamin D status.

The creatinine measurement in the 24-hour urine is used to determine the percentage ratio of the creatinine height index, one of the most important tests to detect protein deficiency, particularly skeletal muscle catabolism. The following formula is used:

Percent creatinine-height index

$$= \frac{\text{24-hr creatinine excretion of patient}}{\substack{\text{24-hr creatinine excretion expected for normal} \\ \text{person of same height (obtained from} \\ \text{a standard table)}}} \times 100$$

The 24-hour urine creatinine is related to lean body mass by the conversion, lean body mass (kg) = 21.0 + 21.5 (percent creatinine per 24 hours). Creatinine clearance is also a frequent determination. The formula is as follows:

$$\text{Creatinine clearance} = \frac{\text{urinary creatinine (in mg/dl)}}{\text{serum creatinine (in mg/dl)}}$$
$$\times \text{volume of urine (in ml/min)}$$

The urea nitrogen in the 24-hour urine is used to assess the degree of hypermetabolism and actual metabolic expenditure. During stress, approximately 15% of the calorie expenditure is provided by amino acid oxidation. The urine urea nitrogen represents the end product of protein metabolism. Estimated nitrogen balance can be calculated to assess nutritional therapy by the following formula:

$$\text{Estimated nitrogen balance} = \frac{\text{protein input (in grams)}}{6.25}$$
$$- [\text{24-hr urine urea nitrogen (in grams)} + 4]$$

For the purposes of nutritional assessment, the addition of 4 to the urine urea nitrogen generates a useful value for total nitrogen output when the patient has daily stools.

Immunologic Response

The immunologic response is determined by the total lymphocyte count and the reaction to skin-test antigens. The total lymphocyte count is used as a measure of cellular defense mechanisms (immunocompetence) as well as visceral protein status. It is calculated as follows:

Total lymphocyte count

$$= \frac{\text{percent lymphocytes} \times \text{white blood cells}}{100}$$

The patient also may be skin tested with one or more intradermal skin tests: streptokinase-streptodornase, mumps, *Candida albicans*, dilute tetanus toxoid, and purified protein derivative. The goal is to assess the immunologic response (or, more commonly, delayed hypersensitivity or cellular immunity). If the patient has an intact immune response and has been exposed to the antigen previously, a positive reaction will be noted. The induration is measured in millimeters at 24 and 48 hours. A normal response is a 15-mm wheal in 24 to 48 hours to any one of the antigens. A response of 10 mm to 15 mm indicates mild impairment in immunologic response, 5 mm to 10 mm indicates moderate impairment, and less than 5 mm signifies severe immunoincompetence. *Anergy* is the term usually used to signify the inability of a patient to respond with a positive reaction to any one of the battery of skin antigens. The presence of adequate immunologic response is demonstrated by a positive reaction. The positive reaction or cutaneous response after injection of the antigen presents clinically as an area of induration that is the result of cellular infiltration of T lymphocytes and macrophages. Erythema has no significance in the response, because it only indicates vasodilatation.

The physical examination and nitrogen balance are the most valuable assessment parameters in the acutely ill patient. Anthropometrics, skin tests, and laboratory tests to include the creatinine-height index, albumin, and transferrin are helpful on admission and during the convalescent phase.

Prescription and Prognosis

One of the goals of nutritional assessment is to organize patient variables into categories that will quantitate the degree of clinically relevant malnutrition and associated clinical risk and allow patient outcomes for therapy to be identified. A simple means to differentiate patients and perhaps one of the most widely used is the selection of maintenance or repletion therapy. *Maintenance therapy* can be administered by the enteral route (the gastrointestinal tract) or the enteral plus peripheral venous routes. Central vein cannulation is not needed. *Repletion therapy* can be given by three routes: enteral, enteral plus peripheral venous, or central venous. As a general rule, patients with rapidly progressive or severe undernutrition need repletion therapy, whereas patients with slowly progressive or mild undernutrition need maintenance therapy.

Blackburn et al.[7] have suggested one organization of categories. Three syndromes are identified: marasmus, kwashiorkor-like, and a mixture of the two. *Marasmus* is a variant of undernutrition characterized by decreased body weight, decreased creatinine-height index, and, when severe, delayed immunologic response. The visceral proteins are preserved at the expense of the lean muscle mass. In the *kwashiorkor-like syndrome,* visceral protein is depleted. The syndrome is characterized by decreased serum proteins (albumin and transferrin), decreased total lymphocyte count, and delayed immunologic response. It is a protein deficiency without a major calorie deficit. Anthropometric measurements are intact, whereas the visceral proteins are depleted. A mixed type of marasmus-kwashiorkor picture is usually seen in the hospital setting. Patients present with skeletal muscle and visceral protein wasting, depleted fat stores, immunoincompetence, and vitamin and mineral deficiencies.

Buzby et al.[12] have developed the *Prognostic Nutritional Index.*[33] The index is formulated as a predictor of outcome and is based on albumin (Alb), transferrin (TFN), triceps skinfold (TSF), and the number of skin tests reactive (DH). The following formula is used:

Prognostic Nutritional Index (percent predicted risk)

$$= 158\% - 16.6 \ (\text{Alb, in g/dl}) - 0.78 \ (\text{TSF, in mm})$$
$$- 0.2 \ (\text{TFN, in mg/dl}) - 5.8 \ (\text{DH})$$

Patients are correctly classified by outcome 80% of the time; the remaining 20% are false positives, in which a poor outcome has been predicted but not realized.

Nutrition and Diet

The patient's normal and recent protein and calorie intakes are assessed. Actual monitoring of all intake is the most accurate method. The rate of the protein and calorie undernutrition is assessed by the patient's daily intake of protein and calories.[19] *Undernutrition* is a state of rapid progression with a daily intake of less than 30 g of protein and 1000 calories. The rate of progression will be more severe if associated problems such as fever, infection, or malabsorption are present.

Systems for assessing protein and calorie status do not take into account the significant variations in body build. Skeletal weight may vary by as much as 50% in individuals of the same height, as do the skeletal muscles. There is also great variation with age.

The patient's calorie needs are calculated. A simple method for supplying calorie needs is to provide 25 to 35 calories/kg/day for maintenance and 45 calories/kg/day for nutritional repletion. However, a more accurate method is to calculate the basal energy expenditure (BEE) first and then, based on that value, calculate the maintenance or nutritional repletion therapy. The BEE is calculated using the Harris-Benedict equation, which follows:

Men:

$$\text{BEE} = 66 + (13.7 \times \text{weight}) + (5 \times \text{height}) - (6.8 \times \text{age})$$

Women:

$$\text{BEE} = 655 + (9.6 \times \text{weight}) + (1.7 \times \text{height}) - (4.7 \times \text{age})$$

Using the basal energy expenditure calculated, the total calories needed for 24 hours can be calculated for those patients who only need maintenance therapy and for those patients who need nutritional repletion therapy:

Maintenance therapy:

$$\text{BEE} \times 1.22 = \text{calories/24 hr}$$

Nutritional repletion therapy:

$$\text{Oral: BEE} \times 1.54 = \text{calories/24 hr}$$
$$\text{IV: BEE} \times 1.76 \text{ to } 2.0 = \text{calories/24 hr}$$

If no extraordinary nutritional demands are placed on the patient and only maintenance is needed, the protein requirement is estimated to be 0.8 g/kg ideal body weight. If there are additional nutritional demands and repletion therapy is needed, the level of protein intake can be adjusted according to the blood urea nitrogen level,[7] or the following formulas can be used for nitrogen intake per 24 hours (6.25 g nitrogen = 1 g protein):

$$\text{Maintenance: } \frac{\text{Calories/24 hr}}{300} = \text{grams nitrogen/24 hr}$$

$$\text{Repletion: } \frac{\text{Calories/24 hr}}{150} = \text{grams nitrogen/24 hr}$$

Nutritional Support

The guidelines for the critically ill patient's nutritional requirements have been formulated by many researchers, but a great deal of research remains to be done before specific baseline requirements can be determined. Nutritional requirements parallel the degree of stress on the patient (Fig. 36–2).

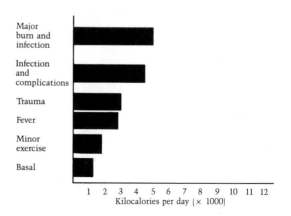

Figure 36–2

Nutritional support required for the average adult.

Kinney *et al.*[27] suggest a change in the calorie-nitrogen ratio from a normal of 200 calories to 300 calories/g of nitrogen in the active uninjured state to 100 calories to 150 calories (in some circumstances, 75 calories to 150 calories)/g of nitrogen in the injured state. Dudrick *et al.*[17] suggest daily supplements of about 12 g to 24 g of nitrogen and 2500 calories to 4000 calories for people who have major illnesses. Moore[32] suggests 200 mg of nitrogen and 50 calories/kg of body weight daily. Wilmore[45] recommends 15 g of nitrogen and 2000 calories/m²/day for thermally injured patients. Curreri *et al.*[15] have developed the following formula for the ideal calorie intake of burn patients that considers the person's individual differences (TBSA stands for total body surface area):

25 calories × kilograms of body weight + 40 calories

× percent TBSA burned = calorie intake

In general, for critically ill patients, nutritional repletion requires 2700 calories to 3500 calories/day and 1.5 to 3 times the recommended daily allowances of essential vitamins and minerals. Nutritional maintenance usually requires 2000 calories to 2700 calories and about 0.7 times the recommended daily allowances.

With stress, the body's nutritional needs may be met by oral means, tube or intravenous feedings, or by a combination of these methods.

NURSING DIAGNOSES, PATIENT OUTCOMES, AND PLAN

The preceding material on physiology, pathophysiology, nursing assessment, and diagnostic tests guides the nurse in establishing nursing diagnoses, patient outcomes, and the plan for the patient with altered nutrition.

NURSING CARE PLAN SUMMARY *Patient with Altered Nutrition*

NURSING DIAGNOSIS

1. Altered nutrition: less than body requirements related to anorexia, malabsorption, or hypermetabolism (exchanging pattern)

Patient Outcomes	Nursing Orders
1. The metabolic stress on the patient will not be increased by environmental stimuli.	1. If possible, work with the patient in drawing up the plan of care and scheduling procedures. A. Use analgesics as needed. B. Use relaxation techniques and music therapy. C. Provide for the longest periods of sleep possible. D. Carry out all nursing procedures with a minimum of stress. E. Maintain the patient's muscle mass by a planned exercise program. F. For burn patients, maintain a warm environment and cover the burned areas with heat shields.
2. The patient will meet nutritional and caloric needs by the oral intake of food.	2. In collaboration with the nutritionist, pharmacist, and physician, assess the patient's nutritional requirements. A. Assess the patient's eating habits: food preferences, former eating habits, traditions, and preferences about mealtimes and about the amount of food to be served. B. Assess the patient's threshold for smells and taste: (1) If the threshold for a sweet taste is elevated, increase the sugar intake as appropriate. (2) If beef and (occasionally) pork taste bitter, encourage the consumption of poultry, fish, eggs, and cheese. C. Consult with a nutritionist about the patient's diet during a staff conference. D. Help select the patient's meals. E. Involve the patient's family in selecting food and in feeding. If a problem arises, ask the family to bring some of the patient's favorite foods. F. Give the patient a calorie-containing beverage rather than water to take with medications and to assuage thirst. G. Add polycose to liquids and sprinkle on foods. H. Keep a running tabulation of the calories taken in and those still to be eaten. I. Make rounds during mealtimes to assess the patient's eating.
3. Anorexia will be diminished.	3. If pain is a problem at mealtimes, give the patient an analgesic 30 minutes before eating. Check for anorexia or gastric distress after the analgesic has been given.

(continued)

NURSING CARE PLAN SUMMARY *Patient with Altered Nutrition* *Continued*

Patient Outcomes	Nursing Orders
	Remember that narcotic analgesics further delay gastric emptying.

Remember that narcotic analgesics further delay gastric emptying.
A. Do not schedule laboratory tests, physical therapy, and painful procedures at mealtimes.
B. Try to make mealtimes more social (*e.g.*, by staying with the patient or having a family member present).
C. Be aware that the following drugs may depress the appetite: digitalis, atropine, phenothiazine tranquilizers, antihistamines, iron and potassium salts, theophyllin, salicylates, antibiotics (especially tetracycline and erythromycin), quinidine, and procainamide.
D. Give mouth care every 4 hours as needed. Do not routinely use lemon and glycerine, because they are drying. Use a solution that is half hydrogen peroxide and half water.
E. Give the patient liquid-diet supplements. Make them more palatable by doing the following:
   (1) Using various flavors
   (2) Chilling them
   (3) Serving them as ice cream, popsicles, snow cones, puddings, or sauces
F. If applicable, provide an alcoholic beverage before meals as ordered to enhance appetite and add calories.

4. The patient will meet nutritional needs by liquid supplementation through tube feeding.

4. Assist in the feeding.
A. Assist in the nasoenteric tube feeding. Use a small feeding catheter or tube, such as a Dobhoff tube.
   (1) Keep the head of the patient's bed elevated 30° at all times.
   (2) Check the placement of the tube every 8 hours or before feeding.
   (3) Administer the feeding by a constant infusion pump or, in some instances, by gravity.
   (4) Start at a prescribed rate and gradually increase (*e.g.*, begin infusion with an isotonic formula at a rate of 50 ml/hour for 24 hours and increase rate in 25 ml/hour increments over a 24-hour to 36-hour period until prescribed total is reached).
B. Assist in the jejunostomy feeding of the patient. Jejunostomy feeding will usually be given by continuous drip. Occasionally, a patient will tolerate intermittent jejunostomy feedings without diarrhea. Intermittent delivery of formula into the jejunum can result in less efficient absorption of nutrients, even though the patient does not experience diarrhea. Monitor the patient closely for inadequate weight gain and symptoms of nutrient deficiency.
   (1) Postpone the feeding until the site is verified by a radiograph.
   (2) Observe for signs of peritonitis.
   (3) As ordered, begin with 200 ml of a warm feeding every 2 hours on even hours.
   (4) If diarrhea begins, consult with the physician about the following protocol:
      a. Discontinue the feedings for 24 hours.
      b. Begin the feeding schedule again, but increase the amounts more slowly.
      c. If the diarrhea has not abated, 30 minutes before a feeding give the patient tincture of belladonna (10 drops) or a Lomotil tablet or Paragoric (5 ml) if ordered.
   (5) Refeed the fistula drainage every 2 hours on odd hours.
   (6) Monitor for symptoms of "dumping syndrome," which is diaphoresis, hypotension, and acute diarrhea associated with delivery of formula. If these symptoms occur, consider continuous jejunal feeding.
C. Monitor for mechanical obstruction of the catheter lumen or gastrointestinal complications (vomiting, bloating, diarrhea, or cramping). If complications present, reduce the flow or the concentration of the feeding, consult with the physician, and supplement with peripheral intravenous fluid. Advance the flow rate more slowly on the second attempt.

(continued)

NURSING CARE PLAN SUMMARY *Patient with Altered Nutrition* *Continued*

Patient Outcomes	*Nursing Orders*
	D. Assess the patient's inability to assimilate a large nutrient load: hyperglycemia, glycosuria, hyperosmolar coma, hyperkalemia, hypercalcemia, hypermagnesemia, hyperaminoacidemia, and azotemia. If necessary, reduce the flow and consult with the physician.
5. In the event the patient's calorie needs cannot be met by the methods previously outlined, the protein calorie needs will be met by peripheral venous or central total parenteral nutrition therapy.	5. Support and monitor the patient during the insertion of the central line as follows:
	A. If the line is to be inserted into the subclavian vein, have the patient lie supine in a slight (15°) Trendelenburg position and place a small roll between the shoulders so that they can drop, thus making the vein more accessible.
	B. If the needle or catheter becomes detached from the syringe or tubing, ask the patient to hold his or her breath, ask the patient to do the Valsalva maneuver, or apply firm pressure to the abdomen. If an air embolism is suspected, look for the following signs: the patient becomes unconscious, the pulse is weak or absent, and a sloshing murmur is heard over the right side of the heart. Put the patient exhibiting such signs on the right side with feet up and head down. Notify the physician for an emergency evacuation of air from the heart.
	C. After insertion of the catheter, monitor for a possible pneumothorax. The fluid administered should be a 5% dextrose-in-water solution until the site is verified by a chest radiograph.
	D. If the chest radiograph does not establish that the catheter is in the superior vena cava, innominate vein, intrathoracic subclavian vein, or right atrium, withhold the total parenteral nutrition solution until the physician has been notified.
	E. After insertion of the catheter, observe for respiratory distress, chest pain, pneumothorax, tingling fingers, numbness of the arm, or an allergic reaction (increased pulse, headache, nausea, and vomiting).
	F. Maintain a continuous flow with an intravenous pump.
	(1) Check the order daily. The physician will order gradual increments until the desired amount is reached. The same procedure may be used in discontinuing the solution, because suddenly stopping the hypertonic infusion may produce an insulin rebound and hypoglycemia. However, the solution may be stopped for several hours without problems in moderate to well-nourished, well-hydrated patients.
	(2) Calculate the number of drops per minute and check the flow every hour if an infusion pump is not available.
	(3) Attach to an electronic continuous volumetric infusion administration set.
	G. Initiate therapy gradually. The nonacute adult receives 1 L of solution in first 24 hours. Regular insulin may be needed. Measure blood glucose 2 hours before second liter is to start. Two liters of solution are given in the second 24 hours.
	H. Be aware that the position of the patient may alter the drip rate. If the administration of the solution gets behind schedule, do not speed it up (the percentage hourly increase should be determined and carefully monitored; 10% to 20% increase is usual). A too rapid administration may produce hyperglycemia and hyperosmolar nonketotic coma.
	I. Monitor the urine for glycosuria every 6 hours to make sure that the patient's glucose tolerance is not exceeded at normal rates of infusion. Obtain a blood glucose for glycosuria 2+ or greater. Older patients and stressed patients may have a lower renal threshold and will have glycosuria with a normal blood glucose. When the blood sugar is above 200 mg/dl and the glycosuria is 3+ or greater, the renal threshold is exceeded, leading to an osmotic diuresis. However, patients who have decreased circulating volumes and a decreased renal perfusion may have extremely high levels of blood glucose and a low level of urine sugar. Water continues to be drawn into the

(continued)

NURSING CARE PLAN SUMMARY   *Patient with Altered Nutrition*   *Continued*

Patient Outcomes	*Nursing Orders*

intravascular space and excreted, resulting in hypertonic dehydration. The number of osmols in the intravascular space increases (hyperosmolar state) with increases in serum electrolytes, blood urea nitrogen, and blood sugar levels (even to more than 1000 mg/dl). The patient becomes progressively more lethargic and confused in a process that ends in coma and death. The treatment is insulin therapy and free water, usually given as a 5% dextrose-in-water solution.

J. As ordered, administer insulin for glycosuria subcutaneously or intravenously. Insulin may be added to the nutrient solution in patients who are mildly hyperglycemic but well hydrated. As the level of endogenous insulin rises, the insulin supplementation should decrease, as the following table shows:

GLYCOSURIA	INSULIN SUPPLEMENTATION
1+	None
2+ (often occurs for 24–72 h while higher insulin levels are developed)	None
3+	5 U
4+ (blood sugar check is the accepted protocol in many critical care units)	10 U

   (1) Use a fresh urine specimen for testing.

   (2) If the patient is receiving cephalothin, aspirin, or amino acids (total parenteral nutrition solution) use Testape for the urine test, because false-positive results are obtained with Clinitest tablets.

K. Stop infusion per physician order. The following is a common protocol: slow gradually over a 24-hour period; infuse 5% dextrose-in-water solution in 0.33% saline with 20 mEq KCl for several hours after solution has ceased in order to prevent hypoglycemia.

L. Remember that sudden glucose intolerance with or without a fever is a cardinal sign of sepsis in the trauma patient.

M. Monitor the following physiologic parameters:

   (1) Check the patient's vital signs every 4 hours. If the patient has a fever, notify the physician, change the entire intravenous line to the insertion site, change the total parenteral nutrition solution, and have cultures tested.

   (2) Check the fluid intake and output every 8 hours.

   (3) Weigh the patient daily.

   (4) Chart the condition of wounds daily.

   (5) Have the appropriate laboratory work done daily until the patient's condition has stabilized.

   (6) Check the serum electrolyte levels daily until stable, then three times a week.

   (7) Check the blood sugar, blood urea nitrogen level, prothrombin time, complete blood count, platelet count, and serum calcium, phosphorus, and magnesium levels.

   (8) Check the serum and urine osmolality and serum protein levels.

   (9) Monitor nutritional parameters as follows and per the physician's order: nitrogen balance twice a week, total lymphocyte count weekly, and anthropometrics, serum transferrin, and skin tests every 3 weeks.

N. Keep the solution sterile.

   (1) Inspect the bags and the solution for a cloudy appearance.

   (2) Return to laminar flow for addition of medications before hanging solution.

(continued)

NURSING CARE PLAN SUMMARY *Patient with Altered Nutrition* Continued

Patient Outcomes	Nursing Orders
	(3) Refrigerate the bottle or bag (at 4°C) until it is used. (It should not be kept longer than 24 hours.)

(4) Always clean the cap with an isopropyl alcohol solution before opening the bag.

(5) New bottles of fluid should be hung at least every 12 hours.

(6) Do not add drugs to the solution unless agreed on with the physician. Check the compatibility with the pharmacist.

(7) Check the bag for the patient's name, date, additives, preparation time, expiration time, and rate of administration.

O. Prevent infection acquired through the skin and administration lines by taking the following precautions:

(1) If possible, set up for a catheter insertion in the treatment room or the operating room.

(2) Order enough gowns, masks, and gloves for those involved in inserting the catheter.

(3) Maintain sterile conditions during the insertion.

(4) Before the insertion, determine whether the hair should be removed.

(5) Prepare the insertion site with acetone, tincture of iodine, and alcohol. For example, use a 1% iodine in 70% alcohol solution, allow it to dry 30 seconds to 2 minutes, then wash it off with a 70% isopropyl alcohol solution. Using friction, work from the center of the site to its periphery.

(6) If the patient has sensitive skin, use an iodophor skin preparation. It should not be washed off; it should be allowed to dry.

P. Monitor the insertion site.

(1) Inspect the site every 24 hours or whenever the dressings are changed. Observe for inflammation, phlebitis, or purulence.

(2) If the anchoring sutures become dislodged, notify the physician. With proper care, the site may be used for 30 days. In thermally injured or septic patients, the site is changed every 3 days.

(3) Observe the following infection-control policy: At least once every 2 days, clean the site with acetone to remove the tape debris, iodophor agent, and alcohol. Pay particular attention to the small parts of the catheter, including the plastic needle guard.

(4) Apply an iodophor ointment to the site.

(5) Cover the site with an occlusive dressing:

　a. Cover the site with gauze (two or three sponges).

　b. Use benzoin on the surrounding skin.

　c. Form an occlusive dressing with Elastoplast and adhesive tape (not paper tape).

　d. Tape all connections.

　e. Anchor the filter and the intravenous tubing.

(6) Record the data on the outside of the dressing and in the nurses' notes.

Q. Monitor the intravenous lines.

(1) Use an in-line filter between the catheter and the tubing according to the recommendations of the hospital's infection control committee.

(2) Stabilize the filter with tape so that the tubing cannot be dislodged from the filter.

(3) Change the entire administration set every 24 to 48 hours (the time is currently under investigation).

(4) Scrub the tubing and connections with an iodophor agent before and after changing the administration set.

(5) Always clamp the tubing of the central venous catheter with a smooth hemostat while changing the administration set. The patient should lie flat while the tubing is changed.

(6) Do not measure the central venous pressure or draw or give blood with the line. Some authorities agree that antibiotics, fat emulsions, and other compatible medications may be piggybacked upstream of the final filter.

(continued)

NURSING CARE PLAN SUMMARY *Patient with Altered Nutrition* Continued

Patient Outcomes	Nursing Orders
	Others say an inviolate line is desirable (although not always practical) and sometimes can be obtained by placing compatible medications such as hydrocortisone, heparin, and cimetidine directly into the total parenteral nutrition solution. (Research is now under way to ascertain the safety of using the total parenteral nutrition line for these measurements.)
	(7) At the first sign of infection, suspect a catheter-related sepsis. Evaluate all peripheral intravenous sites for erythema and pustulence. Consider urinary tract infection.
	R. Educate the patient and family about the advantages of parenteral nutrition therapy and the principles of asepsis.

IMPLEMENTATION AND EVALUATION

The provision of nutritional support must be evaluated for its effectiveness. Part of the evaluation is to determine the protein and calorie intake of the patient and how this intake corresponds to the patient's weight. Figure 36–3 illustrates one method of monitoring graphically the patient's weight and protein and calorie intake on a daily basis.

Documentation in the patient's record should be organized in a manner consistent with the nursing diagnosis and the report the critical care nurse has received. The pertinent defining characteristics for the nursing diagnosis are a helpful tool for this organization. Kim et al.[25] have identified 21 defining characteristics for the nursing diagnosis category altered nutrition: less than body requirements. These are listed in Table 36–5.

Nutritional support is provided by oral, nasoenteric, or intravenous feedings, or by a combination of these methods.[18] By obtaining essential nutrients, the patient can again generate a host defense response to various invasive agents and stresses. The following sections describe the implementation of enteral, peripheral venous, and central venous alimentation.

Enteral Feedings

If the gastrointestinal tract is functioning, it is used to the maximum. Oral feedings often are combined with tube feedings and intravenous feedings. Central venous total parenteral nutrition is instituted when other methods are not effective.

Basic to oral feedings is an assessment of the patient's nutritional status. Eating is a habit, and critically ill people eat the foods to which they are already accustomed. The quantity of food eaten is also based on one's eating habits. People cannot eat more after they are sick than they ate before (in fact, they eat about 10% less).[42] One may anticipate that an active adolescent patient accustomed to eating vast quantities of food will be able to eat significantly more than a frail elderly patient accustomed to eating small quantities of food. Pain, analgesics, tracheostomies, facial injuries, and general malaise may also limit oral feedings.

Feedings by tube may take the form of nasal catheter, gastrostomy, or jejunostomy feedings. With nasal catheters, small-bore, highly flexible catheters and feeding tubes are used with continuous feedings through an infusion pump. Pediatric feeding tubes or small nasogastric catheters are gently inserted while the patient swallows. When passing the catheter, several things may help accomplish placement: use of a stylet; use of a no. 18 French Levine tube placed parallel to the catheter with the ends of both catheters wedged into half of a gelatin capsule; stiffening of the catheter with ice water; passage of a small catheter through a larger-bore catheter already placed in the esophagus (e.g., rectal tube or endotracheal tube, so that the smaller catheter remains when the larger catheter is withdrawn; use of a guitar string in the lumen of the tube; or use of a straight stainless steel spring guide. Catheters such as the Dobhoff enteric feeding tube are essentially long pediatric feeding tubes with a heat-sealed mercury capsule attached to the end of the feeding tube and several additional side holes placed near the end. The additional length and the mercury tip allow spontaneous passage of the tube through the pylorus into the distal duodenum or upper jejunum. These small tubes can be left in place for extended periods without the complications of larger-bore nasogastric tubes. Large-bore nasogastric tubes are no longer used for feeding because of associated pharyngitis, pulmonary aspiration, gastroesophageal reflex, nasal erosion, esophagitis, esophageal structure rhinitis, parotitis, otitis media, and diarrhea.[23]

Enteral feedings are most commonly used because of simplicity, economic advantages, and the fact that they are well tolerated in most patients. The incidence of upper gastrointestinal bleeding is decreased.[35] Factors that preclude enteral feeding are intractable vomiting, intestinal obstruction, and upper gastrointestinal bleeding.

Intermittent or bolus feeding of isotonic formula into the stomach is preferable in the patient with normal gastrointestinal function. Continuous delivery of isotonic formula into the stomach or jejunum is well tolerated by critically ill patients.

Patients who have not received oral or enteral feedings for as little as a week will have decreased absorptive capacity and may experience some diarrhea. The feeding should only be

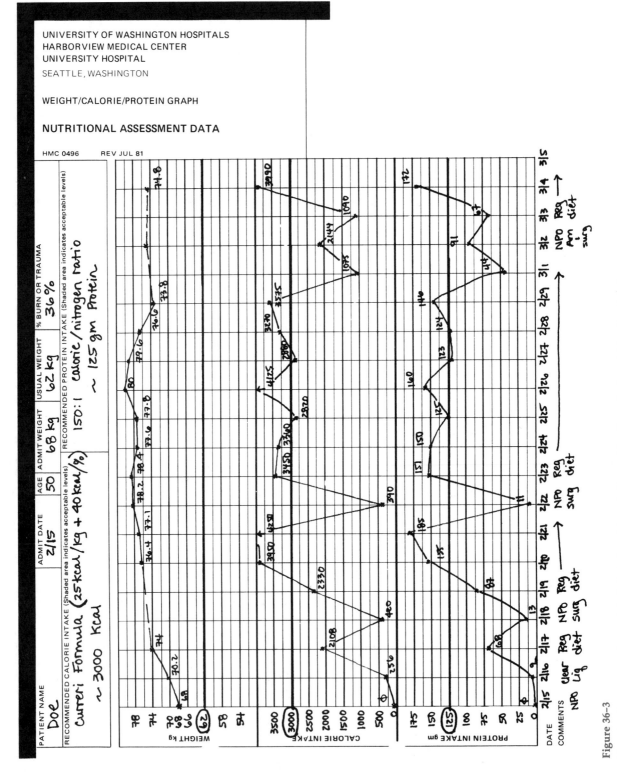

Figure 36-3

Nutritional assessment data: weight/calorie/protein graph. By graphing the patient's weight and protein/calorie intake, the daily record of the variables can be assessed immediately. (Courtesy of J. Williamson, R. D., University of Washington Burn Center.)

Table 36–5
Defining Characteristics for Nursing Diagnosis Category Altered Nutrition: Less Than Body Requirements

Abdominal cramping
Abdominal pain with or without pathologic conditions
Aversion to eating
Body weight 20% or more under ideal for weight and frame
Capillary fragility
Diarrhea or steatorrhea
Excessive loss of hair
Hyperactive bowel sounds
Lack of information, misinformation
Lack of interest in food
Loss of weight with adequate food intake
Misconceptions
Pale conjunctival and mucous membranes
Perceived inability to ingest food
Poor muscle tone
Reported altered taste sensation
Reported inadequate food intake less than RDA
Reported or evidence of lack of food
Satiety immediately after ingesting food
Sore, inflamed buccal cavity
Weakness of muscles required for swallowing or mastication

stopped if the volume of diarrhea is greater than half the volume of delivered formula or if there is difficulty maintaining the patient's hydration or electrolyte status. Kaopectate (a source of fiber) may decrease diarrhea. Diarrhea should decrease or stop within 48 to 72 hours as the absorptive surface of the bowel is enhanced by oral or enteral feeding.

Peripheral Venous Alimentation

If feedings by mouth or tube cannot meet the patient's nutritional needs, parenteral alimentation is added to the therapeutic regimen. Crystalline amino acid solutions and fat solutions can be infused through a peripheral vein. Administration of peripheral parenteral fluids is sometimes termed *protein-sparing therapy* because lean body mass is preserved. It provides protein and calories, decreases insulin levels, and mobilizes the body's own fat as an energy source. The body adapts to the use of nonprotein calories, free fatty acids, and ketone bodies as fuel substrates. Peripheral venous alimentation, therefore, can be used in patients with minimal nutritional deficits and demands and who are not expected to deteriorate.

The fluid administered is essentially isotonic amino acids in 3% to 5% solution mixed with other carbohydrate-free fluids and vitamin, mineral, and electrolyte additives. The solution usually provides 400 calories to 2000 calories/day.

Ten percent fat emulsion may also be administered by peripheral vein, because the solution is essentially isotonic. Calories are supplied in a concentrated form of 9 calories/g up to 1500 calories. Calories may be administered at a rate of 2 g/kg daily. Essential fatty acids and triglycerides that are usually not available are supplied. Fatty acid deficiencies can be avoided by infusing 10% of the calories as fat or using one bottle of fat emulsion three times weekly. Carbohydrate administration accompanies the fat emulsion in order to stimulate the release of insulin. Fat emulsions may also be mixed with glucose and administered through a central vein to provide 30% to 50% of calories administered.

The most common way nutrition by peripheral vein is pro-

vided is with 3 L of fluid daily: two bottles of 500 ml each of fat emulsion (10% intralipid) and two 1-liter bottles of 5% dextrose in 3% to 5% amino acid. The two are infused simultaneous by way of Y-tubing. Approximately 1400 calories and 60 g to 90 g of amino acids are provided.

Central Venous Hyperalimentation

Central venous hyperalimentation (total parenteral nutrition) is a method for delivering carbohydrates, proteins, minerals, vitamins, and trace elements through a central venous catheter. All the patient's nutritional requirements can be met by this method. Originally suggested by Dudrick et al.,[17] the technique provides for the administration of hypertonic glucose and amino acids into a central vein, where the blood flow is high and the solution administered will not be detrimental to the veins. The technique is especially valuable in hypermetabolic patients with apparent nutritional deficits and a negative nitrogen balance of more than 5 g of nitrogen/24 hours. After therapy has been undertaken, measurable nitrogen losses decrease.

Each solution must be administered according to the patient's individual needs, but several guidelines are pertinent for patients in general.[36] Usually for 24 hours each patient receives 2000 ml of fluid, 12 g of nitrogen, and 2400 calories. A 3% to 5% protein hydrolysate or crystalline amino acid solution and a 20% to 25% dextrose-in-water solution make up the basic solution. Water, all necessary electrolytes, trace elements, and vitamins in sufficient quantity to maintain anabolic activity are administered. Electrolyte requirements are met by the delivery of adequate amounts of sodium, potassium, magnesium, chloride, phosphate, sulfate, acetate, and gluconate. Vitamins and trace elements (copper, zinc, manganese, cobalt, and iodine) are added to the solution in appropriate amounts.

An average of 50 mEq of sodium is added to each liter of solution, depending on the patient's acid-base status. Usually sodium is added to the protein hydrolysates as sodium chloride. Another additive is necessary with the crystalline amino acids solution because the amino acids precipitate as a hydrochloride salt and produce acidosis. In such cases, sodium bicarbonate is the additive.

Large amounts of potassium (averaging 40 mEq/1000 calories) are needed to achieve a positive nitrogen balance and to restore the depleted intracellular potassium levels. The body needs up to 250 mEq of potassium/day. Initially, many patients who have suffered trauma are potassium-depleted. Their kidneys cannot conserve both potassium and sodium. Gastrointestinal losses of potassium are high. Protein deamination is associated with potassium loss. Many of the patients are alkalotic; potassium ions have been exchanged for sodium ions in their renal tubules and excreted in their urine in an attempt to conserve hydrogen ions. Although these problems are corrected before total parenteral nutrition is begun, hypokalemia remains a potential problem. Potassium accompanies glucose into the intracellular space and, in the presence of a pre-existing hypokalemia, may produce a lethal dysrhythmia. In any event, further hypokalemia, metabolic alkalosis, and glycosuria are likely to occur. If they do, the physician's assessment of low serum potassium levels will be followed by potassium therapy, not insulin therapy.

The high concentrations of glucose in total parenteral nutrition solutions and enteral formulas stimulate insulin. Phosphorus and potassium move intracellularly. Thus, in the moderately to severely malnourished patient, a normal phosphorus level may decrease rapidly to a level that creates respiratory distress for the patient. Monitor serum phosphorus levels closely. Increase the phosphorus content of the total parenteral nutrition solution as needed. Calcium is administered on the basis of the serum calcium levels, but the administration of phosphorus may produce hypocalcemia. Usually the daily allotment is 4 mEq to 5 mEq/L, or 300 mg. Magnesium deficiency is prevented by the administration of magnesium sulfate (10 mEq to 25 mEq/day).

Trace minerals usually are supplied by the administration of plasma. Zinc deficiency is associated with poor wound healing (it is being studied by many people). Intravenous supplementation is approximately 2 mg to 4 mg/day. Iron therapy is usually given by the intramuscular route. Iron is an important nutrient for bacteria. Iron therapy is usually avoided until the patient is no longer at risk for infection.

Water- and fat-soluble vitamins (a commercial preparation, such as Berroca-C) or a multivitamin infusion is given daily. The body's need for vitamin C has been long established. It is thought that the urinary excretion of water-soluble vitamins is higher after intravenous administration than it is after oral administration. Also, vitamin K (10 mg) is administered intramuscularly once a week, and vitamin B_{12} (250 mEq) is administered intramuscularly usually once a month.

The concentration and quantity of the solution are increased gradually until the desired state is attained. The same care is usually given to discontinuing the solution. Nitrogen and carbohydrate are administered simultaneously to increase the use of nitrogen. Wound healing, one of the primary purposes of alimentation, is associated with cell synthesis and repletion. Thus, intracellular components are needed in great supply, and a deficiency in any nutrient is readily apparent. The potential complications of central venous hyperalimentation are listed in Table 36–6.

Overfeeding

Overfeeding the patient may lead to long-term problems, especially problems associated with pulmonary and liver dysfunction. Feeding hypertonic glucose as the only source of nonprotein and nonfat calories substantially increases the carbon dioxide output ($\dot{V}CO_2$); the result is a respiratory quotient greater than 1.0.[2–4] Because this rise in $\dot{V}CO_2$ increases the ventilatory load, it is difficult to wean patients with chronic pulmonary disease from assisted ventilation. Respiratory work, as shown by a respiratory quotient over 1.0, is excessive, because the body is attempting to preserve homeostasis.

Liver dysfunction is characterized by increased enzymes and bilirubin. The precise etiology of the liver dysfunction is not known. It is thought that, because glucose oxidation to carbon dioxide and water is limited under stress, a glucose infusion greater than 4 mg/kg/minute results in increased lactic acid production and lipogenesis.[31] Because the fat is not cleared from the liver, excess triglyceride and glycogen storage, hepatomegaly, and impaired structural and secretory function result. Liver abnormalities improve if the proportion of nonprotein calories is adjusted so that 20% to 40% is fat and 60% to 80% is carbohydrate and the total caloric intake is held below maintenance requirements.[37]

Table 36–6
Potential Complications From Central Venous Hyperalimentation

Air embolism
Brachial plexus injury
Cardiac dysrhythmias
Cardiac tamponade
Catheter clotting
Catheter embolism
Catheter misplacement
Central venous thrombosis
Electrolyte abnormalities
Hemothorax
Hydrothorax
Hyperglycemia
Hyperosmolar nonketotic hyperglycemia
Hypoglycemia
Hypophosphatemia
Pneumothorax
Sepsis
Subclavian artery injury
Subcutaneous emphysema
Tension pneumothorax

SUMMARY

Nutritional support has become a vital component of critical care therapy today. Because protein synthesis, resistance to infection, and wound healing depend on adequate protein and calorie intake, no other form of therapy can be effective if nutritional deficits remain. It is only by careful assessment and monitoring of therapy that nutritional support may be provided.

DIRECTIONS FOR FUTURE RESEARCH

A wealth of critical care nursing knowledge can be obtained from research for patients with altered nutrition. Sample research questions[28] follow:

1. Which indicators most accurately reflect the nutritional status of the critically ill patient?
2. What are effective noninvasive techniques of evaluating hydration status of patients in critical care areas?
3. What are the effects of various methods of administration of nutritional alimentation (*e.g.*, route, rate, temperature or absorption, gastrointestinal motility, patient comfort, and the prevention of complications)?
4. Which position is most effective in preventing aspiration in patients with feeding tubes?
5. What are the most effective ways of managing critically ill patients with diarrhea?
6. What are the most effective interventions for preventing elimination problems in patients with dietary alterations and restrictions?

REFERENCES

1. Apelgren, K. N., Rombeau, J. L., Twomey, P. D., *et al.* Comparison of nutritional indices and outcome in critically ill patients. *Crit. Care Med.* 10(5):305, 1982.
2. Askanazin, J., Carpentier, Y. A., Elwyn, D. H., *et al.* Influence of total parenteral nutrition on fuel utilization in injury and sepsis. *Am. Surg.* 191:40, 1980.

3. Askanazin, J., Rosenbaum, S. H., Michaelson, B., *et al.* Respiratory changes secondary to the high carbohydrate load of T.P.N. *J.A.M.A.* 243:1444, 1980.

4. Askanazi, J., Weissman, C., Rosenbaum, S. H., *et al.* Nutrition and the respiratory system. *Crit. Care Med.* 10(3):163, 1982.

5. Bistrian, B. R., Blackburn, G. L., Hallowell, E., *et al.* Protein status of general surgical patients. *J.A.M.A.* 230:858, 1974.

6. Bistrian, B. R., Blackburn, G. L., Vitale, J., *et al.* Prevalence of malnutrition in general medical patients. *J.A.M.A.* 235:1567, 1976.

7. Blackburn, G. L., Bistrian, B. R., Maini, B. S., *et al.* Nutritional and metabolic assessment of the hospitalized patient. *J. Parent. Enteral Nutr.* 1(1):11, 1977.

8. Blackburn, G. Hyperalimentation in the critically ill patient. *Heart Lung* 8(1):67, 1979.

9. Blackburn, G. L. Protein metabolism and nutritional support. *J. Trauma* 21:707, 1981.

10. Boles, J. M., Garre, M. A., Youinou, P. Y., *et al.* Nutritional status in intensive care patients. Evaluation in 84 unselected patients. *Crit. Care Med.* 11(2):87, 1983.

11. Bruya, M. A., and Severtsen, B. Evaluating the effects of music on electroencephalogram patterns of normal subjects. *J. Neurosurg. Nurs.* 16(2):96, 1984.

12. Buzby, G. P., Mullen, J. L., Hobbs, C. L., *et al.* Prognostic nutritional index in gastrointestinal surgery. *Am. J. Surg.* 139:160, 1980.

13. Cahill, G. Starvation in man. *N. Engl. J. Med.* 282:669, 1970.

14. Cannon, W. B. *Bodily Changes in Pain, Hunger, Fear and Rage.* New York: Appleton, 1929.

15. Curreri, P. W., Richmond, P., Marvin, J., *et al.* Dietary requirements of patients with major burns. *J. Am. Diet. Assoc.* 65(4):415, 1974.

16. Cuthbertson, D. P. The disturbance of metabolism produced by bony and nonbony injury with notes on certain abnormal conditions of bone. *J. Biochem.* 24(2):1244, 1930.

17. Dudrick, S. J., Wilmore, D. W., Vars, H. M., *et al.* Long-term parenteral nutrition and growth development, and positive nitrogen balance. *Surgery* 64:134, 1968.

18. Echenique, M. M., Bistrian, B. R., and Blackburn, G. L. Theory and techniques of nutritional support in the ICU. *Crit. Care Med.* 10(8):546, 1982.

19. Elwyn, D. H. Nutritional requirements of adult surgical patients. *Crit. Care Med.* 8:9, 1980.

20. Gump, F. E., and Kinney, J. M. Oxygen consumption and caloric expenditure in surgical patients. *Surg. Gynecol. Obstet.* 137:199, 1973.

21. Gump, F. E., Long, C. L., Geyir, J. W., *et al.* The significance of altered gluconeogenesis in surgical catabolism. *J. Trauma* 15:704, 1975.

22. Gump, F. E., Long, C. L., Killian, P., *et al.* Studies of glucose intolerance in septic injured patients. *J. Trauma* 14:378, 1974.

23. Heymsfield, S. B., Horowitz, J., and Lawson, D. H. Enteral Hyperalimentation. In E. Beck (ed.), *Developments in Digestive Disease.* Philadelphia: Lea & Febiger, 1980.

24. Hill, G. L., Blackett, R. L., Pickford, J., *et al.* Malnutrition in surgical patients: An unrecognized problem. *Lancet* 1:689, 1977.

25. Kim, M. J., McFarland, G. K., and McLane, A. M. *Pocket Guide to Nursing Diagnosis* (3rd ed.). St. Louis: C. V. Mosby, 1989.

26. Kinney, J. M., Jeejeebhoy, K. N., Hill, G. L., *et al. Nutrition and Metabolism in Patient Care.* Philadelphia: W. B. Saunders, 1988.

27. Kinney, J. M., Long, C. L., and Duke, J. H. Energy Demands in the Surgical Patient. In C. L. Fox and G. C. Wahas (eds.), *Body Fluid Replacement in the Surgical Patient.* New York: Grune & Stratton, 1970.

28. Lewandowski, L. A., and Kositsky, A. M. Research priorities for critical care nursing: A study by the American Association of Critical Care Nurses. *Heart Lung* 12(1):35, 1983.

29. Light, G. A., Love, D. M., Benson, D., *et al.* Music in surgery. *Curr. Res. Anesth. Analg.* 33:258, 1954.

30. Locsin, R. The effect of music on the pain of selected post-operative patients. *J. Adv. Nurs.* 6:19, 1981.

31. Lowry, S. F., and Brennan, M. F. Abnormal liver function during parenteral nutrition: Relation to infusion excess. *J. Surg. Res.* 26:300, 1979.

32. Moore, F. D. La maladie post-operative: Is there order in variety? The six stimulus-response sequences. *Surg. Clin. North Am.* 56:803, 1976.

33. Mullen, J. L., Gertner, M. H., Buzby, G. P., *et al.* Implications of malnutrition in the surgical patient. *Arch. Surg.* 114:121, 1979.

34. Nev, J., Wendell, C., Kien, C. L., *et al.* Calculator-assisted monitoring of nutrition, fluids, and electrolytes. *Crit. Care Med.* 10(7):461, 1982.

35. Pingleton, S. K., and Hedzima, S. K. Enteral alimentation and gastrointestinal bleeding in mechanically ventilated patients. *Crit. Care Med.* 11:13, 1983.

36. Salmond, S. W. Monitoring for potential complications of total parenteral nutrition administration. *Crit. Care Q.* 3(4):21, 1981.

37. Saunders, R. Hepatic dysfunction during hyperalimentation. *Arch. Surg.* 113:504, 1978.

38. Schlichtig, R., and Ayres, S. M., *Nutritional Support of the Critically Ill.* Chicago: Yearbook Medical Publishers, 1988.

39. Siegel, S. H., Goldwyn, R. M., and Friedman, H. P. Patterns and process in the evolution of human septic shock. *Surgery* 70:232, 1971.

40. Taylor, D. B. Music in general hospital treatment from 1900 to 1950. *J. Music Ther.* 18(2):62, 1981.

41. Walesby, R. K., Goode, A. W., and Bentel, A. H. Nutritional status of patients undergoing valve replacement by open heart surgery. *Lancet* 1:76, 1978.

42. Wilmore, D. Nutrition and metabolism following thermal injury. *Clin. Plast. Surg.* 1:603, 1974.

43. Wilmore, D., Mason, D., and Pruitt, B. A., Jr. Insulin response to glucose in hypermetabolic burn patients. *Ann. Surg.* 183:314, 1976.

44. Wilmore, D., Orcutt, T. W., Mason, A. R., *et al.* Alterations in hypothalamic function following thermal injury. *J. Trauma* 15:697, 1975.

45. Wilmore, D. W. *The Metabolic Management of the Critically Ill.* New York: Plenum, 1977.

Diabetic Ketoacidosis

Angela Pruitt Clark

DIARIES, JOURNALS, AND LETTERS

Diaries, journals, and letters are valid tools for self-growth. They are personal books in which creativity, play, and self-therapy interweave, foster, and complement each other. They become safe places in which to explore thoughts, ideas, and feelings.

Create a ritual with your diary, journal, or letters. Each of these records helps you track your daily rhythms and bodymind connections. Remember that there is no correct way to do this; just let your own creativity flow. These are your records, and you can individualize them as you wish. Be creative, for these records become treasure troves of new patterns and possibilities. Choose a special bound book that is easy to use and that has eye and touch appeal. You might even purchase a special pen, pencil, or colored writing instrument that can add to your writing ritual.

Diaries can be free-form or structured. Structured diaries or records increase your strengths and self-confidence and help shape new images of health behaviors. These new images and behaviors occur because you are enhancing your awareness of your patterns. If you are trying to shape new life-style behaviors, diaries are very useful in weight management, exercise, smoking cessation, or in overcoming addiction. People who keep some form of written record (*e.g.,* frequency, inner reactions and moods, habit cues, and patterns of eating, exercise, smoking, and alcohol or drug use) have the greatest success at changing life-style patterns. These are also the people who avoid total collapse into old life-style patterns.

Journals are a longer written record that reflect more aspects of life. Using a journal is more involved than keeping a diary. Develop different sections and divisions in your journal, such as people, events, community activities, dreams, intuition, and so forth. When journaling, let your inner experiences flow without judgment. If it seems right, take some of your inner fears, worries, fantasies, or dreams into your imagery process and see what appears. Then record your experience.

Letters can be used as a cathartic process to express love, support, anger, disappointment, and other deep emotions. Letters can help you achieve a sense of peace with unresolved or difficult situations. You can address body parts, offspring, deceased family members, or friends. Letters can be full of insight and represent an attempt to come to terms with crisis, to enter it fully, to explore the meaning it contains, and to try to find a personal path through the labyrinth of adversity.

Through the process of letter writing, old emotional wounds can finally be healed. Letters can contain thoughts and feelings that you have kept inside of you, maybe for decades. The letter is to be kept and reread until you feel the emotion has been quieted. Then you can choose to keep it or create a special ritual in which it may be torn up, burned, or buried.

LEARNING OBJECTIVES

After reading this chapter, the nurse should be able to do the following:

1. List in the order of importance the primary patient care objectives for the patient with diabetic ketoacidosis.
2. List the most common causes of diabetic ketoacidosis.
3. List the subjective and objective assessment data for diabetic ketoacidosis.
4. State how the nursing process will be used.
5. Teach the patient and family the essentials they need to know for safe and thorough self-care after the acute phase has passed.

CASE STUDY

Mr. V. M., a 21-year-old college senior, was found unconscious in his apartment by his girlfriend. She called an ambulance. Mr. M. was taken to the emergency room of a nearby hospital, where he was immediately admitted to the intensive care unit.

The information obtained from Mr. M.'s girlfriend revealed that Mr. M. had complained of nausea and had been coughing for several days. She did not know whether he had had a fever or if he had notified his physician.

Mr. M.'s mother was notified. She arrived at the hospital within 15 minutes. She said that her son had been a diabetic since he was 11 years old and that his condition was fairly well controlled. He had been taking one injection of NPH insulin per day, and on the average he had four or five insulin reactions per month. He had not been following his diet well since he moved into his own apartment a year ago. He had a blood glucose monitoring machine and had been taught to use it. However, his mother suspected he only rarely checked it at home.

Mr. M.'s past medical history included many hospitalizations for diabetes-related conditions. His mother said that he had attended diabetic education classes held at a hospital when he was 17 years old. Mr. M.'s current medications included NPH insulin. His mother said that her son was allergic to pork and thus must use insulin obtained from beef sources.

Physical examination at the time of his admission to the critical care unit showed that Mr. M was acutely ill. The following information was obtained:

General observations: Acutely ill white man with rapid, deep respirations. Intravenous fluids: 0.9% normal saline solution given in the left antecubital vein (started by the emergency medical service)

Vital signs: Blood pressure: 96/70 mm Hg in supine position, right arm; heart rate, 110; sinus tachycardia; respirations, 36/minute and deep; temperature, 101.8°F rectally; height, 6 feet; weight, 160 lb

Integument: Pale except for very flushed face; skin turgor poor; skin dry

Head: No abnormalities noted; no lacerations

Eyes: Pupils equal and reactive to light; sclera clear; fundi, grade I retinopathy; ocular pressure shown by palpation to be reduced

Ears: Tympanic membranes intact and clear

Nose: Flaring of nares

Mouth: Mucous membranes dry and pink

Neck: Supple; no neck vein distention; no bruits; no lymphadenopathy

Chest: Vesicular breath sounds in left lung; right lung has bronchovesicular breath sounds; slight dullness in right lower lung; crackles in anterior and posterior right lower lung

Cardiovascular system: Sinus tachycardia (110 beats/minute); PMI fifth intercostal space at midclavicular line; poor capillary refill; extremities cool; first and second heart sounds normal; no murmurs

Abdomen: Distended; bowel sounds absent; no palpable masses

Genitourinary system: Bladder distended; genitals normal; testes descended with no masses

Extremities: Intravenous line in left arm; full range-of-motion exercises possible; no edema or cyanosis; all pulses present

Neurologic responses: No response to commands; deep tendon reflexes 0 to 1+

The following laboratory data were obtained immediately:

Blood glucose level: 650 mg/dl

Serum acetone: Strong (4+ reaction at 1:16 dilution in plasma)

Complete blood count: White blood cells, 19,000/mm³; neutrophils, 70%; lymphocytes, 26%; hemoglobin, 16 g/dl; hematocrit, 58%

Arterial blood gases: pH, 6.9; PaO_2, 98; O_2 saturation, 95%; $PaCO_2$, 20; calculated HCO_3^-, 3.75; measured HCO_3^-, 5; base excess, −29;

Electrolytes: sodium, 129 mEq/L; chloride, 93 mEq/L; carbon dioxide, 5 mM/L; potassium 5.1 mEq/L

Other: Blood urea nitrogen, 30 mg/dl; creatinine, 0.8 mg/dl; cholesterol, 235 mg/dl

Chest radiograph: Shows a diffuse infiltrate in the right lower lobe that appears to be pneumonia

Clinical Presentation of Case Study

Patient was admitted to intensive care unit. Several actions were taken at once.

6:30 P.M.

Mr. M. arrived with an intravenous route established. A 0.9% normal saline solution was given at 200 ml/hour. Hypotension (blood pressure, 96/70 mm Hg) was noted, and check of Mr. M.'s vital signs every 30 minutes was ordered. The stat blood glucose on Mr. M.'s admission was 650 mg/dl, and regular insulin (beef) (100 U by intravenous push) was given. Blood glucose checks every hour were ordered. An infusion pump was prepared with additional regular insulin, and it was piggybacked into the intravenous line. A rate of 6 U/hour was established. Monitor leads were attached to the patient; a continuing sinus tachycardia with no ectopic beats was noted. To relieve abdominal distention, a sump nasogastric tube was inserted and connected to low suction. A Foley catheter was inserted, and 870 ml of urine was obtained. The urinalysis revealed the following data: pH, 5; specific gravity, 1.036; glucose, 5%; and acetone strong. A sputum specimen was obtained by tracheal suctioning, and sputum and urine cultures were requested.

7:30 P.M. (Second Hour)

Penicillin was given for the pneumonia while results of the culture were awaited. A second blood glucose test showed 602 mg/dl. The electrolyte levels were sodium, 130 mEq/L; potassium, 5 mEq/L; chloride, 93 mEq/L; carbon dioxide, 5 mM/L. The arterial blood analysis showed pH of 6.9, PaO_2 of 97, $PaCO_2$ of 21, and HCO_3^- of 5.

Because of Mr. M.'s pH and low $PaCO_2$, sodium bicarbonate was given. Vital signs revealed a slight temperature decrease (to 101°F rectally) and a blood pressure increase (to 100/70 mm Hg). Mr. M.'s neurologic responses continued to be depressed. His Kussmaul's respirations continued. Ultrasonic nebulizer mist therapy was administered every 6 hours for 20 minutes.

8:30 P.M. (Third Hour)

Potassium was 4.2 mEq/L; blood glucose was 542 mg/dl; urine output for the last hour was 320 ml; and bowel sounds were still absent. Family members visited and asked whether they could see Mr. M. again. The nurse gave them a summary of Mr. M.'s condition. They seemed to be relieved but said they had been through similar experiences with Mr. M. many times before, and they did not worry about his dying in a coma as they previously had. They asked to be allowed to return during the night and were assured that they could.

11:30 P.M. (Sixth Hour)

Potassium was 3 mEq/L, reflecting an intracellular potassium shift. Potassium phosphate was added to the intravenous fluids.

4:30 A.M. (Tenth Hour)

Blood glucose was 402 mg/dl, and blood pressure was 112/74 mm Hg. Temperature was 100.6°F rectally. Arterial blood pH was 7.1. Hourly check of vital signs was continued.

10:30 A.M. (Sixteenth Hour)

Arterial blood pH was 7.31. Carbon dioxide (venous) rose to 13. Infusions were continued.

12:30 P.M. (Eighteenth Hour)

Mr. M. slowly regained consciousness. The nurse told him where he was and why. Her explanation seemed to satisfy him. Family were allowed to visit him. Blood glucose was 355 mg/dl. Hourly blood glucose checks were continued. Urine volume averaged about 100 ml/hour. Blood pressure was 120/76. Sinus tachycardia continued. Bowel sounds are still absent.

3:30 P.M. (Twenty-first Hour)

The patient was oriented to time and place. Blood pressure was 122/76; heart rate, 108; respirations, 24; and temperature, 99.6°F orally. Arterial blood gas analysis showed pH 7.34 and a serum PCO_2 of 18. Blood glucose was 315 mg/dl.

5:30 P.M. (Twenty-fourth Hour)

Blood glucose was 266 mg/dl. Urine acetone was trace. Intravenous infusion of insulin was discontinued to avoid a hypoglycemic reaction. Intravenous solution was changed to a 5% dextrose in 0.45% normal saline solution at 100 ml/hour.

7:30 P.M. (Twenty-sixth Hour)

Blood glucose was 230 mg/dl. Regular insulin (25 U intramuscularly) was given. A sliding-scale administration of regular insulin was ordered, based on blood glucose levels to be done every 4 hours. Bowel sounds were present. Nasogastric tube was removed. Clear liquids were given by mouth and were tolerated without nausea.

9:30 P.M. (Twenty-eighth Hour)

Crackles were still present in right lower lung. Temperature was 99.4°F orally. Penicillin was continued. Chest radiograph showed some clearing of the infiltrate. Sputum culture showed *Streptococcus pneumoniae* (pneumococcus), which was sensitive to the antibiotic being given.

3:30 A.M. (Next Day)

Mr. M. was well oriented to his environment and could remember the events that led to his hospitalization. Mr. M. was put on an 1800-calorie American Diabetes Association (ADA) diet. Hydration state was satisfactory, as indicated by clinical signs. Blood glucose was 154 mg/dl. Sliding-scale administration of insulin was continued.

11:00 A.M.

Mr. M. was transferred from the intensive care unit to a medical nursing unit. Vital signs were as follows: blood pressure, 130/78 mm Hg; heart rate, 100; respirations, 18; temperature, 99.2°F orally. His mother was waiting for him in his new room.

Fourth Day

Mr. M. was again given NPH insulin (36 U every morning); sliding-scale administration of insulin was stopped. Mr. M. was interviewed by a member of the diabetic teaching team, who assessed Mr. M's knowledge of diabetes. Mr. M said that he had become careless about checking his blood glucose level and did not understand the significance of acetone in urine. He did not rotate injection sites systematically; in fact, he had never used the abdomen as a site. Mr. M. and his teacher planned his teaching. He was to be instructed by a registered nurse, a pharmacist, and a dietitian during his hospitalization.

He was encouraged to perform self-blood glucose monitoring to be done at home three to four times a day. He was educated about glycosalated hemoglobin (also called hemoglobin A_{1C}), a blood test that reflects the mean value of blood glucose for the previous 4 to 6 weeks. He was advised to have this checked every 3 months. Mr. M. was taught about the ADA diet and allowed to practice choices in the hospital.

Ninth Day

Mr. M. was discharged from the hospital. He was to take NPH insulin (36 units subcutaneously every morning), and he was to follow a 2000-calorie ADA diet. He was to be contacted for follow-up care by a member of the diabetic teaching team within 3 days. He had an appointment to see his physician in 5 days and was to bring records of self-blood glucose checks.

REFLECTIONS

Nurses often care for people with a chronic disease. Do they really grasp the significance of the disease to the patient? An acute illness may cause the patient unexpected problems, but the illness is generally short in duration. A chronic illness such as diabetes mellitus is a permanent one, and it affects many areas of a person's life.

The nurse must consider what having diabetes means to the patient. Often the diabetic may act in ways that reflect feelings of guilt, anxiety, or fear. Many adult diabetics have said that they felt they had lost control over their bodies. One man with diabetes said that he lived in constant fear of having an insulin reaction when he was alone. One woman said that having diabetes meant to her that she might lose a leg or foot.

The physiologic effect of stress on human beings is well known. It has been established that stress can elevate the blood glucose level and, in fact, can lead to a significant degree of hyperglycemia in some people. Stress is a high-risk factor in cardiovascular disease, which is one of the main complications of diabetes mellitus. One interesting research study found that progressive relaxation training significantly lowered glucose levels in a group of type II diabetics.[19]

The role of the critical care nurse with regard to the patient with a chronic disease is multifaceted. The nurse must be knowledgeable and skillful in order to maintain life. However, the nurse must remember that patients must learn to cope with the disease and its complications for the rest of their lives. The nurse needs communication skills to help in counseling the patient and family. The use of diabetic education teams for hospitalized patients and their families is highly recommended. The person with a chronic disease needs every possible opportunity to learn good self-care. Identifying what the patient needs to learn and using a nursing assessment tool before the teaching sessions are valuable.

ANATOMY AND PHYSIOLOGY

The pancreas contains three main types of cells: alpha cells, beta cells, and delta cells. The alpha cells secrete glucagon, a substance that elevates blood glucose levels. The beta cells produce insulin, a powerful hypoglycemic agent. The delta cells appear to contain somatostatin, which can inhibit both insulin and glucagon secretion.[10]

Insulin

Insulin, a small protein, is made of 51 amino acids formed in two separate chains.[7] About 50 U of insulin is produced daily. The stored insulin awaits a stimulus for its release. Glucose is the major stimulus of insulin secretion and release. When the glucose level rises (as it does after a meal), the pancreas immediately begins to produce and secrete insulin.

Insulin acts primarily to facilitate the movement of glucose into the cell for use by the cell. It increases the rate of glucose transport from the blood stream through the cell membrane. Because the glucose molecule is too large to enter the cell pores by simple diffusion, it must be carried in by a transport process. Some glucose can enter the cell without insulin, but only in small amounts. When insulin is present, the transport rate is 10 times greater.[10] It is apparent that if insulin moves glucose intracellularly, it decreases the amount of glucose circulating in the blood stream.

Once insulin is secreted into the blood, it has a half-life of only about 6 minutes, so that it is cleared from the circulation in 10 to 15 minutes. The insulin that is not used is degraded by the liver and kidneys. This rapid removal is an important mechanism when insulin is not needed.[10]

Some cells (e.g., the cells in the brain, liver, and nervous tissue) do not need insulin to transport glucose. Other cells that do not need insulin to transport glucose are the cells in the renal tubules and the erythrocytes. Those cells collectively make up a very small percentage of the total body mass.

Besides increasing the glucose metabolism rate and decreasing the blood glucose concentration, insulin increases glycogen storage in the tissues. The stored glycogen can be converted to glucose if it is needed for energy.

Carbohydrate Metabolism

Glucose is the body's primary source of energy. One obtains exogenous glucose by eating nutrients, principally carbohydrates. Endogenous glucose is obtained from the conversion of stored glycogen to glucose and by gluconeogenesis from amino acids and other substances.

When carbohydrates are eaten, they are broken down into monosaccharides, or simple sugars. The monosaccharides are absorbed from the small intestine into the intestinal capillaries and are transported to the liver by the portal vein.

The fate of nutrients is decided in the liver, and it depends on what the body needs at the time. Generally, about 50% of the glucose (the main monosaccharide) is used immediately to meet the body's energy needs. Some glucose is stored in reserve as adipose tissue by conversion to fats. The remainder is stored as glycogen in the skeletal muscles and the liver to be converted to glucose if needed.

Carbohydrate is the body's preferred source of energy—its active fuel. The proper use of fat and protein is dependent on an adequate intake of carbohydrate. The body can, however, use the fat and protein to provide energy if absolutely necessary.

Fats as a Source of Energy

Fats can become the major supplier of energy on demand by oxidation of the fatty acids and glycerol. Fats, a concentrated form of stored energy, provide 9 calories/g; proteins and carbohydrates provide 4 calories/g.

A dangerous situation arises when large amounts of fat are used instead of carbohydrates. This situation results in the production of intermediate byproducts—ketoacids—which are acidic. The primary acids—acetoacetic acid and beta-hydroxybutyric acid—accumulate in the blood stream and are responsible for the metabolic acidosis that follows. Diabetic ketoacidosis is discussed later in the chapter. Ketoacids are not totally undesirable. Although the body cannot tolerate large amounts of ketoacids, muscle and kidney cells can use them in reasonable amounts as nutrients.

Hormones

Besides insulin, several other hormones affect carbohydrate metabolism. Hormones that can raise glucose levels are called counterregulatory hormones. These include glucagon, epinephrine, cortisol, and growth hormone.[4,18] These hormones are able to elevate the blood glucose level by various means; thus, they may be considered antagonistic to insulin. Hypoglycemia can cause the secretion of all these hormones.

Insulin Resistance

It appears that obese people have some degree of insulin resistance. Surprisingly, many obese diabetics have been found to have high insulin levels (hyperinsulinemia). Weight loss is accompanied by an increase in the number of insulin receptors.[17]

ETIOLOGY AND INCIDENCE

Diabetes mellitus is a chronic, usually hereditary, disease characterized by an abnormally high blood glucose level and the urinary excretion of some of that glucose. All or part of the body's ability to use carbohydrates has been lost because of a deficiency in insulin or a decrease in the efficiency of insulin. There are more than 10 million diabetics in the United States. The number is increasing rapidly.

A system for classifying types of diabetes was developed in 1979. The new terms are type I (insulin-dependent diabetes mellitus, IDDM) and type II (non-insulin-dependent diabetes mellitus, NIDDM). Type I replaces the old category of juvenile-onset diabetes and is most common in children, but it may occur at any age. Type II consists of two subtypes that include obese NIDDM and nonobese NIDDM. Type II roughly replaces the term maturity-onset diabetes. Table 37–1 compares types I and II.

The insulin deficiency in diabetes appears to be polygenic. The oldest theory is that of beta-cell dysfunction, with inadequate amounts of insulin being secreted. This appears to be the primary problem in type I diabetes. It is thought that one inherits the tendency to develop diabetes. A decrease in insulin activity has been seen in children after viral infections. The virus destroys some of the beta cells in children, who probably

Table 37–1
Comparison of Type I and Type II Diabetes Mellitus

	TYPE I	TYPE II
Onset	Abrupt with acute symptoms	Mild
Pathology	Insulinitis leading to complete destruction of beta cells	Hypertrophy initially; then later degeneration
Genetics	HLA association; familial tendency	No HLA association; strong familial tendency
Possible antecedents	Virus	Obesity
Immune systems	Islet cell antibodies present; other immune disease may be in family	Islet cell antibodies absent
Exogenous insulin requirements	Always	Rare

inherit the genetic susceptibility to respond to the virus. It is clear that the major susceptibility to type I diabetes is closely associated with the HLA histocompatability system.[5] The basement-membrane thickening seen in diabetes has received much research attention. An excessive amount of glucagon, the hormone that is antagonistic to insulin inaction, has been found in many young type I diabetics. Insulin may be destroyed by antibodies and may be a factor for some individuals.

Type II diabetes mellitus has a different etiology. Current research has found that the primary dysfunction is at the cell receptor sites. A deficiency in both quality and quantity of insulin receptors is present, thus providing a lack of entry of glucose into the cell.

PSYCHOPATHOPHYSIOLOGY

Diabetes has many serious complications. Diabetics who are admitted to the critical care unit often already have one or more of the complications. Generally, the duration of diabetes correlates with the extent of the complications, but there are exceptions.

COMPLICATIONS OF DIABETES

Macrovascular or macroangiopathic disease is one of the major complications of diabetes. It is seen most frequently in the person with type II diabetes. Lipid deposition and medial calcification of the vessel are common. The complication may be manifested in coronary artery disease and arterial insufficiency to the central nervous system or extremities or other large vessels. Atherosclerotic heart disease is the leading cause of death in diabetics. Gangrene has been found to be about 150 times more common in the diabetic in the fifth decade of life than in a nondiabetic of the same age.

Microangiopathy is most often seen in the type I diabetic. It is characterized by thickening of the vascular basement membrane. It is often manifested in the patient by retinopathy or nephropathy. Diabetic retinopathy is the leading cause of blindness in the United States. Diabetics also have a higher incidence of cataracts. Nephropathy can be seen in many renal conditions (*e.g.*, glomerulosclerosis, tubular nephrosis, or renal failure). Renal failure is a common cause of death in the type I diabetic.

Diabetics appear to have a greater predisposition for infections than have nondiabetics, although the studies are limited. Infection commonly triggers an episode of ketoacidosis and, hence, must be looked for when acidosis appears.[3]

Many neurologic complications occur in a person who is diabetic. Neuropathy can be manifested in numerous ways (*e.g.*, diabetic neurogenic bladder, atrophy of the extremities, orthostatic hypotension, and neurotrophic foot ulcer). Impotence is probably the most common symptom of neuropathy in male diabetics. Possibly up to 60% of male patients will become impotent.[8]

Abnormal skin lesions can be a complication of diabetes. The term *diabetic dermopathy* is generally used to refer to the presence of reddish-brown papular spots on the shins that may have an erythematous border. Crusts and scar tissue may form. Another, more severe skin lesion is *necrobiosis lipoidica diabeticorum*. It is an ulcerating and necrotic process, and it may be quite difficult to control.

DIABETIC KETOACIDOSIS

Diabetic ketoacidosis (DKA) is an acute metabolic condition that occurs in uncontrolled hyperglycemia. It is life-threatening and can rapidly lead to severe dehydration, electrolyte disturbances, and death if not recognized and treated. A minimum of 4000 deaths from DKA occur in the United States each year.[2] No substantial reduction in mortality has been seen in the past 25 years.[13] The following are possible causes of DKA: infection, a common cause, which increases the metabolic rate; interruption of insulin administration, which can result in an imbalance between insulin and glucose; a major emotional crisis, which can cause hyperglycemia; a decrease in the usual amount of exercise; increased food intake over a period of time; and undiagnosed diabetes, presenting in DKA.

Diabetic ketoacidosis develops when there is a deficiency of insulin and an excess of counterregulatory hormones. The insulin deficiency begins the process of ketoacidosis because insulin is not available to transport glucose into the cell through the cell membrane. The glucose concentration of the blood increases and will continue to do so if the condition is not treated. When the renal threshold for resorption of glucose is reached, some of the glucose is excreted in the urine. The threshold varies; in many people, it is about 170 mg/dl. The hyperglycemic state initiates an osmotic diuresis, drawing fluid from intracellular and interstitial spaces into the intravascular compartment.

Four counterregulatory hormones (sometimes called *stress hormones*) are also responsible for much of the pathogenesis of DKA. These are glucagon, epinephrine, cortisol, and growth hormone. When increased secretion of these hormones is sustained, hyperglycemia continues.[13]

In search of energy from noncarbohydrate sources, the body begins to break down large amounts of fat to obtain glucose. Fat is broken down into glycerol and fatty acids. With the exception of brain tissue, almost all cells can use fatty acids for energy.[10] The glycerol is released and is converted to glucose. The fatty acids are further processed and converted to acetylcoenzyme A (acetyl-CoA) by the liver. Acetyl-CoA unites with a substance called *oxaloacetate* before it is transferred to peripheral tissues to be used for energy production. If the cycle were allowed to progress normally, the eventual outcome would be carbon dioxide, water, and energy (stored as adenosine triphosphate and creatine phosphate).[10]

Lipolysis increases, partly because insulin normally inhibits lipase. Free fatty acids are released, and their oxidation results in excess amounts of acetyl-CoA. Acetyl-CoA accumulates because it is in excessive amounts relative to the available oxaloacetate. As mentioned, this situation increases the number of ketone bodies or ketoacids (acetoacetic acid and beta-hydroxybutyric acid). Acetone is found in the patient's urine and is detectable on the breath; it is a spontaneous breakdown product of acetoacetic acid.[13]

Hyperglycemia and ketonemia can lead to a critical loss of water, electrolytes, and calories in the three body compartments. The osmotic diuresis is severe. Sodium, potassium, chloride, magnesium, and phosphate are apt to be lost, but the laboratory measurements may not show a decrease in these substances, primarily owing to the dehydration and hemoconcentration. Hemoconcentration can develop along with a decrease in the vascular volume and, hence, a decrease in the circulatory competence. Polyuria results from the large water loss because the tubular capacity to resorb glucose is exceeded; approximately 15 ml of water is needed to excrete 1 g of glucose. If nausea and vomiting are present, they will contribute further to the loss of fluid and electrolytes.

A metabolic acidosis with excess hydrogen ion concentration results from the ketosis, and death will occur if the condition is not treated. Some physicians think that the pH of the cerebrospinal fluid is a more accurate index of the degree of acidosis and coma. Mental confusion and coma occur when the cerebrospinal fluid falls below pH 7.15. Cerebral edema is a complication of the fluid therapy when treatment is started.

Compensatory mechanisms occur in buffering substances, the renal system, and the lungs. The respiratory center is stimulated, and the patient begins to breathe deeply and rapidly in an effort to blow off excess carbonic acid as water and carbon dioxide. (This type of respiration is called Kussmaul's respirations.) The kidneys increase their excretion of hydrogen ions by the secretion of ammonia, which is then excreted as ammonium chloride. The kidneys also excrete ketones (ketonuria).

NURSING PROCESS

ASSESSMENT

The diagnosis of DKA is usually made without much difficulty. If the patient is a known diabetic, the process is easier. Every patient in a coma should have a blood glucose test done.

Unique causes of coma in diabetes are hypoglycemia (insulin reaction, insulin shock), hyperosmolar nonketotic coma, lactic acidosis, and DKA. A blood glucose test will quickly rule out hypoglycemia. Hyperosmolar coma is similar to DKA, but it lacks the acidotic component. Hyperglycemia is present but not metabolic acidosis (see Chap. 38). Lactic acidosis may also be present in the patient with DKA.

The diagnosis of DKA should be based on the patient's clinical picture, history (if one is available), and laboratory findings.

Clinical Manifestations

The patient with DKA appears acutely ill. Significant dehydration is manifested by dry skin with poor turgor, thirst, soft eyeballs, and possibly even wrinkled corneas. The mucous membranes in the conjunctival and oronasopharyngeal areas are dry. Polyuria, with bladder distention if the patient is comatose, is noted. Crackles may be present (as in the Case Study), but they may not be heard because of the dehydration. A pleural friction rub may be present; it disappears on rehydration.

The signs of DKA related to the acidotic state are mental changes ranging from confusion to coma, an acetone odor to the breath, and a flushed face. The flush is probably due to superficial vasodilatation secondary to the increase in carbonic acid. Fever and dehydration may be other causes of the flush. Kussmaul's respirations occur in about 75% of patients.

Abdominal pain may result from sodium loss or possibly from a neuropathy. Fluid loss may also be a cause. Vomiting frequently is present. Deep tendon reflexes may be diminished or absent. They return after treatment.

Often the nurse can tentatively diagnose DKA after making a few quick, astute observations. Kussmaul's respirations, acetone breath, and severe dehydration are important signs.

Diagnostic Tests

Many diagnostic tests are helpful. Obviously, tests of the blood glucose levels, the blood and urine ketone levels, and the arterial blood gases must be done immediately. Hyperglycemia up to 2000 mg/dl and glycosuria up to 5% may be seen. The usual blood sugar range is 300 to 800 mg/dl. Fifteen percent of the patients will have blood sugars of less than 350 mg/dl.[13] Arterial blood gases usually reveal an acidotic arterial pH. The PaO_2 may be normal, because DKA is not a respiratory system problem. The bicarbonate concentration will be reduced.

Leukocytosis is generally present. It may be as high as 30,000/mm³. It reflects hemoconcentration and stress, but not necessarily infection. The carbon dioxide combining power (a venous blood sample) is expected to be low. It reflects the decrease in alkaline reserve.

NURSING DIAGNOSES, PATIENT OUTCOMES, AND PLAN

The preceding material on anatomy, physiology, nursing assessment, and diagnostic tests guides the nurse in establishing nursing diagnoses, patient outcomes, and the plan for the patient with DKA.

NURSING CARE PLAN SUMMARY   *Patient With Diabetic Ketoacidosis*

NURSING DIAGNOSIS

1. *Altered metabolic process (hyperglycemia) related to insufficient insulin to meet metabolic needs (exchanging pattern)*

Patient Outcomes	Nursing Orders
1. The patient will achieve a blood glucose level below 250 mg/dl.	1. Assess, treat, and evaluate the patient's blood glucose level. A. Give the patient regular insulin as ordered (50 U to 200 U intravenously, intramuscularly, or subcutaneously). For the intravenous push route, give 50 U or less every minute. B. With the intravenous infusion pump, do the following: (1) Check the dose carefully. (2) Maintain sterile technique. (3) Check the pump periodically to make sure the proper dose is being delivered. C. Be aware that as much as 20% of the insulin may be bound to the tubing and bottle or bag. More binding occurs when lower doses of insulin are used. In time, the equipment can become saturated with insulin. Therefore, changing the equipment decreases the amount of insulin the patient receives, and keeping the same equipment increases it. As much as 44% to 47% of the insulin may be bound.[22] D. To avoid inactivation, do not mix the insulin with sodium bicarbonate. E. Evaluate the patient's blood glucose levels every 30 to 60 minutes. (1) Check the patient's blood glucose at the bedside with a portable meter every hour. (2) Notify the physician when the patient's blood sugar level reaches 250 to 300 mg/dl. F. Use urine testing for evaluation *only* if blood glucose measures are not available. It is considered unreliable. Blood testing is the standard of care today. A well-equipped critical care unit should have a bedside glucose meter to check stat glucose levels. Bedside blood glucose monitoring requires only a fingerstick, not a venous sample.[1]
2. The patient will not develop hypoglycemia.	2. Observe, assess, and treat the patient for hypoglycemia. A. Know the following signs and symptoms of hypoglycemia: (1) Excitability (2) Diaphoresis (3) Tremors (4) Increased heart rate (5) Dilated pupils (6) Headache (7) Seizures (8) Decreased blood pressure B. Know that sympathetic nervous signs may be diminished or absent in the long-term diabetic (*e.g.,* one who has had diabetes for 20 years). C. Change to a 5% glucose solution in the intravenous infusion when the patient's blood glucose level reaches 250 mg/dl. D. Determine the patient's blood glucose level if hypoglycemia is suspected. E. Treat hypoglycemia with a 50% dextrose in water solution. F. Observe the patient for the Somogyi phenomenon—the rebound effect. The nurse should do the following: (1) Suspect that the Somogyi phenomenon occurs when the patient has alternating periods of hyperglycemia and hypoglycemia. (2) Know that the Somogyi phenomenon occurs when hypoglycemia causes a physiologic compensation that elevates the blood glucose levels (*i.e.,* the release of growth hormone, ACTH, and glucagon) and thus causes hyperglycemia. (3) Know that the cycle is made worse if the physician increases the dosage of insulin (as often happens) to treat the rebound hyperglycemia. The correct treatment is to decrease the insulin.

(continued)

NURSING CARE PLAN SUMMARY   *Patient With Diabetic Ketoacidosis   Continued*

Patient Outcomes	Nursing Orders

	G. Watch the patient for signs of insulin resistance.
	  (1) Evaluate the patient's blood glucose levels relative to the amount of insulin given.
	  (2) Take into consideration the patient's usual dose of insulin.
	  (3) Give the patient hydrocortisone if insulin resistance is severe.

NURSING DIAGNOSIS

2. *Actual fluid volume deficit related to osmotic diuresis (exchanging pattern)*

Patient Outcome	Nursing Orders

The patient will have no signs and symptoms of dehydration.	1. Observe, assess, and treat the patient.
	  A. Assess for the state of hydration as follows:
	    (1) Note skin turgor and hydration status, eyeball tone, and the condition of mucous membranes.
	    (2) Check urine output every hour.
	    (3) Check and regulate intravenous rate every hour.
	    (4) Note the status of Kussmaul's respirations.
	    (5) Examine for a pleural friction rub.
	    (6) Check the specific gravity of urine.
	  B. Give the patient intravenous fluids as ordered.
	    (1) Give a 0.9% or 0.45% normal saline solution.
	    (2) Maintain the sterility of the intravenous line.
	    (3) Check the infusion site every 4 hours for signs of phlebitis, infiltration, or infection.
	  C. Assess the patient's cardiovascular functioning.
	    (1) Check vital signs every 30 to 60 minutes or as needed.
	    (2) Check central venous pressure to help evaluate venous tolerance of high volumes of fluids.
	    (3) Evaluate venous system. Check the patient's heart rate and look for distended neck veins and peripheral or sacral edema.
	    (4) Carry out continuous cardiac monitoring.
	    (5) Evaluate all pulses every 2 hours.
	    (6) Observe the patient for congestive heart failure, especially the elderly patient.
	  D. Record information about the patient's fluid intake and output and vital signs on the flow sheet.
	  E. Give the patient fluids by mouth when tolerated.
	    (1) Evaluate the patient with regard to peristalsis (check for presence of bowel sounds).
	    (2) Offer patient fluids that are high in potassium (*e.g.,* beef broth, orange juice, and oatmeal gruel).
	  F. Monitor the patient for signs of cerebral edema and a reduced level of consciousness. Have a lumbar puncture tray and an osmotic diuretic, such as urea or mannitol, available.

NURSING DIAGNOSIS

3. *Altered electrolyte balance related to osmotic diuresis (exchanging pattern)*

Patient Outcomes	Nursing Orders

1. The patient will not demonstrate signs or symptoms of hypokalemia or hyperkalemia.	1. Assess and treat the patient's potassium status.
	  A. Know the signs of hypokalemia, which are as follows:
	    (1) Muscle weakness
	    (2) Decrease in peristalsis (evidenced by ileus or distention)

(continued)

NURSING CARE PLAN SUMMARY   *Patient With Diabetic Ketoacidosis*   *Continued*

Patient Outcomes	Nursing Orders
	(3) Decrease in blood pressure
	(4) Weak pulse
	(5) Dysrhythmia
	(6) Respiratory arrest
	(7) Electrocardiographic changes: a prolonged QT interval, a depressed T wave, and prominent U waves.

   B. Know the signs of hyperkalemia, which are as follows:
     (1) Dysrhythmias: heart block, ventricular fibrillation, and cardiac arrest
     (2) Intestinal disturbances (diarrhea and nausea)
     (3) Electrocardiographic changes: peaked T waves, absence of P wave, and wide QRS interval
   C. If the initial potassium level is low (it rarely is), give potassium chloride (20 mEq to 40 mEq/L) intravenously after initial hydration.
   D. If the initial potassium level is normal, give potassium chloride (20 mEq to 40 mEq/L) 1 to 4 hours after fluid therapy is begun.
   E. If the initial potassium level is high, withhold potassium.
   F. Carry out continuous cardiac monitoring.
   G. Give fluids high in potassium by mouth when the patient is able to tolerate them.

2. The patient will not demonstrate signs or symptoms of hyponatremia.

2. Assess and treat any sodium deficiency.
   A. Look for the following signs of hyponatremia:
     (1) Abdominal cramps
     (2) Diarrhea
     (3) Apprehension
     (4) Increased heart rate
     (5) Diaphoresis
     (6) Cyanosis
     (7) Seizures
   B. Give sodium chloride in the initial intravenous fluid replacement as ordered.
   C. Evaluate the results of electrolyte studies, and notify the physician of any significant or unexpected changes.

NURSING DIAGNOSIS

4. *Altered acid-base balance related to acidic metabolic byproducts (exchanging pattern)*

Patient Outcome	Nursing Orders
The patient will regain normal acid-base status.	1. Assess the patient and treat severe acidosis.

   A. Check the relevant serum laboratory data: pH, bicarbonate, base deficit, or presence of acetone.
   B. Check the serum and urine acetone if ordered. (The urine should be taken from the catheter tubing with a sterile syringe.)
   C. Assess the depth of the patient's coma.
   D. Give sodium bicarbonate for severe acidosis.
     (1) Give the sodium bicarbonate by intravenous push or add it to the intravenous solution.
     (2) Give 1 amp (44 mEq) of sodium bicarbonate initially.
     (3) Monitor the patient's pH, bicarbonate level, and carbon dioxide content.
     (4) Observe the patient for any increase in acidosis.

NURSING DIAGNOSIS

5. *High risk for complications of DKA related to other body systems (exchanging pattern)*

Patient Outcomes	Nursing Orders
1. The patient will not demonstrate signs or symptoms of respiratory complications.	1. Assess and evaluate the patient's pulmonary status.

   A. Assess the patient's respiratory status by doing the following:
     (1) Note any decrease in Kussmaul's respirations.

(continued)

NURSING CARE PLAN SUMMARY   *Patient With Diabetic Ketoacidosis*   Continued

Patient Outcomes	*Nursing Orders*
	(2) Auscultate the lungs.
	(3) Check for pulmonary edema or congestive heart failure.
	B. Evaluate the patient's gas exchange, noting PaO_2 and $PaCO_2$.
	C. Give the patient oxygen as needed.
	D. Perform tracheal suctioning as needed.
2. The patient will not demonstrate signs or symptoms of urinary complications.	2. Assess and evaluate the patient's urinary system.
	A. If the patient is comatose, insert a Foley catheter under sterile conditions.
	B. Give the patient catheter care every 8 hours.
3. The patient will not demonstrate signs or symptoms of gastrointestinal complications.	3. Assess and evaluate the patient's gastrointestinal system.
	A. Insert a nasogastric tube if the patient is vomiting or has abdominal distention.
	B. Auscultate the patient's abdomen for bowel sounds every 2 hours to decide whether to give fluids by mouth.
	C. Check the patient's intake and output every hour.
	D. Give the patient mouth care every 4 hours.
4. The patient will not demonstrate signs or symptoms of infection.	4. Assess and evaluate the patient's body defense systems.
	A. Observe the patient for signs of infection.
	B. If the patient has an infection, give antibiotics as ordered.
	C. Turn the patient every 1 to 2 hours.
5. The patient will maintain psychosocial integrity.	5. Assess and evaluate the patient's psychosocial integrity.
	A. Listen to the patient.
	B. Learn what having diabetes means to the patient.
	C. Allow the patient to make some decisions about care and, thus, have some control over the illness.
	D. Include the patient's family in the patient's care and education.
6. The patient will not demonstrate signs or symptoms of neurologic complications.	6. Assess and evaluate the patient's neurologic system.
	A. Note the degree of coma.
	B. Check vital signs every 30 to 60 minutes or as needed.

NURSING DIAGNOSIS

6. *Knowledge deficits related to prevention of further episodes of DKA and to health maintenance (knowing pattern)*

Patient Outcomes	*Nursing Orders*
1. The patient will discuss the etiologies and prevention of DKA.	1. Find out what the patient and family know about preventing DKA.
	A. Assess their readiness to learn more.
	B. Discuss with them the following causes of hyperglycemia:
	(1) Infections. Ensure that when at home the patient will be able to determine the presence of an infectious process and take proper care of any wound.
	(2) Increased food intake
	(3) Emotional stress
	(4) Inadequate amounts of insulin
	(5) Nonadherence to treatment recommendations
2. The patient will demonstrate an adequate self-care knowledge base.	2. Evaluate the patient's self-care ability and self-evaluation habits.
	A. Make sure patients know how to check blood glucose levels and how to give themselves insulin. The patient must understand the following:
	(1) The need to rotate the site of administration
	(2) The onset, peak, and duration of the type(s) of insulin prescribed
	(3) The complications of insulin therapy: insulin reaction, lipodystrophy (atrophy, hypertrophy), and allergy.
	B. Discuss the following signs and symptoms of hyperglycemia and hypoglycemia with the patient:
	(1) Hyperglycemia: thirst, weakness, flushed face, glycosuria, acetonuria, and polyuria

(continued)

NURSING CARE PLAN SUMMARY Patient With Diabetic Ketoacidosis Continued

Patient Outcomes	Nursing Orders
	(2) Hypoglycemia: nervousness or excitability, weakness, headache, diaphoresis, and behavior changes
	C. Discuss the emergency treatment for hypoglycemia. Many commercial preparations will provide about 10 g of glucose to treat reactions. In addition, various fruit juices or colas can be used in the conscious patient.
	D. Discuss the relationship of illness to diabetes. Patients should be told to do the following:
	(1) Notify the physician if they consistently have acetone in their urine or elevated blood glucose.
	(2) Try to take liquids if they are unable to eat solid food.
	(3) Do not omit insulin. (The physician may change the dosage to regular insulin or to a sliding-scale administration of insulin if the patient has an infection. An infection increases the patient's need for insulin.)
	E. Instruct the patient and family about the ADA diet. The nurse should do the following:
	(1) Assess the patient's eating habits.
	(2) Discuss with the patient the diet to be followed if he or she becomes ill.
	F. Discuss with the patient the following main complications of diabetes mellitus:
	(1) Macrovascular disease
	(2) Microvascular disease
	(3) Neuropathy
	(4) Infections
	(5) Visual problems

IMPLEMENTATION AND EVALUATION

Diabetic ketoacidosis must be treated if the patient is to survive. Because DKA is life-threatening, early diagnosis and management are needed. The chief components of the nursing and medical treatment are insulin therapy, fluid replacement, electrolyte replacement, antiacidosis therapy, and management of the symptoms. Use of a flow sheet (Table 37–2) to record and correlate the laboratory values and replacement factors is helpful.

Insulin Therapy

Insulin therapy is perhaps the cornerstone of treatment. Without it, the pathologic cycle cannot be stopped. Before 1972, it was traditional therapy to give very large doses of insulin in DKA. Part of the rationale for the large doses was to treat the insulin resistance seen in DKA. However, since that time, numerous studies have compared the large doses of insulin (e.g., 100 U in intravenous bolus) with small doses of insulin, given intermittently or in a continuous infusion. Over 20 research studies have now documented the value of small doses of insulin in the treatment of DKA.[13]

There are various recommendations for routes: intravenous, intramuscular, subcutaneous, or a combination of two of these. The blood glucose level generally decreases at a fairly predictable level of about 75 to 100 mg/dl/hour.[13] Certainly, there are individual exceptions to this. One study found that the subcutaneous and intramuscular routes were slower in lowering glucose than intravenous routes and reached a peak between 2 and 3 hours after injection.[12] Some physicians prefer to give all insulin intravenously, but a key point in recent trends is to avoid the large-dose therapy. The intravenous route is preferred. The subcutaneous route should be avoided if the patient is markedly hypotensive, dehydrated, or in shock, because of poor absorption.[6]

Monitoring the patient's blood glucose levels is imperative. At about 250 to 300 mg/dl, the danger of hypoglycemia necessitates decreasing the insulin dose.[21]

A continuous insulin infusion using an infusion pump is commonly piggybacked into an intravenous line. Generally about 5 U to 10 U/hour of regular insulin is given.[2] Albumin may be used to bind the insulin to it to keep it from adhering to the glass and tubing. Use of the infusion pump ensures that the patient receives the prescribed dose and results in a more predictable drop in blood glucose. The patient in DKA is treated with regular insulin; once the initial hyperglycemic crisis is over, the patient will likely be returned to one or more kinds of the other insulins.

The biologic half-life of insulin is less than 9 minutes,[14] a fact that should be considered when administering intravenous insulin. There are no detectable differences between diabetic and nondiabetic individuals in insulin half-life calculation. If 100 U is administered as an intravenous bolus, 10 minutes later in the average patient, only 50 U will still be circulating. One exception is the patient with impaired renal function, which can extend the serum half-life of insulin, because the kidneys normally excrete insulin.[14]

Insulin resistance may be present in some patients. If insulin resistance is present, circulating antibodies counteract some

Table 37-2
Flow Sheet for Diabetic Ketoacidosis

VITAL SIGNS

Time	BP	HR	R	T	Urine Output	Level of Consciousness	Other

LABORATORY VALUES

Time	Blood Glucose	Acetone Dilution	pH	PCO$_2$	HCO$_3$	Na	K	Cl	CO$_2$	Other

TREATMENT

Time	Insulin	Type Intravenous Fluid	Amount	Cumulative Amount	K	Bicarbonate	Other

of the effect of the insulin. Insulin must saturate the antibody before the effect of the insulin can be seen.[22] If insulin resistance is present, much higher doses of insulin are given, and the total amount may be in the thousands of units. There is recent evidence that the phenomenon of insulin resistance resolves during treatment in most patients.[13] In a recent study, the average amount of insulin administered for severe ketoacidosis was a total of 550 U.[7]

The patient is carefully evaluated during the insulin therapy. Blood glucose evaluations are done every hour. After the first few hours of treatment, insulin may be given on a sliding scale, with the dosage based on the blood glucose level. Insulin is inactivated when the pH is above 7.5. Thus, some inactivation may be seen when bicarbonate therapy is used.

Hypoglycemia (insulin shock, insulin reaction) is one of the main complications of insulin therapy. It may follow rigorous treatment of DKA, and it can lead to permanent damage of the central nervous system. The clinical manifestations of hypoglycemia are a response to stimulation of both the central nervous system and the sympathetic nervous system. The term *neuroglycopenia* is used to describe the state in which there is decreased glucose to the brain during hypoglycemia.[5] Vasomotor nerves lose their ability to maintain vessel tone and size, leading to vasodilatation and hypotension. A shock state can ensue if the hypoglycemia is untreated. Because the myocardium needs adequate amounts of glucose, cardiac functioning may be affected. The signs and symptoms of hypoglycemia include diaphoresis, excitability, dilated pupils, blurred vision, fall in blood pressure, weakness, pallor, and behavioral changes. Several studies have documented cognitive functioning problems during hypoglycemia.[11,15]

Hypoglycemia can usually be avoided by stopping the insulin infusion when the blood glucose level reaches 250 to 300 mg/dl. An intravenous solution containing 5% glucose should be administered at this point in the treatment.

Fluid Replacement

Rapid rehydration is needed to maintain vascular tone and metabolic functioning. Large amounts of fluids are given initially and as long as needed. The average fluid deficit is 3 L to 5 L of water in an adult.[9] Isotonic normal saline solution (0.9%) is the initial fluid of choice despite its hyperosmolarity.[9] One half normal saline solution (0.45%) may be given because it is less hyperosmolar for some patients. Generally, 1000 ml to 2000 ml is given in the first 2 hours or so.[21] Up to 10 L of fluid is the average volume to be administered in the first 12 hours. Some authorities calculate fluid losses and replace fluids accordingly. One formula estimates the average losses at 100 ml of water/kg of body weight.[13] Monitoring the blood pressure is a useful guide for fluid replacement. After the first few hours, the fluid will probably be changed to 0.45% normal saline solution. Because more water than sodium is lost owing to osmotic diuresis, extra free water will be needed in the form of a 5% dextrose-in-water solution or a 0.45% normal saline solution. By this time, the extent of the patient's hyperosmolar state can be determined and the types of fluids should be selected with this in mind. Lactated Ringer's solution may be used to minimize the chloride load and avoid hyperchloremia.[9,21] A 5% glucose solution should be given before hypoglycemia is likely to occur. After insulin therapy, glucose is metabolized, and because there is no available glycogen, glucose is needed.

Alkalinizing solutions, such as sodium bicarbonate and sodium lactate, are occasionally used for severe acidosis. These solutions must be administered with caution because they can produce alkalosis or can contribute to the development of spinal fluid acidosis.[13] The use of sodium lactate can lead to lactic acidosis.

Cerebral edema is a rare but often fatal complication of DKA and is seen a few hours after therapy is begun. A dramatic neurologic change preceding a respiratory arrest may be seen.[16] Cerebral edema should be suspected in a patient with deterioration 3 to 10 hours into the treatment regimen, which is reflected in increasing stupor or coma with signs of increased intracranial pressure.[21] The cause is unknown, but an osmotic disequilibrium does occur between plasma glucose and intracerebral glucose. Cerebral edema and hypoxia are associated with this condition.[9] A recent study[16] of possible predictors for cerebral edema failed to implicate treatment variables such as the rate of hydration, tonicity of intravenous fluids, the use of bicarbonate, or the rate of correction. The researchers concluded that prevention of DKA is the most important goal to avoid intracerebral complications.

Electrolyte Replacement

Replacement of lost electrolytes is another major therapy. Losses of sodium, potassium, chloride, magnesium, phosphate, and calcium are seen in the patient with DKA, and the primary concern is replacement of these elements. They may be added to the intravenous solutions, but some are not always replaced.

Sodium and chloride are replaced with a 0.45% or 0.9% normal saline intravenous solution given rapidly. The therapy is monitored by serum electrolyte studies.

Calculation of potassium replacement is difficult. The serum potassium level does not reflect the patient's true status because most potassium is normally intracellular. In DKA, the total body amount of potassium is deficient. However, the patient may present with high, low, or even normal serum potassium levels. When insulin and fluid administration are instituted, potassium is rapidly moved back into the cell, and a life-threatening hypokalemia can ensue. It usually occurs after 1 to 4 hours of treatment, but it may occur earlier.[13] Giving potassium before insulin is begun is potentially lethal.[21] Potassium replacement should be carefully evaluated using the serum potassium level. If the level is high initially, obviously no potassium is needed. In fact, to give the patient potassium would endanger the patient and make the patient susceptible to cardiac dysrhythmias. If the potassium level is normal, potassium chloride (20 mEq–40 mEq/L) may be given after the initial hydration therapy.[21] If the patient's potassium level is low on admission (it is low extremely rarely), potassium replacement is begun immediately. Potassium phosphate may be given as a form of potassium replacement because it also treats phosphate depletion and may help in oxygen transport to tissue.[21] Potassium should only be given with extreme care to any patient with anuria.[21] The electrocardiogram is a useful guide to the patient's potassium level (see Nursing Diagnosis 3).

After the acute phase is over, the oral route of administering potassium is a safe one if the patient is able to tolerate liquids. Orange juice, beef broth, or other fluids high in potassium can be given.

Magnesium replacement is controversial. Some feel it is

rapidly restored once the patient resumes eating.[13] Others suggest intravenous replacement in addition to multivitamins.[2]

Antiacidosis Therapy

Alkali therapy to counteract the metabolic acidosis is usually reserved for severe acidosis only. The carbon dioxide content can serve as a guide for the degree of acidosis. A pH of less than 7 indicates acidosis severe enough for sodium bicarbonate therapy.[9,21]

There has been a trend in recent years to give sodium bicarbonate cautiously. Opposition to bicarbonate administration is based on its contribution to lactic acidosis.[21] When 2,3-DPG is low, a sudden rise in pH may reduce oxygen release to the tissues (shifting the oxygen dissociation curve to the left) and predispose the patient to lactic acidosis.[21] Careful evaluation of potassium levels is imperative because bicarbonate treatment can produce hypokalemia[20] and metabolic alkalosis.[21]

Management of Symptoms

Other medical and nursing treatments of DKA may be instituted, depending on the needs of the individual patient. The treatments include dextran, plasma, or whole-blood replacement in severe hypovolemic shock. Vasopressors may be used in peripheral vascular collapse. Antibiotics are prescribed if an infection is present. Gastric intubation is used if vomiting or distention is present.

EVALUATION OF OUTCOMES

The nursing and medical management of the patient with DKA can be evaluated by the patient outcomes. The nursing orders should be continually scrutinized to determine if they are contributing to the best possible patient outcomes.

SUMMARY

Diabetic ketoacidosis is a life-threatening condition that can occur in the patient with diabetes mellitus. The mortality is 1.5% to 15%. The critical care nurse needs to assess the patient quickly, using knowledge of the pathophysiology, anticipated patient problems, and medical management. Diabetic ketoacidosis leads to severe dehydration, metabolic acidosis, and electrolyte depletion. Medical and nursing management is aimed at correcting these disorders and providing the discharge teaching, which aims at preventing the recurrence of DKA.

DIRECTIONS FOR FUTURE RESEARCH

Nurses need to investigate the effects of specific nursing interventions used in caring for the patient with DKA. Possible research questions may include the following:

1. What is the relationship of knowledge about etiologies of DKA to the incidence of it?
2. How accurate are nurses in blood glucose monitoring techniques? How important is it to practice this skill regularly?
3. What are the earliest clinical signs for nursing assessment of hypokalemia?
4. What are the most reliable nursing assessment findings to detect fluid overload for the elderly patient who is receiving high volumes of intravenous fluids?
5. What is the relationship between relaxation exercises and blood glucose levels?

REFERENCES

1. American Diabetes Association: Bedside glucose monitoring in hospitals. *Diabetes Care* 13:1, 1990.
2. Carroll, P., and Matz, R. Uncontrolled diabetes mellitus in adults: Experience in treating diabetic ketoacidosis and hyperosmolar coma nonketotic coma with low-dose insulin and a uniform treatment regime. *Diabetes Care* 6:6, 1983.
3. Cassey, J. Host Defenses and Infections in Diabetes Mellitus. In M. Ellenberg and H. Rifkin (eds.), *Diabetes Mellitus: Theory and Practice* (3rd ed.). New York: Medical Examination Publishing Co., 1983.
4. Cryer, P. Glucose Homeostasis and Hypoglycemia. In J. Wilson and D. Foster (eds.), *William's Textbook of Endocrinology* (7th ed.). Philadelphia: W. B. Saunders, 1985.
5. Cudworth, A., and Gorsuch, A. Autoimmunity and Viruses in Type I (Insulin-Dependent) Diabetes. In M. Ellenberg and H. Rifkin (eds.), *Diabetes Mellitus: Theory and Practice* (3rd ed.). New York: Medical Examination Publishing Co., 1983.
6. Davidson, J. *Clinical Diabetes Mellitus: A Problem-Oriented Approach.* New York: Thieme, 1986.
7. Davidson, M. Insulin Therapy. In K. Sussman, B. Draznin, and W. James (eds.), *Clinical Guide to Diabetes Mellitus.* New York: Alan R. Liss, 1987.
8. Ellenberg, M. Diabetic Neuropathy. In M. Ellenberg and H. Rifkin (eds.), *Diabetes Mellitus: Theory and Practice* (3rd ed.). New York: Medical Examination Publishing Co., 1983.
9. Foster, D., and McGarris, J. The metabolic derangements and treatment of diabetic acidosis. *N. Engl. J. Med.* 309:3, 1983.
10. Guyton, A. *Textbook of Medical Physiology* (7th ed.). Philadelphia: W. B. Saunders, 1986.
11. Hoffman, R., Speelman, D., Hinnen, D., et al. Changes in cortical functioning with acute hypoglycemia and hyperglycemia in type I diabetes. *Diabetes Care* 12:3, 1989.
12. Kitabchi, A., Matteri, R., and Murphy, M. Optimal insulin delivery in diabetic ketoacidosis (DKA) and hyperglycemic, hyperosmolar nonketotic coma (HHNC). *Diabetes Care* 5(suppl 1):78, 1982.
13. Kriesberg, R. Diabetic Ketoacidosis, Alcoholic Ketosis, Lactic Acidosis, and Hyporenimemic Hypoaldosteronism. In M. Ellenberg and H. Rifkin (eds.). *Diabetes Mellitus: Theory and Practice* (3rd ed.). New York: Medical Examination Publishing Co., 1983.
14. Larner, J. Insulin and Oral Hypoglycemic Drugs. In A. Gilman, L. Goodman, T. Rall, et al. (eds.), *The Pharmacological Basis of Therapeutics* (7th ed.). New York: Macmillan, 1985.
15. Reaven, G., Thompson, L., Nahum, D., et al. Relationship between hyperglycemia and cognitive function in older NIDDM patients. *Diabetes Care* 13:1, 1990.
16. Rosenbloom, A. Intercerebral crisis during treatment of diabetic ketoacidosis. *Diabetes Care* 13:1, 1990.
17. Salans, L., Kittle, J., and Hirsch, J. Obesity, Glucose Intolerance. In M. Ellenberg and H. Rifkin (eds.), *Diabetes Mellitus: Theory and Practice* (3rd ed.). New York: Medical Examination Publishing Co., 1983.
18. Shade, D., and Eaton, P. Hormonal Interrelationships. In M. Ellenberg and H. Rifkin (eds.), *Diabetes Mellitus: Theory and Practice* (3rd ed.). New York: Medical Examination Publishing Co., 1983.
19. Surwitt, R., and Feinglos, M. The effects of relaxation on glucose tolerance in non-insulin dependent diabetes. *Diabetes Care* 6:2, 1983.
20. Sussman, K. Diabetic Ketoacidosis. In K. Sussman, B. Draznin, and W. James (eds.), *Clinical Guide to Diabetes Mellitus.* New York: Alan R. Liss, 1987.
21. Unger, R., and Foster, D. Diabetes Mellitus. In J. Wilson and D. Foster (eds.), *William's Textbook of Endocrinology* (7th ed.). Philadelphia: W. B. Saunders, 1985.
22. Weber, S., Wood, W., and Jackson, E. Availability of insulin from parenteral nutrient solutions, *Am. J. Hosp. Pharm.* 34:353, 1977.

38

Hyperosmolar Coma

Angela Pruitt Clark

SPIRITUALITY AND HEALTH

Once persons discover that their own consciousness can play a major role in their health, they may decide that they can "create their own reality" in matters of health, totally structuring and determining whatever happens. Thus, many persons claim that we are "100% responsible" for everything that occurs in our health. Some go further. They assert that good health correlates with "being spiritual"; that is, if we are attuned and aligned with our idea of the "Absolute," we should never get sick.

These assertions demonstrate a marked hubris of consciousness—an arrogant, narcissistic presumption that we can tell the universe what to do. The slightest bit of reflection shows the emptiness of these beliefs. Consider the health histories of the spiritual geniuses who crop up in history from time to time. Two of the most well-known spiritual teachers of this century died from cancer—J. Krishnamurti of India and Japan's Suzuki Roshi, who established the San Francisco Zen Center. If the spiritual giants are not immune from illness and sometimes grotesquely painful deaths, how can we presume to be?

An avalanche of modern evidence shows clearly that human consciousness *can* affect the body in positive ways; about this, there is no doubt. To extend this to the claim of total, absolute control of everything that happens in our health is unjustified. There is no scientific or historical justification for this point of view.

Those nurses who understand the concepts of psychobiologic unity need always to bear these limitations in mind. We will confront patients from time to time who experience a sense of failure when their psychologic and spiritual lives seem to be on track but they get sick anyway. They may feel guilty, as if they did not "try hard enough." We can remind them that even the greatest spiritual achievers get sick, frequently with the same illnesses that affect the rest of us. Bearing this in mind can allay guilt and anxiety, and it can contribute to the emotional peace of our patients.

LEARNING OBJECTIVES

After reading this chapter, the nurse should be able to do the following:

1. Describe the causative and precipitating factors in hyperosmolar coma.
2. Discuss the pathophysiology of hyperosmolar coma.
3. After reading Chapter 37, differentiate the patient with hyperosmolar coma from the patient with diabetic ketoacidosis on the basis of the clinical manifestations and expected laboratory data.
4. Identify and list (in the order of importance) the patient care objectives for the patient with hyperosmolar coma.
5. Teach the diabetic patient with hyperosmolar coma and the family what they need to know to prevent complications.

CASE STUDY

Mrs. S.W., a 66-year-old retired teacher, was taken on a stretcher from a nearby convalescent center to the hospital. The charge nurse in the convalescent center had noticed early that afternoon that Mrs. W., who had become more and more difficult to arouse, had become semicomatose.

Mrs. W. was examined by the physician in the emergency room. Using a report from the convalescent center, the results of the physical examination, and the laboratory data, the physician made a tentative diagnosis of hyperosmolar coma, and he ordered initial therapy. Mrs. W. was transferred to the critical care unit.

Mrs. W.'s daughter and son-in-law were able to give information about Mrs. W. Also, Mrs. W.'s medical records from the convalescent center had been sent with her to the hospital.

Mrs. W. had recently been treated in the same hospital for coronary insufficiency and mild congestive heart failure. Her current medications were digoxin (Lanoxin), furosemide (Lasix), and propranolol (Inderal).

Two weeks ago, Mrs. W. had been discharged from the hospital and transferred to the convalescent center to regain her strength and ability to care for herself. Her family said that she had suggested the transfer and had seemed to accept the need for it (she lived alone). Mrs. W. was known to have had diabetes for 10 years. She controlled the disease by diet therapy alone.

The following information was gathered in the physical examination:

General observations: Acutely ill white woman; no intravenous line; some dyspnea; when admitted, patient receiving oxygen by nasal cannula

Vital signs: Blood pressure, 96/70 in supine position, left arm; heart rate, 116; sinus tachycardia with occasional ectopic beats, primarily premature ventricular contractions; respirations, 32 and deep; no acetone breath; temperature, 100.2°F rectally; height, 5 feet 7 inches; weight, 140 lb

Integument: Skin tone and turgor poor; skin very dry to touch; no lacerations or breaks in skin; scar on left ankle

Head: No masses; no abnormalities

Eyes: Pupils equal and reactive to light: eyeballs soft; sclera clear; no retinopathy

Ears: Membranes clear; no discharge

Nose: Flaring of nostrils on inspiration; no discharge

Mouth: Pink; mucous membranes very dry

Neck: No lymphadenopathy; no bruits or neck vein distention

Chest: Vesicular breath sounds; no crackles or rhonchi

Cardiovascular system: Normal first and second heart sounds; no third or fourth heart sound; no murmur; apical thrust; poor capillary refill; patient pale

Abdomen: Distended; liver nonpalpable; bowel sounds absent

Genitourinary system: No discharge; bladder distended

Extremities: Pulses present; some pedal edema bilaterally; no cyanosis; no diabetic foot lesions

Neurologic responses: Deep tendon reflexes grade 1; no response to verbal stimuli

The following laboratory data were obtained immediately:

Blood glucose level: 1156 mg/dl

Plasma ketones: Negative

Serum osmolality: 356 mM/liter

Complete blood count: White blood cells, 9000; hemoglobin, 16.3 g; hematocrit, 60%

Electrolytes: Sodium, 146 mEq/L; potassium, 4.5 mEq/L; chloride, 103 mEq/L; carbon dioxide combining power, 18

Arterial blood gases: pH, 7.33; PaO_2, 90 mm Hg; $PaCO_2$, 33 mm Hg

Urinalysis: Negative except for 5% glucose

Other data: Blood urea nitrogen, 70 mg; cholesterol, 289 mg

Chest radiograph: Negative; some cardiomegaly

Clinical Presentation of Case Study

When Mrs. W. was admitted to the intensive care unit, the nurse immediately began an assessment and examination. The following intravenous fluids were started: a 0.45% normal saline solution infused at a rate of 300 ml/hour, and regular insulin (10 U by intravenous push) for the elevated blood glucose level. It was felt that she was hypotensive because she was dehydrated, but that she was not in hypovolemic shock. A Foley catheter was inserted, and 1100 ml of urine was obtained.

3:15 P.M. (Second Hour)

Blood pressure was 100/74. Apical heart rate increased to 128. There were no clinical signs of heart failure, except the sinus tachycardia. Intravenous fluid rate was 300 ml/hour (no increase). Blood glucose level was 804 mg/dl. Regular insulin was administered (5 U by in-

travenous push into tubing medication additive site). No improvement in skin turgor or mucous membranes was observed. An insulin infusion was started at 5 U/hour of regular insulin.

5:15 P.M. (Fourth Hour)

Sinus tachycardia 140. Lanoxin (0.25 mg by intravenous push). Blood glucose 630 mg/dl. Regular insulin continued.

6:15 P.M. (Fifth Hour)

Heart rate decreased to 124. Electrolytes: sodium, 134; potassium, 3.9. Blood glucose level was 501 mg/dl. Serum osmolality was 338 mM/L.

9:15 P.M.

The family visited. Mrs. W. was still unconscious. Potassium level decreased to 3.6. Potassium chloride was added to intravenous line.

12:15 A.M. (Tenth Hour)

Blood glucose level was 379 mg/dl. Mrs. W. was partly aroused when she was spoken to. Infusion of 0.45% normal saline solution was decreased to 200 ml/hour.

4:15 A.M. (Fourteenth Hour)

Mrs. W. was awake and asking for daughter. Daughter was not in family room. Mrs. W. assured by the nurse that daughter had been present all evening. Patient seemed satisfied with that information.

5:15 A.M.

Blood glucose level was 315 mg/dl. Regular insulin was continued via an infusion pump.

9:00 A.M. (Second Day)

Patient was taking fluids by mouth as tolerated. Bowel sounds were present, and there was no distention. Blood glucose level was 260 mg/dl. Insulin was discontinued. Intravenous therapy was changed to 5% dextrose-in-water solution. Serum osmolality was 308 mM/L.

3:00 P.M.

Blood glucose level was 174 mg/dl. Mrs. W. was transferred from the intensive care unit to a nursing unit. Sixteen hundred calorie soft American Diabetes Association (ADA) diet was taken without difficulty.

Third Day

Teaching about diabetes was begun by teaching team made up of a nurse, a pharmacist, and a dietitian. Blood glucose level was 164 mg/dl. Patient was told that they would attempt to control her diabetes with diet and moderate exercise.

Fifth Day

Patient was still complaining of some weakness. Vital signs were stable. Glucose level was responding to diet.

Sixth Day

Patient was discharged to daughter's home and was instructed to see physician in 2 days for follow-up care. Patient and daughter were encouraged to contact the teaching team if they had questions.

REFLECTIONS

Hyperosmolar coma (HOC) demonstrates vividly the interrelatedness of mind and body. One's mental acuity changes with changes in osmolality. As intellectual functioning deteriorates, a vicious cycle may become established. Patients may forget to take insulin or oral hypoglycemics, or may become oblivious to their deteriorating physical condition. As the person's judgment fails, self-care also fails. This is usually disastrous, because to prevent a diabetic crisis, the diabetic must pay close attention to detail. Hyperosmolar coma is associated with elderly patients generally; thus, there may be other physiologic reasons for changes in mental acuity. Thus, in diabetes, body and mind must function as a unit. What the patient thinks and perceives affects the course of the disease, and as HOC demonstrates, the disease can adversely affect the patient's thoughts and perceptions. Diabetes mellitus demonstrates the interrelatedness of mind and body, an essential concept for nurses to consider.

DEFINITION

Hyperosmolar coma (hyperosmolar nonketotic coma) is a complication of diabetes mellitus that can be manifested as an acute illness. The mortality in HOC is high; it is generally thought to be 40% to 60%.[12] Some large medical centers have reported a lower mortality rate.[11] Unfortunately, HOC is often not diagnosed early enough to be treated successfully. It occurs mainly in the type II diabetic, and it is an emergency condition. Hyperosmolar coma occurs also in the nondiabetic. Like diabetic ketoacidosis (DKA), HOC can lead to severe dehydration with loss of electrolytes, and, if untreated, it can lead to death.

INCIDENCE AND ETIOLOGY

The incidence of HOC is the same in men and women,[14] and it is one sixth the incidence of DKA (Table 38–1). Hyperosmolar coma is seen primarily in people 60 years of age and older. Most people who develop HOC have type II diabetes or develop diabetes at the same time that they develop HOC.

Two thirds of patients with HOC will have no previous history of diabetes, yet most will have mild type II diabetes on recovery.[4] After the acute phase of HOC, the diabetes can usually be controlled by diet and oral hypoglycemic drugs.[16] In some cases, diabetes is not present, and it never develops.[14] Rarely, a child with type I diabetes presents in HOC.[14]

Some writers feel that a primary antecedent event for many of the people is related to thirst. Either they cannot recognize thirst or cannot express their need for water.[11]

Numerous factors precipitate or accompany HOC. These factors increase the person's need for insulin beyond the amount that can be produced. The factors may be divided into three groups: certain acute or chronic diseases, certain medical procedures, and the use of certain drugs. The three groups are discussed in the following paragraphs.

Acute or Chronic Conditions

The following conditions have been noted to precipitate or accompany HOC:

- Previously undiagnosed diabetes[18]
- Severe burns (often treated with large amounts of glucose)[11]
- Diabetes insipidus[11]
- Thyrotoxicosis[11]
- Dehydration[18]
- Acute pancreatitis[14]
- Central nervous system damage[18]
- Gastrointestinal bleeding[11]
- Protracted diarrhea[11]
- Gram-negative pneumonia[10]
- Uremia[8]
- Acute pyelonephritis
- Acute myocardial infarction[15]
- Subdural hematoma[8]
- Arterial thrombosis[2]
- Heat stroke[17]
- Pulmonary embolus[15]
- Stress[17]
- Urinary tract infection[18]

Most of the conditions that precipitate or accompany HOC are acute illnesses. It most frequently occurs when an intercurrent illness increases glucose production secondary to stress hormones but also impairs the ability to drink fluids.[17] The precoma phase is longer in HOC than in DKA, and often patients have had polyuria for over a week in HOC.[14]

Table 38–1

Comparison of Hyperosmolar Coma and Diabetic Ketoacidosis

FACTOR	HYPEROSMOLAR COMA	DIABETIC KETOACIDOSIS
Age	Older adult, usually over 50	Any age
Diabetic status	Usually type II diabetic—may be undiagnosed	Often a known diabetic, usually a type I diabetic
Hyperglycemia	Frequently over 1000 mg/dl	Generally less than 1000 mg/dl
Ketosis; acidosis	No ketosis; if acidosis present, it is lactic or renal	Yes
Severe dehydration	Yes	Yes
Acetone breath	No	Yes
Serum sodium	Usually high (may be normal or low)	Usually low
Insulin as treatment	Not as much needed as in DKA, usually less than 100 U	Large amounts needed

Medical Procedures

The following medical procedures are associated with HOC:

- Hemodialysis or peritoneal dialysis (involving the use of a hyperosmolar dialysate)[16]
- Hypothermia[11]
- Nasogastric tube feedings with high-calorie mixtures[17]
- Intravenous hyperalimentation[17]
- Prolonged mannitol diuresis[11]
- Intravenous 5% dextrose solutions[13]
- Intravenous 50% dextrose solution[13]

Drugs

The following drugs have been known to cause or accompany HOC:

- Diphenylhydantoin (Dilantin)[11]
- Thiazide diuretics[11]
- Steroids[17]
- Mannitol[2]
- Propranolol (Inderal)[11]
- Immunosuppressive drugs[2]
- Diazoxide[11]
- Glucagon
- Furosemide (Lasix)[11]
- Ethacrynic acid (Edecrin)
- Azathioprine[16]
- Sodium bicarbonate (large amounts in infusion)[8]
- Alcohol intoxication
- Cimetidine[11]

PSYCHOPATHOPHYSIOLOGY

Hyperosmolar coma is a comatose or near-comatose state that is characterized by a significant degree of hyperglycemia, hyperosmolarity, hypernatremia, and dehydration. If acidosis is present, it is usually due to an accompanying lactic or renal acidosis.

The principles of physiology discussed in Chapter 37 are valid for HOC as well. The stressors just listed increase the body's need for insulin. The person who develops HOC does not have enough insulin to cope with the stressor. Because insulin is not available to help transport glucose into the cell, the blood glucose concentration rises.

Hyperglycemia develops because of a decrease in the peripheral utilization of glucose by muscle and liver cells and also because the liver increases its glucose production as a result of glycogenolysis and glyconeogenesis. The endogenous production of glucose by the liver in the type II diabetic can reach large quantities—up to 1000 g/day.[11]

The range of hyperglycemia is about 600 mg to 2800 mg/dl or higher. The normal renal threshold for glucose (about 170 mg/dl) is quickly exceeded, and glycosuria ensues, with a dramatic loss of water and electrolytes. The depletion causes severe dehydration and leads to hypovolemia and hemoconcentration. With the decrease in volume, renal blood flow is decreased, and a prerenal azotemia that leads to further hyperglycemia occurs. Renal insufficiency is probably present in all patients with HOC.

The normal range for serum osmolality is 280 mM to 300 mM/L. When a patient's osmolality level is higher than 310 mM/L, he or she shows some signs of confusion. At a level of 325 mM/L and above, coma may occur. In HOC, the osmolality level is at least 350 and averages 380 mM/L.[18]

Hyperglycemia and the osmotic diuresis it brings cause such an increased volume of urine through the distal convoluted tubules and collecting tubules that the kidney can no longer maintain a water balance. Severe dehydration in all three body compartments follows. People so affected lose water and electrolytes, but they lose relatively more water than electrolytes.

Failure to maintain adequate renal function can occur either from previous kidney disease or secondary to dehydration. This drops the glomerular filtration rate and may lead to remarkably high glucose levels.[11]

The serum sodium levels in HOC are frequently high and contribute to the hyperosmolar state.[14] The serum sodium levels may be low or low normal, reflecting the dilution of serum sodium in the water osmotically obligated to glucose. There is a decrease in the serum sodium of about 2.7 mEq/L for every 100 mg/dl of blood glucose.

The absence of ketosis distinguishes HOC from DKA. The mechanism by which ketosis is suppressed is unknown.[17,18] Insulin is known to inhibit lipolysis, but other factors are unexplained.

NURSING PROCESS

ASSESSMENT

Prompt diagnosis of HOC is critically important. A delay can mean death for the patient. Because the symptoms may resemble those of many other conditions, HOC is often not suspected until it is too late. The most common misdiagnosis is cerebrovascular accident.[8] Remember, the patient is usually over 60 years of age.[11]

The diagnosis is based on clinical signs and symptoms and information obtained from the history (if one can be taken) and from laboratory tests. The nurse who understands HOC will be more apt to consider its presence in the acutely ill, dehydrated patient.

Clinical Manifestations

The histories of patients with HOC usually note an insidious onset (a few days or weeks) of thirst and polyuria, which they tried to satisfy by eating a high-carbohydrate diet.[14] Patients with HOC may be stuporous or comatose on admission, probably with severe dehydration, an altered state of consciousness, and other neurologic disturbances.

Severe dehydration is shown by such clinical signs as decreased skin turgor, dry skin, thirst, and soft eyeballs. Hypotension is present, and hypovolemic shock can be a complication of the dehydration.

The respirations in HOC may be rapid but not acidotic, as are the Kussmaul's respirations in DKA. The breath does not smell of acetone.[11]

The central nervous system dysfunction can be manifested in hallucinations or vestibular disturbances. Approximately 25% of patients have some seizures.[14] Dehydration accounts for the depressed state of consciousness.[17]

Gastric stasis and ileus occur in over 50% of patients. Nausea, vomiting, and abdominal discomfort are common assessment findings.[11]

Diagnostic Tests

Several diagnostic tests are indicated in HOC. The tests that should be done immediately are a blood glucose test, a urinalysis to test for the presence of glucose and ketones, and determinations of the blood ketone level (to rule out DKA), the arterial blood gas measurements, and the serum osmolality.

Although the range of hyperglycemia can be extreme (600–2800), typically the blood glucose level is at least 600, with an average of 1000 mg to 1200 mg/dl.[17,18] Glucose values as high as 4800 have been reported.[11] The blood glucose level in HOC is higher than that in DKA. A high degree of glycosuria is present. If the blood glucose level is high and serum ketones are absent, HOC should be considered first.

The patient with pure HOC (no DKA or lactic acidosis) is not acidotic, but often such a patient has a slight degree of metabolic acidosis. An average pH of 7.26 has been found in patients with pure HOC.[2]

The serum osmolality test is the most important test. In HOC, a reading of over 350 mM/L is obtained.[18] The osmolality of body fluids can be calculated with the use of an osmometer or one of several formulas.

Other helpful tests are the blood urea nitrogen and electrolyte levels and a white blood cell count. In HOC, the blood urea nitrogen level is elevated, averaging about 87 mg/dl.[2,17] Leukocytosis is significant and not particularly helpful in ruling out DKA. Electrolytes are lost in the osmotic diuresis, but the water imbalance may cause high, low, or normal electrolyte readings. Hypernatremia is usually seen, averaging 145 mEq.[14] A sodium range of 119 mEq to 188 mEq has been seen.[14] Serum potassium levels may be high, low, or normal, but there is a total body deficit.[6,18] The plasma bicarbonate level averages about 17 mEq/L.[18]

NURSING DIAGNOSES, PATIENT OUTCOMES, AND PLAN

The preceding material on etiologies, nursing assessment, and diagnostic tests guides the nurse in establishing nursing diagnoses, patient outcomes, and the plan for the patient with HOC.

NURSING CARE PLAN SUMMARY *Patient With Hyperosmolar Coma*

NURSING DIAGNOSIS

1. *Acute hyperosmolality related to hyperglycemia and hypernatremia (exchanging pattern)*

Patient Outcome	Nursing Orders

The patient will regain a normal serum osmolality level.	1. Assess, treat, and evaluate the patient's serum osmolality.
	  A. Observe the patient for effects of the hyperosmolarity.
	    (1) Check urine output every hour.
	    (2) Note skin turgor, eyeball tone, and the condition of the mucous membranes.
	    (3) Check and regulate intravenous rate every hour.
	    (4) Note ventilation status.
	    (5) Examine for a pleural friction rub.
	    (6) Check the specific gravity of the urine.
	    (7) Calculate serum osmolality levels as needed.
	  B. Give the patient intravenous fluids as ordered.
	    (1) Use a volume expander (*e.g.*, dextran) for hypovolemic shock.
	    (2) Use a 0.45% normal saline solution (0.9% normal saline may be ordered). Rapid infusion rates are typical.
	    (3) Maintain the sterility of the intravenous line.
	    (4) Check the infusion site every 4 hours for signs of phlebitis, infiltration, and infection.
	    (5) Check the intravenous line every hour.
	  C. Monitor blood glucose levels at least every hour, preferably at the bedside.
	  D. Monitor serum sodium levels.
	  E. Evaluate blood pressure every hour or more often as needed.
	  F. Consider the age of the patient (usually over 60 years) when assessing effects.
	  G. Evaluate level of consciousness continuously.

(continued)

NURSING CARE PLAN SUMMARY *Patient With Hyperosmolar Coma* *Continued*

NURSING DIAGNOSIS

2. *Altered electrolyte balance related to hypernatremia and hypokalemia (exchanging pattern)*

Patient Outcomes	Nursing Orders

1. The patient will not demonstrate signs or symptoms of hypokalemia.	1. Assess and treat the patient's potassium status.
	  A. Know the signs and symptoms of hypokalemia (see Chap. 37, Nursing Diagnosis 3, p. 700).
	  B. Know the signs and symptoms of hyperkalemia (see Chap. 37, Nursing Diagnosis 3, p. 701).
	  C. If the initial potassium level is low (it rarely is), give potassium chloride (20 mEq to 40 mEq/L) immediately.
	  D. If the initial potassium level is normal, give potassium chloride (20 mEq to 40 mEq/L) 1 to 4 hours after fluid therapy is begun.
	  E. If the initial potassium level is high, withhold potassium.
	  F. Carry out continuous cardiac monitoring.

2. The patient will not demonstrate signs or symptoms of hypernatremia.	2. Assess and treat the patient's sodium status.
	  A. Know the signs and symptoms of hypernatremia, because this may occur quickly once fluid therapy is begun (see Chap. 35, Nursing Diagnosis 5, p. 662).
	  B. Know that hyperlipemia (common in older patients) may cause a falsely low level of serum sodium.[11]
	  C. Give sodium chloride in the initial intravenous fluid replacement as ordered, usually 0.45% NaCl.
	  D. Evaluate results of electrolyte studies, and notify the physician of any significant and unexpected changes.
	  E. Sodium bicarbonate is not appropriate for treatment of HOC. The patient is not acidotic or ketotic.[8]

NURSING DIAGNOSIS

3. *Altered thought processes related to hyperosmolality (knowing pattern)*

Patient Outcome	Nursing Orders

The patient will be alert and oriented before discharge.	1. Assess and treat the patient's altered level of consciousness.
	  A. Evaluate the patient's neurologic status.
	  B. Determine the patient's Glasgow Coma Scale score as frequently as needed.
	  C. Determine the patient's vital signs as needed.
	  D. Monitor osmolality levels, and evaluate for the expected level of consciousness.
	  E. Orient the patient to time, place, and person.
	  F. Provide emotional support to the patient and family during periods of confusion.

NURSING DIAGNOSIS

4. *Altered metabolic processes (hyperglycemia) related to decreased use of glucose (exchanging pattern)*

Patient Outcome	Nursing Orders

The patient will regain a normal blood glucose level, at least under 200 mg/dl.	1. Evaluate the patient's blood glucose level.
	  A. Remember that the person with HOC is sensitive to insulin.
	  B. Give the patient regular insulin as ordered (10 U to 25 U intravenously, subcutaneously, or intramuscularly).
	    (1) For the intravenous push route, give insulin over 1 minute.

(continued)

NURSING CARE PLAN SUMMARY *Patient With Hyperosmolar Coma* Continued

Patient Outcome	Nursing Orders
	(2) With an intravenous infusion pump do the following:
	a. Check the dose carefully. Usually 5 U to 10 U/hour is given, or 0.1 U/kg/hour.
	b. Maintain a sterile technique.
	c. Check the pump periodically to make sure the proper dose is being delivered.
	(3) Be aware that as much as 20% of the insulin may be bound to the tubing and bottle or bag. More binding occurs when lower doses of insulin are used. In time, the equipment can become saturated with insulin. Therefore, changing the administration set decreases the insulin dose, and keeping the same set can increase the amount of insulin the patient receives. As much as 44% to 47% of the insulin may be bound.[19]
	C. Evaluate the patient's blood glucose levels at least every hour. Blood testing is the standard of care today. A well-equipped critical care unit should have a bedside glucose meter to check stat glucose levels. Bedside blood glucose monitoring requires only a fingerstick, not a venous sample.[1]
	D. Notify the physician when blood glucose levels are down to 250 mg to 300 mg/dl.
	E. Observe the patient and assess for hypoglycemia.
	(1) Know the following signs of hypoglycemia:
	a. Excitability
	b. Perspiration
	c. Tremors
	d. Increased heart rate
	e. Dilated pupils
	f. Headache
	g. Seizures
	h. Blood pressure that is normal initially and then decreases
	(2) Know that sympathetic signs may be diminished or absent in the long-term diabetic (*e.g.,* one who has had diabetes for 20 years).
	(3) Add a 5% glucose solution intravenously when the patient's blood glucose level reaches 250 mg/dl.
	(4) Determine the patient's blood glucose levels if hypoglycemia is suspected.
	(5) Treat hypoglycemia with a 50% dextrose-in-water solution.
	F. Use urine to evaluate glucose status *only* if blood glucose measures are unavailable.

NURSING DIAGNOSIS

5. *Knowledge deficit about HOC, dehydration, and prevention related to acute onset of illness (knowing pattern)*

Patient Outcome	Nursing Orders
The patient will verbalize an understanding of HOC, the need to avoid dehydration states, and strategies for prevention of future episodes of HOC.	1. Assess baseline knowledge of patient and family and initiate teaching related to the following:
	A. Teach the causes of HOC, dehydration, and hyperglycemia.
	B. Teach the signs and symptoms of hyperglycemia.
	C. Teach strategies to prevent future episodes of HOC (repeat episodes of HOC are common).[18]
	D. Evaluate the patient's self-care abilities and available support systems. Remember that most patients are likely to be elderly.
	E. Refer the patient to community resources as needed.

(continued)

NURSING CARE PLAN SUMMARY   *Patient With Hyperosmolar Coma*   *Continued*

NURSING DIAGNOSIS

6. *High risk for complications of HOC related to other body systems and age (exchanging pattern)*

Patient Outcome	*Nursing Orders*
The patient will not develop complications of HOC related to the respiratory, urinary, gastrointestinal, immune, or psychosocial systems.	1. See Chapter 37, Nursing Diagnosis 5, page 701. (Note that Kussmaul's respirations generally are not present in patients with HOC.)

IMPLEMENTATION AND EVALUATION

It is obvious from the high mortality in HOC that prompt diagnosis and treatment are essential. The chief components of therapy are fluid replacement, insulin therapy, electrolyte replacement, and management of other symptoms as needed. Because the treatment of HOC closely resembles that of DKA, the reader will probably find it helpful to read the discussion of treatment in Chapter 37. The flow sheet in that chapter can be adapted to the patient with HOC and can be used as a record of treatment. Nursing and medical interventions are lifesaving.

Fluid Replacement

Rehydration is the main component of therapy.[18] Because patients with HOC are severely dehydrated, prompt initiation of rehydration therapy is of primary importance. There are wide variations of opinion regarding the best combinations of water and electrolytes for replacement. Usually more fluid replacement is needed for HOC than for DKA. Rapid administration of large volumes of fluid is begun—6 L in the first 12 hours and another 5 L over the next 24 hours.[18] The first 2 L or 3 L are given rapidly, even to elderly individuals with uncertain cardiac function.[17]

If the patient shows signs of hypovolemic shock or vascular collapse, a plasma expander (*e.g.*, dextran) is used initially. Isotonic normal saline solution may be used at the same time. Albumin or whole blood is occasionally ordered. After the blood pressure is stabilized, large volumes of hypotonic electrolyte solutions are administered. Most authorities prefer to use 0.45% normal saline solution, but some use full-strength saline solution. Dextrose solutions are not used early in the treatment.[14,16,17]

Because most patients with HOC are elderly, their cardiovascular and renal tolerance of high-volume fluid replacement must be assessed. Monitoring the patient's blood pressure and urinary output will help in managing rehydration.

A complication of fluid therapy is a secondary or latent shock state of dehydration. As the hyperosmolar state improves and the blood glucose level falls rapidly, the interstitial and cellular spaces begin to pull in water, which leads to an intravascular hypotension.

Fluids are given by mouth when the patient is able to tolerate them and when bowel sounds are present.

Insulin Therapy

Chapter 37 discusses the methods of administering insulin and gives other information about insulin that is relevant to the treatment of HOC.

The amount of insulin needed in HOC is less than that needed in DKA (because acidemia and ketonemia are not present in HOC), but insulin is nevertheless essential. The blood glucose level will fall somewhat with rehydration alone, partly because hypertonicity inhibits the release of insulin from the pancreas. The goal of insulin therapy is a gradual decrease in hyperglycemia and hyperosmolality.

Patients with HOC have been shown to be more sensitive to insulin than are patients with DKA.[16] Thus, patients with HOC may respond to much smaller doses than would be expected. A total of 100 U to 150 U may suffice. An initial dose of 10 U of regular insulin is usual.[14,18] Further doses of regular insulin are based on continued blood glucose readings.

Low-dose treatment appears to be as effective as high-dose treatment in HOC. It decreases the likelihood of hypoglycemia and may be simpler to manage.[7,10,11] Thus, after the initial dose, additional insulin is typically given in low doses with an infusion of 0.1 U/kg/hour until the glucose level is down to 250 mg/dl.[18] This can average about 5 U to 10 U/hour.[17]

The biologic half-life of regular insulin is about 10 minutes. When insulin is given intravenously, the response is immediate. If a bolus is given, in 10 minutes only one half the total insulin remains. When insulin is given subcutaneously, it is absorbed more slowly and its half-life is about 4 hours. Intramuscular injections are absorbed faster than are subcutaneous injections, but obviously intramuscular injections are "slower" than are intravenous injections. The half-life of insulin given intramuscularly is about 2 hours.[5] Insulin is degraded by the liver and kidneys.[9]

After the acute phase of HOC, the patient usually does not require insulin to treat the diabetes; it can be controlled by diet. Some patients need oral hypoglycemics.[16,18]

It is imperative to avoid hypoglycemia. Careful monitoring of the serum glucose levels and observation of the patient are also essential. Intravenous glucose should be administered, and insulin should be stopped when the blood glucose level nears 250 mg/dl.[18]

Electrolyte Replacement

Sodium replacement is done with a normal saline infusion. Parenteral replacement of potassium is considered after hydration begins to shift potassium back into the cells, lowering the serum potassium level. Potassium chloride or potassium phosphate may be added to the intravenous solution. Knowing the serum potassium levels and using cardiac monitoring should help the physician to decide about potassium replacement. Profound potassium losses have been seen.[18]

Evaluation

Nursing and medical interventions for the patient with HOC can be evaluated by patient outcomes. The nursing orders may need to be altered as the patient's condition changes.

SUMMARY

Nonketotic hyperosmolar coma, a comatose condition usually seen in the type II diabetic, has a high mortality. It is similar to DKA with regard to the physiologic alterations, except for the acidosis seen in DKA. Some insulin reserve is present in the patient with HOC contributing to the prevention of lipolysis and thus ketosis. The main problems of HOC are severe dehydration, hyperosmolality from glucose and sodium, and electrolyte alteration. Treatment is focused on correcting these problems and, thus, restoring equilibrium.

DIRECTIONS FOR FUTURE RESEARCH

Nurses need to investigate the effects of specific nursing interventions in caring for the patient with HOC. Some possible research questions follow:

1. What is the effectiveness of the "buddy system" among elderly patients to prevent self-care deficits such as dehydration?
2. How can nurses correlate the level of consciousness with serum osmolality to improve assessment skills?
3. What physiologic cues to hyperglycemia might be recognized by an elderly person?
4. How reliable and accurate are nurse's skills in performing blood glucose monitoring techniques? How important is it to practice this skill? How often?

REFERENCES

1. American Diabetes Association. Bedside glucose monitoring in hospitals. *Diabetes Care* 13:1, 1990.
2. Arieff, A., and Carol, H. Cerebral edema and depression of sensorium in nonketotic hyperosmolar coma. *Diabetes* 23:525, 1974.
3. Arieff, A., and Flets, P. *Hyperosmolar Coma*. Kalamazoo, MI: Upjohn, 1974.
4. Bivins, B., Hyde, G., Sachatello, C., *et al.* Pathophysiology and management of hyperosmolar hyperglycemic nonketotic dehydration. *Surg. Gynecol. Obstet.* 154:543, 1982.
5. Boshell, B. *Diabetes Mellitus Case Studies*. New York: Medical Examination Publishing Co., 1976.
6. Carroll, P., and Matz, R. Uncontrolled diabetes mellitus in adults: Experience in treating diabetic ketoacidosis and hyperosmolar nonketotic coma with low-dose insulin and a uniform treatment regimen. *Diabetes Care* 6:579, 1983.
7. Davidson, J. *Clinical Diabetes Mellitus: A Problem Oriented Approach*. New York: Thieme, 1986.
8. Davidson, M. Insulin Therapy. In K. Sussman, B. Draznin, and W. James (eds.), *Clinical Guide to Diabetes Mellitus*. New York: Alan R. Liss, 1987.
9. Guyton, A. *Textbook of Medical Physiology* (7th ed.). Philadelphia: W. B. Saunders, 1986.
10. Kitabchi, A., Matteri, R., and Murphy, M. Optimal insulin delivery in diabetic ketoacidosis (DKA) and hyperglycemic nonketotic coma (HHNC). *Diabetes Care* 5(suppl. 1):78, 1982.
11. Matz, R. Coma in the Nonketotic Diabetic—Hyperosmolar Nonketotic Coma (HNKC) in the Diabetic. In M. Ellenberg and H. Rifkin (eds.), *Diabetes Mellitus: Theory and Practice*. New York: Medical Examination Publishing Co., 1983.
12. Podolsky, S. (ed.). *Clinical Diabetes: Modern Management*. New York: Appleton-Century-Crofts, 1980.
13. Podolsky, S. Management of diabetes in the surgical patient. *Med. Clin. North Am.* 66:1361, 1982.
14. Prockop, L. Hyperosmolar Hyperglycemic Nonketotic Diabetic Coma. In L. Rowland (ed.), *Merritt's Textbook of Neurology*. Philadelphia: Lea & Febiger, 1989.
15. Sommers, M. Nonketotic hyperosmolar coma. *Crit. Care Nurs.* 3: 58, 1983.
16. Sussman, K. Diabetic Ketoacidosis. In K. Sussman, B. Draznin, and W. James (eds.), *Clinical Guide to Diabetes Mellitus*. New York: Alan R. Liss, 1987.
17. Unger, R., and Foster, D. Diabetes Mellitus. In J. Wilson and D. Foster (eds.), *William's Textbook of Endocrinology* (7th ed.). Philadelphia: W. B. Saunders, 1985.
18. Vignati, L., Asmal, A., Black, W., *et al.* Coma in Diabetes. In A. Marble, L. Krall, R. Bradley, *et al.* (eds.), *Joslin's Diabetes Mellitus* (12th ed.). Philadelphia: Lea & Febiger, 1985.
19. Weber, S., Wood, W., and Jackson, E. Availability of insulin from parenteral nutrient solutions. *Am. J. Hosp. Pharm.* 34:353, 1977.

39

Hyperthyroidism and Thyroid Crisis

Christine A. Kessler   Cathie E. Guzzetta

AFFIRMATIONS

Affirmations are strong, positive statements that acknowledge that something is already so or could be so. Affirmations can help you change your perceptions and beliefs. If you believe an affirmation to be true, then your perceptions selectively reinforce it because you change your self-talk. Your mind is constantly engaged in active thought processing because of your constant self-dialogue. Self-talk even operates in your dreams while you sleep. What are you reinforcing moment by moment? If your thoughts are hopeful and optimistic, your body responds with confidence, energy, and hope. If, on the other hand, negative thoughts dominate, your body responds with tightness, uneasiness, and an increase in breathing, blood pressure, and heart rate, just to name a few changes. Affirmations are statements that you select to affirm your intention and choices. Affirmations can help you do the following:

- Increase clarity of goals that help you exercise your options.
- Assume more responsibility for your actions, thoughts, beliefs, and values.
- Identify what is true for you, and then the truth can manifest in helpful behaviors.
- Increase your empowerment.
- Envision a new way of being.
- Clarify goals and actions, and assist in self-evaluation.

Set aside time each day to use affirmations and reflect on aspects of your spiritual self. As you read the following phrases, allow your imagery process to evolve:

- I am a spiritual being whose life is full of value, meaning, and direction.
- I share my life with others to allow deeper understanding about my life, to solve old conflicts, and be with painful moments from a new perspective.
- I am in the present moment to be with my love, compassion, worry, fear, hope, faith, and grief.
- I operate from the perspective that life has meaning, direction, and value.
- I feel a part of life and living.
- I recognize that the different roles of my life are expressions of my true self.
- I feel, at some level, a connection with some power higher than myself and a connection with the universe.

LEARNING OBJECTIVES

After reading this chapter, the nurse should be able to do the following:

1. Describe the normal synthesis and secretion of thyroid hormone.
2. Describe the transport and metabolism of thyroid hormone.
3. Describe the hypothalamic-pituitary-thyroid control system.
4. Identify the clinical manifestations of hyperthyroidism.
5. Describe the basic thyroid function tests used in the diagnosis of hyperthyroidism.
6. Contrast the major medical and surgical treatments of hyperthyroidism.
7. List the physiologic and psychologic stressors that may precipitate or accompany thyroid crisis.
8. List the modalities of treatment for thyroid crisis.
9. Describe priority nursing diagnoses, patient outcomes,

nursing orders, implementation, and evaluation of a patient in thyroid crisis.

CASE STUDY

Mr. S.R., a 32-year-old grocery store stockclerk, was taken to the hospital by his mother because of progressive confusion, an elevated temperature, and vomiting and diarrhea for 2 days. He was examined by the emergency room physician and nurse. His temperature was 105.2°F rectally, his pulse was 180/minute and irregular, his respirations were 40/minute, and his blood pressure 100/40. Orthostatic hypotension was also considerable. The patient was agitated and disoriented to time, place, and person. He was immediately admitted to the intensive care unit.

Mr. R. had been well until age 28, when he was diagnosed as being hyperthyroid (with Graves' disease) and was given methimazole (Tapazole). Three months later, he underwent a subtotal thyroidectomy. Subsequently, his antithyroid medications were discontinued, and he did well.

Mr. R.'s mother said that her son had had a great deal of emotional trauma in the past 2 months; he was getting a divorce. He had a healthy 3-year-old daughter. Recently, he had moved back into his mother's house. Mr. R.'s mother had noticed a decrease in her son's weight, a dramatic swelling of his neck, and noticeable trembling of his fingers. He had refused to seek medical attention until he developed a severe sore throat. He consulted his family physician, who treated the sore throat with penicillin. His symptoms grew worse, and his mother sought additional medical help.

On examination, the patient was found to be diaphoretic, warm, and flushed, and he had poor tissue turgor. He was noted to have fine, silky hair. Proximal muscle weakness was observed in his upper and lower extremities. Upon examination, the eyes had a conjugate gaze, but the lids were retracted, producing a startled expression. The patient's tongue showed signs of dehydration, and white tonsillar patches and pharyngeal erythema were noted. The jugular neck veins were normal, and the trachea was midline. A large asymmetric goiter five times the normal size with a large right lobe was observed. A thyroidectomy scar was present. The patient had a thrill and an audible bruit over the entire gland. Crackles were heard in the left lung base. The patient had an irregularly irregular rhythm; the point of maximal impulse was at the fifth left intercostal space, midclavicular line. No third or fourth heart sounds, murmurs, or rubs were heard. Hyperactive bowel sounds were heard; the liver and spleen were not palpable. All pulses were equal and full. No cyanosis, clubbing, or edema was seen. The patient had a rhythmic finger tremor.

Admission diagnostic studies were ordered and done. A throat culture was also done. Blood gas samples were drawn while Mr. R. received oxygen through a face mask (6 L/minute). The results of the blood gas studies, which were corrected for the increase in temperature, were as follows: PaO_2, 121 mm Hg; oxygen saturation, 98.4%; pH, 7.45; $PaCO_2$, 32 mm Hg; plasma HCO_3^-, 21 mEq/L; base deficit, -1.

The chest film showed mild cardiomegaly without heart failure. Evidence of right middle lobe pneumonia was also noted. The electrocardiogram showed a supraventricular tachycardia with frequent premature atrial contractions, premature junctional contractions with occasional aberration (lead 2), and left ventricular hypertrophy.

The presumptive diagnosis of acute thyroid crisis was made, and appropriate therapy was instituted. Mr. R. was given crushed propylthiouracil (PTU) (200 mg through a nasogastric tube every 4 hours) to help reduce the overproduction of thyroid hormone. One hour later, he was given intravenous sodium iodide (1 g every 8 hours) to prevent the release of thyroid hormone from the thyroid gland. He was initially given propranolol (Inderal) (2 mg intravenously) to block sympathetic nervous system overactivity. Four liters of 5% dextrose and 0.45 normal saline with potassium chloride and multivitamins were given over 24 hours, followed by 3 L a day to combat the patient's dehydration, hypokalemia, and vitamin deficiency. Because of the

acute crisis and the probable reduction in adrenocortical reserve, Mr. R. was given intravenous hydrocortisone (50 mg every 6 hours). Intravenous potassium penicillin G (2.5 million units every 6 hours) was given to combat the infection. A hypothermia blanket was used to suppress the temperature. Continuous cardiac monitoring was begun.

Clinical Presentation of Case Study

Second Day

By the end of the second day after his admission, Mr. R. was combative and restless, although less confused and disoriented. The results of the admission laboratory studies were hemoglobin, 15.2 g; hematocrit, 36%; white blood count, 14,000/mm³; sodium, 133 mEq/L; potassium, 4.7 mEq/L; calcium, 13.0 mg/100 ml; chloride, 98 mEq/L; alkaline phosphatase, 200; serum glutamic pyruvate transaminase, 50; total bilirubin, 2 mg/100 ml; fasting glucose, 97 mg/100 ml; blood urea nitrogen, 40 mg/100 ml; creatinine, 2.1 mg/100 ml. The thyroid function test results were abnormal. The throat culture showed beta-hemolytic streptococci. The resting pulse was 160, respirations were 30, blood pressure was 110/60, and temperature was 102°F rectally. The propranolol dosage was changed to 40 mg orally every 6 hours.

Third Day

The third day after Mr. R.'s admission, he was oriented to time, place, and person. He remained anxious, nervous, and combative, and he was abusive toward those caring for him. His resting pulse had decreased to 110 without ectopy, his respirations to 24, and his rectal temperature to 100°F. His blood pressure rose to 126/78.

The nursing staff became increasingly anxious about Mr. R.'s physical and verbal abuse. The primary care nurse held a short conference with the healthcare team. It was decided that the primary care nurse would discuss Mr. R.'s behavior with him and that together they would plan his care.

Fourth Day

During the fourth day, Mr. R. was less anxious and more cooperative. One outcome of the planning conference was that his 3-year-old daughter was allowed to visit. Mr. R.'s spirits seemed to improve. His nasogastric tube was removed, and he was put on a high-protein, 4000-calorie diet with supplemental feedings. His hydrocortisone therapy was discontinued, and he was given oral prednisone (20 mg/day). Oxygen therapy was discontinued. Mr. R. was transferred to a "step-down" unit.

Fifth Day

On the fifth day after his admission, Mr. R.'s oral temperature was 98°F, his resting pulse was 100, his respirations were 18, his blood pressure was 128/76. The prednisone dosage was reduced to 10 mg/day. He began to ask questions about his illness and treatment. Mr. R.'s primary care nurse answered his questions honestly and in terms Mr. R. easily understood. Together, Mr. R. and his nurse discussed his teaching care plan.

Seventh Day

During the seventh day, Mr. R. was transferred to a general medical floor. His medications were penicillin, propranolol, PTU, and Lugol's solution. The Lugol's solution was discontinued the next day. His prednisone and intravenous infusion were discontinued.

On Mr. R.'s transfer to the general medical floor, the primary physician told Mr. R. and his mother about the possible choices for therapeutic thyroid control. He did not recommend further thyroid surgery because of the high incidence of technical problems associated with reoperation. He recommended that Mr. R. be treated with radioactive iodine (^{131}I). The nurse-physician team began discharge teaching that covered principles of home care and information about emotional stress, infection, and future ^{131}I therapy.

Discharge

The nurse explained to Mr. R. the indications for and dosage and side-effects of his discharge medications (PTU and propranolol). He was discharged without further complications.

Readmission

Three months later, Mr. R. was readmitted to the hospital in a euthyroid state for ^{131}I therapy. An appropriate dose of ^{131}I was given 7 days after PTU was discontinued. Seven days after Mr. R. had received ^{131}I therapy, he was again given PTU, which he was to take for 2 to 3 months. At the time of his discharge, Mr. R. had normal thyroid function tests and no symptoms of acute thyrotoxicosis. He was to remain under close medical supervision and monitoring for evidence of treatment-induced hypothyroidism.

REFLECTIONS

Physicians and nurses have long observed that periods of psychologic stress often precede the onset or exacerbation of underlying endocrine disease. Thyroid disease is no exception. However, it is well known that hyperthyroidism may itself cause significant psychologic symptoms. Agitation, anxiety, paranoia, and depression are observed frequently during the course of illness. Indeed, absence of behavioral aberrations points away from a diagnosis of thyroid crisis.

Is the emotional instability associated with hyperthyroidism a cause or an effect? Does emotional stress worsen hyperthyroidism, or does the hyperthyroid state itself result in psychologic disturbances? In either case, what physiologic mechanisms are involved? Although answers to these questions remain elusive, it is postulated currently that these behavioral manifestations probably relate to underlying excesses in adrenergic activity.

Mr. R.'s case history clearly illustrates the body-mind-spirit continuum. One might speculate about whether Mr. R.'s hyperthyroid state affected his marriage or whether the emotional impact of his pending divorce affected his hyperthyroid state. In any case, stress certainly may have altered his immune function, precipitating his bout of pneumonia. Pneumonia is one of many known physiologic triggers for thyroid crisis in the hyperthyroid patient.

Depending on the severity of the disease and on their personality, hyperthyroid patients are often hyperactive, tense, and restless. They tend to be extremely sensitive, crying at a slight provocation. They may be depressed and have feelings of impending disaster. Their irritation and agitation may precipitate family quarrels and conflicts. Their speech may be rapid, excitable, and high-pitched. They may complain that they have lost control of their thoughts or that their ideas run together in a frightening way. Their accelerated mental activity may lead to fears of insanity, disorientation, or delusions. They may have visual and auditory hallucinations.

It is well known that physiologic stressors (*e.g.,* infection [especially pulmonary infections], trauma, surgery, or prolonged exposure to cold) can increase the rate of thyroid stimulating hormone (TSH) secretion and can precipitate acute thyrotoxicosis in a patient with underlying hyperthyroidism. Acute hyperthyroidism may also be precipitated by vascular accidents, diabetic ketoacidosis, adrenocortical insufficiency, pulmonary embolism, radiographic contrast studies, postirradiation thyroiditis, premature withdrawal of antithyroid drugs, ether anesthesia, toxemia in pregnancy and childbirth, and too vigorous palpation of the thyroid gland in the uncontrolled thyrotoxic patient.[2,3,16,22,25,44,53] Also, it is postulated that emotional stressors may precipitate or trigger the disease. Emotional shock during combat, prolonged worry, divorce, and loss of esteem, a loved one, or a job often occur before hyperthyroidism develops.

The preceding discussion of cause and effect leads to a discussion of the following popular assumptions about disease:

- A disease is primarily either functional or organic in origin (*i.e.,* either the mind or the body is at fault).
- A disease is a process that affects primarily either the mind or the body.
- Therapy should, therefore, be directed toward the mind (should be psychotherapeutic) or toward the body (should be traditionally medical or surgical), depending on whether mind or body is primarily at fault in the particular disease.

These assumptions are so ingrained in people's thinking that they often escape attention. They operate unconsciously, but they determine in major ways people's attitudes toward patients and illness.

The concerns of critical care nurses must, however, transcend the traditional assumptions of physiology, of how things happen. They must begin to question the basic assumptions about disease. Mainly, they must strive to see beyond the "either/or" of the assumptions. Disease is not a state of malfunction of *either* the mind *or* the body. Critical care nurses must try to discover the psychobiologic unity that operates in every person in every disease process.

ANATOMY OF THE THYROID GLAND

The thyroid gland, which has an average weight of 20 g, is a relatively vascular organ. The organ is not unique to the mammalian species, having been found in starfish and earthworms.[17,26] It is located below the larynx anteriorly and on either side of the trachea (Fig. 39-1). It comprises two lobes joined by an isthmus. The thyroid gland is made up of round follicles whose walls are composed of cuboidal epithelium. Their lumina are filled with a colloid that contains *thyroglobulin*, a protein specific to the thyroid. The four parathyroid glands are located on the posterior surface of the lateral lobes of the thyroid gland. The recurrent laryngeal nerves lie between the trachea and esophagus, just medial to the lateral lobes.

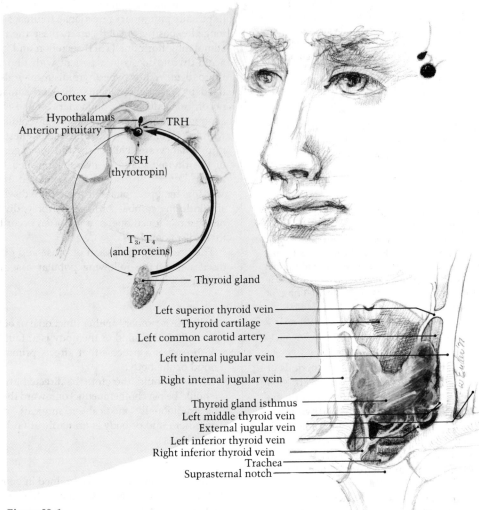

Figure 39–1
The thyroid gland and the hypothalamus-pituitary-thyroid control system.

SYNTHESIS AND SECRETION OF THYROID HORMONE

The main function of the thyroid gland is to secrete the thyroid hormones *triiodothyronine* (T_3) and *thyroxine* (T_4) into the circulatory system as a means of stimulating the metabolic processes of virtually all body cells. In addition, T_3 and T_4 are synergistic with many hormones, among them growth hormone, to promote normal growth and maturation of the person, especially of the skeletal and central nervous systems.

The quantitative and qualitative synthesis of thyroid hormones depends on the entry of iodine into the thyroid. *Iodine* enters the thyroid from the blood stream in an inorganic form that is derived primarily from iodine ingested from medications, water, and food. The average daily requirement of iodine is 100 μg to 200 μg.[18] This amount is needed to replace the iodine lost in the urine. The principal dietary sources of iodine are bread, iodized salt, seafood, milk, and eggs. Because iodine is deficient in the soil of inland regions (*e.g.,* the Great Lakes region) the dairy products and eggs produced in those areas contain less iodine than do those in coastal regions.[18,23] Dietary iodine is converted rapidly to iodide in the stomach and upper small bowel. Iodide is then actively transported from the blood into the thyroid gland, where it is oxidized to elemental iodine in the follicular cells.

Iodide is removed from the blood primarily by the thyroid gland and the kidneys, which compete for plasma iodide. Because renal clearance depends largely on glomerular filtration and is not affected by plasma hormones or iodide concentrations, the kidneys are generally a passive competitor. Changes in the rate of iodide entry into the thyroid gland relative to the rate of urinary excretion are therefore controlled primarily by the thyroid gland.

TRANSPORT AND METABOLISM OF THYROID HORMONE

The formation of thyroid hormone is described in Figure 39–2. Approximately 90% of the active thyroid hormone entering the circulatory system is in the form of T_4; the remainder is in the form of T_3.[23] When T_3 and T_4 enter the blood, they are almost entirely bound by plasma proteins (*i.e.,* mainly by *thyroxin-binding globulin* [TBG] and in small amounts by prealbumin and albumin).

Normally, less than 0.1% of the thyroid hormone is free or unbound in the plasma.[23] Only the unbound hormone is

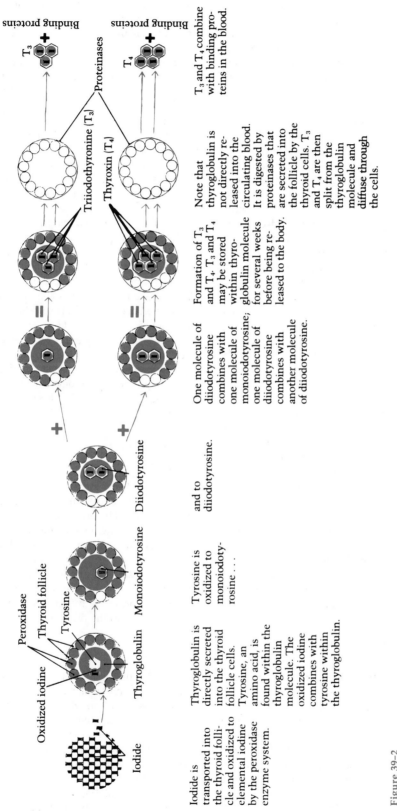

Figure 39-2
Formation of thyroid hormone.

physiologically active and available to the tissues. The metabolic state of the patient, therefore, correlates more precisely with the concentration of free hormone than with the total concentration of hormone in the plasma (bound hormone plus unbound hormone).

The ability of TBG to combine with T_4 is much greater than its ability to combine with T_3.[23] Because T_3 is less firmly bound to plasma proteins, it enters cells more rapidly. Moreover, much of the remaining free T_4 is converted to T_3 in the liver and peripheral tissues. It is therefore believed that T_3 may be the most active thyroid hormone.[23]

Essentially all the metabolic activities of the tissues are increased under the influence of thyroid hormones. The overall metabolism of cells is accelerated. It is now known that thyroid hormones have an additive effect on adrenergic (catecholamine) activity. The exact nature of this synergistic relationship, however, is not understood. It has been reported that hyperthyroid patients have more beta-adrenergic receptor-binding sites in cardiac muscle than do euthyroid patients, which could account for the augmented adrenergic myocardial response observed in the setting of normal serum norepinephrine and epinephrine levels. It has also been suggested that, because thyroid hormones function similarly to catecholamines, they may act as pseudocatecholamines, producing the adrenergic hyperactivity and metabolic acceleration seen in thyrotoxicosis and thyroid crisis.[35]

The mitochondria of most cells increase in size, and large numbers of intracellular enzymes are stimulated by thyroid hormones. As a result, the basal metabolic rate is increased, and the rate of use of foods for energy is increased. Carbohydrate and fat metabolism is increased. Protein synthesis and protein catabolism are increased. The growth rate is increased, and mental activities are excited. Thyroid hormones also increase oxygen requirements and heat production.

An insufficiency in thyroid hormone production in early life can greatly stunt growth and mental development (a condition known as *cretinism*). In adult years, hypothyroidism will cause metabolic processes to slow and impair thermoregulation (cold intolerance).

Another hormone secreted by the thyroid gland is calcitonin. Calcitonin is produced by parafollicular cells and is released in response to high serum calcium levels. It works to reduce circulating calcium levels by inhibiting calcium resorption from bones and reabsorption by the kidneys. Its effects in humans are relatively weak and pose few pathologic consequences.[55]

CONTROL OF THYROID HORMONE

The synthesis and release of T_3 and T_4 are controlled by the anterior pituitary hormone TSH (also known as thyrotropin). The main functions of TSH are to increase the size and secretory activity of the thyroid gland, increase the rate of iodine trapping into the thyroid gland, increase the number of thyroid cells, and increase the proteolysis of the thyroglobulin in the follicles, resulting in the release of T_3 and T_4 into the blood.

Thyroid-stimulating hormone, like many other hormones, increases the quantity of cyclic 3',5'-adenosine monophosphate (cyclic AMP) in the thyroid cell.[20] *Cyclic AMP* is an intracellular hormonal mediator. The hormone, in this case, TSH, combines with a receptor specific for the particular type of stimulating hormone at the membrane of the target cell (the thyroid cell). Once combined with the receptor, the hormone activates the enzyme adenyl cyclase, which is found within the membrane. This enzyme catalyzes the chemical reaction, which results in the generation of cyclic AMP. Cyclic AMP is responsible for many cellular functions, such as altering the permeability of the cell membrane and initiating the synthesis of specific intracellular chemicals. The type of effect that occurs as a result of cyclic AMP depends on the character of the specific cell. An increase of cyclic AMP within a thyroid cell, for example, will increase thyroid hormone formation. A similar increase in the beta cells of the islets of Langerhans will increase insulin secretion.

Actual release of TSH from the anterior pituitary is under hypothalamic supervision. A negative-feedback mechanism, formed by the hypothalamus-pituitary-thyroid control system, exerts ultimate control over the rate of thyroid hormone secretion. Circulating levels of T_4 and T_3 are noted within the hypothalamus. Decreased levels of thyroid hormones prompt the hypothalamus to release thyrotropin-releasing hormone (TRH). Thyrotropin-releasing hormone circulates to the anterior pituitary gland through hypothalamic-hypophyseal portal vessels, where it stimulates the production and release of TSH. Consequently, TSH stimulates the thyroid production and release of T_3 and T_4. As plasma levels of T_3 and T_4 increase, TRH release by the hypothalamus is reduced, along with a subsequent decrease in TSH secretion. Stimulation of the thyroid gland is thus reduced (see Fig. 39–1).[26,55]

Another potent trigger for TRH release is cold. To maintain body temperature, thyroid hormones are secreted to increase the metabolic processes responsible for generating heat. Both physiologic and psychologic stressors can increase the rate of TRH release, although the precise mechanism for this is not understood.

HYPERTHYROIDISM (GRAVES' DISEASE)

Hyperthyroidism (thyrotoxicosis) represents the physiologic response of the body to an excessive functional activity of the thyroid gland. Hyperthyroidism has a number of etiologies (Table 39–1).[7] The most common form, *Graves' disease* (also known as Parry's disease and Basedow's disease), is characterized by a diffuse enlargement of the thyroid gland (goiter).

Graves' disease occurs seven to nine times more frequently in women than in men, often in people in their thirties and forties[23,45] and rarely in children. There is a distinct familial predisposition to the disease.

Etiology

The exact cause of Graves' disease is not known.[18] It is likely that there is no one cause of the entire syndrome. Recently, Graves' disease is thought to be associated with thyroid-stimulating immunoglobulins. Such thyroid-stimulating antibodies have been detected in the majority of patients with Graves' disease. One of the thyroid-stimulating immunoglobulins, *long-acting thyroid stimulator* (LATS), can be detected in about 60% to 80% of patients.[18,30] Long-acting thyroid stimulator is capable of stimulating the release of thyroid hormone and increasing the activity of cyclic AMP. Long-acting thyroid stimulator has been established as one immunoglobulin of the IgG class synthesized by the lymphocytes and is believed to be an antibody to some component of human thyroid tissue.

Table 39–1
Causes of Hyperthyroidism in Order of Frequency

Graves' disease
Toxic multinodular goiter
Toxic uninodular goiter
Thyroiditis (inflammatory or neoplastic)
Drug-induced
    Excessive pharmacologic thyroid hormone intake
    Excessive iodine intake, with underlying multinodular goiter, thyroid adenoma (known as
        Jodbasedow effect)
Tumors with circulating thyroid stimulators: hydatidiform mole, choriocarcinoma, embryonal
        carcinoma of the testis. (These secrete human chorionic gonadotropin, which has
        TSH-like effects.)
TSH-secreting pituitary tumor
Thyroid carcinoma
Stuma ovarii (teratomas of the ovary), which secrete ectopic thyroid hormone

Graves' disease may, therefore, be caused by an autoimmune phenomenon. Serum LATS titers, however, do not correlate well with the presence or absence or the severity of hyperthyroidism, so it is unlikely that LATS alone plays a direct causative role.[18]

Pathophysiology

Graves' disease is characterized by the triad of diffuse toxic goiter, infiltrative ophthalmopathy, and pretibial dermopathy. The thyroid gland enlarges, becoming more vascular and developing a rubbery consistency. This hyperplasia of thyroid gland parenchymal cells is due to incessant ectopic stimulation.

The thyrotoxicosis of Graves' disease is caused by an excessive rate of thyroid hormone synthesis and release. The disease is also associated with lymphatic hyperplasia and infiltration and occasionally with enlargement of the spleen and thymus. Also, fatty infiltration and fibrosis of the liver, loss of body tissue, decalcification of the skeleton, and degeneration of the skeletal muscles may be found.

The ophthalmopathic changes in Graves' disease are caused by inflammation and infiltration of the orbital contents with lymphocytes and mast and plasma cells. The orbital muscles are generally involved, causing lid retraction, protrusion of the globe (the classic "staring" expression), lid lag, or loss of upward or lateral gaze.[35]

THYROID CRISIS

Thyroid crisis (or thyroid storm) is a syndrome characterized by exaggerated manifestations of hyperthyroidism, including fever and cardiovascular, gastrointestinal, metabolic, and central nervous system problems. Without treatment, death is a certainty within 72 hours. The difference between severe hyperthyroidism and thyroid crisis is not clear. McArthur[31] says that thyroid crisis is a state in which the patient can no longer tolerate the strain imposed by thyrotoxicosis and finally reaches a point where hyperthyroidism is "life-endangering." To date, there are no universally accepted criteria to define thyroid crisis.[46,50] The difference is of little consequence, because treatment for both is the same.

Before 1930, 70% of all deaths from thyrotoxicosis were due to thyroid crisis after thyroidectomy.[53] Because the hyperthyroid patient is now given iodide, antithyroid, and beta-adrenergic receptor-blocking drugs before surgery, thyroid crisis after thyroidectomy is rare (see Nursing Diagnosis 1).[55]

Although "surgical storm" after thyroidectomy is no longer a problem, "medical storm" is common. It occurs in patients with untreated or inadequately treated disease and usually manifests within 2 months to 4 years after diagnosis of hyperthyroidism.[18,30] It is not uncommon for thyroid crisis to develop suddenly in a patient who has never been diagnosed as hyperthyroid.

Thyroid crisis is nearly always precipitated by or associated with psychologic stressors or some concurrent pathophysiologic process, or it may be precipitated by a physiologic stressor (see Reflections). The amount of TBG may also be reduced after surgery or stress, resulting in an increase in both the proportion and the absolute concentration of free T_3 and T_4 in the plasma.

NURSING PROCESS

ASSESSMENT

A complete biopsychosocial assessment is completed on all patients suspected of thyrotoxicosis or thyroid crisis. The patient's associated or precipitating disease or problems should be identified. It is important to obtain information about the patient's thyroid history and the type and amount of associated medications. Physiologic and psychologic stressors that may have precipitated the event should be identified (see Reflections). The clinical picture of Graves' disease varies with the person, the severity of the disease, the age of the patient, and the presence of underlying disease.

Skin and Appendages

The skin is velvety, moist, and warm as a result of cutaneous vasodilatation. There is excessive sweating and heat intolerance. The skin changes are usually seen in the legs or feet. They are commonly called *nonpitting myxedema, pretibial myxedema,* or *pretibial dermopathy.* The affected area is usually raised and thickened with an orange-peel appearance and it may be pruritic and nodular (Fig. 39–3). Excessive melanin pigmentation is frequent as a result of a hypersecretion of ACTH secondary to the accelerated metabolism of cortisol. The nails are soft and friable, and the middle edge of the nail may detach from its base (oncyholysis). Clubbing of the fingers and toes is occasionally noted. The hair is fine, silky, and easily

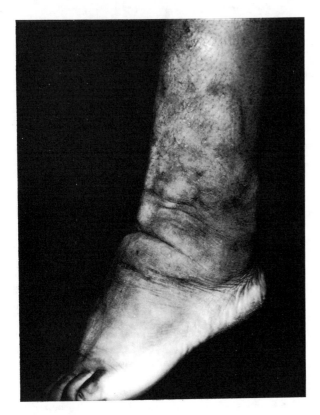

Figure 39–3
Pretibial myxedema.

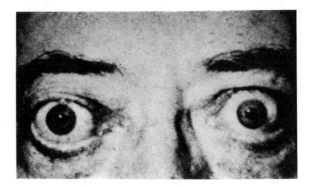

Figure 39–4
Exophthalmos.

broken; often it does not hold a curl. There may be hair loss on the temporal scalp.[45]

Eyes

A stare or "frightened" facies is characteristic of Graves' disease. The person has wide eyes, with lid retraction revealing a white rim of sclera above the iris. In addition, there may be abnormal protrusion of the eyeballs (due to fatty deposits behind the globe), lid lag, infrequent blinking, and difficulty in gazing upward or laterally (Fig. 39–4).[45] Such patients have marked photophobia and will be observed to have a furrowed brow due to continual squinting to reduce the light in their eyes.[18] These signs are believed to be due to overstimulation of the sympathetic nervous system, muscle weakness, congestion, and edema.

Thyroid Gland

The thyroid gland is the only endocrine gland accessible to physical examination. It is evaluated by inspection, palpation, and auscultation. The gland is inspected for asymmetry and enlargement of one or both lobes. It is palpated from behind, from the front, and from beneath. The normal thyroid gland is barely palpable or not palpable by the examining fingers. A diffuse toxic goiter may be lobular and asymmetric. Auscultation of the thyroid gland is accomplished by lightly placing the diaphragm of the stethoscope over the thyroid. Normally, no sound is heard. In thyrotoxicosis, a bruit is often heard directly over the gland; it is caused by the increased

blood flow. In severe cases, a thrill may be felt over the upper lobes. A thrill or bruit is highly suggestive of hyperthyroidism.

Cardiovascular System

The hyperthyroidism of Graves' disease has a dramatic effect on the cardiovascular system. The hypermetabolism and the need to dissipate excess heat produce increased circulatory demands. There is an increase in stroke volume and heart rate associated with a decrease in peripheral vascular resistance and an increase in local blood flow to the tissues. Cardiac output may therefore be increased as much as two times normal. Clinically, resting tachycardias are generally observed. Palpitations, a frequent complaint, are caused by an increase in the force of contraction. Atrial fibrillation or other atrial dysrhythmias are common, especially in elderly patients. Systolic heart murmurs, a loud first-heart sound, and a widened pulse pressure due to a rise in the systolic pressure and a decrease in the diastolic pressure may be noted. Cardiac enlargement, mild edema, and high-output cardiac failure are occasionally present.[15]

Muscular Function

Because the rate of protein catabolism is greater than the rate of protein synthesis, there is a net degradation of tissue protein that results in a negative nitrogen balance, weight loss, muscle loss, and hypoalbuminemia. Thus, there is an increase in free amino acids and a decrease in the amount of tissue and muscle protein. The patient often demonstrates proximal muscle weakness, evidenced by difficulty arising from a sitting or squatting position.

Respiratory function can be affected by muscle loss, producing a decrease in vital capacity and dyspnea.[25] Furthermore, the increased use of oxygen and the formation of carbon dioxide can cause an increase in the rate of respirations. As respiratory function deteriorates in severe cases, hypoventilation, hypercapnia, and respiratory failure can occur.[25]

Central Nervous System

The nervous system is most often affected, producing accelerated mental activity (see Reflections). Patients are likely to become extremely nervous, hyperactive, anxious, or paranoid, and experience mood swings. They may be chronically tired and yet unable to sleep. An important sign of hyperthyroidism is a fine, rhythmic muscle tremor of the hands, tongue, or eyelids (when the eyelids are slightly closed).[35,45]

Gastrointestinal Tract

Although hyperthyroidism causes a great increase in appetite, patients typically lose weight. They are incapable of consuming sufficient calories to meet the increased metabolic demands. Gastrointestinal motility and food absorption are increased. Occasionally, anorexia, nausea, vomiting, diarrhea, and abdominal pain are experienced.

Thyrotoxicosis commonly alters liver function tests, raising levels of bilirubin, alkaline phosphatase, and transaminases. Accompanying congestive heart failure may be contributory to this. Conversely, serum cholesterol and triglyceride levels may be somewhat reduced owing to increased production and clearance of both. Hyperglycemia may be accentuated in the diabetic patient, and insulin requirements may be increased.[35,45,55]

Endocrine System

The half-life of cortisol is shortened by hyperthyroidism. Consequently, ACTH secretion is increased. Hyperthyroidism also increases the level of sex hormone-binding globulin, which lowers circulating levels of free estrogen. Amenorrhea and infertility may be a problem in some women. Although free testosterone levels increase in men, extragonadal conversion of androgens to estrogen is increased causing gynecomastia, decreased libido, and impotency in males.[26]

Skeletal System

Serum calcium levels may rise as a result of bone resorption, and large amounts of calcium and phosphorus may be lost in the urine and stool. Excessive losses may be associated with demineralization of the bone and pathologic fractures (especially in the elderly).[26]

THYROID CRISIS

The clinical picture of a patient in *thyroid crisis* is a result of an abrupt and life-threatening exacerbation of thyrotoxic manifestations and a significant increase in general cellular function. The compensatory mechanisms of peripheral vasodilatation and diaphoresis no longer are adequate to dissipate the excess heat production. As a result, fever, considered the sine qua non of thyroid crisis, usually ranges from 101°F to 105.8°F. Profuse sweating is frequent, with fluid loss up to 4 L in 24 hours not uncommon. Nausea, vomiting, and diarrhea may occur. Excessive thyroid hormone may produce hyperglycemia due to adrenergic precipitation of gluconeogenesis, glycogenolysis, and relative insulin resistance. Diarrhea or hyperdefecation may herald the onset of thyroid crisis. This, along with vomiting and diaphoresis, may precipitate hypokalemia and severe dehydration.[4,35,49] Hyponatremia may occur if the patient drinks large amounts of water because of thirst from sweating, vomiting, or diarrhea. Hypercalcemia may occur from demineralization of bone.

Reflexes are generally exaggerated in thyroid crisis. The increased central nervous system metabolism may cause severe agitation, restlessness, anxiety, and psychotic behavior, and

the patient's condition may progress to extreme weakness, disorientation, coma, and death.

Hypotension may be caused by extreme vasodilatation. Supraventricular tachycardias, with rates near or above 200 beats/minute, are present in nearly 100% of acutely thyrotoxic patients. Atrial fibrillation with a rapid ventricular response occurs in 30% of patients. Tachycardia is often accompanied by some degree of heart failure or pulmonary edema that is refractory to usual therapy (*e.g.*, digitalis). Occasionally, cardiac output may be increased to the point of high-output failure. A reduction of adrenocortical reserve may be observed.[18] The patient may complain of abdominal pain. The liver is frequently enlarged, and mild jaundice may be seen. The latter is a poor prognostic sign.

APATHETIC THYROTOXICOSIS

Apathetic thyrotoxicosis is an unusual form of hyperthyroidism that is misdiagnosed frequently. The patient is elderly, generally in the seventh decade or older, is lethargic, and exhibits slowed mentation and placid apathetic facies. These patients may develop thyroid crisis without the usual hypermetabolic manifestations. Fever is an uncommon presenting symptom and makes diagnosis difficult. The patient may quietly lapse into coma and die. Proximal muscle weakness and excessive weight loss are usual. However, the typical eye signs of exophthalmos, stare, and lid lag are absent; instead, blepharoptosis (drooping upper eyelid) is common. Many times, these patients are monosymptomatic. Their disease may be manifested solely by cardiovascular disturbances—most often rapid atrial fibrillation with heart failure. The pathogenesis of apathetic thyrotoxicosis is not fully understood, but it should always be considered in an elderly patient who presents with refractory atrial fibrillation and accompanying heart failure in whom no underlying cardiac pathology is known.[26,46]

THYROID TESTS

There are many tests of thyroid functioning and hormone homeostasis. No one test is completely reliable because of the exogenous and endogenous factors that can complicate the findings. The interpretation of each test is dependent on an understanding of the individual patient and the psychophysiologic mechanisms and clinical manifestations of each illness state.

Radioactive Iodine Uptake Test and Scan

The radioactive iodine uptake (RAIU) test is commonly used to assess thyroid functioning. Radioiodine (^{131}I or ^{123}I) mixes with endogenous iodide and indicates the percentage of iodide entering and leaving the thyroid. A trace of ^{131}I is given orally (usually 5 μc to 10 μc), and the amount of ^{131}I taken up by the thyroid is measured with a gamma counter placed over the gland. The RAIU varies inversely with the amount of endogenous iodide, and it can be correlated with the functional state of the thyroid. In the patients with hyperthyroidism, for example, both the peak uptake and the rate of uptake of ^{131}I are greater than in the euthyroid person. The uptake of ^{131}I is reduced in hypothyroidism or when a high level of inorganic iodide is present in the plasma as a result of a large intake of iodine, which is found in high amounts in some foods, cough syrups, lozenges, gargles, vitamins, drugs, and various radiographic contrast media.[55]

Serum T_4 Concentration Test

The serum T_4 concentration test is used to assess the hormonal concentration and binding in the blood. It is measured by the ability of T_4 to displace radiolabeled T_4 from a protein mixture containing TBG. The normal range for T_4 is 4 μg to 12 μg/100 ml. The value may also be expressed as "T_4 by displacement" (T_4D). Serum T_4 levels may be elevated by factors that increase the concentration of binding proteins without indicating hyperthyroidism. An increase in the concentration of binding proteins is noted in pregnancy, neonates, hepatitis, porphyria, and with oral contraceptive use. A depression of serum T_4 also may occur when the concentration of binding proteins is low (Table 39–2). A decrease in the concentration of binding proteins is seen in acromegaly, nephrosis, chronic liver disease, critical illness, iodine starvation, and with steroid use.[55]

Serum T_3 Concentration Test

Serum T_3 concentrations may be measured by radioimmunoassay; they are abbreviated T_3 (RIA). Serum T_3 is measured by its ability to displace labeled T_3 from anti-T_3 antibodies when compared with that of a known quantity of T_3. Normal values are 75 ng to 195 ng/100 ml.

T_3 Resin Uptake Test

The T_3 resin uptake (T_3RU) test is an indirect measurement of free T_3 that reflects the quantity of TBG in the blood stream and the amount of thyroid hormone attached to it. Generally, TBG is never fully saturated with thyroid hormone; a large percentage of binding sites remain free to combine with any additional hormone available. The greater the amount of thyroid hormone present in the blood, the fewer the number of sites available for binding with a radioactively labeled thyroid hormone test reagent. The T_3 resin uptake is measured by adding a known amount of T_3 labeled with ^{131}I (hence, the name of the test) to a certain volume of the patient's serum. The serum is then absorbed on a resin sponge. Any free TBG in the serum will bind with the radioactive T_3. When there is nearly complete binding of the proteins by endogenous thyroid hormones (as seen in the hyperthyroid person), there is little opportunity for the exogenous radioactive T_3 to bind with protein. The radiolabeled T_3 therefore remains unbound in the tested serum sample and is absorbed by the resin sponge. The result is a high level of T_3RU, indicating hyperthyroidism. Conversely, in the hypothyroid person, the T_3RU is low because the exogenous T_3 labeled with ^{131}I attaches to the large quantity of the patient's unbound serum TBG. Less labeled T_3 remains to be absorbed by the resin sponge because it is bound to the patient's own proteins. The T_3RU is also affected by factors that increase and decrease the concentration of binding proteins. The normal range for the T_3RU is 25% to 35%.[8,18]

Free T_4 Index

The T_3RU test just described is capable of measuring the proportion of free hormone in the blood. It does not, however, differentiate primary alterations in the hormone concentration from primary alterations in hormone binding.

Table 39–2
Differential Laboratory Findings in Conditions With Elevated Serum T_4 Levels

CONDITION	RAIU	T_4	T_3RIA	T_3RU	FT$_4$I	TSH RESPONSES TO TRH INJECTION
Hyperthyroidism*	↑	↑	↑	↑	↑	Absent
Increased binding proteins						
TBG excess	Normal	↑	↑	↓	Normal or slightly ↑	Normal
Dysalbuminemic hyperthyroxinemia	Normal	↑	Normal to slightly ↑	Normal	↑	Normal
Thyroxine therapy† (euthyroid patients)	↓	↑	Normal	↑	↑	Absent or blunted
Drug therapy						
Amiodarone	↓	↑	Normal	↑	↑	Normal
Propranolol	Normal	↑	Normal	↑	↑	Absent or blunted
Acute psychiatric illness or euthyroid sick syndrome‡	Normal	↑	Normal or ↓	↑	↑	Normal or slightly blunted
Anti-T_4 antibodies	Normal or ↓	↑	Normal§	Variable	Variable	Normal
Resistance to thyroid hormone‖						Normal or exaggerated

* Some hyperthyroid patients have normal T_4 concentrations with elevated T_3RIA—so-called T_3 toxicosis.

† Many patients taking L-thyroxine have normal T_4 concentrations. Hyperthyroid patients taking thyroxine have elevated T_3 RIA.

‡ Most acute-phase psychiatric patients and sick patients do not have elevated T_4 concentrations.

§ Assumes double antibody assay. If anti-T_3 antibodies are present as well, T_3 RIA is elevated.

‖ This includes rare patients with peripheral resistance to thyroid hormone who are clinically euthyroid or hypothyroid. Although hormone levels are elevated, the hormones are not active.

T_4: thyroxine concentrations; T_3RU: T_3 resin uptake; FT$_4$I: free thyroxine index ($T_4 \times T_3$ RU); RAIU: radioiodine (^{123}I) uptake of thyroid gland; TSH: thyroid-stimulating hormone or thyrotropin; TRH: thyrotropin-releasing hormone.

(Modified from Daniels, G. Thyroid function testing: An approach to ordering and interpreting tests. *Consultant* 26(1):83–111, 1986; with permission.)

In hyperthyroidism, the concentration of binding proteins does not increase proportionately with the elevated thyroid hormone concentration. The concentration of both total (bound and free) thyroid hormone and free thyroid hormone increases, but the increase in free thyroid hormone is relatively much greater than the increase in the total hormone concentration, so that the *proportion* of free hormone increases. When T_3RU is used to evaluate thyroid disorders, abnormal values are presumed to be the result of a primary alteration in the concentration of the hormone (*i.e.*, a high level of T_3RU is presumed to be the result of a primary increase in the concentration of thyroid hormone). It is known, however, that abnormal T_3RU values, similar to those obtained in primary thyroid disease, may also be produced when the TBG concentration is abnormal.[8,55]

To distinguish primary alterations in hormone binding from hormone concentration, the *absolute concentration of free thyroid hormone* is calculated. The absolute concentration of free hormone is the product of the proportion of free hormone and the total concentration of the hormone. For example, the value of T_3RU can be expressed as a ratio of the T_3RU value of the patient's serum to the value obtained from the control specimen (the T_3RU ratio). The product of the T_3RU ratio and the serum T_4 concentration yields the absolute concentration of free T_4 (free T_4 index [FT_4I] or T_4–T_3RU index). If the concentration of TBG is altered, the FT_4I index remains normal. Conversely, primary alterations in thyroid hormone concentration produce an abnormal FT_4I index. As a result, the FT_4I index provides an important means of determining whether a change in the total concentration of the hormone is due to a change in the production rate of thyroid hormone or a change in hormone binding, and it plays an important role in differentiating hypothyroidism and hyperthyroidism from euthyroid states.

The TRH Stimulation Test

The TRH stimulation test is used to assess thyroid function. After the intravenous administration of TRH, the serum TSH rises in 10 minutes, peaks in 15 to 30 minutes, and then falls.

The TSH response leads to a rise in T_3 90 to 150 minutes after the administration of TRH.[24] The test may be useful in assessing pituitary reserve, hypothyroidism, and thyrotoxicosis. In thyrotoxicosis, the TSH response is flat.[24] Normal TSH values are less than 3.5 $\mu U/ml$.[24]

Radioactive Iodine Suppression Test

The radioactive iodine (RAI) suppression test is another test of thyroid functioning. In the euthyroid person, RAIU is suppressed after the administration of exogenous thyroid hormones. The person receives T_3 or T_4 hormones orally and then is given ^{131}I. The RAIU by the thyroid gland is measured, and in all cases of hyperthyroidism, the decline in RAIU normally induced by the suppressive effects of the thyroid hormones does not occur. The test helps to differentiate patients with hyperthyroidism from those with "high normal" RAIU levels.[8]

Thyroid Scan

Thyroid imaging localizes sites of technetium-99m or RAI accumulation in the thyroid gland. The scan is used to determine the overall size of the thyroid. It is also used to define areas of increased function ("hot" areas) and areas of decreased function ("cold" areas). A nodule that is palpable and appears cold on the scan demonstrates a decreased uptake of the isotope and may be malignant. Conversely, a functioning nodule that is more active than the surrounding tissue and that appears hot on the scan is not likely to be malignant. Thyroid scans are primarily indicated for patients suspected of having thyroid cancer or those with thyroid nodules.

NURSING DIAGNOSES, PATIENT OUTCOMES, AND PLAN

The preceding material on anatomy, physiology, nursing assessment, and diagnostic tests guides the nurse in establishing nursing diagnoses, patient outcomes, and the plan for the patient with thyroid crisis.

NURSING CARE PLAN SUMMARY *Patient With Thyroid Crisis*

NURSING DIAGNOSIS

1. Altered cardiac output related to hypermetabolic responses that may result in low blood pressure, heart failure, and dysrhythmias (exchanging pattern)

Patient Outcome	Nursing Orders
1. The patient will respond therapeutically to medications that inhibit thyroid function and adrenergic activity. 　A. Heart rate will return to premorbid levels.	1. Assess the patient's cardiovascular status: heart rate and rhythm, quality of heart sounds (murmurs or gallop rhythms), and blood pressure. The degree of hypotension (if possible, ascertain orthostatic hypotension) and pulse pressure should be determined. Continued electrocardiographic monitoring is essential. 2. Assess rate, depth, regularity, and effort of respirations; auscultate the lungs for

(continued)

NURSING CARE PLAN SUMMARY   *Patient With Thyroid Crisis*   *Continued*

Patient Outcome	Nursing Orders

Patient Outcome

B. Dysrhythmias will be minimized or abolished.

C. Evidence of heart failure will abate.

D. Thyroid function tests will reach normal levels.

Nursing Orders

crackles and evidence of heart failure; monitor the results of blood gases; and note acral and circumoral color (for presence of cyanosis).

3. Assess the results of the thyroid function tests.

4. Administer antithyroid medications *immediately* after the physician has made the diagnosis and ordered the drugs (Table 39–3).

   A. Give 200 mg of PTU by mouth every 4 hours (or 900 mg to 1200 mg/day). Methimazole (Tapazole) may be used instead of PTU by giving an initial dose of 90 mg to 120 mg followed by 40 mg daily. If the patient is unable to swallow or to cooperate, the nurse should crush the medications and administer them through a nasogastric tube. Methimazole is capable of maintaining stability in solution form and may be administered rectally.

     Antithyroid drugs inhibit one or more stages of hormone synthesis. They block the synthesis of T_3 and T_4 by acting on the peroxidase complex. The production of thyroid hormones is then reduced, and the patient can be made euthyroid until the natural course of the disease carries it into remission. The response to these drugs may take days to weeks to occur.[5,37,42]

   B. Observe the patient for the following adverse reactions to antithyroid therapy: skin rashes, gastrointestinal symptoms, arthralgias, fever, and hepatitis. Agranulocytosis, a rare but serious complication, is usually preceded by a sore throat or some other localized or generalized infection. The condition will disappear when the drug is withdrawn. A low-grade fever or "physiologic" leukopenia is the principal side effect of both antithyroid medication and untreated thyrotoxicosis, but it is not generally an indication for discontinuing the medication.

   C. Thionamides should not be withdrawn abruptly because they can precipitate thyroid crisis.[6]

5. Administer medications that inhibit the release of thyroid hormone (see Table 39–3).

   A. In the clinical setting of thyroid crisis, iodide may be given in the form of sodium iodide (1 g intravenously every 8 to 12 hours) or Lugol's solution (30 drops of saturated solution of potassium iodide by mouth or nasogastric tube).

   B. Do not administer iodide therapy for at least 1 hour after the administration of antithyroid medications. Iodides given in large doses transiently inhibit the synthesis of thyroid hormone. They are also useful in reducing the vascularity and causing involution of the thyroid gland. More important, they effectively inhibit the release of thyroid hormone by retarding the proteolysis of thyroglobulin. The response to iodide is usually rapid and dramatic, frequently occurring within the first 24 hours of therapy (as opposed to antithyroid medication, which may not show evidence of clinical benefit for days or weeks). Because iodides increase the storage of thyroid hormone within the gland, they may unfortunately delay the therapeutic response of subsequently administered antithyroid hormones and cause an accumulation of iodide in the thyroid that might be used to synthesize additional thyroid hormone. As a result, iodide is best given after the administration of antithyroid hormones.[23,48] Iodides are useful primarily in preparing patients for subtotal thyroidectomy or for acute surgical emergencies. They are often used to treat patients with impending or actual thyroid crisis. Because its inhibitory effect on the thyroid gland is transient and unpredictable, long-term iodide therapy is not recommended.

   C. Observe the patient for any adverse reactions to iodide therapy (skin rash or skin lesions, salivary gland inflammation, conjunctivitis, rhinitis, and eosinophilia).

6. Suppress adrenergic overactivity.

   A. Identify the contraindications to beta-adrenergic receptor-blocking drugs, such as asthma or other bronchoconstrictive disorders, cardiac failure (except when cardiac insufficiency is caused by sinus tachycardias), sinus bradycardia, atrioventricular heart block, pregnancy (because of

(continued)

NURSING CARE PLAN SUMMARY   *Patient With Thyroid Crisis*   *Continued*

Patient Outcome	Nursing Orders

	propranolol's ability to increase uterine activity), and severe thyrocardiac disease.
	
	B. Administer propranolol in the following dosages to block beta-adrenergic activity:
	  (1) Oral dosage: 20 mg to 80 mg is given every 4 to 6 hours.
	  (2) Intravenous dosage: 2 mg to 10 mg is titrated slowly at a rate less than 1 mg/minute and repeated every 3 to 4 hours, as necessary.
	    Because catecholamines or pseudocatecholamines contribute to the symptoms of hyperthyroidism, adrenergic antagonists that block beta-adrenergic receptor sites are used in the treatment of hyperthyroidism and thyroid crisis. Propranolol (see Table 39-3) is used to control the manifestations of sympathetic overactivity, such as palpitations, sweating, heat intolerance, tremor, nervousness, and eyelid retraction[4,9,37,38,39] by blocking the catecholamine response at the receptor site. Propranolol is useful in decreasing the heart rate and the cardiac work and to abort early thyroid crisis.[5,18,26,30] Propranolol has also been found to block the conversion of T_4 to T_3 and, therefore, slightly decrease serum T_3 levels.[49,52,56]
	    Propranolol must be used carefully because adrenergic activity may be necessary in some patients for optimal cardiac functioning. Abolition of sympathetic drive may result in, or contribute to, cardiac decompensation. If propranolol is used to treat a patient who has cardiac failure, the patient must first be digitalized.[45] Long-term administration of beta-adrenergic blocking drugs is not recommended, however, because of the high incidence of heart failure.[11,52] Other adrenergic antagonists that deplete tissues of their catecholamine content (*e.g.*, resperine and guanethidine sulfate) are used occasionally.
	
	7. Assess the patient for the following signs of therapeutic control of sympathetic overactivity after the administration of propranolol: reduction of heart rate, palpitations, sweating, heat intolerance, tremor, tension, agitation, and psychomotor activity.[13]
	8. Administer hydrocortisone, 100 to 300 mg/day intravenously, to prevent adrenal insufficiency due to hypermetabolism and accelerated cortisol degradation. Steroids appear to reduce the peripheral conversion of T_4 to T_3 and may be beneficial in thyroid crisis, although steroid replacement therapy is still controversial.[55]

NURSING DIAGNOSIS

2. *Ineffective thermoregulation related to the hypermetabolic state and resultant hyperthermia (exchanging pattern)*

Patient Outcome	Nursing Orders
The patient will experience a normalization of body temperature and increased tolerance to ambient temperature.	1. Assess the patient's rectal temperature, the degree of diaphoresis and dehydration, the temperature and condition of the skin, and the degree of peripheral vasodilatation. 2. Use a hypothermia blanket to reduce temperature. One may also attempt to apply ice packs to the axilla and groin. Excessive thyroid hormones cause severe lipolysis and free fatty acid production. Fatty acids oxidize to produce an overabundance of thermal energy that cannot be dissipated by vasodilatation alone and cause fever and increased oxygen consumption. 3. Administer antipyretics as ordered by the physician. Do not use aspirin to reduce fever, however, because it can theoretically reduce the binding of T_3 and T_4 with thyroid-binding proteins and can therefore raise the level of free thyroid hormones in the plasma.[30]

(continued)

NURSING CARE PLAN SUMMARY *Patient With Thyroid Crisis* *Continued*

Patient Outcome	Nursing Orders
	4. Make sure the patient's bed clothes are not too warm or constricting.
	5. Monitor fluid intake and output. Ensure that diaphoretic fluid losses, which may be as high as 4 L in 24 hours, are replaced orally or intravenously.
	6. Notify the physician if shivering occurs. Shivering increases the metabolic rate and body temperature. Muscle relaxants such as chlorpromazine may be ordered to combat the shivering.
	7. Change damp clothing and linen frequently to promote patient comfort and skin intactness. Give frequent tepid sponge baths as needed.

NURSING DIAGNOSIS

3. *Ineffective coping (individual) related to excessive anxiety, as manifested by irritability, insomnia, and decompensation of interpersonal relationships (choosing pattern)*

Patient Outcome	Nursing Orders
1. The patient will experience reduced anxiety and enhanced adaptive coping mechanisms. A. The patient will verbalize fears, anxieties, and concerns regarding illness, behavior, and hospitalization. B. The patient's degree of nervousness, emotional lability, and hyperkinesis will return to previous levels. C. The patient will demonstrate an optimal balance of rest and activity, reporting improved sleep patterns. D. The patient will learn and practice relaxation techniques twice a day for 20 minutes. E. The family will ventilate their concern and anxiety regarding the patient's condition.	1. Assess the patient's level of consciousness, nervousness, and emotional stability (*e.g.*, mood swings and psychosis), noting subtle changes. 2. Encourage patients and families to express feelings and concerns. 3. Reorient and confirm reality as necessary. Make sure there is a clock and calendar in the room if the patient is confused. 4. Promote a quiet, tranquil environment as much as possible. Reduce all stimuli to a minimum. Give nursing care in a calm, consistent way. 5. Identify for patients' small gains in physical status. Some patients believe they have lost psychologic control and are going "crazy." Provide frequent reassurances and point out improvements.[11] 6. Assist the patient with diaphragmatic, slow, rhythmic breathing (see p. 36). Have the patient practice this breathing for several minutes.[21] After these breathing exercises, assist the patient with some method of relaxing body muscles. The head-to-toe relaxation script found on page 36 can be used. While patients are relaxing, encourage them to image the medications they are receiving, suggesting to them that the medications are flowing through the blood stream to affect all cells and organs. Suggest that the medications are reducing thyroid hormone production and are slowing down all body processes, resulting in a slower heart rate, lowered temperature, more muscle strength, and a calm, relaxed emotional state. 7. Provide sedatives as ordered and required. 8. Reassure the patient and family that any irritable behavior is primarily disease-related and may be controlled with appropriate therapy. 9. See Nursing Diagnosis: Ineffective Individual Coping, Chapter 8.

NURSING DIAGNOSIS

4. *High risk for self-injury related to fatigue, tremor, osteoporosis, and exophthalmus (exchanging pattern)*

Patient Outcome	Nursing Orders
1. The patient will not experience self-injury as defined by the following: A. The patient will be able to identify factors that increase the potential	1. Evaluate and prevent situations that place the patient at high risk for self-injury. A. Assess the patient's psychophysiologic response to activities. Explain factors that increase the potential for injury. B. Clear the environment of potential obstacles and hazards of mobility.

(continued)

NURSING CARE PLAN SUMMARY   *Patient With Thyroid Crisis*   *Continued*

Patient Outcome	Nursing Orders

Patient Outcome

for injury and engage in behaviors that minimize the risk of injury.

B. There will be no incidence of accidental injury related to tremor or falls.

C. The patient will experience increased, safe mobility.

D. The patient will exhibit increased activity tolerance (*e.g.*, less exertional dyspnea).

E. There will be no evidence of preventable corneal damage.

Nursing Orders

C. Assist the patient with the following activities:
   (1) Range-of-motion exercises
   (2) Simple activities such as bathing and eating
   (3) Ambulation
D. Increase activities as tolerated.
   (1) Schedule patient activities to conserve energy.
   (2) Coordinate activities with other health team members.
   (3) Schedule uninterrupted periods of rest.
   (4) Anticipate the patient's daily needs to minimize energy expenditure. Protein degradation that exceeds protein synthesis produces weakness in all muscle groups.
   (5) Avoid fatiguing the patient with frequent monitoring routines.
E. If the patient has severe exophthalmos, protect the eyes from irritants and injury.
   (1) Shield the eyes from excessive dust, light, and so-forth with eyeglasses or eye patches.
   (2) If eyelids cannot close completely, moisten cornea and conjunctiva with isotonic eye drops. Cover or tape eyelids shut at night.
   (3) Provide cool, moist compresses to soothe irritated eyes.
   (4) Examine the corneas frequently for clarity and intactness.
   (5) Instruct the patient to report any changes in visual acuity.

NURSING DIAGNOSIS

5. *Altered nutrition: less than body requirements related to increased gastric motility, protein catabolism, and hypermetabolism of tissues (exchanging pattern)*

Patient Outcome

1. The patient will achieve an adequate nutritional status to meet the metabolic demands of the body, as demonstrated by the following:
   A. The ability to achieve and maintain an ideal body weight
   B. A resolution of abdominal cramping
   C. A return to a normal defecation pattern
   D. Verbal and behavioral evidence of increased physical stamina

Nursing Orders

1. Evaluate the patient's nutritional status and implement appropriate therapy.
   A. Assess the patient's signs and symptoms of gastrointestinal disturbance (*e.g.*, anorexia, nausea, vomiting, diarrhea, increased hunger, and abdominal pain or tenderness). Auscultate bowel sounds for hypermotility.
   B. Assess the patient's degree of catabolism by monitoring daily weight (variance from ideal body weight), degree of fatigue, and presence of weak or wasted musculature.
   C. Monitor serum albumin, hemoglobin, and white blood cell count, because these parameters provide valuable information about the patient's nutritional status. It is important to remember that serum albumin levels take 3 days to mirror improvement or decay in the patient's nutritional status.
   D. Provide a well-balanced diet, high in carbohydrates and proteins with up to 4000 calories a day.
      (1) Avoid foods high in roughage, such as raw fruits and vegetables, to reduce diarrhea.
      (2) Give supplemental vitamins.
      (3) Administer thiamine, riboflavin, vitamin B_{12}, and vitamin C as ordered. Vitamin absorption may be impaired because of the increased gastrointestinal motility, and vitamin deficiencies may occur because of the hypermetabolism.[11,17,18]

(continued)

NURSING CARE PLAN SUMMARY *Patient With Thyroid Crisis* *Continued*

NURSING DIAGNOSIS

6. *Fluid volume deficit related to diaphoresis, vomiting, diarrhea, or gastric suctioning (exchanging pattern)*

Patient Outcome	*Nursing Orders*

The patient will not experience signs and symptoms of fluid volume deficit, such as dry skin or mucous membranes; decreased urinary output; hypotension (especially orthostatic hypotension); weak, thready pulse; rapid, shallow respirations; flat neck veins; or reduced central venous or pulmonary capillary wedge pressure.	1. Evaluate the patient's volume status, and implement the appropriate therapy.
	  A. Assess the patient for signs and symptoms of dehydration, such as dry skin and mucous membranes (tissue signs may take 24 hours to manifest); decreased urinary output; orthostatic hypotension; weak, thready pulse; rapid, shallow respirations; and flat neck veins. Fluid depletion can occur because of severe diaphoresis, vomiting, diarrhea, and gastric suctioning.
	  B. Monitor the central venous pressure or pulmonary capillary wedge pressures as appropriate.
	  C. Monitor the vital signs frequently.
	  D. Carefully measure the intake and output.
	  E. Weigh the patient daily.
	  F. Monitor the urine specific gravity every shift. Elevation of urine concentration indicates a decreased extracellular fluid volume.
	  G. Carefully assess the effects of medications such as propranolol, which may further reduce blood pressure.
	  H. Replace fluids intravenously as ordered by the physician.
	  I. Treat nausea and vomiting or diarrhea as ordered by physician.

NURSING DIAGNOSIS

7. *Altered electrolyte balance related to vomiting, diarrhea, nasogastric suctioning, and bone demineralization (exchanging pattern)*

Patient Outcomes	*Nursing Orders*

1. The patient will not experience signs and symptoms of hypokalemia.	1. Assess the patient for signs and symptoms of hypokalemia.
	  A. Signs and symptoms of hypokalemia include malaise, anorexia, nausea and vomiting, leg cramping, shallow respirations, decreased blood pressure, weak pulse, electrocardiographic U waves, and ventricular ectopic beats. Hypokalemia may result from vomiting, nasogastric suctioning, and diarrhea or from diuretic therapy.
	  B. Monitor serum potassium levels.

2. If hypokalemia does occur, the patient will respond therapeutically to potassium replacement.	2. Administer intravenous potassium slowly or by oral preparations as ordered by the physician.

3. The patient will not experience signs and symptoms of hypercalcemia (a rare occurrence).	3. Assess the patient for signs and symptoms of hypercalcemia.
	  A. Signs and symptoms of hypercalcemia include fatigue, drowsiness, depression, lethargy, disorientation, muscle weakness or hypotonicity, polyuria, deep bone pain, anorexia, nausea and vomiting, constipation, thirst, stupor or coma, electrocardiographic evidence of a shortened QT interval, or cardiac dysrhythmias. Degradation of bone may cause hypercalcemia.
	  B. Monitor serum calcium levels.

4. The patient will not experience pathologic bone fractures.	4. Implement safety precautions to prevent fractures.[25] Demineralization of bone can cause pathologic bone fractures.
5. The patient will tolerate passive (active) range-of-motion exercises.	5. Administer passive range-of-motion exercises every 2 hours. When the patient is stable, teach and supervise active range-of-motion exercises. Bed rest and inactivity contribute to breakdown of bone.[25]
6. If hypercalcemia does occur, the patient will respond appropriately to therapy to reduce serum calcium levels.	6. Anticipate the following therapy for hypercalcemia: administration of diuretics, sodium bicarbonate, phosphate and glucocorticoids (inhibits calcium absorption), enediaminetetraacetic acid (lowers calcium by chelation), or dialysis.

(continued)

NURSING CARE PLAN SUMMARY   *Patient With Thyroid Crisis   Continued*

NURSING DIAGNOSIS

8. *Knowledge deficit about medical regimen and future prophylactic care related to insufficient knowledge about thyroid illness (knowing pattern)*

Patient Outcomes	Nursing Orders
1. The patient and significant others will be able to verbalize an understanding of the following: 　A. Anatomy and physiology of the thyroid gland 　B. Pathophysiology of thyrotoxicosis 　C. Physiologic and psychologic stressors that precipitate or are associated with thyrotoxicosis 　D. Clinical signs and symptoms of thyrotoxicosis 　E. Importance of medical follow-up care 　F. Indications, dosage, frequency, and adverse side-effects of antithyroid drugs 　G. Indications, dosage, frequency, and adverse effects of beta-adrenergic blocking drugs	1. Assess the patient's readiness to learn. Include the patient and family in the teaching sessions. 　A. Explain the anatomy and physiology of the thyroid gland. 　B. Discuss the pathophysiology of thyrotoxicosis. 　C. Discuss the physiologic and psychologic stressors that precipitate or are associated with thyrotoxicosis (see Reflections). 　D. List the clinical manifestations of thyrotoxicosis. 　E. Discuss the need for medical follow-up in the future. 　F. Explain the indications for and the dosage, frequency, and adverse side-effects of antithyroid medications. The patient must understand the following: 　　(1) The need for maintaining daily therapeutic blood levels 　　(2) The importance of seeking medical attention at the first sign of any local or generalized infection, which may herald the approach of the serious complication of agranulocytosis 　G. Explain the indications for and the dosage, frequency, and adverse side-effects of propranolol therapy.
2. The patient will be able to discuss the rationale regarding possible future treatment with ^{131}I or subtotal thyroidectomy.	2. Discuss possible future treatment with ^{131}I therapy or subtotal thyroidectomy as appropriate.
3. The patient will be able to describe the manifestations of hypothyroidism and the need to seek medical assistance for this condition.	3. Instruct patient and family members to report possible signs of hypothyroidism, which may occur after thyroid gland ablation by surgery or [131]I (the latter may not precipitate hypothyroidism for up to 10 years after therapy). Manifestations of hypothyroidism (which are usually insidious) include exceptional fatigability; dry, cool, scaly skin; hair loss; a puffy face; periorbital edema; and cold intolerance.
4. The patient will be able to discuss the importance and benefits of practicing relaxation techniques after discharge.	4. Discuss the benefits of continuing to practice relaxation techniques after discharge.

IMPLEMENTATION AND EVALUATION

A high index of suspicion should be present with regard to any patient who presents with unexplained cardiac decompensation or atrial dysrhythmias.[8,18,20] Also, laboratory findings may reveal increases in RAIU, T_4, FT_4I, T_3RIA, and T_3RU. The seriousness of the situation, however, demands that treatment be instituted even before the results of laboratory measurements are available. The presumptive diagnosis of thyroid crisis is based on the history, the clinical findings, and sound medical judgment.[50]

The treatment of thyroid crisis requires taking certain immediate measures to counteract the harmful effects of hypermetabolism. Because of the long half-life of T_4 (7 to 8 days) and T_3 (36 hours), acute medical interventions must continue for at least a week after initial diagnosis of thyroid crisis. The therapy is directed toward the following[50]: diagnosing and treating any associated or precipitating disease or problem, inhibiting the synthesis and release of excess quantities of thyroid hormone, reducing the metabolic effects of excessive thyroid hormone and sympathetic overactivity, and providing general supportive therapy.

Graves' disease is often characterized by periods of exacerbation and remission. No clinical criteria are universally useful in predicting medical remission early in the course of treatment.[35] Because the cause of Graves' disease is not known with certainty, there is no ideal way to treat the disease; thus, the basic approach to treatment remains controversial.[53] There are two basic approaches. However, in the long-term treatment of patients with Graves' disease associated with thyrotoxicosis or thyroid crisis, both approaches are aimed primarily at reducing the overactivity of the thyroid gland. The first approach involves the use of long-term antithyroid medication that prevents the overproduction of thyroid hormone. The second approach attempts to ablate a portion of the thyroid by means of RAI or by subtotal thyroidectomy.

Overview of Medical Regimen

In the *first approach,* long-term medical therapy using *antithyroid drugs* has been limited, for the most part, to patients under 40 years of age.[8,18,30,53] Because thionamide drugs (PTU or methimazole) inhibit the synthesis but not the release of thyroid hormone, the thyroid gland must first be depleted of its hormonal stores before there is a reduction in the supply of hormone at the tissue level. This may take days to weeks to occur. Once the patient becomes euthyroid, the antithyroid dosage is reduced to the lowest therapeutic level.

The patient should then be given daily thyroid hormone therapy to prevent the development of hypothyroidism, which may develop as a result of prolonged use of antithyroid medication.[8,18,53] The undesirable consequences of hypothyroidism (*e.g.,* ophthalmopathy and enlargement of the thyroid gland) may thus be avoided. Thyroid replacement therapy combined with the long-term use of antithyroid medication is, however, controversial. Hypothyroidism can be prevented simply by adjusting the dosage of the antithyroid medication. Perhaps more important, medical follow-up is essential to assess the patient's ability to take the appropriate drugs faithfully.

The length of therapy is difficult to predict; it may depend simply on the spontaneous course of the disease. Frequently, patients are treated from 12 to 24 months before medications are discontinued. In general, patients who have been symptomatic less than 1 year or who have small goiters that quickly diminish in size during antithyroid therapy are more likely to have permanent remissions after adequate medical therapy.[5,26,42] The overall rate of remission after prolonged antithyroid medication is about 15% to 50%.[42] The recurrence rate of hyperthyroidism after medical treatment is increasing, however, probably because larger amounts of iodine have been added to daily foods.[54]

The *second major approach* to the treatment of hyperthyroidism is the destruction of functional thyroid tissue, which limits the amount of thyroid produced. The destruction is accomplished either by ^{131}I therapy or by surgery. Therapy with ^{131}I, which was introduced in 1941, eliminates thyroid tissue by radiation necrosis of the thyroid follicle cells and replaces it with interstitial fibrosis.

The administration of ^{131}I is a simple, painless, bloodless, and inexpensive procedure. The early fears about the possible carcinogenic and harmful genetic effects of ^{131}I therapy have not been realized.[10,18,41] Therapy with ^{131}I is not generally recommended, however, for patients who are pregnant or who have childbearing potential.[18,53] It is also not recommended for patients who cannot be adequately observed medically throughout their lives.[23,30]

Radioactive iodine is effective in 100% of cases: 75% to 80% of patients become euthyroid after the initial dose, and the remaining 20% to 25% become euthyroid after a second treatment.[51] Because the patient should be euthyroid before the administration of ^{131}I, the patient is given antithyroid medication until thyroid function tests are normal. Antithyroid therapy is then discontinued for several days before and after the administration of ^{131}I to allow ^{131}I to accumulate in the thyroid, and it is administered once again to maintain a eumetabolic state until ^{131}I exerts its effect (usually weeks to months).

The major side-effect of ^{131}I therapy for hyperthyroidism is hypothyroidism.[36] Most patients treated with ^{131}I become hypothyroid at some time in their lives. It is essential that the patient be educated about the problem and that thyroid replacement therapy be instituted as soon as the patient becomes euthyroid.[34,51] Because hypothyroidism may develop insidiously (up to 10 years after therapy), and cause irreversible damage, the use of thyroid medication after ^{131}I therapy cannot be overemphasized. The lifetime replacement of thyroid hormone in therapeutic doses is simple and inexpensive, and it is not associated with untoward metabolic or allergic effects.

Before ^{131}I therapy was introduced, subtotal thyroidectomy was the treatment of choice for hyperthyroid patients. Surgery is still recommended for children, adults with childbearing potential, patients who refuse ^{131}I therapy, those with secreting thyroid carcinoma, and pregnant women who do not respond to antithyroid medication.

Preoperatively, patients should be rendered euthyroid to prevent thyroid crisis. This is accomplished by use of beta-adrenergic receptor-blocking drugs[47] and a 2- to 4-month course of a thionamide drug with the addition of iodides during

Table 39-3
Drugs Used in the Treatment of Hyperthyroidism

DRUG	FUNCTION	ADVERSE EFFECTS
Thionamides Propylthiouracil Methimazole (Tapazole)	Block synthesis of T_3 and T_4 by acting on the peroxidase complex	Hypothyroidism resulting in goiter and ophthalmopathy, skin rash, gastrointestinal symptoms, arthralgias, fever, hepatitis, agranulocytosis, "physiologic" leukopenia
Iodides Lugol's solution Sodium iodide	Inhibit release of thyroid hormone; cause involution and reduce vascularity of thyroid gland	Skin rash or skin lesions, salivary gland inflammation, conjunctivitis, rhinitis, eosinophilia Not recommended for long-term use Response unpredictable if given before administration of antithyroid drugs May delay the therapeutic response of subsequently administered antithyroid medication Iodine may accumulate in gland to be used for synthesis of additional thyroid hormone
Beta-adrenergic Receptor-Blocking Drugs Propranolol (Inderal)	Control peripheral manifestations of sympathetic overactivity by blocking catecholamine response at receptor site	Cardiac arrest, cardiac failure, bradycardia, hypotension, acute respiratory problems

the final 2 or 3 weeks before surgery. Iodide is an antithyroid compound when used for short-term therapy (see Table 39-3) and it is useful in reducing the vascularity of the gland before surgery.

The surgery involves removal of most of the thyroid tissue, leaving only a small remnant in place. The remnant left behind will, it is hoped, produce enough thyroid hormone to allow the patient to maintain a euthyroid state. The surgery eliminates both the hyperthyroidism and the goiter of Graves' disease.

Most patients achieve a euthyroid state after surgery. The mortality associated with the surgery is extremely low (less than 0.1%).[43,55] Complications include wound infections, transient tetany (due to damage to parathyroid glands), and hemorrhage leading to respiratory obstruction.[23] Recurrent hyperthyroidism persists in 2% to 8% of patients, who will at some time require therapy with antithyroid medication or [131]I.[55] In the presence of excessive TSH secretion or ectopic stimulation of the thyroid gland (e.g., LATS), the thyroid remnant may again hypertrophy (as was the problem in Mr. R.'s case). The complication of hypothyroidism can be expected to develop in 8% to 10% of all patients.[1,55] Damage to the recurrent laryngeal nerve during surgery can produce permanent vocal cord paralysis in approximately 0.6% of patients.[33,34,47,55] Permanent hypoparathyroidism is a severe complication, occurring in up to 3% of patients.[1,43,55] It is induced iatrogenically by the inadvertent removal of parathyroid tissue or by impairment of the blood supply of the parathyroid gland during surgery.

Because the long-term treatment of hyperthyroidism in Graves' disease remains controversial, it is important that the approaches be offered to the patient in a clear and understandable way.

SUMMARY

Thyroid crisis is a life-threatening exacerbation of thyrotoxicosis, and it is an acute emergency condition. The critical care nurse who understands the pathophysiology, clinical manifestations, complications, and objectives of care is equipped to play an essential role in caring for the patient in thyroid crisis.

DIRECTIONS FOR FUTURE RESEARCH

1. What are the effects of practicing relaxation techniques on adrenergic hyperactivity of patients with thyroid crisis?
2. What nursing activities are important in assisting the patient with thyroid crisis to conserve energy?
3. What is the most effective method of long-term follow-up, teaching, and support of the hyperthyroid patient?
4. Can long-term psychologic support and therapy reduce the number and length of exacerbations of hyperthyroid patients?
5. What is the safest and most efficient way to correct hyperthermia in the patient with thyroid crisis?

REFERENCES

1. Beahrs, O. H., and Sakulsky, S. B. Surgical thyroidectomy in the management of exophthalmic goiter. *Arch. Surg.* 96:512, 1968.
2. Blum, M., Kranjac, T., Park, C., *et al.* Thyroid storm after cardiac angiography with iodinated contrast mediums. *J.A.M.A.* 235:2324, 1976.
3. Bullas, J. B., and Pfister, S. Hyperthyroid crisis. *Crit. Care Nurs.* 4:98, 1984.
4. Bybee, D. Saving lives in thyroid crisis. *Emerg. Med.* 19:20, 1987.
5. Cooper, D., and Ridgway, E. Clinical management of patients with hyperthyroidism. *Med. Clin. North Am.* 69:953, 1985.
6. Coulombe, P., Dussault, J., and Walker, P. L. Catecholamine metabolism in thyroid disease. *J. Clin. Endocrinol. Metab.* 44:1185, 1977.
7. Davies, A. G. Thyroid physiology. *Br. Med. J.* 2:206, 1972.
8. de los Santos, E. T., and Mazzaferri, E. L. Thyroid function tests: Guidelines for interpretation in common clinical disorders. *Postgrad. Med.* 85:333, 1989.
9. Dial, P., and Hastings, P. R. The use of a selective beta-adrenergic receptor blocker for the preoperative preparation of thyrotoxic patients. *Ann. Surg.* 196:633, 1982.
10. Dobyns, B. M., Sheline, G. E. Workman, J. B., *et al.* Malignant and benign neoplasms of the thyroid in patients treated for hyperthyroidism: A report of the cooperative thyrotoxicosis therapy follow-up study. *J. Clin. Endocrinol. Metab.* 38:976, 1974.
11. Evangelisti, J. T., and Thorpe, C. J. Thyroid storm: A nursing crisis. *Heart Lung* 12:184, 1983.
12. Fatourechi, V., and Gharib, H. Hyperthyroidism following hypothyroidism: Data on six cases. *Arch. Intern. Med.* 148:976, 1988.
13. Feely, J., Forrest, A., Gunn, A., *et al.* Propranolol dosage in thyrotoxicosis. *J. Clin. Endocrinol. Metab.* 51:658, 1980.
14. Forfar, J. C., Muir, A. L., Sawers, S. A., *et al.* Abnormal left ventricular function in hyperthyroidism. *N. Engl. J. Med.* 307:1165, 1982.
15. Fowler, N. O. Hyperthyroidism: How to recognize it from circulatory signs. *Consultant* 4:25, 1976.
16. Freeman, M., Giuliani, M., Schwartz, E., *et al.* Acute thyroiditis, thyroid crisis and hypocalcemia following radioactive iodine therapy. *N.Y. State J. Med.* 69:2036, 1969.
17. Genuth, S. M. The Thyroid Gland. In R. M. Berne and M. N. Levy (eds.), *Physiology.* St. Louis: C. V. Mosby, 1983.
18. Greer, M. A. Disorders of the Thyroid. In J. H. Stein (ed.), *Internal Medicine.* Boston: Little, Brown, 1983.
19. Greer, M. A., Kammer, H., and Bouma, D. J. Short-term antithyroid drug therapy for the thyrotoxicosis of Graves' disease. *N. Engl. J. Med.* 297:173, 1977.
20. Guyton, A. C. *Textbook of Medical Physiology.* Philadelphia: W. B. Saunders, 1986.
21. Guzzetta, C. E., and Dossey, B. M. *Cardiovascular Nursing: Bodymind Tapestry.* St. Louis: C. V. Mosby, 1984.
22. Hanscom, D., and Ryan, R. J. Thyroid crisis and diabetic ketoacidosis. *N. Engl. J. Med.* 257:697, 1957.
23. Harrison, T. R., Thorn, G., Adams, R., *et al.* (eds.). *Principles of Internal Medicine* (11th ed.). New York: McGraw-Hill, 1988.
24. Jackson, I. M. D. Thyrotropin-releasing hormone. *N. Engl. J. Med.* 306:145, 1982.
25. Johnson, D. Pathophysiology of thyroid storm: Nursing implications. *Crit. Care Nurs.* 3:80, 1983.
26. Kabadi, U. M. Thyroid disorders and the elderly. *Compr. Ther.* 15:53, 1989.
27. Klein, I., Trzepacz, P., Roberts, M., *et al.* Symptom rating scale for assessing hyperthyroidism. *Arch. Intern. Med.* 148:387, 1988.
28. Larsen, P. R. Salicylate-induced increase in free triiodothyronine in human serum. *J. Clin. Invest.* 51:1125, 1972.
29. Locke, W. Management of hyper- and hypothyroid conditions. *Postgrad. Med.* 125:118, 1982.
30. Mathewson, M. K. Thyroid disorder. *Crit. Care Nurs.* 7:74, 1987.
31. McArthur, J. W. Thyrotoxic crisis. *J.A.M.A.* 134:868, 1947.
32. Menendez, C. E., and Goldzieher, J. W. Modern laboratory diagnosis of thyroid disease. *Tex. Med.* 72:66, 1976.
33. Moosman, D. A., and DeWeese, M. S. The external laryngeal nerve as related to thyroidectomy. *Surg. Gynecol. Obstet.* 127:1011, 1968.
34. Mountain, J. C., Stewart, G. R., and Colcock, B. P. The recurrent laryngeal nerve in thyroid operations. *Surg. Gynecol. Obstet.* 133:978, 1971.

35. Nicoloff, J. Thyroid storm and myxedema coma. *Med. Clin. North Am.* 69:1005, 1985.

36. Nofal, M. M., Beierwaltes, W. H., and Patno, M. E. Treatment of hyperthyroidism with sodium iodide [131]I. *J.A.M.A.* 197:605, 1966.

37. O'Neil, J. R. Thyroid crisis. *Nursing '87* 17:33, 1987.

38. Peden, N. R., Gunn, A., Browning, M. C., *et al.* Nadolol and potassium iodide in combination in the surgical treatment of thyrotoxicosis. *Br. J. Surg.* 69:638, 1982.

39. Peden, N. R., Isles, T. E., Stevenson, I. H., *et al.* Nadolol in thyrotoxicosis. *Br. J. Clin. Pharmacol.* 13:835, 1982.

40. Ross, D. S. Subclinical hyperthyroidism: Possible danger of overzealous thyroxine replacement therapy. *Mayo. Clin. Proc.* 63:1214, 1988.

41. Safa, A. M., Schumacher, O. P., and Rodriquez-Antunez, A. Long term follow-up results in children and adolescents treated with radioactive iodine (^{131}I) for hyperthyroidism. *N. Engl. J. Med.* 292:167, 1975.

42. Sakiyama, R. Common thyroid disorders. *Am. Fam. Physician* 38:227, 1988.

43. Schwartz, S. I., Hume, D. M., and Kaplan, E. L. Thyroid and Parathyroid. In S. I. Schwartz (ed.), *Principles of Surgery* (5th ed.). New York: McGraw-Hill, 1989.

44. Shafer, R., and Nuttall, F. Acute changes in thyroid function in patients treated with radioactive iodine. *Lancet* 2:635, 1975.

45. Spaulding, S., and Lippes, H. Hyperthyroidism: Causes, clinical features and diagnosis. *Med. Clin. North Am.* 69:937, 1985.

46. Tibaldi, J., Barzel, U., Albin, J., *et al.* Thyrotoxicosis in the very old. *Am. J. Med.* 81:619, 1986.

47. Toft, A. D., Irvine, W. J., Sinclair, I., *et al.* Thyroid function after surgical treatment of thyrotoxicosis. *N. Engl. J. Med.* 298:643, 1978.

48. Toth, E. L., Mant, M. J., Shivji, S. Propylthiouracil-induced agranulocytosis: An unusual presentation and a possible mechanism. *Am. J. Med.* 85:725, 1988.

49. Tucker, S. M., Canobbio, M. M., Paquette, E. V., *et al.* Hyperthyroidism: Thyroid crisis (storm, thyrotoxic crisis). *J.E.N.* 15:352, 1989.

50. Urbanic, R. C., and Mazzaferri, E. L. Thyrotoxic crisis and myxedema coma. *Heart Lung* 7:435, 1978.

51. Utiger, R. D. Treatment of Graves' disease. *N. Engl. J. Med.* 298:681, 1978.

52. Utiger, R. D. Beta-adrenergic-antagonist therapy for hyperthyroid Graves' disease. *N. Engl. J. Med.* 310:1597, 1984.

53. Waldstein, S. S., Slodki, S. J., Kaganiec, I., *et al.* A clinical study of thyroid storm. *Ann. Intern. Med.* 52:626, 1960.

54. Wartofsky, L. Low remission after therapy for Graves' disease: Possible relation of dietary iodine with antithyroid results. *J.A.M.A.* 226:1083, 1973.

55. Werner, S. C., and Ingbar, S. H. (eds.). *The Thyroid.* (5th ed.). New York: Harper & Row, 1986.

56. Wiersings, W., and Touber, J. The influence of β-adrenoceptor blocking agents on plasma thyroxine and triiodothyronine. *J. Clin. Endocrinol. Metab.* 45:293, 1977.

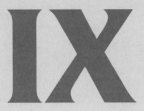

IX

The Critically Ill Adult After Trauma

RECOGNIZING MY UNIQUE QUALITIES

How often do you recognize and validate your unique qualities of being a critical care nurse? Take time each day to acknowledge and affirm to yourself the unique aspects that you bring into your own life and the lives of others:

- I am a risk taker.
- I am caring.
- I am a critical thinker.
- I am self-aware.
- I am assertive.
- I am an active listener.
- I facilitate healing in self and others.
- I avoid power struggles.
- I use time and resources wisely.
- I value the clarity of my decisions.
- I recognize the healing purposes of my work.
- I respect and love myself and my colleagues.
- I am an advocate for nursing.
- I am future-oriented.

40

Trauma Assessment

Cornelia Vanderstaay Kenner

RELAXATION AS MEDICINE

Ms. D was a 39-year-old multitrauma patient recently admitted to the Special Care Unit. From report, I learned that Ms. D continued to have pain despite medication and would scream and cry despite increased levels of medication. On assessment, I found that Ms. D was experiencing discomfort as well as stress and anxiety from the accident and hospitalization. She stated that she was having a problem coping with the situation and wanted enough medication to "knock her out" until she was well.

I worked with Ms. D to cope with the present situation and to promote relaxation. When morphine was administered, I told her that the medication was being given and that soon she would have less pain and feel more relaxed. I promoted relaxation by having her close her eyes, focus on slowing her breathing, and having her relax each part of her body slowly. She was asleep in 10 minutes. It was the first sleep she had experienced in 10 hours. During the day, I continued the same techniques, which produced relaxation and sleep within a few minutes. She began to request help to relax without the medication and would experience the same levels of relaxation. Some of the nursing staff were present as we had just finished repositioning her in traction and I began the relaxation exercise. She was snoring in less than 2 minutes, and the staff was amazed. Was this the same woman who 5 hours earlier had been screaming? They had observed my technique, and I shared my methods with them.

The techniques used were documented in the patient care plan and demonstrated by the nurse giving report to the next nurse. At present, Ms. D is still a patient in the Special Care Unit, but it is much quieter now and she is able to visit with her family without the effects of high-dose medication.

Pam Davis, RN, BSN, RNC, CCRN
Special Care Unit
Maine Medical Center
Portland, Maine

LEARNING OBJECTIVES

After reading this chapter, the nurse should be able to do the following:

1. Calculate the trauma scale for an injured patient.
2. Identify the important points in the history of the accident.
3. List the steps in the primary and secondary surveys.
4. Assess and monitor a patient who has had a MAST suit applied.
5. Perform a preflight assessment for a patient to be transferred to the regional trauma center by air ambulance.

EMERGENCY MEDICAL SYSTEMS

Emergency medical systems have had a great impact on the morbidity and mortality in prehospital care. In one study, for example, a review of statistics before and after implementation of a trauma care system at the paramedic level revealed that the ultimate survival of patients arriving at the emergency department with open intra-abdominal vascular trauma and a blood pressure greater than 60 mm Hg had significantly increased.[1] Before the paramedic system, 3 of 21 patients survived, whereas after implementation of the paramedic system, 11 of 22 patients survived.

Survival is also greatly increased when patients receive care in a regional trauma center rather than in a community hospital. Trunkey[19] states that death from trauma has a trimodal distribution. The first peak of deaths occurs in the first seconds or minutes after injury. Only a few of these patients can be saved. The second peak from deaths occurs within 2 hours after injury. A significant number of these patients can be saved with accurate prehospital and initial hospital care. The third peak of deaths occurs days to weeks after injury.

Of first importance is care at the accident site. Speed alone is not the primary consideration. Identification of the problem and appropriate and immediate care before and during transit will bring a viable patient to a well-equipped, well-staffed hospital for definitive care. Appropriate on-site care increases the chances that the patient's life can be saved. To a large extent, the fate of the injured person depends on the initial care. Emergency medical care has been taken out of the realm of the haphazard and inexperienced and is moving toward an organized and sophisticated system of care. The essential components of emergency medical care include communications, evacuation and transportation by ground and air ambulance, categorization of hospitals, education of and practice for personnel (e.g., lay groups, emergency medical technicians and paramedics, firefighters, police, physicians, nurses, and respiratory therapies), and program evaluation. Prehospital emergency care takes a multifaceted approach that includes system design; selection of personnel; provision for a rapid response to emergencies through good distribution of equipment and personnel; safe transportation to the hospital by well-trained personnel, good equipment, and enough vehicles; and standardized algorithms for therapy.

Emergency Care

The initial assessment and management of the injured patient are dependent on a systematic evaluation by a well-educated team whose roles are defined and who have planned for all contingencies. Pre-established guidelines and protocols are a necessity. Each team member must know and respect the duties and responsibilities of other team members. Accurate communication, both oral and written, is vital so that changes in the patient's condition can be readily observed and assessed.

Predictors of Injury Severity

Although patients with severe injuries are best cared for in highly specialized treatment facilities, patients with lesser injuries do not require such care and may be treated in a general hospital. It then becomes a problem in assessment to determine rapidly which patients have a more severe injury. Of the many tools available, two seem to have the widest use. The *injury severity score*[2,13] is based on anatomic indices, is useful in grading the majority of trauma, is widely used in research, and is correlated with outcome. However, it is best used as a retrospective tool, because it cannot be calculated accurately until the full extent of injury is known and any surgical intervention is completed. The *trauma score*[3,15] consists of a set of data points that can be collected at the scene of the accident and used on a continuing basis for reassessment. It has been developed in an attempt to get the right patient to the right hospital at the right time. It comprises a series of cardiopulmonary functions and the three neurologic functions of the Glasgow Coma Scale. Each data point in the score is given a number. High numbers are for normal functions, and low numbers are for impaired functions. The Glasgow Coma Scale is reduced by about one third its value before computation. The severity of injury can then be expressed by a sum of the numbers; the highest score is 16, and the lowest is 1.

Triage

In many hospitals, triage is a nursing function. Triage comes from the French word meaning "to sort." *Triage* is a sorting of patients so that priorities of care can be established. It is a preliminary screening of patients to assess their needs and care priorities. Before any patient arrival is the development of a system that outlines who will triage, what protocols and policies will be followed, and where triage will be performed.

NURSING PROCESS

ASSESSMENT

History

Information about the accident and pertinent historical details will greatly facilitate both the initial and ongoing assessments of the patient. Patterns of injury are common with different types of accidents, so the history will alert the trauma team to be particularly cognizant of certain areas. Figure 40–1 shows a sample patient assessment form suitable for recording patient data.

Chief Complaint

Patients should be asked to describe what has happened to them and why they have sought medical assistance. A surprising amount of information can be obtained in only a few words (e.g., "I had terrible chest pain before I lost control of my car.").

History of Present Illness

Even before the patient arrives at the hospital, obtaining the history of the accident should be begun by using the radio report from the emergency medical technicians or the telephone report from the medical team at the transferring facility. The nurse should obtain the history as soon as possible. The major points can be gathered, if necessary, while the physical examination is being performed. The history may be difficult to obtain from a severely injured patient, but much information can be gathered from bystanders, family, and friends. Even when the patient is severely injured, the trauma team should persevere in history taking and combine a systematic examination with careful, meaningful questions.

Information should be recorded in the patient's record about the accident. The circumstances surrounding the accident should be detailed in an orderly fashion. Details to be included are when the accident occurred, the patient's position at the time of the accident, any subsequent displacement, whether the patient struck or was struck by an object, and information about any penetrating object (e.g., type, size, length, caliber, or angle of penetration). Information about any treatment that has been rendered before admission should be obtained as well.

Past Medical History

Information about the patient's past history should include pertinent medical and surgical history (e.g., cardiovascular, pulmonary, renal, metabolic, or neurologic disorders), current medications, immunizations, and allergies and drug sensitivities. It is far too easy in the stress of the situation to overlook details. For example, the patient with a history of cardiovascular disease involved in a motor-vehicle accident may have suffered a concomitant myocardial infarction.

History of the Physiologic Subsystem

The history of the physiologic subsystem involves gathering data pertinent to the particular systems involved and how those systems function in the part of the body traumatized. It is also important to identify the type of accident and the mechanism of injury, because injuries follow different patterns depending on the type of accident. As examples, three types of accidents involved with moving vehicles are described in the following sections: pedestrian, motorcycle, and driver injuries.

Pedestrian Injuries. Severe deformities can result from the high-velocity forces sustained by pedestrians who are struck by a motor vehicle. Usually the pedestrian has been struck from the side by the bumper with direct trauma to the lower extremities. The pedestrian may be thrown up against the hood or windshield with a resultant skull fracture and head injury. As the pedestrian falls to the ground, a secondary impact occurs.

Motorcycle Injuries. Motorcycle injuries are associated with a higher degree of morbidity and mortality than automobile driver accidents. The group most at risk are young men between the ages of 15 and 25 who have had their motorcycles for less than 1 year. Injuries are hard to classify and often include more than one area. Patients should be suspected of having spinal cord and intracranial injuries until proven otherwise.

Automobile Accidents. Injuries to those within the automobile are far more significant if seat belts and shoulder harnesses have not been worn. Although penetration-resistant laminated windshields and padded dashboards have helped decrease injuries, the forces sustained within the accident are significant enough to cause severe injury. Additionally, older-model cars do not have the safety features built into more recent models. McSwain[14] has identified three primary types of accidents: frontal head-on impact, rear impact, and side impact.

Before a *head-on collision,* the car and driver are moving at the same speed. Once the car stops, the person continues to move forward at the original speed. In order to reach the dashboard, windshield, or steering wheel column, the driver follows one of two pathways: upward over the steering wheel or downward under the steering wheel. If the person moves in an upward direction, the momentum is up over the dashboard into the windshield. Cervical spinal injuries are possible and can be severe. A secondary, often simultaneous impact occurs as the person's chest hits the steering wheel or dashboard. If the speed of the car at impact was 30 miles/hour, the momentum of the 150-lb driver is 205 lb/second. The average force required to stop the driver in one hundredth of a second is 20,500 lb, a tremendous force. If the driver stops more slowly the average force required to stop him would be correspondingly smaller. The momentum of the body must be absorbed before the body can come to rest. The energy from crashing is usually absorbed by the skeleton. Weak points in the structure are injured more frequently than strong points. On stopping, the person who has moved down under the steering wheel will continue to move forward with his knees in front of the body. The knees strike the dashboard and stop. The skeletal weak points in the lower extremities are the joints. Possible injuries are posterior dislocation of the knee, fracture dislocation of the ankle, fractured tibia, and other long-bone fractures. During impact, although the motion of the lower extremities has stopped, the upper part of the body continues forward. Usually the head or upper part of the chest strikes the dashboard or windshield and stops the body. As the pelvis moves forward after the femur has stopped moving, additional force is placed on the head of the femur. A distal posterior fracture dislocation is the likely result.

In a *rear-end collision,* the car at rest suddenly gains forward momentum. The parts of the person's body that are in contact with the car also gain momentum and are accelerated. The parts of the body not in contact with the car are pulled along by the accelerated parts. However, the two are not simultaneous, and strong forces result within the body.

In a *side impact,* the lateral motion of the colliding car or truck is transmitted to the car. The person moves in a lateral motion against the door of the car. As the chest is compressed from the side, ribs may be fractured and the underlying lung contused. In the lower extremities, as the femur is compressed, the force against the acetabulum may be so great that the femur head is driven through the acetabulum into the retroperitoneal space.

Therefore, information about the accident should include what happened, what structures were involved, what damage occurred to the car, what part of the car was damaged, the direction of the car's impact, and the final resting position of the car compared with where the impact occurred.

Activities of Daily Living and Social and Personal History

Questions related to the patient's activities of daily living and the social and personal systems have been described. Specifically related to *activities of daily living* are questions about nutrition and hydration, sleep and rest patterns, exercise habits, and especially alcohol or drug or narcotic consumption.

Exploring the *social system* involves questions related to the cultural beliefs involving accidental injury and to the socioeconomic impact of injury. Many groups see accidents as happening because of something negative that has been done. The question "What have I done to deserve this?" is common.

Specific questions related to the personal system involve the uniqueness of the person and how the trauma affects the personhood of the patient. The injury may have an impact on the patient's self-esteem, self-confidence, self-acceptance, and body image. Decreased ability to function or loss of a limb has a catastrophic, sudden impact. Patients usually feel very vulnerable to being injured and, as such, are quite ready to explore ways to prevent injury to themselves and to their loved ones. Once the initial crisis is past, it is an excellent time for patients to recognize and incorporate safety and prevention methods into their life-style.

PRIMARY SURVEY

The *primary survey* is the first examination of the patient and essentially includes the ABCs of cardiopulmonary resuscitation. At the same time, perfusion to the brain and tissues is assessed by the level of consciousness and peripheral circulation. The primary survey, then, is a rapid (about 30 seconds) assessment of cardiopulmonary function.

Name _____ Date _____
Transport mode _____ Time _____
T _____ P _____ R _____ BP _____ Trauma score _____
Chief complaint: _____
_____
HISTORY OF ACCIDENT: _____
_____
TRAUMA: Single _____ Multiple _____ Site _____
   Abrasion _____ Laceration _____ Hematoma _____ Puncture _____ Poss Fx/Dis _____
BLEEDING: Site _____
   Minimal _____ Moderate to steady _____ Hemorrhage _____ Occult _____
BURN: Site _____
PAIN: Minimal _____ Constant _____ Moderate _____ Severe _____
   Description _____
HISTORY: Cardiac _____ Diabetes _____ Neurological _____ Pulmonary _____
   Hypertension _____ Epilepsy _____ Other _____
CURRENT MEDICATIONS: _____
   Taken at _____
IMMUNIZATIONS: Yes _____ No _____ Last tetanus toxoid _____
ALLERGIES: _____
PRIOR TREATMENT: Oxygen _____ IV fluids _____ Sandbags _____ Dressing _____
   Splint _____ Ice _____ Medications _____ Other _____
GENERAL APPEARANCE: _____
_____
VITAL SIGNS: Temp _____ Pulse: Rate _____ Quality _____
   Blood pressure _____ Respirations: Rate _____ Quality _____
SKIN: Normal _____ Pale _____ Cyanosis _____ Jaundice _____ Dry _____ Moist _____
   Edema _____ Turgor _____ Rash _____ Ecchymosis _____ Abrasions _____
   Lacerations _____ Other _____
HEAD AND NECK: _____
NEUROSENSORY:
   L.O.C. _____ Coma score _____
   Oriented to time _____ Place _____ Person _____
   Verbal
     No response _____ Clear _____ Slurred _____ Appropriate _____ Confused _____
     Inappropriate words _____ Incomprehensible sounds _____
   Eye opening
     Spontaneously _____ To speech _____ To pain _____ None _____
   Motor response
     Obeys _____ Purposeful _____ Semi-purposeful _____ Localizes _____
     Flexion _____ Extension _____ Flaccid _____
   Weakness/Paralysis
     Site _____
NOSE AND MOUTH: _____
CHEST:
   Aeration: Rate _____ Rhythm _____ Pattern _____
   Chest wall _____ Lungs _____
   Artificial airway _____ Chest tubes _____

Figure 40–1

Sample assessment sheet.

SECONDARY SURVEY

The *secondary survey* is a more complete examination of the patient. It is a rapid, hands-on assessment that should take only a few minutes to complete. There are two primary objectives: to assess and treat life-threatening injuries, and to identify injuries that require emergency treatment and stabilization. After the secondary survey, a thorough diagnostic evaluation can be performed. The following sections describe the assessment steps for the secondary survey in a head-to-toe assessment.

General Overview

In order to make a more accurate assessment of the patient as a person and to obtain an impression of the effect of the trauma on the patient, several factors are noted immediately on beginning to care for the patient. These are degree of distress; odor of breath, clothes, skin, and urine; body position and spontaneous activity; speech (normal, slurred, or absent); affect, mood, and thought organization; and appearance (facial expression, general nutrition state, hygiene, and manner of dress).

Head, Neck, and Face

Only the most pertinent points are assessed. The guiding principles are look, feel, and listen. The following are assessed:

- Cervical spinal integrity assessment includes asking the patient whether he hurts and moving the examiner's hand

CIRCULATORY: AP _____ R.P. _____ B.P. _____
PMI _____ Neck veins _____

Heart sounds: S$_1$ _____ S$_3$ _____ murmurs _____ S$_2$ _____ S$_4$ _____

Peripheral pulses: carotid   brachial   radial

             R   _____   _____   _____

             L   _____   _____   _____

                     femoral   tibial   pedal

             R   _____   _____   _____

             L   _____   _____   _____

EXTREMITIES:
  Impairments
    Circulatory _____
    Soft tissue _____
    Neurological _____
  Deformities
    Fractures _____
    Dislocation _____

LABORATORY:
  Hgb _____ Hct _____ RBC _____ WBC _____ Na _____ K _____ CO$_2$ _____ Cl _____
  BUN _____ Glucose _____ PT control _____ pt _____ PTT control _____ pt _____ Urine _____

DIAGNOSTIC:
  ECG _____
  CT scan _____
  Other _____

Figure 40-1 *(Continued)*

down the cervical spinal area for any tenderness, spasm, or deformities. A cervical spinal injury is suspected in all patients in whom one is possible with the mechanism of injury and in all unconscious patients with head injury. The patient's neck should be splinted until an injury is ruled out by radiographic examination. Figure 40-2 shows a radiograph of a patient with a cervical fracture.

- Level of consciousness and coma scale. As the patient moves about on the examining table or stretcher, intracranial pressure levels will not change significantly.
- Pupil size, shape, equality, reactivity to light, and symmetry; eye position; visual acuity; orbital ecchymosis; and red conjunctivae
- Scalp depressions, contusions, or lacerations. Blood loss is estimated.
- Mastoid process and orbits for collected blood. A blue tympanic membrane indicates blood collection behind the membrane.
- Discharge from nose or ears. Any fluid present is tested for the presence of sugar.
- Facial bone deformity. The patient's bite is assessed. The mouth is checked for drainage, obvious lacerations, foreign bodies, and broken teeth.
- Pertinent cranial nerves
- Respiratory pattern
- Any response or posturing to painful stimuli

Chest

Any potential chest injuries are treated immediately. Assessment is often performed simultaneously with treatment. Time is not wasted waiting for further diagnostic study if life-threatening chest injuries are present. Whether the paramedic, physician, or nurse is performing the secondary survey, the points of assessment are the same. The following areas should be assessed:

- Neck veins are assessed for filling. If possible, the patient is placed at a 30° angle. If neck veins are distended, the patient is likely in pump failure from tension pneumothorax, myocardial contusion, air embolism, pericardial tamponade, or

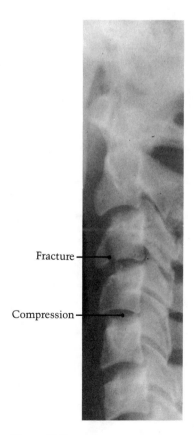

Fracture —

Compression —

Figure 40-2
Radiograph showing cervical spinal fracture.

myocardial infarction (Table 40–1). If the neck veins are flat, the patient is likely in hypovolemic shock and in need of volume replacement.

- The trachea is assessed for position and motion.
- The clavicular area is felt for pain, hematoma, deformity, and subcutaneous emphysema.
- The sternum and rib cage are felt for pain, tenderness, deformity, and symmetry.
- Chest symmetry during breathing. With paradoxic movement, the patient likely has a flail chest. With asymmetric movement, the patient likely has a pneumothorax or hemothorax.
- The chest wall is assessed for intactness or contusions.
- Breath and heart sounds. The examiner should listen for absent or reduced breath sounds, bronchial sounds where vesicular sounds should be, adventitious sounds, muffled heart sounds, murmurs, and extra heart sounds.
- Peripheal pulses are assessed for rate, rhythm, and quality.
- An electrocardiogram (ECG) should be obtained.

With hypovolemia, two large-bore peripheral lines are placed for volume replacement. A MAST suit is applied for patients with massive pelvic fracture and intra-abdominal hemorrhage, continuing blood loss, and systolic blood pressure less than 70 mm Hg to 100 mm Hg. Open chest wounds should be covered with petrolatum, gauze, and tape. A flail chest should be splinted with a sand bag, an intravenous bag, or a similar weight. A tension pneumothorax must be treated immediately. A needle or intravenous catheter inserted in the second intercostal space in the midclavicular line or in the fourth intercostal space laterally on the affected side will relieve the pressure.

Abdomen

Assessment of the abdomen in a conscious patient, especially after blunt trauma, may help pinpoint the injury. The following steps are recommended:

- Any trauma below the fourth to fifth intercostal space should be considered as potential thoracoabdominal injury.
- Contusions, lacerations, masses, increased vascularity, and distention. Any distention should be monitored with serial measurements to assess any increase. Notify physician immediately of any increase.
- Femoral, tibial, and pedal pulses
- The patient should be asked to point to any area of pain or discomfort. Auscultate for bowel sounds and then lightly palpate all four quadrants of the abdomen. Palpation should be started in nontender areas and moved toward the area of pain. The patient's sides should be inspected for any discoloration caused by bleeding into the peritoneal cavity. Point tenderness, guarding, rigidity, softness, and muscle spasm should be assessed (Fig. 40–3).
- If palpation over symphysis pubis or ischium elicits any complaints of pain, notify physician and be suspicious of possibility of pelvic fracture, lumbar spine fracture, or bladder trauma.

Back

- Spinous processes. The examiner's hand is run under the patient's back and the spinal processes are felt. A separation or compression (usually at the L1-L2 level as depicted in Fig. 40–4) often can be felt as a difference in spacing. Adequacy of sphincter tone can be assessed on rectal examination.
- Any obvious wounds
- Bilateral level of sensory and motor loss

Pelvis

- The iliac crest and symphysis pubis should be felt gently. Any pain or abnormal movement is noted.
- The urinary meatus should be checked for the presence of blood.

Table 40–1
Pump Failure

LIFE-THREATENING POSSIBILITY	CLINICAL SIGNS
Tension pneumothorax	Trachea deviated away from injury
	Absent or unilateral breath sounds
	Hyperresonance or tympany on injured side
	Cyanosis
Myocardial contusion	History of extrication from motor vehicle
	Dysrhythmias associated with myocardial infarction
Air embolism	Penetrating trauma or fractured ribs that may lacerate lungs
	Altered sensorium and local or lateralizing neurologic signs present in patient with chest injury and no sign of head injury
Pericardial tamponade	Patient in shock, no evidence of blood loss
	High central venous pressure
	Narrow pulse pressure
	Decreased blood pressure
	Distant and muffled heart sounds
	Paradoxic pulse
	Radiograph shows bigger heart, and fluroscopy shows diminished cardiac pulsation
Myocardial infarction	Chest pain, pallor, tachydysrhythmias, bradydysrhythmia, extra systoles, gallop rhythm, pulmonary rales, diaphoresis

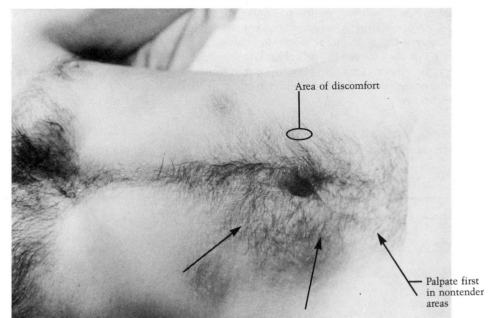

Figure 40-3

Abdominal assessment. If patient complains of pain or discomfort, palpate first in nontender areas and move toward the area of pain. Assess point tenderness, guarding, rigidity, and muscle spasm. Any pain in the splenic region should be reported to the physician. The spleen should not be palpated or percussed, because the injured spleen is fragile and might rupture.

- The rectum should be assessed for the presence of blood and for sphincter control.

Extremities

Assessment of the extremities is important in preventing loss of both life and limb. A significant amount of blood can be lost externally or hidden internally. Each extremity should be checked and then compared with the other. The following points are important:

- Color, size, length, temperature, and symmetry of extremities
- Brachial, radial, femoral, popliteal, and pedal pulses
- Deformities. Any areas of crepitus should not be pressed; the physician should be notified.

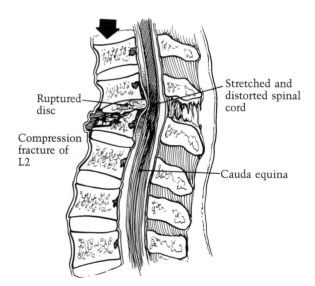

Figure 40-4

Compression fracture of first lumbar vertebrae.

- Open wounds and closed trauma
- Sensation and motion
- Reflexes
- Position and range of motion

Diagnostic Tests

Further study is performed as indicated by the patient's condition. Blood is drawn for complete blood count, serum electrolytes, blood glucose, blood urea nitrogen, creatinine, amylase, type and crossmatch, platelet count, prothrombin time, partial thromboplastin time, and toxicology screen. Arterial blood gases are often assessed. A urine specimen is sent for analysis. Radiographs often include cervical spine, skull, face,

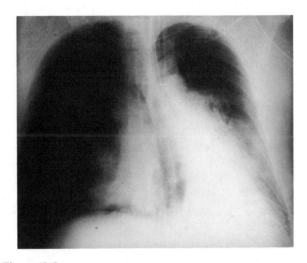

Figure 40-5

Radiograph of patient with tension pneumothorax showing increased volume of air that is producing pressure. With clinical signs of distended neck veins, deviated trachea, hyperresonance, decreased blood pressure, and cyanosis, the physician will perform chest decompression with a needle or intravenous catheter and not wait for a diagnostic radiograph.

chest, abdomen, intravenous pyelogram, and cystogram. Figure 40–5 documents the presence of tension pneumothorax on radiograph. Other diagnostic tests often ordered by the physician include paracentesis, peritoneal lavage, computed tomographic scan, and arteriography.[9] Although tests other than arteriography are being used, it is still an excellent tool for visualization.

NURSING DIAGNOSES, PATIENT OUTCOMES, AND NURSING ORDERS

The preceding material on anatomy, physiology, nursing assessment, and diagnostic tests guides the nurse in establishing nursing diagnoses, patient outcomes, and the plan for the patient with trauma.

NURSING CARE PLAN SUMMARY   The Patient With Trauma

NURSING DIAGNOSIS

1. *Impaired gas exchange related to obstructed airway (exchanging pattern)*

Patient Outcomes	Nursing Orders

1. The patient should maintain an adequate airway.	1. Assess consciousness.
	A. Call for help.
	B. Position the patient properly.
	C. Establish airway.
	    (1) Do head tilt and chin lift.
	    (2) Do head tilt and neck lift.
	    (3) Do jaw thrust.
	D. Perform mouth ventilation.
	E. Clear esophageal airway.
	F. Perform abdominal thrusts.
	G. Do tonsil suction.
	H. Refer to Chapter 16 for details of intubation.

2. The patient should demonstrate adequate oxygenation.	2. Assess arterial blood gases.

NURSING DIAGNOSIS

2. *Decreased cardiac output related to hemorrhage, shock, or traumatic condition (exchanging pattern)*

Patient Outcomes	Nursing Orders

1. Cardiac output will return to normal range.	1. Open airway.
	A. Ensure breathing.
	B. Maintain circulation.
	C. Carry out definitive therapy.[4,5]
	D. Apply pressure to hemorrhaging sites. External hemorrhage is best controlled by direct finger pressure on the bleeding wound or vessel. Application of pressure to major pressure points may also be used. A tourniquet is used only when too few medical personnel are available to institute higher-priority measures. If the exposed vessel is accessible, it can be ligated. Wounds should not be probed, because probing may dislodge a clot. The nurse should observe the nasogastric and Foley catheter drainage and measure the girth of the neck, abdomen, and thighs, as indicated, to watch for an increase in size.
	E. Perform a rapid assessment to determine the presence of critical injuries and to establish priorities. The following should be differentiated:
	    (1) Injuries or conditions that interfere with vital physiologic function and thus are an immediate threat to life
	    (2) Injuries that are not an immediate threat to survival
	    (3) Injuries that produce occult damage

(continued)

NURSING CARE PLAN SUMMARY   *The Patient With Trauma*   *Continued*

Patient Outcomes	*Nursing Orders*

Nursing Orders

F. Assess for a spinal fracture. All patients should be treated as though they had a fracture until proven otherwise.

G. Place patient in recumbent position.

H. Begin oxygen by nasal prongs.

I. Assess and record blood pressure, pulse, respiration, skin condition, urinary output, and sensorium every 15 to 30 minutes or more often if indicated.

J. Restore an adequate circulating volume. Ringer's lactate solution is given initially in amounts up to 2 L and then continued at the rate of 10 ml to 25 ml/kg/hour. Signs of adequate resuscitation are listed in Table 40–2. Blood is replaced as indicated by the degree of loss.

K. Have a clot sent to the blood bank for typing and crossmatching for 6 U to 8 U.

L. Send samples for a complete blood count, amylase, arterial blood gases, and urinalysis.

M. Obtain electrocardiogram and monitor continuously.

N. Place Foley catheter unless blood is present at meatus or a perineal or scrotal hematoma is present.

O. Monitor intake and output.

P. Place a nasogastric tube unless vascular injury is present.

Q. Perform a complete physical examination.

R. Cover any open wounds.

S. Splint fractures.

T. Elevate legs if necessary. Deep Trendelenberg position interferes with respiratory exchange, but passive leg raising may be beneficial. However, study of normal volunteers has shown that passive leg raising does not produce a sustained effect on stroke volume.[8]

U. Apply MAST suit per physician order to control internal hemorrhage, immobilize fractures, or provide an autotransfusion.
   (1) Unfold MAST suit and lay it on the stretcher. Attach foot pump and open stopcocks.
   (2) Place patient on MAST suit so that the upper section is just below the lowest rib. Wrap and secure Velcro on both legs.
   (3) Using foot pump, inflate all three chambers simultaneously until Velcro crackles or air comes through relief valves and systolic blood pressure is stable.
   (4) Close stopcocks, and remove hose and pump.
   (5) Recheck and monitor blood pressure (parameter by which blood pressure is controlled while hemorrhage is controlled by trouser pressure).

V. Once condition is stable, the MAST suit is deflated over a period of 15 to 30 minutes as ordered.
   (1) The suit essentially provides an autotransfusion of about 2 L of blood; the reverse is true when it is removed.
   (2) Before removal of the suit, have two intravenous infusions running.
   (3) Obtain baseline vital signs.
   (4) Deflate the abdominal portion.
   (5) Monitor vital signs for 5 to 10 minutes. If pulse increases and blood pressure decreases, infuse 100 ml to 200 ml of intravenous fluid.
   (6) Deflate one leg of the suit. Monitor vital signs for 5 to 10 minutes. If one sees signs of shock, administer intravenous fluid until patient stabilizes.
   (7) Deflate the other leg. Monitor vital signs for 30 minutes.

2. The patient will be free of complications.

2. Use adjunct parameters as ordered.
  A. Set new priorities.
  B. Administer tetanus prevention.

(continued)

NURSING CARE PLAN SUMMARY   *The Patient With Trauma*   *Continued*

NURSING DIAGNOSIS

3. *Altered tissue perfusion related to trauma (exchanging pattern)*

Patient Outcome	*Nursing Orders*

The patient should demonstrate a stable physiologic response.	1. Monitor for stable physiologic response in the following areas:
	  A. Monitor apical heart beat for rate and heart sounds every 30 minutes.
	  B. Monitor temperature, apical and radial pulses, respirations, and blood pressure as indicated.
	  C. Assess mental status every hour.
	  D. Monitor hourly urine output. Notify physician if it is less than 0.5 to 1 ml/hour.
	  E. Assess respiratory system, including rate, rhythm, breath sounds, and presence of adventitious sounds every hour.
	  F. Connect ECG monitor and set alarms for 30 beats above and below baseline. Notify physician of any abnormalities.
	  G. Obtain a 12-lead ECG as indicated.
	  H. Note arterial pressure measurement on the monitor and monitor every 30 minutes. Check the pressure with a cuff every 2 hours. If an arterial line is not present, check the pressure every 30 to 60 minutes as indicated. Notify physician for pressure less than 90 mm Hg.
	  I. Draw arterial blood gases as indicated. Monitor oxygenation.
	  J. Measure pulmonary artery and central venous pressure every hour.
	  K. Observe for any other signs of peripheral vasoconstriction.
	  L. If ordered, measure the pulmonary capillary wedge pressure and cardiac output by thermodilution every 4 hours.
	  M. Every 15 minutes, check orifices for bleeding. Mark dressings.
	  N. If a vascular injury is present, note the color and presence of pulse in distal extremity. Use Doppler.
	  O. If the possibility of injury exists, perform serial assessments of neck, abdomen, or extremities with tape measure.
	  P. Monitor and assess trends in laboratory data.
	  Q. Weigh daily.
	  R. Determine the patient's temperature during surgery. Postoperative rise in temperature is often related to the drop in temperature during surgery.

NURSING DIAGNOSIS

4. *High risk for injury (cervical spinal fracture) related to forces exerted during hyperflexion, hyperextension, or compression injury (exchanging pattern)*

Patient Outcome	*Nursing Orders*

The patient will be treated as having a spinal cord injury until a fracture can be ruled out by radiographic examination and the patient will be free from additional injury.	1. Maintain patient in supine position during assessment. Support head to prevent twisting of neck.[7]
	  A. Use a semirigid collar for patients with suspected cervical injury.
	  B. Use a long spinal board for patients with suspected vertebral fractures.
	2. Assess neurologic status.
	  A. Establish level of consciousness. Use Glasgow Coma Scale.
	  B. Identify level of neurologic deficit.
	    (1) Record sensation.
	    (2) Record muscle strength.
	    (3) Record reflexes.
	  C. Repeat neurologic examination frequently.
	  D. Check rectal sphincter tone and perianal sensation.
	3. Order radiographs of the following per physician order:
	  A. Cervical vertebrae

(continued)

NURSING CARE PLAN SUMMARY   *The Patient With Trauma*   *Continued*

Patient Outcome	*Nursing Orders*
	(1) Obtain lateral cervical spine radiograph first. All seven cervical vertebrae must be seen. This may require firmly pulling the shoulders down and a lateral swimmer's view.

    (1) Obtain lateral cervical spine radiograph first. All seven cervical vertebrae must be seen. This may require firmly pulling the shoulders down and a lateral swimmer's view.
    (2) If lateral view is normal, obtain an anteroposterior view.
    (3) Obtain open-mouth (odontoid) view for conscious patients.
  B. Thoracic vertebrae
    (1) Obtain lateral and anteroposterior views.
    (2) View all 12 vertebrae.
  C. Lumbar vertebrae
    (1) Obtain lateral and anteroposterior views.
    (2) View all five vertebrae.
4. Provide initial care per orders.
  A. Immobilize the patient. Protective devices (*i.e.*, cervical collar, spinal board) must not be removed until radiographs are obtained.
  B. Administer intravenous fluids.
  C. If movement is necessary, log roll patient.
  D. Catheterize bladder.
  E. Use nasogastric intubation.
  F. Administer corticosteroids.
5. Assess respiratory status.
  A. Maintain patency of airway.
    (1) Use jaw thrust.
    (2) Apply suction.
    (3) Administer supplemental oxygen.
    (4) Monitor arterial blood gases.
    (5) Use nasotracheal intubation.
  B. Assess respiratory effort.
  C. Assess circulation and treatment of hemorrhagic shock. Hypotension and a slow pulse may not indicate blood loss from some other injury.
  D. Assess general medical status.
    (1) Obtain description of accident
    (2) Obtain information about patient's medical history and present drug therapies.
    (3) Perform general physical examination.

REASSESSMENT

Treatment of the trauma patient requires reassessment on a continuing basis. Initially, many conditions may not be apparent or may not have developed.

The magnitude of blood loss can generally be assessed from the response to rapid administration of Ringer's lactate and the avoidance of uncrossmatched blood.

A quick and thorough assessment of the chest for such lower airway problems as hemothorax, pneumothorax, tension pneumothorax, and pericardial tamponade is rapidly undertaken, and the problems are treated. Initially, thoracoabdominal injuries take precedence over orthopedic and most neurologic injuries. An orderly examination of the patient and appropriate radiographs are instituted as the therapy of shock continues. The response to the initial use of Ringer's lactate permits the assessment of severe or continuing blood loss. Such an approach eliminates the contributions of gastric dilatation, obstructing respiratory or cardiovascular lesions, or pain to the picture of shock from blood loss.

Vascular injuries are seen frequently with penetrating trauma, but they may occur as a result of blunt trauma either associated with fractures or as an isolated problem secondary to the fracturing of atheromatous plaques. Table 40–2 gives guidelines for adequate signs of fluid resuscitation. Assessment is important and should begin with a baseline examination.

Table 40–2

Clinical Assessment: Signs of Adequate Resuscitation

Increased blood pressure and decrease pulse to within a normal range
Increased sensorium
Urine output greater than 0.5 ml/kg/hr
Improved peripheral perfusion
Preload increased, *i.e.*, central venous pressure, 3 cm H_2O–8 cm H_2O and pulmonary capillary wedge pressure, 4 mm Hg–12 mm Hg
Improved cardiac output, greater than 3.5 L/min
Increased pH

In particular, the presence or absence of pulses and bruits is noted. The presence of a cold, pulseless extremity with threatened viability constitutes an acute emergency, and valuable time is not wasted with sophisticated diagnostic studies. The surgeon often consults a vascular surgeon. Distal pulses may be palpable in the presence of proximal injuries, including complete occlusion. Potential vascular injuries are not probed or digitally examined because uncontrollable hemorrhage may ensue if a clot is inadvertently dislodged. Doppler examination is used to determine distal flow. The appearance of a bruit may indicate an arteriovenous fistula or external compression of the vessel because of soft-tissue swelling. Its disappearance may be misleading if a clot forms between the two injured vessels. If the extremity is not in jeopardy, arteriography and venography are used by the surgeon before surgery.

Orthopedic injuries initially have a low priority in the polytrauma patient with life-threatening problems. Any splinting done in the field should be maintained in all cases of fracture or dislocation. Extensions that can be added to emergency department stretchers facilitate stabilization of the extremity. When it is necessary to delay surgical attention to an open fracture, the bones are splinted and the wound is covered with sterile dressings and left intact. Antibiotics are begun.[16] Frequent assessment of the circulation to the digital segment of the injured limb is performed and recorded. Thorough examination is performed at the time of operation. In most instances, dislocated joints are reduced rapidly. Frequently, reduction is accomplished under local anesthesia in the emergency department. Radiographs are usually taken before and after reduction. Neurovascular monitoring by the nurse before and after reduction is mandatory.

The assessment of hand injuries is made under sterile conditions. The extent of skin loss and injury is determined by inspection. Damage to tendons, nerves, and arteries is best assessed by a functional examination of the digits without wound probing. Bleeding from the wound is controlled by pressure and elevation. There is not an attempt to clamp arteries. Amputated parts are cleansed under sterile conditions, wrapped in a sterile, saline-soaked gauze, placed in a sterile plastic bag, and then covered with ice or refrigerated until surgical replantation. Radiographs of both the amputated and remaining parts are obtained to assess the extent of bone and joint damage.

MAST Suit

The MAST suit (pneumatic antishock trousers, MAST trousers, military antishock trousers, or pneumatic compression device) is a commonly used adjunct in the management of shock. The trauma team must assess patients for the need for application of the suit and the response to application. The MAST suit is used to restore blood pressure in patients with systolic blood pressures below 70 mm Hg to 100 mm Hg, improve tissue circulation, and control internal hemorrhage. The response to application of the MAST suit is assessed by the reason for application. For example, the patient's blood pressure is the parameter used for assessing restoration of blood pressure. An increase in blood pressure or a systolic pressure of approximately 110 mm Hg is usually the desired outcome. In hemorrhage control, the parameter assessed is usually trouser pressure. Because bleeding cannot be seen, an indirect parameter must be assessed and monitored.

With the application of the MAST suit, compression on the legs and abdomen squeezes blood out of the venous and capillary systems and returns it to the heart, brain, and lung circulation. Increased pressure on the arterial system increases peripheral resistance and prevents pooling of blood. The external pressure produced by the MAST suit is complementary to the body's release of norephinephrine and epinephrine. It is as if the patient received an instant blood transfusion of up to 200 ml or 30% of the blood volume from the abdomen and lower extremities. In other words, it is thought that the patient receives an *autotransfusion*. Importantly, this autotransfusion can occur within 1 to 3 minutes, whereas a transfusion of blood or an infusion of Ringer's lactate solution may require at least 15 to 30 minutes.

Emotional Impact

Patients are often in a state of panic and disbelief. New things happen before they are able to assimilate what has just transpired. The physician relies on the nurse to assess the need for and to carry out these interventions. On admission, the patient is often in dire distress, and all the mental and physical capacities of the physician are focused on the patient's condition. The physician expects the nurse to share the assessment and diagnosis process, just as the physician will do with the nurse. The two roles are dependent on one another; as such, the nurse and physician working together can provide better patient care than when they are working separately.

The power of the resolution of panic is well recognized by all working in emergency situations, but it is rarely implemented in the actual critical patient situation. Just as the patient has trouble thinking clearly, it is quite possible that the team members have trouble thinking clearly unless situations have been role-played previously and algorithms have been provided.

Swearingen,[18] an orthopedic surgeon in Colorado, noted over a period of time that some injured skiers brought down off the mountain slopes were not in such a state of panic as many other skiers and did not have as much pain. On further investigation, he found out that these skiers had been rescued by one particular team. On even more investigation, he found out that this team used simple but very effective skills when finding the injured skiers. They used touch, relaxation measures, and generally helped the person through the experience. By the time the skiers were in the rescue station, they were ready to start dealing with the effects of the injury and their recovery.

Perhaps no one is as aware of the importance of helping someone deal with panic as a former patient. Cousins[6] writes of an experience with another human being and how, as a bystander turned responder, he helped that human being deal with panic:

Similarly, being in a speeding ambulance with the siren in full cry can be harmful and even devastating in itself. This is not to ignore or minimize the need for prompt care; it is only to emphasize the need to give at least as much attention to the patient's emotional needs as to his or her physical condition.

Let me cite a specific. . . . The paramedics, working systematically and methodically, were attending to their duties but no one was talking to the man. He was ashen and trembling. I looked at the cardiograph monitor. It revealed what is termed a tachycardia—a runaway heart rate. The intervals on the monitor were irregular. I also looked at the

Table 40-3

Sample Instruction Sheet to Be Given to Patient (and Family) Who Can Be Sent Home but Must Be Carefully Observed for Potential Head Injury

You have had a head injury that is not severe enough to require hospitalization, but be sure to follow these guidelines:

1. Be sure someone (family or friend) stays with you. They should be sure that you stay alert. They should check your breathing and pupils every 2 hours for 12 hours and then every 4 hours for the next 12 hours.
2. Take only aspirin for headache or discomfort. Consult the emergency department before taking any other medicines you may have at home.
3. Take only clear cold liquids for 8 hours (no milk). For the next 24 hours, you may take reduced amounts of food.
4. Have limited activity for 24 hours. Do not go to work.
5. In a small number of cases, signs of serious injury may appear later; return for your appointment.
6. If any of the following things happen, you should consult the emergency department immediately:
   A. Nausea or vomiting
   B. Unusual sleepiness or difficulty awakening. (Someone should be sure you stay alert. You should be awakened from sleep every 2 to 3 hours during the period of sleep or during the first night.)
   C. One pupil much larger or different from the other; peculiar movements of the eyes or difficulty in focusing (blurred vision)
   D. Weakness, paralysis, or numbness of arms or legs, peculiar gait, stumbling
   E. Mental confusion or disorientation (excessive drowsiness, inattentiveness, incoherent thought, change in personality, inability to concentrate, stupor)
   F. Irregular or labored breathing
   G. Persistent dizziness

paramedics, who, true to their training, were efficiently attending to the various emergency procedures. But no one was attending to the patient's panic, which was potentially lethal.

I put my hand on his shoulder. "Sir," I said, "You've got a great heart."

He opened his eyes and turned toward me. "Why do you say that?" he asked in a low voice.

In Oliver Wendell Holmes' phrase, I "rounded the sharp corners of the truth" with my reply. "Sir," I said, "I've been looking at your cardiograph and I can see that you're going to be all right. You're in very good hands. In a few minutes, you'll be in one of the world's best hospitals. You're going to be just fine."

"Are you sure?" he asked.

"Certainly. It's a very hot day and you are probably dehydrated. The electrical impulses to the heart can be disrupted when that happens. Don't worry. You'll be all right."

In less than a minute, the cardiograph showed unmistakable evidence of a slowing down of the heartbeat. The gaps between the tall lines began to widen; the rhythm began to be less irregular. I looked at the man's face; the color began to return. He propped up his head with his arms and looked around; he was taking an interest in what was happening.

Patient Education

The nursing role in trauma assessment is truly multifaceted. Perhaps no one else on the trauma team is expected to perform in so many different roles. The patient educator may be called on to instruct anyone from the severely traumatized patient to the patient who will be sent home with instructions. It is the responsibility of the nurse to make a quick assessment of the patient's and family's general understanding and present the information at a level they can understand. Written instruction sheets for patients who will be sent home are an invaluable aid (Table 40-3).

Air Transportation

Over the past several years, patient transport by air ambulance has become an accepted procedure. Assessment is important before, during, and after flight (Fig. 40-6).

Helicopters are usually used for initial rapid transport in much the same way as mobile critical care units are used over shorter distances. They tend to be noisy and have high vibration and turbulence levels. Both helicopters and fixed-wing aircraft are used for patient transfer over longer distances to

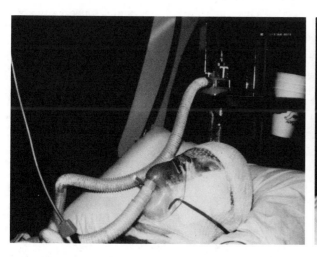
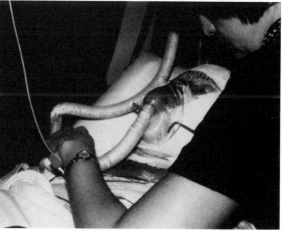

Figure 40-6

Critically ill patient being transported by air ambulance to regional center. (*A*) Patients with potential pulmonary injury should receive supplemental oxygen. (*B*) Although space is limited, the nurse performs a continuing clinical assessment. A portable bedside monitor is used to visualize the electrocardiogram, and the Doppler is used to hear the pulse and blood pressure.

Table 40–4
Aircraft Characteristics

AIRCRAFT	ALTITUDE	AIR SPEED	RANGE	RUNWAY DISTANCE
Rotary wing				
Helicopter	10,000 ft	120 mi/hr	150 mi	50 ft^2
Fixed wing				
Propeller	25,000 ft	200 mi/hr	1000 mi	3000 ft
Jet	40,000 ft	500 mi/hr	1300 mi	4000 ft

the regional trauma center after stabilization at the local hospital (Table 40–4 compares aircraft characteristics).

Fixed-wing aircraft require landing strips, whereas rotary-wing aircraft may land anywhere, commonly on the hospital's parking lot. Jet-propulsion aircraft fly at altitudes between 20,000 and 45,000 feet and can avoid turbulent weather. Propeller aircraft fly at lower altitudes and may not be able to fly over turbulent weather. The aircraft cabin should be pressurized so that the pressure in the cabin is equivalent to that at a lower altitude. Because helicopters fly at lower altitudes, pressurization is not needed; as a matter of fact, helicopters used as air ambulances rarely fly at a greater altitude than 1000 feet. The physiologic effects on the transported patient are primarily determined by the altitude of the air ambulance and are described in the following sections. The nurse must be aware of the potential pathophysiologic effect on the patient, prevent as much of the effect as possible, and continually assess the patient's status during flight.

Oxygenation

As the actual or cabin altitude varies, the partial pressure of oxygen varies. Dalton's law predicts the change. It states that *the pressure exerted by a mixture of nonreacting gases is equal to the sum of the partial pressures of the separate components.* At sea level (760 mm Hg), normal inspired oxygen tension is 159 mm Hg, providing an alveolar oxygen tension (PaO_2) of 107 mm Hg. At 8000 feet (560 mm Hg), inspired oxygen tension is 116 mm Hg, providing a PaO_2 of 59 mm Hg. Therefore, ambient pressure at 8000 feet is considered the maximum cabin altitude that provides adequate inspired oxygen tension levels for normal passengers (Table 40–5). Injured patients, especially those who already have a compromised respiratory situation, are in a particularly precarious position and need supplemental oxygen even at a pressure that is satisfactory for normal passengers. Take, for example, the patient with chest injury and pulmonary contusion with a resulting large shunt fraction and marginal arterial oxygenation. Shock and blood loss hinder oxygen availability at the tissue level still more. Any reduction in available oxygen will result in an even greater decrease in

arterial oxygenation and a potentially life-threatening situation. Therefore, all patients with chest injury should be transported with 100% oxygen delivered by mask or endotracheal tube. Patients with ocular injuries will also need supplemental oxygen because of the high oxygen use by the retina.

Gas Volume Changes

As the pressure of a gas decreases, the volume increases. This relationship is stated as Boyle's law: *At a constant temperature, the volume of a gas varies inversely with the pressure.* During ascent from sea level to a cabin altitude of 8000 feet, a volume of gas will expand approximately 50%. During descent, a similar contraction of volume is expected. It is important that the nurse predict these changes and prevent any serious complications that may result.

Air in any body cavity can enlarge and precipitate problems. Patients with even a small pneumothorax should not be transported by air until they have undergone either a closed-tube thoracotomy or a needle decompression. A Hemlich valve of the flutter type or waterseal drainage should be attached. Because any intra-abdominal air will expand, placement of a nasogastric catheter is mandatory to prevent acute gastric dilatation, vomiting, and subsequent aspiration. In patients suspected of having air embolism after a chest injury, increased altitude can cause an exacerbation of clinical signs and symptoms. Air bubbles in the cerebral circulation can enlarge. The nurse should assess the patient for altered sensorium, paresthesias, and paralysis.

Problems with ear blockage or sinus squeeze usually occur on descent. Normally, equilization of middle ear air volume occurs through the eustachian tube. With trauma and swelling around the eustachian tube orifice, the eustachian tube may remain closed. Usually air exits through the eustachian tube without difficulty on ascent, but because the air in the middle ear contracts on descent, the tympanic membrane may retract as a middle ear vacuum develops. Damage to the tympanic membrane or ossicles may occur. A similar situation exists with the sinuses, and sinus wall rupture may occur. Valsalva maneuvers may clear this mechanical obstruction.

Table 40–5
Oxygen Changes at Increased Altitudes

ALTITUDE LEVEL	ATMOSPHERIC OXYGEN (mm Hg)	ALVEOLAR OXYGEN (mm Hg)	ARTERIAL OXYGEN (mm Hg)
Sea level	159	107	98
2000	148	96	86
4000	137	84	80
6000	125	71	64
8000	116	59	55

Air-volume changes in patient care equipment must also be assessed and problems prevented. Changes in the endotracheal tube cuff may produce injury to the tracheal wall on ascent or leakage of air on descent. Large-volume, low-pressure endotracheal tube cuffs (and fluid-filled Foley catheter balloons) will negate problems of malfunction due to alterations in gas volume. Gas-volume variation in intravenous fluid administration may alter infusion rates, and constant assessment is required on ascent and descent to maintain desired flow rates. Air splints for stabilization of extremity fractures may produce circulatory impairment due to tourniquet effect with expansion of air unless vented during ascent.

Acceleration and Deceleration

The rapid attainment of adequate speed for takeoff and the steep climb after takeoff may produce physiologic effects by volume redistribution. A similar but lesser effect may occur from speed reduction on landing. A patient with hypovolemia or cerebral edema may suffer deterioration of that condition with redistribution of intravascular volume. Proper positioning of the patient can minimize the effects of acceleration or deceleration forces. The head-forward position is better to prevent cerebral congestion, and the feet-forward position is better to prevent cerebral hypoperfusion.

Relative Humidity

Evaporative losses from the patient increase during air travel owing to the decreased relative humidity. Compensation by providing warm humidified air aids in preventing dry respiratory secretions. The patient has an increased need for fluids. Careful assessment of intake and output during flight is necessary, because increased fluid administration may be needed on long flights. Moist protective wound dressings to decrease evaporative wound losses and moist eye pads or artificial tears for cornea protection in comatose patients are important considerations for local care to prevent further injury from the dry atmospheric conditions.

SUMMARY

Assessment of the traumatized patient is a challenge to everyone on the health team. With the polytrauma patient especially, maintenance of vital functions is essential. The assessment process is a systematic evaluation of the patient's injuries to determine the urgency of therapy and to identify hidden injuries. The primary survey identifies immediate life-threatening injuries. An obstructed airway is a grave danger to the traumatized patient. It probably causes more deaths than does any other malfunction. In the secondary survey, high-priority injuries are identified.

REFERENCES

1. Aprahavin, H. R., Thompson, B. M., Towne, J. B., *et al.* The effect of a paramedic system on the mortality of major intra-abdominal vascular trauma. *J. Trauma* 23(8):687, 1983.
2. Baker, S. P., O'Neil, B., Heddon, W., *et al.* The injury severity score: A method for describing patients with multiple injuries and evaluating emergency care. *J. Trauma* 44:187, 1974.
3. Champion, H. R., Gainer, P. S., and Yackee, E. J. A progress report on the trauma score in predicting a fatal outcome. *J. Trauma* 26:927, 1986.
4. Chaudry, I. H., Sayeed, M., and Baue, A. E. Depletion and restoration of tissue ATP in hemorrhagic shock. *Ann. Surg.* 108:208, 1974.
5. Condon, R. E. Post-splenectomy sepsis in traumatized adults. *J. Trauma* 22:169, 1982.
6. Cousins, N. The Healing Heart: Antidote to Panic and Helplessness. New York: Norton, 1983.
7. Demetriades, D. Cardiac wounds: Experience with 70 patients. *Ann. Surg.* 203:315, 1986.
8. Gaffney, C. V., Bastian, N. C., Thal, E. R., *et al.* Passive leg raising does not produce a significant or sustained autotransfusion. *J. Trauma* 22:190, 1982.
9. Gomez, G. A., Alvarez, R., and Plasencia, G. Diagnostic peritoneal lavage in the management of abdominal trauma: A reassessment. *J. Trauma* 27(1):1, 1987.
10. Hammond, B. B., Gough, J. E., Allison, E. J., *et al.* Case review: Flail chest. Management implications for emergency nurses. *J. Emerg. Room Nurses* 13:330, 1987.
11. Hartford, J. M., Fayer, R. L., and Shaver, T. E. Transection of the thoracic aorta: Assessment of a trauma system. *Am. J. Surg.* 151:224, 1986.
12. Hebler, R. F., Ward, R. E., Miller, P. W., *et al.* The management of splenic injury. *J. Trauma* 22:492, 1982.
13. Keene, A. R., and Cullen, D. J. Therapeutic scoring system: Update. *Crit. Care Med.* 11:1, 1983.
14. McSwain, N. E. The management of multiple injury. *Emerg. Med.* 16(4):56, 1984.
15. Morris, J. A., Auerbach, P. S., and Marshall, G. A. The trauma score as a triage tool in the pre-hospital setting. *J.A.M.A.* 256:1319, 1986.
16. Nelson, R. M., Benitz, P. R., and Newell, M. A. Single antibiotic use for penetrating abdominal trauma. *Arch. Surg.* 121:153, 1986.
17. Stevens, S., and Becker, K. How to perform a picture perfect respiratory assessment. *Nursing '88:* January, 1988.
18. Swearingen, R. L. A humanistic approach to the management of fractures. *Today's Clinician:* February, 1978.
19. Trunkey, D. The value of trauma centers. *Am. Coll. Surg. Bull.* 67:5, 1982.

41

Abdominal Trauma

Kathleen MacKay White   *Cornelia Vanderstaay Kenner*

LETTING GO

What gives meaning to your life? What is your purpose in being alive? Exploring meaning and purpose is at the core of the ordinary process of peaceful being. Taking time for yourself is a must. Relaxation, imagery, and music can facilitate your receptiveness to new possibilities. They may also assist you in the process of releasing your worries, fears, pain, and attachment to the ego.

To learn the skills, you must have daily practice in letting go of attachments to what is right and wrong, what is good and bad. Each time you hear your inner voice judging yourself for what you are doing wrong or that you aren't working hard enough, release the judging; just listen, and be ready for the next moment of listening, of being in the present moment. Being present in silence to listen to your inner wisdom is essential for peace in your life and work. The practice of releasing your ordinary fears and emerging with awareness and openness for the present moment is the healing. This is also the skill that assists you in being more present when caring for others during recovery from illness or when assisting another during death.

LEARNING OBJECTIVES

After analyzing and synthesizing the information in this chapter, the reader should be able to collect the appropriate information about the patient who has had abdominal trauma, assess the injuries, assist and collaborate with the physician, make the nursing diagnoses, plan interventions for the patient, implement the plan, and evaluate the patient responses to care. The nurse should be able to do the following:

1. Compare and contrast the initial findings and the patient's clinical course with regard to the type of abdominal injury.
2. Identify the physiologic mechanisms of shock.
3. Determine the positive findings in abdominal paracentesis and peritoneal lavage.
4. Assess the extent of injury of a patient who has had a gunshot wound.
5. Determine the priorities for a patient with abdominal trauma.

CASE STUDY

Mr. T., a 28-year-old man, was admitted to the emergency room on an ambulance stretcher. He had been rabbit hunting, and while he was climbing over a fence, his .22-caliber rifle had discharged. The bullet struck his right thigh. During the trip to the hospital, the ambulance driver lost control of the vehicle, and the ambulance was in an accident.

According to Mr. T.'s wife, before the accidents, Mr. T. was in excellent health. He had not been drinking, nor had he taken any medications for 12 hours before his injury. She also said that after the ambulance accident, Mr. T. had complained of pain in his right thigh and abdomen. She said that Mr. T. had no known allergies and that his last tetanus booster was about 5 years ago. Mrs. T. seemed to be a reliable informant.

The paramedics who had attended Mr. T. at the scene of the accident noted that he was pale, his skin was cool, his blood pressure was 90/60 mm Hg, his pulse was 120 and faint, and his respirations were 24 and nonlabored. Mr. T. was restless, and he complained of thirst and abdominal pain. Abdominal palpation revealed guarding. He had a gaping wound on the lateral aspect of his right thigh, moderate, nonpulsatile bleeding, and obvious debris in the wound. Mr. T was oriented with regard to time, place, and person; he answered questions appropriately but somewhat irritably. The paramedics treated Mr. T. immediately for shock, giving him Ringer's lactate solution. Before moving Mr. T., the paramedics stopped the bleeding in his thigh wound by direct pressure and a compression bandage. Stability of the femur was achieved by splinting the leg with minimal manipulation.

During his trip to the hospital, Mr. T. became apathetic. He complained of feeling exhausted and chilly, and then he became difficult to arouse. An oral airway was inserted and oxygen was administered during the trip.

Emergency Room Examination

The following observations were made during the emergency room examination:

General appearance: A well-developed, well-nourished man admitted on a stretcher.

Respiratory system: Spontaneous breathing with an airway in place. Rate 28 and depth increased. Chest excursions symmetrical bilaterally. Breath sounds normal with no rales or wheezes.

Cardiovascular system: Carotid pulse thready, regular, and 120. Radial and femoral pulses not palpable. Systolic blood pressure 80 (diastolic pressure was not obtainable). Capillary refill in nailbeds slow. Big toe was cool to touch. ECG showed sinus tachycardia but no dysrhythmias.

Neurologic system: Patient extremely difficult to arouse by verbal command. Pupils equal in size; reacted briskly with consensual response. Eye movements spontaneous and random. Painful stimuli applied to sternum evoked prompt avoidance response. No pathologic reflexes present. Tendon reflexes 2+ in all extremities, except the right, which was deferred.

Gastrointestinal system: No penetrating injuries to abdomen. No abdominal distention. Bowel sounds absent. Gastric contents, obtained by way of nasogastric tube, negative for blood.

Integument and musculoskeletal system: Skin cold, ashen to cyanotic; circulation response to pressure blanching very sluggish. Peripheral pulses imperceptible. Right thigh swollen; tissue about the open wound appeared crushed and nonviable. Compound fracture of the femur in midportion of diaphysis.

Genitourinary system: Genitalia appeared normal. Catheterization and urinalysis showed no hematuria.

Emergency Room Management

An oral airway remained in place. Mr. T. was appraised as being in hypovolemic shock. A large-bore (16-gauge) catheter was inserted into his right arm. The intravenous infusion into his left antecubital vein was continued. Blood samples were obtained for a complete blood count, electrolyte, glucose, urea, and amylase studies, and typing and crossmatching. A radial artery puncture was performed for arterial blood gas analysis.

Fluids were given rapidly (2 liters of Ringer's lactate solution given in 45 minutes). After the rapid infusion of fluids Mr. T. showed a transient improvement, as indicated by his improved sensorium (he responded to his name and to commands), a rise in blood pressure (to 100/60 mm Hg), and a decrease in pulse (to 100). No urine was obtained. During the improvement in Mr. T.'s hemodynamic state, the circulation to the right lower extremity was verified. His pedal pulses could be heard with the Doppler relative flow ultrasonic amplifier.

The results of bilateral peritoneal flank taps were negative for non-clotting blood. Consequently, a peritoneal lavage of 1 L of Ringer's lactate solution was begun. The results were negative.

Mr. T.'s thigh wound was irrigated repeatedly with several liters of normal saline solution. Exploration of the wound, ligation of vessels, and removal of foreign materials were postponed until the wound could be inspected adequately during surgery. Packing the wound with sterile gauze and applying hand pressure brought the bleeding under control. A Thomas splint was used to stabilize the femur.

As prophylaxis, Mr. T. was given 0.5 ml of tetanus toxoid booster and started on 2 g of cephalothin sodium (to be given intravenously six times an hour). A Levine tube was placed.

Continued monitoring showed no urinary output. Mr. T.'s abdomen was not distended, and his bladder was not palpable. A new catheter was inserted, but urine was not recovered from his bladder. An intravenous pyelogram showed no excretion of contrast media from either kidney. Angiography confirmed the presence of bilateral renal artery thrombus secondary to disruption of the intima of the renal arteries.

Surgery

Exploratory surgery was carried out. It revealed bilateral renal artery thrombosis with no pulsations in the artery distal to the point of trauma. The area of intimal injury in the right renal artery was resected, and the renal artery was anastomosed. Pulsatile flow through the arterial tree was good. The traumatized area in the left renal artery was resected, and an incontinuity vein graft was inserted to bridge the defect. Pulsatile arterial flow was reestablished.

The thigh wound was incised and debrided widely, and the necrotic tissue was removed. Muscle tissue that was considered nonviable was also removed. Foreign material and blood clots were removed by irrigation to avoid a nidus for infection. The wound was left open to drain. A Steinmann pin was inserted under strict aseptic conditions. Balanced surgical traction using a Thomas splint with a Pearson attachment and 25 pounds of weight was to be employed postoperatively to stabilize the fractured femur.

When Mr. T. arrived in the critical care unit, his vital signs were T 97, P 98, R 18. His respirations were easy and even. He was awake, and his responses were appropriate. The arterial pressure monitor registered his blood pressure at 100/68. Analysis of an arterial blood sample taken from the radial artery catheter site showed PaO_2 97 mm Hg, pH 7.41, $PaCO_2$ 39 mm Hg, and delta base + 1. Mr. T.'s peripheral pulses were strong, and his urine was pink. He was receiving 1000 ml of Ringer's lactate solution, and his third unit of whole blood was running.

Clinical Course

Mr. T. remained in the critical care unit 7 days, and then he was transferred to the surgical unit. He had no complications. His vital signs remained stable, he was alert, and his urinary output was normal. He began to eat and drink. Supplemental alimentation had been discussed, but it was not needed because his protein and calorie intake was satisfactory. Sepsis was identified as a potential problem, and the medical team gave meticulous wound care and was alert to the environmental factors that could produce wound contamination. Mr. T. was given the same attentive care on the surgical unit. Mr. T. and his family were receptive to all teaching programs, and they helped with several volunteer projects. Mr. T. was discharged 6 weeks after his injury.

REFLECTIONS

Although there are times when the instability of the patient becomes the highest priority, there are also many times when trauma patients can be stabilized quickly and the examination and studies can be performed in a more orderly fashion. When time and the priorities allow, the nurse should seize the opportunity to carry out a very important step in trauma care: explanations of what has happened and of what is about to occur. Not only do patients need to know about what will happen procedurally, but they also need to know what sensations they will experience. The process is called *sensory education.*

Sensory education and systematic desensitization are similar processes. However, the former evolved from nursing and the latter from the psychological discipline. Differences in intent and terminology therefore exist, while procedurally and in outcome, the result is virtually identical in that the patient is less anxious during treatment. The notion of sensory education or sensory information has been most widely developed and published by Johnson and her colleagues.[31] Sensory education carries patient education beyond the typical boundaries of procedural explanations. It provides what is probably more important to the patient, namely, how the treatment is going to feel, smell, sound, or taste, and what he or she can expect to experience (the key word) in the new or threatening event. The usual process of explaining procedures to patients identifies what medically is going to be done and why, but normally details about the private experience are not dealt with, leaving the patient potentially anxious and fearful. In looking experimentally at the effects of sensory information, Johnson and colleagues provide a variety of convincing data. The techniques were used in controlled experimentation with patients about to undergo cholecystectomy, laboratory-induced ischemic pain, cast removal, pelvic examination, and endoscopy. By a variety of subjective and objective measures, the sensory-conditioned patients responded better to treatment, even to the extent of significantly decreasing postoperative hospital days. When relaxation was added to sensory education, the results of Johnson and colleagues were consistently superior.

The nurse explains to the patient the importance of understanding how a new procedure will feel and what to expect. The session is presented as a time for information giving and, if possible, is preceded by a relaxation exercise. In all probability, it will help to tell patients that the session will allow for less pain or help them cope. First, breathing instructions are coupled with focusing on relaxation of the major muscle groups with the intention of synchronizing the total system and blotting out room noises. The patient is taken on an imaginary trip through the x-ray procedure. Emphasis is placed on the patient's participation. One of the best ways to present the information is to use an audiotape played by cassette recorder. Tape-recorded instructions are valuable because they provide a standardized format, controlling for variations in instructions and individual voice inflections; they provide a means of automating the process, since individually administered relaxation instructions are not feasible in a busy emergency department/critical care unit; they provide the opportunity for independence, autonomy, and self-reliance in a situation in which passive dependency is reinforced; and they offer a protocol for systematic investigation. Typical statements on the tape are, "The steel table feels cold and hard when you move onto it. In the x-ray room, the technicians put a light on over you and it's warm and feels good, but it's pretty bright. The sound of the machine moving is like a door closing. The smell is a lot like that of a hospital, rubbing alcohol and disinfectant." The total approach is to balance an honest description, which allows the patient to predict the experience, with a simultaneous downplaying of emotionally laden words and expressions.

The goals are to desensitize patients to fearful events, to give them alternate words and emotions for their fear and discomfort, to make them aware beforehand of the sensations they will perceive, and generally to carry them through the procedure in a relaxed state.

ETIOLOGY AND INCIDENCE

Trauma accounts for approximately 150,000 deaths annually in the United States, is the fourth leading cause of death, and is the leading cause of death in persons under the age of 44.[9] Trauma is the cause of almost 50% of deaths in the under-4 age group and of 80% of the deaths in the 15- to 24-year age group.[39] Trauma is known as the disease of the young.[57]

The economics of trauma is staggering. There are more than 70 million nonfatal injuries per year, of which 10.5 million involve disability beyond the day of the accident. Trauma patients make up almost 25% of an emergency department's census and one third of all hospital admissions, and they occupy approximately 12.5% of hospital beds at any given time.[39] With an estimated loss of more than 4 million years of future work life, the direct and indirect economic losses are estimated to be between $75 and $100 billion annually.[9]

To appreciate the frequency of specific causes of trauma, refer to Table 41–1, the Committee on Trauma statistics on the major causes of trauma deaths in the United States. To anticipate the frequency of specific types of injuries likely to occur as the result of a motor vehicle accident, refer to Table 41–2.

Although abdominal trauma occurs less frequently than trauma to the head, chest, and extremities, it is accompanied by these injuries 70% of the time. When abdominal injury is accompanied by other injuries, the mortality rate increases according to the number of associated injuries: abdominal injury alone, 13% mortality; abdominal and chest injury, 40% mortality; abdominal, chest, and head injury, 87% mortality. Abdominal organs are vulnerable to the injuring mechanisms of blunt, penetrating, crushing, compressive, and decelerative trauma that result from motor vehicle accidents, industrial accidents, gunshot and knife wounds, sports, fights, and falls. Penetrating injury affects the small bowel and liver most frequently, whereas blunt trauma most often injures the liver and spleen.

Table 41–1

Major Causes of Trauma Deaths in 1982 in the United States

TYPE OF INJURY	TOTAL DEATHS	FREQUENCY (%)
Motor vehicle	44,786	30
Firearms	32,988	22
Falls and jumps	13,013	9
Drowning	7353	5
Poisoning	7226	5
Burns	5904	4
Suffocation, hanging	6000	4
Cutting	2791	3
Carbon monoxide	2791	2
Other	22,895	15

(Committee on Trauma, Commission of Life Sciences, National Research Council, Institute of Medicine. *Injury in America*. Washington, DC: National Academy Press, 1985.)

Table 41-2
Frequency of Various Injuries in Motor Vehicle Accidents

LOCATION OF INJURY	FREQUENCY (%)
Extremities	34
Head and neck	32
Chest	25
Abdomen	15

(Waller, J. A. *Injury Control: A Guide to the Causes and Prevention of Trauma.* Lexington: Lexington Books, 1985, p. 222.)

PATHOPHYSIOLOGY

Blunt and Penetrating Abdominal Trauma

The spleen, liver, and colon are injured more often because they are close to the abdominal wall. The pancreas, located deep in the abdominal cavity, is well protected by the stomach, colon, and diaphragm, so it is injured much less often. The colon may be injured by penetrating trauma or by blunt injury; for example, in an automobile accident, the steering wheel may compress the bowel against the vertebral column with the result that a loop of intestine is first closed off, then ruptured by forceful, continued compression.

Deceleration forces, particularly in motor vehicle accidents and falls, may tear organs from their points of fixation. For example, the liver may be torn from the inferior vena cava, the spleen from the splenic pedicle, the bladder from the bladder neck, and the kidney from the renal artery and vein.[36] In-driven fractures are known for injuring certain organs, with the spleen vulnerable to a left lower rib fracture, the liver to a right lower rib fracture, the kidney to a posterior floating rib fracture, and the bladder to a pelvic fracture. A patient who has one or more of these fractures should be evaluated carefully; a force strong enough to produce a fracture is strong enough to produce an intra-abdominal injury.

Trauma is managed according to the general category, blunt or penetrating. The reason for the distinction is that blunt trauma often is complicated by associated injuries that may make both diagnosis and identification of the involved organs more difficult. One of the most important factors in positive patient outcome in multiple injury is prompt recognition of intra-abdominal trauma.

In blunt trauma, solid organs such as the spleen, liver, and kidney tend to be injured. Hollow organs, such as the colon and bladder, are also vulnerable to blunt trauma, especially when they are distended.[55] With a blunt injury, an exploratory laparotomy may seem the most logical solution, but exploratory laparotomy, which is relatively safe for a healthy person, may be extremely risky for a patient with multiple injuries. These patients frequently have associated injuries to their cardiorespiratory system, nervous system, or musculoskeletal system.[11] They also may be inebriated or suffering from a head injury, and therefore are unable to verbalize symptoms such as pain. If abdominal trauma is suspected in a patient, the physician carefully weighs the risks of operating against the risks of not operating. Subjecting the patient to surgery and its risks is a decision that has not become routine.

With penetrating injuries, there are usually no associated head or chest injuries and, therefore, fewer factors to complicate a decision to operate. In general, laparotomy is the treatment of choice. However, there are exceptions. With stab wounds, because the results of routine exploratory laparotomy are often negative, the patient is assessed carefully and thoroughly before surgery is performed. Fixed organs tend to be more vulnerable to stab wounds. The colon may escape penetration by the knife blade because of the bowel's ability to "slide out of the way."[25]

The nurse who has cared for a patient with multiple abdominal injuries who has then developed complications probably knows how frustrating these injuries can be with regard to nursing care and the patient's recovery. Probably the most notable feature of abdominal trauma is that it can be extremely difficult to manage. There are many reasons:

1. Injuries to the abdominal structures subject the patient not only to hemorrhage or organ death, but also to the release into the peritoneal cavity of potent digestive enzymes that produce additional injury by digesting the neighboring organs.
2. The virulent bacterial contents of the bowel may be spilled into the peritoneal cavity, thus subjecting even uninjured structures to bacterial invasion and cell death. Sepsis is a particular danger when this occurs.
3. The release of some organ excretions, even ones that are not enzymatic, may result in collections of fluid that provide excellent culture media for the development of abcesses.
4. Abdominal trauma often involves the loss of the patient's digestive functions and, depending on severity, may result in a continuing catabolic state where nutritional deficits can be severe.

Splenic Injury

The spleen is injured more often than any other abdominal organ; it is involved in more than 25% of all intra-abdominal injuries.[55] Located in the left upper quadrant near the abdominal wall and under the diaphragm, the spleen is partly protected by the left lower ribs, but it is also vulnerable to these ribs when they are fractured. Twenty-five percent of patients who have a splenic injury have a fracture of the left lower rib. Splenic injuries are to be suspected in any type of blunt trauma, particularly after motor vehicle accidents, falls, bicycle accidents, and blows received in vigorous contact sports.

The danger of splenic injury is directly related to the spleen's high vascularity. The spleen is the most vascular organ in the body; it is perfused by more than 350 liters of blood per day. Small splenic tears and lacerations and ruptured splenic hematomas are sources of persistent and profuse bleeding into the peritoneal cavity. Massive amounts of blood may be lost into the intra-abdominal spaces, resulting in severe and sometimes fatal hypovolemic shock. Evidence of such bleeding depends on the amount of blood lost and the extent of peritoneal contamination.

Two types of injury occur after blunt trauma: splenic rupture and subcapsular hematoma. Rupture of the splenic parenchyma is the most common injury (occurring 85% to 90% of the time), and it is an emergency. Subcapsular hematoma occurs in 10% to 15% of cases; it involves trauma to the splenic tissue with subsequent local bleeding that is arrested by the thick (1- to 2-mm) capsule surrounding the spleen. The result is formation of a hematoma between the spleen and the capsule. The hematoma prevents immediate intraperitoneal bleeding, but it may be only temporarily benign. The capsule may yield to the expanding hematoma, and then the spleen ruptures. Delayed rupture may not occur for as long as 1 week to 10 days, during which time few if any signs or symptoms occur. It occurs very rarely and is now primarily attributed to delayed recognition of the rupture.[26]

Over the past decade, the therapeutic trend has moved away from splenectomy as the only treatment of choice in splenic trauma.[29] In the past, the risk associated with splenic repair (postoperative hemorrhage) was believed to outweigh any benefits that a preserved spleen could provide. Now, however, the spleen is recognized as an important immunologic structure that has a role in the production of opsonins, IgG, and tuftsin, all of which are necessary for combating encapsulated bacteria.[10] Also, alveolar macrophages, the phagocytic cells of the pulmonary alveoli, display depressed function in postsplenectomy patients. The asplenic patient has an exaggerated risk for early as well as delayed infection, and is vulnerable to overwhelming postsplenectomy sepsis (OPSS).[41] This syndrome is characterized by the rapid onset of a fulminating infection that can occur immediately or several years later (it has been known to occur 13 days to 25 years later) and carries a mortality rate as high as 80%. In half the cases, the offending organism is *Diplococcus pneumoniae*, with *Hemophilus influenzae* and *Neisseria meningitidis* accounting for the remainder of the infections. When the immunologic function of the spleen is combined with its role in filtering old red blood cells, platelets, and particulate matter, and with its role as a blood reservoir (contributing 150 ml of blood to the circulation in response to sympathetic stimulation), splenic preservation becomes a high priority in trauma management.[42,47]

Creative methods of repairing the spleen and securing hemostasis have been reported and include suture repair bolstered by omentum, application of topical hemostatic agents, and wrapping with absorbable mesh. These methods have increased the splenic preservation rate from 50% to 67%.[32,38,42]

With the diagnostic accuracy of abdominal computed tomography (CT), nuclear scan, ultrasound, and arteriography, attention has recently been directed toward nonoperative management of patients with splenic trauma.[7] In an experience with 832 splenic trauma patients in six trauma centers, one study showed that surgery could be avoided successfully (98% of the time in children, 83% of the time in adults) as long as no hemodynamic instability occurred, there were no associated abdominal injuries, and there were no extra-abdominal conditions that precluded ongoing abdominal assessment.[8]

Liver Injury

The overall mortality in liver trauma (approximate average, 10% to 15%) is attributable to massive intra-abdominal bleeding that occurs immediately after the injury, as well as to the late complications of delayed rupture, gastrointestinal bleeding, and sepsis.[55] The mortality rate is related to the severity of the liver injury and the number of intra-abdominal organs injured. For example, the mortality rate for patients with stab wounds of the liver is low (about 1%), but if significant liver trauma is associated with injuries to more than five intra-abdominal organs or if major hepatic resection is required, the mortality rate rises precipitously (to about 40% to 50%). Injury to the liver alone is usually classified I to V with I being the least (Table 41–3). Trauma to the liver may result in three types of injury:

1. The liver capsule may rupture. This is the most common type of liver injury, and it results in loss of blood and bile into the peritoneal cavity and is immediate evidence of peritoneal contamination.
2. A subcapsular hematoma may form. Like a hematoma of the spleen, it may be essentially undetectable on the patient's admission to the hospital, only to rupture spontaneously several days later. Bleeding from the delayed rupture can be fatal.
3. An intrahepatic hematoma may form. This too is an occult injury that can cause major complications later, with extensive tissue necrosis, abscess formation, and erosion of hepatic vessels with bleeding into the bile ducts (hemobilia). When this occurs, large amounts of blood can be lost through the bile ducts, which drain into the duodenum, producing massive and sometimes fatal gastrointestinal bleeding.

Most liver injuries requiring surgery can be managed by simple techniques such as electrocautery, hemostatic agent application, simple suture repair, or perihepatic drainage. Complex liver injuries, however, carry a greater risk for hemorrhagic shock and higher mortality rates. In the past, surgical repair for complex injuries usually involved deep parenchymal suturing or formal hepatic lobectomy. In recent years, however, there has been a trend toward nonresectional techniques that involve hepatotomy with direct vessel ligation and limited debridement. Class V injuries remain the most difficult and

Table 41–3
Classification of Hepatic Injuries

CLASS	TYPE OF INJURY	SHOCK	MORTALITY
I	Capsular avulsion Parenchymal fracture < 1 cm deep		
II	Parenchymal fracture 1–3 cm deep Subcapsular hematoma < 10 cm diameter Peripheral penetrating wound		
III	Parenchymal fracture > 3 cm deep Subcapsular hematoma > 10 cm diameter Central penetrating wound	38%	25%
IV	Lobar destruction Massive central hematoma	46%	46%
V	Retrohepatic vena cava injury Portal vein injury Extensive bilobar disruption	85%	80%

can require emergency thoracotomy for the treatment of shock, perihepatic packing (usually with large laparotomy packs) when coagulopathy occurs after surgical repair, and early placement of caval shunts to prevent portal hypertension. The most frequent postoperative complications of 210 complex liver trauma patients reported by Cogbill et al.[8] were coagulopathy (16%), severe hyperpyrexia (11%), intra-abdominal abscess (9%), prolonged biliary leak (8%), late hemorrhage (7%), and hypoglycemia (4%). In another study[3] sepsis occurred in 12% of the patients and was associated with splenectomy, liver packing, colon injury, massive blood transfusion, and open (Penrose) drains.[3]

The surgical repair of all liver injuries once mandated placement of Penrose drains for the purpose of preventing perihepatic fluid collections and abscess formation. It is now believed that Penrose drainage is unnecessary and perhaps detrimental for class I or II injuries, and it is no longer recommended.[8] It is extremely important in complex liver injuries, however, to provide drainage of blood, plasma, and bile, but the drainage systems should be closed, such as Jackson-Pratt drains. Class IV and V injuries sometimes require large sump drains to allow the egress of blood and necrotic hepatic tissue.

With hemostasis and, where appropriate, adequate drainage, most liver injuries heal rapidly. The liver itself regenerates rapidly, but the healing process is impaired in the presence of bile. Although the exact mechanism is not known, the production of fibrinous exudate, the development of granulation tissue, and the production of the scar itself are impaired.

Liver Function During Shock

During shock and circulatory failure, the liver is at great risk. The primary chemical workhouse of the body, nearly 30% of the body's total blood flow, reaches the liver through the splanchnic circulation, three quarters of which originates in the portal system, with the remainder coming from the hepatic arteries. Both during and after shock, the findings in portal vein blood are hypoxia, hypercarbia, acidosis, elevated blood lactate, elevated ammonia, decreased portal oxygen saturation, and elevated portal venous pressure.

Liver Failure

When there is extensive damage, such as from high-velocity gunshot wounds, severe liver edema with necrosis and fibrosis formation may occur, followed by liver dysfunction and eventual liver failure. The edema, necrosis, and fibrosis interfere with the important complex functions of the liver by obstructing its two vascular systems, the portal system and its own blood supply system. (Together these systems circulate 1500 ml of blood/minute.) The obstruction not only compromises the function of individual liver cells, it also produces mechanical obstruction of blood flow through the portal system, resulting in a cascade of complications for the liver as well as the entire body.

Venous blood that leaves the abdominal organs (intestines, esophagus, stomach, and spleen) circulates through the portal system into the liver, where it undergoes complex metabolic changes. The most important of these processes are as follows:

- Carbohydrate metabolism, including gluconeogenesis and glycogen storage

- Protein metabolism, including the manufacture of most of the plasma proteins and detoxification of ammonia to form urea for excretion
- Fat metabolism, including the formation of lipoproteins and phospholipids
- The manufacture of important clotting factors, including fibrinogen, prothrombin, and factor VII
- The removal by the reticuloendothelial system (Kupffer's cells) of 99% of the bacteria that entered the portal system from the gut
- The formation of lymph
- The breakdown and disposition of bilirubin
- The manufacture of bile, which is necessary for digestion

In an extensive injury, all the functions just listed are affected. Blood flow through the hepatic vasculature is reduced, causing death to the liver cells. Carbohydrate metabolism is reduced, ammonia and bilirubin accumulate in the blood, and the manufacture of clotting factors, plasma proteins, lymph, and bile is severely impaired. Also, blood flow through the portal system is obstructed, resulting in portal hypertension. Bacteria accumulate and grow in the portal system as phagocytosis by the Kupffer cells is impaired. Increasing pressure in the portal system (from a normal of 8 to 30 mm Hg) causes fluid to shift from the vasculature into the interstitial and abdominal spaces (resulting in ascites). The fluid that transudates is almost pure plasma; it contains 80% to 90% as much protein as does normal plasma. The transudation, in addition to the reduced production of plasma proteins by the damaged liver, produces a profound loss of normal plasma oncotic pressure, followed by severe hypovolemia as fluid is lost (as edema) to the interstitial spaces. The increasing pressure in the portal system eventually causes passive congestion of the organs it drains (the spleen, intestines, and esophagus). The pressure causes dysfunction of these organs, just as it does of the liver.

In the later stages of liver failure, the patient shows jaundice, from the loss of the liver's ability to break down bilirubin; edema, from the loss of plasma proteins; volume depletion, from the loss of the plasma oncotic pressure; hemorrhagic tendencies, from the loss of the liver's ability to manufacture clotting factors; anemia, leukocytopenia, and thrombocytopenia from hypersplenism; and fever and sepsis from bacterial invasion through the unguarded portal system.

Small Bowel Injury

The small bowel can be injured by both penetrating and blunt trauma. It is the organ most commonly injured in penetrating trauma. Typically in blunt trauma that occurs in an automobile accident, a sudden forceful blow to the midabdomen by a steering wheel forces the bowel against the vertebral column. When the bowel is compressed suddenly, the intraluminal pressure rises quickly. If the loop of bowel is pinched closed by the vertebral column or other structures, rupture results. Two other mechanisms are also common: crushing or pinching of the bowel between the spine and a blunt object, usually the steering wheel, and a tangential shearing force exerted on an immobile portion of the bowel.

With small bowel injuries, surgery usually consists of simple suture repair. However, when perforation, rupture, thrombosis, or necrosis is extensive, the surgeon must undertake bowel resection and anastomosis. Postoperatively, the patient has a number of gastrointestinal tubes—namely, nasogastric, gastrostomy, or jejunostomy—which are designed to decompress the bowel, reduce tension on the suture lines, and drain the small bowel secretions, enzymes, blood, and bile. Nasogastric suction is maintained for 5 to 7 days. Ample Penrose drainage is included to ensure the removal of fluid and prevent abscess formation. Skin excoriation due to drainage must be prevented. Suction is maintained on the duodenostomy tubes until peristalsis returns. The tube is then placed to dependent drainage for about 2 weeks.

Complications that occur postoperatively can cost a great deal in terms of time, morbidity, and patient morale and comfort. Immediately postoperatively, large extracellular volume deficits may occur as a result of edema and the translocation of fluid into a nonfunctional "third space" in the injured bowel wall and irritated peritoneum. Electrolyte imbalances can be severe when gastrointestinal suction and decompression are prolonged. If large amounts of the small bowel have been removed, malabsorption syndromes may result, making normal nutrition difficult to achieve. Finally, poor blood supply to the repaired bowel, infection, tension on the suture lines, or distal obstruction can cause fistulas to form in the small bowel, peritoneal cavity, or drain tracts. When this occurs, the mortality increases, since leakage of the small bowel contents into the peritoneal cavity increases the probability of sepsis. Attention to the details of supplemental nutrition has greatly decreased the incidence and complications previously seen with small bowel fistulas.

Renal Injury

Most renal injuries are the consequence of blunt trauma, but about one fourth of renal admissions are for penetrating injuries that involve the kidney or urinary bladder. A major blunt injury to the kidney or other genitourinary structure is usually accompanied by an injury to another abdominal organ. Consequently, the sign of an injury to the other organ often masks the renal injury and delays or prevents its diagnosis. Because the incidence of renal injuries is third only to the incidence of splenic and liver injuries, the health team must have a high index of suspicion of renal trauma and must diligently assess all patients who have abdominal trauma.[5,11]

The kidney responds to blunt trauma with contusions, hematomas, stellate tears, lacerations, fractures, and avulsions of either pole or diffuse rupture and fragmentation (Fig. 41–1). Much like the spleen, the kidney is covered by a capsule that may arrest bleeding and so cause the formation of a subcapsular hematoma. These hematomas, however, do not tend to expand but rather resolve spontaneously over a period of weeks.

High-velocity gunshot wounds of the kidney deserve special mention because of the complications that can occur postoperatively. The temporary cavity formed by a high-velocity missile produces crushing trauma to renal tissue several centimeters from the wound tract. The crushed renal tissue may seem viable at the time of repair, but later may deteriorate because of microthrombus formation, internal elastic tissue breakdown, hemorrhage, acute inflammation, and thrombotic occlusion of the small vessels with eventual anoxia, necrosis, or bleeding. Profuse hematuria and delayed bleeding, evidenced by falling serial hematocrit and hemoglobin levels,

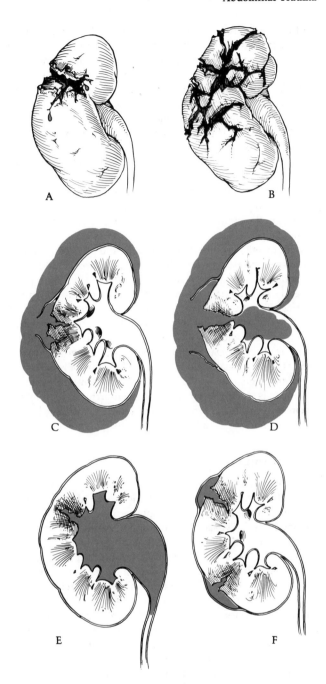

Figure 41–1

Examples of renal injuries. (*A*) Capsular rupture. (*B*) Fragmentation. (*C*) Hematoma from cortical laceration. (*D*) Hematoma from cortical laceration with renal pelvis laceration. (*E*) Renal pelvis hematoma. (*F*) Subcapsular hematomas from cortical laceration.

signal the presence of this type of delayed development. Nephrectomy is often required.

Tears or lacerations in the outer parenchyma that do not invade the collecting system (the calyx) usually cause minimal bleeding and can be treated with suture repair or Penrose drainage. Once the collecting system has been invaded, however, extravasation of urine into the peritoneal spaces or around the kidney provides an excellent environment for bacterial growth and invites infection and abscess formation. Suture repair of the renal parenchyma or of the collecting system, and ample Penrose drainage of extravasated urine, are necessary. If there is extensive damage to the upper collecting system (the calyx or the upper ureter), a nephrostomy tube may be inserted to drain urine from the calyx until the edema subsides and healing has begun. In this way, the perils of an obstructive nephropathy may be avoided.

After blunt trauma to the kidney, most patients (80%) do not require surgery. Bed rest, forced fluids, monitoring of vital signs, blood tests, and antibiotic therapy are the usual therapeutic measures needed and are followed by clearing of the hematuria and loss of the flank pain. Failure of the conservative approach is indicated by sustained or rising fever, increased leukocytosis, persistent or increasing pain and tenderness in the kidney region, and evidence of secondary renal hemorrhage.

With extensive blunt kidney trauma, the physician usually selects a surgical approach. More serious injuries are indicated by shock requiring blood transfusion, increasing flank mass or tenderness, damage or occlusion visualized on arteriogram, and significant extravasation seen on intravenous pyelogram (IVP). With simple stab wounds of the kidney, conservative treatment with close observation is seen. With gunshot wounds, the physician usually chooses exploration. However, indications for renal exploration, nephrectomy, or renal repair continue to be a subject of controversy. When nephrectomy is done, it is usually because of renal hemorrhage. Many physicians now try to prevent or control renal hemorrhage before exploration in order to improve the salvage rate.

Bladder Injury

Most bladder injuries are the result of blunt trauma of considerable force, usually from automobile accidents. Twenty percent of bladder injuries are intraperitoneal and 80% are extraperitoneal. Typically, intraperitoneal rupture occurs when the bladder is distended and full, and a substantial blow is delivered to the lower abdomen. A full bladder is more susceptible to injury than an empty one. The pressure of the blow is transmitted to the dome of the bladder, structurally the weakest portion of the bladder wall. Rupture in this location allows urine to escape into the peritoneal cavity, and it may produce a serious peritonitis. Besides intraperitoneal rupture, the bladder is vulnerable to extraperitoneal rupture when torn by in-driven fragments of a fractured pelvis (usually the symphysis pubis or the superior or inferior rami). Although this type of injury is not attended by the perils of peritoneal contamination, there may be blood loss or extravasation of urine into the surrounding tissue.

After surgical repair of the bladder, decompression to ensure continuous drainage of urine and to prevent accumulation of urine (which might interfere with wound healing) is provided by a suprapubic cystostomy tube in males and a urethral catheter in females. Bladder drainage is maintained for 10 to 14 days.

Ureteral Injury

Injuries to the ureter are rare, and they are hard to detect early in their course.[5] Sometimes they are discovered during a diagnostic workup for another injury (usually an IVP), but more often they are not recognized until flank pain, fever, and infection develop.

Injured ureters are repaired by debridement and reanastomosis. When the ureteral injury is determined, reconstructive repair must be carried out to prevent hydronephrosis from ureteral stricture and to drain the intra-abdominal collections of extravasated urine; the potential of postoperative stricture is great. All gunshot wounds are stented because of the potential infection from associated colon trauma and overall extent of injury, whereas stab wounds heal well without a stent. On rare occasions, patients who have suffered extensive penetrating trauma will have lost large segments of the ureter. In these patients, complicated reconstructive surgery involving anastomosis of the viable end of the ureter to the other ureter (ureteroureterostomy), reimplantation of the ureter into the bladder (ureteroneocystostomy), or mobilization of the kidney with its short viable ureter closer to the bladder for reimplantation may be undertaken.

Renal Pedicle Injury

Because of the magnitude of blood flow into and out of the kidney, an injury to the renal pedicle (artery and vein) must be treated immediately to save the patient's kidney (and sometimes the patient's life). Pedicle injuries are caused five times more often by penetrating trauma than by a blunt, decelerating force. In high-speed motor vehicle accidents, the sudden halt in rapid forward motion exerts a shearing force on the vessels of the renal pedicle. The layers (intima, media, adventitia) of the vessel's walls may be sheared, torn, or even completely avulsed from the relatively mobile kidney as the kidney continues its forward motion away from the more stationary aorta. Renal arteries that are torn or damaged can easily thrombose, resulting in rapid ischemia or death of the kidney. A laceration or avulsion of the renal pedicle is life-threatening in that it may involve the loss of massive amounts of blood.

Colon Injury

The colon may be injured by both blunt and penetrating trauma, but penetrating injuries are more frequent. Injuries to the colon can be more serious than injuries to the small bowel, because the contents of the colon are more virulent and its blood supply is less abundant. Because of the virulence of the spilled contents of the colon, it is extremely important that intravenous antibiotics be administered as soon as possible.[52]

Recently, the trend with penetrating colon injuries has been toward the avoidance of colostomy.[14] Primary repair and intra-abdominal placement are usually undertaken with minor tissue injury, few associated injuries, minor fecal contamination, injuries less than 6 hours old, and a stable patient. When the preceding favorable conditions for placement of the injured colon back into the abdomen are not present, exteriorization of the colon suture lines may be performed.[56] Technical details that enhance success of exteriorization include adequate debridement, mobilization of the injured section of colon, and postoperative maintenance of moisture (petroleum jelly gauze or saline soaks). The exteriorized colon is usually replaced in the abdominal cavity about the tenth postoperative day. Gunshot wounds are much more likely to cause extensive injury than stab wounds. They are usually the injuries that require resection. However, at least half the patients will heal with exteriorization, and the patient is not subjected to colostomy or to the risk of intraperitoneal leak that may attend primary repair. For patients who have more severe injuries, are unstable, have associated injuries, or have head injuries, a temporary colostomy is usually done.

With a diverting colostomy and delayed closure, the virulent colonic contents are diverted from the wound so that the anastomosis is protected and decompression is ensured.[54] The movement of fecal material is under control, and the danger from leakage, peritoneal contamination, and stress on the repaired segment of bowel is minimized. A diverting colostomy has two stomas (double barreled); one is located proximal to the wound to divert fecal material from the wound, and the other represents an exteriorization of the area of wounded colon. The ideal diverting colostomy should provide immediate complete diversion of the fecal stream, be constructed so that it can be easily closed, be free from postoperative complications, and be aesthetically acceptable to the patient and produce minimal psychological distress. Depending on the extent of bowel damage, the colostomy may be closed as early as 2 to 3 weeks after injury or as late as 1 year after injury. Although some questions have evolved concerning the high morbidity associated with temporary colostomy, a recent report has shown much lower incidence of complications when details are carefully observed.[54] Patients received a preoperative barium enema and preoperative mechanical bowel preparations, and some patients received preoperative antibiotics. After bowel anastomosis and peritoneal closure, most patients had delayed closure of the subcutaneous tissue and skin in an effort to prevent infection. No drains or wound antibiotics were needed.

Postoperative complications are usually related to continued fecal soiling of the peritoneal cavity. Also, abscess formation, small bowel obstructions, bowel ischemia, gangrene, and stenosis can all result from the continued inflammatory process.[30] In these cases, another operation for abscess drainage, relief of obstruction, resection of more bowel, colostomy revision, and intra-abdominal irrigation with antibiotic solutions may be necessary.

Pancreatic Injury

Because of its rather protected retroperitoneal location, the pancreas is not often injured. Penetrating trauma is the most frequent cause of pancreatic injury, accounting for 70% to 80% of all cases.[55] Although the overall mortality is low, the morbidity for pancreatic injuries can be very high, owing to the chemical peritonitis that follows leakage of potent pancreatic enzymes into the peritoneal cavity. The mortality increases when there are associated injuries (usually the spleen, vena cava, or stomach, which are close to the pancreas).

Although the initial mortality for penetrating trauma is higher than that for blunt trauma, the complication rate is higher in blunt trauma because greater organ disruption usually occurs. The pancreas is particularly vulnerable to decelerating accidents because its retroperitoneal location and immobility make it unable to withstand decelerating, shearing stresses. As digestive enzymes are leaked by the injured pancreas into the peritoneal cavity, the signs and symptoms of peritonitis begin to appear. There are three basic mechanisms: impact forces concentrated to the right of the vertebral bodies, with the head of the pancreas crushed (also associated with hepatic lacerations, duodenal rupture, and biliary tract avulsion); impact concentrated at the midline, with pancreatic transection (associated injuries are frequently not present); and impact concentrated to the left of the vertebral bodies, with distal pancreatic contusions and lacerations (splenic injury is a frequent accompaniment).

Under normal circumstances, pancreatic secretions are inactive; they have no proteolytic activity until they are activated in the duodenum. A direct vascular injury, however, can activate trypsin and other substances which, in turn, activate the pancreatic enzymes. Activation of pancreatic enzymes results in autodigestion of the pancreas and surrounding tissues and varying degrees of edema, hemorrhage, coagulation necrosis, and fat necrosis. If the blood flow to the pancreas is reduced 40% to 60%, the resulting ischemia can convert edematous pancreatitis into hemorrhagic pancreatic necrosis. In both cases, large amounts of fluid may be lost, either as transudation from the swollen, edematous pancreas or as actual blood lost from a hemorrhagic pancreatitis.

During the low-flow state, probably because of the lack of adenosine triphosphate (ATP), deranged transmembrane potential, and drastically reduced blood flow, potassium and magnesium leave the cell, and calcium and sodium enter the cell. Ion shifts result in the loss of cellular and organellar volume control. Damage to lysosomal membranes probably occurs, and release of proteolytic enzymes leads to widespread cellular damage. The cell dies, releasing potentially toxic factors which then damage other cell membranes. The myocardial depressant factor that has been much talked about but never actually isolated has been thought to be of pancreatic origin. Additionally, because the pancreas has an important role in maintaining hepatic energy metabolism and both splanchnic and celiac blood flow, it has a prime role in the microcirculatory problems of the shock state.

Pancreatic injury due to penetrating trauma is approached with immediate exploration and operative repair. With blunt injury, however, the approach is more difficult for the surgeon to select. The procedure used for pancreatic injury depends on the type of injury. It ranges from simple drainage for laceration to a *roux-en-Y* pancreaticojejunostomy for pancreatic transection. In all cases, however, the single most important factor in the patient's recovery is adequate drainage of the leaking enzymes. Resection of devitalized tissue and wide drainage of the retroperitoneal space are employed. Because ductal reanastomosis is not possible, the surgeon must provide some means of ducting pancreatic secretions.

A pancreatic fistula results when a disrupted pancreatic duct does not heal and continues to pour enzymes into a fistulous tract that communicates with the peritoneal cavity and, sometimes, even with the abdominal wall. A pancreatic pseudocyst is a collection of pancreatic secretions surrounded by a fibrous wall. Not only is the collection of fluid an excellent medium for bacterial growth and abscess formation, it also produces an obstruction to the flow of enzymes through the ductal system.

Pelvic Fractures

Pelvic fractures have a mortality rate of 5% to 20%, which is usually the result of associated injuries and pelvic hemorrhage. Intra-abdominal organ injury accompanies pelvic fracture in 36% to 55% of the patients. Major pelvic bleeding occurs in about 3% to 5% of all fractures but accounts for one-half the mortality. Actively bleeding patients who have been involved in a pedestrian accident have a particularly high mortality. A great deal of soft-tissue injury as well as bone injury from the fractured pelvic ring (the pubic rami and ischium, ilium, sacrum, pubic symphysis, and sacroiliac joints) can be present. If the ilium is fractured, the internal iliac vein can be torn, with resulting extensive retroperitoneal hemorrhage.[27] Massive blood loss may require replacement of as many as 12 to 20 U of blood, and it is usually the underlying cause of profound shock. In one study of 245 patients with pelvic fracture, 50% to 60% of patients with unstable pelvic fracture required 4 or more U of blood; 30% to 49% required greater than 10 U.[13] However, many pelvic fractures can be mild and the healing course relatively benign. The fractures may even be difficult to detect by radiographs because the bones move very little and only a crack can be seen.

Trunkey and associates[57] have discussed pelvic fractures following crushing blunt trauma and have categorized them as either unstable or stable fractures (Fig. 41–2). The most serious bone injury of the pelvis is the comminuted, or crushing, fracture. It is classified as a type I injury, and it involves three or more structures of the pelvic ring. Usually such a fracture is unstable, and it involves extensive soft-tissue injury and hemorrhage.

Another kind of unstable fracture, a type II injury, has four variants: a fracture characterized by actual or potential displacement of the hemipelvis toward the head; an undisplaced diametric fracture (a *diametric* fracture is one in which the fracture extends anteriorly through the rami or symphysis and posteriorly through the sacrum, sacroiliac joint, or ilium, resulting in displacement of the hemipelvis); the sprung pelvis, or the "open book" (the posterior structures are intact, like the spine of a bound book, while the anterior structures are fractured and opened, like the pages of a book); a fracture of the acetabulum (such a fracture may be further complicated by dislocation of the head of the femur and, in some cases, may require surgical fixation). These fractures are the most common fractures associated with pelvic hemorrhage, both arterial and venous.

Any fracture of the symphysis is likely to injure the bladder or the urethra. As a matter of fact, 10% of patients who have pelvic fractures have an associated bladder injury. The mechanism is purely anatomical. The anteroinferior surface of the bladder is contiguous with the pubic bones and is not covered with peritoneum. The triangular ligament, or urogenital diaphragm, is stretched across the pubic arch, through which the membranous urethra passes. If blood is found in the urine, rupture of the bladder must be considered. Rectal injuries are less common and are most likely caused by a fracture of the ischium.[45]

With pelvic hemorrhage, the patient receives multiple transfusions in the hope of tamponading the pelvic hematoma. The surgeon decides whether or not to operate based on preoperative arteriographic visualization of the sites of arterial bleeding in the fractured pelvis; the size and rapidity of enlargement of a palpable, expanding hematoma; the severity and location of trauma (positive correlation between the number of fractures, degree of displacement, and need for laparotomy; bladder perforation; and positive needle paracentesis and lavage.

Early skeletal fixation limits bleeding by rigidly controlling movements of the pelvic hematoma and limiting motion of

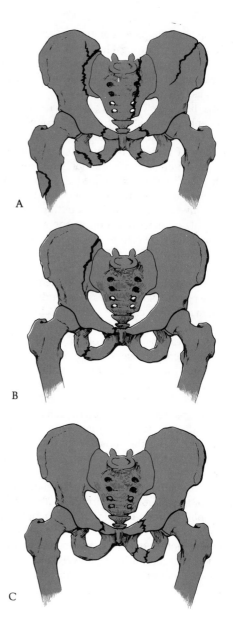

A

B

C

Figure 41–2

Unstable and stable pelvic fractures. (*A*) Type 1 injury. Unstable fracture involving three or more structures of the pelvic ring. (*B*) Type 2 injury. (*C*) Type 3 injury. Stable fracture. These are usually isolated fractures (*e.g.,* fractures of the pubic rami), and patients are treated with bed rest and gradual mobilization.

the fracture fragments. Stability is provided without interference with other surgical procedures, and early rehabilitation is enhanced. Other methods used to control persistent hemorrhage are Military Anti-Shock Trousers (MAST) trousers, embolization, suture ligation, hypogastric artery ligation, temporary aortic cross-clamping, and pelvic packing. During the procedure, the patient's blood may be autotransfused if there is no fecal, urinary, or other contamination.

Hemorrhagic Shock

Many patients with abdominal trauma arrive in the emergency room in a state of shock, often from blood loss. The shock state must be assessed and managed before specific abdominal injuries are determined.

A succinct description of shock is difficult, because so many factors interact. One classical description is also a very simple one: *Shock* is a low-flow state with poor tissue perfusion. More recently, shock has been defined as insufficient delivery of oxygen to organs and tissue; the amount of oxygen delivered does not meet the oxygen demand of the organs and tissue. Too little blood reaches the microvasculature, the oxygen deficiencies build, and organ failure results.

Classification of Types of Shock

Basically, shock results from a defect in one or more of the following: the pump, the fluid pumped, the arterial vessels, or the venous bed capacity. The following classification of shock is based on the hemodynamic changes that occur in shock, and it is commonly used in clinical practice[49]:

1. Volume decrease (hypovolemia)
   a. Whole blood loss
   b. Plasma volume loss
   c. Extracellular fluid loss
2. Changes in resistance of vessels (distribution shock)
   a. Decrease in resistance
      (1) Spinal anesthesia
      (2) Neurogenic reflexes
   b. Septic shock
      (1) Change in peripheral resistance
      (2) Change in venous capacitance
3. Cardiogenic shock
   a. Pump failure
      (1) Coronary thrombosis
      (2) Cardiac dysrhythmias
      (3) Severe valvular disease
   b. Decreased venous inflow (decreased preload, obstructive shock)
      (1) Mediastinal shift
      (2) Cardiac tamponade
      (3) Pulmonary embolism
      (4) Tension pneumothorax

The classification is extremely practical, because the patient may have a number of problems, and the principal cause of the patient's shock may not be the most obvious problem. For example, the patient who has been injured in a motor vehicle accident may be in shock not only from blood loss and inadequate volume, but also from cardiac failure caused by tamponade.

Shock from volume decrease, or hypovolemia, may be caused by the body's loss of blood, plasma, or water. Blood loss may be external, such as in a severe laceration, or internal, such as in a pelvic fracture or a ruptured spleen. Plasma loss may be internal and external, such as in multiple draining wounds, or internal, such as in peritonitis. Water loss may be from water deprivation, in which electrolytes become concentrated in a decreased amount of body water, or from the actual loss of volume, water, and electrolyes from the body, such as in vomiting and diarrhea.[49]

Hemorrhagic shock is a type of hypovolemic shock. It results from external or internal blood loss. External blood loss is a visible loss, and it can be measured. Common causes of external blood loss are severe lacerations, gunshot wounds, and stab wounds. Internal blood loss is a hidden loss, and it is difficult to quantify. Common causes of internal blood loss

are a ruptured spleen, liver, or vena cava.[44] Blood loss may be unrecognized or underestimated, especially when internal losses are concealed. Retroperitoneal hemorrhage can cause a shock state in excess of the amount of blood lost, perhaps due to the involvement of autonomic ganglia and renal ischemia.

Severity and duration of hypoperfusion are important variables. In the previously healthy person, acute mild hypovolemia (10% to 20% of blood volume lost) may be spontaneously corrected. Uncorrected moderate hypovolemia (20% to 30% of blood volume lost) can lead to organ malfunction. Acute severe hypovolemia (30% to 50% of blood volume lost), if untreated, can lead to cell damage and death.

With rapid blood loss to half the volume normally present, exsanguination and cardiac arrest are highly likely. The patient loses consciousness, has a rapidly declining blood pressure, and quickly becomes pulseless and apneic—clinical death. If resuscitation is started earlier than about 10 minutes of pulselessness, the stage may still be reversible. Because the heart responds well to volume replacement, the arrest is highly resuscitable. Actually, cardiac arrest in the form of electromechanical dissociation occurs frequently. Ventricular fibrillation can also occur.

After blood loss, the hematocrit, which at first remains unchanged, begins to decrease, probably because of the transcapillary refill mechanism. Plasma from the extracellular fluid compartment refills the intravascular space. The mechanism of hemodilution and transcapillary refill after hemorrhage is based on the Starling hypothesis: The reduction in the hydrostatic pressure in the capillaries (because of hypotension and arterial vasoconstriction) results in a shift of the pressure gradient to encourage passage of fluid from the tissue extracellular space into the capillary bed.

The low flow state produces many cellular alterations. Because of tissue hypoxia, anaerobic cellular metabolism increases. If hyperventilation is great enough in terms of compensatory mechanisms, the pH may not be much reduced. During resuscitation, acidosis is at first more severe, because the accumulated acids are being washed out of the body tissues. Catecholamine release decreases insulin levels and results in hyperglycemia. Glucose transport is affected. Bleeding induces a hypercoagulable state, which can be followed later by a generalized coagulability. Acutely, the brain is most vulnerable to the low-flow state. Initially manifested as an alteration in consciousness or confusion, the neurologic damage can be severe and irreversible. Once cerebral blood flow is significantly reduced (cerebral perfusion pressure to less than 50 mm Hg), stupor and coma result.

Hemodynamics

Mean arterial blood pressure is determined by cardiac output and systemic vascular resistance according to the following formula:

$$MAP = CO \times SVR$$
$$80 = 6 \times 13$$
$$80 = 4 \times 20$$
$$80 = 2 \times 40$$

where *MAP* is mean arterial pressure in mm Hg, *CO* is cardiac output in L/minute, and *SVR* is systemic vascular resistance, measured in Woods units. Hemorrhagic shock threatens cardiac output because volume loss (often called "preload" deficit) threatens cardiac filling. If cardiac output is threatened to the extent that mean arterial pressure falls and the pressure receptors are stimulated, the sympathetic nervous system will attempt to restore cardiac output first by increasing heart rate, as seen in the following formula:

$$CO = SV \times HR$$
$$6 = 80 \times 75$$
$$6 = 60 \times 100$$
$$6 = 40 \times 150$$

where *CO* is cardiac output in L/minute, *SV* is stroke volume in ml/beat, and *HR* is heart rate.

Tachycardia is therefore a response that occurs early in hemorrhagic shock, evidence that the sympathetic nervous system has intervened to support cardiac output, and therefore blood pressure. Meanwhile, additional compensatory mechanisms, including increased myocardial contractility, aldosterone, and antidiuretic hormone (ADH) secretion to increase circulating blood volume, and vasoconstriction to decrease venous capacitance, work to support cardiac output. When cardiac output finally falters, systemic vascular resistance increases in the final attempt to sustain perfusion pressure.

Although the sympathetic nervous system may at least temporarily achieve a mean arterial pressure greater than 70 mm Hg, the marginal and falling cardiac output, along with the increasing SVR, threaten the periphery with insufficient delivery of oxygen to tissue. Tissue ischemia occurs and, if severe and prolonged, results in multiorgan system failure.

First kidney and lung failure occurs, followed by cerebral and cardiac failure. Stagnation and hypoxia at the tissue level transform aerobic metabolic pathways to anaerobic ones. Increasing quantities of lactic acid are produced, the base bicarbonate level falls, acidosis progresses, and the serum potassium level increases to the point of cardiac arrest.

Stages of Shock

Hemodynamic changes produce several levels, or stages, of shock, namely, early, middle, and late shock. During the early stage of shock, arterial blood pressure and cardiac output decrease, but they are restored to normal by the body's compensatory mechanisms. The early stage of shock is characterized by increased cardiac activity. In the middle stage of shock, the compensatory mechanisms are no longer effective, and extrinsic support must be given. The middle stage is characterized by increased cardiac activity that tends to progress to a stage in which myocardial contractile function is depressed. In the late (sometimes called irreversible) stage, compensatory mechanisms are nonexistent, and total failure of the body systems is imminent.

Early cardiac failure is manifested by the development of a decreased mean arterial pressure without a change in cardiac output in the face of an elevated central venous pressure. Failure of the cardiovascular system produces low cardiac output, peripheral pooling of blood, minimal tissue perfusion, the translocation of protein into the extracellular extravascular spaces, and metabolic alterations. Some patients go through the syndrome of cardiac failure more rapidly or more slowly than others.

Mechanism of Fluid Change

The work of Shires and associates[49-51] on resuscitation with Ringer's lactate solution has revolutionized the treatment of hemorrhagic shock. Initially, their research recognized that despite blood replacement, many people in clinical shock died, and many of those who lived had damaged kidneys and even renal failure. Investigations were made of several aspects of the extracellular fluid (ECF) and the actual mechanism operating at the cellular level.

Early in their studies, Shires and associates noted that the extracellular fluid volume loss was greater than anticipated. They postulated that the mechanism for the extracellular fluid loss included a tremendous shift of sodium and water into the intracellular compartment. In such a shift, the cell membrane loses its integrity in that the membrane potential decreases significantly and the sodium pump is no longer efficient. Normal concentrations of sodium and potassium are altered, and significant increases occur in the intracellular sodium and extracellular potassium levels. In essence, the cell becomes leaky, and protein moves into the cell, resulting in increased oncotic pressure and intracellular swelling. The water in the intracellular compartment rises, but the total body water remains the same. An internal shift redistributes, or translocates, extracellular fluid into the intracellular compartment.

Later, the results of successful laboratory studies were utilized in the management of patients who were transferred to the trauma facility in hemorrhagic shock. Their treatment centered on the administration of Ringer's lactate solution as well as whole blood. The use of a balanced salt solution and blood returned the extravascular space to normal and significantly decreased the incidence of renal failure.

Deficiency of Adenosine Triphosphate

Since the breakthrough of Shires and associates, many other researchers have sought to explain the complex systemic interrelationships. Cellular alterations are varied, interrelated, and progressive. In tissues that are not well perfused with oxygen and are without adequate substrates, changes occur in the energy pathways. Intracellular and extracellular levels of lactate rise, because not enough oxygen is present to oxidize lactate to carbon dioxide and water. Rather, anaerobic pathways produce large quantities of lactic acid and little adenosine triphosphate (ATP).

Work with the experimental shock model in the awake, bled rat demonstrated a deficiency of ATP within the cell and the reversal of mortality in hemorrhagic shock with the administration of ATP.[6] Treatment seemed to correct the intracellular accumulation of sodium and water. Significantly, the fact that intracellular concentrations of ATP may be brought to levels three times greater than normal shows that ATP does cross the cell membrane.

A mechanism that begins with alteration of the cellular membrane and a decrease in the membrane potential has been proposed. The sequence is as follows: Intracellular sodium and extracellular potassium rise, sodium and potassium ATPase is activated, ATP is used, and stimulation of the mitochondria is followed by a decrease in cyclic adenosine monophosphate (AMP). Concomitant with the decrease in cyclic AMP are a change in the insulin response, changes in the end results of many hormones, a further decrease in metabolic capability, a decreased production of ATP, and the breakdown of lysosomes.[6] Eventually, as the process continues, sodium enters the mitochondria, the ATP levels are reduced, and swelling occurs in the mitochondria, endoplasmic reticulum, and the cell in general.

Fluid and Electrolyte Abnormalities

Predictably, fluid and electrolyte abnormalities persist for extended periods of time. Sodium and water increase and potassium decreases intracellularly for 5-day periods and longer. In severely stressed patients sodium and water levels in the intracellular spaces may be increased for 10 to 20 days after surgery.

Antidiuretic hormone acts to increase the retention of free water by the kidney. The actual mechanism by which ADH increases permeability to water in the distal convoluted tubule and collecting ducts is not understood. One theory is that ADH increases the diameter or number of pores in an area of the cell membrane (not in the total area available for diffusion). By osmosis, the water flows through the pores and into the extracellular fluid of the renal medulla, which is hypertonic because of the countercurrent mechanism active in the loop of Henle. Thus, the intratubular fluid is no longer as hypotonic as it was after the active transport of solute out of the ascending limb of the loop, but it has the same osmotic concentration as the extracellular space. Systemic absorption is completed by the blood flowing through the vasa recta. The stimuli primarily responsible for ADH secretion are decreased vascular volume and increased plasma osmolarity. When the effective vascular volume diminishes, decreases in arterial pressure or central venous pressure stimulate receptors, which, in turn, transmit impulses to the central nervous system and produce the release of ADH. Further loss of volume in the urine is prevented by the increased water absorption produced by ADH. When the osmolarity or concentration of solute in the plasma is increased by even a small percentage, osmoreceptors near the supraoptic nuclei induce the release of ADH. The free water resorbed decreases the osmolarity (dilutes the solutes in the plasma). In both processes, inhibition is by a feedback system.

An important mineralocorticoid is aldosterone. Resorption of sodium into the extracellular fluid is stimulated. The process is governed to a large extent by angiotensin II, which stimulates the zona glomerulosa of the adrenal gland to synthesize and release aldosterone. Although the effects of aldosterone appear relatively slowly and do not peak for several hours, a fine control is exerted over extracellular fluid volume and potassium secretion. Every resorbing epithelium in the body responds to the hormone. Because sodium, accompanied by water and anions, is resorbed and not lost, extracellular osmolality and therefore volume are maintained. Acid–base balance and potassium metabolism are affected by the hormone in the distal tubule. The magnitude of potassium secretion depends on sodium resorption, because potassium moves passively into the tubular fluid according to the electrochemical potential gradient. When large amounts of aldosterone are present, sodium resorption in the distal tubule is stimulated and potassium is excreted. Partially through exchange of potassium and hy-

drogen ions in the tubule, sodium is retained, resulting in decreased serum levels of potassium and hydrogen. Logically, urinary sodium levels decrease, and urinary potassium and hydrogen ion levels increase (Chap. 33). These changes produce a change—the decrease in the ratio of urinary sodium to urinary potassium—that is often used as a clinical indicator. The process leads to metabolic alkalosis, because increased acidification of the urine results from both hypokalemia and a specific but unidentified effect of aldosterone on the tubular acidification mechanisms.[51]

The endorphins appear to play an integral role in the low-flow state. Released by the pituitary gland during stress, these endogenous opiate-like compounds have a significant effect on the circulation. Endorphins also have a potential effect on many physiologic (as well as psychologic) functions, because receptors have been found in the central nervous system, heart, liver, kidneys, and intestines. Although unproven, it is possible that these compounds are responsible for changes in the sodium-potassium pump and the resulting reduced skeletal muscle transmission potential.[1]

Ballistics

Injury and death by gunshot wounds has become an American epidemic.[58] With close to 30,000 deaths per year, gunshot wounds are second only to motor vehicle accidents in injury-induced fatalities, taking more lives in two years than the entire Vietnam War and more than all deaths to date due to acquired immunodeficiency syndrome (AIDS). There are 50 million handguns in this country and more than 2.5 million new handguns sold legally in the United States each year. It is believed that the escalation of gunshot wounds will continue, fueled by easy access to arms and ammunition, by serious crime and drug wars, and by domestic disputes inflamed by our high-stress society. Meanwhile, the improvements in emergency care and transport will salvage more victims of gunshot wounds, presenting the emergency and critical care units with patients whose wounds are multiple and more severe.[59]

When dealing with a victim of gunshot wounding, the clinician is better able to anticipate the severity of the injury if the factors that contribute to wounding are understood.

Mechanisms

The extent to which a missile creates injury depends on the occurrence of any combination of three wounding mechanisms:[16,19,20] tissue crush, cavitation, and combustion.

Tissue Crush

When a bullet penetrates, tissue is injured by crushing and cutting mechanisms. The severity of injury is often related to what structures have been penetrated.

Figure 41–3 illustrates the many injuries that can result from only one missile. Entrance and exit wounds, however, do not always plot the path of the bullet, and clinicians are warned that bullets may take unexpected trajectories, deflect off and fragment bone, or penetrate a vessel, thereon embolizing to locations remote to the visible wounds. When a bullet fails to exit, one can only speculate as to its path and final location.

The tissue crush inflicted by a penetrating missile results in

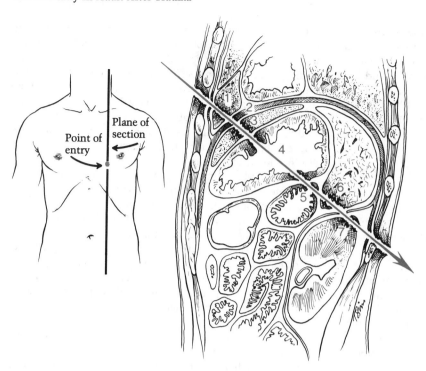

Figure 41–3

Left parasagittal section showing a multiorgan injury produced by one bullet: (*1*) lung, (*2*) diaphragm, (*3*) liver, (*4*) stomach, (*5*) jejunum, (*6*) spleen, and (*7*) kidney.

microcirculatory disruption at best and obliteration of arterial blood flow at worst, both of which threaten the supply of oxygen to that tissue. The tissue around the wound tract undergoes hypoxic injury, as evidenced by a reduced production of high-energy phosphates (ATP) and by the accumulation of lactate.[2] Survivability of the tissue and organ is determined by the extent of the hypoxic injury.

Cavitation

A second injuring mechanism, cavitation, can be a major factor in the severity of a gunshot wound due to a bullet with high kinetic energy. If the energy of the penetrating bullet is transmitted to the tissue, the tissue will be hurled away from the bullet's path. This phenomenon of transmission of energy from the missile to the tissue can best be illustrated by observing a propelled object striking a stationary object. An example is what happens when a cue ball (a missile) that has been set in motion by a cue stick (a weapon) hits an eight ball (a tissue). The cue ball stops, and the eight ball, having received the cue ball's kinetic energy, is set in motion. This is what happens mechanically when the kinetic energy of a missile is transmitted to tissue.

Experiments performed with blocks of gelatin used to simulate human tissue have shown how kinetic energy affects the surrounding tissue. As the missile penetrates, it produces a permanent wound tract and temporary displacement of the tissue away from the tract. The phenomenon has often been described as a shock wave that surrounds the missile path and radiates from it. A temporary cavity is created that may be much larger than the missile's path; the size depends on how much kinetic energy the missile had to begin with and how much of it was transmitted to the tissue.[19,20] The volume of the temporary cavity may be as much as 15 times the volume of the missile, and the pressure exerted against the walls of the cavity may be as much as 100 times atmospheric pressure.

Although the lifetime of the cavity is only 5 to 10 msec, the rapid, forceful expansion of the cavity can damage muscle, injure nerves, rupture blood vessels, and fracture bone, even when these structures may have been in a position outside the direct path of the bullet. Furthermore, the pressure of the cavity itself is subatmospheric, allowing air and any contaminants in the air to be drawn into the depths of the cavity and to contaminate the whole of the missile tract.

Kinetic Energy. Because the amount of cavitation is related directly to the amount of kinetic energy transmitted to the tissue, the extent of injury may be anticipated if one knows the kinetic energy of the wounding missile. The *kinetic energy* (*KE*) is defined as

$$KE = \frac{1}{2}mv^2$$

where *KE* is kinetic energy, *m* is mass, and *v* is velocity.

The kinetic energy of a missile is proportional to the product of its mass and the square of its velocity. As the energy formula shows, velocity is an important determinant of kinetic energy. Thus, if two missiles have the same velocity but one has twice the mass of the other, the more massive missile has twice as much kinetic energy. However, if two missiles have the same mass but one has twice the velocity of the other, the faster missile has four times more kinetic energy.

The energy formula is illustrated by the following example for the .22 short bullet (the .22 short is the smallest handgun bullet made and is fired from a .22 caliber gun, the barrel of which is .22 inch in diameter):

Because the weight of one .22 shot is 29 grains, the mass is

$$1.286 \times 10^{-4} \frac{\text{lb} \cdot \text{sec}^2}{\text{ft}}$$

The kinetic energy of a .22 shot is

$$KE = \tfrac{1}{2}mv^2$$

$$= \tfrac{1}{2}\left(1.286 \times 10^4\ \frac{\text{lb} \cdot \text{sec}^2}{\text{ft}}\right)\left(1045\ \text{ft/sec}\right)^2$$

$$= 70\ \text{ft} \cdot \text{lb}$$

Although there is great potential for wounding owing to the transmission of energy to tissue, a high kinetic energy bullet will not cause significant cavitation if it is aerodynamic and nondeforming. A nondeforming bullet may simply "cut" as it penetrates and exit with much of its speed, and thus much of its energy, still remaining. For the transmission of energy and cavity formation to occur, the bullet design must be such that it deforms or flattens when it enters.[21,53] Various bullet designs have been created with this end in mind. For example, bullets with a hollow-point nose expand in a mushroom effect while passing through the tissues. This flattening out of the bullet causes it to give up greater amounts of its kinetic energy to the tissue. Soft-nosed and flat-nosed bullets undergo a similar effect when passing through tissue.

Besides the mushrooming effect, two other factors tend to increase the transmission of energy and cause greater injury due to cavity formation:

1. The bullet's angle of yaw at the time it hits the body. *Yaw* is the deviation of deflection of the nose of the bullet from its straight, "nose first" line of flight. Instead of striking the body nose first, the bullet strikes the body at an angle. The greater the angle of yaw, the more kinetic energy imparted to the tissue.
2. The density of the tissue. The greater the density of the tissue the bullet passes through, the more kinetic energy the tissue absorbs. The size of the temporary cavity depends on the specific gravity of the tissue and its cohesiveness and elasticity.[40] These two properties tend to counteract expansion of the wound tract. Thus, tissues that are more cohesive and more elastic have greater resistance to injury. For example, although the energy absorbed by both the liver and muscle tissue may be essentially identical, the temporary cavity and the resultant permanent wound tract are larger in the liver than in muscle tissue.[16,22]

The principle of greater speed for greater injury is the basis of the magnum handguns.[8,59] The .357 and the .44 magnum bullet have essentially the same caliber as the .38 special bullet and the .45 automatic bullet, respectively. The difference is in the kinetic energy. The magnum bullet contains more gunpowder, which propels the bullet at a greater speed, thus capitalizing on the velocity advantage shown in the kinetic energy formula. (The kinetic energy of various types of handguns is shown in Table 41–4.) Cavity formation and tissue destruction by a magnum bullet are usually greater than those inflicted by the regular .38 or .45 bullet.

Although magnums cause greater injury because of their greater bullet speed, the increase over other handguns is very small compared with the relative speed of high-powered rifles. The dramatic difference between the speed and kinetic energy of handgun bullets and the speed and kinetic energy of high-powered rifle bullets can be seen in Table 41–4.

Table 41–4
Kinetic Energy of Selected Handgun and Rifle Bullets

BULLET	WEIGHT (grains)	MUZZLE VELOCITY (ft/sec)	MUZZLE ENERGY (ft · lb)
Handgun			
.22 short	29	1045	70
.25 automatic	50	810	73
.357 magnum	158	1410	695
.38 special	158	855	256
.44 magnum	240	1470	1150
.45 ACP	230	850	370
Rifle			
222 Remington	35	3020	1114
243 Remington	100	2960	1945
30-30 Winchester	150	2390	1902
30-06 Springfield	150	2920	2839
308 Winchester	150	2820	2648

The size of the temporary cavity produced by a high-velocity missile can be grasped if one considers the destruction caused by a 150-grain deforming bullet. A deforming bullet with an impact velocity of 2500 ft/second perforates an 8-inch thigh and exits at a velocity of 1500 ft/second. During its travel through the tissue, the bullet will have expended 1331 foot pounds of energy [$.5(150/7000) \times 1/32.2(2500^2 - 1500^2)$ = 1331 ft · lb], creating a temporary cavity with a maximum diameter of 12 to 15 inches. This explains why nerves, vessels, and bones that are distant from the bullet's path may be injured. Lethal injury may occur to structures that seem remote to the bullet's path.

High-velocity missile wounds of the head are usually fatal, owing to the pressure that develops in the skull when a temporary cavity forms. The skull is a closed, rigid structure, and it cannot accommodate a large, expanding temporary cavity. The high pressures produced by the cavity result in the loss of skull integrity.

Combustion

A third mechanism of wounding is combustion, caused by the cloud of hot gas and burning powder present at the muzzle immediately after firing and extending outward 1 to 3 feet. Although combustion is a factor in tissue injury only when the gun is in physical contact with the skin, massive and lethal injury can be produced when the gas from a shotgun enters the wound. Once inside the body, the gas and powder continue to expand and burn, causing a severe injury by internal combustion. If the shotgun wound is to the head, a wound similar to that of high-powered rifle injuries results, not from the cavity formation but from the combustion of the powder. Patients with contact wounds made by a shotgun to the head, chest, or abdomen often do not survive long enough to be taken to the hospital. Internal combustion in contact wounds inflicted by handguns inflicts little additional injury because the amount of gas is less. A characteristic wound is produced, however, by a handgun held in contact with skin that overlies bone. The gas is trapped between the bone and skin and it expands, making the skin balloon out away from the bone. If the elasticity of the skin is exceeded, a stellate tear of the skin is produced.

When the contact wound is not over bone, the subcutaneous tissues are able to yield sufficiently and a stellate entry tear does not occur.

Shotguns

Shotguns have characteristics that distinguish them from handguns and rifles.[23] Although shotgun shells, like handgun bullets, are fired at a relatively low velocity, the shotgun "bullet" is usually a shell containing many round lead pellets instead of a single slug. These pellets are designed to form a dense pattern to enhance the hunter's chance of hitting small game with one firing. The pellets (Fig. 41–4) usually range in size from 0.08 inches in diameter (for the no. 9 shot) to 0.33 inches (for the 00 buckshot). The shell may contain from 200 small pellets to 9 pellets (in 00 buckshot); the number depends on the size of the pellets and the gauge of the gun. An obvious danger of a shotgun blast is that one shell contains many individual missiles. It has been observed that being shot once with a shotgun that takes 00 shot can be equivalent to being shot nine times with a .32 caliber handgun.

Besides the pellets, the shell contains gunpowder and a plastic or paper wad that separates the powder from the pellets. When the shotgun is fired, the powder does not explode or detonate; rather, it burns with great speed, creating an expanding volume of hot gas to drive the wad and pellets forward (without the wad, the hot gases would melt and deform the pellets). Because the wad is heavy and flat, it quickly loses momentum in the air and falls to the ground about 6 feet from the end of the shotgun barrel. The pellets, meanwhile, are ejected out the end of the barrel in a pattern that initially is dense but that gradually widens the farther the pellets travel from the gun.

The extent of injury produced by shotgun pellets depends in large part on the distance from the weapon at the time of wounding.[16,59] At less than 6 feet, all combinations of shotgun shells and gauges produce a tight, dense pattern. Damage is extensive, with pulverizing and crushing of the tissues, because the pellets hit the body almost like a single mass. At 3 to 6 feet, the single entrance wound is 1.5 to 2 inches in diameter, and it shows "scalloping" of the edges. At distances closer than 12 inches and with contact wounds, the single round entrance wound is 0.75 to 2 inches in diameter. Extensive contamination occurs because shotgun wadding, bits of clothing, skin, hair, and burning and unburnt powder are driven into the wound. Not until the distance is greater than 8 to 10 yards do the pellets separate from the main mass and produce the characteristic speckled appearance of a shotgun wound. The damage that occurs then is more the result of the mass and velocity of each individual pellet. Because the pellets are round, they are not particularly efficient in retaining speed and energy over extended ranges. At 40 yards, the shot has lost more than 50% of its original energy. The greater the distance, the less likely it is that any one pellet will do extensive damage by itself.

If the distance is close, the wad may contribute to the wounding. In contact wounds, the wad is propelled into the body through the large single entrance wound. If the distance is more than 10 to 15 feet, the wad will have separated from the pellets and will not enter the body, but it may mark the body or leave an impression on the skin before it falls to the ground.

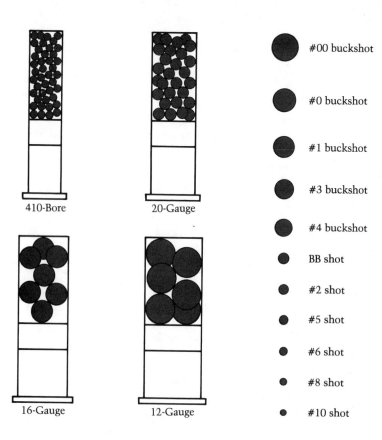

410-Bore   20-Gauge

16-Gauge   12-Gauge

#00 buckshot

#0 buckshot

#1 buckshot

#3 buckshot

#4 buckshot

BB shot

#2 shot

#5 shot

#6 shot

#8 shot

#10 shot

Figure 41–4

Structure of shotgun shells with various gauge and pellet loads. The gauge of a shotgun is determined by how many barrel-sized lead balls it takes to make a pound. For example, it takes 20 balls the size of a 20-gauge shotgun barrel to weigh a pound. Similarly, it takes only 12 balls the size of a 12-gauge shotgun to weigh a pound.

Table 41–5
Clinical Picture Exhibited by Patient in Shock

	PUMP FAILURE	DECREASED VOLUME	DECREASED RESISTANCE
Urinary output	↓	↓	Normal to ↓
Blood pressure	↓	↓	↓
Cardiac output	↓	↓	Normal to ↓ (early ↑)
Central venous pressure	↑	↓	Normal to ↓
Temperature	Normal	↓	↑ or ↓
Peripheral vascular resistance	↑	↑	↓

NURSING PROCESS

ASSESSMENT

The initial assessment of the patient who has sustained abdominal trauma should take into consideration the emergency priorities: First, establish the airway, breathing, and circulation; and then assess the respiratory, cardiac, and circulatory systems. The abdominal trauma is not assessed until these systems are assessed or supported and the patient's condition is stabilized. Identification of blunt intra-abdominal injury depends essentially on frequent abdominal examination, peritoneal lavage, laboratory studies, radiograph procedures, and other studies the physician may order.

Clinical Manifestations

The presence of the low-flow state is evidenced by decreased mentation and level of consciousness, reduced urinary output (renal constriction), increased pulse, faint peripheral pulses (reduced pulse pressure), peripheral vasoconstriction, cool clammy skin (compensating vasoconstriction), decreased cardiac output and blood pressure, and metabolic acidosis (Table 41–5). The administration of Ringer's lactate solution, besides being a therapeutic measure, is a clinical means to assess the pre-existing degree of blood loss. The solution is administered at a rapid rate so that in a period of 30 minutes, 1000 to 2000 ml is given intravenously.

Three classical responses to Ringer's lactate infusion have been described.[50] With less than 10% volume loss and without continued loss, the blood pressure returns to normal after 1 to 2 L and it stabilizes even if the patient initially had marked hypotension. If correlated with measurements of the blood volume, the degree of pre-existing blood loss would be shown to be relatively minimal. With severe blood loss and continuing hemorrhage, the response in vital signs (with elevation of blood pressure and decrease in pulse) after rapid intravenous infusion is transient. Whole blood that has been typed and crossmatched is administered. With patients who do not respond to the initial 1 to 2 L of Ringer's lactate solution, uncrossmatched type O, Rh negative, or type-specific blood is administered. In this group of patients, the prognosis is poor unless immediate surgical intervention can correct the problem (Table 41–6).

Blood loss may be unrecognized or underestimated, especially when internal losses are concealed. In internal blood loss, serial assessments of the significant body parts and physiologic parameters must be made so that a gross estimate of bleeding may be made. Retroperitoneal hemorrhage can cause a severe shock state in excess of the amount of blood lost,

Table 41–6
Clinical Picture Exhibited by Patient According to Degree of Blood Loss

	MILD (<750 ml)	MODERATE (750–1500 ml)	SEVERE (>1500 ml)
Sensorium	Oriented to time, place, person	Remains oriented; words slurred	Disoriented
Pulse	Rate, 110–120; quality full to decreased	Rate, 120–150; quality, decreased and variable	Rate, greater than 150; quality, weak
Blood pressure	Normal to low (10–20%) decrease, but may be slightly increased as compensatory mechanism	Decreased 40–50 mm Hg below normal (20–40% decrease)	Systolic less than 80; diastolic may not be heard
Urinary output	35–50 ml/hr	20–35 mg/hr	Less than 20 ml/hr
Color	Pale	Pale	Mottled
Capillary refill	Circulation return may be slightly slowed	Circulation return slowed	Circulation return very slowed; skin pale both before and after; large differences between rectal and big toe temperature
Response to Ringer's lactate infusion	Blood pressure returns to normal after 1 IL	Blood pressure increase and pulse decrease is transient; blood is needed	No response to RL; uncrossmatched or type-specific blood is needed

perhaps because of the involvement of autonomic ganglia and renal vessels.

Penetrating Trauma

The patient suffering from penetrating trauma may have a wide variation in injuries. For example, he or she may be moribund from hemorrhage after a shotgun wound at close range or may have only a superficial injury from a knife wound that did not penetrate the peritoneal cavity.

Even before the patient arrives, if possible, historical facts about the injury should be ascertained. For example, the paramedics should be asked about the type of weapon used, the blood lost at the scene and en route to the hospital, and the time lapse between the injury, first response, and arrival at the hospital.

The patient should be examined carefully, turned, and every possible wound should be noted. One patient, for example, was found to be in profound shock, but the only wound was an innocuous looking stab wound of the back. During surgery this wound was found to extend into the vena cava.

The penetrating abdominal trauma index (PATI) is helpful in the evaluation of the significance of associated injuries. This is an anatomical severity index score based on the number of organs injured and the severity of the individual injuries.

If the patient has suffered penetrating trauma from a stab wound, the surgical team uses the following assessment parameters to determine a surgical or nonsurgical approach:

- Clinical assessment
- Signs of peritoneal injury
- Ileus
- Evidence of visceral injury, such as evisceration or blood in the stomach, bladder, or rectum
- Results of local wound exploration
- Results of peritoneal lavage

Some centers suggest that selective observation can be used in the assessment and management of certain more minor bullet wounds of the abdomen.

Nurses who understand the mechanisms of missile wounding and the variables that determine the extent of injury are better equipped to assess the patients' wounds. The following approach indicates the direction of and priorities in the assessment.

If possible, it should be determined what type of weapon was used. If a high-velocity hunting rifle was used, the internal injury may be much more extensive than if a handgun was used. A person wounded by a .45 caliber bullet that has a hollow-point design probably has a more extensive internal wound that does the person injured by the lower-powered, solid-point .22 caliber handgun, the type commonly used in domestic arguments.

Injury to major vessels by any missile, large or small, slow or fast, may produce profound levels of shock due to blood loss. One study reported a high incidence of vascular injury in patients admitted in shock after a gunshot wound to the abdomen; 50% of the patients in shock died from the injury.[18]

The patient's blood pressure should be determined immediately. Systolic pressures of less than 80 that do not respond to the rapid administration of 2000 ml of blood indicate that 30% of the total blood volume has been lost and that immediate operative intervention is required.

If possible, the examiner should locate both the entrance and the exit wounds and plot mentally the structures that lie between these two points. This will indicate the complications to be anticipated and the steps that may be taken by the physician. (However, it must be noted that the examiner can often be in error when trying to determine which is an entrance or an exit wound. A forensic pathologist is really the person to make the determination.) If there is no obvious exit wound, the examiner should palpate for the missile. Often it is found to lie subcutaneously, having spent its energy without exiting. The examiner should be aware of wounds that have no exit; these wounds have received all the energy the missile could transmit.

Blunt Trauma

If the patient has suffered blunt abdominal trauma, a careful history and physical examination are of utmost importance. This history will often tell the mechanism of injury, be it a blow, a seat belt restraint, or rapid deceleration. A description of the patient's position in the car before a motor vehicle accident, the presence or absence of shoulder straps and seat belts, and details of how the patient was removed from the vehicle are all points that will help determine the type and extent of injury. If the patient is alert, he or she can be most helpful in explaining how the accident occurred, as well as any reaction to the physical examination, especially the description of pain. However, as many as one-fifth of patients have injuries with no signs or symptoms.

It is apparent why blunt abdominal trauma carries a higher mortality than penetrating trauma. A patient who has sustained a blunt abdominal trauma usually has an associated injury. If the patient has an associated chest injury, pain and irritation of the diaphragm caused by a hemothorax may produce peritonitis-like abdominal rigidity and guarding. The pain of fractures of the lower ribs or pelvis may mask the signs of peritonitis. The patient may be unconscious as a result of shock or alcohol intoxication. Finally, a patient who has a spinal cord injury at the thoracic level or above may have a flaccid abdominal wall, sensory loss, and no abdominal pain, even in the presence of an intra-abdominal injury.

Once a description of the accident has been obtained, the next step is to evaluate the patient for the following signs and symptoms of peritoneal irritation: abdominal wall rigidity; guarding; generalized pain or tenderness; abdominal distention and loss of bowel sounds; rebound tenderness; a localized point of maximal tenderness; pain on movement or coughing; splinting of the abdominal muscles and thoracic breathing; or unexplained shock.

All the signs and symptoms are the result of irritation of the peritoneal membranes by spilling bowel contents, digestive enzymes, urine, bile, or blood into the peritoneal cavity. The onset of peritonitis may be insidious, because blood does not always irritate the peritoneum and because small bowel lacerations may be nearly painless if the leakage is minimal. Therefore, continuous, careful assessment must be carried out so that occult injuries are detected as soon as possible.

Blood Pressure

Continuous assessment of patients with occult abdominal injuries is essential to early detection of these injuries. Besides the continuous monitoring of the patient for peritoneal signs, serial measurements of the patient's blood pressure can be used to provide very useful information. Many patients who have multiple injuries are admitted to the hospital in varying degrees of shock.

Hypotension may be absent in persons until 20% to 30% of blood volume has been lost; because of compensatory vasoconstriction, arterioles and veins constrict in skin, muscles, kidneys, and the splanchnic bed, while coronary and cerebral vessels dilate.

Patients whose hypotension is the result of mild volume loss or neurogenic causes usually respond promptly to the rapid infusion of 500 to 1000 ml of Ringer's lactate solution. However, patients who have multisystem injuries and whose blood pressure responds transiently to vigorous fluid resuscitation therapy and then returns to hypotensive levels should be strongly suspected of having continued occult bleeding. When the source of bleeding is not visible, the most likely cause is progressive hemoperitoneum. For this reason—and also because slow bleeding that progresses to ever-deepening shock is always a danger in the normotensive patient—serial measurement of blood pressure is a valuable part of the assessment approach. If the blood pressure is falling rapidly, the nurse must monitor it so that any trends become apparent immediately.

Diagnostic Tests

Several laboratory tests are helpful in gathering evidence of the presence and location of intra-abdominal injuries. In blunt trauma, a serum amylase is obtained initially and at 6-hour intervals. The serum amylase level may become elevated whenever amylase leaks into the peritoneal cavity, where it is freely absorbed into the blood. Such a spill of amylase may result from direct pancreatic trauma or from injury to the upper small bowel and duodenum (where the pancreatic enzyme is secreted into the bowel by way of the pancreatic duct), with leakage of amylase-containing fluid from the injured bowel into the peritoneal cavity. Hyperamylasemia that occurs immediately after trauma may thus also indicate a second injury—small bowel perforation. A rise in the amylase level caused by a significant and direct pancreatic injury may not occur until 12 to 24 hours after the injury.

The hemoglobin and hematocrit levels give little information about acute blood loss, but they do show a decline 6 to 8 hours after the acute episode. Because of the fluid shifts that occur after trauma, the levels are difficult to interpret, and they are generally not used as the only guide to fluid and blood replacement.

It is commonly believed that a blood leukocyte count of more than 15,000/mm³ suggests that a solid viscus has been ruptured, but this belief is beginning to be questioned. White blood cell counts of more than 25,000/mm³ may occur in rupture of the spleen and (occasionally) in rupture of the liver.

Other diagnostic studies needed are crossmatching, blood urea nitrogen, blood sugar, electrolytes, and urinalysis. A chest radiograph, erect and flat films of the abdomen, and a lateral view of the abdomen should be taken. Usually an infusion intravenous pyelogram is needed. Although arteriography is still considered important, computed tomography (CT) has become a primary diagnostic aid (Fig. 41–5).[37]

CT was reported to have a sensitivity of 89%, specificity of

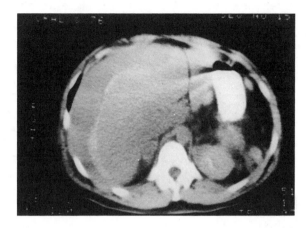

Figure 41–5

CT scan of a 21-year-old man who was clearing dead wood from a tree with a chain saw when he fell. He arrived at the hospital with multiple injuries. CT scan revealed a subcapsular hepatic hematoma. During laparotomy, bleeding from a major tear was controlled.

98%, and accuracy of 97% in the evaluation of penetrating trauma to the back and abdomen,[43] but it was unreliable in the detection of bowel or diaphragmatic injuries. Many physicians recommend that CT be performed before arteriography or surgery whenever an abscess, pseudoaneurysm, or aortoenteric fistula is suspected. CT is rapid, sensitive, and noninvasive for detecting or excluding postoperative complications. Sonography and CT remain the first diagnostic tools for evaluating suspected biliary complications.

Paracentesis and Peritoneal Lavage

Two diagnostic tools that have been of great help in detecting intra-abdominal injury are paracentesis and peritoneal lavage. In paracentesis, an 18-gauge, short-bevel spinal needle is attached to a syringe and inserted through the abdominal wall, which has been prepared and anesthetized (locally). The technique is accurate in about three-quarters of patients. Figure 41–6 shows where the needle is inserted. An attempt is then made to aspirate any free intraperitoneal blood (nonclotting) that may be present as a result of intra-abdominal injury. Because different areas of the abdomen may be aspirated, the procedure is often called a "four-quadrant tap" or a "bilateral flank tap." A bilateral tap is considered as accurate as a four-quadrant tap. The aspiration of even a small amount of nonclotting blood is considered a positive tap and evidence of an intra-abdominal injury that requires an exploratory laparotomy. A paracentesis that fails to aspirate blood is not definitive; that is, it does not indicate that the patient's abdomen has not been injured.[57] Other diagnostic procedures must be used to prove that there is not an injury.

The following problems are associated with paracentesis and must be considered whenever the procedure is undertaken[49]:

- An intra-abdominal blood vessel may inadvertently be entered. If it is, the aspirated blood does clot, which differentiates it from blood from the peritoneum, which does not clot.
- An accidental puncture of the intestine may occur. However,

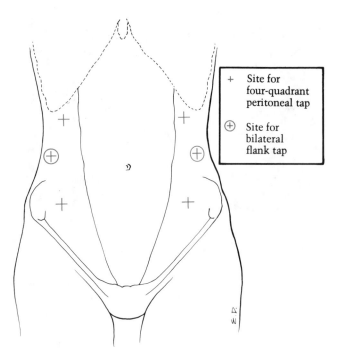

Figure 41-6
Anatomical sites for paracentesis.

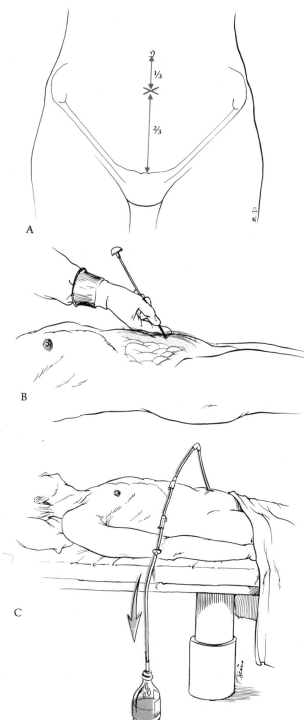

Figure 41-7
Peritoneal lavage. (*A*) Anatomical site for the percutaneous insertion of a lavage catheter. (*B*) After penetration of the peritoneum and removal of the trocar, the lavage catheter is inserted. (*C*) After lavage, the solution is infused into the peritoneal cavity and the patient is moved from one side to the other; the lavage fluid is siphoned out of the peritoneal cavity.

it happens rarely, and when it does happen, it is relatively harmless because the opening made by the 18-gauge needle is small, seals off quickly, and usually does not allow the bowel contents to leak.

- Accidental puncture of the rectus abdominis sheath may produce a large hematoma of that muscle.
- Free intraperitoneal blood that settles in the posterior aspects of the abdomen may not be accessible to the needle, thus giving a false-negative result.

If the following precautions are taken, the problems of paracentesis may be minimized:

- Peritoneal taps should be avoided in the patient whose bowel is distended significantly.
- Peritoneal taps should be avoided in areas of scar, where the bowel may be fixed to the abdominal wall.
- Care should be taken to insert the needle at the proper site, namely, lateral to the rectus abdominis sheath.

Peritoneal Lavage

Peritoneal lavage is more accurate (97%) than paracentesis and gives fewer false-negative results. It is sometimes used for the assessment of penetrating trauma from stab wounds as well as blunt trauma.[25] Peritoneal lavage is also performed on victims of stab wounds who are stable and have a nontender abdomen in order to rule out intra-abdominal injury and to avoid laparotomy. The procedure is unreliable for detecting retroperitoneal injuries. In peritoneal lavage, a peritoneal dialysis catheter is inserted and advanced into the peritoneal cavity (Fig. 41-7). If no blood or fluid is aspirated, 1 L of a balanced saline solution is infused rapidly into the peritoneal cavity. The patient is turned from side to side (except the patient who has a pelvic fracture or who for some other

reason cannot be turned), the empty intravenous bottle or bag is positioned below the patient's abdomen, and the fluid is siphoned out of the peritoneal cavity. The fluid that is collected is evaluated for the presence of red and white blood cells, amylase, bacteria, and bile. The criteria for positive peritoneal lavage[49,55] are gross blood in the lavage fluid or one or more of the following:

1. Red blood cell count of more than 100,000/mm[3]
2. White blood cell count of more than 500/mm[3]
3. An elevated amylase or bilirubin level
4. The presence of bacteria or bile

Like paracentesis, peritoneal lavage has some disadvantages. Accidental puncture of intra-abdominal structures may occur. Injuries to the retroperitoneal space cannot be evaluated, because the space does not communicate with the peritoneal cavity and therefore is inaccessible to the lavage fluid. Sometimes the insertion of the peritoneal catheter may cause enough abdominal bleeding to produce false-positive results. This problem can be prevented by using a local anesthetic preparation that contains epinephrine (to constrict the locally traumatized vessels).

Also, percutaneous peritoneal lavage using an 18-gauge needle and Seldinger technique to pass an No. 8 French lavage catheter over a guidewire have been found to be as safe as and quicker than conventional trocar insertion of a No. 12 French dialysis catheter.[48]

Lavage is contraindicated in the following patients:

- Patients who have a history of many operations, because adhesions increase the likelihood that the bowel will be penetrated and that the lavage fluid will be trapped, making its return difficult.
- Pregnant patients (because of possible danger to the fetus).
- Patients who have extensive missile injuries of the abdomen.

ASSESSMENT PARAMETERS OF SPECIFIC ORGAN INJURY

Spleen

Splenic bleeding may be detected by several assessment parameters. A history of injury, however slight, to the left upper quadrant (LUQ) followed by pain in the LUQ should raise the staff's index of suspicion. Varying degrees of hypovolemia may be present, with such signs as tachycardia, hypotension, and syncope. The patient may have difficulty breathing as intraperitoneal blood collects under and irritates the diaphragm. In 50% of the patients, Kerr's sign is present (*i.e.,* pain that is referred to the left shoulder tip because blood is irritating the diaphragm). Occasionally, the patient may have to be placed in Trendelenburg's position for Kerr's sign to be elicited. Muscular rigidity and guarding in the LUQ may occur in association with the LUQ pain.

Other parameters are important in assessing splenic injury. Arteriography is a very useful technique. Peritoneal lavage is helpful in documenting the presence of intraperitoneal blood. Radiographs may show such positive diagnostic signs as an elevated left hemidiaphragm, an enlarged spleen, gastric displacement, or hemorrhage into the gastrosplenic ligament (which separates the spleen and stomach). Leukocytosis of 15,000 to 25,000/mm[3] is common, as are declining hematocrit and hemoglobin values, shown by serial determinations. In any event, a history that suggests splenic trauma followed by serial assessments of the patient's condition is a prerequisite to diagnosing both acute and delayed splenic trauma.

Renal Injury

The presence of a renal injury may be revealed by pain, flank tenderness, and hematuria. The presence of a posterior bruise over the ribs or flank or a mass in the loin indicates the possibility of trauma to the kidney. The signs of blood loss vary according to the extent of the injury. Bowel sounds may be absent because of a reflex ileus. Fractures of the lumbar vertebrae or lower ribs may also be associated with kidney injury. Urinary tract injury may be suspected when trauma is followed by pain, flank tenderness, or hematuria.

Urine samples are collected from the conscious patient as a midstream specimen and from the unconscious patient as a catheter specimen. The placement of a catheter may cause microscopic hematuria. If the patient cannot void, gentle placement of a No. 16 Foley catheter should not aggravate the existing injury. However, if even a drop of blood is seen at the meatus, catheterization should not be performed until the patient is evaluated by the physician. Additionally, in patients with pelvic fractures, any difficulty with catheterization should make the nurse immediately suspicious of disruption of the bladder neck or urethra.

The presence of hematuria is helpful in detecting renal injury, but its absence does not mean that the kidney is free of injury. In about 15% of patients who have a renal injury, the urine is free of red blood cells.[49,55] Furthermore, urine that seems on visual inspection to be free of blood may actually contain blood. Urine does not look pink until it contains more than 500 red blood cells per cubic millimeter (gross hematuria). Detection of red blood cells in quantities less than 500 per cubic millimeter (microscopic hematuria) requires microscopic examination. The presence of as few as 10 red blood cells per cubic millimeter of urine is considered abnormal.

The presence of gross or microscopic hematuria necessitates further investigation.[5] With an intravenous pyelogram (IVP), dye that has been injected into the peripheral vein circulates to the kidney, where it can be shown by radiograph to be concentrated by the kidney and excreted into the collecting system. Dye concentrated in the uninjured areas of the kidney will cause those parts of the kidney to be seen on a radiograph when done. Areas of kidney that are injured will not be able to concentrate the dye and therefore will not be seen on the radiograph. Furthermore, if the collecting system has been lacerated, the concentrated dye can be seen to leak (extravasate) from the uninjured areas. Radiographs are taken at intervals of 1, 2, 3, 4, 5, 10, 15, and 30 minutes after injection of the dye, in order to record the progress of the concentrated and excreted dye into the calyces, ureters, and bladder. Injury in any of those areas will be shown by dye extravasation or by obstruction of the dye's progress through the system.

False-negative results may occur. In an effort to prevent false negatives, the physician may order that a higher dose of the contrast medium be given. Indications for infusion or large-dose excretory IVP include macroscopic or microscopic hematuria, pain in the abdominal side or back, tenderness with muscular guarding, and a flank or abdominal mass.[3] If an IVP does not visualize a kidney on one side, arteriography, a more accurate procedure, is indicated. Especially in gunshot wounds, fractured pelvis, and bladder involvement, IVP is followed by a retrograde cystogram.[40]

Signs and symptoms of bladder rupture include lower abdominal pain, inability or difficulty in voiding, and hematuria. Occasionally, extraperitoneal rupture permits urine to dissect

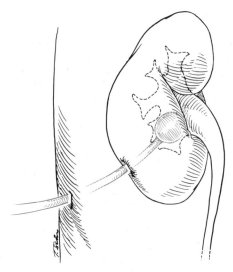

Figure 41–8
Placement of nephrostomy tube frequently seen after renal surgery.

along the fascial planes and enter the thighs or ascend into the abdominal wall. In intraperitoneal rupture, signs of peritonitis develop within 24 hours (sooner if the urine is infected). A retrograde cystogram is ordered to determine the location of bladder tears. Because urine leaks continuously from the tear, operative repair must be carried out as soon as possible.

Renal Pedicle Injury

A history of deceleration accompanied by signs of massive blood loss is strong evidence of a laceration of an intra-abdominal vessel, particularly the renal pedicle. Because profound hemorrhagic shock usually accompanies an injury to the renal pedicle, the diagnostic procedures done right before the operative repair are greatly limited. Flank mass and pain are rare, and hematuria may be absent. Often, most of the blood is lost into the retroperitoneal space, and so the blood loss is not detected by the usual physical examination of the abdomen. If the systolic blood pressure is greater than 90, an emergency IVP may be performed with minimal difficulty to define the injury more clearly. A preoperative IVP also gives vital information about the functioning of the uninjured kidney when removal of the injured kidney is seriously considered. Although an arteriogram would permit a more accurate diagnosis, the patient's unstable condition usually does not allow enough time for it to be done.

Intimal damage of one renal artery that results in renal artery thrombosis poses special problems in the early assessment period. Because total renal functioning can be assumed by the uninjured kidney, few (or no) symptoms of the thrombosis and renal ischemia may be present immediately after the injury. Flank pain, along with a history of injury, may make up the whole clinical picture. The thrombosis is found days, weeks, or even months later, when the patient returns to the physician with symptoms of secondary hypertension from the release of renin and angiotensin.

Liver Injury

To reduce the morbidity and mortality in liver trauma, it extremely important to make careful serial assessments of the patient's condition. The early signs and symptoms of complications may thus be assessed and treatment started as soon as possible. Patients who have blunt trauma to the right upper quadrant and who have no immediate problems should be watched for several days for delayed rupture. It is important to watch for the signs and symptoms of peritoneal irritation because blood or bile may collect. Hemobilia is caused by arterial hemorrhage into the biliary tract and classically presents with a triad of symptoms: upper or lower gastrointestinal hemorrhage, obstructive jaundice, and colicky abdominal pain. In the patient who has had liver repair, drainage from the Penrose drains and suction drains should be evaluated carefully for evidence of blood or purulence. If biliary drainage continues in copious amounts, a biliary fistula is suspected.

Small Bowel Injury

Signs of peritoneal irritation can be surprisingly few immediately after rupture of the ileum or jejunum. The pH of the bowel contents at this point is neutral to the peritoneal cavity and the small bowel fluid is relatively sterile.

However, rupture of the duodenum causes fulminant signs and symptoms of peritoneal irritation because the pH of the duodenal contents is highly alkaline to the peritoneal membranes. Irritating substances such as bile and pancreatic enzymes are also highly concentrated in the duodenal contents. When the blunt injury produces a retroperitoneal injury, minimal signs and symptoms are produced even with duodenal rupture. In such a case, the retroperitoneal and not the intraperitoneal spaces are contaminated by the duodenal secretions, and the classic signs of intra-abdominal injury may be absent.

In duodenal trauma, with or without associated pancreatic injury, the most common physical finding is minimal abdominal tenderness. With duodenal injury, the patient becomes worse after a 6-hour period of observation. Early suspicions of rupture are best confirmed or excluded by an emergency gastrointestinal series with Gastrografin (because peritoneal lavage is unreliable in detecting retroperitoneal involvement). If the diagnosis is delayed for more than 24 hours, retroperitoneal dissection of air on a radiograph may become obvious (because it extends upwards). Unfortunately, with such findings, mortality and morbidity are greatly increased.

The assessment of small bowel injury depends heavily on a history of severe blunt injury to the upper abdomen or lower chest, abdominal pain located in the periumbilical areas or radiating to the shoulder tips, testicular pain, positive paracentesis or lavage (if the injury is not retroperitoneal), and a rising or elevated serum or urine amylase level. An abdominal radiograph that reveals free intra-abdominal air is the strongest evidence of small bowel rupture.[57]

Colon Injury

The signs of intra-abdominal contamination and peritoneal irritation develop very rapidly. Peritoneal lavage reveals the presence of blood and fecal material. On rectal examination, the presence of bleeding is suggestive of injury, and palpation of a bony spicule is diagnostic of injury. Radiographs are an important diagnostic tool in assessing free intraperitoneal air that has escaped through perforations or tears of the colon.

Pancreas

Actual injury to the pancreas can be occult, often producing the first physical signs and symptoms 12 to 24 hours after the initial injury. Physical signs can be deceptively minimal because of the protected retroperitoneal position. Sometimes, the injury may be detected before physical signs and symptoms occur, through the use of paracentesis or peritoneal lavage. Laboratory procedures may reveal the presence of an elevated amylase level. A serum or urinary amylase level that is elevated immediately after injury and that stays elevated (or persistently rises), as shown by serial determinations, strongly suggests pancreatic injury and malfunction.

Nonspecific signs and symptoms that are seen are pain, tenderness, guarding, fever, and paralytic ileus. In patients with isolated blunt pancreatic trauma, manifestations typically appear slowly, even days to months later when a pseudocyst is formed.

Sonography and CT scan have changed the diagnostic techniques for acute pancreatitis radically. CT scan is preferable to sonography when the imaging is for an acutely inflamed pancreas.

Postoperatively, the nurse must assess the patient for potential complications: inadequate control of pancreatic secretions, hemorrhage, inadequate control of external drainage at the site of injury, persistent fistulas, abscess formation, and pseudocyst formation. Continued postoperative elevation of the urinary or serum amylase is an important indicator to continue nasogastric suction even in an asymptomatic patient. Signs and symptoms of pseudocyst include pain, fever, ileus, nausea, vomiting, and anorexia. If an abdominal mass is palpated or determined by sonogram or CT scan, the area is surgically drained to prevent rupture and spillage of the contents into the peritoneal cavity.[60]

Although pancreatic drainage is not the major problem of small bowel drainage, the patient's skin should be assessed and protected. (An appliance pouch with Karaya seal or even aluminum paste is beneficial. Dressings should not be used, because a skin reaction will result from the fluid in the dressing, even in the presence of relatively bland pancreatic juice.)

Pelvic Fractures

The physician may determine the presence of a pelvic fracture by palpating the pubic rami and pressing simultaneously on the iliac crest. The technique is particularly good in determining fractures of the iliac crest and sacral region.

The fractures are seen on radiograph. Uncontrolled sites of bleeding are visualized on arteriography (selected arteriography is used for localization of bleeding and for transcatheter embolization with Gelfoam). Diagnostic peritoneal lavage is not accurate in discriminating intraperitoneal from extraperitoneal hemorrhage in the face of pelvic hemorrhage.

The key assessment parameter to determine associated urologic injury is blood in the urine. Because many urologic structures are in the pelvic area, any abnormality found makes an intravenous pyelogram, a retrograde cystogram, and a urologic evaluation imperative. If the patient voids urine that is not bloody, the chances of having a urologic injury are greatly reduced.

NURSING DIAGNOSES, PATIENT OUTCOMES, AND PLAN

The preceding material on anatomy, physiology, nursing assessment, and diagnostic tests guides the nurse in establishing nursing diagnoses, patient outcomes, and plans for the patient with abdominal trauma.

NURSING CARE PLAN SUMMARY   Patient with Abdominal Trauma

NURSING DIAGNOSIS

1. *Decreased cardiac output related to blood loss and hemorrhagic shock (exchanging pattern)*

Patient Outcome	Nursing Orders

1. The patient should demonstrate a stable physiologic response.	1. Monitor the patient's temperature, apical and radial pulses, respirations, and blood pressure as indicated.
	   A. Monitor the apical heartbeat for rate and heart sounds every 30 minutes.
	   B. Assess the respiratory system, including rate, rhythm, breath sounds, and presence of adventitious sounds every hour.
	   C. Assess the patient's mental status every hour. Monitor the hourly urinary output. Notify the physician if it is less than 0.5 to 1 ml/Kg/hr.
	   D. Connect the ECG monitor and set the alarm for 30 beats above and 30 beats below the baseline rates. Notify the physician of abnormalities.
	   E. Obtain a twelve-lead ECG as indicated.

(continued)

NURSING CARE PLAN SUMMARY   *Patient with Abdominal Trauma*   *Continued*

Patient Outcome	*Nursing Orders*
	F. Note the arterial pressure measurement on the monitor every 30 minutes. Check the pressure with a cuff every 2 hours. If there is no arterial line, check the arterial pressure with a cuff every 30 to 60 minutes as indicated. Notify the physician of a systolic pressure less than 90 mm Hg.
	G. If ordered, draw arterial blood gas samples from the arterial line every 4 hours. Monitor oxygenation.
	H. Look for any signs of peripheral vasoconstriction every hour.
	I. Once the patient's condition is stable, the MAST trousers may be systematically and sequentially deflated over a period of 15 to 30 minutes as ordered.
	(1) The trousers were once believed to improve blood pressure during hemorrhagic shock by extremity compression and thus "autotransfusion" of approximately 2 U of blood. Studies have shown, however, that the improvement in blood pressure is due to an increase in systemic vascular resistance. When the trousers are removed, the SVR will fall, which removes the support for the patient's blood pressure. Removal therefore must be accomplished slowly and with adequate volume replacement.[15]
	(2) Before removing the trousers, have two intravenous infusions running.
	(3) Obtain baseline vital signs.
	(4) Deflate the abdominal portion of the trousers.
	(5) Monitor the vital signs for 5 to 10 minutes. If the patient's pulse increases and blood pressure decreases, administer 100 to 200 ml of intravenous fluid until the vital signs stabilize (about 10 minutes).
	(6) Deflate one leg of the trousers. Monitor the vital signs for 5 to 10 minutes. If the patient's pulse increases and the blood pressure decreases, administer intravenous fluid until the pulse decreases and the blood pressure increases.
	(7) Deflate the other leg of the trousers. Monitor the vital signs for 30 minutes.
	J. Measure pulmonary artery and central venous pressures every hour.
	K. If ordered, measure the pulmonary capillary wedge pressure and cardiac output with thermodilution technique.
	L. Every 15 minutes, check for bleeding from orifices or dressings. Mark the dressings.
	M. If there is a vascular injury, note the color and pulse in the distal extremity every 15 minutes. Use the Doppler.
	N. If there is a possibility of injury, perform serial assessments of the structure with a tape measure. (Use a tape measure that does not stretch when it is wet.)
	O. Monitor and assess the trends in the laboratory parameters.
	P. Weigh the patient daily.
	Q. Determine the patient's temperature during surgery. A postoperative rise in temperature is often related to the drop in temperature during surgery.
	R. Administer multiple blood transfusions:
	(1) See Chapter 44.
	(2) Administer fresh blood every 3 to 4 U.
	(3) Monitor clotting studies.

NURSING DIAGNOSIS

2. Fluid volume deficit related to injury and loss of blood (exchanging pattern)

Patient Outcomes	*Nursing Orders*
1. The patient will regain or maintain an adequate oxygen-carrying capacity by means of a blood transfusion.	1. In the emergent situation, initiate therapy with Ringer's lactate solution and have blood typed and crossmatched. If the patient does not respond, if possible use type-specific blood rather than low-titer O negative blood. The blood group

(continued)

NURSING CARE PLAN SUMMARY *Patient with Abdominal Trauma* *Continued*

Patient Outcomes	Nursing Orders

determination takes 5 minutes, and the crossmatch procedure takes 45 minutes. The whole blood is typed but not crossmatched. Do not allow blood to stand at room temperature. If blood cannot be used immediately, return it to blood bank. Blood should be maintained at a constant temperature of 2 to 6°C, and this temperature can be found only in the blood bank, not in the medicine refrigerator.

A. Check the blood type against the patient's name and blood type according to the established protocol.

B. Inspect blood before administration. Send back to blood bank if the bag has been damaged or an abnormal appearance is noted.

C. Assess degree of volume deficit and anticipate replacement (Table 41-6). Communicate potential patient need to blood bank technician.

D. In administration (for 1 U given in less than 3 hours or multiple units administered over a short period of time), use a heat exchanger or a warming apparatus or place the tubing in a pan of warm water. Under no circumstances should cold blood be administered through a central line. When the blood temperature is below 92°F, cardiac dysrhythmias begin to occur: prolongation of the S-T segment, distorted QRS complexes, peaked T waves, premature ventricular contractions, bradycardia, and cardiac standstill.

E. If physician uses a nylon-mesh filter change it after every third unit.

F. Use a pressure apparatus as needed for rapid transfusion. Do not squeeze the bag.

G. For rapid administration as ordered by the physician, packed red blood cells may be reconstituted with saline solution to a 500-ml volume. Observe the patient's clinical and laboratory findings; hypofibrinogenemia and hypoalbuminemia have been noted during massive transfusions with packed red blood cells diluted with saline solution.

H. Do not obtain blood from the band until it is needed, and infuse it within 2 hours. If the blood is warmed, administer it immediately.

I. Obtain baseline information before transfusion—lung sounds, skin color, urine color, and pain status—and observe the patient continuously during the first 50 ml of blood transfusion. Administer blood at no more than 50 drops per minute for the first 2 minutes. Observe and monitor the vital signs every 30 minutes during the transfusion and for 2 hours after it.

J. In the case of multiple transfusions, for every 2 units of blood 9 days old or more, if possible give 1 unit that is less than 48 hours old.

K. During massive transfusion of packed red blood cells or whole blood, anticipate the need for transfusion of platelets and fresh frozen plasma (which contains all the protein constituents of plasma and all the active labile clotting factors). Because the depletion of plasma and clotting factors differs according to individuals, the patient's bleeding status and clotting screen are monitored, and platelets and plasma are given accordingly. As a rule of thumb, with every 10 units of rapidly transfused blood, 2 to 3 units of platelets and 2 to 4 units of fresh frozen plasma are needed.

L. If blood is to be administered to a patient who cannot handle an increased potassium load, transfuse with blood less than 5 days old.

M. If old blood is given, monitor for the signs of hyperkalemia. If hyperkalemia occurs, the treatment includes the use of insulin and glucose to drive the potassium intracellularly. Hyperkalemia is not anticipated unless renal functioning is impaired or unless the blood is given at a rate greater than 100 to 150 ml/minute.

N. Monitor for pulmonary edema and thrombophlebitis.

O. If ordered, administer 10 ml of calcium gluconate (or 44 mEq of calcium chloride) for every 3 units of blood administered rapidly. Do not add calcium to the blood. Monitor the patient for dysrhythmias with an ECG. If the patient needs 10 to 20 U of blood, call the physician before administering calcium to avoid excessive calcium therapy.

P. Know that the patient may exhibit a transitory jaundice after multiple transfusions. If the production of bilirubin is greater than 500 to 900 mg/

(continued)

NURSING CARE PLAN SUMMARY   *Patient with Abdominal Trauma*   *Continued*

Patient Outcomes	Nursing Orders
	day, the normal liver cannot excrete all the pigment load. Both the indirect and direct serum bilirubin levels are elevated. In the 24 hours after transfusion, approximately 10% of the transfused blood undergoes hemolysis. Thus with multiple transfusions, the pigment load is often exceeded and the bilirubin level increases. Also, particularly after retroperitoneal hemorrhage, the breakdown of blood produces the same sequence, and the patient exhibits jaundice.
	Q. Observe for signs of hepatitis after about 6 weeks. Although the testing protocol for hepatitis antigen has decreased the incidence of hepatitis, the risk remains.
2. The patient will not experience a transfusion reaction.	2. Reactions may take place at the beginning of the transfusion, during, or after it. At any untoward sign, stop the transfusion, change the tubing, start the saline solution, and notify the physician. Observe for the following reactions:
	A. A pyrexial reaction, which is the most common one, but which cannot be distinguished from early hemolytic reaction. The cause of a pyrexial reaction is usually not known, but it may be related to the components of the donor's blood, such as the white blood cells or the platelets. Observe for chills, a rise in temperature, nausea, vomiting, headache, and muscle pain.
	B. Allergic reactions occur in 2% to 3% of patients who receive transfusions. Observe for hives, rash, and itching. If ordered by the physician, administer an antihistamine and continue the transfusion.
	C. Bacterial reactions are now extremely rare. Observe for fever, chills, pain, hypotension, and shock. Anticipate treatment for septic shock.
	D. Incompatibility reactions occur once in every 15,000 to 20,000 transfusions. The nurse should:
	(1) Observe for an inappropriately severe aching pain, particularly in the flank, shoulders, back, or hamstrings, a burning pain in the infusion arm, or a constricting pain in the chest; a very tense or anxious feeling; nausea and vomiting; hemoglobinuria; an increase in temperature, pulse, and respirations; headache and chills; and oliguria.
	(2) Monitor vital signs every 15 minutes for 2 hours after transfusion reaction is noted.
	(3) Save all the transfusion equipment and return it to the laboratory.
	(4) Save the urine.
	(5) Monitor the fluid intake and output hourly.
	(6) As ordered by the physician, administer fluid therapy at sufficient volume to maintain the urinary flow at 50 ml/hour. The fluid ordered is usually Ringer's lactate solution. Sodium bicarbonate is ordered to alkalinize the urine and to prevent precipitation of hemoglobin in the tubules. Mannitol is often administered to maintain the urinary flow.

NURSING DIAGNOSIS

3. *High risk for impaired gas exchange related to atelectasis (exchanging pattern)*

Patient Outcomes	Nursing Orders
1. The patient should demonstrate adequate respiratory status.	1. Explain the following procedures to the patient and have them carried out:
	A. Deep breathing once every hour: The patient inhales slowly and evenly, holds breath for three seconds, and exhales normally. This exercise is repeated five times.
	B. Coughing once every hour: The patient takes several deep breaths and then coughs. The abdomen is splinted with hands or pillow.
	C. Assessing the patient's recent smoking history.
2. Oxygenation and ventilation parameters should be within normal limits.	2. Administer 40% to 50% oxygen for approximately 6 hours after transfusion. Temporary hypoxemia is due to general anesthetic, loss of surfactant, airway closure, microatelectasis, and shunting.[4]

(continued)

NURSING CARE PLAN SUMMARY   *Patient with Abdominal Trauma*   *Continued*

Patient Outcomes	Nursing Orders
3. Breath sounds and chest radiograph will indicate clear lungs.	3. Use the incentive spirometer.

NURSING DIAGNOSIS

4. *Impaired gastrointestinal function related to trauma response or surgical procedure (exchanging pattern)*

Patient Outcome	Nursing Orders
1. The patient should show signs of returned gastrointestinal functioning, ileus will disappear, and bowel sounds will become active.	1. Explain the procedure of gastric intubation and its purpose.

1. Explain the procedure of gastric intubation and its purpose.
   A. Maintain the patency of the nasogastric tube. Check the functioning of the suction machine, check the nasogastric tube for kinks or obstruction, and check the connections. Pin the tube to the bed sheet. Irrigate the nasogastric tube with 20 to 30 ml of saline solution every 2 hours.
   B. Record and check the drainage.
   C. Observe for and report any nausea or vomiting. To ameliorate any symptoms
      (1) Avoid a sudden change in the patient's position.
      (2) Maintain the patency of the nasogastric catheter.
      (3) Keep the room well ventilated.
      (4) Keep odors to a minimum.
      (5) Apply an ice collar to the patient's neck.
      (6) Administer antiemetic medications as ordered.
      (7) In a calm voice, tell the patient how the medicine will help. Plan a rest period for the patient after the injection. If vomiting occurs,
         • Turn the patient's head to the side and downward.
         • Support the patient's forehead.
         • Have an emesis basin available.
         • Have a suctioning machine available.
      (8) Following emesis:
         • Remove the vomitus.
         • Help the patient freshen up with a cool, wet washcloth and give mouth care.
         • If necessary, change the bed linens.
         • Provide a period of rest.
         • Remember that often the best relief for nausea is vomiting.
   D. Give mouth care every 2 hours. Have the patient use mouthwash and apply a Chapstick or mentholatum to the lips.
   E. Lubricate the nares with a water-soluble lubricant to prevent dryness and irritation.
   F. Change the tape daily.
   G. Auscultate for bowel sounds.
   H. Check the patient's abdomen for distention and report passage of flatus.

NURSING DIAGNOSIS

5. *Pain related to trauma (feeling pattern)*

Patient Outcome	Nursing Orders
1. The patient will experience a reduction of pain to within a manageable or tolerable level and will have increased comfort.	1. Assess patient's pain with regard to the following: A. Onset B. Duration C. Type

(continued)

NURSING CARE PLAN SUMMARY   *Patient with Abdominal Trauma   Continued*

Patient Outcome	*Nursing Orders*
	D. Intensity
	E. Location
	2. Administer pain medication as ordered. Assess effectiveness.
	3. Allow the patient to express what makes the pain better and what makes it worse.
	4. Reassure patient, and help relieve other sources of discomfort including fear and anxiety. Both fear and anxiety will increase release of pancreatic enzymes, producing more pain.
	5. Assist the patient to assume positions of comfort.

NURSING DIAGNOSIS

6. *Altered gastrointestinal stability related to blunt trauma with potential multiple injuries (exchanging pattern)*

Patient Outcomes	*Nursing Orders*
1. Any findings will be assessed rapidly and managed.	1. Look for a localized area of pain or tenderness, generalized pain, pain on movement or coughing, abdominal distention or rigidity, decreased or absent bowel sounds, rebound tenderness, and increased abdominal size.
	A. Do not palpate or percuss the spleen or liver because it may be fragile and might rupture.
	B. Look for indications of liver trauma, including an elevated white blood cell count, elevated serum glutamic-oxaloacetic transaminase and serum glutamic-pyruvic transaminase levels, and an increased serum bilirubin level.
	C. Note the drains and tubes and know the purpose of each one. Protect the patient's skin from drainage and maintain sterility (Fig. 41–8).
	D. Keep the drains covered with a sterile plastic colostomy bag to protect the wound and collect drainage.
	(1) Liver injuries: one or more large (1-inch) Penrose drains, posterolateral site, gravity drainage, or silastic suction drains; drains left in place 5 to 10 days and slowly advanced/removed over a three-day period, possible T tube to drain common duct.
	(2) Renal injuries: nephrostomy tube, ureterostomy tube.
	(3) Small bowel injury: Penrose drainage; protect skin from excoriation.
	(4) Pancreatic injury: Penrose drainage, sump tube connected to 100 mm Hg suction.
	E. Sutures are removed when enough collagen has been laid in the wound. The time of removal varies according to the patient and the injury. Also, the rate of healing varies in different people, in different parts of the body, and under different conditions. The tensile strength is at or near normal levels at the end of the first month, and it very slowly increases during the next 2 years.
2. The patient will demonstrate healing without any undue complications.	2. Observe for pancreatitis by noting any nausea, vomiting, increased temperature, severe abdominal pain, and rigid abdomen.
	A. Measure all drainage every 8 hours. Record and report any abnormal amounts.
	B. In an injury of the spleen, observe closely for an occult liver injury.
	C. Observe, record, and report any of the following signs of infection: fever, liver pain, an enlarged and tender liver, chills, anorexia, nausea, vomiting, diaphoresis, increased alkaline phosphatase, and an elevated white blood count (18,000 to 20,000 mm³).
	D. Observe for hemobilia by noting any colicky pain, melena, hematemesis, and mild to severe jaundice.
3. The patient should maintain hepatic stability after a liver resection.	3. Assess the patient. The following are considered normal postoperative findings:
	A. A normal blood ammonia level.

(continued)

NURSING CARE PLAN SUMMARY *Patient with Abdominal Trauma* *Continued*

Patient Outcomes	Nursing Orders

Nursing Orders

B. A normal prothrombin time.

C. An increased transaminase level.

D. An increased alkaline phosphatase level.

E. Mild, transient jaundice.

   (1) Monitor carefully if the physician orders analgesics, major tranquilizers, or hypnotics that are normally detoxified by the liver.

   (2) Administer albumin if ordered.

   (3) If the prothrombin time is abnormal, administer vitamin K as ordered.

   (4) Administer whole blood or platelets if they are ordered.

   (5) Increase the patient's calorie and protein intake.

   (6) Observe the intravenous site. Encourage the patient to take nourishment by mouth.

F. If hepatic failure is a threat, take steps as ordered to prevent hyperammonemia, control active bleeding, remove blood from the gastrointestinal tract, and decrease bacterial flora in the gastrointestinal tract. The cause of the encephalopathy seems to be the failure of the diseased liver to detoxify or remove the metabolic products of dietary protein.

   (1) Anticipate that the patient will have an endotracheal tube inserted and will be placed on mechanical ventilation. In hepatic failure with hypoxia and hypercapnia, the cerebral blood flow does not increase reflexly. In the presence of alkalosis, the nondiffusible ammonium ion is converted to toxic diffusible free ammonia. Thus, even small derangements in the arterial oxygen and carbon dioxide levels must be corrected.

   (2) Administer vasopressin (Pitressin) for active bleeding if ordered.

   (3) Perform gastric lavage if ordered.

   (4) Administer magnesium sulfate (15 ml) for catharsis if ordered.

   (5) Give tap water enemas twice daily if ordered.

   (6) Administer neomycin, kanamycin, chloramphenicol, or tetracycline as ordered. The usual therapy is neomycin sulfate (1 g every 4 hours).

   (7) Administer diuretic therapy as ordered.

   (8) Administer potassium salts with diuretic therapy as ordered (the increase in blood ammonia accompanying diuretic therapy is thought to be associated with hypokalemia). Remember that the patient is abnormally sensitive to central nervous system depression.

   (9) Decrease the patient's protein intake to 50 g/day or less as ordered.

  (10) Encourage the patient to eat carbohydrates, because glucose inhibits the bacterial production of ammonia.

  (11) With the dietitian, plan frequent small feedings. Teach the patient to eat slowly and chew thoroughly.

  (12) Use an ice collar for nausea.

  (13) Give mouth care before meals. If the patient's gums bleed easily, use a soft toothbrush or swabs or a gauze pad. Use extreme care, and do not agitate the patient.

  (14) Plan rest periods for the patient.

  (15) Record the patient's fluid intake and output.

  (16) Weigh the patient daily.

  (17) Use padded siderails and keep them in the up position.

  (18) Protect the patient from infection.

  (19) Assess the patient's clinical degree of jaundice daily.

  (20) Observe the stool for consistency and for the presence of blood.

  (21) Prevent pressure areas by turning the patient every hour, by using an alternating pressure mattress, and by putting foam rubber or sheepskin protectors under the pressure areas.

  (22) Use small-gauge needles for injections. Apply pressure to the injection site for 5 minutes after injecting the medication.

  (23) Shave male patients daily and with extreme care.

  (24) Elevate edematous extremities, keeping each distal part higher than the proximal part.

  (25) If the patient complains of pruritus, bathe with sodium bicarbonate or

(continued)

NURSING CARE PLAN SUMMARY *Patient with Abdominal Trauma*   Continued

Patient Outcomes	Nursing Orders
	cornstarch (no soap) and use a soothing lotion. Keep the fingernails short.
	(26) If ordered, administer medications, such as lactulose. Lactulose is administered in doses of 25 to 30 ml three times a day to achieve a stool pH of 5.5 or less. In all likelihood, the colon bacteria convert the lactulose into lactic acid and acetic acid. In the presence of acid, the free ammonia diffusing into the gut is converted into the nondiffusible ammonium ion and excreted. A mild diarrhea is produced.

NURSING DIAGNOSIS

7. *Altered bowel elimination related to temporary externalization of bowel with colostomy (exchanging pattern)*

Patient Outcomes	Nursing Orders

1. The patient should establish a functioning bowel.	1. Observe and record the first passage of flatus and drainage from the temporary colostomy. Auscultate for bowel sounds.
	   A. Determine which stoma is from a proximal loop and which from the distal loop. Be aware that single-use bags may be used if the drainage is minimal and infrequent. Change the bag as needed.
	   B. Know that drainage bags are used if the drainage is profuse and frequent.
	   C. If the stoma is too large for the bag, cut a larger opening in the bag. If the stoma is still too large, use a colostomy belt.

2. The patient will not experience any complications.	2. Consult with the physician about the coverage for the stoma in the early postoperative period.
	   A. The dressings are usually impregnated with petroleum jelly or an antibiotic, such as neomycin or gentamicin.
	   B. Keep the stoma and the surrounding skin clean. Wash the skin with soap and water as it is soiled and keep it dry.
	   C. Determine whether the skin needs an adhesive or protective preparation.
	   D. Order colostomy bags, preferably with a karaya seal. Keep an extra bag on hand, and change the bag as needed.
	   E. Apply Stomadhesive wafers to the surrounding skin to protect it. Bags or dressings will adhere to the adhesive rather than to the skin.

3. The patient will have minimal psychological distress.	3. Explain to the patient and family the purpose of the colostomy and how it works. The patient should be told that the colostomy is temporary.
	   A. With the patient or a member of the family, select foods from the bland, low-fiber menu. Add new foods one at a time to determine whether they cause flatulence.
	   B. Notice when the patient wants to participate in the colostomy care.
	   C. Secure the dressings before the patient begins ambulation. Assure the patient that the dressings will be secure during ambulation.

NURSING DIAGNOSIS

8. *Anxiety related to length of time in unit and continuing unknown prognosis (feeling pattern)*

Patient Outcome	Nursing Orders
The patient should begin to verbalize anxieties.	See Nursing Diagnosis: Anxiety, p. 111.

(continued)

NURSING CARE PLAN SUMMARY   *Patient with Abdominal Trauma*   *Continued*

NURSING DIAGNOSIS

9. *High risk for ineffective individual and family coping related to acute illness and critical care unit (choosing pattern)*

Patient Outcome	Nursing Orders
The patient and family will be able to express feelings and cope with patient's acute illness.	See Nursing Diagnosis: Ineffective Individual and Family Coping, p. 112.

IMPLEMENTATION AND EVALUATION

Priorities in the implementation and evaluation of life-threatening emergencies due to severe trauma, regardless of the organs involved, include: establishing an adequate airway, insuring ventilation, and controlling hemorrhage and shock. The approach to all injured patients should be practical and systematic, to ensure that these priorities are carried out in an efficient, if not automatic, manner. Then the extent and type of injury can be further determined.

Reassessment of the patient with possible intra-abdominal injury must become a permanent part of the patient's ongoing care. Conditions in the abdomen can develop many days after the patient's initial injury. For this reason, the nurse must remain alert to even the most subtle findings, to identify early an occult injury that may have been missed and organ disruption that is delayed. Evaluation for postoperative complications of bleeding, intra-abdominal infection, and poor wound healing follow. It is only with early identification that these sequelae may be managed in such a way that major dysfunction can be averted.

In the effort to treat hemorrhagic shock, it must be remembered that the treatment can create its own problems. The complications of blood transfusions, coagulapathies, transfusion reactions, and electrolyte imbalances, to name a few, added additional system dysfunctions to organs already insulted by the initial trauma. It is important to recognize the pros and cons of each form of volume replacement in hemorrhage, so that new problems can be identified and managed early in the course of the patient's care. Minimizing the adverse effects of the different therapies makes it possible to concentrate on the physiologic consequences of the shock itself, which spares few systems and targets some more than others. Maintenance of the patient's respiratory and renal systems and prevention of infection take priority in the posthemorrhage stage of care.

Probably the most difficult stage in the care of the patient with multiple injuries, for the patient, his family, and the health care team, occurs when the patient's acuity remains high and problems fail to resolve. Multiple procedures must be performed in the effort to reverse persistent problems such as abscesses, poor wound healing, and gastrointestinal dys-function. Multiple trips to the radiography department and to the operating room get translated into feelings of hopelessness over problems that seem never to change, much less resolve. Repeated invasion of the patient tends to press him beyond his limits, at a time when physiologically he is the most stressed and exhausted. The patient and family will need great support in dealing with the discouragement.[46] The health team will need to gather renewed strength to persevere in the attempt to reverse the complications and to keep alive in the patient the hope that things will get better.

Volume Replacement

Fluid resuscitation of shock or hemorrhage begins with insertion of large-bore intravenous catheters or needles into at least two extremities for the infusion of fluid. When trauma involves areas below the diaphragm, one of the catheters is placed in the arm so that injury to large veins in the abdominal cavity or pelvis will not result in loss of infused fluid. Such mechanical precautions allow accurate evaluation of the magnitude or severity of shock or blood losses. Two liters of lactated Ringer's solution is administered rapidly until the blood pressure, pulse, and clinical condition of the patient stabilize or until blood is ready for administration. Blood for type and crossmatch as well as hemoglobin, hematocrit, and other blood chemistries is drawn at the time the intravenous fluids are begun.

It is commonly believed that additional volume support may be gained by elevating the legs to a 45° to 60° angle, a modified Trendelenburg position. The underlying concept is that gravity causes a central translocation of leg venous blood (450 to 750 ml) and an increase in filling pressure, cardiac output, and arterial pressure. The technique has come under closer scrutiny, since the desired results have not been borne out in studies on normal subjects.[24] Further investigation in a hypovolemic model should help clarify the situation.

The type of fluid to be given, electrolyte (crystalloid) solution or colloid, has been the source of much controversy.[12,28,35] Because of its low molecular weight, crystalloid solution has been found to exit the vascular space quickly, resulting in volume expansion effects that are sometimes transient, and threatening the patient with the consequences of interstitial edema. Since crystalloid must be given in three times the volume of colloid infusions, there has been concern that crystalloid could easily cause volume overload in the circulation. Colloid, with its high molecular weight, has more sustained volume expansion effects and minimizes tissue edema by offering increased oncotic pressure to the vascular spaces. A lesser volume of colloid is required to restore hemodynamic stability.[34]

Proponents of crystalloid have long advocated the cost effectiveness of crystalloids over colloids, as well as the reduced side effects. Colloid solutions have been shown to disturb blood type and crossmatch procedures, to cause platelet disturbance and coagulopathy, to depress the levels of free ionized calcium, to depress the levels of immunoglobulins, and to induce allergic reaction in a small percentage of patients. Further investigations, comparing crystalloid to colloid, have continued to support crystalloid solutions.[34,51] Since shock results in a severe contraction of the interstitial fluid compartment, crystalloid, even in large volumes, is the ideal solution for replacement. The administration of large volumes has not been found to increase the risk for pulmonary complications. Meanwhile, colloid can cause rapid, unpredictable increases in cardiac filling pressures, inducing high pulmonary artery and pulmonary capillary pressures, and resulting in hydrostatic pulmonary edema. Shires et al, whose research on hemorrhagic shock led to the development of Ringer's lactate, found that animals resuscitated with blood alone had an 80% mortality; with blood and supplemental plasma had a 70% mortality, and with blood and Ringer's lactate had a 30% mortality.

Ideally, salt replacement solutions should resemble extracellular fluid, which has a pH of 7.4 and electrolyte concentrations in mEq/L of 140 for sodium, 4 for potassium, 109 for chloride, 27 for total base, and 3 for calcium. Normal saline solutions have more sodium and chloride and none of the other electrolytes, and the pH is 6.0. With lactated Ringer's solution, the electrolytes resemble extracellular fluid and the pH is 6.5. In mEq/L, the electrolytes are 130 for sodium, 4 for potassium, and 3 for calcium. The ratio of lactate to chloride is 28:109; therefore, it is called a "balanced" salt solution. More bicarbonate need not be administered, because the lactate is converted rapidly to bicarbonate. Normosol resembles Ringer's solution, except that the pH is 7.4 and there is no calcium.

The goal of colloidal therapy is restoration of volume and flow. The concept of therapeutic hemodilution is aimed at the following: expanded plasma volume, decreased viscosity of the blood at low flow rates, and dispersed aggregated cells for single-file perfusion through capillaries. Evaluative criteria for titration of therapy in the critical care unit are targeted at altering increased viscosity of blood at low flow rates, low pressures, increased hematocrit, increased viscosity of suspending medium, and separation of cell and plasma flow in branched systems due to low flow rate.

Much work is being done on hemoglobin solutions as oxygen-delivering resuscitation fluids; once perfected, their implementation should revolutionize fluid therapy.[17]

Drugs

In hemorrhagic shock, drugs are almost never needed; volume restoration will suffice. Any drugs the physician selects are used only as adjuncts and must be administered carefully in titrated doses.

Although prolonged use of vasoconstrictors is contraindicated, their brief use to prevent cardiac arrest and maintain arterial blood pressure while volume therapy is being initiated is accepted in some institutions. Norepinephrine, administered through central line by meticulous titration, is probably the drug of choice in these situations. The drug tends to sustain cerebral perfusion pressure and protect the brain by increasing extracerebral peripheral resistance and to maintain coronary artery perfusion and prevent cardiac arrest by maintaining diastolic blood pressure.

Several drugs may be used to improve cardiac function. Glucagon clinically acts as a cardiac stimulant and improves cardiac contractility (ATP is converted to cyclic AMP). Digitalis is helpful in patients with pre-existing cardiac disease to improve their hemodynamics when hemorrhagic shock is not helped by other means. Digitalis is not helpful in patients with previously normal hearts. Vasodilators may have a place in the treatment of the rare patient in irreversible shock whose peripheral vascular resistance is increased.[1] Here, vasodilatation will reduce myocardial oxygen consumption by reducing peripheral resistance and cardiac wall tension. Blood supply to the cardiac muscle may improve. Tachycardia and a decreased perfusion pressure during diastole, however, may result. In these selected instances, vasodilator therapy has been combined with blood volume expansion.

Inotropic drugs (epinephrine, dopamine in low doses, dobutamine, and isoproterenol) may cause dysrhythmias and are contraindicated. Although the force of cardiac contraction is increased, heart rate and automaticity are also increased and set the stage for dysrhythmias. Isoproterenol is a pure beta-receptor agonist and decreases organ perfusion by dilating blood vessels in the skin and muscles.

SUMMARY

Patients with abdominal trauma evidence a wide range of conditions. Hypovolemic shock states often accompany abdominal trauma and range in severity and duration from moderate, transient blood loss (which may be quickly treated by blood volume restoration) to severe, prolonged hypoperfusion resulting in unresponsiveness to therapy, death of cells, and cardiac arrest. Members of the health team must be diligent in assessing and managing patient problems. Nurses work as members of the team and have responsibilities in every area of the hospital: emergency department, operating room, recovery room, and critical care unit. Because the patient moves from one area to another, transfer of information and coordination of care become a primary nursing responsibility.

DIRECTIONS FOR FUTURE RESEARCH

Areas for nursing research are prevalent in trauma nursing. Even the fundamental areas in trauma nursing have not been well researched. Viable topics in prehospital care include documentation, information relay systems, assessment parameters for viability and recovery, protocol determination and implementation, and identification of potential candidates for organ donation. Time often does not permit the type of educational program seen with the cardiac patient before open heart surgery, but nurses do need to identify the type and quantity of preparatory information that should be imparted to the patient. Rehabilitation of the patient with abdominal trauma starts with admission, and it is important to identify the effect of early initiation of nursing measures (*e.g.*, passive range of motion exercises, body positioning, sleep/rest periods) on successful rehabilitation.[33]

Once nurses practicing in care delivery settings as well as nurses associated with educational programs identify relevant, researchable questions and begin to implement systematic investigations, nursing care will become more and more founded in science. Many hospital administrators believe they have a responsibility to help nurses in these studies. They see research as a priority in the acute care setting, and believe nurses should have budgeted time, funds, appropriate educational programs or conferences, consultants, and library/secretarial assistance.

REFERENCES

1. Albert, S. A., Shires, G. T., III, Illner, H., and Shires, G. T. Effects of haloxone in hemorrhagic shock surgery. *Surg. Gynecol. Obstet.* 155:326, 1982.

2. Almskog, B. A., Heljamoe, H., Hosselgren, P. O., Hordstrom, G., and Seeman, T. Local metabolic changes in skeletal muscle following high energy missile injury. *J. Trauma* 22:382, 1982.

3. Bender, J. S., Geller, E. R., Wilson, R. F. Intra-abdominal sepsis following liver trauma. *J. Trauma* 29:1140, 1989.

4. Breslin, E. H. Prevention and treatment of pulmonary complications in patients after surgery of the upper abdomen. *Heart Lung* 10:510, 1981.

5. Cass, A. S. Immediate radiologic and surgical management of renal injuries. *J. Trauma* 22:361, 1982.

6. Chaudry, I. H., Sayeed, M. M., and Baue, A. E. Depletion and restoration of tissue ATP in hemorrhagic shock. *Arch. Surg.* 108:208, 1974.

7. Cogbill, T. H., Moore, E. E., Jurkovich, G. J., Morris, J. A., Mucha, P., and Shackford, S. R. Nonoperative management of blunt splenic trauma: A multicenter experience. *J. Trauma* 29:1312, 1989.

8. Cogbill, T. H., Moore, E. E., Jurkovich, G. J., Feliciano, D. V., Morris, J. A., and Mucha, P. Severe hepatic trauma: A multicenter experience with 1,335 liver injuries. *J. Trauma* 28:1433, 1988.

9. Committee on Trauma, Commission of Life Sciences, National Research Council, Institute of Medicine: *Injury in America*, Washington, D.C.: National Academy Press, 1985.

10. Condon, R. E. Post splenectomy sepsis in traumatized adults. *J. Trauma* 22:169, 1982.

11. Cox, E. F. Blunt abdominal trauma. *Ann. Surg.* 199(4):467, 1984.

12. Cross, J. S., Gruber, D. P., Burchard, K. W., Singh, A. K., Moran, J. M., and Gann, D. S. Hypertonic Saline Fluid Therapy Following Surgery: A Prospective Study, *J. Trauma* 29:817, 1989.

13. Cryer, H. M., Miller, F. B., Evers, B. M., Rouben, L. R., and Seligson, D. L. Pelvic fracture classification: Correlation with hemorrhage. *J. Trauma* 28:973, 1988.

14. Dang, C. V., Peter, E. T., Parks, S. N., and Ellyson, J. H. Trauma of the colon: Early drop-back of exteriorized repair. *Arch. Surg.* 117:652, 1982.

15. Dickerman, J. D. Traumatic asplenia in adults, a defined hazard. *Arch. Surg.* 116:361, 1981.

16. DiMaio, V. J. M. Penetration and perforation of skin by bullets and missiles: A review of the literature. *Am. J. Forensic Med. Pathol.* 2(2):107, 1981.

17. De Venuto, F. Hemoglobin solutions as oxygen delivering resuscitation fluids. *Crit. Care Med.* 10:238, 1982.

18. Duncan, A. O., Phillips, T. F., Scalea, T. M., Maltz, S. B., Atweh, N. A., and Sclafani, S. J. A. Management of transpelvic gunshot wounds. *J. Trauma* 29:1335, 1989.

19. Fackler, M. L. Ballistic injury. *Ann. Emerg. Med.* 15:1451, 1986.

20. Fackler, M. L. Wounds ballistics: A review of common misconceptions. *JAMA* 259:2730, 1988.

21. Fackler, M. L., Surincha, J. S., Malinowski, J. A., et al. Bullet fragmentation: A major cause of tissue disruption. *J. Trauma* 24:35, 1984.

22. Fackler, M. L., and Malinowski, J. A. The wound profile: A visual method for quantifying gunshot wound components. *J. Trauma* 25:522, 1985.

23. Flint, L. M., Cryer, H. M., Howard, D. A., et al. Approaches to the management of shotgun injuries. *J. Trauma* 24:415, 1984.

24. Gaffney, F. A., Bastian, B. C., Thal, E. R., Atkins, J. M., and Blomquist, C. G. Passive leg raising does not produce a significant or sustained autotransfusion effect. *J. Trauma* 22:190, 1982.

25. Goldberger, J. H., Bernstein, D. M., Rodman, G. H., and Suarez, C. A. Selection of patients with abdominal stab wounds for laparotomy. *J. Trauma* 22:476, 1982.

26. Goris, R. J., and Draaisma, J. Causes of death after blunt trauma. *J. Trauma* 22:141, 1982.

27. Grieco, J. G., Perry, J. F. Retroperitoneal hematoma following trauma: Its clinical importance. *J. Trauma* 20:733, 1980.

28. Gross, D., Landau, E. H., Assalia, A., Krausz, M. M. Is hypertonic saline resuscitation safe in "uncontrolled" hemorrhagic shock? *J. Trauma* 28:751, 1988.

29. Hebeler, R. F., Ward, R. E., Miller, P. W., and Ben-Menachem, Y. The management of splenic injury. *J. Trauma* 22:492, 1982.

30. Ivatury, R. R., Zubowski, R., Psarras, P., Nallathambi, M., Rohman, M., and Stahl, W. M. Intra-abdominal abscess after penetrating abdominal trauma. *J. Trauma* 28:1238, 1988.

31. Johnson, J. E., Rice, U. H., Fuller, S. S., and Endress, P. M. Sensory information: Instructions in a coping strategy and recovery. *Res. Nurs. Health* 11:4, 1978.

32. Lange, D. A., Zaret, P., Merlotti, G. J., Robin, A. P., Sheaff, C., Barrett, J. A. The use of absorbable mesh in splenic trauma. *J. Trauma* 28:269, 1988.

33. Lewandowski, L., and Kositsky, A. M. Research priorities for critical care care nursing: A study by the American Association of Critical-Care Nurses. *Heart Lung* 12:35, 1983.

34. Maier, R. V., Carrico, C. J. *Developments in the Resuscitation of Critically Ill Surgical Patients*. Chicago: Year Book Medical Publishers, Inc., 1986.

35. Mattar, J. A. Hypertonic and hyperoncotic solutions in patients. *Crit. Care Med.* 17:297, 1989.

36. Mattox, K. D. Abdominal venous injuries. *Surgery* 91(5):497, 1982.

37. Meyer, D. M., Thal, E. R., Weigelt, J. A., and Redman, H. C. The role of abdominal CT in the evaluation of stab wound to the back. *J. Trauma* 29:1226, 1989.

38. Millikan, J. S., Moore, E. E., Moore, G. E., and Stevens, R. E. Alternatives to splenectomy in adults after trauma. *Am. J. Surg.* 144:711, 1982.

39. National Center for Health Statistics: *Current Estimates from the National Health Interview Survey*. Hyattsville, MD: United States, Series 10, #141, DHHS Publication # (PHS) 82-1569, 1981.

40. O'Connel, K. J., Clark, M., Lewis, R. H., et al. Comparison of low- and high-velocity ballistic trauma genitourinary organs. *J. Trauma* 28:S139, 1988.

41. O'Neal, B. J., and McDonald, J. C. The risk of sepsis in the asplenic adult. *Ann. Surg.* 194:775, 1981.

42. Pickhardt, R., Moore, E. E., Moore, F. A., McCroskey, B. L., and Moore, G. E. Operative splenic salvage in adults: A decade perspective. *J. Trauma* 29:1386, 1989.

43. Rehm, C. G., Sherman, R., and Hinz, T. W. The role of CT scan in evaluation for laparotomy in patients with stab wounds of the abdomen. *J. Trauma* 29:446, 1989.

44. Rivkind, A. I., Siegel, J. H., and Dunhma, M. Patterns of organ

injury in blunt hepatic trauma and their significance for management and outcome. *J. Trauma* 29:1398, 1989.

45. Robertson, H. D., Ray, J. E., Ferreri, B. T., and Gathright, J. B. Management of rectal trauma. *Surg. Gynecol. Obstet.* 154:161, 1982.

46. Schilpp, A. M., and Levesque, J. Helping the patient cope with the sequelae of trauma through the self-help group approach. *J. Trauma* 21:135, 1981.

47. Schwartz, P. E., Sterioff, S., Mucha, P., Melton, J. L., and Offord, K. P. Postsplenectomy sepsis and mortality in adults. *J.A.M.A.* 248:2279, 1982.

48. Sherman, J. C., Delaurier, G. A., Hawkins, M. L., Brown, L. G., Treat, R. C., and Mansberger, A. R. Percutaneous peritoneal lavage in blunt trauma patients: A safe and accurate diagnostic method. *J. Trauma* 29:801, 1989.

49. Shires, G. T., Jones, R. C., Perry, M. O., et al. Trauma. In S. S. Schwartz (ed.). *Principles of Surgery.* New York: McGraw-Hill, 1984.

50. Shires, G. T., Williams, J., and Brown, F. Simultaneous measurement of plasma volume, extracellular fluid volume, and red blood cell mass in man utilizing I^{131}, S^{35} O_4, and Cr^{51}. *J. Lab. Clin. Med.* 55:776, 1960.

51. Shires, G. T. *Principles of Trauma Care.* New York: McGraw-Hill, 1985.

52. Strate, R. G., and Grieco, J. G. Blunt injury to the colon and rectum. *J. Trauma* 23:384, 1983.

53. Sykes, L. N., Champion, H. R., and Fouty, W. J. Dum-dums, hollow-points, and devastators: Techniques designed to increase wounding potential of bullets. *J. Trauma* 28:618, 1988.

54. Thal, E. R., and Yeary, E. C. Morbidity of colostomy closure following colon trauma. *J. Trauma* 20:287, 1980.

55. Thal, E. R., McClelland, R. N., and Shires, G. T. Abdominal trauma. In G. T. Shires (ed.), *Principles of Trauma Care.* New York: McGraw-Hill, 1985.

56. Thompson, J. S., and Moore, E. E. Factors affecting the outcome of exteriorized colon repairs. *J. Trauma* 22:403, 1982.

57. Trunkey, D. D. Massive abdominal trauma. In J. D. Hardy (ed.), *Critical Surgical Illness.* Philadelphia: W. B. Saunders, 1980.

58. Waller, J. A. *Injury Control: A Guide to the Causes and Prevention of Trauma.* Lexington, VA.: Lexington Books, 1985, p. 222.

59. White, K. M. Injuring mechanisms of gunshot wounds. *Crit. Care Nurs. Clin. North Am.* 1:97, 1989.

60. Wilford, M. E., Foster, W. L., Helvorsen, R. A., and Thompson, W. M. Pancreatic pseudocyst: Comparative evaluation by sonography and computer tomography. *Am. J. Radiol.* 140:53, 1983.

42

Extremity Trauma

Connie A. Walleck   *Cornelia Vanderstaay Kenner*

DREAM LOG

Dreams, combined with nonsleep imagery, are powerful sources of inner knowledge and interpretation of feelings and symptoms. There are ways to get more involved in your dream life. It is possible to learn how to direct the "storyline" and outcomes of your dreams to some extent. When you do this, it is called *lucid dreaming*. Guidelines for **lucid dreaming** are as follows:

- Ask yourself frequently during the day if you are dreaming, and look for evidence to prove to yourself that you are not. LaBerge* suggests reading something, looking away, and then reading it again. If it reads the same way twice, you are probably not dreaming.
- Tell yourself that you want to recognize a nighttime dream the next time one occurs.
- As you prepare to go to sleep remind yourself that you want to recognize that you are dreaming when you begin to do so. This is the same technique as reminding yourself during the day to fill your car with gas on the way home.
- If you awaken during the night from a dream, imagine returning to it immediately. This may be enough to allow you to dream lucidly when you return to sleep.
- Practice this exercise as often as possible over several nights, and record your results in your log as soon as you awaken.

Keeping dream logs can add to your insight and self-confidence and improve physical and mental health. The reason this occurs is that more of your creative self is revealed to you. A dream log is similar to the intuition log (p. 501). In your dream log, notice people, animals, locations, colors, patterns, and associated feelings. Some dreams are easy to figure out; others take time. Then there are other dreams that are very obscure in their meaning. Just be with all the dreams that surface, and over time new insight will be gained.

Another helpful technique to influence your dream life is to record positive affirmations to yourself on a tape recorder and play them before you go to bed. It is also helpful to play affirmations on awakening in the morning because these thought forms get into conscious awareness and affect your self-image throughout the day. Thus, as you go to bed, the positive thoughts are still in conscious awareness and continue into your sleep states. Entries in your dream log might include the following:

- What is a title that pops into your mind about this dream?
- Do your dreams have repetitive themes and messages?
- Is there a message that applies to events in your life right now?
- Is this an ordinary dream, or is it spectacular?
- What are the emotions that come forward in the dream (gentleness, anger, action, and so on)?
- Who are the characters in the dream?
- Did you like the ending to the dream?
- Do you want to have this dream again? If you do, how do you want to change the ending?
- Can you give yourself positive affirmations about this dream before sleep or upon rising in the early morning?

* LaBerge, S. *Lucid Dreaming*. New York: Ballantine Books, 1985.

LEARNING OBJECTIVES

After reading this chapter, the nurse should be able to do the following:

1. Assess and monitor a fractured extremity in a person who has an associated nerve injury and in a patient who has not.
2. Monitor preoperatively and postoperatively the patient who has a vascular injury.
3. List the clinical signs in a patient with fat emboli.
4. Define two clinical situations in which imagery or therapeutic touch would prove useful in the management of a patient with orthopedic trauma.
5. Outline the observations made by the nurse for a patient receiving a blood transfusion.

CASE STUDY

Mr. T., a 21-year-old Mexican-American man, presented to the emergency department after a motorcycle accident. Immediately after the accident, Mr. T. had complained of severe pain in his right thigh. He had a profuse hematoma of his right thigh, a gaping wound on the lateral aspect of his right thigh, moderate nonpulsatile bleeding, and obvious debris in the wound. Crepitus was noted over his right femur as an incidental finding, and the position and angulation of the thigh seemed abnormal. Before moving Mr. T., the paramedics stopped the bleeding in the thigh wound by direct pressure and a compression bandage. Stability of the femur was achieved by splinting the leg with minimal manipulation.

On admission to the emergency department, Mr. T. had a blood pressure of 100 mm Hg systolic by palpation, pulse of 130/minute, and gross hematuria. His hematocrit was 28% and his central venous pressure (CVP) was 3 cm H_2O. Urine output was 50 ml for the first hour. A basic workup showed a major disruption of the right kidney; an open grade II comminuted, displaced subtrochanteric fracture of the right femur; open grade II severely comminuted fractures of the right distal tibia and fibula with major soft-tissue loss; and left talar neck fracture. His right thigh was swollen, and the tissue about the open wound appeared crushed and nonviable. In the midportion of the diaphysis, the compound fracture of the femur could be noted. During the assessment, the intactness of circulation to his right lower extremity was verified, because his pedal pulses could be heard with the Doppler. Mr. T. was not allergic to penicillin and had had his last tetanus booster about 5 years before.

Mr. T.'s thigh wound was irrigated repeatedly with several liters of normal saline solution. Exploration of the wound, ligation of vessels, and removal of foreign materials were postponed until the wound could be inspected adequately under sterile conditions during surgery. Packing the wound with sterile gauze and applying hand pressure brought the bleeding under control. A Thomas splint was used to stabilize the femur during Mr. T.'s trip to the operating room.

At surgery, an abdominal laparotomy was performed, and the right inferior renal pole was amputated. During the procedure, a large retroperitoneal hematoma was identified in the pelvis and felt to be secondary to retroperitoneal tissue disruption associated with the kidney injury. Simultaneous with laparotomy, the fractures of the tibia and fibula were debrided and stabilized with a Hoffman device. The thigh wound was incised and debrided widely, and the necrotic tissue was removed. Muscle tissue that was considered nonviable was also removed. Foreign material and blood clots were removed by irrigation to avoid a nidus for infection. No associated vascular or peripheral nerve injury seemed to be present with any one of the fractures. At this point in the procedure, Mr. T.'s general condition deteriorated. His blood pressure was 82/48 mm Hg, pulse 134 beats/minute, and CVP 2 cm H_2O. Because of Mr. T.'s unstable condition, the surgeon decided to change his plan to fix the subtrochanteric fracture internally.

Instead, a Steinmann pin was inserted under strict aseptic conditions. Balanced surgical traction using a Thomas splint with a Pearson attachment and 25 pounds of weight was to be employed postoperatively to stabilize the fractured femur. The wound was left open to drain.

When the primary nurse received Mr. T. in the critical care unit, she noted that he had received an additional 500 ml of Ringer's lactate and 3 U of whole blood because his condition had become unstable. Communication with the surgeon led to the assessment of hypovolemia related to blood loss that was now corrected.

The next day Mr. T. told his primary nurse how worried he was about his leg. He let her know that he felt so anxious he was almost consumed with worry. Several years before his accident, an uncle had been injured in a similar mishap. The uncle had suffered a lifelong handicap following osteomyelitis and nonunion. Mr. T. stated that he was afraid he would meet the same fate.

On trauma rounds that afternoon, the primary nurse discussed Mr. T.'s concerns with the other members of the team. It was decided to involve Mr. T. more in the healing process. A form of imagery would be used to help facilitate wound healing. Such involvement would also give Mr. T. control over one aspect of his own care and prevent feelings of helplessness and psychological immobility. Mr. T. responded readily to the interventions. He was much more comfortable and began to believe he would have an uneventful recovery. One week later he was transferred to the orthopedic unit, where the nurses continued the original plan. Four weeks later he was discharged from the hospital. He returned to full-time work in 2 months.

REFLECTIONS

Fear of the unknown, powerlessness, helplessness, and anxiety all contribute to the stress experienced by the patient with extremity trauma. It is generally agreed that the experience of being in a critical care unit is individually interpreted and translated by patients depending on their life history patterns, psychological makeup, and situational events (see Chap. 8). Stress is influenced greatly by such factors as fear, anxiety, and anticipation. These factors may indeed account for more variance in perception of the experience than the extent of the injury itself.

Although it is not known how decreasing stress levels can influence the outcome of bone fractures, the body's electromagnetic fields may be involved. When a bone breaks, an electrochemical current develops and continues to flow until bone repair is completed. If the current stops flowing before healing is complete, the result is nonunion, a failure of the bone to heal. Bassett[3] and Brighton et al[6,7,27] have demonstrated healing by stimulating the fracture site with small electrodes and minute currents. Bassett has shown the effectiveness of pulsing electromagnetic fields of selected pulse character to influence the actual healing process. Brighton et al have shown improvements by using capacitatively coupled devices that are portable and relatively insensitive to positioning errors, and they have demonstrated healing of nonunited bones as long as 20 years after the fracture.

Medicine and nursing are just now approaching the level of sophistication at which the disciplines can collaboratively study the entire electromagnetic field of the body and what affects it. It is possible that the work in therapeutic touch[16,26,30,38] actually attempts to affect the body's electromagnetic field. Therapeutic touch is directed toward a conscious use of self in the patient interaction. Not only therapeutic touch, but touch itself, when introduced into the nurse–patient interaction, may facilitate the communication process, decrease levels of anxiety, and reinforce a component of security—all of which decreases the stress levels of the patient. Today what is known is that stress causes a physiologic shift toward catabolism, and that the relaxation response causes a shift in the opposite direction.[23] In the future the benefits of decreasing stress by manipulation of the electromagnetic fields will become more clear.[46]

ETIOLOGY

Trauma is the number one killer of Americans between the ages of 1 and 44 and the number one killer of all Americans. Trauma kills more than 150,000 per year and permanently disables 400,000 others.[53] Seventy-five percent of all trauma involves the extremities.[15,24] There are over 6 million fractures or dislocations in the United States each year. This represents over 30% of all days of restricted activity due to injuries of all types. The hand or function of the hand is involved one third of the time.[21] Patients may suffer permanent functional impairment that prevents their return to a previous level of employment.

Vascular injury may occur alone from blunt or penetrating trauma or may be associated with a fracture. Arterial injuries are associated infrequently with fracture and dislocation. Sher[39] found an incidence of 2.8% of associated arterial and fracture/dislocation injuries. When associated with orthopedic trauma, vascular compromise is most likely to occur from open fractures and gunshot wounds, supracondylar fractures of the humerus or femur, femoral shaft fractures, and knee dislocations.

Peripheral nerve injuries may accompany fracture/dislocation or vascular injury. In one series,[25] 35% of patients with vascular injury to the axilla also had evidence of injury to the brachial plexus, and these patients had the most severe and permanent disabilities.

PSYCHOPATHOPHYSIOLOGY

Injury to the extremities may involve any combination of the following: bone, cartilage, ligaments, muscles, soft tissues, blood vessels, nerves, and the skin. In the following sections, three of the most hazardous injuries will be discussed: fractures, vascular injury, and associated peripheral nerve injury.

Fractures

A fracture of the bone occurs when either *direct* or *indirect* forces placed on the bone exceed its elasticity and thus cause deformation (Fig. 42–1). The normal continuity of bone or cartilage is interrupted. Fractures may be closed or open.

Open Fractures

Open fractures are an entity unto themselves. A primary objective of care of open fractures is the prevention of infection and the encouragement of bone union. The causes of open fractures range from laceration to a crushing injury. By definition, *open fractures* communicate with the external environment and thus are contaminated with microorganisms, have soft-tissue injury, and possibly contain a foreign body. As in all forms of trauma, the greatest variable is the severity of the initial accident and the resulting damage to bone, skin, blood

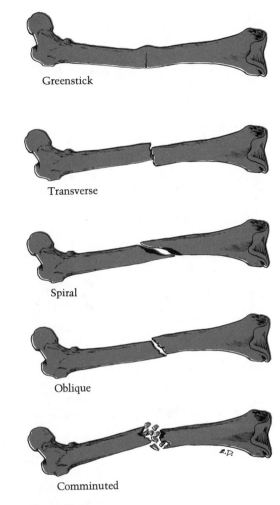

Figure 42–1

Common types of fractures.

Greenstick

Transverse

Spiral

Oblique

Comminuted

vessels, nerves, muscles, and tendons. Added to the problems of the initial injury are the possible complications of decreased circulation, infection, osteomyelitis, delayed union, and nonunion.

Open fractures are often associated with severe bleeding. Fractures of the femoral shaft and proximal tibia are the most common. The blood is lost from the torn muscles and bony fragments as well as from an artery or vein cut by a sharp bony fragment.

Healing

Once the extravasated blood around the end of the bone clots, healing begins (Fig. 42–2). Fracture healing is intimately related to the process of revascularization across the fracture gap. Refer to Chapter 3, Case Study 1, for imagery and bone healing. An aseptic inflammatory response is soon apparent with blood vessel dilatation, resulting in a hyperemia and a local increase in temperature. Increased capillary permeability permits protein and granulocytes to leak out into the tissue and produces edema. Both ecchymosis and swelling result. Organization of the blood clot is rapid (36 to 48 hours), in that the conversion of fibrinogen to fibrin forms a meshwork of fibers that later collects albumin, globulin, fibrinogen, and

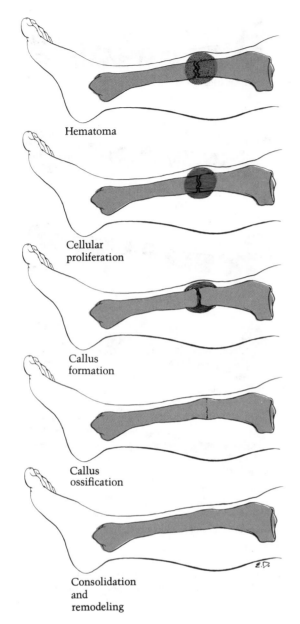

Figure 42–2

Progression of fracture healing.

The process takes place both around the bone fragments and at a distance. Thus an irregular bridge, or callus, is built from one bone fragment to another. At first, the callus is composed of fiber bone, but later it is absorbed and remodeled with osteal bone according to the stresses and strains that have occurred. This major contribution of soft-tissue blood supply and external callus formation is made in the first 6 to 8 weeks after injury.

Acute Compartment Syndrome

Compartment syndrome is defined as elevated interstitial pressure within a space defined and limited by a fascial envelope.[13] If the interstitial pressure is high enough, it will increase the venous pressure, reduce the local arteriovenous gradient, diminish the local blood flow, and reduce tissue oxygenation. This chain of events may result in temporary or permanent ischemia and damage to the soft-tissue structures within that compartment. Any patient with an extremity injury, whether caused by penetrating or blunt trauma, should be considered at risk for the development of compartment syndrome.[47] Certainly, blunt trauma, with its resulting contusion and hemorrhage within the compartment, often produces elevated tissue pressures.[9]

Figure 42–3 illustrates the four fascial compartments of the lower leg. Any of the compartments can contain tightly swollen muscle that becomes compressed and ischemic. Transverse or comminuted fractures, whether from a direct blow or sustained in a motor vehicle accident, often have considerable soft-tissue contusion and result in acute compartment syndrome. Pieces of torn muscle can also act with fascial tears in a ball valve mechanism and close an already swollen compartment. Hypotension increases the susceptibility to increases of compartment pressure.[12]

Fat Embolism

Fat embolism most commonly occurs 12 to 72 hours after a fracture of a long bone, although it can be seen as soon as 1 hour or less after the injury.[5] It causes approximately 5000

other extravasated cells. Granulation tissue thus invades the clot, and reticuloendothelial cells remove the debris. The pH of the tissue fluid around the bone fragments decreases so that some of the calcium goes into solution. New capillaries grow into the blood clot, and fibroblasts follow the pattern established by the fibrin meshwork. The torn edges of periosteum, endosteum, and bone marrow produce cells that help form new bone.

After 2 weeks, the alkaline phosphatase concentration increases around the bone fragments, and the pH of the tissue rises. Because calcium is then no longer soluble, calcium salts precipitate in the meshwork. Osteoid tissue is produced by the bone-forming cells, collagen is formed from fibroblasts, ground substance is formed from myxoplasts, and cartilage is formed from chondroblasts. Calcium salts and ground substance are deposited onto and around the collagen meshwork.

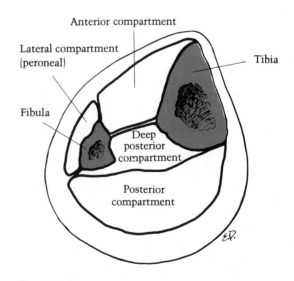

Figure 42–3

Cross section of compartments in the middle third of the leg.

deaths per year. It is manifested as the posttraumatic respiratory distress syndrome of skeletal trauma. The earliest signs are an elevation of pulse, temperature of above 100°F, and a falling PaO_2. Although the condition may occur in people of any age, it occurs most commonly in people aged 20 to 30 (among whom the tibia and the femur are the long bones most commonly fractured) and in people aged 70 to 80 (among whom the hip is the long bone most commonly fractured). Fat embolism also occurs with extensive trauma, burns, infection that develops after cardiac resuscitation, bypass procedures, renal transplantations, diabetes, and alcoholism.

It is commonly accepted that fat embolism results in hypoxemia, probably produced by fat globules that occlude the pulmonary circulation. After mechanical trauma, pressure in the long bones that have a high fat content is increased. The veins within the bones are prevented from collapsing because they adhere to the bony framework. Fat droplets are forced into the bloodstream through the open veins. The signs and symptoms observed depend on the body system affected. The lung is the primary filter, and embolism results in parenchymal damage as well as increased pulmonary vascular resistance that affects the patient's cardiovascular status. Embolism may also be observed as a central nervous system aberration and as petechiae in the skin.

Two other mechanisms for fat embolisms have been proposed. The first focuses on biochemical changes in the body after fracture. Fat droplets arise within the circulated blood as a result of the metabolic response to injury. In severe stress, the stability of the body's emulsified fat (neutral triglycerides and phospholipids) is lost. The small fat particles coalesce and form microglobules that are large enough to be trapped in the lung capillaries. These fat microglobules then act as emboli and block the capillaries. The other mechanism implicated in fat embolism addresses the result of catecholamine and corticosteroid release as a response to stress. The hormones act on the serum lipids to mobilize tissue stores of fats that act as emboli after their release into the circulation. It is possible that all three postulates play a part in fat embolism.

In any event, the particles act as emboli in the lung and set up a response that may result in the adult respiratory distress syndrome.[21] The patient may suffer from cor pulmonale, direct lung damage inflicted by the free fatty acids, vasospasm, and airway constriction from the vasoactive amines from the fracture site, platelet amines, and the histamine locally released.

Vascular Injury

Traumatic damage to a large artery or vein that supplies blood most often results from a penetrating injury. The vascular injury may be complicated by an associated fracture or dislocation. In an accident, the force imparts a tremendous amount of energy to the tissues:

Energy = ½ mass × velocity squared

The heat dissipated is likely to injure a vessel even though the vessel has not been touched directly.

Three categories of patients with vascular injury have been identified.[8] Category 1 consists of patients with obvious life-threatening vascular injuries (*e.g.*, the patient in hemorrhage shock). These patients require immediate surgery. Category 2 consists of patients in whom an obvious vascular injury endangers a limb, but the injury is not life-threatening. The physician will have time to have arteriography performed before taking the patient to surgery. Category 3 consists of patients with injuries near major vessels, but an injury to the vasculature is not immediately apparent. Here, arteriography is vital in determining the presence of a vascular injury.

The patient may also form a pseudoaneurysm, a hole in an artery that is a contained hematoma. The pseudoaneurysm gets bigger and bigger until it ruptures. This is one of the most common causes of delayed hemorrhage. When the initial clot lyses in about 48 hours, the patient may start to bleed severely.

Popliteal Artery Involvement

Injury of the popliteal artery results in amputation of the affected extremity more often than any other arterial injury. Adjacent injuries, small-vessel thrombosis, and muscle necrosis are the major deterrents to limb salvage. During the last two decades, reported amputation rates for civilian popliteal artery injuries have been in the range of 20% to 30%.[36,44] Single muscle or stab wounds uncommonly result in amputation, but shotgun wounds and blunt trauma cause limb loss in one third or more of such injuries. There are several factors related to the success of vascular surgery for popliteal artery trauma: the delay before establishment of blood flow must be as short as possible, because there is poor collateral blood flow to the leg below the knee; and patients with a penetrating injury have a greater chance for limb salvage than those with blunt trauma.[34]

Fracture dislocations of the knee threaten limb viability.[4,54] The popliteal vessels are fixed above by the adductor muscles and below by the soleus; the genicular collaterals are fragile and easily torn. A posterior dislocation of the knee is likely to injure the artery. These delicate vessels maintain some distal perfusion after occlusion of the normal popliteal artery but are easily obliterated by swelling.[44] The paucity of resilient and high-flow channels about the knee increases the necessity to prevent distal small-vessel thrombosis after traumatic popliteal artery occlusion. It is easy for knee instability to be overlooked in multiple injuries. Sudden severe and perhaps irreversible limb ischemia may be the first indication that popliteal artery thrombosis caused by stretch damage to the artery has supervened.

Peripheral Nerve Injury

A frequent concomitant of trauma is an injury to one or more peripheral nerves (Fig. 42–4), especially when associated with a vascular injury. Open fractures are described in the literature as the classic predisposing problem, but the cause may as well be a closed fracture or a crushing, blunt, or penetrating injury.

Injuries may be caused directly or indirectly. For example, a sharp object (*e.g.*, a knife or the end of a splintered bone) may damage a nerve directly. An injury may occur from edema or hemorrhage, resulting in ischemia or nerve compression. Later, the injury may become apparent because of neural entrapment in scar tissue or callus formation during bone healing.

A high-velocity projectile missile has a destructive effect over a considerable distance from the missile's path. Damage results from the release of large amounts of energy in the tissues. The injuries to the nerves are often unrecognized, and the nerve deficit is not identified.[47] Nerve bundles suffer vary-

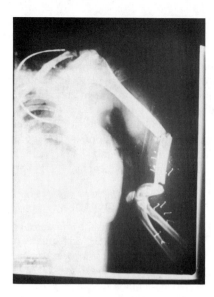

Figure 42–4
Patient with multiple fractures, vascular injury, and associated peripheral nerve involvement.

ing degrees of damage, ranging from a loss of conductivity to complete severance and paralysis. A concussion to the nerve may cause sensory loss and paralysis that lasts just a few days. If the return of function is fast, the injury has been a concussive one from the pressure transmitted by the blast effect. But the return of functioning can be delayed for weeks. If the nerve is completely severed, complete paralysis and a sharply defined loss of deep sensitivity are present.

Essentially, a peripheral nerve comprises hundreds of axis cylinders enclosed in endoneural tubes. The axis cylinder in the center of the axon is continuous with the nerve cell itself, and a thin membrane covers both. Myelin envelops the cylinder and, in turn, is surrounded by a sheath of Schwann cells, which are essential for regeneration. The endoneurium (a loose, fibrous tissue) separates one fiber from another, and the perineurium (a thin, strong connective tissue sheath) encases groups of fibers (fascicles). The fascicle is usually composed of both motor and sensory axons. The epineurium is the outer covering of the nerve.

Nerve injuries are classified according to the damage and the recovery time. A *first-degree injury* is usually the result of a contusion or prolonged compression. Functioning returns in 1 week to 4 months. Although no actual break in continuity is present, the conductivity of the axis cylinders is decreased or blocked. Structurally, the axon is intact, although segmental damage can be present. The return of sensation is first noted and is followed by the return of motor power.

In a *second-degree injury,* several of the axis cylinders are severed and degenerate. Recovery is preceded by Wallerian nerve degeneration of the distal segment. Because the proximal end of the nerve degenerates to the nearest node of Ranvier, the axon in the distal segment is not in contact with the nerve cell itself. Thus, for 3 to 7 days after the injury, the distal segment degenerates into fragments and the myelin sheath is digested by the Schwann cells. As part of the process, Schwann cells proliferate and nerve regeneration is initiated by growth

of the proximal axon down the Schwann cell encasement at the rate of 1 to 2 mm a day, or about 1 inch per month. The Schwann cells layer fresh myelin around the nerves, and the distal nerve segment swells to about twice its original size. The entire process takes about 30 days. Generally, sensation returns before motor functioning does. Sensation returns first in the area proximal to injury, but the sensation is not normal at first. For example, tingling sensations or paresthesias are common responses to stimulation. These responses tend to travel down the length of the nerve as growth proceeds (Tinel's sign).

In a *third-degree injury,* the internal structure of the nerve is disorganized. The endoneural tube around the cylinder remains intact, even though all the tubes are no longer intact.

In a *fourth-degree injury,* the continuity of the epineurium is disrupted and the nerve shrinks to a slender thread.

In a *fifth-degree injury,* the nerve is completely severed. Because there is no continuity of the epineurium, there is nothing to guide regeneration. The involved muscles are totally paralyzed. Surgical repair is mandatory. It may be done immediately, or it may be delayed for 2 to 6 weeks. If the wound is not contaminated excessively and if the nerve ends can be approximated satisfactorily, repair at the initial wound closure is often the treatment of choice. Some surgeons decide on delayed repair because in time the extent of damage is clearly demarcated and the supporting axon structures (the perineurium and the epineurium) have thickened and increased the tensile strength. Interfascicular suture is attempted. The return of functioning is problematic because the undulating, twisting growth of nerve fibers from one fascicle to another forms various new plexuses throughout the length of the nerve. Factors that play a significant role in the quality and the quantity of regeneration are the type of injury, the age of the patient, the level of injury, the duration of the injury, the alignment of nerve ends, a tension-free anastomosis, and any associated injuries.[51]

An alternate classification of peripheral nerve injuries entails description of neurapraxia, axonotmesis, and neurotmesis. In *neurapraxia,* the axon is structurally intact with no anatomic disruption of the nerve fiber, but transmission is decreased. In some areas of the axon there may be demyelination. In *axonotmesis,* the axon is disrupted, but the supporting structures (*e.g.,* the epineurium, the perineurium, and the Schwann cell tubes) are intact. In *neurotmesis,* nerve fibers and their sheaths of connective tissue are transected.

Prognosis

Nerve fibers vary in size. The motor nerve fibers are the largest and most heavily myelinated ones. The fibers concerned with proprioception and cutaneous sensation are next in size, and the pain fibers and the fibers of the autonomic nervous system are small. The large, heavily myelinated fibers conduct impulses at a faster rate.

Nerve lesions may be complete or incomplete. Overall functioning can be decreased, or one type of conduction deficit can be more apparent than another (*e.g.,* there may be more motor loss than sensory loss). In general, motor dysfunction is more common than sensory dysfunction. The patient may not be able to move a body part, yet may feel pain in that part. Motor nerves seem to be damaged more easily than sensory nerves because they are larger and conduct impulses more rapidly. An analogous phenomenon is present in the sensory nerves with regard to touch and pain; that is, the patient may lose the sense of light touch and yet retain the sense of pain.

Injuries of the brachial plexus and of the nerve trunks proximal to the extremities (*e.g.*, the ulnar and the sciatic nerves) usually have a poor prognosis. Movements that require fine muscle control are often not recoverable. Such sensations as proprioception in small joints and two-point discrimination are slow to recover and often remain abnormal. Light touch and proprioception are frequently maintained, even though a small number of sensory fibers are present. Lower extremity injuries are more susceptible to high-energy, blunt trauma, which results in nerve gaps. This pathophysiologic process makes healing less likely. The sciatic and tibial nerves carry the worst prognosis.[54]

Physical and Psychological Immobility

In the patient with extremity trauma, the wait is long in the critical care unit. The process of healing is slow. Physical immobility affects psychological immobility, and psychological mobility affects physical mobility.[20,45] The two are related and interconnected. For the patient with nerve injury, the burden of waiting is great, to see what nerves will regenerate or to determine when the body is at a point at which secondary nerve repair may be performed. The fracture that could not be internally or externally fixed early after trauma confines the patient to bed in skeletal traction. Although fractures and associated nerve injury have a low priority in determining the emergent conditions that must be attended in initial care, they have an overwhelming impact on the quality of the patient's life and are far higher in his priority ranking.

Psychological immobility is seen in the critical care unit and is used by patients as a temporary defense mechanism. Based on life experiences, patients have defense mechanisms that have worked for them in the past. Confined to the critical care unit, their bodies filled with tubes, they do not have control over themselves or their destiny, and they are no longer able to respond constructively nor to assess the significance of the threat to themselves. They may have concerns that seem out of proportion to others. Most of the threats are very real to them.[23] One of the dangers of this temporary situation is that the situation will become permanent, and the patients will not be able to cope. They will become emotional cripples. In their overwhelming fears, forces may impinge on them, precipitated by their interpretation of the illness; the environment, which is so intense that the patient feels intimidated; or adaptation to a new overpowering role.

Changes in body image contribute to psychological immobility. People have a mental picture of their bodies, and this picture or image is how they perceive themselves. Body image is important in how people value themselves and how secure they feel. With an alteration (real, feared, or imagined) in body image, people may lose their ability to make decisions and function independently. At first, the patient may be in a state of shock and may even dissociate himself or herself from what has happened. Next, as reality is viewed and realized, the patient may retreat. The patient retreats emotionally, because physical retreat is not possible. This retreat gives the patient time to assess the situation and identify support measures. The patient should not be hurried through this time because it acts as a protective mechanism. When ready, the patient proceeds through the last two stages: acknowledgment and reconstruction. Here the body image is adapted, and the patient copes with the changes.

NURSING PROCESS

ASSESSMENT

After the initial trauma assessment and treatment of such conditions as upper airway obstruction, hemorrhage, shock, and neurologic injuries, the injured extremity is assessed.[2,24,32] First, the neurovascular functioning is assessed with regard to circulation, sensation, and motor power. (People who have gunshot wounds and open fractures are particularly likely to have problems.) Then the local skin trauma and soft-tissue injury are assessed, noting whether the injury is open or closed, the degree of bleeding, the degree of contamination, and the extent of injury. Finally, the bone injury is assessed. The initial examination establishes the level of functional abnormality and a baseline by which progressive changes can be evaluated.[50]

The classic clinical parameters for extremity injury are known as the five Ps: pain, pulselessness, pallor, paresthesia, and paralysis.[45] The patient's circulation is assessed by palpating the distal pulses and evaluating capillary refill, color, and temperature. Clinical signs that suggest arterial injury are looked for; for example, if the ischemia is severe enough, an excruciating pain or (sometimes) a glove-like anesthesia is present. Penetrating injuries in the region of a major blood vessel or nerve are explored by the surgeon, if evaluation of the individual patient suggests that it would be desirable. Sensation in the injured area is assessed by touch and pinprick. Motor power is assessed as good, poor, or absent. Movement of the arms or hand grip is a satisfactory indicator for the arms, and dorsiflexion or bending the knees up is a satisfactory indicator for the feet.

Historical details are important, and as with every other form of trauma, they include the who, what, when, where, why, and how of the accident. The details and circumstances include the environment in which the accident took place. Particularly if there is an open wound, information is gleaned about the initial wound contamination. Knowing the time of the accident gives some clues about how much time bacteria have had to proliferate in the wound.

Fractures

The amount of blood loss associated with the fracture depends on the structures in the particular bone, the type of fracture, and how much blood flow to the fractured extremity is increased after an injury. A vascular injury may also accompany the fracture. Assessment of the site itself entails comparison of the injured side with the uninjured side with regard to appearance and size. When measured with an accurate tape measure, the circumference of the injured extremity can be used as an indicator of blood loss; each 1-inch increase in circumference indicates a 1-unit loss of blood (Table 42-2):

Table 42-1
Open Fractures

CLASSIFICATION	ASSESSMENT
First degree	Little to no contused tissue. Punctured from inside out. Low-energy forces cause spiral or oblique fracture. Bacterial contamination negative.
Second degree	No damage to deep structures. Lacerated skin and soft tissue. Moderate energy forces cause comminuted or displaced fracture. Moderate contamination.
Third degree	Damage to deep structures. Lacerated skin and soft tissue. High-energy forces cause significantly displaced fracture. Heavily contaminated.
Fourth degree	Total amputation or partial contamination.

Assessment parameters for the fracture are instability, pain, deformity, shortening, rotation, ecchymosis, swelling, and crepitus reflex splinting. The site should not be palpated for crepitus, but crepitus should be documented if it is felt. Every fracture is carefully assessed as to whether it is open or closed. If any doubt exists, it usually is treated as an open fracture (Table 42–1). With positive fracture signs, further evaluation includes two plane radiographs at the fracture site taken perpendicular to each other.

The patient must be considered as an entity, and his whole body should be checked systematically. For example, an injury to the shoulder might be accompanied by an injury of the brachial plexus or the radial nerve and artery. An injury of the shaft of the humerus can injure the radial nerve. A fractured elbow can cause problems with the radial artery and median nerve. In a crushing injury of the forearm, functioning of both hand and forearm must be assessed.

Injuries of the lower extremities are associated frequently with significant problems. At particular risk is the elderly woman who has a fractured hip and many associated geriatric problems. Fractures about the knee may be accompanied by significant popliteal artery damage. Evaluation of the pulses and an arteriogram are important because many patients who have injured arteries may have satisfactory distal pulses. Dislocations of the knee are notorious for being associated with damaged popliteal arteries, and the surgeon routinely orders an arteriogram following reduction of the dislocation. Injuries of the tibial plateau are associated with the anterior compartment syndrome.

Compartment Ischemia

Any bone or vascular injury may lead to compartment ischemia. Incorrect deflation of the legs of military antishock trou-

sers has even led to the syndrome.[9] Anterior compartment syndrome in the lower extremity is most commonly observed, but any muscle compartment in the body may be affected. Increased pressure in a closed compartment leads to ischemia and eventually necrosis (Fig. 42–5). It is the responsibility of the nurse to monitor the injured extremity and report immediately to the orthopedic surgeon any findings that suggest compartment syndrome (Table 42–3). The situation must be treated as an emergency if the patient is to retain function.

Forearm

In the forearm, there are three basic compartments: volar, mobile wad, and dorsal. The *volar compartment* consists of the flexors and pronators of the forearm and wrist. The *mobile wad* separates the volar from the dorsal compartment. The compartment is small and consists of the brachioradiales, ex-

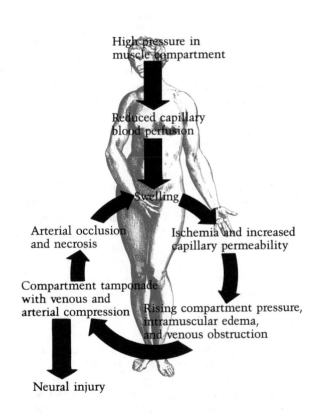

High pressure in muscle compartment

Reduced capillary blood perfusion

Swelling

Arterial occlusion and necrosis

Ischemia and increased capillary permeability

Compartment tamponade with venous and arterial compression

Rising compartment pressure, intramuscular edema, and venous obstruction

Neural injury

Figure 42-5

Sequence of increased compartment ischemia. Clinical manifestations are related to the amount of pressure within the compartment.

Table 42-2
Fractures and Blood Loss

BONE WITH CLOSED FRACTURE	POSSIBLE HIDDEN BLOOD LOSS (ml)
Humerus	500 to 1000
Elbow	250 to 750
Radius/ulna	250 to 500
Pelvis	750 to 6000
Femur	500 to 3000
Tibia/fibula	250 to 2000
Ankle	250 to 1000

(Strange, J. M., and Kelly, P. M. Musculoskeletal injuries. In V. D. Cardona, P. D. Hurn, P. J. Bastnagel-Mason, et al (eds.). *Trauma Nursing: From Resuscitation Through Rehabilitation.* Philadelphia: W. B. Saunders, 1988.)

Table 42-3

Monitoring Parameters for Potential Compartment Ischemia

Subjective
  Pain
  Pain with passive stretch
  Paresthesia, anesthesia
  Decreased sensation to pinprick and two-point discrimination
Objective
  Decreased motor function
  Increased compartment pressure
  Tightness and weakness are variable findings and difficult
    to assess
  Normal skin perfusion and pulses

tensor carpi, radiales brevis, and longus muscles. The muscles of the *dorsal compartment* are supplied by a continuation of the radial nerve.

Lower Extremity

Anterior compartment syndrome is the most common. Bleeding results in tightness and tenseness that produce paralysis. Initially, the syndrome is manifested by decreased sensation to light touch on the dorsum of the foot. Pain with passive stretch of the muscles is a cardinal sign of ischemia. The deep peroneal nerve controlling dorsiflexion of the ankles and toes could be affected. The parameters to be assessed are the patient's ability to dorsiflex the toes and to feel sensation in the dorsal web space between the first and second toes. As in all compression syndromes, the surgical treatment is opening of the compartment.

Compression in the other three compartments of the leg is less common than in the anterior compartment. Compression of the lateral compartment is unusual. The lateral compartment contains the peroneal muscle group and the superficial peroneal nerve. Assessment parameters include the loss of eversion power and sensory loss of the dorsum. Compression in the posterior compartment is even more rare. Assessment parameters include the functioning of the soleus and the gastrocnemius muscles. In the deep posterior compartment are the posterior tibial nerve, artery, and vein, the tibialis posterior muscle, and the long toe flexors. Assessment parameters include the tone of the toe flexors and plantar sensation.

Often all four fascial compartments require decompression. Decompression is usually recommended for pressures in the range of 30 to 40 mm Hg; however, the critical point for the development of ischemia is assessed in relationship to the patient's diastolic blood pressure. The measurement of intracompartmental pressures is advocated by some orthopedic surgeons to determine if patients need decompression by fibulectomy or fasciotomy.[33] In fasciotomy, each of the four fascial compartments of the leg is opened widely. Wound healing occurs usually by second intention. The wounds are covered with wet saline dressings to prevent dessication, with wet to dry dressing changes being done every four hours. An alternate treatment is several days of elevation of the leg followed by delayed primary suturing and skin grafting.

Vascular Injury

Although most major vascular wounds not associated with orthopedic trauma are caused by acts of violence, each year an increasing number of injuries result from blunt trauma, mainly motor vehicle accidents. Penetrating wounds of the extremities caused by bullets or knives are obvious and in such situations are readily diagnosed by the surgeon.

Determination of an arterial injury is extremely important. Irreversible changes from muscle ischemia occur in 5 to 8 hours. Amputation may be the unfortunate result of incomplete assessment. Vascular injuries are particular problems for the general surgeon. If possible, a vascular surgeon is consulted. The nurse is in a position to assist in the initial assessment and to monitor the patient carefully.

Vascular injuries are suspected when the patient demonstrates any of the following: a diminished or absent distal pulse; persistent bleeding; a large hematoma that increases in size; wounds that are close to a major vessel; an aberration in functioning of a nerve that is in close anatomic position to the vessel; a bruit or thrill from partial thrombosis of an A-V fistula; alteration in skin color, warmth, and capillary refill; ischemic pain in the extremity; and abnormal motor or sensory function. The presence of a normal distal pulse does not mean that an artery has not been damaged. Because of collateral circulation, a normal pulse may be palpated. Most likely, a "soft clot" has formed through which pulsations but not blood may pass. Arteriography is considered to be 97% sensitive

Table 42-4

Common Peripheral Nerve Injuries Associated With Fractures

NERVE	FRACTURE	ASSESSMENT FINDINGS
Radial	Humerus	Motor: Wrist drop, weakness of wrist extensors and fingers Sensory: Loss over base of thumb and sometimes over dorsal web space
Median	Distal radius	Motor: Weakness of thumb opposition Sensory: Loss over volar aspect of index, middle, radial half of ring fingers
Axillary	Shoulder dislocation	Motor: Weakness of shoulder abduction Sensory: Loss may be over lateral aspect of upper arm and shoulder
Peroneal	Fibula neck	Motor: Foot drop, weakness of foot and toe dorsiflexors Sensory: Loss in web space
Sciatic	Hip dislocation	Motor: Weakness of plantar flexion Sensory: Loss over sole of foot

and 90% specific, with only a 2.7% failure rate.[44] It is particularly useful in patients who have associated skeletal injuries and scattered bullet wounds of the extremities.

Blood loss is also not necessarily a determinant of the severity of the injury. Hemorrhage from an arterial tear may be profuse, whereas a transected artery may clamp down to stop blood loss.

It is important to monitor the quality of the pulse with the Doppler. The same nurse should listen for the character of the pulsatile flow at the same place in the extremity to note any changes. The normal pulse is heard as a triphasic signal. With obstruction, there is a change to a biphasic sound. If the obstruction is severe, a monophasic sound is heard.

Surgical exploration is usually performed when there are many penetrating wounds in the vicinity of a major artery. Arteriography is used routinely to determine what patients are candidates for surgery.[25,34,40] If a major artery in an extremity is injured, direct repair reconstruction of the artery or grafting is usually needed to prevent the loss of function or amputation. Ligation and amputation are no longer accepted procedures under normal conditions.

Peripheral Nerve Injuries

A careful neurologic examination including sensory and motor components is part of the examination of an injured extremity. A peripheral nerve may be contused, stretched, or severed.[37] If all function is absent, the damage cannot be assessed by clinical examination. The extent of injury remains undetermined until time of surgery or until what can heal has healed. Table 42–4 shows the five most likely peripheral nerve injuries

associated with dislocation and fracture. More complete assessment of nerve involvement is discussed in the following paragraphs.

In the upper extremities, there are five major nerves: the median, ulnar, radial, axillary, and musculocutaneous nerves.

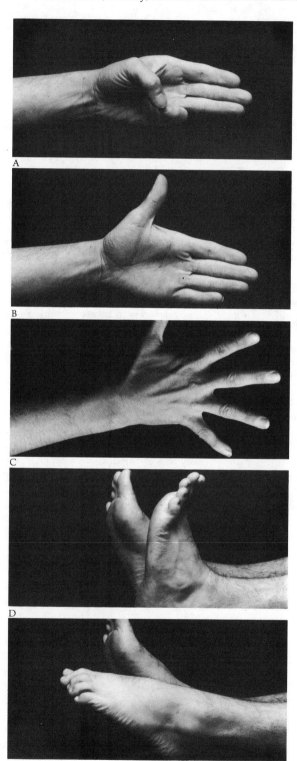

Figure 42–7

Monitor motor functioning to identify associated peripheral nerve involvement. (*A*) Assessment of median nerve. (*B*) Assessment of radial nerve. (*C*) Assessment of ulnar nerve. (*D*) Assessment of peroneal nerve. (*E*) Assessment of tibial nerve.

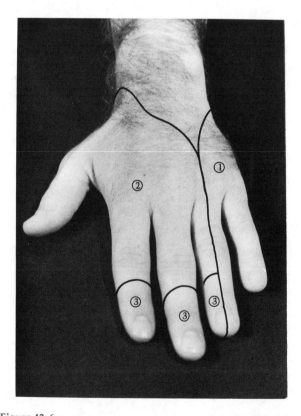

Figure 42–6

Dorsal view of the hand with the areas supplied by the (*1*) ulnar, (*2*) radial, and (*3*) median nerves outlined.

The area of the dorsal aspect of the hand supplied by the median, ulnar, and radial nerves is shown in Fig. 42–6. Involvement of the median nerve results in both motor loss and sensory loss, namely, motor loss of wrist and finger flexion, loss of forearm pronation and finger-thumb opposition, and sensory loss in the palmar aspects, including the thumb, index finger, middle finger, and radial half of the ring finger. Assessment is made of the patient's ability to oppose the thumb and little finger and to flex the wrist. Involvement of the ulnar nerve results in motor and sensory loss over the ulnar border of the hand, the ulnar side of the ring finger, and the little finger. Assessment is made of the patient's ability to abduct these fingers. Involvement of the radial nerve results mainly in a motor loss (Fig. 42–7). Most of the extensor muscles of the elbow, forearm, and hand are innervated by the radial nerve, and involvement results in wrist drop. Sensory loss includes the dorsal web space between the thumb and index finger. Assessment is made of the patient's ability to hyperextend the wrist and fingers. Involvement of the axillary nerve results in a sensory loss in the skin over the deltoid muscle and in a motor loss of the deltoid muscle. Assessment entails abduction of the arm at the shoulder. Involvement of the musculocutaneous nerve results in a sensory loss on the radial side of the forearm and a motor loss of the biceps brachii, brachialis, and coracobrachialis muscles. Assessment is made of the patient's ability to flex the arm at the elbow.

In the lower extremity, involvement of the peroneal nerve results in foot drop, because the anterior tibial peroneal and toe extensor groups are not innervated. Assessment entails the patient's ability to dorsiflex the foot. Involvement of the tibial nerve is assessed by asking the patient to plantarflex the ankle and noting if he or she is able to flex and extend the toes.

Diagnostic Studies

Blood is drawn for an arterial blood gas analysis, hematocrit and hemoglobin, type and crossmatch, electrolytes, glucose, chemistry profile, and coagulation studies. The radiograph is the fundamental tool of the surgeon. At least two views, an anteroposterior and a lateral, including the distal and proximal joints, are taken of the extremity. Radiographs of the opposite extremity are used for comparison. Computed tomographic (CT) scanning is now being used effectively, especially for fractures that are difficult to see on radiograph.[28] It is particularly valuable in assessment of penetrating wounds of the extremity in proximity to a major vessel, knee dislocations, and fractures associated with abnormal pulses.[35] Electromyography is used to assess peripheral nerve dysfunction.

Arteriography is a valuable tool to characterize the nature of vascular injury and to define vascular anatomy.[36] However, if the limb is without blood flow, no time is lost obtaining diagnostic studies before operative intervention. The arteriogram is a diagnostic tool, and the patient must be assessed further if the arteriogram does not fit completely with the clinical picture.[41,43] For example, if definite physical signs of vascular trauma are present, a negative arteriogram cannot rule out a significant vascular injury. However, in patients with no clinical evidence of vascular trauma, a completely negative arteriogram does reliably rule out vascular injury.[39,43]

NURSING DIAGNOSES, PATIENT OUTCOMES, AND PLAN

The preceding material on anatomy, physiology, nursing assessment, and diagnostic tests guides the nurse in establishing nursing diagnoses, patient outcomes, and plans for the patient with extremity trauma.

PATIENT CARE PLAN SUMMARY *Patient With Extremity Trauma*

NURSING DIAGNOSIS

1. *Decreased cardiac output related to shock and blood loss (exchanging pattern)*

Patient Outcomes	Nursing Orders
1. The patient will regain or maintain a cardiac output within normal limits. 2. The patient will be free from clinical signs and symptoms of shock.	See Nursing Diagnosis 1, Chapter 41, p. 777.

NURSING DIAGNOSIS

2. *Actual fluid volume deficit related to injury and loss of blood (exchanging pattern)*

Patient Outcome	Nursing Orders
1. The patient will regain or maintain an adequate oxygen-carrying capacity by means of a blood transfusion.	See Nursing Diagnosis 2, Chapter 41, p. 778.

(continued)

PATIENT CARE PLAN SUMMARY   *Patient With Extremity Trauma*   *Continued*

Patient Outcome	*Nursing Orders*
A. The patient's circulating blood volume will be reestablished (Table 42–4). B. The patient will not experience a transfusion reaction.	

NURSING DIAGNOSIS

3. *Neurovascular compromise related to the forces exerted during injury (exchanging pattern)*

Patient Outcomes

1. The patient's extremity will remain viable.

Nursing Orders

1. Assess and reassess extremity.
   A. Control bleeding.
   B. Maintain pressure and elevation.
   C. Observe and monitor extremity closely for cyanosis or mottling. Feel the extremity for coolness, especially as compared with the uninjured extremity.
   D. Measure compartmental pressure as ordered.
   E. Prepare for intracompartmental pressure measurement. Assemble equipment.
      (1) For continuous monitoring:
         a. Betadine skin preparation solution
         b. Local anesthetic/syringes
         c. Continuous indwelling monitoring catheter
         d. Transducer set-up
         e. Sterile heparinized saline
         f. Suture
         g. Dressing materials
      (2) For one-time measurement:
         a. Betadine skin preparation solution
         b. Local anesthetic
         c. 18-gauge spinal needle
         d. Water manometer set
         e. Sterile saline solution
   F. Start procedure:
      (1) For continuous monitoring:
         a. Position extremity and prepare skin by cleansing.
         b. Catheter is introduced into the compartment through a small skin incision using an introducer.
         c. Catheter is connected to a preflushed monitoring system.
         d. The monitor and transducer are zero balanced and the initial pressure is recorded.
         e. The catheter is sutured into place and a sterile dressing is applied.
      (2) For one-time pressure measurement:
         a. Position extremity and prepare the skin.
         b. Area is anesthetized.
         c. Spinal needle is attached to a water manometer and the system is flushed.
         d. The needle is inserted into the fascial compartment.
         e. The pressure is measured as the distance from the insertion site to the top of the manometer as measured in centimeters. (Centimeters of water pressure are converted to millimeters of mercury by dividing the centimeters of water by 1.36.)
         f. The pressure is recorded and the needle is withdrawn. A sterile dressing is applied to the insertion site.
   G. Palpate major peripheral pulses, noting force and quality. Use the Doppler if necessary.

(continued)

PATIENT CARE PLAN SUMMARY   *Patient With Extremity Trauma*   *Continued*

Patient Outcomes	*Nursing Orders*
	H. Test for capillary refill by pinching the nailbed and noting any delay in the return of color. (Normal CRT less than 2 sec.) I. Observe while the patient extends the fingers or toes actively (or do it passively if the patient is not able). If there is no pain and capillary refill is adequate, circulation should be adequate. J. Splint the extremity as needed. K. Test and monitor for distal loss of sensation. L. Test and monitor for motor loss. Monitor functioning for associated peripheral nerve (Fig. 42–7).
2. The patient will experience no permanent dysfunction.	2. If the patient has had an incomplete amputation, splint the attached portion and, if possible, cool the devitalized portion. If the patient has had an amputation and replantation is possible, the nurse should[39]: A. Assist with stabilization of patient's condition; for example, administer intravenous fluids, tetanus prophylaxis, and antibiotics. B. Cleanse the stump with saline and control the bleeding. C. Wash the amputated part thoroughly in isotonic saline (preferably Ringer's lactate). D. Wrap the part in sterile gauze moistened with solution of aqueous penicillin (100,000 units in 50 ml Ringer's lactate). E. Wrap the stump in a similarly moistened towel. F. Place the amputated part in a plastic bag and an insulated cooling chest filled with crushed ice for transportation to the regional center. G. Do not use any antiseptics or other solutions; float the part in a bag of solution or freeze it.

NURSING DIAGNOSIS

4. *Impaired skin and skeletal integrity related to traction and immobilization after extremity trauma (exchanging pattern)*

Patient Outcomes	*Nursing Orders*
1. The patient should demonstrate proper healing while in an immobilizing device (Hoffman apparatus, splint or cast). 2. The patient will be free from complications from cast application.	1. Use care when moving the patient. A. While the plaster is wet, use the palms of hands when moving. B. If the cast is in the perineal area, use plastic to protect it. 2. Perform a neurovascular check every hour for 48 hours and then every 8 hours. Observe the patient's pulse, color, temperature, sensation, active and passive mobility, and edema. The physician should be notified of any abnormalities. A. If bleeding occurs, mark the cast and monitor the patient. B. Notify the physician of any painful areas under the cast that are still present when the cast is elevated. C. Teach the patient isometric exercises and help the patient do them every 2 hours. D. Pad the edges of the cast to make the patient comfortable.
3. The patient will maintain skin traction.	3. Use no more than 8 to 10 pounds of weight as ordered. Make sure weights hang freely. Apply tincture of benzoin to the skin first, then moleskin, and then the traction device. The device should be secured with an elastic bandage wrap.
4. The patient will maintain proper body positioning.	4. Support the foot or the hand to avoid a position of extreme flexion or extension. A. Support the lower leg with a pillow. B. If the patient tends to slip down to bottom of bed, elevate the lower portion of the bed 1 foot. C. Avoid putting pressure on the peroneal nerve over the head of the fibula. D. Inspect the area around the Achilles tendon.
5. The patient will maintain skeletal traction.	5. Prepare the patient for surgery: A. Clean the operative site by sudsing it repeatedly. Leave the suds on 5 to 10 minutes. B. Clean the site for 10 to 30 minutes. C. Remove hair from the site (if possible with a depilatory).

(continued)

PATIENT CARE PLAN SUMMARY   *Patient With Extremity Trauma*   *Continued*

Patient Outcomes	*Nursing Orders*
	D. Cover the site with a sterile dressing.
	E. Provide for patient education.
6. The patient will tolerate the discomfort of an external fixation device as evidenced by self-report.	6. Before setting up traction, make sure that all clamps are functional, lubricate the pulleys, and make sure that the ropes are not frayed.
	A. Position the patient so that the ropes and pulleys maintain an appropriate pull on the long axis of the bone.
	B. Keep the ropes unobstructed and the weights hanging free. Secure and wrap the knots with adhesive tape.
	C. After traction is set up, take a Polaroid picture of the apparatus and put the picture at the head of the bed.
	D. Compare the injured extremity with the normal one with regard to size, color, temperature, blanching, numbness, and motor activity eight times every hour, then four times every 2 hours, and then once every 4 hours.
	E. Explain the traction apparatus to the patient and family, using pictures and diagrams. Educate the patient about what movements are permitted and what ones are restricted.
	F. Keep the patient's shoulders and hips in alignment.
	G. In an affected extremity, maintain a neutral position with a trochanter roll, sandbags, or a footboard.
	H. Maintain the integrity of the patient's skin by massaging the bony prominences every 8 hours, turning the patient every 2 hours if possible (with assistance), and using a sheepskin, an air pressure mattress, a flotation pad, an egg crate mattress, or a low air-loss bed.
	I. Observe for pressure areas, particularly areas at the edges of the splint and under the splint. Use a mirror attached to a long handle to inspect the body parts that are not immediately visible.
	J. Keep the popliteal space, tibial tuberosity, malleolar areas, and the head of the fibula free of pressure.
	K. Keep the bed dry and wrinkle-free.
	L. Use analgesics and comfort measures to relieve pain.
	M. Perform range-of-motion exercises of all extremities three times a day.
	N. Inspect and clean the pin site every 8 hours. Use hydrogen peroxide and then betadine. Instruct the patient in care of the pin when he is able to take the responsibility.
7. The patient will be free of infection at the pin sites.	7. Check the integrity of the external fixator at least every 8 hours.
	A. Do not pull on the device because this may loosen it or tear the soft tissue around the pin insertion sites.
	B. Perform neurovascular assessments on the involved extremity at least every hour for the first 24 hours and then every 8 hours.
	C. Check the pin insertion sites and cleanse them every 4 hours. Note any signs and symptoms of infection including redness, swelling, or drainage at the pin sites.
	D. Teach the patient and family to care for the external fixator.

NURSING DIAGNOSIS

5. *Impaired physical mobility related to extremity trauma and fracture (moving pattern)*

Patient Outcomes	*Nursing Orders*
1. The patient should demonstrate increased mobility.	1. Help the patient actively exercise the unaffected areas every 2 hours with assistance (*e.g.*, gluteal setting exercises, knee bends, straight leg-raising exercises, and ankle flexion exercises). Set the number of repetitions.
	A. After a conference with the physician, encourage isometric exercises of the affected area.
	B. Encourage the patient to take fluids. Find out what the patient likes to drink and set up a "beverage schedule" with the patient. It should be specific; for example, orange juice, 120 ml at 9:00 A.M.

(continued)

PATIENT CARE PLAN SUMMARY   *Patient With Extremity Trauma*   Continued

Patient Outcomes	Nursing Orders
	C. Encourage the patient to eat a well-balanced diet.
	D. Keep the patient as active mentally and physically as possible. Change the patient's position and have the patient cough and deep-breathe every 2 hours with assistance. Use an incentive spirometer.
2. The patient should be free of any complications from the hazards of the bed rest.	2. Observe for signs of thrombophlebitis (tenderness, swelling, pain on dorsiflexion of the foot), especially in the calf. If ordered, administer prophylactic "minidose" heparin to prevent thrombophlebitis.
3. The patient should not exhibit thrombophlebitis.	3. Apply antiembolic stockings. Have two pairs. Rotate them daily, and keep one pair washed.
	A. Keep all pressure off the calf and the heel or possible pressure areas.
	B. Do not raise the knee gatch routinely.
	C. Refrain from dangling the patient's legs.
	D. After a consultation with the physician, encourage the patient to get out of bed as soon as possible and encourage early ambulation. Plan the patient's schedule carefully, and slowly increase the activity level each day. For example, the first day the patient may take three steps, the next day six steps, and the next day ten steps. Evaluate the patient's pulse and tolerance so that the activity level can be decreased if necessary.
	4. Apply alternating calf compression device if available.

NURSING DIAGNOSIS

6. *Pain related to anxiety and extremity trauma (feeling pattern)*

Patient Outcomes	Nursing Orders
1. The patient will remain relatively comfortable.	1. Assess pain with regard to potential associated injury. Once the fracture is immobilized, the pain should be reduced significantly. Continued severe pain is likely to be associated with arterial insufficiency.
2. The patient will be able to describe pain so that pain associated with extremity trauma complications will be identified.	2. Monitor for potential vascular injury, compartment syndrome, associated peripheral nerve involvement, tight cast, inadequate fracture immobilization, migration of traction pin, infection of pin tract and fracture site, pressure sores under the cast, or venous thrombosis.
	A. Pad the cast edges with abdominal dressings or similar material. Petal the cast edges with small pieces of adhesive tape.
	B. Maintain elevation to decrease swelling.
	C. Position the patient with pillows to prevent any sudden jerking caused by the weight of the cast.
	D. Use sufficient help when moving the patient.
3. The patient will be able to cooperate and thus enhance any pain relief measures administered.	3. Assess the pain and check the time of the patient's previous analgesic injection.
	A. Perform nursing comfort measures, such as giving a back rub, changing the patient's position, and providing clean bed linens.
	B. Speak in a calm voice and work efficiently and carefully.
	C. Keep the sheet tight and brush away any plaster crumbs from the cast.
	D. Protect the skin from drainage.
	E. Administer analgesics if ordered. Narcotics often blunt the assessment parameters and frequently are not ordered.
	F. In the low-flow state, absorption is irregular, and analgesics should be administered intravenously in small doses. The time interval may be continuous titrated drip or from 30 minutes to 3 hours depending on the quantity of the last dose, the patient's size, and the degree of pain.
	G. Note the presence of respiratory depression associated with pain. Relieve the pain as much as possible. The usual protocol is the administration of small amounts of intravenous analgesics titrated against the patient's respiratory rate and depth, nursing comfort measures, and techniques used to achieve the relaxation response.

(continued)

PATIENT CARE PLAN SUMMARY *Patient With Extremity Trauma* *Continued*

NURSING DIAGNOSIS

7. *Impaired gas exchange related to fat embolism (exchanging pattern)*

Patient Outcomes	*Nursing Orders*

1. The patient will be free from signs of pulmonary failure as evidenced by a $PaO_2 > 80$ mm Hg, a $PaCO_2 < 45$ mm Hg, normal breath sounds, and a clear chest radiograph.

1. Keep a high index of suspicion about all patients who have fractures, especially fractures of the long bones (Fig. 42–8).
   A. Prevention is the best treatment. Use adequate emergent splinting, handle the patient with major skeletal injuries gently, and elevate the injured limbs.
   B. Know about laboratory tests the physician might order. In about 50% of patients, the serum lipase level is elevated and free fat is found in the urine.
   C. Make an overall assessment based on the following:
      (1) *Mental signs:* lucid interval; dyspnea; restlessness; confusion; obstinacy.
      (2) *Physical signs:* increased temperature; increased respirations; increased pulse; changing neurologic status (weakness, spasticity, incontinence); petechiae, especially on upper chest on the lateral aspects of the chest and axilla; edematous patches on fundi.
      (3) *Laboratory signs:* PaO_2 60 to 70 mm Hg; chest radiograph changes; decreased platelet count; decreased hemoglobin level; lipiduria; increased serum lipase level; ECG changes; venous fat droplets; positive skin biopsy.
   D. Place thromboembolic stockings on the patient to reduce venous stasis.
   E. If ordered, administer low-dose heparin.
   F. If ordered, administer corticosteroids.
   G. If the patient has an increased erythrocyte sedimentation rate and thrombosis, administer low-molecular-weight dextran if ordered.
   H. Be aware that intravenous alcohol is sometimes ordered.

2. The patient should receive immediate therapy if fat embolism occurs.

2. Assess and monitor the patient's respiratory status, looking for an increased respiratory rate, dyspnea, decreased oxygenation shown by serial arterial blood gas measurements, and changes shown by serial chest radiographs.
   A. Assess and monitor the patient's cardiovascular status, looking for an increased pulse, decreased blood pressure, right- or left-sided heart failure, and any of the following ECG changes:
      (1) An inverted T wave
      (2) A prominent S wave in lead 1, which suggests myocardial and right ventricular failure
      (3) A prominent Q wave in lead 3
      (4) Depressed RS segment
      (5) A right bundle branch block
      (6) Dysrhythmias, which are common and often fatal
   B. Assess and monitor the patient's neurologic status, looking for restlessness, confusion, a refusal to cooperate, and an elevated temperature.
   C. Look for decreased hemoglobin levels.
   D. Look for petechial hemorrhages on the chest, shoulders, and axilla. Petechial hemorrhages may also be seen on the abdominal wall and extremities, on the palate, in the subconjunctival region, and on funduscopic examination (manifested as macular edema, hemorrhage, or emboli in the vessels). Use the following chart to make an overall assessment:
      (1) *Mental signs:*
         a. Restlessness
         b. Confusion
         c. Obstinacy
      (2) *Physical signs:*
         a. Increased temperature
         b. Increased respirations
         c. Increased pulse
         d. Changing neurologic status (weakness, spasticity, incontinence)
         e. Dyspnea
         f. Petechiae, especially on upper chest on the lateral aspects of the chest and axilla
         g. Edematous patches on fundi

(continued)

PATIENT CARE PLAN SUMMARY   *Patient With Extremity Trauma*   *Continued*

Patient Outcomes	*Nursing Orders*
	(3) *Laboratory signs:*
	a. PaO$_2$ 60 to 70 mm Hg
	b. Chest radiograph changes
	c. Decreased platelet count
	d. Decreased hemoglobin level
	e. Lipurea
	f. Increased serum lipase level
	g. ECG changes
	h. Venous fat droplets
	i. Positive skin biopsy
	E. If a fat embolism is diagnosed, center the treatment first on respiratory management. Oxygen is administered at the first sign of restlessness and cyanosis.
	(1) Monitor the following assessment parameters continuously and record the information gathered hourly until further notice:
	a. Level of alertness and responsiveness
	b. Temperature, pulse, respirations, and blood pressure
	c. ECG
	d. Respiratory, cardiovascular, and neurologic systems
	(2) Place thromboembolic stockings, or alternating-calf compression devices on the patient to reduce venous stasis.
	(3) If ordered, administer low-dose heparin (10 to 50 mg intravenously every 6 to 8 hours), which is thought to clear lipemic plasma and to stimulate lipase activity.
	(4) If the patient has an increased erythrocyte sedimentation rate and thrombosis, administer low-molecular-weight dextran (1000 ml every 1 to 3 days) if ordered. It alters platelets and decreases intimal adhesions.
	(5) Be aware that intravenous alcohol is sometimes ordered (alcohol is a lipase inhibitor).

IMPLEMENTATION AND EVALUATION

The principles of wound management must be followed. The fracture site is covered with a sterile moist dressing and splinted until it can be shaved and debrided through an extension of the wound. Cold is applied, the extremity is elevated to reduce swelling, and any exposed tendons are covered with a wet saline dressing. Intravenous fluid is never infused into the fractured extremity. Every effort is made to prevent infection. Open fractures are not probed in the emergency room. Examination and debridement are done under sterile conditions by the physician in the operating room.

Aseptic conditions are maintained. Antibiotics (commonly first-generation cephalosporins) are administered. In some instances, cultures are done before and after debridement. Tetanus prophylaxis is given.[18] Surgery is performed within 6 to 8 hours of the injury under optimal conditions.

Maintaining anatomic position, the extremity is splinted above and below the fracture to align the fracture and to immobilize the bone fragments. Splints are used to prevent motion of the fracture; increased pain; further damage to muscles, nerves, and blood vessels; conversion of a closed fracture to an open one; restriction of blood flow to the injured extremity; and increased bleeding into the soft tissues.

To stabilize temporarily a fracture distal to and including the knee or elbow, an air splint may be used for short periods of time. The splint is inflated to an internal pressure of 30 mm Hg or to the point at which external pressure compresses the splint 0.5 inch. For a fracture of the humerus or shoulder, a sling is used. For a fracture of the femur, a traction splint (*e.g.,* a Thomas splint) is used to overcome muscle spasms. Preparations are made for the application of a cast, wound debridement, skeletal traction, internal fixation, or external fixation.[10,11,12,14,42]

Six to eight U of blood can be sequestered in the thigh. Without appropriate splinting, a large number of patients will bleed so much into the thigh that they reach a moribund condition. The thigh normally has a cylindrical shape, but with a fractured femur, the thigh acquires a spherical shape. Because the volume of a sphere is approximately one-half larger than the volume of a cylinder, the patient with an untreated femoral fracture can easily have an internal hemorrhage that requires large volumes of blood replacement.

In the polytrauma patient, most orthopedic surgeons strongly consider internal fixation. If multiple injuries are present in a single extremity, the priority of treatment is given to stabilization of all fractures.[10,24,32] The overall goals are soft-tissue healing, bone healing, good alignment, good range of motion, and minimal complications.

In severe wounds and extensive soft-tissue injury, the wound is usually kept open. In particular, most physicians will keep open an injury caused by a rotary lawn mower or gunshot and any injury that is questionable. If the dressing is dry and the wound is not draining, a delayed primary closure is performed in 5 to 7 days. The extremity is elevated 30° to 45° postoperatively. The wound is again debrided in 4 to 5 days, and the bone is stabilized.

For patients with a second-degree peripheral nerve injury, physical therapy and some type of positioning and splinting are important to maintain the paralyzed area during the regeneration process. Otherwise, permanent functional abnormalities are likely to ensue. Prompt corrective measures are not necessary, and other injuries (for example, vascular injuries) have greater priority. If a tendency toward contracture is not present, splinting is often omitted.

Each patient must be treated as an individual. The decision about treatment is made after assessing the patient's fractured bone, foreign material, and damaged tissue.[24] The nurse must be prepared to assist with whatever treatment approach the physician chooses and should be able to answer the patient's and the family's questions. The possible treatment approaches are as follows:

- Primary closure or cover by suture or split-thickness skin graft
- Delayed primary closure or cover by suture or split-thickness skin graft
- Secondary closure or cover by suture or split-thickness skin graft
- Healing by granulation or secondary intention

Internal Fixation

Early internal fixation with rigid immobilization can stabilize the fracture immediately and restore the stability of the frame.[52] Rather than immobilization with skeletal traction, surgeons are increasingly using internal fixation. Healing occurs by intramedullary callus formation, because internal fixation sacrifices the external callus response for immediate rigid fracture immobilization. Anatomic reduction realigns some of the bone's vascular channels that were disrupted by the fracture. Once revascularization begins, vascular elements proliferate along with the restored channel. New cancellous bone is formed along the channel in a process called *primary vascular bone healing*. The process proceeds with the re-formation of trabeculae across the fracture site and cannot occur if there is any motion at the fracture site. It can occur only with the rigid immobilization and bony compression produced by the internal fixation.

Particularly in the polytrauma patient, there are many reasons for the surgeon to select early internal fixation: through stable fixation, the limb is painless; early manifestations of fracture disease are prevented; the patient is more mobile in bed; care in the unit is facilitated because the skeletal fraction device is not needed; and the patient mentally does not feel as ill, and psychological aberrations are prevented.

Rigid internal fixation uses bony compression to enhance immobilization and should be done before swelling is evident. Because the new bone is weaker without the implant than bone allowed to heal with callus and ossification, the implant is left in place until sufficient bony strength has been achieved. To allow for normal stress patterns on healed bone, the implant is removed at a later time. At all times, the nurse must keep

a high index of suspicion about all patients who have fractures, especially fractures of the long bones (Fig. 42–8).

Arterial Repair

Emergency care entails, first, the use of simple digital pressure.[2] Then with the patient under anesthesia, devitalized tissue is debrided and an incision is made to allow proximal and distal visualization of the injured vessel.

Some surgeons may use surgical sympathetomy, sympathetic blockade, or mechanical dilatation and the application of magnesium sulfate to prevent arterial spasm.[22] During the procedure, the proximal and distal segments are injected with about 10 ml of a balanced salt solution containing 1:10 solution of heparin to prevent thrombosis. (Some surgeons use systemic heparinization.) If a clot is present in the segment, a balloon-type (Fogarty) catheter or a small suction catheter is used to dislodge and retrieve the clot and establish flow.

The type of repair depends on the extent and type of injury. It may be a lateral repair, an end-to-end anastomosis, or a graft. Because the wound may be contaminated, a greater saphenous vein graft rather than a synthetic graft generally is used.

Besides the usual monitoring done in a critical care unit, the patient must be monitored with regard to blood pressure,

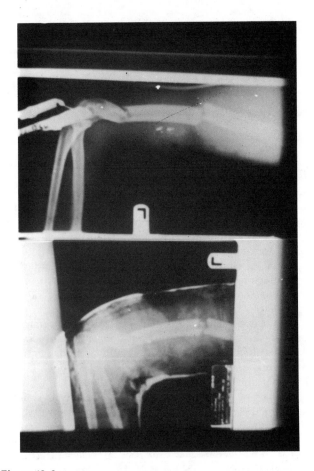

Figure 42–8

In patients with fractures of the long bones, the nurse should maintain a high index of suspicion for fat embolism and implement preventive nursing actions.

temperature and color of the skin, and distal pulses. The Doppler is an invaluable aid.

Blood Replacement

Replacement of the blood that was lost may be lifesaving. Table 42–5 lists findings with actual blood loss. Although whole blood is needed when the patient is bleeding actively or has lost whole blood within the last 24 hours, fractionalization or component therapy is used for specific purposes, and it is standard practice in trauma centers. Transfusions may take any of the following common forms: whole blood, packed red cells, platelet concentrates, cryoprecipitate, fresh or fresh-frozen plasma, aged plasma, and leukocyte preparations (leukocyte-poor red cells or leukocyte-rich preparations).

The main purpose of administering whole blood is to increase oxygen delivery at the tissue level, particularly in the patient who is hemorrhaging massively. Stored blood becomes a greater percentage of circulating blood volume. For example, when 50% of the blood volume has been lost and 10 U of blood transfused, only 28% of the patient's original red blood cells and plasma remain; and when 20 U of blood have been transfused, only 11% of the original red blood cells and plasma remain. Because the oxygen content of arterial blood depends primarily on the hemoglobin concentration, increasing the hemoglobin is vastly superior to administering oxygen with regard to transporting oxygen to the tissue level. Tissue function is closer to normal when the hematocrit is kept above 35%. One unit of whole blood or 1 U of packed cells raises the hematocrit 3 percentage points. A significant increase in blood loss and defective coagulation at the operative site has occurred in patients whose hematocrits were below 20%.

Stored Blood

Several changes occur during the storage of blood. The changes begin within 24 hours after donation and continue through the 35 days the blood can be used for administration; the blood is considered outdated after 35 days.[17] Potassium levels increase proportionally with the age of the blood (30 to 40 mEq/L in 3-week-old blood), making hyperkalemia a potential problem. In an acidotic patient who has renal impairment, the potassium increase could lead to a fatal dysrhythmia. In rare instances, rapid transfusion into an acidotic patient may require alkalinization.

Stored blood does not contain ionized calcium, since the citrate binds the calcium. Because of a fear that the reduction in calcium not only would cause hypocalcemia but also would augment the effects of the hyperkalemia on the myocardium, many physicians order intravenous calcium during massive transfusions. However, it is generally accepted that the syndrome is rarely seen clinically, and most patients are closely monitored for any signs rather than given unneeded prophylaxis. Most authors agree that citrate intoxication does not occur at transfusion rates below 1 U of blood every 5 minutes in an adult whose circulation is intact and whose liver is functioning.

Stored blood has a lower pH than blood circulating in a person. The citrate used for preservation lowers the pH, and anaerobic metabolism occurs in stored blood. The longer blood has been in storage, the greater are the amounts of lactic and pyruvic acids contained.

In patients who have hepatic insufficiency, the ammonia increase in aged blood may precipitate hepatic coma. In those patients, the administration of aged blood must be avoided. Washed or frozen-thawed red cells are preferred for these patients.

Platelets are significantly affected by storage. After 48 hours of storage, blood is devoid of functional platelets. If blood is transfused within 6 hours of donation, the platelets are viable, but the platelets' function is severely impaired after only a few minutes of refrigeration. From 6 to 48 hours after donation, the blood may be used in thrombocytopenia associated with massive transfusions (a single transfusion of more than 2500 ml or a number of transfusions that total 5000 ml or more in a 24-hour period), but the use of platelet concentrates is the preferred approach. In general, the greater the amount of whole blood transfused, the greater the platelet deficit in both function and quantity. In the traumatized patient, two other factors that affect the platelets are present. Tissue trauma and shock increase the platelet consumption, and in the hemorrhaging patient, massive transfusions may produce a dilutional thrombocytopenia. In addition to the platelet deficiency, stored blood is deficient in most of the factors necessary for blood coagulation, namely, factors V, VIII, and IX. These factors deteriorate 50% within 7 days after donation. Fresh-frozen plasma is administered to replete these factors when large quantities of stored blood are administered. Fibrinogen and other stable factors are retained in stored blood.

Table 42–5
Actual Fluid Volume Deficit Related to Blood Loss: Mild, Moderate, and Severe

NURSING DIAGNOSIS	FINDINGS	ASSESSMENT
Actual fluid volume deficit (mild) related to blood loss	10% to 20% blood volume lost, pH normal Decreased perfusion to bone, muscle, feet, and skin	Subjective: Feels cold and thirsty Objective: Postural *tachycardia* and hypotension, collapsed neck veins, concentrated urine, skin: *cool, pale, moist*
Actual fluid volume deficit (moderate) related to blood loss	20% to 40% blood volume lost pH decrease with decreased base bicarbonate Decreased perfusion to liver, colon, and kidneys	Subjective: Thirst Objective: tachycarida, hypotension, *oliguria* (output should be greater than 0.5 ml/kg each hour)
Actual fluid volume deficit (severe) related to blood loss	40% blood volume lost Severe pH decrease with decreased base Bicarbonate and increased $PaCO_2$ Decreased perfusion to brain and heart	Subjective: Confusion, feelings of agitation, stupor, coma Objective: Decreased sensorium, tachycardia, hypotension, rapid deep respiration, and dysrhythmias

Left Shift of the Oxyhemoglobin Dissociation Curve

A shift of the oxygen dissociation curve to the left is particularly significant in decreasing the oxygen available at the tissue level. The transfusion of stored blood contributes to the shift. With a left shift, the affinity of hemoglobin for oxygen is increased so that the hemoglobin holds the oxygen more tightly and less oxygen is available at the tissue level. Decreased body temperature, increased pH (alkalosis), and a decrease in 2,3-diphosphoglycerate (2,3-DPG) all contribute to the left shift.

The ability of the red blood cells to accept and release oxygen is controlled by 2,3-DPG, a glycolytic intermediate and the most abundant phosphate in the cell. The red cell glycolytic rate, red cell survival, delivery of oxygen, and concentrations of ATP and 2,3-DPG are interdependent. Reduced hemoglobin preferentially binds 2,3-DPG and so significantly lowers its own affinity for oxygen. Blood that is stored in an acid medium has red blood cells that are deficient in 2,3-DPG. When these red blood cells are transfused into a patient, the affinity of hemoglobin for oxygen is increased. In order to have more 2,3-DPG available and to make the blood less acid, citrate-phosphate-dextrose (CPD) has been adopted in the United States as the preservative for stored blood products. The initial pH of blood stored in CPD is 7.2, and levels of 2,3-DPG are high enough for satisfactory oxygen delivery at the tissue level for about a week. At about 14 to 21 days, pH has decreased to about 6.5 to 6.8.

Although the initial pH is higher and deterioration is slower in CPD-stored blood than in the preservative used previously, acid-citrate-dextrose, the levels of 2,3-DPG still diminish and produce a left shift in transfused patients. For example, 9-day-old blood is considered deficient in 2,3-DPG. When it is used for transfusions, correction of the cellular deficiency takes 24 hours. Thus, in the hemorrhaging patient, a ratio of 1:2 is preferred; that is, for every 2 pints of blood that are older than 9 days, 1 pint that is less than 2 days old should be transfused.

Bleeding Diathesis

Multiple clotting defects induced by massive transfusions, trauma, and complications may produce an uncontrollable bleeding. The danger increases with each unit of blood administered. In particular, a bleeding diathesis may be produced when platelets and clotting factors are reduced by 70% or after the replacement of approximately 5 L of blood. Platelets are transfused as single-donor pooled units or multiple-donor pooled units. Although the risk of hepatitis is greater, multiple donor packs are transfused. A single unit raises the platelet count of a normal person (70 kg) approximately 5000 platelets/mm^3.

Intravascular hemolysis, a life-threatening complication of blood transfusions, usually results from incompatibilities involving the ABO blood-group system. Because the hemolyzed donor red blood cells release hemoglobin into the plasma, the plasma is tinted a reddish pink. Haptoglobin, a plasma protein of the albumin type, is able to bind 125 to 150 mg of free hemoglobin per deciliter of plasma. Bound hemoglobin is not filtered into the urine. However, if large amounts of hemoglobin are released as a result of the hemolysis of many red blood cells, the hemoglobin-binding capacity of haptoglobin is exceeded, and free hemoglobin is filtered into the urine, turning the urine red or pink. If the urine is acidic or if the hemoglobin has been in the plasma for longer than 24 hours, the iron in the hemoglobin is oxidized from the ferrous state to the ferric state or, in other words, from hemoglobin to methemoglobin. Because methemoglobin is brown, the urine is a brownish color.

Hepatitis B

This form of hepatitis was previously known as "serum hepatitis." The primary route of transmission is through blood products or inoculation of the virus through skin or mucous membranes. The hepatitis B surface antigen (HBsAg) has been found not only in blood but also in other body fluids such as urine and stool; however, infectivity of a given excretion or secretion is likely related to how much serum or blood is present. Current epidemiologic evidence demonstrates that transmission may also occur through saliva of an infected person.

The exact incubation period is unknown and is probably related to the dose of the virus, but it is thought to be up to 180 days after exposure, with an average of 2 to 3 months. The clinical picture of hepatitis B is similar to that of hepatitis A, except the onset may be more gradual. Joint pains and hives can occur in some individuals before the onset of jaundice. Patients with hepatitis B are not as "infectious" as patients with hepatitis A, because stool and urine are not sources of hepatitis B infection. Owing to the occasional progression to chronic hepatitis and cirrhosis, the prognosis in hepatitis B infection is less favorable than infection with hepatitis A. A definitive diagnosis of hepatitis B is made by demonstration of the HBsAg. This was previously called *hepatitis-associated antigen* and frequently is called *HAA*. The antigen may be found in the blood for several weeks before the onset of symptoms of the disease and may persist for weeks or months. The hepatitis B surface antigen may be evident in the blood of asymptomatic carriers and remain present for years. Infectivity appears to correlate best with the presence of the "e antigen." Because this test is not routinely available, all blood from HBsAg-positive individuals must be considered as potentially infectious.

Non-A, Non-B Viral Hepatitis

This form of the disease may be caused by more than one agent, and it occurs most frequently after blood transfusions. It is probably responsible for approximately 75% or more of posttransfusion hepatitis. Available data suggest that the incubation period is about 5 to 10 weeks. The infection resembles hepatitis B more than hepatitis A in its clinical and epidemiologic patterns, and chronic active hepatitis may occur after acute illness.

Transmission of the disease by routes other than parenteral inoculation probably does occur, but at a lower frequency. Personnel must use caution at all times when handling blood or blood products regardless of their origin. It is not known whether immune serum globulin is an effective preventive measure for this type of hepatitis.

Autotransfusion

Because of concerns about the transmission of blood-borne infections such as hepatitis B; hepatitis non-A, non B; and acquired immunodeficiency syndrome (AIDS), the collection and reinfusion of the patient's own blood has become a popular method of intravascular volume replacement. The advantages of using autologous blood include the following: the blood is readily available, it is always compatible with the recipient's blood, and it is cost effective. Autotransfused blood does not need to be typed or crossmatched, which avoids time delays and errors. The risk of hemolytic and febrile reactions—resulting from isosensitization to the leukocytes, platelets, and red cell antigens—is minimized. Other hematologic advantages are that the blood has a normal pH and a normal potassium concentration. One final advantage is that autotransfusion offers a viable alternative to persons whose religious convictions do not allow them to receive homologous blood transfusions.

There are a few limitations on the type of patient who should be considered for autotransfusion. Any patient who is septic, has renal or liver failure, has primary carcinoma, or has a severe coagulopathy should not receive autologous blood. Another major concern when using autotransfused blood is the risk of embolization from blood that may clot during the collection phase. The potential for bacterial transmission must also be considered in the trauma patient. Closed autotransfusion systems, scrupulous technique, and the use of the appropriate antibiotics can decrease this risk.[33]

There are many autotransfusion systems available for use. The Bentley autotransfusion system is a closed system; a cannister receptacle that collects the blood is hooked to a vacuum source for suction. From the collection cannister, a tubing is hooked to a pump to send the blood back to the patient through an intravenous line. The Pleur-evac collection device is an intermittent autotransfusion device. This method requires the use of a chest drainage system with the autotransfusion option and a disposable collection bag. The blood is collected through the chest tube and drained into the disposable bag. When it is time to reinfuse the blood, the disposable bag is removed from the drainage device, blood tubing is attached, and the blood is reinfused. The blood must be reinfused within 4 hours of collection. Cell savers also use the principle of autotransfusion; they not only collect the blood that has been shed but also wash the cells.

Nursing considerations when using an autotransfusion system include establishing a water seal and ensuring that the appropriate amount of suction is being applied. Frequent monitoring of the amount of blood in the collection chamber is important to prevent severe hemorrhage from occurring and to make sure that the reinfusion process is done within the appropriate time limit. Accurate recording of intake and output during the entire process and for several hours after is necessary.

Acquired Immunodeficiency Syndrome

Exposure to the human immunodeficiency virus (HIV) through blood transfusions has been clearly linked to AIDS. Since 1987, all blood has been tested for the HIV virus, but the test is not 100% accurate. There is widespread public fear of acquiring AIDS from blood transfusions infected with the virus. Reassurance to the patient and family about the low risk is important to help allay their fears.

SUMMARY

Extremity injuries demand prompt attention. The threat of loss of life from hemorrhage or loss of limb from blood loss, pressure, or ischemia is a real danger. Bone, vessels, nerves, and soft tissue may be involved. Any further trauma must be minimized by aggressive, appropriate interventions. The incidence of complications occurring in this patient population is high but can be minimized by strict adherence to the extremity salvage protocol and attentive daily clinical care.

DIRECTIONS FOR FUTURE RESEARCH

The critical care nurse is a pivotal person in the coordination of care for the patient with extremity trauma. The members of the trauma team rely on the nurse to be sure that all communication is shared and important assessment findings are made known to the team. The nurse should be careful about the details of care and not let anything fall through the cracks; prevention is the best treatment. The role of coordinator of activities and facilitator of patient care forms the basis for a large area of nursing research.

Clinical questions include the following[31]:

1. How can the functions of the trauma team members be best facilitated or coordinated?
2. What are some of the clinical indices that differentiate pain from anxiety?
3. What nonpharmacologic measures are most effective in relieving pain?
4. What measures are effective in helping patients maintain basic stress-reduction techniques?
5. What are the most effective ways of promoting optimum sleep-rest patterns and of preventing sleep deprivation?
6. What is the effect of selected measures (*e.g.*, body positioning, passive range of motion) on successful rehabilitation?

In addition to researching the current nursing and medical therapies, attention should focus on prevention of extremity trauma. How can the safety of automobile occupants be increased? How can severe injuries to the lower extremities be reduced by redesigned bumpers and hood profiles? What are the effects of public education programs on reducing injury? These and other questions must be addressed.

REFERENCES

1. Achterberg, J. and Lawlis, F. *Bridge of the Body and Mind.* Champaign, IL: Institute for Personality Testing, 1985.
2. Atkins, J. M., Roberts, B. G., and Thai, E. R. Emergency medical systems. In A. H. Giesecke (ed.), *Anesthesia for the Surgery of Trauma.* Philadelphia: F. A. Davis, 1976.
3. Bassett, C. A. The development and application of pulsed electromagnetic fields (PEMFs) for ununited fractures and arthrodeses. *Orthop. Clin. North Am.* 15(1):61, 1984.
4. Beitz, D. Algorithm for critically injured patients. *J. Trauma* 17: 55, 1977.
5. Bucholz, R. W., Lippert, F. C., Wenger, D. R., and Ezaki, M. *Orthopedic Decision Making.* Philadelphia: B. C. Decker, 1984.
6. Brighton, C. T. and Pollock, S. R. Treatment of nonunion of the tibia with a capacitivity coupled electric field. *J. Trauma* 24(2): 153, 1984.

7. Brighton, C. T. The semi-invasive method of treating nonunion with direct current. *Orthop. Clin. North Am.* 15(1):33, 1984.

8. Brink, B. E. Vascular trauma. *Surg. Clin. North Am.* 51(1):189, 1977.

9. Brotman, S., Browner, B. D., and Cox, E. F. Mast trousers improperly applied causing a compartment syndrome in lower extremity trauma. *J. Trauma* 22(7):598, 1982.

10. Brooker, A. New techniques in fracture management. *Surg. Clin. North Am.* 63(3):607, 1983.

11. Browner, B. D., Kenzora, J. E., and Edwards, C. C. The use of modified Neufield traction in the management of femoral fractures in polytrauma. *J. Trauma* 21(9):777, 1981.

12. Brumback, R. J. and Blick, S. S. Compartment syndrome. In M. J. Yaremchuck, A. R. Burgess, and R. J. Brumback (eds.), *Lower Extremity Salvage and Reconstruction: Orthopedic and Surgical Management.* New York: Elsevier, 1989.

13. Burgess, A. R. and Brumback, R. J. Early fracture stabilization. In R. A. Cowley, A. Conn, and A. M. Dunham (eds.), *Trauma Care. Volume 1: Surgical Management.* Philadelphia: J. B. Lippincott, 1987.

14. Byrd, H. S., Cierny, G., and Tebbetts, J. B. The management of open tibial fractures with associated soft tissue loss: External pin fixation with early flap coverage. *J. Plast. Reconstr. Surg.* 68(1):373, 1981.

15. Chan, D., Kraus, J. F., and Riggins, R. S. Patterns of multiple fractures in accidental injury. *J. Trauma* 13:107, 1973.

16. Clark, P. E. and Clark, M. J. Therapeutic touch: Is there a scientific basis for the practice? *Nurs. Res.* 33(1):37, 1984.

17. Collins, J. A. Pertinent recent developments in blood banking. *Surg. Clin. North Am.* 63(2):483, 1983.

18. Committee on Trauma. American College of Surgeons. A guide to prophylaxis against tetanus in wound management. *Bull. Am. Coll. Surg.* 57(12):23, 1972.

19. Committee on Trauma. Guidelines for management of amputated parts. *Bull. Am. Coll. Surg.* 67(10):12, 1982.

20. Diers, D. The effect of nursing interaction on patients with pain. *Nurs. Res.* 21(5):41, 1972.

21. Evans, C. M. The fat embolism syndrome. In Marvin H. Myers (ed.), *The Multiply Injured Patient with Complex Fractures.* Philadelphia: Lea & Febiger, 1981.

22. Flint, L. M. and Richardson, J. D. Arterial injuries with lower extremity fracture. *Surgery* 93(1):5, 1983.

23. Frank, J. Mind–body relationships in illness and healers. *Int. Acad. Prevent. Med.* 11(3):46, 1975.

24. Freeland, A. E. and Highes, J. L. Early management of the severely injured extremity. In J. D. Hardy (ed.), *Critical Surgical Illness.* Philadelphia: W. B. Saunders, 1980.

25. Graham, J. M., Mattox, K. L., Feliciano, D. V., and DeBakey, M. E. Vascular injuries of the axilla. *Ann. Surg.* 195(2):232, 1982.

26. Heidt, P. Effects of therapeutic touch on anxiety level in hospitalized patients. *Nurs. Res.* 30:32, 1981.

27. Heppenstall, R. B., Brighton, C. T., Esterham, J. L., and Becker, P. Clinical and roentgenographic evaluation of nonunion of the forearm in relation to treatment with DC electric current. *J. Trauma* 23(8):740, 1983.

28. Hubbard, L. F., McDermott, J. H., and Garrett, G. Computed axial tomography in musculoskeletal trauma. *J. Trauma* 22(5):388, 1982.

29. Kim, S. Pain: Theory, research and nursing practice. *Adv. Nurs. Sci.* 2:43, 1980.

30. Kreiger, D. *The Therapeutic Touch: How to Use Your Hands to Help or Heal.* Englewood Cliffs, NJ: Prentice Hall, 1979.

31. Lewandowski, L. A. and Kositsky, A. M. Research priorities for critical care nursing. *Heart Lung* 12:35, 1983.

32. Markison, R. E. Trauma to the extremities. In D. D. Trunkey and F. R. Lewis (eds.), *Current Therapy of Trauma—2.* Philadelphia: B. C. Decker, 1986.

33. Martin, E., Harris, A., Johnson, N., *et al.* Autotransfusion systems (ATS). *Crit. Care Nurse* 9(7):65, 1989.

34. McCabe, C. J., Ferguson, C. M., and Ohinger, L. W. Improved limb salvage in potential artery injuries. *J. Trauma* 23(11):982, 1983.

35. Mendonca, T. M. and Metos, A. N. Arterial injuries associated with trauma to the knee. *Am. J. Surg.* 147(2):210, 1984.

36. Moss, C. M., Veith, F. J., Jason, R., and Rudavsky, A. Screening isotope angiography in arterial trauma. *Surgery* 86(6):881, 1979.

37. Omer, G. E. Physical diagnosis of peripheral nerve injuries. *Orthop. Clin. North Am.* 12:207, 1981.

38. Randolph, G. L. Therapeutic and physical touch: Physiological response to stressful stimuli. *Nurs. Res.* 33(1):33, 1984.

39. Sher, M. H. Principles in the management of arterial injuries associated with fracture dislocation. *Ann. Surg.* 182(5):630, 1975.

40. Siminek, K. R., Levine, B. A., Gaskill, H. V., and Root, A. D. Reassessment of the role of routine operative exploration in vascular trauma. *J. Trauma* 21(5):339, 1981.

41. Smith, F. L., Lim, W. N., Ferris, E. J., and Casali, R. E. Emergency arteriography in extremity trauma: Assessment of indications. *Am. J. Radiol.* 137:803, 1981.

42. Smith, P. J., Lowenstein, P. W., and Bennett, J. E. Surgical options to the repair of lower extremity soft tissue wounds. *J. Trauma* 22(5):374, 1982.

43. Snyder, W. H., Thai, E. R., Bridges, R. A., *et al.* The validity of normal arteriography in penetrating trauma. *Arch. Surg.* 113:424, 1974.

44. Snyder, W. H. Vascular injuries near the knee. *Surgery* 91(5):502, 1982.

45. Strange, J. M., and Kelly, P. M. Musculoskeletal injuries. In V. D. Cardona, P. D. Hurn, P. J. Bastnagel-Mason, *et al.* (eds.), *Trauma Nursing: From Resuscitation Through Rehabilitation.* Philadelphia: W. B. Saunders, 1988.

46. Swearingen, R. L. A humanistic approach to management of fractures. *Today's Clinician,* February 21, 1978.

47. Tscherne, H. and Gotzen, L. (eds.), *Fractures with Soft Tissue Injury.* Berlin: Springer-Verlag, 1984.

48. Twedt, B. Control of pain in orthopedic patients. *R.N.* 38:39, 1975.

49. Virgin, C. E., Mooney, V., Leslie, M. R., *et al.* Orthopedic pain. *Contemp. Orthop.* 1(5):56, 1979.

50. Webb, K. J. Early assessment of orthopedic injuries. *Am. J. Nurs.* 74:1048, 1974.

51. Weinstein, L. Trauma. *N. Engl. J. Med.* 289:1293, 1973.

52. Whittaker, R. P., Heppenstal, B., Menkowitz, E., and Monique, F. Comparison of open versus closed rodding of femurs utilizing a Simpson rod. *J. Trauma* 22(6):461, 1982.

53. Withers, B. F. and Baker, S. P. Epidemiology and prevention of injuries. *Emerg. Med. Clin. North Am.* 2:701, 1984.

54. Yaremchak, M. J. Special injuries. In M. J. Yaremchuk, A. R. Burgess, and R. J. Brumback (eds.), *Lower Extremity Salvage and Reconstruction: Orthopedic and Surgical Management.* New York: Elsevier, 1989.

43

Burn Injury

Elizabeth I. Helvig   *Cornelia Vanderstaay Kenner*

PURPLE AND BLUE AS HEALING COLORS

Mrs. B. was a burn victim. The extent of her injuries included second-degree and third-degree burns on her hands, arms, chest, and face. She had no signs of inhalation injury and was not intubated or on the ventilator.

My experience with burn patients has been very limited. I was never eager to learn, finding it too emotionally difficult for me to implement burn care. Then, when I was introduced to techniques of relaxation and guided imagery, I thought it was a perfect outlet for me to help care for these patients.

When I was asked to help with a dressing change, I gowned up and went into the room with much reluctance. As I was holding the patient's arm, I wondered how I might introduce these techniques to this lady. I started with simple breathing techniques. Then she said, "When I think of the colors purple and blue, it makes me feel better." That was my cue. I took that and incorporated it into breathing and imagery. I said, "Okay, Mrs. B., focus on the ceiling or close your eyes and imagine and feel the color blue surrounding you, cool and vibrant. Then take a slow, deep breath and breathe in the color that's all around you. Your body is filled with the color blue, reaching to the ends of your toes. Now, slowly breathe it all out, as it comes out from your lips and into the air around you it has turned purple. A beautiful hue of purple now surrounds you. It's soft and comforting, floating all around you."

I continued to use these colors with various images and breathing. Before we knew it, the dressing changes were over. I then encouraged her to use these images whenever she felt bad. The patient's nurse, realizing the value of these images, immediately added this intervention to her care plan. Identifying what things help patients feel better or what activities they enjoy and incorporating them into nursing interventions can enhance the meaning and the outcome of the therapy.

Kim Tierney, RN, CCRN
Special Care Unit
Maine Medical Center
Portland, Maine

LEARNING OBJECTIVES

After reading this chapter, the nurse should be able to do the following:

1. Obtain quickly the pertinent details of the accident and the patient's medical history.
2. List the important facts surrounding the accident.
3. Assess the patient's injuries systematically.
4. Calculate the extent of injury.
5. According to appearance, differentiate first-degree, partial-thickness, deep partial-thickness, and full-thickness burns.
6. Describe the types of hospitals in which burn patients with various areas, depths, and extents of injury can be treated successfully.
7. Identify the clinical and laboratory criteria that show adequate resuscitation from burn shock.
8. Derive nursing diagnoses, plan nursing interventions, and evaluate the patient's response to treatment.
9. Correlate burn wound sepsis with the results of surface cultures, biopsy reports, and therapy.
10. Assess early clinical signs and prevent complications.
11. Identify the important aspects of patient care after the application of heterograft.
12. Write a paragraph describing positioning and exercises needed for a patient who has limited range of motion in the hand.
13. Be cognizant of the possible psychosocial responses of the patient and integrate appropriate interventions into the care delivery system.
14. Provide for patient and family education.

CASE STUDY

Mr. S. was admitted to the critical care burn unit with a 65% total body surface area (TBSA) burn. He was 28 years old, a policeman, married, and the father of two children. He had been assigned to the police department's project at the local community center and had been burned while he was cleaning a shower stall with gasoline. The fumes had ignited, probably because of a nearby hot water heater. He did not become unconscious. When he got out of the building, he rolled in the grass to put out the fire. He was transferred to the regional burn center in a ground ambulance, arriving at 3 P.M., 1 hour after he was burned.

Mr. S.'s initial assessment for airway involvement and life-threatening trauma was negative. His vital signs were T 97.2°F (36.2°C), P 140, R 28, and BP 140/70. His burn was calculated as a 65% TBSA partial-thickness and full-thickness injury that covered his face, upper chest, arms, and parts of his legs and back. Based on the extent of his burn and his weight (77 kg), his fluid resuscitation was calculated to be 20,020 ml for the 24-hour period after the injury. Fifty percent of that amount (10,000 ml) was to be infused in the next 6 hours and 45 minutes, 25% (5000 ml) in the second 8-hour period, and 25% in the third 8-hour period.

Blood samples were drawn for arterial blood gases, serum electrolytes, serum chemistry, complete blood count, carboxyhemoglobin, and typing and crossmatching. A Foley catheter and a nasogastric catheter were placed.

Mr. S.'s history indicated that he did not have a pre-existing disease. On physical examination, he was noted to have singed nasal hairs and reddened mucous membranes. His carboxyhemoglobin level was 6%. His arm burns were circumferential, and they were clinically classified as full-thickness injuries. Radial pulses had decreased to 1+. Bowel sounds were absent.

On 40% oxygen, Mr. S.'s arterial blood gas measurements were PaO$_2$ 138, pH 7.63, PaCO$_2$ 15, bicarbonate level 24.5, and delta base −3. His blood review showed hemoglobin 13.3 gm/dl hematocrit 39.6 percent, red blood cells 5.1 × 10^6/mm^3, and mean corpuscular volume 78.

Clinical Presentation

2/8 4:00 P.M. (postburn hour 2)

Mr. S. was alert and oriented, with a urinary output of 50 ml/hour. His vital signs were T 99.2°F (37.3°C), P 130, R 22, BP 100/70, and CVP 3 cm H$_2$O. His cardiorespiratory assessment showed an adequate airway, a normal sinus rhythm, a productive cough, and no rales or wheezes. He had no signs of progressive respiratory involvement indicative of inhalation injury. The bronchoscopic examination showed no mucosal exudate, ulceration, or erythema. Humidified oxygen therapy continued to be 10 L, administered by face tent. Positive-pressure breathing was ordered to be given every 6 hours. External heat was maintained by a heat shield. Preventive antacid therapy was given every 2 hours, with Amphojel and Maalox alternating (30 to 60 ml). A gastrointestinal assessment showed Mr. S. to have a dark-brown drainage in his nasogastric tube and abdominal distention. His right and left radial pulses were palpated at 1+, and they were heard with the Doppler. A clinical examination revealed no numbness, tingling, or decreased motor activity. Ringer's lactate solutions (IV's numbered 3 and 4) were given in the right arm and the left leg, respectively.

5:00 P.M. (postburn hour 3)

Morphine sulfate (10 mg intravenously) was administered before wound care was begun. Explanations were given before the treatment was started. The nurse helped Mr. S. relax with deep breathing techniques. During tubbing, Mr. S. complained of numbness in his hands; his pulses were barely palpable.

6:00 P.M. (postburn hour 4)

Mr. S. was alert, with a urinary output of 48 ml/hour and clearing of the hematuria. His vital signs were T 101°F (38.3°C), P 130, R 28, BP 100 with the Doppler, and CVP 3 cm H$_2$O. Ringer's lactate solutions (Nos. 7 and 8) were given. Mr. S. complained of numbness in both hands that was decreased somewhat after exercise. His pulses were not palpable, but they were heard with the Doppler. During the family's visit, the nurse stayed at the bedside.

8:00 P.M. (postburn hour 6)

Mr. S. was alert, with a urine output of 55 ml/hour. His vital signs were T 101.8°F (38.7°C), P 130, R 26, BP 100 with the Doppler, and CVP 4 cm H$_2$O. He had a normal sinus rhythm. A urine test for sugar was negative. Ringer's lactate solutions (Nos. 9 and 10) were given. Examination of his arms revealed decreased sensation, increased discomfort in his hands, and an occasional skipped radial pulsation with the Doppler.

9:00 P.M. (postburn hour 7)

Mr. S. was alert, with a urinary output of 50 ml/hour. His vital signs were T 101.8°F (38.7°C), P 156, R 32, BP 96 with the Doppler, and CVP 4 cm H$_2$O. Arterial blood gas measurements on 40% O$_2$ were PaO$_2$ 108, pH 7.41, PaCO$_2$ 33, and delta base −2. Evaluation of Mr. S.'s arms showed decreased motor activity and a deep, aching pain. With the use of the Doppler, the flow was detectable for 5 or 6 seconds and then undetectable for 2 or 3 seconds. Bilateral escharotomies of his forearms and distal upper arms were performed. Bleeding was controlled with pressure. The bulging underlying edematous tissue was covered with silver sulfadiazine, and to minimize edema, Mr. S.'s arms were wrapped with Kerlix gauze fitted with 24-hour positioning splints and elevated above the level of his heart.

10:00 P.M. (postburn hour 8)

Mr. S. was alert, with a urinary output of 60 ml/hour. His vital signs were T 102°F (38.8°C), P 140, R 24, BP 90 with the Doppler, and CVP 4 cm H$_2$O. His urine was dark yellow. Bowel sounds were absent; gastric pH was 6 and antacid therapy was continued. Ringer's lactate solutions (Nos. 11 and 12) were given, and the rate was recalculated at 625 ml/hour.

Midnight (postburn hour 10)

Mr. S. was alert, with a urinary output of 50 ml/hour. His vital signs were T 101°F (38.3°C), P 110, R 24, BP 82 with the Doppler, and CVP 3 cm H$_2$O. Morphine sulfate (10 mg intravenously) was administered for pain and coordinated with deep breathing.

6:00 A.M. (postburn hour 16) 1st postburn day

Mr. S. was alert, with a urinary output of 60 ml/hour. His vital signs were T 101°F (38.3°C), P 100, R 24, BP 90 with a Doppler, and CVP 5 cm H$_2$O. Mild hoarseness was noted. His arterial blood gas measurements on 40% oxygen were PaO$_2$ 110, pH 7.38, PaCO$_2$ 33, and delta base −2. The blood test results were RBC 6.72 × 10^6/mm^3, Hgb 21.2 g/dl, Hct 60.5%, WBC 18,900/mm^3, glucose 164 mg/dl, Na 140 mEq/L, K 4 mEq/L, Cl 105 mEq/L. Ringer's lactate solutions (Nos. 16 and 17) were given. Ice chips were taken orally. Mr. S.'s escharotomies were oozing, so small bleeders were cauterized and the dressings were changed. The ophthalmologist noted that the epithelium of Mr. S.'s right eye had improved and that his eyelids, although swollen, were only mildly involved.

10:00 A.M. (postburn hour 20)

Mr. S. was alert, with a urinary output of 50 ml/hour. His vital signs were T 101.2°F (38.4°C), P 116, R 20, BP 94 with the Doppler, and CVP 5 cm H$_2$O. His hoarseness had not increased. His arterial blood gas measurements on 40% O$_2$ were PaO$_2$ 114, pH 7.53, PaCO$_2$ 27, and delta base −4. Mr. S.'s wounds were wet and weeping. Deep breathing techniques and morphine sulfate (10 mg intravenously) was administered before wound care was given by the bedbath procedure.

The open method of therapy was maintained, with a slight modification—light-mesh dressings were applied over the silver sulfadiazine.

Noon (postburn hour 22)

Mr. S.'s plasma volume was calculated to be 3789 ml, and his hematocrit was 46%. Administration of 8 units of replacement plasma was anticipated.

2:00 P.M. (postburn hour 24)

Mr. S.'s mental status and urinary output were unchanged. His vital signs were T 101.2°F (38.4°C), P 140, R 24, BP 94 with the Doppler, and CVP 8 cm H_2O. His hoarseness had increased slightly. He complained of thirst and was given ice chips. His resuscitation therapy with 20,000 ml of Ringer's lactate solution was completed, and resuscitation therapy for the fourth 8-hour period was begun with aged plasma. The blood test results were RBC $5.35 \times 10^6/mm^3$, Hgb 17 g/dl, Hct 47.9%, WBC 8100/mm^3, and platelets 215,000/mm^3.

6:00 P.M.

Mr. S. was alert. He asked about patient care procedures and showed that he understood the explanations. He asked whether his family could remain with him for a short time after visiting hours. He said that he was very tired and that it was painful for him to move. Mr. S.'s wife later told the staff that Mr. S. feared for his life but felt he was going to live.

10:00 P.M.

Monitoring of Mr. S.'s physiologic status showed no abnormalities. Mr. S. complained of being cold, and his over-the-bed heater was turned up. He took clear liquids in small amounts. His total body edema had increased as anticipated, and his joint movement was minimal because of the edema. His care was planned so that his rest periods were as uninterrupted as possible.

2/10 8:00 A.M. (2nd postburn day)

Mr. S.'s vital signs and general condition remained stable. He slept for long periods during the night and was given pain medication once. He was alert, with a urinary output of 68 ml/hour. His vital signs were T 100°F (37.7°C), P 148, R 22, BP 116/92, and CVP 7 cm H_2O. On cardiorespiratory examination, a loud S_4 and wheezes were noted. On ECG, he had a sinus tachycardia. His bowel sounds were active, so his nasogastric tube was removed. He was able to take a clear liquid diet without nausea. His daily nutritional needs were calculated to be 4525 calories and 189 g of protein. After a nutritional assessment, his diet was planned. A small nasogastric feeding tube was placed so that he could be given high-protein calorie supplements.

10:00 A.M.

Mr. S. was bathed in the hydrotherapy tub. He was not submerged in the water, but was placed horizontally on a plinth over the tub. He was then sprayed gently with filtered tap water and washed gently with Betadine.

Noon

Mr. S.'s vital signs were T 100°F (37.7°C), P 140, R 24, BP 100/94, and CVP 10 cm H_2O. His arterial blood gas measurements on 40% oxygen were PaO_2 123, pH 7.47, $PaCO_2$ 29, and delta base -1. Mr. S.'s wife helped him with his liquid diet. At a relatively quiet time, he listened to audiotapes that helped him learn the relaxation response and helped him visualize the experience of the wound care procedure.

10:00 P.M.

Mr. S. was given an analgesic intravenously before his dressings were changed. He initiated deep relaxation breathing by himself. Because his albumin level was low, he received 2 units of aged plasma.

2/11 (3rd postburn day)

Mr. S.'s vital signs were stable. No respiratory involvement was noted. His arterial blood gas measurements were essentially unchanged. Mr.

S. was able to see without difficulty. He listened to audiotapes before his wound care procedure. With the assistance of the tapes, he was able to imagine both sensory and procedural aspects of wound care while he maintained a relaxed state. He was able to generalize the response and to relax after wound care. Serum sodium level had decreased to 129 mEq/L, so additional sodium was added to his nasogastric feedings. Wound biopsies were taken.

8:00 P.M.

Mr. S. developed an increased respiratory rate, tachycardia, and confusion. His urine output dropped to 20 ml/hour. He responded to intravenous fluid administration. His topical therapy was changed to Sulfamylon. He was scheduled for surgery.

2/12-2/14 (4th-6th postburn days)

Mr. S. was taken to surgery for excision and application of homograft. The areas of full-thickness injury were excised tangentially and wrapped with elastic wraps until stasis had occurred. Homograft was applied to burned areas. Postoperatively, Mr. S. developed metabolic acidosis and tachycardia with a drop in urine output. Fluid administration reestablished adequate urine output. Two units of blood were infused. Two days after this procedure the patient returned to the operating room. The homograft was found to be well adhered to all of the graft bed except the left leg. Donor skin was taken from the lower chest and abdominal areas. The homografts were removed and sheet grafts were applied to Mr. S.'s hands with 1.5:1 meshed grafts applied to full-thickness areas on his upper chest and arms. The homograft on his right leg was undisturbed because it was well adhered to the wound. Homograft on his left leg was poorly adhered so the area was washed thoroughly and new homograft was applied.

6:00 P.M.

The sheet grafts were rolled every 30 to 60 minutes initially to prevent accumulation of exudate beneath the grafts. The arms were kept elevated on pillows to minimize edema. Mr. S. was alert and eager to see his family. At 6 P.M., tube feedings were resumed.

2/15-2/16 (postburn day 7-8) (postoperation day 1-2)

Mr. S. sustained a urinary output of 40–50 ml/hour. His vital signs were normal. His lungs were clear and he had active bowel sounds. His hemoglobin was 10.4 g/dl, so he was given 2 U of packed cells. Sheet grafts continued to be rolled every 1–2 hours; meshed grafts remained intact beneath dressings; donor areas remained covered with a synthetic dressing. Partial-thickness wounds were being dressed twice daily. Mr. S.'s legs were wrapped with an elastic bandage to the groin and he was encouraged to sit in a chair for 2 hours with arms elevated on a pillow-covered over-bed table in front of him.

2/17-2/19 (postburn day 9-11) (postoperation day 3-5)

Dressings over meshed-graft areas were soaked with saline and removed gently. The graft take was 75%. Homografts were applied to areas where the autografts did not take. Dressings over all wounds were changed twice daily. Chest radiograph showed some infiltrates. A regimen of frequent coughing, turning, and ambulation with legs wrapped was implemented.

2/20-3/3 (postburn day 12-23) (postoperation day 6-7)

The areas of partial thickness injury (face, arms, legs, and back) were healing. Full range of motion was maintained by gentle exercise 2 to 3 times daily. Until 3/1 Mr. S.'s antibiotic therapy was intravenous gentamicin and ticarcillin. On 3/1 Mr. S. had an episode of low temperature of 95.6°F (35.3°C) rectally, increased pulse, and decreased urine output. His white count was 4500/mm^3, with a segmented-to-nonsegmented ratio of 15:54. Blood cultures were done; the results were negative. The sensitivity reports from a tissue biopsy taken from his left leg showed *Pseudomonas* to be resistant to gentamicin and ticarcillin. Mr. S. was started on amikacin and ceftazidime based on sensitivities. Sulfamylon was applied to the left leg. Mr. S. continued to receive a high-protein, high-calorie diet supplemented by enteral feedings to meet daily caloric goals. He was weighed daily and had lost 1 kg during hospitalization.

3/4–3/5 (postburn day 24–25) (postoperation day 18–19)

Mr. S.'s donor sites have healed completely. He was being ambulated and exercised vigorously to prepare for a postoperative period of bed rest. Mr. S.'s spirits improved. He could visit for longer periods with his family, and he began to talk more about going home. To prepare Mr. S. for surgery on 3/5 he was given 1 U of packed cells because his Hgb was 11.5 g/dl and his hematocrit was 36.3%. In surgery, homografts on his legs were removed and all open areas were covered with meshed autografts and wrapped with occlusive dressings. Re-cropped donor sites on his lower chest and abdomen were covered with a synthetic dressing.

3/6–3/9 (postburn day 26–29) (postoperation day 1–4)

Mr. S. was maintained on bed rest with legs elevated postoperatively. His family spent long periods of time with him. His complaints stemmed from donor site pain and joint tightness. He met caloric requirements through hospital diet supplemented by cans of high-protein feedings, milkshakes, and puddings. Nursing and rehabilitation therapists worked with him each morning and afternoon to maintain range of motion in his hands, upper extremities, and shoulders. His legs were maintained in proper alignment.

3/10–3/20 (postburn day 30–40) (postoperation day 5–15)

Mr. S. was moved to an intermediate care unit. He began ambulation with legs wrapped to the groin. Legs and arms continued to be elevated when sitting or lying. He spent most of his time in the physical medicine department, exercising and rebuilding his muscle tone. He spent significant periods with the occupational therapist working on fine motor function of his hands. The synthetic dressing on a small area of donor site was replaced with Silvadene when some erythema in the area developed.

3/20–25 (postburn day 40–45)

Healed wounds and donor sites were being moistened with hand lotion many times a day and Mr. S.'s chief complaint was itching. He was measured for pressure garments. Until they arrived his arms, legs, and trunk were fitted with tubular elastic dressings to maintain compression. Small open areas were painted with mercurochrome and covered. He was discharged from the hospital. His rehabilitation care had only begun; besides his home care, he came to the physical medicine department for therapy every day for 1 month, then three times a week and, later, two times a week for a 3-month period. He was also seen in the clinic once a week for 2 months. He may still undergo surgical procedures for contracture release and other plastic surgical needs. Fully realizing that the effects of burn injury will last for a lifetime, Mr. S. acted maturely and expressed a desire to help others in a similar predicament. He became a founding member of the local chapter of Burns Recovered, an organization to help burn patients and their families adjust to the aftermath of burn injury.

REFLECTIONS

Many issues are addressed in the treatment of a victim of trauma such as burn injury. One such issue constantly associated with burn injury is pain. Pain is a complex phenomenon, a highly personal and subjective experience, and comprises physiologic (physical or body) and psychological (emotional or mind) aspects. The physiologic aspects are not often as severe as anticipated, whereas the emotional aspects may be pronounced. Each has its own set of causes and characteristics, but each is also dependent on the other. Treatment in one realm changes these characteristics, affects the other realm, and influences the overall experience.

The physical treatment of burn pain alone has proved less than adequate. The duration and intensity of the pain are such that emotional aspects are brought into play for almost all patients. History, adjustment, what has been learned about pain, and the individual's own ways of dealing with pain are important in patient perceptions of pain. Two patients may have the same depth, extent, and location of burn and yet have different amounts of pain. Refer to Chapter 3, Case Study 2, for decreasing pain with burns.

ETIOLOGY AND INCIDENCE

A burn injury is a complex form of trauma. In general, the patient with a major burn suffers the same alterations in body functioning that other trauma patients do, but such patients exhibit the most extreme response. In a burn injury, every body system is likely to go awry.

It is estimated that there are more than 2 million burn injuries in the United States every year. Between 70,000 and 108,000 people are hospitalized every year for acute burn injuries, and the mortality is 6000 per year.[9,80] Many of those who survive have debilitating problems. The rehabilitation period is seven times as long as the hospitalization period—and the person may never be able to return to his or her former life-style.

PSYCHOPATHOPHYSIOLOGY

Burn injury results in a coagulation necrosis of the cellular elements of the epidermis and dermis. Blood vessels are disrupted or thrombosed, and cells are destroyed. Early in the inflammatory response, leukocytes and platelets adhere to the blood vessel endothelium. Microvascular permeability changes also occur, allowing plasma and water to leak from the microvasculature. As capillary permeability increases, plasma leaks out from the microvasculature, primarily into the burned area. Local and systemic changes result.

Depth of Injury

The depth of injury is primarily determined by the intensity and duration of heat exposure. Normal protective functions of the skin are lost in relation to the depth of injury. Because the exact depth of injury is difficult to ascertain, especially at the time of admission, many centers differentiate wounds only as *partial-thickness* injuries (Fig. 43–1) and *full-thickness* injuries

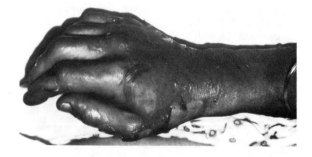

Figure 43–1
Partial-thickness burn injury.

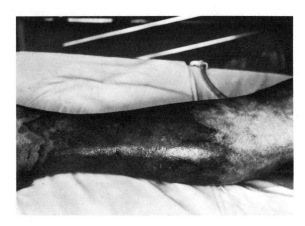

Figure 43–2
Full-thickness burn injury.

(Fig. 43–2). The estimates are modified as the wound evolves. Clinically, most wounds are not entirely partial-thickness or full-thickness, but are mixtures; frequently the center area is full-thickness surrounded by partial-thickness injury. Traditionally, the depth of burn injury has been described in degrees (*i.e.*, first-degree, second-degree, and third-degree burns) (Table 43–1).

Extent of Injury

The severity of injury is related to the extent of burn more than the depth of burn. For a rapid determination, the Rule of Nines (Fig. 43–3) is used. For a more precise determination, the Lund and Browder system (Fig. 43–4) provides an alternate means for estimation. Each side of the burn patient's hand equals roughly 1% of his total body surface area (TBSA); therefore the palm may be a useful guide in determining the size of small burned areas such as those seen with splash injuries.

Not every hospital has facilities to care for massively burned patients. The American Burn Association has developed the following criteria for patients who should be transferred to a Burn Unit or Burn Center. These guidelines are also taught in the Advanced Burn Life Support Course[2]: a burn of 10% or more in a person less than 10 years or over 50 years of age; a burn of 20% or more in a person 10 to 50 years of age; a burn involving the hands, face, eyes, ears, feet, and perineum; an inhalation injury; an electrical injury; and a burn associated with extenuating problems, such as soft-tissue injury, fractures, other trauma, or significant preexisting health problems.

Fluid Changes

Burn shock, a low-flow state, is characterized by reduced circulating blood volume and decreased cardiac output. Cardiac output plummets after a burn injury. All compensatory hemodynamics occur at the expense of adequate wound and skin perfusion. In order to maintain arterial pressure and venous return, peripheral and splanchnic bed vasoconstriction occurs, shunting blood from the extremities and intestines to the heart, brain, lungs, and kidneys. The decreased blood flow causes decreased oxygenation. Cellular hypoxia results in cellular changes, accumulation of lactic acid, and development of metabolic acidosis. The magnitude of the response is proportional to the extent and depth of the injury and the patient's physiologic status at the time of injury.

Two responses to the decrease in cardiac output are pertinent: the early response and the response associated with the volume decrease. Because resuscitation is based on the response to the volume decrease and the early response is related to the myocardial depressant factor, the response to volume depletion is discussed first.

Table 43–1
Depth of Burns

BURN	CAUSE	AREA OF INVOLVEMENT	CLINICAL PICTURE	HEALING TIME
First degree	Sunburn, flash burn	Epidermis	Red, dry, painful	A week or less
Second degree (partial-thickness)	Flame, flash, hot liquids, hot objects, chemicals			
Superficial		Epidermis, some dermis	Pink or mottled red, very painful, edematous, moist blisters	10–14 days
Deep		Epidermis, most of dermis	Pale, mottled, relatively dry, edematous, waxy white; little to no pain; clinically indistinguishable from third degree	30–60 days by reepithelialization from elements in hair follicles if infection does not convert; may be grafted
Third degree (full-thickness)	Flame; prolonged contact with hot liquids, hot objects, and chemials; electricity	Epidermis, dermis, subcutaneous tissue	White, cherry red or black eschar; dry, edematous, visibly thrombosed blood vessels; insensitivity to pinprick and pain; any hair present removed painlessly and effortlessly	Skin grafting always required, since healing can occur only with wound contraction from the epithelium of the wound margin 10–14 days for graft vascularization and donor size reepithelialization

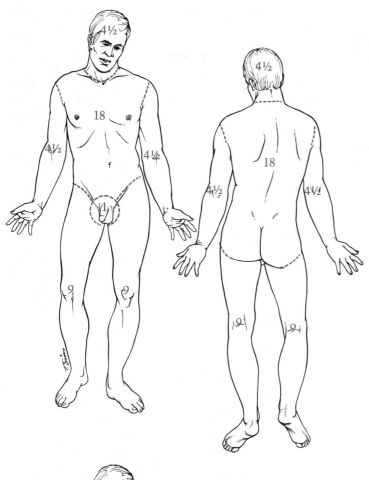

Figure 43-3

The Rule of Nines. This method for rapid approximation of the extent of injury is most useful for triage purposes.

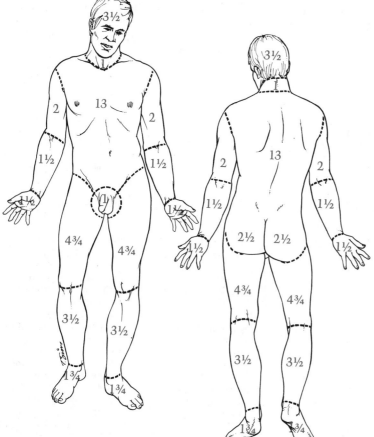

Figure 43-4

The Lund and Browder method is useful for the accurate determination of injury. After the burned area is calculated, the unburned area should be calculated.

Fluid Volume Deficit

The most significant physiologic change that follows burn injury is capillary leak, which leads to sequestration of fluid in the injured area and results in a decrease in the volume of circulating fluid. Soon after the injury, large amounts of isotonic fluid are translocated from a functional space into a nonfunctional one. Edema is most prominent in or directly surrounding the burned tissues; however, edema formation can also be found in nonburned tissue, including the lung.[24] Edema formation in a small wound is maximum at about 8 to 12 hours after injury.[25] In a large injury, fluid volume decrease (translocation) is greatest during the first 12 hours and continues for 18 to 24 hours after injury.[7]

Normally, the capillary and venular walls are permeable only to electrolytes and water. However, after a burn injury, the vasculature is permeable also to the plasma proteins. Another phenomenon connected with increased capillary permeability is that the colloid osmotic pressure is no longer effective in maintaining compartment equilibrium. Demling's research[25] suggests only a small transient increase (less than 8 hours) in permeability in the soft tissues (skin, fat, muscle). He writes that the increased net transvascular fluid flux that occurs in soft tissues is caused, in large part, by severe hypoproteinemia after burn injury.[25] Hypoproteinemia enhances edema formation by decreasing the plasma-to-interstitial-oncotic-pressure gradient.

With the use of electrophoresis, the protein concentration of burn wound edema fluid has been determined to be remarkably similar to the protein concentration of plasma. Molecules of high molecular weight have been found in the edema fluid. The leaking of large molecules is demonstrated by the fact that the edema fluid contains proportionately as much globulin as albumin. Fibrinogen has been found at levels of 3 g/dl. Despite the clinical use of many different types of resuscitative methods, the increased permeability persists until sealing occurs, approximately 18 to 30 hours after injury.[59]

Aldosterone is released from the adrenal cortex and produces maximal sodium and water reabsorption with a decrease in the urinary sodium level. Antidiuretic hormone is released from the posterior pituitary, and it produces maximal water reabsorption in the distal renal tubules. The result is oliguria, with an increased urine concentration and a decreased sodium concentration.

Also, a process similar to that seen in hemorrhagic shock is present. The transmembrane potential is decreased from a normal of −90 mV to −70 to −80 mV. This change (perhaps due to reduction of cell-membrane adenosine triphosphatase [ATPase] secondary to tissue ischemia) causes a shift in sodium, and in turn water, into the intracellular space.[25] Cell swelling results, particularly in skeletal muscle cells, 30 to 60 minutes after the burn.[5]

Myocardial Depressant Factor

Investigators have attributed the direct effect of burn injury on cardiac output to a circulating myocardial depressant factor (MDF). It has been suggested that the amount of MDF released or formed is related to the degree of injury and that in patients with burns greater than 65% TBSA, the MDF may be the primary limiting factor in response to fluid therapy.[59] Newer research suggests that the release of oxygen-derived free radicals from ischemic myocardium may mediate cardiac dysfunction after thermal injury.[40]

Late Phase of Edema Formation

Clinically, edema can be observed to increase slowly for 2 to 2½ days after the burn. Baxter[6] suggests the following explanations for the late phase of edema, when deeper tissues that have not been damaged contain the greatest portion of the sequestered fluid: the edema of surrounding tissues may result from the effects of histamine, bradykinins, or other amines released in response to the injury; and because of nonproteolytic changes in collagen, these deeper areas may have an increased affinity for sodium and water and essentially act like a sponge.

Edema after a burn injury is different from other kinds of edema in that it is viscous or gel-like. It is thought that this kind of edema is due to its high concentration of fibrinogen. Because of the gel-like state, local lymphatics and venules are occluded, and drainage of the damaged area is blocked, resulting in extension of edema both in depth and laterally.

Beginning approximately 36 hours after the burn, potassium is excreted in large amounts in the urine because of respiratory alkalosis, high aldosterone levels, and a high urinary output. Although serum potassium levels may remain in the normal to low-normal range, the intracellular deficit may be quite high. As a matter of fact, as much as 80 to 200 mEq of potassium must be administered daily to maintain the total body potassium levels.

The mobilization of burn edema begins after the second day. The time varies, but usually the edema is mobilized by the tenth to fourteenth postburn day.

Evaporative Water Loss

When the vapor barrier of the skin is lost because of injury, the amount of water lost through evaporation increases 4 to 15 times normal. If the burn wound is covered with a piece of plastic, drops of condensed water vapor are visible in a few minutes. The mean loss is estimated at 1.5 ml/kg/TBSA and may be as high as 3.5 ml/kg/TBSA. The loss of water from partial-thickness injuries is as significant as that from deeper injuries, because it is proportional to the TBSA.

Hematologic Alterations

After a major burn injury, the patient demonstrates changes in red blood cell mass, white blood cells, platelets, and fibrinogen. In the early postburn period in patients who have injuries greater than 40% TBSA, the hematocrit usually reaches 50% to 70% and remains elevated until the plasma volume is restored. Thus an elevated hematocrit is an expected finding. Serial increases in the hematocrit are used in some burn units as one of the indicators of inadequate fluid resuscitation.

The initial red blood cell destruction (of 3% to 15% of the red blood cell mass) is produced by the insult and is followed by a progressive anemia (3% to 9% daily loss of the red blood cell mass for about 2 weeks). Previously, mobilization of burn wound edema was thought to expand the blood volume so that the hemoglobin concentrations only appeared to be low. This is not true; in actuality, a profound anemia exists. The severity of the anemia correlates directly with the extent of the injury. Initially, it was postulated that the anemia was caused by a microangiopathic condition, probably produced by an unidentified plasma factor. In the original work,[52] red blood cells from burn patients transfused into normal subjects had a normal half-life, whereas red blood cells from normal subjects transfused into burned patients showed a significantly reduced half-life. Thus, it seems clear that the anemia probably is not intrinsic, nor is it caused by the injury; it is probably produced by a circulating factor or an environmental problem that produces a defect in the red cell membrane (possibly due to the altered metabolic response). In any event, the injured patient needs frequent transfusions of packed red cells to correct the anemia and to maintain the hematocrit between 35% and 40%.

White blood cell adhesiveness and entrapment in edema fluid may produce an early leukopenia, which tends to be a poor prognostic sign. Neutrophil function is particularly important, because as function decreases, the number of bacteria in the eschar increases. By the third postburn day, the oxygen consumption of white blood cells decreases by 50% unless ascorbic acid is administered and the patient's nutritional needs are met.

Through the first 5 postburn days, the patient exhibits accelerated platelet destruction and a progressive thrombocytopenia. Platelet counts then rise to normal or elevated levels. Platelet adhesiveness, hypercoagulability, and increased blood viscosity are present. Platelets and leukocytes aggregate and produce a progressive vascular thrombosis. Thrombin times are prolonged, but prothrombin times and partial thromboplastin times are variable.

Initially, plasma levels of fibrinogen decrease largely because of sequestration within the burn wound. During the first 6 postburn hours, fibrinogen concentrations in burn wound edema reach levels of 28% of the plasma concentration. By 36 to 48 hours after the burn, the plasma fibrinogen measurements are at nearly normal levels, and then rise rapidly to elevated levels.[5] Elevations in fibrin split products (FSP) accompany the changes in fibrinogen levels, with elevated levels of FSP seen first in the edema fluid and later in the plasma. It is thought that FSP elevations in the first 10 to 14 postburn days are secondary to coagulation in the extracellular edema fluid rather than to abnormal intravascular coagulation.

Clotting factors V and VIII are elevated four to eight times normal, and they remain elevated for 2 to 3 months.

Respiratory System Changes

After injury, the initial stability of the pulmonary blood volume is followed by a change in the venous pulmonary vasculature. Pulmonary engorgement occurs as a result of increased pulmonary blood volume and vascular resistance. These changes are compounded by any additional injury.

Carbon Monoxide Poisoning

Impaired gas exchange related to anoxia (from consumption of oxygen by the fire itself) and carbon monoxide poisoning is the leading cause of death at the scene of a fire. Carbon monoxide is produced by the incomplete combustion of carbon-containing materials. The gas is colorless, odorless, tasteless, and nonirritating.

Inhalation of carbon monoxide can produce significant hypoxemia. Carbon monoxide has an affinity for hemoglobin 200 times that of oxygen,[39,72] thereby displacing oxygen at available binding sites. Even after exposure to low levels of

carbon monoxide, carboxyhemoglobin levels may be elevated. Serum oxygen (PaO_2) levels may not be affected because they reflect oxygen dissolved in the plasma and not total oxygen content of the blood.[16] Carbon monoxide shifts the oxygen dissociation curve to the left, further reducing cellular availability of oxygen.[38]

Direct Injury

Inhalation of superheated air (>300°F/149°C) produces tissue damage and necrosis in the upper airway but not in the lower airway.[61] The lower airway is protected by laryngeal reflexes and the tremendous heat-exchanging efficiency of the oropharynx and nasopharynx.[16] Only with the inhalation of steam (with its heat-carrying capacity being 4000 times that of dry air) can heat damage reach the bronchiole level.[16,61]

Smoke Inhalation

Lower airway injury results from the introduction of toxic chemicals into the lungs. After closed-space injuries, inhalation of the products of incomplete combustion frequently leads to chemical pneumonitis. Both natural materials and plastics produce noxious gases. Aldehydes and the oxides of nitrogen and sulphur are damaging to the airway. The burning of plastics produces hydrochloric acid, hydrogen cyanide, and benzene, all of which are potentially lethal to cells.

Initially ciliary action and surfactant are lost. The mucosa becomes edematous,[89] and bronchospasm from mucosal irritation may occur.[16] With mucosal ulceration and shedding, exudate and epithelial casts accumulate in the airways, and both microatelectasis and macroatelectasis result.[89] Lung compliance is reduced within 12 hours by increased extravascular lung water and lymph flow.[38] Inhalation injury impairs pulmonary function by increasing resistance to breathing, altering the distribution of inspired air, and decreasing the diffusion of gases across alveolar membranes. Severe cases of the syndrome proceed to death with irritation, edema, tracheobronchitis, necrotizing bronchiolitis, pneumonitis, hyaline membrane formation, intra-alveolar hemorrhage, and alveolar pulmonary noncardiac edema.

Pneumonia

Bronchopneumonia may be superimposed on other respiratory problems at any time. After injury, neutrophils move into the lungs, producing oxygen-free radicals and proteolytic enzymes. These irritants contribute to edema formation. The combination of protein-rich edema, debris, and the immunosuppression that accompanies burn injury creates an ideal environment for bacterial proliferation.[37] The incidence of pneumonia increases with increasing burn size up to 90% TBSA burn.[73]

Bacterial pneumonia may occur from 3 to 15 days postinjury. Early colonization is often due to airborne staphylococci. Some authors note a close relationship between endotracheal aspirate cultures and wound flora in the presence of a mechanical airway (tracheotomy or endotracheal tube).[72] Other researchers are evaluating the possibility that translocation of gram-negative bacteria occurs across the gut mucosa after a period of ischemia (burn shock) and subsequently colonizes the lung fields.[23,62] Lower airway complications may also be associated with aspiration injuries.

Stress

The burned patient undergoes many severe physiologic and psychological stresses. The injury itself produces fear and pain, and the victim has numerous anxieties. Powerlessness, depersonalization, fear of the unknown, dependency, change in body image, disfigurement, loss of function, and even death are possibilities that may confront the patient day by day.[4,74]

Often during the period of hospitalization, the stress and pain alter the patient's defenses for an indefinite period of time. Regression and denial are often present, and they seem to be protective mechanisms. The stages of grief are frequently seen, and the denial stage tends to be prolonged. A commonplace occurrence is that the patient does not seem to realize the extent of the injury. Denial may be an adaptive protective mechanism patients employ. Watkins et al[82] have identified a continuum of seven stages involving both cognitive and affective processes in adaptation to burn injury. They include: survival anxiety, during which the patient is fearful as he considers the issues of survival and death; the problem of pain, during which the patient concentrates on his physical and psychological pain, distress, and helplessness; the search for meaning, in which he strives to find an acceptable explanation for why the injury occurred; investment in recuperation, in which the patient focuses his attention on and measures his progress in procedures and tasks required of him; acceptance of losses, in which the patient begins to comprehend and seek legitimization despite long-term and permanent losses sustained; investment in rehabilitation, in which the patient focuses on regaining the functions specific to his or her own unique life-style; and reintegration of identity, as he or she weighs the significance of his injury and reestablishes an identity and sense of self.

Pain

Pain is a common denominator in the critical care unit. It is a daily companion of the patient. Everyone who has had even a small burn remembers the pain associated with it. If a small burn can cause a great deal of pain, what must be the pain caused by a burn over a large part of the body?

The patient's pain varies according to the depth and extent of injury, the type of therapeutic measures used, the patient's individual response to pain, and the patient's anxieties and fears. For the family, the waiting, feelings of helplessness, and sorrow in watching their loved one suffer often make their pain unbearable. To the staff, the patient's pain brings many anxieties. In their skilled hands lie many techniques to help relieve the discomfort. But what of the pain they must inflict on the patient during such procedures as bathing and debriding of the wounds? Even in the most skilled hands, such procedures bring anguish. Some patients cannot tolerate the pain, and they attack the staff verbally, calling them unkind inflictors of pain, and thus bring more distress to the staff.

It is generally agreed that pain, even in the acute situation, is cognitively mediated (i.e., translated and interpreted by each individual depending on life history patterns, psychological make-up, and situational events). Experimental evidence shows that pain is influenced greatly by such cognitive factors

as fear, anxiety, and anticipation. Choinière et al[18] evaluated the pain of 42 adult burn patients. A conservative wound care approach was used, with twice-daily dressing changes. An average of 6.5 mg morphine was given intramuscularly before wound care. Anxiety and depression levels were assessed (using the State-Anxiety and Beck Depression Inventories) just before a painful procedure such as hydrotherapy or physiotherapy. Immediately after the procedure, patients were asked to recall and rate their levels of pain during the therapy. Their pain was assessed later in the day during a time at rest. Pain rating was done using the McGill Pain Questionnaire and a Visual analogue scale. Generalizations about the group revealed a population whose anxiety and depression levels were comparable to that found in other medical/surgical patients. It was found that anxiety and depression levels usually increased with time. Patients with higher anxiety and depression levels tended to rate their at-rest pain as higher; however, their evaluation of procedural pain was not higher than the pain reported by the others in the study population. Therefore, psychological methods of intervention (behavior modification, stress reduction techniques, and hypnosis) may be of value to some patients to help them deal with day-to-day pain.

Average pain at rest was relatively mild. Pain associated with dressing changes showed a wide degree of variation, with daily fluctuations of pain in each patient. Pain scores did not decline steadily with time; some patients suffered as much in later phases of treatment as they did in earlier stages.[18] Pain at the injury site may be replaced by significant suffering related to mobilization, donor site pain, and itching sensations.[18] Causalgia and dysesthesias may develop, especially in wounds that heal through granulation and in donor sites that have been cropped multiple times.[55] Because of this variation from patient to patient, it is important that health care workers solicit feedback from patients concerning their pain experiences so that treatment may be individualized. When nurses' scoring of patients' pain has been compared with patients' scoring of their own pain, nurses were found to overestimate or to underestimate the patients' burn pain frequently.[45,67]

Pain is a complex physiologic phenomenon that is perceived peripherally and transmitted to the brain centers. The psychological impact of pain can be mild (e.g., in cases of moderate and short-lived pain), or it can be devastating (e.g., the chronic, agonizing pain of patients who have intractable trigeminal neuralgia, which drives some of them to suicide).

The current leading theory of pain perception allows for, and attempts to account for, variations in pain experience. This theory, the gate control theory, postulates a neural mechanism in the dorsal horns of the spinal cord that acts as a gate, modulating sensory input before it evokes pain perception and behavioral response. In essence, smaller-diameter fibers transmit nerve impulses from peripheral nerves to T cells in the dorsal horns. When the output of the T cells reaches or exceeds a critical level, a signal occurs that triggers the system responsible for pain perception. However, transmission can be inhibited either by stimulation or activity of the larger, faster-transmitting fibers or by descending fibers from the brain. Thus, central nervous system activity, such as emotion, memories of prior experience, attention, and so forth, can exert influence over sensory input to open or close the pain "gate." In other words, psychological factors influence pain response and perception by acting on the gate control system.

Research on endorphins identifies further processes. The

endorphins, literally the "morphine within," are proteins that serve as a natural means of pain suppression on activation. The endorphins, identified by several groups of investigators, appear to be released by the brain—particularly the pituitary gland is implicated. They seem to be modulators of the signals between nerve cells, and they act specifically on the same nerve receptors that are affected by other opiates. Non-opiod transmitters such as norepinephrine and seratonin may also play a role in pain modulation.[50]

To date, endorphins have been implicated as the pain-relief mechanism in acupuncture, transcutaneous nerve stimulation, and in the so-called placebo effect. Apparently, the variability among patients in reported pain intensity for any given condition is due to differences in endorphin activity. Because the endorphins appear to be related to the patient's expectations, which can be considered to include a host of factors (past experiences, emotional predisposition, psychological make-up), offering a treatment that allows the possibility of some patient control over physiology (such as patient-controlled analgesia) even for minimal anxiety relief, should greatly enhance these expectations.

The end result may well entail a rallying of the patient's defenses against pain. An unfortunate side effect of drugs that suppress pain is the inhibition of endorphin release, such that greater dependency on the drugs seems to be coupled with a declining ability to use endogenous means of pain control. The actual effect of one on the other has not been identified yet.

Pain should be viewed as an initial physical insult that, finally, has spiritual repercussions. These repercussions vary, ranging from temporary ego dissolution ("I am so small and my pain is so large") to psychosis if the pain is severe and unrelenting and if the patient sees no hope of escape from it ("The only escape from my overwhelmingly real pain is to leave reality"). Pain diminishes the sufferer's sense of worth. It forces dependence and helplessness on the sufferer—and with a vengeance. The sufferer is not only rendered helpless, as in a major body burn, but is also in agony while being helpless.

The use of hypnosis or self-directed visualization can help some patients gain a sense of mastery over their pain. In those who are receptive, it may prove valuable, in that the patient remains fully conscious and capable of communicating and cooperating, and some patients benefit from a posthypnotic suggestion.[79]

Whereas most patients are alert at the time of burn injury, some state that they experienced no pain at first. Choinière *et al*[18] found that 37% of the patients in his study reported a pain-free period immediately after the injury. Whereas variations in depth of injury may account for some discrepancy, Choinière notes that it is common for victims of extensive injuries to be less responsive to pain, perhaps owing to physiologic and emotional shock.

It is demeaning to patients to be judged by others to be "intolerant" of pain, "unable to cope with pain," "liking their morphine," or "infantile" in handling pain. Nurses (and others) know too little about the physiology of pain to be judgmental. Visual analogue and graphic rating scales may be used reliably to help patients express their perceptions of their pain as it relates to a variety of activities throughout the day.[78] A proper approach is to regard pain as an existential experience that has physiologic roots—as an example of the body–mind–spirit continuum.

Metabolic Response to Injury

The metabolic response to burn injury has three facets (see Chap. 36): hypermetabolism, severe protein wasting, and weight loss.[84] Mediated by a significant catecholamine response and other hormonal changes, the metabolic rate shows a rapid linear increase from its normal resting metabolic expenditure to a peak (hypermetabolic) rate that is about twice normal in patients with burns of 40% to 50% or greater body surface area burns.[13] Caloric expenditures and protein catabolism are greater and more sustained after burn injuries than in any other physiologic condition.[66] This hypermetabolic state is marked by increased cardiac output and high oxygen consumption. At this maximal physiologic state, energy expenditures cannot increase further in response to additional stresses. As the wound closes, metabolic rate and oxygen consumption return to normal.[10]

The amount of protein in the body decreases mainly, it is thought, from the catabolism of skeletal muscle. Amino acids are converted to glucose, and nitrogen and other intracellular constituents are lost. Weight loss greater than 20% of the preburn weight may be expected in patients who have an injury greater than 40% TBSA, unless attention is given to caloric support.[21,28] The problem is related to sex, body build, preburn nutritional status, severity of injury, and complicating factors. If the patient has a loss in body weight greater than 10% of preburn weight and a loss of body water, the ability to perform work is decreased. If a patient loses one fourth to one third of protein mass or 40% to 50% of body weight, death is likely. Increases in body protein and in body weight do not usually occur until wound closure.

A caloric intake of 5000 calories per day in burned patients stabilizes the condition of the red blood cell so that a normal concentration of intracellular sodium is maintained. It has been suggested that thermal burn injury either inhibits the active transport mechanism of red blood cells or produces a defect in the red blood cell membrane, and that the inhibition or defect may be reversed by the maintenance of a positive energy balance. The functioning of red blood cells may reflect the functioning of other body cells, and thus intracellular sodium concentrations may reflect the effectiveness of nutritional support.

Wilmore *et al*[85] demonstrated that blood flow to a burned extremity is increased and, furthermore, the increased blood flow is not related to the extremity's aerobic metabolic demands. In the body's response to injury, the healing wound has top priority. Although the uninjured extremity does not use glucose, the healing wound does. The hyperdynamic systemic response appears essential to maintaining the circulatory and metabolic needs of the healing wound.

The body routinely will break down even uninjured tissue to supply energy, substrate, and micronutrients to the healing wound. In an effort to enhance repair, the body increases both blood flow to the wound and the temperature of the injured surface. The glucose that is synthesized by the liver is used primarily by granulation tissue.

Underlying the patient's metabolic response to the burn injury is the response to stress. Physiologically, sympathetic stimulation, adrenergic activity, and energy needs are increased, so that the body fuels are used rather than stored.[13] Many different mechanisms figure in the stress phenomenon. The greater the stress, the greater the response. Afferent neuronal signals such as pain, hypoxia, hypotension, fear and anxiety, in addition to humoral stimuli (prostaglandins, interleukin 1, and complement factors) alter the central nervous system functioning.[66] A reset phenomenon of the hypothalamus[13] causes increased adrenergic stimulation with release of catecholamines, growth hormone (GH), beta-endorphins, and adrenocorticotropic hormone (ACTH).[66] The ACTH stimulates the adrenals to produce cortisol, and the catecholamines stimulate the pancreas to produce glucagon.

In the early phases of burn shock, insulin levels decrease, and the burn patient may develop hyperglycemia in response to the catecholamines. After resuscitation, insulin level increases to normal (relative to the metabolic rate), yet hyperglycemia may still develop.[13] This phenomenon may be due to the peripheral tissue's resistance to insulin in the presence of high levels of catecholamines, or from the marked gluconeogenesis.[13]

As a result of these metabolic changes, the burned patient exhibits a significant tendency toward catabolism: glycogenolysis, gluconeogenesis, and ureagenesis rather than synthesis of protein.[13] Increased glucagon and catecholamines increase lipolysis; however, burned tissues preferentially use glucose over fat. Without exogenous glucose, the patient mobilizes proteins from skeletal and visceral stores. This process can result in significant weight loss and immunologic compromise.[32] Once support levels of protein and calories are attained, protein synthesis and anabolism are possible. Substrate flow is affected, the negative nitrogen balance and weight loss are decreased, and wound healing improves. Hypermetabolism continues until wound closure.

Formerly, it was accepted that the hypermetabolic response was due to the increased caloric expenditure needed to provide for the evaporation of water. However, further definitive work has identified other important factors.[88] It was shown that a raised metabolic rate in burn patients was not the direct result of water evaporation. The investigation showed prevention of evaporative water loss by covering the injured area with an impermeable piece of plastic film for periods up to 12 hours did not significantly reduce the patient's oxygen consumption. Studies by Wilmore et al.[84,85] demonstrated that the evaporative water loss was not primary in the metabolic response, but that the increased energy production was related to the reset of metabolic activity. The thermally injured person produces great quantities of heat as a consequence of the injury, and such a person is internally warm, not externally cold. Increased water loss is a means to transfer the heat generated.

Hematemesis

Hematemesis of small amounts of coffee-ground material in the first 48 hours after a burn injury is characteristic of hemorrhagic gastritis. Congested gastric capillaries rupture and produce the blood. The congestion and irritation may set the stage for further acute gastroduodenal disease. Patients may also develop bleeding from peptic ulcer disease, disseminated intravascular coagulation, and gastric erosion from a nasogastric tube.

Stress Ulceration

With the advent of prophylactic antacid therapy and H_2 blocker administration, stress ulceration (acute gastroduodenal disease or Curling's ulcer)[56] and bleeding are rarely seen. Previously, stress ulceration was seen at autopsy in about 25% of all burn patients. Its presence was usually heralded by a massive hematemesis of bright red blood or the passage of tarry stools. Perforation was the initial sign in about 10% of patients.

In an effort to determine the incidence and natural history of stress ulceration, Czaja and associates[22] performed early and serial gastroduodenoscopies in 32 patients who had thermal injury. In areas of intense superficial mucosal injury, after the first 72 postburn hours, 22% of patients had a gastric ulcer and 28% had a duodenal ulcer.

The cause of stress ulceration is not known; early ischemia and adrenal hormone secretion appear to play a significant role. Hyperacidity and pre-existing ulcer disease do not seem to be causative factors. Sepsis acts as an added stress. Other possible causative factors are elevated corticosteroid levels; decreased gastroduodenal blood flow (hemoconcentration, elevated catecholamine levels, and hypovolemia); the lytic effect of regurgitated chyme; and a quantitative or qualitative change in mucus.[31]

Sepsis

In sepsis, the most significant complication in the acute phase of burn injury, one or more of the following problems may be found: burn wound sepsis, pneumonia, suppurative thrombophlebitis, closed-space infection, urinary tract infection, prostatitis, or infection in any part of the body. The use of invasive procedures and monitoring devices increases the likelihood of infection.[53]

The Burn Wound

The burn wound is the most frequent source of infection. Loss of skin is loss of the body's first line of defense against microorganisms. The burn wound may contain three zones: the zone of coagulation, the zone of stasis, and the zone of hyperemia. The *zone of coagulation* is the part of the wound that received the greatest heat and is characterized by cell death, microvascular thrombosis, and occlusion of local blood supply. Immediately adjacent to this zone is the *zone of stasis,* in which initial cell damage and impaired blood supply is reversible barring complications of hypoxia, hypovolemia, wound desiccation, and infection. Peripheral to the zone of stasis is the *zone of hyperemia,* which is characterized by vasodilatation and increased blood flow.[69,87] Though initially free of major bacterial contamination except for gram-positive organisms found in sweat glands and hair follicles, the destroyed tissue is an excellent culture medium, and bacteria proliferate and colonize the wound within about 48 hours.[53] If infection is not controlled in areas of partial-thickness injury, a progressive tissue necrosis converts the wound into a full-thickness injury.

In a series of investigations in the animal model, Order et al.[65] demonstrated the vascular characteristics of the burn wound. In partial-thickness injury, the body's ability to elicit an inflammatory response is maintained beneath the damaged tissue. Underlying blood vessels begin to form new canals in areas of partial-thickness injury approximately 2 days after the burn, and the process is completed at approximately 7 days. A full-thickness injury is characterized by arterial occlusion and the absence of an inflammatory response. Coagulation necrosis is manifested clinically as thrombosed blood vessels. The tissue under the eschar remains without a blood supply until granulation tissue develops, a process that begins approximately 14 days after the injury and is completed approximately 21 days after the injury. The established capillary network in mature granulation tissue enables the phagocytic cells to congregate at the site of infection, producing a resistance to infection.

Bacterial colonization of the burn wound usually occurs between the 5th and 25th day after the injury, but may occur within 24 hours. Three types of colonization have been described: supraeschar, intraeschar, and intrafollicular. *Supraeschar colonization* is defined as bacterial growth on the wound, *intraeschar colonization* is defined as growth within the wound, and *intrafollicular colonization* is defined as growth within the hair follicles. Intrafollicular colonization emanates from bacteria trapped at the time of the burn injury.[77]

Infection in the burn wound can be caused by a variety of organisms. Early after the injury, the organisms are likely to be gram-positive, and later, even in the first week, the organisms are likely to be gram-negative (*Pseudomonas, Klebsiella, Enterobacter, Escherichia coli,* and *Serratia*). Transferable resistance to antibiotics has been reported with several organisms. Other opportunistic organisms, such as *Candida, Phycomycetes, Aspergillus,* and certain viruses, may cause significant problems.

After bacterial colonization of the wound and invasion of the adjacent subcutaneous tissues, the infectious process reaches systemic proportions. The proliferation and active invasion of the burn wound by 100,000 or more microorganisms per gram of tissue is commonly defined as *burn wound sepsis.* The definition is based on the work of Teplitz and associates[77] with the animal model, using *Pseudomonas aeruginosa* as a prototype. Supraeschar and intrafollicular colonization were followed by intraeschar colonization. Invasion of the nonviable–viable interface was followed by invasion of viable tissue and systemic spread through the lymphatics and blood.

Full-thickness wound biopsy is the method used most to quantitate bacterial colonization and to determine the predominant organism(s) and antibiotic sensitivities.[8] A small piece of an entire thickness of eschar and its underlying tissue is excised, or a punch biopsy of the eschar is taken and the number of organisms per gram of tissue is determined. A rapid frozen section may be sent for immediate histologic examination to identify invasion into viable tissue. Preliminary results on routine cultures that demonstrate growth at a 10^4 dilution suggest the need to treat the patient for sepsis; the assumption is that bacteria have continued to proliferate and are at invasive levels by the time the laboratory reports are received. The wound biopsy can be used to evaluate the progression or regression of bacterial growth and thus the effectiveness of therapy.

Monitoring by surface-culture techniques alone is not satisfactory; the correlation between surface colonization and deep tissue colonization is poor. Contact plates help predict what organism is likely to cause problems, but contact plates have several disadvantages: a contact plate is likely to identify a variety of organisms, topical antimicrobial therapy changes the surface flora, and bathing may change the bacterial count, because the mechanical agitation breaks up the colonies. Similar problems are present with the capillary gauze and swab culture techniques.

Blood cultures have limited usefulness early in the pathologic process of sepsis. Blood cultures are positive only a small portion of the time the patient is clinically septic; however, when the cultures are made of a terminally ill patient, a high percentage are positive. For example, in one study,[54] blood cultures were positive in only 4% of patients, although 13% died with sepsis; 19% demonstrated clinical signs, and 27% had burn wound biopsy cultures that showed more than 10^4 organisms per gram of tissue.

Host Defense Mechanisms

Burn trauma is accompanied by significant abnormalities in the host's defense system (see Chap. 45). The altered inflammatory response and the defect in the capacity of neutrophils to kill bacteria seem to be more significant than the humoral defects.

The inflammatory reaction stimulated by the damaged cells of the burn is seen immediately after injury. Oxygen free radicals, produced by polymorphonuclear leukocytes, are an early mediator of inflammation.[44] The complement system is activated to produce C3a and C5a, which increase vascular permeability, stimulate the release of histamines and serotonin, and serve as chemoattractants.[60] The arachidonic acid cascade produces vasoactive and chemoattractive substances, including thromboxane, prostaglandins, and leukotrienes.[44] Research is being conducted currently to evaluate the feasibility of mediating the negative effects of the inflammatory response in order to restrict edema formation, decrease thromboxane-stimulated platelet adhesiveness and vasoconstriction, and reduce pain.

Nonspecific resistance to infection is one of the most important components of immunity. Significant abnormalities are found to be present in neutrophil functioning. Neutrophil function is significantly depressed in patients who suffer 40% or greater total body surface area burns.[37] Studies have shown that, preceding and accompanying the septic process, there is a reduction in the results of the nitroblue tetrazolium test, which measures the intracellular capacity of neutrophils to kill bacteria.[5] The chemotactic index that measures the attraction of white blood cells has also been found to be depressed. Burn wound sepsis occurs when the ability of phagocytic cells to migrate to the wound and to kill ingested bacteria is depressed.

Noncirculating phagocytic cells found in the reticuloendothelial system also function to remove bacteria, cellular debris, and other particulate matter from the circulation. The activity of this system is significantly depressed with defective clearing ability,[60] which may be related to a fibronectin deficit[86] seen immediately after injury and again in burned patients who become septic.[32]

The complement system is important in antibacterial defense as a result of stimulation of leukocyte chemotaxis and opsonization.[32] It may be activated by interaction with IgM or IgG or by substances such as endotoxins.[86] Many burned patients have defects in complement levels.[32]

Cellular and humoral immunity is also impaired in the burn patient, with the activities of the T-cell system being more depressed than the activity of the B-cell system.[86] This defective cell-mediated immunity has been observed for years with prolonged survival of homograft skin. In addition, many burn patients are unable to mount delayed hypersensitivity skin reactions (anergy).[86]

Wound Healing

Contracture Formation

Burn scars go through three stages of development. In the immature stage there are many fibroblasts,[44] and fibrosis is minimal. In some wounds, even at this early stage, the collagen fibers are oriented in parallel bands; these wounds do not become hypertrophic. In other wounds the collagen at this stage is disoriented, forming whorls and nodules; these wounds have a tendency to develop hypertrophic scars. Early increased microcirculatory blood flow has also been associated with hypertrophic scar formation.[41] In the semi-mature stage there is decreased vascularity, the fibrosis is more pronounced, and the collagen is more organized. The mature stage is characterized by fewer capillaries and fibroblasts and increased fibrosis.[1] The longer the wound takes to heal, the greater the tendency for development of hypertrophic scarring. The reduced circulation in scars results in thin skin, which may break down or blister after minor trauma. Healing of this skin is slow.

Contractures of the scars are common, especially across flexed joints because of the patient's tendency toward flexion when at rest. Efforts to maintain full extension of these joints may be hampered by scar shortening, tightness, and pain.

Current therapy is based on information gathered from studies of granulation tissue.[36] If the fibers of collagen develop parallel to the direction of stress, the nodular swirls are not as likely to form. Thus therapy aims to maintain extension and to encourage parallel fibers of collagen by proper positioning, splinting, exercising, and using traction. However, it must be emphasized that although prevention is the best therapy, because of the nature of the burn injury, not all deformities are preventable. Care must always be individualized for the patient.

Proper positioning—including avoiding positions of comfort and pressure areas early in the course of the burn injury—maintains functional range of motion and proper body alignment, decreases edema, and prevents deformities and decubitus ulcers. Contracture formation may occur across any joint. The hand that suffers deep burns is particularly vulnerable. Surgical release may be necessary, preferably after scars reach maturity. Neck and axillary contractures are also common. Once contractures have developed, stretching or a combined operative and rehabilitative approach to contracture release is associated with an excellent chance of restoring function and mobility.[48]

NURSING PROCESS

ASSESSMENT

A complete health history and physical examination are essential to determine the status and appropriate problem list of any trauma victim. The burned patient may have suffered severe associated injuries, so such a patient must first be assessed as any other trauma patient. Even the massively burned patient will not die in the first few minutes from burn, but may die from an obstructed airway or an open chest injury. The initial assessment after burn injury then entails certain specifics.

History

The history of being burned in a *closed space* or of *excessive smoke inhalation* alerts the team to pay particular attention to respiratory functioning. The physical findings on admission may be negative, and serious respiratory embarrassment may develop later. Table 43–2 outlines historical data.

The type of burning agent should be documented:

- If the history of *chemical burn* is given, the immediate treatment is washing with copious amounts of water.
- If the body has become the conduit for *electric current*, a tremendous amount of damage has occurred. This is not immediately visible, so the usual formulas and treatments for external burns do not apply.
- Flame, hot liquid, steam, a hot object, or tar should be specified.

The *circumstances surrounding the injury* give information of possible other injuries, possible depth of burn, and possible extensive involvement of underlying tissues. Whether the patient lost consciousness should be noted.

The history of *pre-existing disease* alerts the team to possible alterations in reactions to treatment and complications. Of particular importance would be data concerning any history of cardiovascular, pulmonary, renal, metabolic, or neurologic disorders.

Also included are a detailed drug history and any history of alcohol intake or narcotics use. The tetanus immunization and any history of drug sensitivities are documented.

Clinical Manifestations

The initial assessment is derived from the collection of subjective and objective data concerning assessment of impaired gas exchange, inadequate cardiac output, and impaired tissue perfusion (Table 43–3). Assessment and initial care are often performed simultaneously (Fig. 43–5). A decreased arterial

Table 43–2
History of the Accident

Time and place
Burn incident
    Cause of injury
    Length of exposure
    Temperature
Circumstances surrounding injury
    Events before, during, and after
    Presence of smoke and time exposed
    Closed-space involvement
    Accidental or deliberate, inflicted by self or another person
    Condition of others involved in accident
    Presence of alcohol or drugs
    Medical history

Table 43–3

Nursing Diagnoses Formulated From Initial Assessment

NURSING DIAGNOSIS	CLINICAL SIGNS	PLAN
Potential for complications related to associated injuries	History of trauma, bleeding, fractures, neurologic damage (especially spinal injury)	Treat for trauma, monitor, initiate measures to stabilize, immobilize
Impaired gas exchange 1. Related to obstructed airway and burn edema	Increased respirations, singed nasal hairs, alteration in consciousness, burns of the face and neck, hoarseness, cough, drooling	Maintain airway, suction if appropriate; elevate head; oxygen, with FIO_2 of 1.0; prepare for endotracheal intubation and mechanical ventilation
2. Related to carbon monoxide poisoning	Alteration in consciousness, combative behavior, history of injury in enclosed space, carboxyhemoglobin > 15%, hypoxemia, cherry red color on unburned areas	Maintain airway; oxygen with FIO_2 of 1.0; prepare for endotracheal intubation and mechanical ventilation
3. Related to lower airway obstruction and smoke inhalation	Carbonaceous sputum; respiratory insufficiency with obstructed airway; history of smoke inhalation; history of unconsciousness associated with injury; red swollen buccal membranes; progressive rales and rhonchi; arterial oxygenation < 80 mm Hg	Maintain airway; elevate head; oxygen, with FIO_2 of 1.0; maximal inspiratory maneuver; cough and deep breathe; monitor; start intravenous infusion; prepare for endotracheal intubation and mechanical ventilation
Decreased cardiac output related to fluid changes and shock syndrome	Alteration of consciousness; decreased urinary output; tachycardia (blood pressure may be normal to high early postburn, then low); cutaneous burn > 20%; metabolic acidosis; increased hemoglobin and hematocrit; decreased to absent bowel sounds; increased blood sugar	Start Ringer's lactate infusion through large peripheral line; continue to orient; monitor sensorium, urine, vital signs every 30 minutes to 1 hour; place Foley catheter; calculate extent of burn and fluid requirements; sugar acetone determination (SAD) every 4 hours
Pain related to exposed cutaneous nerve endings and fear/anxiety	Subjective complaints	Provide care in calm, efficient manner; give direct explanations to patient; cover burn with clean sheet or room-temperature sterile saline compresses; cover wound with topical antimicrobial agent as soon as possible; assist pateint with deep breathing techniques; administer low-dose intravenous analgesics as ordered
Decreased to absent bowel sounds related to ileus and stress response	Decreased bowel sounds, vomiting, cutaneous burn > 20%	NPO, place nasogastric catheter and attach to intermittent suction
Decreased tissue perfusion in extremities related to peripheral burn wound edema and circumferential full-thickness burn injury	Progressive loss of pulses both by palpation and by Doppler; deep, throbbing muscle pain	Elevate burned extremity above level of heart; apply positioning splints and encourage active exercise at least hourly; monitor pulse with Doppler at least every 30 minutes; prepare for escharotomy
Potential for wound infection related to environmental contamination and lowered resistance	Presence of cutaneous burn, cellulitis	Maintain clean environment and use sterile equipment; administer tetanus prophylaxis; wash wound at bedside, in shower, or in tub; debride gently; cover wound with topical antimicrobial agent

Table 43–4

Carbon Monoxide Poisoning

CARBOXYHEMOGLOBIN LEVEL	CLINICAL SIGNS AND SYMPTOMS
15%–20%	Headache, dyspnea, confusion, diminished vision, making coordinated movements difficult
20%–40%	Nausea, further diminished vision, poor judgment; any movement produces rapid fatigue
40%–60%	Confusion, hallucinations, ataxia, collapse, stupor, coma, situation still reversible with treatment
60% and above	Rapid deterioration and death

oxygenation is often seen before resuscitation is initiated. The reason for this decrease is not known, but restoration of the cardiac output improves the oxygenation. Serial determinations of arterial oxygen levels indicate a pulmonary tract injury or declining left-sided heart output.

Impaired Gas Exchange

With carbon monoxide (CO) poisoning, the patient is clinically hypoxic, restless, and confused (Table 43–4). The patient may complain of headache, visual changes, weakness, or nausea,[16] or may demonstrate diminished coordination[39] or difficulty with short-term recall. The skin or buccal membranes may have a cherry red coloring. Carbon monoxide poisoning must always be suspected in a patient who is hypoxic, restless, and confused, even though several hours have passed since the accident; the half-life of CO on room air is about 4 hours.[39] In a study by Clark et al[19] in which the data from 108 smoke inhalation victims were compiled, carbon monoxide was responsible for a "profound hypoxic stress reflected in the metabolic acidosis present in more than 50% of our patients." This metabolic acidosis is evident even when blood volume appears adequate.[26] In severe poisoning stupor, ECG changes, coma, and death may occur.

Upper airway injury may progress to total airway obstruction. All patients with burns about the lower face and neck, singed nasal hair, red and dry buccal mucosa, or soot in the sputum must be monitored closely. The immediate cause of respiratory distress is often laryngeal edema or spasm, and accumulation of mucus. Suctioning not only helps to clear the secretions but also to evaluate the extent of involvement. The signs of impending obstruction are not apparent for several hours and may occur as late as 18 to 24 hours after injury when edema maximizes. Clinical signs of airway narrowing include increasing hoarseness, brassy cough,[72] inability to handle secretions, dyspnea, and stridor.[63] The nurse should ask the patient questions at least every 15 minutes, assessing the sound of the patient's voice for increasing pitch and hoarseness.

Signs of true pulmonary injury are rarely apparent until about 24 hours postburn; however, inhalation of certain chemicals can lead to the immediate development of pulmonary edema.[16,38] Fifty percent of patients with lower airway injury have both a negative physical examination and a negative chest radiograph on admission. Inflammatory changes occurring during the first 24 hours often cause acute respiratory distress syndrome changes by the first postburn day. The following parameters are used for assessment:

- History of closed-space confinement during the fire
- Known inhalation of smoke or noxious gas
- History of loss of consciousness
- Clinical signs of upper airway obstruction
- Soot in the oropharynx
- Carbonaceous sputum
- Carboxyhemoglobin levels greater than 15%, hypoxemia, and hypercarbia
- Widening of the A-a gradient
- Brassy cough
- Cyanosis, rales, hoarseness, and increased secretions

The nurse should consult with the physician about any positive findings[43,63] from the bronchoscopic examination (mucosal blisters, massive nasal edema or erythema, and mucosal hemorrhage and ulceration in the upper airway), a positive xenon scan (unequal scintillation density, a clearance time of greater than 90 seconds, and an impairment in ventilatory function with significant airway obstruction),[63,73] alterations shown by spirometry, flow-volume loops, and the single breath nitrogen test, and alterations in the residual volume.

Circumferential full-thickness burns of the chest limit the movements of the thorax (Fig. 43–6). The patient shows increasing signs and symptoms of respiratory distress, because the tight eschar prevents adequate movement of the chest and proper oxygenation. Assessment parameters to watch for and monitor are increased work of breathing; rapid, shallow breathing; and respiratory distress. An escharotomy allows the chest to expand, and it alleviates the signs and symptoms.

Table 43–5
Fluid Therapy Formulas for Estimation of Resuscitative Fluid Requirements

	PARKLAND FORMULA	HYPERTONIC RESUSCITATION	MODIFIED BROOKE
Crystalloids	4 ml Ringer's lactate /kg/% burn	250 mEq sodium/L; 100 mEq Cl/L; 200 mEq lactate/L; up to 3500 ml limit isotonic salt solution is given orally during the second 24 hours	2 ml RL/kg/% burn
Colloids	0.3–0.5 ml/kg/% burn to maintain plasma volume during the second 24 hours		0.3–0.5 ml/kg/% burn during the second 24 hours
D₅W	About 2000 ml during the second 24 hours, adjusted to maintain serum sodium in normal range	None	The amount given during the second 24 hours is adjusted to maintain an adequate urinary output
Assessment criteria	Clear, lucid sensorium; urinary output 30–50 ml/hour; pulse < 120/minute; CVP < 5 cm H₂O; PCWP within normal limits; normal temperature	Urinary output adjusted to 30–40 ml/hour	Urinary output 30–50 ml/hour; clinical criteria for shock resuscitation

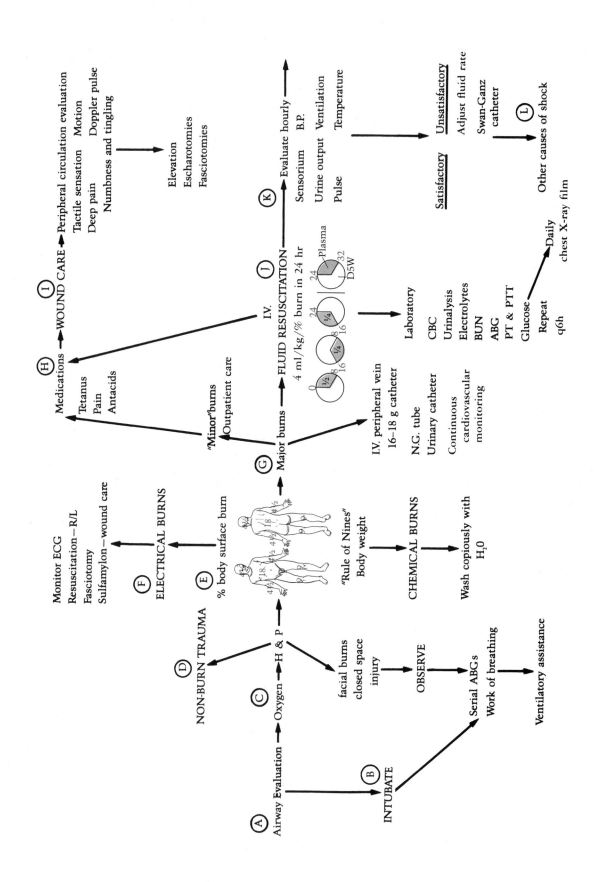

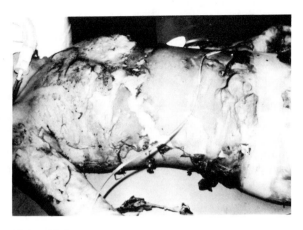

Figure 43-6
Circumferential full-thickness burns of the chest.

Decreased Cardiac Output

The hemodynamic response with low cardiac output and shock is a direct manifestation of the type of injury and magnitude of tissue destruction. The burn patient in shock may not have all the classical signs of shock (*i.e.*, reflexly the blood pressure may be maintained at low-normal levels because of peripheral vasoconstriction and edema). Therefore, assessment signs for shock (and later for the relief of shock) are necessarily different for the burn patient than for other trauma patients. The primary signs to monitor are sensorium and urinary output. Other signs are pulse, temperature, bowel sounds, acid–base status, and cardiac output.

Fluid resuscitation for shock can be administered according to several different formulas.[5,7,58] The important thing is to understand the assessment criteria for adequate resuscitation

(Table 43–5). Initially, the extent of injury must be assessed and the patient's accurate weight must be determined in order to calculate the fluids.

Decreased Tissue Perfusion

Once fluid therapy has been initiated, the underlying tissues swell. Areas of circumferential full-thickness burn are inelastic and cannot swell. They thus remain contracted and increase the peripheral edema. The tight band of eschar acts like a tourniquet and impairs venous return and arterial flow.

Peripheral circulation is constantly assessed. Pulses are palpated, and the ultrasonic Doppler flowmeter is used to listen for arterial flow. Clinical signs monitored include numbness, decreased sensation, and decreased motor activity; decreased capillary refill; and cyanosis. The best clinical signs of arterial insufficiency in burned extremities are a decreased to absent distal pulse as measured by Doppler and a throbbing, deep, aching pain. In several burn centers, various methods are being investigated to measure directly and monitor intracompartmental pressures.

Diagnostic Tests

Baseline laboratory determinations are made of complete blood count, electrolytes, glucose, blood urea nitrogen, carboxyhemoglobin level, clotting tests, and blood type and crossmatch. If there is a possibility of pulmonary damage, arterial blood gases are drawn. Aspirate from the nasogastric tube is tested for pH and the presence of blood. A urinalysis and spot test for glucose are made.

An initial chest radiograph is made and followed serially as determined by the patient's condition (at least daily). Additional diagnostic tests, such as spirometry, bronchoscopy,

Figure 43–5
Assessment and initial care. (*A*) Evaluate both upper and lower airway. Early facial swelling and hoarseness are indications for intubation. Carbonaceous sputum and mucosal redness should be evaluated further (xenon scan, bronchoscopy, and careful observation). (*B*) Nasotracheal intubation is preferred. Use largest size soft cuff tube possible (8.0 mm is minimum for bronchoscopy). (*C*) Oxygen (100%) administered at 10 L/min (if not contraindicated by COPD) compensates for the low flow state and enhances elimination of carboxyhemoglobin. (*D*) Continue to evaluate ventilation by breathing pattern (rate and work) and serial blood gases (ABG). Evaluate and treat non-burn trauma preferentially to burn (except for resuscitation). Do not close lacerations in burn tissue except on the face. Avoid operation when possible until resuscitation is complete. Internal fixation of fractures and simultaneous excision of small burns may be indicated. (*E*) Rule of Nines is sufficient for initial care and resuscitation. Rule does not apply to children. Ignore first degree burns in all calculations. (*F*) Initiate good urine flow (50–100 ml/hr) with Ringer's lactate *rapidly*. If urine is pigmented, give 25 g mannitol IV; then add 1 to 2 amps (40–80 mg) NaHCO$_3$ and 12.5 g mannitol to each liter Ringer's lactate. Maintain urine flow (100–150 ml/hr). Fasciotomy (not escharotomy) is necessary because of muscle swelling. Topical agent of choice is Sulfamylon—better absorption. (*G*) Major burn: burns greater than 15 percent body surface area, or smaller burns with inhalation injury, associated trauma, advanced age, or involvement of face, hands, feet, or genitalia. (*H*) Tetanus prophylaxis: Tetanus booster is mandatory. Give Hyper-tet only when immunization is deficient. Pain medications: Use IV route only in major burns; only small doses required if I (*below*) is followed. Antacids: Empty stomach with NG tube; give 30 to 60 ml every 2 hours adjusting by gastric pH to keep above 5.5. Do not give H$_2$ blockers. (*I*) Remove all clothing, wash gently, and apply cool, moist N/S dressings to relieve pain until definitive wound care is initiated. (*J*) Resuscitate solely with Ringer's lactate, 4 ml/kg/% burn given during the first 24 hours. One half (2 ml/kg/% burn) is given during the first 8 hours (calculated from time of injury); the other half is given during the following 16 hours. The plasma (½ ml/kg/% burn) is given over the next 4 to 6 hours. After that only D5/W at 1 ml/kg is usually required. Changes in these guidelines may be necessary with inaccurate assessment of burn surface area, inhalation injury, delayed fluid therapy, missed injuries, or liver disease. (*K*) Resuscitation evaluation: Normal cerebration and urine output of 0.5 to 1.0 ml/kg/hr (all ages), with normal ventilation, should be established within 2 to 4 hours. Expect pulse faster than 110/min; blood pressure normal to high for age; temperature increase to 37.5°C; PaO$_2$ greater than 70 mm Hg; pH increase to 7.4; normal EKG except S-T segment elevations; all other laboratory values should remain normal. Unsatisfactory resuscitation: Increase fluid administered rate to 5.5 ml/kg/% burn. Insert Swan-Ganz catheter for serial pulmonary wedge pressures and cardiac outputs if faster rate is required. Reduce fluids when satisfactory signs are obtained, otherwise proceed to L. (*L*) Unsuccessful resuscitation: Reexamine for all other courses of continued shock (*e.g.*, unsuspected trauma, hemopneumothorax, and gastric dilatation). (Courtesy Gary F. Purdue, M.D., and Charles R. Baxter, M.D., Department of Surgery, Southwestern Medical School, The University of Texas Health Sciences Center at Dallas.)

and xenon lung scan, are ordered by the physician depending on the patient's condition.

Protocol

The patient with a burn injury should receive initial care according to an established protocol and from a well-functioning team. A sample protocol that can be used as a guideline follows:

- Maintain a patent airway.
- Assess and manage any associated life-threatening injuries

according to the trauma protocol. If spinal injury is suspected, apply a cervical collar and backboard before moving the patient.
- Assess for signs of impaired gas exchange related to carbon monoxide poisoning, upper airway obstruction, or inhalation injury. Administer high-concentration oxygen with warm mist by face mask.
- Wash areas of chemical injury with copious amounts of water.[49]
- Remove rings and other jewelry; cut away clothing.
- Initiate fluid therapy according to the crystalloid resuscitation

BURN TRANSFER CHECKLIST

PATIENT NAME _____
AGE _____
DATE & TIME OF BURN _____
TYPE OF BURN: FLAME   SCALD   ELECTRICAL
CHEMICAL   OTHER _____
B/P _____ P _____ R _____ T _____

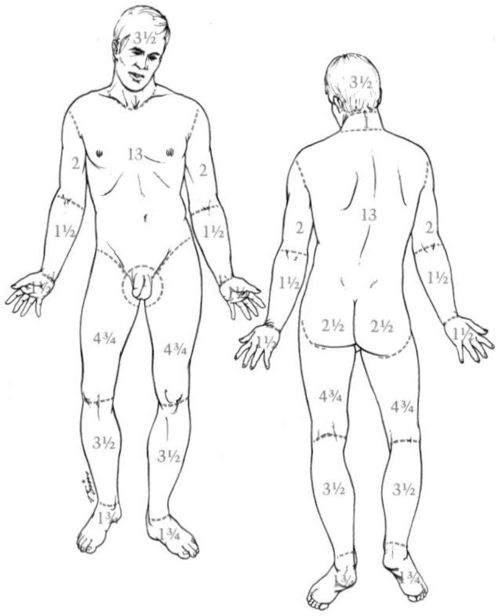

Weight (kg) _____ % Burn _____
FLUID RESUSCITATION
4 ml RL × % Burn × Wt in kg = _____ R/L
RATE OF ADMINISTRATION

| **1st 8 hr** | **2nd 8 hr** | **3rd 8 hr** |
| 1/2 R/L | 1/4 R/L | 1/4 R/L |

Fluid therapy given thus far:

_____ml R/L
Time: _____
Total urine output thus far: _____
Urine output last hour: _____
Other IV fluids given (type & amt.):

Sensorium _____
Signature _____

TIME OF _____A.M.
DATE _____ CALL _____P.M.
REFERRING DOCTOR _____
    AND HOSPITAL _____

PHONE NO. _____
HEART DISEASE	YES	NO
DIABETES	YES	NO
SICKLE CELL ANEMIA	YES	NO
NARCOTIC USER	YES	NO
ALCOHOLIC	YES	NO
ALLERGIES	YES	NO
CLOSED SPACE	YES	NO

ASSOCIATED INJURIES

BLOOD IN URINE	YES	NO
CHEST X-RAY	YES	NO
N.G. TUBE	YES	NO
FOLEY CATHETER	YES	NO
ENDOTRACHEAL TUBE	YES	NO
VENTILATOR	YES	NO
I.V. LINES	YES	NO
(size & site) _____
| CHEST TUBES | YES | NO |
MEDICATION GIVEN   TIME AND ROUTE

WOUND CARE
| 1. Wound cleansing | YES | NO |
| 2. Topical creams | YES | NO |
If yes, specify type _____
| 3. Escharotomy | YES | NO |
If yes, specify location _____
LAB RESULTS: Na _____ K _____ Cl _____
CO_2 _____ BUN _____ Sugar _____
ABG:pH _____ PO_2 _____ PCO_2 _____
Hgb _____ Hct _____ Time drawn _____
INSURANCE DATA:
Policy no.: _____
Type: _____
Workman's Comp? YES _____ NO _____
Physician notified: _____
Refer to: _____
Accept patient: _____

Figure 43–7

Burn transfer checklist. The assessment sheet should be completed by the personnel in the transferring hospital to be sure necessary information is available. (Courtesy Texas Regional Demonstration Program.)

formula as ordered. Monitor for signs of adequate resuscitation.

- Obtain the results of baseline laboratory tests.
- Place nasogastric and urethral catheters.
- Monitor all areas of circumferential full-thickness burn with regard to the need for escharotomy.
- Cover the burn with a clean sheet to decrease the contact with air currents and to promote comfort. Limited areas may be covered with sterile, moist, light dressings.
- Calculate the burn area and weigh the patient.
- Take a history of the accident.
- Administer tetanus prophylaxis as ordered.
- If the patient responds adequately to fluid therapy, administer an intravenous analgesic as ordered. Help the patient with deep breathing relaxation techniques. Work calmly and efficiently while giving simple explanations to the patient. Inform the patient of any sensations he will experience.
- Assess the patient's status with regard to the hospital's facilities. If necessary, have a staff member make arrangements to transfer the patient to a burn center for treatment (Fig. 43–7).

- Clean and debride the wound using aseptic technique.
- Apply topical antimicrobial dressings. (If the patient has a tar burn, apply neomycin sulfate (Neopolycin) dressing. Two applications 24 hours apart may be needed to remove the tar.)
- Apply biologic dressings to areas of partial-thickness injury as ordered.
- Elevate burned extremities above the level of the heart. Consult with the occupational therapist about hand-positioning splints.
- Monitor the urinary sugar every 4 hours to look for pseudodiabetes.

NURSING DIAGNOSES, PATIENT OUTCOMES, AND PLAN

The preceding material on anatomy, physiology, nursing assessment, and diagnostic tests guides the nurse in establishing nursing diagnoses, patient outcomes, and plan for the patient with burn injury.

NURSING CARE PLAN SUMMARY *Patient With Burn Injuries*

NURSING DIAGNOSIS

1. *Decreased cardiac output related to fluid changes and shock syndrome (exchanging pattern)*

Patient Outcomes	Nursing Orders
1. The patient should demonstrate the restoration of normal hemodynamics with a slightly elevated cardiac output.	1. Administer Ringer's lactate (RL) solution according to the following formula as ordered: 2 to 4 ml RL × weight (in kilograms) × percent TBSA burned = ml RL for the first 24 hours. One-half the total amount should be given in the first 8 hours after injury, one-fourth should be given in the second 8 hours after the injury, and one-fourth should be given in the third 8 hours after the injury. Calculate the time for infusion from the time of injury, not from the time therapy is initiated, subtracting any volume given before the fluid calculation is performed. A. Monitor every 30 to 60 minutes for the signs of adequate resuscitation: a clear lucid sensorium, a urinary output of 30 to 50 ml/hour, a pulse that is less than 120, the return of bowel sounds in adults, normal temperature, a normal to slightly alkalotic acid–base status, a pulmonary artery wedge pressure that is normal (or a central venous pressure that is less than 5 cm H_2O), and a normal to slightly elevated cardiac output. B. Calculate the extent of injury. (1) Use the rule of nines for triage and before initiating fluid therapy to approximate fluid therapy. (2) Determine the extent of injury to calculate fluid therapy. (3) After cleansing the wound, make a more accurate calculation of the burned area. Use the Lund and Browder burn chart to calculate the percentage of unburned area, and make sure that the addition equals 100% of the TBSA. Then recalculate the fluid therapy by using the crystalloid formula. C. Weigh the patient on a metabolic scale.
2. The patient's fluid and electrolyte status should be maintained within a normal range.	2. Administer a 5% dextrose in water solution in the second 24 hours as ordered (the amount is determined by the patient's serum sodium level). Assess changes in the fluid and electrolyte balance. A. After fluid resuscitation is completed, administer potassium as ordered. If

(continued)

NURSING CARE PLAN SUMMARY   *Patient With Burn Injuries*   *Continued*

Patient Outcomes	Nursing Orders
	more than 40 mEq of potassium is to be added to a single intravenous infusion, it should be administered by a controlled infusion device, or the hourly quota should be placed in a Volutrol.
	B. Administer magnesium, calcium, zinc, and other medications as ordered later in the burn course.
	C. When the body mobilizes burn edema, closely monitor patients with borderline cardiac and renal function for any signs of congestive heart failure.

NURSING DIAGNOSIS

2. *Impaired gas exchange related to carbon monoxide poisoning, upper airway obstruction, or smoke inhalation (exchanging pattern)*

Patient Outcome	Nursing Orders
The patient should demonstrate adequate respiratory functioning and maintain adequate oxygenation and slight respiratory alkalosis.	1. Assess for signs of hypoxemia. Monitor respiratory rate and rhythm, cough, findings on auscultation, increased work of breathing, arterial blood gas measurements, and spirometric findings. A. Monitor the patient with regard to presence of soot in sputum, respiratory rate and rhythm, cough, drooling, findings on auscultation, increased work of breathing, arterial blood gas measurements, and spirometric findings. B. Notify physician of significant trends.

NURSING DIAGNOSIS

3. *Pain related to burn injury and anxiety (feeling pattern)*

Patient Outcomes	Nursing Orders
1. The patient should not suffer pain unnecessarily.	1. Assess the patient's pain history, anxiety level, and response to pain. A. Educate the patient about painful procedures and the techniques used to decrease pain. Plan approaches to relieve pain; evaluate and document their effectiveness. B. Be gentle and efficient as well as thorough in performing all nursing care procedures. C. Coverage of wounds will reduce pain. Apply biological dressings or topical agents and dressing as soon as possible. D. Administer the analgesic ordered either before hydrotherapy and debridement or after these procedures (when relaxation is possible). Evaluate and document the effect. E. Plan nursing care to facilitate periods of rest and sleep. F. Meet the patient's calculated nutritional needs. G. Help patient make minor changes in positioning to relieve muscle strain secondary to immobility. For example, when abduction boards are used for the arms, remind the patient to move his or her arms from supination.
2. The patient should identify what cluster of techniques gives the most pain relief.	2. Make minor alterations in technique to help the patient maintain proper body alignment and positioning. For example, when abduction boards are used for the arms, remind the patient to move the arms from supination to pronation and back to supination three times every 15 minutes. A. Use environmental comfort measures, such as clean linens and a calm speaking voice. B. Consult with the staff psychologist. C. Keep the patient warm and free from shivering.
3. The patient should learn to achieve the relaxation response.	3. Investigate and use mind–body–spirit techniques to elicit self-control and the relaxation response. Help the patient learn imagery techniques at a relatively quiet time at first and then help the patient implement the techniques before, during, and after wound care. Refer to Chapter 3, Case Study 2.

continued

NURSING CARE PLAN SUMMARY   *Patient With Burn Injuries*   Continued

4. *Altered peripheral perfusion related to peripheral burn wound edema and circumferential full-thickness burn (exchanging pattern)*

Patient Outcome	*Nursing Orders*
The patient should maintain adequate circulation in all areas of full-thickness burn.	1. Assess the depth of the wound. Although the exact depth cannot be determined for several days, clinical assessment may be used early to identify probable areas of full-thickness injury. The injuries are usually not entirely full-thickness or partial-thickness; they are of different depths. The thickness of the skin varies with the patient's age and from one area of the body to another. With similar heat exposure, an area on the back of the hand might well be full-thickness, whereas an area on the back (which tends to have thicker skin) might be partial-thickness.

   A. Elevate any burned extremities above the level of the heart. Encourage active exercise for 5 minutes of every hour. Consult with an occupational therapist to determine the desirable degree of hand motion (making a fist may exacerbate injury to the hand).

   B. Monitor the patient with full-thickness burns of the extremities for signs of impaired circulation.

   C. If the patient's circulation is severely impaired, prepare for escharotomy (the longitudinal incision will be made laterally and medially through the entire thickness of the eschar) (Fig. 43–8). The nurse should have at hand:

      (1) Gauze sponges, iodophor solution
      (2) Scalpels or electrocautery unit
      (3) Sterile gloves
      (4) Gauze dressings, fine-mesh gauze, and elastic wrap bandage
      (5) Topical antibiotic, as ordered

   D. Control bleeding by direct pressure.

   E. After escharotomy, monitor circulation, maintain hemostasis, and prevent infection. Keep a topical antimicrobial agent and light dressings over the site.

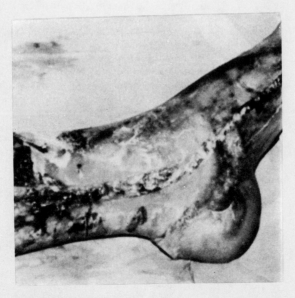

Figure 43–8
Escharotomy site.

continued

NURSING CARE PLAN SUMMARY   Patient With Burn Injuries   Continued

---

NURSING DIAGNOSIS

5. Altered nutrition: less than body requirements related to the metabolic response after burn injury (exchanging pattern)

Patient Outcome	Nursing Orders

The patient's calculated nutritional needs should be met.	1. Refer to Chapter 36 for the protocol (1 g of nitrogen is needed for each 150 calories).
	  A. Institute nutritional support as ordered, usually by the third day.
	  B. Administer vitamins, including ascorbic acid, as ordered.

NURSING DIAGNOSIS

6. High risk for gastrointestinal bleeding related to stress ulceration and to local gastrointestinal changes and systemic hormonal alterations (exchanging pattern)

Patient Outcomes	Nursing Orders
1. The patient should receive prophylaxis for acute gastroduodenal syndrome. 2. The patient will have no gastrointestinal bleeding, and integrity of the gastrointestinal tract will be re-established.	1. Monitor gastric pH; report pH levels below 6 and buffer as ordered. 2. Test with guaiac all GI residuals and stool.

NURSING DIAGNOSIS

7. High risk for systemic infection related to destruction of tissue and altered host defense mechanisms (exchanging pattern)

Patient Outcomes	Nursing Orders

1. Infection in burned areas should be prevented or controlled.	1. Maintain an aseptic environment.
	  A. Follow the protocols established by the infection control committee.
	  B. Cleanse the wound aseptically two to three times a day using the bedbath, tub, or shower procedure. (Some units, however, do not submerge the patient's wound. They remove the old topical antimicrobial agent and apply the new agent.)
	    (1) Assess the cardiopulmonary status, fluid status, bacterial count, and site of infection before bathing.
	    (2) Explain the cleansing procedure to the patient.
	    (3) About 30 minutes before wound care procedure, make available audiotapes that help the patient use imagery to relax.
	    (4) Prepare room for dressing procedure by ensuring cleanliness and maintaining warmth.
	    (5) Do perineal care before tubbing procedure to reduce wound exposure to perineal-area pathogens.
	    (6) Remove the dressings and the topical antimicrobial agent.
	    (7) Empty urinary drainage tubing and take measures to prevent retrograde urinary flow as patient is moved from bed to stretcher and stretcher to bed.
	    (8) Weigh the patient.
	    (9) Monitor the patient continuously.
	    (10) Help patient get on and off the stretcher by using transfer techniques.
	    (11) Keep the water temperature comfortable—between 100°F and 110°F (38°C to 43.2°C).
	    (12) Keep the environment clean, minimizing splashing of droplets.
	    (13) If the patient has many open wounds, do not submerge him or her. Have the patient lie on a plinth and gently spray the patient with water.

continued

NURSING CARE PLAN SUMMARY   *Patient With Burn Injuries*   *Continued*

Patient Outcomes	*Nursing Orders*
	(14) Use sterile gloves and a fresh sponge for each part of the body burned, washing from areas of lower colonization toward areas of higher colonization.
	(15) Shave the hair in the burned area and the areas around it (never shave eyebrows).
	(16) Limit the patient's time submerged in water to 20 minutes.
	(17) If possible, debride the wounds while cleansing them.
	(18) Apply the topical antimicrobial agent.
	(19) Evaluate the patient's cardiopulmonary status, wounds, temperature, and comfort after his or her return to bed.
	C. Pay particular attention to the body folds (*e.g.*, the axilla, breasts, and perineum).
	D. Cover the sites of invasive devices in the wound with topical gauze dressings. Change the dressings every 8 hours. Prevent cross-contamination among patients.
	(1) Follow universal precautions.
	(2) Use thorough handwashing techniques.
	(3) Clean the equipment each time it is used.
	E. Determine nurse-to-patient ratio by evaluating patient acuity and infection control needs. A one-to-one or two-to-one ratio may be required.
	F. Wear a plastic apron over the scrub clothing.
	G. Maintain clean scrub clothing; change whenever it is soiled or wet.
	H. When turning the patient, try to avoid contamination of upper arms or scrubs. Wash thoroughly to elbows and change to clean clothes as needed.
	I. Elect nurses to the infection control committee. Establish appropriate policies. Determine the feasibility of laminar airflow units and establish protocols about their use.
	J. Obtain appropriate specimens (wound biopsies, blood, urine, and sputum) for bacteriologic monitoring as ordered.
	K. Monitor for positive bacteriologic cultures and development of resistant strains. Notify the physician if any are present.
	L. Do not allow patients whose ears are burned to use a pillow under their heads. Observe ears for signs of inflammation (chondritis): tenderness, swelling, or change in color. Notify the physician if any occur. Monitor for the clinical signs of sepsis: an altered sensorium, decreased urine output, metabolic acidosis, an increased respiratory rate, tachycardia, hyperglycemia or glycosuria, decreased bowel sounds, and a decreasing platelet count.
2. The patient should be free of signs of systemic infection resulting from burn wound sepsis.	2. Avoid wound sepsis.
	A. Monitor for the clinical signs of sepsis: altered sensorium, increased respiratory rate, glycosuria, decreased bowel sounds, and decreasing platelet count.
	B. Maintain all supportive measures to achieve optimal resistance to infection.
	(1) See that the patient's nutritional requirements are met.
	(2) Keep the patient warm.
	(3) Prevent respiratory infections.
	(4) Administer blood as ordered.
	(5) Reduce stress.
	(6) Encourage mobility.
	C. Rotate the topical agents as indicated by how effective each one is.
	D. Administer systemic antibiotics if ordered. Systemic antibiotics cannot reach the viable–nonviable interface and granulation tissue in concentrations high enough to prevent bacterial growth. The systemic route generally is used when there is specific evidence of infection; prophylactic antibiotics are used in a very few burn centers. When ordered, monitor for ototoxicity and nephrotoxicity.
3. The patient should demonstrate bacteriologic control of the septic process in the burn wound and healing of partial-thickness wounds or will	3. Monitor and treat for bacteriologic control of sepsis process as follows.
	A. Wash hands thoroughly before each patient contact.
	B. Apply silver sulfadiazine (1%) as ordered.
	(1) Assess for an allergy to sulfa.

continued

NURSING CARE PLAN SUMMARY *Patient With Burn Injuries*   *Continued*

Patient Outcomes	Nursing Orders
demonstrate a healthy graft bed and a high percentage graft take.	(2) Use aseptic technique.

(continued in Nursing Orders column)

(2) Use aseptic technique.
(3) Apply the drug three times a day; between applications keep exposed wounds white with cream.
(4) Use a nonocclusive dressing if desired.
(5) During wound care remove "pseudo-eschar" proteinaceous gel that may develop on wound surface.
(6) Educate the patient about applying the agent.
(7) Evaluate for leukopenia and development of sulfadiazine-resistant gram-negative bacilli.

C. Apply mafenide acetate (Sulfamylon) (11%) as ordered.
(1) Assess for allergy to sulfa.
(2) Apply a thin layer (1/8 inch) no more than once every 12 hours; leave area exposed.
(3) Assess the patient's pain when the drug is applied to partial-thickness wounds to determine the need for an analgesic.
(4) Monitor for metabolic acidosis, tachypnea, and osmotic diuresis.

D. Apply polymyxin B or bacitracin ointments.
(1) Apply to wound, which should be kept moist.
(2) Evaluate for development of resistant organisms.

E. Apply silver nitrate (0.5%) if ordered.
(1) Before applying silver nitrate, make sure there is no invasive bacterial colonization.
(2) Remove loose, devitalized tissue.
(3) Apply thick (5 cm) bulky gauze dressings, making sure patient is placed in optimal position of function.
(4) Saturate the dressings every 2 to 4 hours with warm solution (be sure that dressings do not dry, raising the concentration of silver nitrate to caustic levels of 2% to 3%), and change them every 12 hours.
(5) Cover the body with a light blanket to decrease evaporation and retain heat.
(6) Conduct active debridement.
(7) Monitor clinically for signs of methemoglobinemia, hyponatremia, hypokalemia, hypocalcemia, and the syndrome associated with decreased serum levels of chloride.

F. Monitor culture results for antibiotic appropriateness and changing sensitivity and resistance patterns of organisms present, and bring to the attention of the physician.

G. Administer systemic antibiotics if ordered. Systemic antibiotics cannot reach the viable–nonviable interface and granulation tissue in concentrations high enough to prevent bacterial growth. The systemic route generally is used when specific evidence of infection is present; prophylactic antibiotics are used in very few burn centers. When ordered, monitor for ototoxicity and nephrotoxicity.

NURSING DIAGNOSIS

8. *Ineffective individual coping related to fear and anxiety (choosing pattern)*

Patient Outcome	Nursing Orders
The patient should demonstrate the ability to cope psychologically with the illness. The patient will talk about what has happened, the effect on his life, and plans for lifestyle changes if needed.	1. See Nursing Diagnosis: Anxiety, p. 111.

continued

NURSING CARE PLAN SUMMARY   *Patient With Burn Injuries*   *Continued*

NURSING DIAGNOSIS

9. *Impaired skin integrity related to burn trauma and the open wound (exchanging pattern)*

Patient Outcomes	Nursing Orders
1. The patient should demonstrate adequate removal of eschar.	1. Remove the eschar.

1. Remove the eschar.
   A. Assess the patient's need for an analgesic.
   B. Clean and debride the burn wound initially.
      (1) Make sure the room is clean.
      (2) Wear a gown, mask, and gloves.
      (3) Wash the wound gently with antimicrobial solution.
      (4) Remove the loose epidermis with a gauze pad, using slight pressure. If necessary, use scissors.
      (5) Do not use scrub brushes.
      (6) Shave the hair from the burned area and the adjacent unburned area. Do not shave eyebrows.
      (7) Leave the blisters on the palms and soles intact.
   C. Have another staff member present to help the patient focus on other thoughts or surroundings during the treatment.
   D. Identify areas of subeschar suppuration by applying gentle pressure to the wound with a gloved hand. Unroof and remove the eschar that has been lysed by bacterial suppuration.
      (1) Use sterile scissors and forceps (Fig. 43–9).
      (2) Be gentle.
      (3) Allow 30 minutes three times a day for debridement.
      (4) Stop the procedure for a few minutes if the patient requests it.
   E. Control the bleeding with direct pressure.
   F. Cut only dead tissue—there should be minimal bleeding. Control small bleeders with direct pressure.
   G. To remove the remnants of eschar and dermal debris, use wet-to-wet or wet-to-dry dressings (Fig. 45–10).
      (1) Apply large-pore expandable dressings (Kerlix) that have been wet with saline solution or antibiotic solution.
      (2) Assess the patient's need for pain medication.
      (3) Remove the damp dressing (wet-to-wet) or allow the dressing to dry and gently remove the dry dressing (wet-to-dry) as the physician orders.
      (4) Use a steady motion (the removal is painful).
      (5) Reapply the dressing.
   H. If Travase (an enzymatic debriding agent) is ordered, be aware that
      (1) Travase may be used during the first 24 postburn hours.
      (2) Travase is used when the quantitative biopsy report is less than 10^4 bacteria per gram of tissue.

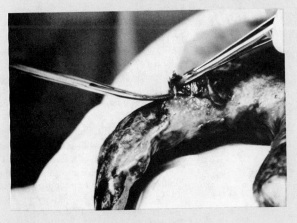

Figure 43–9
Burn wound debridement.

continued

NURSING CARE PLAN SUMMARY   *Patient With Burn Injuries*   Continued

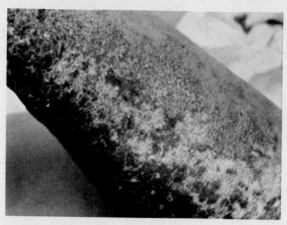

Figure 43–10
Typical burn wound that would benefit from the use of wet-to-dry dressings.

Patient Outcomes	Nursing Orders
	(3) The patient must be monitored for sepsis; Travase has no antibiotic properties.[42]
	I. Crosshatching may be needed to allow maximum penetration of the eschar.
	J. Travase should not be used on the face, hands, feet, or ankles or over the tendons.
	K. Fluid loss may occur after the application of Travase. If Travase is used 48 to 72 hours after the burn, the fluid loss will be greater than the normal bleeding. Monitor fluid balance.
	L. The patient's temperature may rise to 102°F to 103°F, but it should return to baseline in a few hours.
	M. The patient may feel pain when Travase is applied to a partial-thickness wound and may require an analgesic.
	N. Transient dermatitis may be noted. It disappears once the wound is clean and Travase therapy is discontinued.
	O. Daily wound care is needed. It consists of the following:
	(1) Daily washing of the wound
	(2) Travase must be activated by moisture.
	(3) The application of silver sulfadiazine-impregnated gauze over the Travase
	(4) Covering the wound with a Kling bandage and wrapping it with Kerlix. The procedure should be repeated twice a day until the wound is relatively clean (usually only a couple of days).
2. The patient should maintain wound coverage after a homograft or heterograft (Fig. 43–11).	2. Cover the wound.
	A. Maintain aseptic technique.
	B. Remove the topical agent and cleanse the wound.
	C. Prepare biological dressings as directed (thaw or reconstitute if not fresh).
	D. Apply a biological dressing in single pieces, the shiny side next to the wound.
	E. Smooth the skin and remove any air pockets with a sterile-gloved hand or with forceps.
	F. Trim the dressing with scissors so that the skin covers the wound and does not overlap it.
	G. Repeat the procedure until the wound is covered.
	H. Cover the dressing with gauze impregnated with antibiotic ointment or cover it first with a fine-mesh gauze and then a light dressing.
	I. Monitor the patient's vital signs for 24 hours after the dressing has been applied (the patient's temperature may be mildly elevated because the wound is covered). A dramatic temperature spike may be indicative of bacteria trapped beneath dressing.
	J. Observe the wound for small accumulations of serous drainage under the biological dressing.

continued

NURSING CARE PLAN SUMMARY   Patient With Burn Injuries   Continued

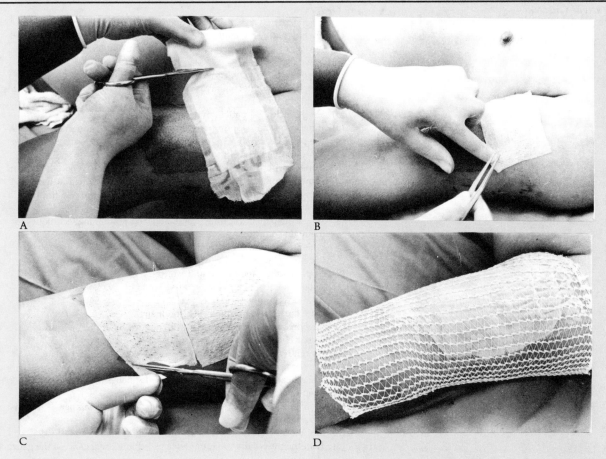

Figure 43–11

Heterograft application. (*A*) Apply the dressing, putting its shiny side next to the burn wound and using aseptic technique. (*B*) Smooth the skin to remove any air pockets. (*C*) Trim the skin in accordance with the wound margin. Avoid overlapping. (*D*) Secure the dressing with an expandable, netlike material.

Patient Outcomes	*Nursing Orders*
	K. Gently pierce the dressing with a sterile needle to drain the serous accumulation and thus enable the dressing to adhere to the wound.
	L. Observe the wound for suppurative drainage or large areas of nonadherent dressing. If any are present, notify the physician, remove the dressing, cleanse the wound, and reapply a new dressing.
	M. Monitor for tissue rejection phenomena. The nurse should look for the following:
	(1) Spotty, raised, edematous granulation tissue
	(2) Increased temperature and pulse
	(3) Irritability
	(4) Anxiety
	(5) Gastrointestinal malfunctioning
3. The patient should demonstrate vascularization of the autograft after wound closure and the healing of donor sites.	3. Care for the graft and donor sites.
	A. Educate the patient and family about preoperative, intraoperative, and postoperative care. Coordinate the educational plan with other health team members. Help the patient learn to visualize how the wound will look after surgery. Refer to psychophysiologic self-regulation, Chapter 3.
	B. Consult with the surgeon and the occupational therapist about any special splints or positioning devices that will be needed at the time of surgery. Plan their use with the operating room nurse.
	C. Immobilize the graft site after surgery. If large, bulky dressings have been applied to immobilize the graft, ask the operating room nurse about special precautions the surgeon may have given.

continued

NURSING CARE PLAN SUMMARY   *Patient With Burn Injuries*   Continued

Patient Outcomes	*Nursing Orders*
	(1) Do not permit the graft to be disrupted by the application of external devices or by movement. Investigate the air-fluidized bed.
	(2) Use a bed cradle.
	(3) Keep the patient comfortable.
	(4) Keep the skin intact in areas of prolonged pressure while the patient is immobilized.
	(5) Keep articles the patient may want within reach.
	(6) If necessary and appropriate, change the family visiting hours so that the patient's family may be close by.
	(7) Discontinue physical therapy and hydrotherapy for 2 to 5 days. Consult with the surgeon and the psychiatrist about when the patient should resume activities. In many units, ambulation with lower extremity grafts is permitted; leg grafts must be supported firmly with elastic wraps or a medicated bandage (Unna's Boot).
	(8) When the patient is prone, use established positioning techniques to maintain comfort and proper positioning; for example, elevate the patient's waist and hips and allow the feet to be positioned over the edge of the mattress.
	(9) Apply elastic bandages to grafts of the legs before permitting the legs to become dependent. New grafts should be wrapped first with Adaptic or antibiotic gauze.
	D. Determine the dressing used on the donor site.
	E. If a gauze dressing has been used on the donor site, do the following:
	(1) Observe it for bleeding.
	(2) Do not remove the single layer of gauze next to the donor site.
	(3) Leave the dressing open to the air.
	(4) Use a heat lamp at a distance of 12 to 18 inches for 24 to 48 hours.
	(5) Keep the patient comfortable.
	(6) Monitor the donor site for a purulent, infected appearance. If there is any, the physician should be notified.
	(7) Resume exercise 24 to 72 hours after surgery.
	(8) Trim the raised, dry areas of gauze as healing occurs and as the gauze separates.

NURSING DIAGNOSIS

10. *Impaired physical mobility related to burn wound edema, pain, and contracture formation (moving pattern)*

Patient Outcomes	*Nursing Orders*
1. The patient should maintain the range of motion.	1. Maintain the patient's range of motion.
	A. Elevate the patient's burned extremities above the level of the heart for approximately 72 hours (Fig. 43–12).

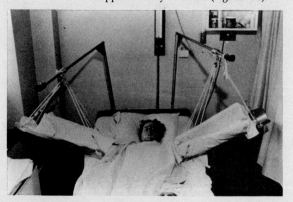

Figure 43–12
Elevation of burned arms in the early postburn period. The trough allows the patient to move and maintain arm comfort.

continued

NURSING CARE PLAN SUMMARY   *Patient With Burn Injuries*   *Continued*

Patient Outcomes	*Nursing Orders*
	(1) After covering the topical antimicrobial agent with a light dressing and flexible, netlike material, suspend the patient's arms on foam wedges, from intravenous poles, or by a substitute means.
	(2) Every hour, discontinue the suspension and encourage active exercise. Apply positioning splints.
	(3) Elevate the patient's bed. If hand dressings are to be used, wrap each finger separately to facilitate movement. If positioning splint is not yet available, place a gauze roll in the palm to help hold the hand in a position of function (Fig. 43–13).
	(4) Elevate the foot of the bed.
	B. With burns of the neck, after 48 to 72 hours, maintain neck hyperextension by having the patient lie on a pediatric mattress that has been put on top of a regular hospital mattress. The patient's position should be changed every hour. Several times a day, a small roll should be placed under the patient's head for short periods. Prism glasses can permit television viewing.
	C. Remember that contracture tends to be a position of comfort.
	D. Keep the patient's shoulders and arms abducted—on abduction boards. The patient's elbows, wrists, hands, (supinated) forearms, and palms should be extended. The distal portions of the arms should not be dependent.
	E. Keep the patient's hips straight and elevated, knees extended, and legs in slight abduction.
	(1) Prevent the patient's knees from falling into the frog-leg position. A trochanter roll and footboard should be used.
	(2) Use foam rubber to relieve pressure and prevent tissue breakdown under the patient's heels and buttocks or along the sides of the feet.
	F. Place a small roll lengthwise against the patient's spine to allow the shoulders to move backward into alignment.
	G. Turn the patient every 2 hours when awake. An air flow bed or another type of bed should be used as needed.
2. The patient will be able to wear the splints.	2. Consult with the occupational therapist about the need for splints. The most common splint is a static splint constructed from thermoplastic material that holds the wrist in 30° extension, the midinterphalangeal joints in 65° flexion, and the proximal and distal interphalangeal joints in full extension (Fig. 43–14).
3. The patient will actively participate in the rehabilitation program.	3. Consult with the physiatrist about an exercise program for the patient. As a rule of thumb, each burned area is taken through the full range of motion five times, at least four times a day. Encourage active exercise and include the activities of daily living. Perform passive exercises gently and do not go past the patient's point of pain.

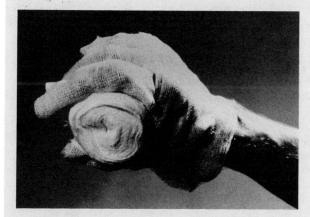

Figure 43–13
If hand dressings are to be used, each finger is wrapped separately.

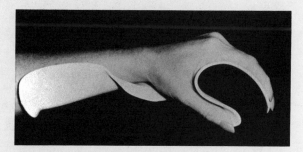

Figure 43–14
Typical static splint for optimal hand positioning.

IMPLEMENTATION AND EVALUATION

Nursing care is directed not only toward the patient's current problems, but also toward potential problems. The prevention of complications is a primary responsibility of everyone on the health team. The following is a list of the most common complications of burn injury:

Fear
Pain
Powerlessness
Depersonalization
Sleep deprivation
Sensory deprivation or
    sensory overstimulation
Burn shock
Myocardial depression
Resuscitation failure
Dysrhythmias
Hypertension
Carbon monoxide poisoning
Upper-airway obstruction
Lower-airway obstruction
Death
Pneumonia
Adult respiratory distress
    syndrome
Pulmonary embolism
Hypermetabolism, protein
    loss, and weight loss
Evaporative water loss
Fever
Oliguric renal failure

High-output renal failure
Acute gastroduodenal
    disease
Gastrointestinal bleeding
Fluid and electrolyte
    imbalance
Liver failure
Stroke
Altered level of
    consciousness
Loss of function
Sepsis
Suppurative
    thrombophlebitis
Disseminated intravascular
    coagulation
Organ necrosis
Allergy
Postoperative complications
Multisystem organ failure
Contractures
Disfigurement
Amputations
Peripheral neuropathy

Resuscitation Phase

The primary goal of initial fluid therapy is the rapid and complete restoration of cardiac output. Many different techniques of calculating fluid therapy are described in the literature. Most use a crystalloid solution without glucose, designed to restore and maintain tissue perfusion, preserve heat-injured but viable soft tissue, and prevent organ ischemia.[26]

Replacement of fluid sequestered as a result of burn injury is the most important part of the initial therapy. Achieving the best physiologic response depends ultimately on the ability of various solutions to restore the intravascular and extracellular fluid volumes and to effect a rapid and complete cardiovascular response. Fluid replacement is dependent on the rate of fluid loss, the total quantity of fluid sequestered, and the composition of the burn edema.[7]

Clinically, burn shock seems to be helped by all the fluid resuscitation regimens. The crucial point is prompt institution of therapy. In general, parenteral treatment is mandatory for all patients who have an injury of more than 20% TBSA, and for elderly patients and for children who have injuries of less than 20% TBSA. What formula is used for fluid resuscitation does not significantly affect the survival of patients who have an injury of less than 40% TBSA. However, the survival of those burned over more than 40% TBSA does depend on the careful selection and evaluation of fluid therapy.

Crystalloid Fluid Therapy

The Baxter or Parkland formula introduced in 1968 calls for crystalloid resuscitation in which specific fluids are administered in the first 32 hours after injury (four time periods of 8 hours each). In the first three 8-hour periods (24 hours), 4 ml/kg/% TBSA burn Ringer's lactate solution (Hartmann's solution) is administered (Fig. 43–5).

Baxter found that crystalloid therapy rapidly restores the functional extracellular fluid compartment deficit within 10% of baseline volumes (the normal volume of extracellular fluid is 20% of body weight). *No further decrease in extracellular fluid volume occurs.* Cardiac output is restored in 12 to 24 hours to 3 L/m². The transmembrane potential is restored, resulting in decreased cell size and decreased intracellular sodium and water. With the restoration of membrane potential and cell integrity, extracellular fluid is kept "pumped" out of the cell, and it accumulates around the cell. Thus the fluid is available for translocation during the late phase of burn edema.

More recently, the modified Brooke formula was introduced, recommending that Ringer's lactate resuscitation be initiated at a rate of 2 ml × weight (kg) × % TBSA burned in the first 24 hours, again with half given in the first 8 hours (Table 43–5). Colloids are infused in the second 24-hour period. Key to this discrepancy is the fact that any fluid resuscitation formula should not be expected to prescribe a strictly calculated volume of fluid. Instead, these formulas should serve as a guide for fluid resuscitation, with the hourly volume being titrated as the patient's clinical parameters dictate. Variability in patient response is most significant in the pediatric and geriatric populations, and in patients with associated injuries or preexisting disease.[70]

As expected, plasma volume levels are not adequately restored by crystalloid therapy. Though discussion continues as to whether or not colloids should be given in the first 24 hours, it is believed by many that because of capillary permeability, colloid therapy also has a minimal effect on plasma volume. Once the capillary permeability is restored (about 24 hours [±6 hours] after the burn), the plasma volume increases by the amount of plasma administered to the patient. The plasma volume measurements, if available, may be used to calculate the deficit. The hematocrit may be used to evaluate the adequacy of plasma restoration; however, the hematocrit is not a useful tool for judging plasma restoration after 48 hours.

Goodwin et al[30] states that the goal of resuscitation is restoration of vital organ function and establishment of hemodynamic stability at the least physiologic cost. In his studies comparing crystalloid and colloid resuscitation after thermal injury, both were found to be equally effective in restoring cardiac output and hemodynamic stability. Though patients resuscitated with crystalloid solutions develop more peripheral edema, gain more weight, and have lower plasma oncotic pressures than patients resuscitated with colloids, colloid solution resuscitation showed no clinical advantages over crystalloid resuscitation when standard clinical indices (urine output, heart rate, and blood pressure) were compared.

Demling expresses concern over the massive edema that develops after crystalloid resuscitation. His work suggests that because *nonburn* tissues appear experimentally to regain normal permeability within about 8 hours of injury, and because hypoproteinemia may accentuate edema formation, colloids begin to be infused in the second 8-hour period.[25,26]

Previously, the mortality for the first 48 postburn hours approached 75%, and death was due largely to the ravages of the low-flow state. Significantly, renal failure was prominent among the terminal conditions. Today it is well established that the "early" renal failure was a result of decreased cardiac output and renal perfusion. Maintenance of urinary output in normal limits (about 50 ml/hour) is a sign of adequate renal perfusion. Without adequate volume therapy, the urinary output is minimal or nonexistent. As volume is replaced, the renal blood flow improves and the urinary volume increases. Hemoglobin or myoglobinuria is indicative of a deep burn; it clears within the first 300 to 400 ml of urinary output without the need for osmotic diuretics. Complications in renal function are usually the result of inadequate fluid and electrolyte replacement. Baxter[6] states that low urinary sodium concentrations (below 20 mg/L) indicate inadequate volume replacement.

The most common reason burn patients have a decreased urinary output is that the calculated amount of fluid is behind schedule. The second most common reason is that the extent of the burn has been underestimated, especially in children. Recalculating the extent of the burn after the initial care has been given helps avoid this error. Other causes of a decreased urinary output are associated injuries, respiratory injury, disseminated intravascular coagulation, myocardial depression, delayed resuscitation, and renal failure.

After the fourth 8-hour period, the fluid administered is a 5% dextrose in water solution. It is administered in amounts that will maintain a normal serum sodium range, usually 2000 to 6000 ml.

The amount of fluid required by each burn patient cannot be determined exactly; frequent laboratory assessments are needed to ascertain the patient's status. In general, 3 to 5 L of water per day are needed to replace the evaporative water losses. This amount is affected significantly by the amount of burn surface exposed to the air, by the wound care, and by the environmental air currents. However, giving too much water quickly leads to water intoxication. The following formula can be used to approximate the patient's water needs:

Square meters × (percent TBSA burned + 25)

= ml evaporative water loss per hour

Acute Phase

After the initial period of burn shock, the goal is closure of the wound. Not until the eschar is removed and the wound is covered by an autograft, or not until a partial-thickness wound is reepithelialized, are the severe derangements resulting from the open wound reversed. There are two main approaches to wound closure: the conservative approach and the aggressive approach.

In the *conservative approach* the wound is covered with a topical antimicrobial agent to prevent and control burn wound sepsis. Hydrotherapy is employed, and debridement is done daily until the areas of partial-thickness injury heal and the areas of full-thickness injury are denuded of eschar and develop granulation tissue. Homografts, heterografts, or both are used as temporary biological coverings to restore the water vapor barrier, decrease the protein loss from the wound, protect the site from infection, relieve pain, allow active joint

functioning, help debride dermal debris, stimulate the growth of epithelium and granulation tissue, and act as a test material before autografting.

Aggressive therapy means surgery or excisional therapy. This approach shortens hospitalization[33,38] and has been made possible by improved patient monitoring techniques. The removal of eschar is followed by autografting (permanently) or the application of a homograft as a temporary biological covering.[14] Staged excisions are performed on patients with large injuries in an attempt to decrease effectively the extent of the burn. For elderly patients in particular, small staged excisions done as limited procedures are beneficial, because the patient's low-reserve cardiovascular system cannot tolerate more extensive procedures. Autografts may be taken during the same procedure or during a second procedure to close the burn effectively.

Excision is first performed 5 days or less after the injury and before significant bacterial colonization has occurred. This provides a closed wound before infection occurs and, especially with burns of a large percent total body surface area, allows donor sites to be recropped as soon as possible.[34] The specific criteria for selecting and further evaluating patients undergoing excisional therapy are being developed. Candidates for excisional therapy are evaluated with regard to age; extent, depth, and location of injury; the presence of associated injuries or illnesses; cardiopulmonary status; bacterial colonization; ability to fight infection (as determined by white blood cell count and other laboratory procedures); clotting factors; and general physiologic status. Table 43–6 lists criteria for nursing evaluation.

Primary excisional therapy entails removal of the full-thickness eschar under anesthesia with a scalpel, knife, electrosurgical cautery, carbon dioxide laser, or dermatome. The area is then covered with a biological dressing or autograft. Tangential excision, a form of excisional therapy, is used to

Table 43–6

Nursing Evaluation Before Excisional Therapy

Response to resuscitation
    Fluid and electrolyte status
    Blood volume
    Cardiac output
    Pulmonary capillary wedge pressure
Status of infection
    Burn wound biopsies
    Temperature
    Antibiotic therapy
    Need for antibiotic prophylaxis
Potential for pulmonary dysfunction
    Clinical assessment
    Arterial blood gases
    Spirometry
    Chest radiograph
Knowledge level of patient and family
    Preoperative protocol
    Recovery room procedures
    Visiting privileges
    Sensory information
Laboratory studies
    Electrocardiogram
    Complete blood count
    Urea and creatinine
    Platelet count
    Clotting studies

decrease morbidity and hypertrophic scarring.[46] The eschar is shaved away layer by layer until viable tissue is reached, as indicated by active bleeding. Substantial blood loss associated with large tangential excisions limits the percent body surface area that may be excised by this method in a single surgery. Fascial excision is removal of tissues (subcutaneous tissue and fat) to the fascial layer. This method has minimal blood loss but results in significant disfigurement in the debrided area. A biological dressing such as heterograft or homograft is then applied to protect the wound from infection until autograft is available.

Autografting

In both the conservative and aggressive approaches, areas of full-thickness injury require the use of an autograft for coverage. Skin grafts can be taken from any area of the body that is not burned and applied to the clean, red vascular bed. Efforts are made when possible to match donor skin to the area requiring grafting (for example, skin for the face is taken from supraclavicular or lower abdominal donor sites when available). The autograft has traditionally been affixed to the wound in the operating room with Steri-strips, sutures, or staples. Currently, research is being done on the application of single-donor fibrin glue to the wound after excision to obtain hemostasis and to promote adherence of the graft to the recipient bed.[75] This seems to be particularly useful in the grafting of difficult recipient sites and areas of cosmetic importance such as the face.[71]

The graft's blood supply is established by both vascular anastomoses and new vascular growth from the graft bed into the graft. During the first day after grafting, a fibrin layer is produced that provides contact for oxygenation and metabolism but not fixation between the graft and the graft bed. During the second day, the fibrin reticulum organizes and advances, and the granulation tissue contains immature fibroblasts and a few open spaces with erythrocytes. Three days after grafting, the granulation tissue is so organized that it is difficult to differentiate the graft from the graft bed by microscopic study. The percentage of graft take is high if the wound has been prepared carefully, infection does not intervene, and pressure and shear forces do not disrupt the graft.

Various depths of skin are used. A full-thickness graft uses the entire depth of skin. It is used for specific areas, such as the eyelids, the tip of the nose, or the hands. Split-thickness grafts are most commonly used; they are transferred to the wound bed in a continuous sheet if enough donor sites are available. If they are minimal, a meshed skin graft is used.[76] Using the Tanner-Vandeput mesher (dermatome), a number of slits are cut so that the skin expands to an area one and one-half to nine times the size of the donor site. Unless very large areas must be covered, the skin is not expanded to a ratio greater than 3:1 (Fig. 43–15). The meshed skin is applied to the clean wound and secured by Steri-strips, staples, sutures, or fibrin glue. The meshed graft is vulnerable to drying and invasion of bacteria through the mesh; therefore, it is covered by a biological dressing, moist antibiotic gauze, or petroleum-based antibiotic that will remain undisturbed for 2 to 3 days while the graft becomes vascularized.

Tissue fluid drains from the wound through the interstices of the graft, eliminating the problem of fluid collection beneath the graft. After vascularization, skin grows across the interstices

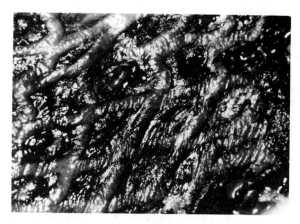

Figure 43–15
Meshed autograft 5 days postburn.

to close the wound. Unfortunately, the healed meshed area has more scarring than does a sheet graft. If possible, the use of the mesh graft is limited to areas where appearance is less conspicuous, such as the back, the abdomen, and the thighs.

Researchers are beginning to look at innovative ways to close the wound. Alexander et al[3] have recommended first the application of meshed autograft expanded three to nine times its size, depending on the size wound to be covered, and next the overlay of 3:1 meshed homograft. In their work, autograft take has ranged from 90% to 100%, and its epithelial outgrowth was twice as fast as that of homograft. Warden et al[81] have recommended a two-stage procedure for excision and autografting. After excision, the wounds are covered with bulky gauze dressings soaked with saline until the next morning. This overnight period is used for patient stabilization to replace red cell mass as well as blood volume and to correct temperature imbalance. Autografting is performed the next morning; the graft bed remains viable because of the moistness and hemostasis provided by the continuous soaks. Burke et al[15] have developed an acceptable artificial dermis. The porous collagen-chondroitin 6-sulfate fibrillar mat material can be prepared commercially. It is applied in the same manner as autograft. When the "artificial skin" is fully vascularized and when donor skin is available, the Silastic sheet covering the artificial dermis is removed and replaced with the patient's own epithelial cells. The thin autografts needed to cover the artificial dermis can be taken at .002 to .003 inch, ensuring a transparent graft and resulting in superficial donor sites[35] that regenerate rapidly and may be recropped frequently if necessary. Availability of the artificial dermis currently is a problem.

Research is currently underway to promote the use of cultured autologous cells to cover burn wounds.[12] Human keratinocytes grown in culture have been used successfully for this purpose. This procedure involves taking cells and plating them in a culture medium to promote growth of thin sheets of skin for reapplication. Techniques to maximize growth in order to accelerate graft availability are undergoing experimentation.[27]

Pain

Within a hospital setting, pain is managed in three phases: anticipation, presence, and aftermath. A complete assessment before intervention is essential. Analgesics complemented by nursing techniques to decrease pain are beneficial. Patient-controlled analgesia has been found to be effective in some burn units. Medications are administered as needed, but it is important that the patient's respiratory status not be compromised. In general, analgesics act by decreasing consciousness, lessening the conduction of impulses over pain fibers, raising the threshold of pain perception, and lessening the awareness of or appreciation of the significance of the pain.

Tranquilizers tend to blunt responses, making a physiologic assessment inaccurate, so they are used as little as possible. Sleep and planned rest periods throughout the day are extremely important. A patient who has a good night's sleep will be able to cope better with the pain and frustration of therapy. Sleep habits and patterns are assessed, and fundamental principles to induce sleep are followed. Procedures and care are planned so that periods of uninterrupted sleep are allowed.

Several investigators have looked at the disparity between staff and patient perceptions of pain.[29,67] The results of these studies clearly indicate that nurses must look carefully at their own biographies, avoid stereotyping of their patients, and focus on the individual's unique pain experience.

Nutrition

Nutritional support of the hypermetabolic burn patient is accomplished through a multidisciplinary approach and daily reevaluation of the patient's metabolic and nutritional status. Energy requirements may be estimated based on indirect calorimetry measures[66] in which consumption and carbon dioxide production rates are evaluated. More often, one of several formulas is used to estimate energy needs. The most popular formulas are variations of the Curreri[21] formula (25 kcal/kg + 40 kcal/% TBSA burn per 24 hours); some suggest that the 40 kcal/% TBSA should be maximized at 50% TBSA.[83] The second most popular formula is the Harris-Benedict equation (Basal Energy Expenditure) multiplied by a variety of energy adjustment factors.[83] Recent work by Cunningham et al comparing indirect calorimetry measurements with predictive equations for 122 patients suggests that two times the predicted resting metabolic rate (RME) was consistently closest to the measured metabolic energy expenditure in burns over 30% TBSA.[20]

Burn patients are placed on a high-protein, high-calorie diet. The calorie-to-nitrogen ratio recommended varies from 100:1 to 150:1.[13] Supplemental oral or tube feedings are used to help patients meet their nutritional needs. Ascorbic acid supplementation is essential for collagen synthesis. Zinc plays a role in wound healing and is also usually supplemented.[66] Daily nutritional goals are set and evaluated based on daily weight, calorie count, protein intake, and biochemical parameters.[13]

Rehabilitation Phase

Rehabilitation begins within 24 hours of admission. With the trend toward survival of people with larger and larger burns, the establishment of new priorities, with attention to quality of life after injury, must focus on maximum physical and psychological recovery.[68] Short- and long-term goals should be set.

Early rehabilitation measures should include surgical decompression of constricting eschar to maintain perfusion of hands and feet. An active exercise plan and attention to correct positioning to minimize deformities should be the responsibility of all who come in contact with the patient. Early ambulation, when possible, helps maintain cardiovascular tone, reduces the incidence of pneumonia, promotes muscle strengthening, reduces joint tightness, and stimulates an overall sense of well-being. Elastic wraps should be applied to extremities before periods of dependence to support circulation and minimize edema and pain.

Burn patients have a tendency to move toward a position of comfort or fetal position. Positioning efforts should focus on antideformity stretch. The burned neck should be fully extended with shoulders abducted to 90°. Elbows are maintained fully extended in supination[68] with the wrist extended 30° to 40°.[11] The metacarpophalangeal joints are flexed with the thumb abducted.[11] Hips and knees must be kept extended, with ankles maintained in 90° of dorsiflexion.[68] Active and active-assisted range of motion is initiated immediately and performed two to four times daily. Splinting may be necessary, especially during periods of sleep or relaxation, to maintain range of motion from day to day.

As the wounds heal and the patient is prepared for discharge, he or she requires instruction in the areas of wound and skin care, management of itching, prevention of exposure to sun and extreme cold, nutrition, wearing of pressure garments, exercise, and emotional adjustments that may be necessary.[64]

After a severe burn injury, reduced physical capacity may result in activity intolerance. The patient may choose decreased involvement in strenuous, rapidly paced, and highly dexterous tasks in favor of lighter and more sedentary activities.[17] Those patients who are usually very active will experience significant disruption of their life-styles. Reintegration into a social role may also require adjustments. Referral to support groups, psychosocial therapy, or vocational rehabilitation services may be beneficial to the burn patient.

SUMMARY

Thermal trauma is unique in its destruction of tissue and the resulting psychopathophysiologic response that ensures. It is well recognized as the most severe type of trauma the human body encounters, and it brings with it the most difficult management problems.

DIRECTIONS FOR FUTURE RESEARCH

Burn care is a multidisciplinary effort. The quality of care is influenced by the knowledge, skill, judgment, and attitudes of those providing care. Research into the details of clinical nursing care delivery are of the utmost importance. Burn care can no longer survive by haphazard or tradition-bound methods. As patients survive larger burn injuries, it is important that nursing look at the rehabilitation outcomes of both the patient and the family in terms of physical and psychological well-being, in order to identify interventions needed during hospitalization to maximize recovery.[47] Also important are investigations into aspects that will affect the great stress on the nurse.

Sample questions[51] relating to some of the most important research areas follow:

1. In light of the persistent personnel shortages in burn nursing, what measures can be taken to prevent or lessen "burnout?"
2. What type of orientation program is most effective in terms of cost, safety, and long-term retention?
3. What types of patient classification systems are the most valid, reliable, and sensitive in determining staffing ratios?
4. What are effective ways of reducing staff stress in burn units?
5. What are effective nursing interventions for patients with impaired communication?
6. What nursing measures are most effective in assessing and relieving anxiety and pain?
7. What nursing measures are most effective in prevention of infections in patients with invasive lines, especially when placed in burned tissue?
8. Does the presence of a clinically oriented clinical specialist improve the quality of patient care?
9. What nursing interventions most effectively minimize stress in the burn patient?
10. What are the effects of various visiting policies for burn units on the physiologic and psychological responses of the patient and family?
11. What types of staff development programs are most effective in preparing the critical care nurse to cope with the ethical, moral, and legal dilemmas surrounding patient care?
12. What techniques are most effective in preventing infections in monitoring lines with stopcocks?
13. What nursing interventions are most effective in assisting the patient with a long-term disfiguring injury?

REFERENCES

1. Abston, S. Scar reaction after thermal injury and prevention of scars and contractures. In J. A. Boswick (ed.), *The Art and Science of Burn Care*. Rockville, MD: Aspen Publishers, 1987.
2. *Advanced Burn Life Support Course* Lincoln, NE: Nebraska Burn Institute, 1987.
3. Alexander, J. W., MacMillan, B. C., Law, E., and Kittur, P. Treatment of severe burns with widely meshed skin autograft and meshed skin autograft overlay. *J. Trauma* 21:433, 1981.
4. Andreasen, N. J. C., Noyes, R., Hartford, C. E., et al. Management of emotional reactions in seriously burned adults. *N. Engl. J. Med.* 286:65, 1972.
5. Artz, C. P., Moncrief, J. A., and Pruitt, B. A. *Burns: A Team Approach.* Philadelphia: W.B. Saunders, 1979.
6. Baxter, C. R. Fluid volume and electrolyte changes of the early postburn period. *Clin. Plast. Surg.* 1:673, 1974.
7. Baxter, C. R. Pathophysiology and treatment of burns and cold injury. In J. E. Rhoads, J. G. Allen, H. N. Harkins, and C. A. Moyer (eds.), *Rhoads Textbook of Surgery*. Philadelphia: J.B. Lippincott, 1977.
8. Baxter, C. R., Curreri, P. W., and Marvin, J. A. The control of burn wound sepsis by the use of quantitative bacteriologic studies and subeschar clysis with antibiotics. *Surg. Clin. North Am.* 53:1509, 1975.
9. Baxter, C. R., and Waeckerle, J. F. Emergency treatment of burn injury. *Ann. Emerg. Med.* 17:1305, 1988.
10. Blackburn, G. Protein metabolism and nutritional support. *J. Trauma* 21:707, 1981.
11. Boswick, J. A. Comprehensive rehabilitation after burn injury. *Surg. Clin. North Am.* 67:159, 1987.
12. Brown, A. S., and Barot, L. R. Biologic dressings and skin substitutes. *Clin. Plast. Surg.* 13:69, 1986.
13. Burdge, J. J., Conkright, J. M., and Ruberg, R. L. Nutritional and metabolic consequences of thermal injury. *Clin. Plast. Surg.* 13:49, 1986.
14. Burke, J. F., Quinby, W. C., Bondoc, C. C., et al. Immunosuppression and temporary skin transplantation in the treatment of massive third degree burns. *Ann. Surg.* 182:183, 1975.
15. Burke, J. F., Yannas, I. V., Quinby, W. C., Bondoc, C. C., and Jung, W. R. Successful use of a physiologically acceptable artificial skin in the treatment of extensive burn injury. *Ann. Surg.* 194:413, 1981.
16. Cahalane, M. and Demling, R. H. Early respiratory abnormalities from smoke inhalation. *J.A.M.A.* 251:771, 1984.
17. Cheng, S. and Rogers, J. C. Changes in occupational role performance after a severe burn: A retrospective study. *Am. J. Occup. Ther.* 43:17, 1989.
18. Choinière, M., Melzack, R., Rondeau, J., et al. The pain of burns: Characteristics and correlates. *J. Trauma* 29:1531, 1989.
19. Clark, W. R., Bonaventura, M., and Myers, W. Part I: Diagnosis and consequences of smoke inhalation. *J. Burn Care Rehabil.* 10:52, 1989.
20. Cunningham, J. J., Hegarty, M. T., Meara, P. A., et al. Measured and predicted calorie requirements of adults during recovery from severe burn trauma. *Am. J. Clin. Nutr.* 49:404, 1989.
21. Curreri, P. W., Richmond, D., Marvin, J. A., et al. Dietary requirements of patients with major burns. *J. Am. Diet. Assoc.* 65:415, 1974.
22. Czaja, A., McAlbany, J. C., and Pruitt, B. A., Jr. Acute gastroduodenal disease after thermal injury. *N. Engl. J. Med.* 291:925, 1974.
23. Deitch, E. A., and Bridges, R. M. Effect of stress and trauma on bacterial translocation from the gut. *J. Surg. Res.* 42:536, 1987.
24. Demling, R. H. Burn edema. Part I: Pathogenesis. *J. Burn Care Rehabil.* 3:138, 1982.
25. Demling, R. H. Fluid replacement in burned patients. *Surg. Clin. North Am.* 67:15, 1987.
26. Demling, R. H. Fluid resuscitation. In J. A. Boswick, Jr. (ed.), *The Art and Science of Burn Care.* Frederick, MD: Aspen Publishers, 1987.
27. deSerres, S., Herzog, S. R., Meyer, A. A., et al. Techniques to accelerate the availability of human keratinocyte grafts. *J. Burn Care Rehabil.* 10:469, 1989.
28. Echenique, M. M., Bistrain, B., and Blackburn, G. L. Theory and techniques of nutritional support in the ICU. *Crit. Care Med.* 10:546, 1982.
29. Fagerhaugh, S., and Strauss, A. *The Politics of Pain Management.* Reading, MA: Addison Wesley, 1977.
30. Goodwin, C. W., Dorethy, J., Lam, V., et al. Randomized trial of efficacy of crystalloid and colloid resuscitation on hemodynamic response and lung water following thermal injury. *Ann. Surg.* 197:520, 1983.
31. Goodwin, C. W., and Pruitt, B. A., Jr. The massive burn with sepsis and Curling's ulcer. In J. D. Hardy (ed.), *Critical Surgical Illness*. Philadelphia: W. B. Saunders, 1980.
32. Hansbrough, J. F., Zapata-Sirvent, R. L., and Peterson, V. M. Immunomodulation following burn injury. *Surg. Clin. North Am.* 67:69, 1987.
33. Heimbach, D. M. Early excision and grafting. *Surg. Clin. North Am.* 67:93, 1987.
34. Heimbach, D. M. The results of early primary excision. *J. Trauma* 21:132, 1981.
35. Heimbach, D., Luterman, A., Burke, J., et al. Artificial dermis for major burns. *Ann. Surg.* 208:313, 1988.
36. Helm, P. A., Kevorkian, C. G., and Lushbaugh, M. Burn injury: Rehabilitation management. *Arch. Phys. Med. Rehabil.* 63:6, 1982.

37. Helvig, E. I., and Herndon, D. N. Airway and pulmonary management of burn patients. *Trauma Quart.* 5:19, 1989.
38. Herndon, D. N., Thompson, P. B., and Traber, D. L. Pulmonary injury in burned patients. *Crit. Care Clin.* 1:79, 1985.
39. Hirsh, H. L. Carbon monoxide poisoning. *Trauma* 30:125, 1988.
40. Horton, J. W., White, J., and Baxter, C. R. The role of oxygen-derived free radicals in burn-induced myocardial contractile depression. *J. Burn Care Rehabil.* 9:589, 1988.
41. Hosoda, G., Holloway, G. A., and Heimbach, D. M. Laser Doppler flowmetry for the early detection of hypertrophic burn scars. *J. Burn Care Rehabil.* 7:496, 1986.
42. Hummel, R. P., Kautz, P. D., MacMillan, B. G., et al. The continuing problem of sepsis following enzymatic debridement of burns. *J. Trauma* 14:572, 1974.
43. Hunt, J. L., Agee, R. N., and Pruitt, B. A., Jr. Fiberoptic bronchoscopy in acute inhalation injury. *J. Trauma* 15:641, 1975.
44. Hurt, A., and Eriksson, E. Management of the burn wound. *Clin. Plast. Surg.* 13:57, 1986.
45. Iafrati, N. S. Pain on the burn unit: Patient *vs* nurse perceptions. *J. Burn Care Rehabil.* 7:413, 1986.
46. Janzekovic, Z. A new concept in the early excision and immediate grafting of burns. *J. Trauma* 10:1103, 1970.
47. Knudson-Cooper, M. What are the research priorities in the behavioral areas of burn patients? *Frontiers in Understanding Burn Injury* 24:S197, 1984.
48. Kraemer, M. D., Jones, T., and Deitch, E. A. Burn contractures: Incidence, predisposing factors, and results of surgical therapy. *J. Burn Care Rehabil.* 9:261, 1988.
49. Leonard, L. G., Scheulen, J. J., and Munster, A. M. Chemical burns: Effect of prompt first aid. *J. Trauma* 22:420, 1982.
50. Levine, J. What are the functions of endorphins following thermal injury? *J. Trauma* 24:S168, 1984.
51. Lewandowski, L. A., and Kositsky, A. M. Research priorities for critical care nursing: A study of the American Association of Critical Care Nurses. *Heart Lung* 12:35, 1983.
52. Loebl, E. C., Baxter, C. R., and Curreri, P. W. The mechanism of erythrocyte destruction in the early postburn period. *Ann. Surg.* 178:681, 1975.
53. Luterman, A., Dacso, C. C., and Curreri, P. W. Infections in burn patients. *Am. J. Med.* 81(1A):45, 1986.
54. Marvin, J. A., Heck, E. L., Leobl, E. C., et al. Usefulness of blood cultures in confirming septic complications in burn patients: Evaluation of a new culture method. *J. Trauma* 15:657, 1975.
55. Marvin, J. A., and Heimbach, D. M. Pain control during the intensive care phase of burn care. *Crit. Care Clin.* 1:147, 1985.
56. McAlhany, J. C., Czaja, A. J., and Pruitt, B. S., Jr. Antacid control of complications from acute gastroduodenal disease after burns. *J. Trauma* 16:645, 1976.
57. McDaniel, J. W. *Physical Disability and Human Behavior.* New York: Pergamon, 1969, p. 138.
58. Monafo, W. W. The treatment of burn shock by the intravenous and oral administration of hypertonic lactated saline solution. *J. Trauma* 10:575, 1970.
59. Moncrief, J. A. Medical progress. *N. Engl. J. Med.* 288:444, 1973.
60. Moran, K., and Munster, A. M. Alterations of the host defense mechanism in burned patients. *Surg. Clin. North Am.* 67:47, 1987.
61. Moritz, A. R., Henriques, F. C., Jr., and McLean, R. The effects of inhaled heat on the air passages and lungs: An experimental investigation. *Am. J. Pathol.* 21:311, 1945.
62. Morris, S. E., Navaratum, N., Townsend, C. M., et al. Bacterial translocation and mesenteric blood flow in a large animal model after cutaneous thermal and smoke inhalation injury. *Surg. Forum* 39:189, 1988.
63. Moylan, J. A., and Alexander, L. G. Diagnosis and treatment of inhalation injury. *World J. Surg.* 2:185, 1978.

64. Neville, C., Walker, S., Brown, B., et al. Discharge planning and teaching programs. *J. Burn Care Rehabil.* 9:414, 1988.
65. Order, S. E., Mason, A. D., Jr., Switzer, W. E., et al. Arterial vascular occlusion and devitalization of burn wounds. *Ann. Surg.* 161:502, 1965.
66. Pasulka, P. S., and Wachtel, T. L. Nutritional considerations for the burned patient. *Surg. Clin. North Am.* 67:109, 1987.
67. Perry, S., Heidrich, G., and Ramos, E. Assessment of pain by burn patients. *J. Burn Care Rehabil.* 2:322, 1981.
68. Petro, J. A., and Salisbury, R. E. Rehabilitation of the burn patient. *Clin. Plast. Surg.* 13:145, 1986.
69. Pruitt, B. A., Jr. Infection: Cause or effect of pathophysiologic change in burn and trauma patients. In Paubert-Braquet, M. (ed.), *Lipid Mediators in the Immunology of Shock.* New York: Plenum Publishing Co., 1987.
70. Rubin, W. D., Mani, M. M., and Hiebert, J. M. Fluid resuscitation of the thermally injured patient: Current concepts with definition of clinical subsets and their specialized treatment. *Clin. Plast. Surg.* 13:9, 1986.
71. Saltz, R., Dimick, A., Harris, C., et al. Application of autologous fibrin glue in burn wounds. *J. Burn Care Rehabil.* 10:504, 1989.
72. Sataloff, D. M., and Sataloff, R. T. Tracheotomy and inhalation. *Head Neck Surg.* 6:1024, 1984.
73. Shirani, K. Z., Pruitt, B. A., Jr., and Mason, A. D. The influence of inhalation injury and pneumonia on burn mortality. *Ann. Surg.* 205:82, 1987.
74. Steiner, H., and Clark, W. Psychiatric complication of burned adults: A classification. *J. Trauma* 17:134, 1977.
75. Stuart, J. D., Kenny, J. G., Lettieri, J., et al. Application of single-donor fibrin glue to burns. *J. Burn Care Rehabil.* 9:619, 1988.
76. Tanner, J. C., Vandeput, J., and Olley, J. F. The meshed skin graft. *Plast. Reconstr. Surg.* 34:287, 1964.
77. Teplitz, C., David, D., Mason, A. D., Jr., et al. *Pseudomonas* burn wound sepsis. I: Pathogenesis of experimental *Pseudomonas* burn wound sepsis. *J. Surg. Res.* 4:200, 1964.
78. Torgerson, W. S. What objective measures are there for evaluating pain? *J. Trauma* 24:S187, 1984.
79. Van der Does, A. J. W. Hypnosis and pain in patients with severe burns: A pilot study. *Burns* 14:399, 1988.
80. Wachtel, T. L. Epidemiology, classification, initial care, and administrative considerations for critically burned patients. *Crit. Care Clin.* 1:3, 1985.
81. Warden, G. D., Saffle, J. R., and Kravitz, M. A two-stage technique for excision and grafting of burn wounds. *J. Trauma* 22:98, 1982.
82. Watkins, P. N., Cook, E. L., May, S. R., et al. Psychological stages in adaptation following burn injury: A method for facilitating psychological recovery of burn victims. *J. Burn Care Rehabil.* 9: 376, 1988.
83. Williamson, J. Actual burn nutrition care practices: A national survey (Part II). *J. Burn Care Rehabil.* 10:185, 1989.
84. Wilmore, D. W. Nutrition and metabolism following thermal injury. *Clin. Plast. Surg.* 1:603, 1974.
85. Wilmore, D. W., Aulick, L. H., Mason, A. D., Jr., and Pruitt, B. A., Jr. Influence of the burn wound on local and systemic responses to injury. *Ann. Surg.* 186:444, 1977.
86. Winkelstein, A. What are the immunological alterations induced by burn injury? *J. Trauma* 24:S72, 1984.
87. Zawacki, B. E. The local effects of burn injuries. In J. A. Boswick, Jr. (ed.), *The Art and Science of Burn Care.* Frederick, MD: Aspen Publishers, 1987.
88. Zawacki, B. E., Spitzer, K. W., Mason, A. P., et al. Does increased evaporative water loss cause hypermetabolism in burn patients? *Ann. Surg.* 171:236, 1970.
89. Zikria, B. A., Budd, D. C., Flock, H. F., et al. What is chemical smoke poisoning? *Ann. Surg.* 181:151, 1975.

44

Multisystem Organ Failure

Connie A. Walleck   *Cornelia Vanderstaay Kenner*

REMINISCING AND LIFE REVIEW

A process basic to your existence is reminiscing and recounting of past events alone or with your friends. Life review is a process of reviewing life and past experiences and imaging events to come, based on previous events. Reminiscence has three parts: memory, experiencing, and interaction with others. Recalling special events in life is not just a simple routine of remembering. It involves creating a healing moment around the remembering process. The following information provides guidelines for facilitating the life review process with a patient during acute illness or if a patient is dying:

- The life review process with a patient begins as you would in reviewing life. Serving as a guide for this patient on his or her healing journey is special for him or her as well as for you.
- Make sure the patient is as comfortable as possible. Start the process by getting the patient to talk about the "old days," first jobs, public figures, personal and national losses, triumphs, and so forth. Use personal items around the patient, such as photos, newspaper clippings, cards, plants, and quilts, to trigger memories. Ask the patient if he or she can remember something special that has happened to him or her such as holidays, vacations, or special events with others. Ask the patient if he or she remembers a time when he or she made a difference in the lives of others. Ask the patient what experiences come forth when he or she remembers these events?
- You do not have to have any answers. The only thing that you need is your compassion, intention, and willingness to share from your heart. Be alert to the patients' needs to be silent with their own thoughts, and be prepared to help them explore memories when they are ready. When the patients ask your opinion, be honest and share what comes.
- Begin to help the patient review important memories of the past and rehearse events coming in the future. This will help ease the potential feelings of isolation that are common around acute illness or crisis, or when the patient is dying. It can help the patient deal with unresolved conflicts and unhealed relationships, emphasize positive aspects of the life one is living, or, if dying, focus on the positive aspects of the life that one has lived.
- Encourage the patient to make decisions about things over which he or she has control, such as medications, treatments, and daily routines. If the patient is dying, does he or she have any special requests about a funeral, and a will? Whom does the patient wish to receive special personal belongings?
- Include different relaxation and imagery exercises to help the patient practice "letting go of this solidness of the physical body." This letting go helps the patient cope with physical and emotional pain, difficult procedures, and conflicts, or enables him or her to experience death with peace and dignity.
- If death approaches, know that life review and self-reflection will take on immediate forms, such as talking, sitting, being, and maintaining physical contact with holding and touching. Barriers that previously had prevented communication may lift as the burden of the ego is laid aside. If the patient is dying, the final words of this patient to family members or friends and vice versa can take on many healing qualities.

LEARNING OBJECTIVES

After reading this chapter, the nurse should be able to do the following:

1. Taking into consideration the body's altered metabolic response, modify all nursing procedures to minimize stress and provide adequate rest while maintaining the patient's mobility.
2. Use all principles of nursing care to prevent sepsis.
3. Prevent further deterioration of the septic patient's condition, by paying close attention to "total-patient" support.
4. Describe the clinical syndrome of disseminated intravas-

cular coagulation and write a plan of care for a patient who has that syndrome.

5. Adhere to a rigorous schedule to prevent gastrointestinal bleeding. If bleeding ensues, determine the nursing diagnosis and prepare for the various modes of therapy the physician might choose.

CASE STUDY

Mr. T.H., a 22-year-old carpenter, was admitted to the community hospital emergency room with multiple injuries. He had been hit by a car while he was riding his motorcycle. He was noted to be in profound shock and to have the following injuries: bilateral pneumothoraces, a lacerated spleen, a ruptured stomach, a fractured pelvis, an open fracture of the left tibia, and a fracture of the distal radius. After placement of chest tubes, immediate surgical procedures were splenectomy, partial gastrectomy, and debridement of the open fracture. He was given 5 U of blood. He was started on carbenicillin (10 g every 8 hours) and gentamicin (80 mg every 8 hours).

Subsequently, during the next 24 hours, Mr. H. remained hypotensive and his urinary output was less than 15 ml/hour. On his second postoperative day, he returned to the operating suite for a tracheotomy, and he was given 3 U of blood. His intravenous fluids were increased in an effort to increase his urinary output, but it remained minimal. He had no response to the administration of furosemide (120 mg). His blood urea nitrogen level rose to 138 mg/dl and his creatinine level rose to 5.3 mg/dl. On the second postoperative day, he had bleeding and massive swelling in his left pelvic area, and that evening, he had a tonic-clonic seizure. His total intake for the 3 days was 25,500 ml, and his total output was 3000 ml. On the fourth day, he was transferred by air ambulance to the regional trauma center.

Mr. H.'s wife and parents were very distressed during this period, but they understood the explanations given them and they were able to make decisions. They described Mr. H. as an outgoing, active, sports-loving person who had never had any serious health problems.

On his arrival at the trauma center, Mr. H.'s vital signs were T 99°F (rectally), P 120, R 16, and BP 120/70. He was maintained on the volume ventilator, his chest tubes were patent, and bloody mucus was obtained on suctioning. His arterial blood gas measurements on 40% F_IO_2 were PaO_2 159, pH 7.43, $PaCO_2$ 29, and delta base -11. His laboratory test results were hemoglobin 8 g/dl, white blood count 20,000 per mm^3, platelets 75,000 per mm^3, prothrombin time 15 sec (control time was 12), partial thromboplastin time (PTT) 45 sec, fibrinogen 320 mg/dl, sodium 141 mEq/L, potassium 4.8 mEq/L, carbon dioxide combining power 24 mEq/L, chlorides 91 mEq/L, creatinine 5.4 mg/dl, blood urea nitrogen 152 mg/dl, and serum amylase more than 320 Somogyi units. His chest radiograph showed bilateral lung infiltrates. His renal arteriogram showed normal arteries with a decreased flow to the right renal superior pole and a delayed right renal vein flow. A cystogram and a retrograde pyelogram showed a moderate-sized bladder, no tears, and bloody urine from both orifices.

Mr. H.'s initial care included the administration of three units of packed cells, one unit of fresh frozen plasma, vitamin K, prophylactic antacids, and parenteral nutrition; the discontinuance of carbenicillin and gentamicin; the institution of hemodynamic monitoring parameters; and the interaction of dopamine at 3 mcg/kg/minute.

After the initial interval, the primary nurse assessed Mr. H.'s immediate problems and planned his nursing care. In collaboration with the clinical specialist (and as part of the in-depth nursing care plan), the nurse requested consultations with the renal clinical specialist and nurse epidemiologist. A patient care conference was planned for the next morning with the other members of the team.

Clinical Presentation of Case Study

2/13 1:00 P.M.

Mr. H. remained on the volume ventilator at an 1100-ml tidal volume and a 1300-ml sigh. His arterial blood gas measurements on 40% F_IO_2 were PaO_2 88, pH 7.40, $PaCO_2$ 35, and delta base -2. His arterial oxygen tension on 100% oxygen was 450 mm Hg. His chest x-ray film showed basilar infiltrates.

Neurologically, Mr. H. was confused and gave inconsistent responses to verbal commands. His pupils were equal and round, and they reacted to light and accommodation; his disks were flat with no papilledema. On his right side, Mr. H. exhibited continuous rhythmic seizure activity that seemed myoclonic. It was treated with intravenous phenytoin Dilantin—500 mg.

Mr. H. exhibited a small degree of bleeding from his tracheostomy site. His hemoglobin was 10.1 g/dl, platelets 50,000 mm^3, prothrombin time 15.5 sec (control time was 11.5 sec), PTT time 45 sec, and fibrinogen 300 mg/dl. His blood urea nitrogen level rose to 180 mg/dl, and his creatinine level rose to 5.6 mg/dl. Platelet packs, fresh frozen plasma, and vitamin K were administered.

Continuous arteriovenous hemodialysis (CAVHD) was started after the placement of an arterial access and a venous line. The ultrafiltration rate was set at 100 ml/hour and the CAVHD was ordered for 48 hours initially. Mr. H.'s fluid replacement was ordered at one half of the previous hour's total ultrafiltrate.

2:00 P.M.

Mr. H. responded to verbal commands; focal motor activity was absent in his left arm. His jaw and limb reflexes were +3; no posturing was present. Maintenance administration of intravenous Dilantin was ordered (100 mg three times a day).

7:30 P.M.

He was placed on positive end-expiratory pressure (PEEP), 5 cm H_2O, for pulmonary edema.

2/14

T 100.8°F (rectally), P 128, R 10, BP 114/70. Mr. H.'s continuing fluid overload was shown by tachycardia (no murmurs or gallops). The following were noted: central venous pressure of 16 cm H_2O, basilar rales, basilar opacification on chest x-ray film, and pitting dependent edema.

His arterial blood gas measurements on 40% oxygen with a PEEP of 5 were PaO_2 80, pH 7.37, and $PaCO_2$ 40. His lung compliance was 29. Digitalization was begun (0.5 mg at first and then 0.25 mg a day). The exact dosage was to be determined by his serial blood measurements.

His total volume was decreased to 1000 ml, his sigh decreased to 1200, and his respiratory rate decreased to 8. His electrolyte levels were sodium 140 mEq/L, potassium 4.8 mEq/L, carbon dioxide 25 mEq/L and chlorides 88 mEq/L. For several hours, his urinary output was 4 to 6 ml/hour.

Mr. H.'s coagulopathy was resolving. The oozing previously noted during dressing changes stopped, but bloody mucus was still suctioned from the tracheostomy. His hematocrit was 37%, prothrombin time 12.5 sec (the control time was 11 sec) with 79.5% activity. Heparin administration was discontinued. The cause of the coagulopathy could not be determined because the parameters were nondiagnostic. The coagulopathy was thought to be secondary to trauma, a washout coagulopathy, or a carbenicillin platelet dysfunction.

Mr. H.'s left lower leg was significantly swollen, and the anterior portion of the wound was necrotic. His distal pulses remained palpable. Two kinds of gram-negative rods were cultured from the site. His white blood count rose to 21,800 per mm^3, with a shift to the left. The wound was debrided and irrigated with hydrogen peroxide. Systemic antibiotics were given: intravenous tobramycin (80 mg) and aqueous penicillin (2.5 million units followed by 1 million units every 4 hours). His serum amylase level was greater than 640 units.

Mr. H. remained lethargic and responsive to verbal commands. His treatments were explained to him in simple terms, and he tried to help turn himself. His family remained at the hospital during the day and went to a nearby motel at night. During Mr. H.'s visits from his family, the nurse remained at his bedside.

2/15

T 101.8°F (rectally), P 120, R 8, BP 104/68. Mr. H. rested for short periods through the night; he was unable to rest for long periods.

On auscultation, a gallop and basilar rales were heard. Mr. H.'s arterial blood gas measurements were PaO_2 66, pH 7.38, $PaCO_2$ 40.6, and delta base -1. On chest x-ray film, apical clearing was seen, but basilar infiltrates remained. Mr. H. remained on PEEP of 5 cm H_2O, and pancuronium (2 to 4 mg given by intravenous push) was ordered every hour as needed to treat respiratory agitation. A morphine drip of 1 mg/hour was begun to sedate Mr. H. Mr. H.'s chest tubes were removed.

The CAVHD was continued with the ultrafiltration rate decreased to 80 ml/hour. Mr. H.'s electrolyte levels were sodium 135 mEq/L, potassium 4.6 mEq/L, carbon dioxide 26.5 mEq/L, and chlorides 90 mEq/L; his fluid intake was 2000 ml and his output was 1688 ml.

The blood work showed a hemoglobin of 11.9 g/dl, a hematocrit of 34.2%, and a white blood count of 22,300 per mm^3. His prothrombin time was 14.5 sec (the control time was 11.5 seconds), and his PTT was 23 seconds.

At the base of the wound over Mr. H.'s tibia, foul drainage and necrotic tissue were noted. The wound was debrided and irrigated.

Under Bier's block anesthesia, a closed reduction of a Salter II fracture of Mr. H.'s distal radius was carried out. Postreduction films were made, and a splint was applied to Mr. H.'s right arm.

5:00 P.M.

Insertion of a pulmonary artery catheter resulted in a 25% left pneumothorax. A chest tube was inserted in the left anterior axillary line in the second intercostal space.

2/16

T 102.4°F, P 120, R 10, BP 124/80. On auscultation, a grade I holosystolic murmur that was similar to a pericardial rub and basilar rales were heard. Arterial blood gas measurement showed no further deterioration in Mr. H.'s condition. Infiltrates seen on the portable chest x-ray film were thought to be pneumonia. His parenteral nutritional therapy was increased to 2500 ml/day.

2/17–2/18

T 102.6°, P 114, R 10, BP 102/64. Mr. H.'s respiratory status was maintained by the volume ventilator, respiratory paralysis, an FIO_2 of 50%, and a PEEP of 10 cm H_2O. Arterial blood gas measurements were PaO_2 76, pH 7.41, $PaCO_2$ 25, and delta base -3. A tidal volume of 800 ml was selected for ventilation. Mr. H.'s pulmonary artery occlusion pressure (PAOP) was 6. On 2/17 his cardiac output averaged 4.4 L/minute (with a PEEP of 10 cm H_2O), and on 2/18 his cardiac output averaged 9.6 L/minute. Mr. H. remained in the oliguric phase of acute renal failure and continued on his CAVHD at 80 ml/hour. His platelet count fell to 17,500 per mm^3. His serum amylase level was higher than 800 units, and the results of an abdominal sonogram were negative.

2/19–2/20

Mr. H. remained lethargic; his exact level of consciousness was impossible to determine because of his metabolic status and the medications he was taking. His Dilantin dosage was increased to 400 mg/day because the neurosurgeon noted that his Dilantin levels were 2 to 3 μg/ml (therapeutic levels are 10 to 20 μg/ml).

Mr. H.'s sputum culture was positive for a gram-negative bacillus, and his white blood cell count increased to 25,000 per mm^3. His arterial oxygen was 83, and his arteriovenous oxygen difference was 3.22. A chest x-ray film showed that a small pneumothorax persisted. Mr. H.'s primary care physician consulted with members of the departments of infectious disease and pulmonary medicine. His sputum, urine, and blood were recultured, and they were specifically labeled for Candida. Mr. H. was given methicillin (6 g daily) and tobramycin (1.5 mg/kg) after every dialysis. His urinary output approached 200 ml for a 24-hour period.

2/21–2/22

Mr. H.'s urine and sputum cultures were reported positive for Pseudomonas, which was sensitive to tobramycin. After peritoneal lavage, the fluid obtained was blood tinged, straw colored, and not odorous. The laboratory analysis was as follows: serum amylase level 377, white blood cell count 27,000 per mm^3, lymphocytes 24%, polymorphonucleocytes 71%, and red blood cell count 4.5 million per mm^3. Because his serum glucose levels remained at 300 to 400 mg/dl despite increased amounts of insulin, his hyperalimentation fluids were decreased to 2000 ml/day. His platelet count increased to 43,000/mm^3.

2/23–2/24

Weight: 60.5 kg. Mr. H.'s family was acutely aware of his physiologic and psychological traumas, and they sought ways to function within the stressful situation. They assessed their own family situation, and they established priorities. A schedule was made so that a family member would always be at the hospital, except during their sleeping hours. The time away from the hospital was used to run errands and to take care of important business. They were careful to eat well and otherwise take care of themselves so that they would not become ill.

Mr. H. remained on the ventilator. On a PEEP of 10 cm H_2O and an FIO_2 of 50%, his arterial gas measurements were PaO_2 73, pH 7.33, $PaCO_2$ 37, and delta base -6, and his mixed venous blood gas measurements were $P\bar{v}O_2$ 46, pH 7.30, $PvCO_2$ 41, and delta base -6. His pulmonary artery occlusion pressure was 8 to 9, and his cardiac output was 6 to 8 L/minute. His electrolyte levels were sodium 135 mEq/L, potassium 4.3 mEq/L, carbon dioxide 21 mEq/L, and chlorides 90 mEq/L, with an anion gap of 24.

Mr. H. was found to have suppurative thrombophlebitis in his right saphenous vein. On sonography, a sonolucent fluid collection was noted in the right upper quadrant; it measured 8×5 cm.

2/24–2/25

Abdominal surgery was performed because Mr. H. showed further signs of infection (a white blood cell count of 30,000 to 40,000 per mm^3 and a flat plate film of the abdomen was suggestive of an intra-abdominal infection). He was found to have pancreatitis with saponification of the lesser sac and tail of the pancreas and an abscess around the tail of the pancreas. Mr. H.'s pancreas was drained to the left upper quadrant with six 1-inch drains, and a jejunostomy tube was placed. Mr. H.'s highest temperature after surgery was 99°F.

The following day Mr. H.'s arterial blood gas measurements were PaO_2 68, pH 7.36, and $PaCO_2$ 40. His carbon dioxide retention was attributed to the severity of adult respiratory distress syndrome and a significant increase in physiologic dead space. The physician left an order that he could have a lower tidal volume with a faster rate if his $PaCO_2$ became difficult to control.

2/26–2/27

Positive-pressure ventilation was continued, with arterial blood gas measurements of PaO_2 63, pH 7.30, $PaCO_2$ 41.8, and mixed venous blood gas measurements of $P\bar{v}O_2$ 35, pH 7.26, and $PvCO_2$ 50.4. Amber fluid drained through the chest tube. The examination of the chest x-ray film by the radiologist indicated that the subclavian catheter was probably in the chest. The catheter was replaced by a new central line.

Mr. H.'s bacteriologic cultures were negative for gram-positive organisms, but his sputum cultures were positive for Pseudomonas aeruginosa, and his urine cultures were positive for Enterobacter cloacae. Colistin (1.5 mg/kg) was ordered because the Enterobacter was sensitive to tobramycin only at a dosage of 16 U/ml, but it was sensitive to colistin and amikacin at 8 U/ml. On the recommendation of the nurse epidemiologist, isolation procedures were instituted.

2/28–3/1

T 103.4°F, P 130, R 8, BP 100/70. Mr. H. demonstrated increasing response to verbal commands and limited spontaneous response on the left side. His urinary output was measured at 375 to 400 ml over a 24-hour period. His creatinine level was 3.8 mg/dl, but his blood urea nitrogen level remained significantly elevated, reflecting his marked catabolic state. Because of the adult respiratory distress syndrome, the intravenous administration of fluid was not increased, and an occlusion pressure of 7 was maintained. Even though recovery from acute renal failure was slowed by limited fluid administration, no lasting deleterious effect on Mr. H.'s renal functioning was anticipated. An increased anion gap secondary to renal failure and parenteral nutritional therapy was treated with sodium bicarbonate.

3/2–3/3

The F_IO_2 was decreased to 40% without deterioration of the arterial blood gases. Wound cultures from the right tibia showed *Enterobacter*, and the colistin dosage was increased.

3/4–3/7

Temperatures of 102°F to 103°F continued. Mr. H.'s cardiac output was measured at 14.5 L/minute, and his arterial venous oxygen difference was 3.1 to 5.2. His urine cultures were sterile, but *Pseudomonas* continued to be reported from the sputum cultures. The tobramycin therapy was discontinued.

3/8–3/11

Mr. H.'s daily urinary output increased to 500 to 700 ml, with a minimal response to the furosemide challenge. The nephrologist assessed that Mr. H. was slowly entering the diuretic phase, and he decided to continue the CAVHD as long as the blood urea nitrogen level was greater than 100 or the urinary output was less than 2 L/day.

Yellow serous drainage from the tibial wound was noted. Areas of new granulation tissue were present. Colistin therapy was discontinued, and amikacin therapy was begun. (In renal insufficiency, the recommended dosage of amikacin after dialysis is 7.5 mg/kg.)

3/12–3/15

The PEEP was lowered to 3 cm H_2O, and the arterial oxygen tension remained above 80. The caloric intake using both jejunostomy feedings and parenteral therapy was estimated to be 3500 to 3750 calories/day. CAVHD was discontinued.

3/15–3/18

After extensive debridement of the tibial wound, Mr. H.'s temperature spiked to 104.5°F, he had a rash over most of his body, and his serum potassium level rose to above 6 mEq/L. Sodium polystyrene sulfonate (Kayexalate) was used to lower the serum potassium level, and CAVHD was reinstituted. A fungus thought to be *Mucor* was isolated from the tibial wound. Antibiotics and parenteral therapy were discontinued, and intravenous catheters were replaced. Amphotericin therapy was considered but not begun.

Mr. H. became abusive and seemed to be psychotic. Because the staff was unable to protect him from himself, restraints were applied.

3/19–3/22

The fungemia was resolved clinically; the culture reports pointed to *Candida* rather than *Mucor*. Mr. H. had severe diarrhea, which was thought to be secondary to the use of Kayexalate and sorbitol. His volume depletion was particularly apparent from a tachycardia of 180. Normal saline solution was administered at a rate of 50 ml/hour, and paregoric was begun.

Mr. H.'s respiratory rate decreased to 15, and his F_IO_2 was decreased to 40%. His arterial blood gas measurements on 40% oxygen were PaO_2 80, pH 7.37, $PaCO_2$ 33.5; on 100% oxygen, they were PaO_2 375, pH 7.35, and $PaCO_2$ 37.

Mr. H. slept for only short periods during the night and took infrequent naps during the day. He cried easily (he felt best during his visits with his family). He had no memories of his early stay in the critical care unit.

3/23–3/26

Mr. H.'s respiratory status continued to improve, and intermittent mandatory ventilation was started. Jejunostomy feedings were slowly increased. At rest, Mr. H. maintained a position of medial and ulnar denervation, and so a volar positioning splint was applied.

3/27–3/30

Mr. H. felt better day by day, and he slept for long periods during the night. He asked few questions; he seemed to understand the explanations given. His family rearranged their schedules to give them more time away from the hospital so that they could attend to family affairs.

Mr. H.'s blood urea nitrogen level was 24, his creatinine level was 1.6, and the CAVHD was discontinued. Although his blood cultures remained negative, multiple cultures revealed many sites of sepsis. Sputum reports indicated a light growth of *Providentia stuartii* and a heavy growth of *Pseudomonas aeruginosa*, both of which were sensitive to tobramycin. The urinalyses indicated the presence of *Enterococcus* and yeast. The wound cultures from the jejunostomy site indicated the presence of *Bacteroides*, and the cultures from the tibia indicated the presence of *Serratia marcescens*.

Mr. H.'s lung compliance increased slowly. The dead space volume was determined from a Douglas bag collection of expired gas using a Searle respirator and 35% oxygen. The dead space volume was 46.7%—two standard deviations from normal.

A dorsiflexion positioning splint was made for Mr. H.'s left lower leg to relieve pressure on his calcaneus.

3/31–4/6

Mr. H. continued to feel better each day, and he became more and more involved in his care. His family visited him for longer periods, and they offered help to the families of other patients.

The process of weaning Mr. H. from the respirator was begun. His caloric intake was 3000 to 4000; the calories came mainly from jejunostomy feedings. Blood culture reports were positive for *Enterococcus*, which was sensitive to ampicillin and tobramycin.

4/7–4/13

Arterial blood gas values measured on the tracheostomy collar with 40% O_2 were PaO_2 88, pH 7.28, and $PaCO_2$ 28. The blood, sputum, and urine cultures remained positive.

4/14–4/30

Before Mr. H.'s transfer to the general unit, many of the staff came to the unit to meet him. His primary nurse conducted nursing rounds and outlined the plan of care. His respiratory condition stabilized, and his cultures were negative.

Mr. H. went to the physical therapy department daily, and his strength gradually increased. He began to eat well, and he gained weight. Final discharge planning was done by the health team at a staff conference. Because both patient and family education had been an important part of nursing care during his stay in the critical care unit, Mr. H. and his family were well informed and understood much of his rehabilitative care. Mr. H. returned home feeling very fortunate and knowing that he had to make outpatient follow-up visits often and over a long period of time.

REFLECTIONS

Many factors affect the consciousness of the patient who has sustained system failure.[29] Changes in his thoughts and feelings are part of the trauma. The mind as well as the body is affected: to traumatize the body is to traumatize the mind (Fig. 44–1).

A person cannot be bombarded with stimuli for long periods of time and maintain functional integrity. The person may become overwhelmingly tired and irritable.

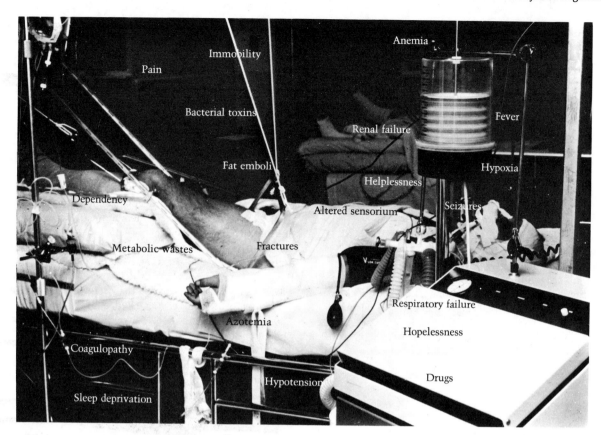

Figure 44–1
Multiple stresses encountered by the patient.

Seemingly minor incidents or aspects of care may seem to be insurmountable problems. The patient's hopelessness may be complete.

The helplessness phenomenon that occurs when a patient feels out of control has far-reaching emotional and biochemical repercussions that have been directly related to the development and exacerbation of disease. Animal analogue studies verify these findings. Once the realization comes that all control has been lost, a person first struggles to re-establish control and then becomes totally passive or gives up. The parasympathetic (giving up) response accompanying this reaction has been associated with rapid physical deterioration. Although the patient cannot establish control over treatment procedures in full measure, some predictability about procedures and their outcomes can serve to protect the patient from total feelings of helplessness. Refer to Chapter 3 for an in-depth discussion of the role of psychophysiologic self-regulation modalities to support patients in this time of crisis. One major goal is to offer patients as much predictability as possible to give them a sense of control and to alleviate some of their anxiety.

ETIOLOGY

The critically ill patient may have many complications. Any organ system affected may exhibit significant alterations, and in turn, other organ systems may be affected. Sequential multisystem organ failure often has more than one etiologic condition. Sepsis is the cause of death in as many as 42% of patients.[12] With sequential failure, for example, the initial insult is often an infection, perhaps in a hypermetabolic patient with undernutrition; then the next insult is hyperdynamic septic shock; then hypodynamic septic shock; then disseminated intravascular coagulation; then renal failure; then gastrointestinal bleeding; then pulmonary failure, and, eventually brain failure and death. With decreased tissue perfusion, there is decreased circulation to all organs and the possibility of multisystem failure. With decreased circulation, there is generalized tissue edema that can lead to any system failure. For example, with respiratory failure, there is hypoxemia, and hypoxemia coupled with decreased tissue perfusion is destructive to the lung tissue itself as well as to other organs. In the brain the tissue edema is produced within a bony box that cannot enlarge. The vessels with low intravascular pressure, such as the capillaries and veins, collapse because the pressure outside the capillaries or veins is greater than the pressure inside. The syndrome is circular:

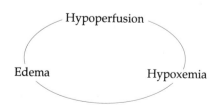

The complications discussed in this chapter are sepsis and septic shock, disseminated intravascular coagulation, and stress ulcers. (The adult respiratory distress syndrome is discussed in Chap. 20, and acute renal failure is discussed in Chap. 33.)

Over 1½ million nosocomial (hospital-acquired) infections occur annually.[22,23] Ten percent are bacteremias and disseminated infections. About 6 to 7 infections per 100 discharges occur.[35] The hospitalized patient has increased susceptibility and is at risk for infection (Table 44–1). Patients in the critical care unit have three times the risk of other hospitalized patients of developing an infection.[10] The urinary tract is the most frequent site of nosocomial infection. Forty-five percent of infections are device-related, and about one-fourth are due to infusion fluids, intravascular catheters, and monitoring devices.[16,39] Nosocomial pneumonia is responsible for 15% of hospital deaths. Up to 60% of critical care patients may develop pneumonia, depending on the severity of the underlying disease.

Septic shock occurs primarily in cases of gram-negative bacteremia, although cases of septic shock have also been reported with gram-positive infections (*e.g.*, toxic shock syndrome), viruses, fungi, rickettsiae, and malaria. It is estimated that there is an incidence of 71,000 to 330,000 patients per year with gram-negative bacteremia. Estimates of septic shock and mortality range from 25% to 50%.[10,22]

PATHOPHYSIOLOGY

Sepsis and Septic Shock

The physiologic alterations that occur with infection range from a minor local inflammatory response to septic shock and even death. Sepsis, the acute systemic response to invading microorganisms, has a constellation of symptoms, physical signs, and laboratory abnormalities. It usually occurs with bacteremia, but not all people who have bacteremia also have septicemia.

The establishment and spread of sepsis is described by the following mechanism. The invading microorganisms get a foothold in damaged tissue and establish a primary lesion there. Sepsis is the result of the interaction between the microorganism and the patient. Different species and strains of microorganisms vary in their ability to produce disease, and patients vary in their ability to resist infection. Pathogenic organisms, including some that seem to be nonpathogenic,

Table 44–1
Antecedent Conditions: Patients at Risk With Increased Susceptibility for Infection

ANTECEDENT CONDITION	PATIENTS AT RISK WITH INCREASED SUSCEPTIBILITY FOR INFECTION
Hospitalization	Urinary tract, skin, respiratory system
Trauma	Burns, abdominal injury
Age	Elderly
Decreased cellular immunity	Organ transplants, undernutrition, cancer
Chronic illness	Diabetes mellitus, cirrhosis, renal failure, chronic lung disease, neurologic disease
Life-style	Alcoholic, drug addict, prostitute, homosexual male, foreign travel

survive and multiply in the patient, producing tissue damage and eliciting an inflammatory response. The patient's hormonal and cellular immunologic capacities may be significantly impaired.

Microorganisms produce sepsis by the invasion of tissues and the elaboration of toxins. From the time organisms and their products enter the extravascular spaces and interact with damaged tissue, the body attempts to localize them by its inflammatory response. Kininogen, a hormone present in all tissues and blood, is activated into kinin, and along with histamine, endotoxin, and other vasoactive substances, it produces a vascular response. Blood flow is slowed by vascular constriction associated with capillary and venular dilatation. Alterations in the endothelial membrane increase permeability and permit extravasation of plasma proteins into the extravascular space and diapedesis of leukocytes. Fibrinogen forms a fibrin network that traps the bacteria. At the cellular level, the A-V oxygen difference is decreased, and local hypoxia occurs. The mechanism for the hypoxia is not known; some authorities have suggested a bypass of the cell, a defect in oxygen transport, or a problem with oxidative phosphorylation.

Sepsis produces vasodilatation and a hyperdynamic state. The blood flow and the cardiac output are increased, and the distribution or the peripheral effectiveness of the blood flow is altered. Histamine released by complement-activated mast cells depletes the intravascular volume by increasing the permeability of the tissues so fluid becomes sequestered in the interstitium. Prostaglandin E_2 (PGE_2) and prostacyclin cause peripheral vasodilatation, lowering the peripheral resistance.[19] This state is known as the hyperdynamic septic shock phase. If compensatory mechanisms fail and the prearteriolar sphincters relax, plasma volume is lost and the patient lapses into the hypodynamic phase of septic shock. The onset is not always abrupt. The blood pressure may either drift down or drop suddenly. There is a release of epinephrine and norepinephrine producing increased peripheral resistance and cardiac rate. Cardiac output is depressed because of the decreased blood volume and venous return. Often problems in other systems are caused by the decreased cardiac output. Multiorgan failure can follow.[4] For example, the patient may suffer a myocardial infarction from decreased myocardial perfusion or he or she may be confused because of the decreased cerebral perfusion. Additionally, the low-flow state may produce not only gastrointestinal problems (especially stress ulcers), but also a dead bowel secondary to venous or arterial thrombosis. The patient would then have distention, absence of normal bowel sounds, and bloody diarrhea.

Broadly speaking, septic shock is primarily a cellular disease. The interactions between the bacterial endotoxin and the cell are both complex and time dependent.[30] Early effects of endotoxin exposure include a reduction in intracellular adenosine triphosphate (ATP) without evidence of mitochondrial dysfunction. However, impairment of the mitochondria may follow within 60 minutes. This latter change represents an irreversible phase of impaired cellular function. The decreased perfusion alters cellular metabolism with glucose metabolism occurring anaerobically, resulting in a lactic acid build-up that produces a metabolic acidosis. Additionally, because less ATP is formed in anaerobic metabolism, less energy is available. This energy deficit changes membrane integrity and allows further fluid shifts to occur intracellularly.

Stagnation in the microcirculation also leads to aggregation of the cellular components and intravascular clotting. As intravascular clotting increases, coagulation factors—platelets, prothrombin, factor V, factor VIII, and fibrinogen—are reduced. If the coagulation factors are used significantly, disseminated intravascular coagulation results.

As cellular death continues, multiple organ system failure occurs. Arteriovenous shunts prevent the delivery of oxygen and nutrients to the vital organs, producing deterioration in their function. Cardiovascular changes may not respond to fluid resuscitation or cardiac support. The release of the myocardial depressant factor causes a negative inotropic effect on the heart. Kidney hypoxia causes greater damage in the cortex than in the medulla. As the cells deteriorate in the cortex, the blood flow may be diverted to the juxtamedullary area. A rapid increase of blood flow to the juxtamedullary area may wash out the osmotic gradient and decrease the kidney's ability to concentrate urine. The glomerular filtration rate falls because blood flow has been diverted from the cortical area to the juxtamedullary area. As the sepsis continues and increasing quantities of platelets and leukocytes aggregate, proteolytic enzymes, vasoactive substances, and endotoxin arrive in the lungs. The patient's ability to oxygenate blood deteriorates, and respiratory failure increases. Endotoxin acts directly on the central nervous system and produces disorientation or coma.

Causative Organisms

As other antibiotics have been developed and as treatment modalities have changed, particularly resistant organisms have arisen and mutated. Before the 1940s, the greatest problem was with *Streptococcus;* in the 1950s, *Staphylococcus;* in the 1960s, *Pseudomonas;* and in the 1970s other gram-negative bacteria and opportunistic organisms. As antibiotics have been developed for each organism, another resistant species has seemingly come to the fore. Often the new organism was one that previously was considered to be not infectious. For example, *Pseudomonas* was once classified as nonvirulent and nonpathogenic. As a matter of fact, at first some hospitals had difficulty identifying *Pseudomonas* as the invading pathogen because their laboratories considered *Pseudomonas* nonvirulent and a normal surface contaminant of laboratory cultures, and so they did not report the presence of the *Pseudomonas.*

Sepsis may be produced by many different organisms. Because gram-negative infections have become more significant, emphasis has been put on them.[36] But gram-positive organisms—as well as polymicrobial and opportunistic organisms—still cause sepsis (Table 44–2). In gram-positive infections, besides group A *Streptococcus, Staphylococcus* may cause necrotizing fasciitis (necrosis of the superficial fascia). A hemolytic *Staphylococcus* and a nonhemolytic *Streptococcus* may work together to cause progressive bacterial synergistic gangrene. An anaerobic *Streptococcus* is often the cause of myositis.

Gram-Negative Organisms

Gram-negative bacteremia occurs in about 1 in every 100 hospitalizations, and it has been calculated to be the cause of about 70,000 deaths each year in the United States.[27] Besides the effects of the numbers of bacteria, gram-negative bacilli contain within their cell walls a lipopolysaccharide called *en-*

Table 44–2
Common Microorganisms Found in Septic Patients

Gram-negative
  Escherichia coli
  Klebsiella pneumoniae
  Enterobacter cloacae
  Pseudomonas aeruginosa
  Serratia
  Proteus
  Bacteroides fragilis
  Hemophilus influenzae
Gram-positive
  Staphylococcus aureus
  Methicillin-resistant *Staphylococcus aureus*
  Pneumococcus
  Alpha- and beta-hemolytic streptococci
Fungi
  Candida

dotoxin. When gram-negative organisms are contained within their normal anatomic environment, the release of endotoxin is not followed by any physiologic derangement. However, once having contaminated other body structures or cavities, these opportunistic bacilli become highly pathogenic and potentially lethal.[36]

Escherichia coli, normally found in the colon, is the most prevalent gram-negative facultative bacterium. Thirty to 40% of gram-negative bacteremias (particularly in the young or in those who have recently had a urinary tract infection) and 85% of uncomplicated urinary tract infections are traceable to *E. coli.* Strains isolated from people outside the hospital tend to be sensitive to many antibiotics, while strains isolated from people inside the hospital tend to be resistant.

Klebsiella pneumoniae causes a large proportion of the respiratory and urinary tract infections. Strains that cause nosocomial infections vary in their sensitivity to antibiotics, but most tend to be resistant. Recent epidemics have occurred with gentamicin-resistant strains. Systemic infections are common. They do not respond to carbenicillin, but they usually respond to cephalothin, cephaloridine, or cephalexin.

Aerobacter species, particularly *cloacae* and *aerogenes,* are notable problems in antibiotic-resistant nosocomial infections. All strains are resistant to cephalosporins, and about one-third are resistant to kanamycin. The antibiotic of choice is usually gentamicin or tobramycin.

Pseudomonas aeruginosa infections are common, and the organism is introduced readily from the environment. It has both exotoxins and endotoxins, as well as protelytic enzymes (in some strains). It is resistant to antibiotics, except gentamicin, carbenicillin, tobramycin, colistimethate, and polymyxin B. A polyvalent vaccine that produces active immunity has been developed and tested, but it is not available for widespread use. In many areas, strains not included in the vaccine have multiplied and caused serious problems. *Pseudomonas* is considered a water contaminant, and it is found wherever water stands or collects. The list of potential reservoirs includes sinks, sink traps, faucet aerators, tracheal catheter rinse solutions, bladder irrigation solutions, disinfectants, nail brushes, ventilators, fluids, local anesthetics, and flowers. It is also frequently found on the hands and clothes of hospital personnel.

Proteus species are often involved in infections of wounds of the urinary and respiratory tracts and in decubitus ulcers, and they may cause gram-negative sepsis. *Proteus* infections are difficult to treat, and antibiotic therapy is usually discussed in terms of indole-positive and indole-negative *Proteus*, that is, by the ability or inability of the *Proteus* organism to form indole from the amino acid tryptophan. Indole-positive *Proteus* organisms have an increased resistance to antibiotics, but fortunately, most *Proteus* infections are caused by indole-negative organisms (meningitis is a notable exception). Indole-negative *Proteus* organisms are usually sensitive to ampicillin and the aminoglycosides (kanamycin and gentamicin). Also, penicillin or the cephalosporins (cephalothin and cephalexin) may be ordered by the physician. In indole-positive *Proteus* infections, the aminoglycosides are the antibiotics of choice, but carbenicillin may be effective. Also usually considered with *Proteus* infections are *Providentia* species, particularly *P. stuartii*, which is often incriminated in postoperative ward infections, pneumonia, urinary tract infections, burn wound sepsis, and septicemia. In a few instances, overgrowth of the organism after therapy with mafenide acetate (Sulfamylon) has caused the death of all the patients in the critical care burn unit. Some species are resistant to all antibiotics, whereas others are occasionally sensitive to carbenicillin and the aminoglycosides.

Serratia marcescens is a motile gram-negative bacillus that is increasingly involved in infections, especially nosocomial infections. The most frequent problems it causes are urinary tract infections, bacteremia, and pulmonary infections. *S. marcescens* also was once considered nonpathogenic. It is a water contaminant and a soil contaminant. The red-pigmented strains are the most visible ones, but most strains are colorless. Most hospital-associated strains are very resistant and they have multiple resistances.

Anaerobic Organisms

The increasing incidence of anaerobic infections, notably those caused by *Bacteroides* and *Fusobacterium* species, warrants a discussion. Quite probably, improved techniques for collecting and processing the specimens have contributed to the increased recognition of them. In some series, *Bacteroides* has specifically been noted in patients who have tumors of the gastrointestinal tract or phlebitis. In fact, some strains may actually contribute to the phlebitis through their ability to degrade heparin and other mucopolysaccharides. Ninety percent of the anaerobic bacteria found in the large intestine are *Bacteroides*. Bacteria of both genera are found in the mouth and in the gastrointestinal, respiratory, and urogenital tracts. The drug of choice with *B. fragilis* is usually clindamycin or chloramphenicol, but *Fusobacterium* is sensitive to most antibiotics, and the use of penicillin is indicated.

Opportunistic Infections

Opportunistic infections are most commonly found in patients whose host defense mechanisms are compromised. The infections may be severe and may even precipitate the person's demise. Infections caused by fungi and even large viruses are considered opportunistic. As with bacterial infections, individual sensitivities must be established. The most common infections are caused by *Candida*, which grows when antibiotics are used; common sites are the mouth (thrush), esophagus, vagina, and cutaneous lesions, which can be treated with nystatin. Systemic fungal infections (which are particularly likely to occur in the kidney) are treated with ampho-

tericin B. The serum creatinine and blood urea nitrogen levels, the urinary pH, and the kidney's ability to concentrate urine must be monitored during treatment with this drug.

Microbial Factors

Microbial patterns of infection are in part determined by microbial density, sources of seeding, microbial virulence and invasiveness, microbial competition, and microbial resistance to therapeutic drugs.

The ability of a microorganism to produce disease varies according to its virulence and its predilection for certain body areas. The term *virulence* refers to the organism's power to invade, and the more virulent organisms are the ones that infect patients a greater percentage of the time. But both virulence and pathogenicity are rather nebulous terms. The microbial world is ever changing, and many organisms that were once considered nonvirulent are now considered virulent.

The use of antibiotics can alter the endogenous microbial flora. Nonpathogenic bacteria may be able to maintain their balance and compete with antibiotic-resistant pathogenic bacteria, but they may be destroyed by antibiotics that allow resistant strains to proliferate. Resistance to antibiotics is most frequently caused by an enzyme the particular bacterium synthesizes. Either the antibiotic is destroyed by the enzyme, or its conformational structure is altered so that ribosomal binding is no longer possible. Resistance also occurs after mutation in a mutant that is able to synthesize drug antagonists or essential metabolites. A common resistant microorganism seen in critical care units is methicillin-resistant *Staphylococcus aureus*.

Different patterns of organisms are seen in different institutions as well as in different parts of the same institution. The hospital's infection control committee knows what organisms are prevalent in the hospital and what their sensitivities are. Often the patterns of medical patients are different from those of surgical patients.[1] Another aspect of bacterial growth is its cyclic variation, which is difficult to identify. Also, emerging pathogenic bacteria are usually seen by large medical centers before they are seen by smaller institutions, because it is particularly in the larger centers that new antibiotics are tested and resistance produced.

The transfer of R factors recently has been implicated in the transfer of antibiotic resistance from one bacterium to another. The resistance is inherent in extrachromosomal pieces of DNA (variously called plasmids, episomes, genetic determinants, or resistance factors). Resistance is usually acquired by the process of transduction, but it may also be acquired by actual mating (conjugation), viral transmission, or transformation (direct entry of DNA). The transfer is usually made after two suitable bacteria come in contact and extend their pili to form a bridge of cytoplasm. The plasmid is replicated in the donor cell and transferred to the recipient cell. (A plasmid consists of two factors, one for drug resistance—the R determinant—and one for transmission of the R determinant—the resistance transfer factor, or RTF.) Both bacteria must have both factors for transfer to occur.

Antecedent Conditions

Hospital areas, including critical care units, are likely places for sepsis to occur. Host defense factors are especially important in hospitalized patients because immune defense mechanisms are depressed in people who are severely ill. Pathogenic organisms, particularly *Staphylococcus* and gram-negative bacteria, are endemic in the hospital, and infections easily spread from their sources to the patient. Common sources of infection are other patients, the staff, the equipment, the air, and any moist areas.[10,23] Control of the environment to prevent cross-contamination is a nursing responsibility. Other predisposing factors are seen in Table 44–1.

Endotoxin

Because the clinical problems caused by gram-negative infections are more prevalent and more severe than those caused by gram-positive infections, much of the literature is devoted to gram-negative infections. It is difficult to decipher the findings of much of the research, because the early research was based on endotoxin. It is now known that the syndrome differs when live bacteria are involved. Also, in the early research on hemodynamics, dogs and cats were the experimental models. The dog's heart is resistant to the early effects of endotoxin, and catecholamines have an inotropic action on the cat's heart, hiding a decrease in cardiac performance.

In all likelihood, the septic shock is initiated by endotoxins from the cell walls of gram-negative bacteria. The endotoxin molecule is a large lipopolysaccharide, and it inactivates or blocks the reticuloendothelial system. The blockade occurs after ingestible particles have saturated the receptor sites in the system, and it prevents further phagocytosis. The body may then be challenged by a minute number of microorganisms and be unable to respond.

Endotoxin has its major effect on the small blood vessels that have sympathetic innervation. Changes are initiated by the endotoxin's acting as a sympathomimetic agent when it combines with antibody and complement. Associated with arteriolar and venular spasm is stagnant anoxia and pooling of blood in the pulmonary, splanchnic, and renal capillaries. The same phenomena as with hemorrhagic shock occur; namely, water and sodium move into the cell, potassium moves out of the cell, aerobic metabolism decreases, and lactic acid increases. But the time sequence may be much quicker in septic shock than in hemorrhagic shock, because the decrease in the formation of adenosine triphosphate results in a decreased synthesis of proteins and immunoglobulins. At the cellular level, the local accumulation of acid produces a relaxation of the arteriolar sphincters, and blood pools in the capillary bed. Plasma leaks into the interstitial fluid because of the increased hydrostatic pressure (Fig. 44–2).

The hemodynamic responses to acute sepsis are complex and time dependent. If the septic insult is sudden and severe, venous return decreases secondary to pooling of blood and a preload dependent hypotension similar to that seen in hypovolemic shock occurs.

After the initial cardiovascular collapse, the characteristics of the circulation change. Arterial tone is reduced, but fluid resuscitation increases the cardiac output despite the low arterial pressures. This hyperdynamic sepsis is characterized by an increased oxygen delivery (DO_2), impaired oxygen extraction, increased lactic acidosis, and depressed ventricular function. Regulation of intraorgan blood flow may be severely impaired.

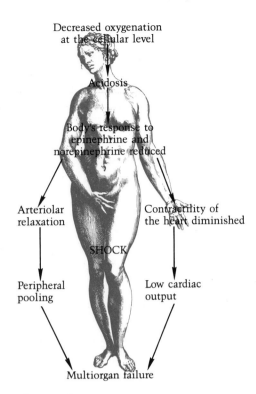

Figure 44–2
Shock syndrome with multisystem failure.

Cardiac Failure

When cardiac failure occurs is a matter of controversy. Some authorities say that cardiac failure occurs during the early or intermediate state of shock, and others say that it is terminal.[34] In any event, the decreased arterial pressure progressively depresses the myocardium, because it results in decreased coronary perfusion pressures and marginal blood flow. It is recognized that at some point pump failure is the chief hemodynamic problem and that decreased venous return (caused by the trapping of blood in the pulmonary and peripheral tissues) is not the chief hemodynamic problem.

The finding of several clinical studies of patients who did not have a pre-existing cardiopulmonary disease was that as the heart failed as a pump, high cardiac output changed to low cardiac output. High central venous pressures and decreased myocardial functioning occurred when left ventricular stroke work values were low. The relationship between the two was a function of time.[21]

Further myocardial depression is added to poor coronary perfusion by the action of the myocardial depressant factor (MDF) that is present in septic shock, as well as in other forms of shock.

Disseminated Intravascular Coagulation

Disseminated or *diffuse intravascular coagulation* (DIC) is a syndrome in which thrombin is generated and fibrin thrombi form within blood vessels, particularly within the microcirculation. As the coagulation cascade is activated, there is a simultaneous activation of the fibrinolytic, complement, and kinin systems. The rate of thrombin generation and the degree of activation of the fibrinolytic system determine the clinical signs.

It is generally accepted that DIC is an intermediary mechanism of disease that complicates the preexisting condition. Pathologic activation of blood coagulation and fibrinolysis results in the syndrome (Fig. 44–3). The primary problem is the generation of excess thrombin with resultant fibrin formation, ischemic tissue damage, and use of clotting factors and platelets. Once DIC occurs, consumption of platelets and clotting factors, plus the anticoagulant properties of fibrin split products (FSPs), creates a potential bleeding problem. The deposition of fibrin in small vessels blocks the capillary flow to organs, resulting in ischemic tissue injury. After the initial clotting and the resultant fibrinolysis, the repolymerization of fibrin and FSPs (paracoagulation) produces a secondary fibrin mesh in the small vessels. Red blood cells are damaged mechanically while they travel through the meshwork, resulting in schistocyte formation and a microangiopathic hemolytic anemia.

Excess Thrombin

Excess thrombin and clinical intravascular clotting may be produced in three ways: the endothelial wall may be injured by such factors as bacterial toxins and activation of the intrinsic clotting system, complement system, or plasmin and the kinin system; tissue injury may cause the release of tissue thromboplastin, activating the extrinsic pathway, and a combination of intrinsic and extrinsic system activation may be operational, as in hemolytic transfusion reactions, in which phospholipids released by the red blood cells indirectly set both pathways in motion. After the formation of excess thrombin, clotting factors are consumed and fibrin deposition occurs. The thrombi are particularly damaging to the microcirculation, and they may result in a consumptive coagulopathy.

Fibrin Formation

As a normal mechanism, the production of thrombin is essential in the conversion of fibrinogen to fibrin. Fibrinogen is composed of three paired chains, called alpha, beta, and gamma chains. Thrombin cleaves the alpha chain and then the beta chain, releasing fibrinopeptides (A and B); it activates factor XIII; and aggregates the platelets. What is left of the fibrinogen is named the *fibrin monomer* (a molecule of low molecular weight). The monomer combines with itself (or polymerizes) to form a gel. The gel is stabilized by factor XIII, forming cross-links between the gamma chains and the alpha chains. The end result is a stable fibrin clot.

As an immediate consequence of intravascular clotting, fibrinogen, platelets, and other coagulation factors are used, and fibrin is formed as small strands and clots. Vascular thrombosis and occlusion may occur at sites of localized trauma or resting sites of emboli. In particular, because circulating fibrin is phagocytized and cleared by reticuloendothelial cells in the liver and spleen, impairment of these cells may allow fibrin deposition in the microcirculation. Ischemic damage is probably seen in the kidney, adrenal glands, lung, liver, and skin.

Secondary Fibrinolysis

After intravascular clotting and fibrin formation, local fibrinolysis is evoked as a homeostatic compensatory mechanism in order to maintain the patency of the microcirculation. Such secondary fibrinolysis elaborates fibrinogen-fibrin degradation and FSPs, whose anticoagulant actions contribute to the severe hemorrhagic diathesis.

Activators act directly on plasminogen or they act on a proactivator in the plasma that in turn acts on plasminogen to produce plasmin (fibrinolysin), a proteolytic enzyme. Many substances that seem to be activators have been isolated from bacteria (streptokinase), urine (urokinase), and tissues, such as the prostate, pancreas, uterus, and, particularly, endothelial cells. Because plasmin is incorporated into the fibrin clot, it can digest the fibrin. Circulating plasmin can digest fibrinogen. Plasmin digests the same proteins that thrombin activates, and it causes fibrinolysis by enzymatically breaking fibrin into fibrin split products (FSPs). Initially, plasmin cleaves the alpha and beta chains of the fibrinogen molecule and later the gamma chains. The fragments (polypeptides) liberated are termed FSPs, and they are named X, Y, D, and E. Fibrinogen reacts with FSPs to form webs of abnormal FSPs and fibrin, which cause the hemolytic phase of the disorder.

Because FSPs are present, any one of several things may happen. The fibrin monomer may react with fibrinogen to form a soluble gel able to be stabilized by factor XIII. Or the

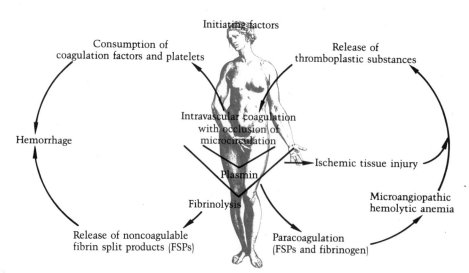

Figure 44–3

Disseminated intravascular coagulation. (Courtesy of James Smith, M.D.)

fibrin monomer may polymerize in the presence of some FSPs (fragments D and E), forming an unstable, abnormal, weak web, and it may react with other FSPs (fragments X and Y), forming unclottable complexes. Plasmin carries on digestion continuously; the products formed vary in size and in characteristics—from slowly clottable fragments to nonclottable fragments. Initially, fragment X is formed, which clots more slowly than fibrinogen but clots completely; further degradation of fragment X produces two nonclottable fragments, Y and D. Fragment Y inhibits the action of thrombin on fibrinogen, whereas degradation of fragment Y produces more D and E fragments, which inhibit the early stages of clotting.

The anticoagulant action of FSPs has been called *antithrombin VI*. Interference with hemostasis involves the following mechanisms[25]:

- Thrombin action is inhibited.
- Fibrin polymerization is inhibited.
- Abnormal polymers with a diminished tensile strength are formed.
- Fibrinogen-fibrin monomer-FSP complexes are formed.
- Thromboplastin generation is inhibited.
- Platelet functioning is inhibited.

Hematologic Abnormalities

Because red blood cells cannot travel through thrombosed vessels, secondary and imperfect fibrin strands from the combination of fibrin and FSPs must be formed before passage. During their movement through the fibrin meshwork, the red blood cells are injured mechanically. The result is a microangiopathic hemolytic anemia characterized by evidence of intravascular hemolysis and by the presence of fragmented red blood cells.

Depression of the platelet count may be caused by platelet use in the fibrin meshwork, adhesion at sites of damaged endothelial surfaces, and aggregation from the effects of endotoxin, thrombin, antigen-antibody complexes, particulate matter, and loose FSP complexes. Coagulation factors are depleted by the continuous formation of thrombi and fibrin. The syndrome is further complicated by anoxic tissue damage to the liver, which impairs synthesis of new factors.

Stress Ulcers

Since fiberoptic endoscopy has become widely used clinically, more patients have been studied and stress ulceration (acute gastroduodenal ulceration) has been better defined.[6] The lesions develop after an initial episode of gastritis. They are acute erosions that generally extend no deeper than the muscularis mucosa. However, the ulcers may also range from deep craters to full-thickness necrosis of the gastric wall (gastromalacia). The most common initial lesion is in the fundus of the stomach, with lesions in the antrum and duodenum occurring later. The amount of bleeding ranges from occult blood in the stool to massive hemorrhage.

Mechanism

The actual mechanism of the syndrome has not been defined. The syndrome is probably the result of a chain of events that involves many factors. The most plausible explanation is based on the concept that a severe stress may cause ischemia of the gastroduodenal mucosa. Because autonomic nervous system activity and circulating catecholamines may open submucosal shunts, the capillary bed of the mucosa would not then receive an adequate blood supply.[24] The resultant mucosal ischemia may be prolonged for hours to days. Increased mucosal permeability results, permitting acid back-diffusion to occur. (Hydrogen ions move into and out of the gastric lumen; the movement outward is named *acid back-diffusion*.) Increased back-diffusion of gastric acid through the gastroduodenal mucosa may contribute to the further disruption of the gastric mucosal barrier (and it may also be one of the reasons for the low initial net acid output). Recent work has shown that actively secreting mucosa is able to withstand the back-diffusion of hydrogen ions better than ischemic mucosa can. Further mucosal membrane damage may be produced by serotonin and histamine, vasoactive amines released from the degranulation of mast cells. Ischemia leads to hypoxia and to a plasma protein leak in the stomach. Regenerative ability in the mucosal cells decreases and focal necrosis results. It has been postulated that after the initial period there may be a period of increased parasympathetic stimulation that produces a relative hypersecretion of gastric acid caused by stimulation of the parietal cells. Most important, the submucosal shunts close and more blood flows through the capillaries of the gastroduodenal mucosa. Engorgement produces even more mucosal injury and necrosis. The result may be ulceration, bleeding, or perforation.

The adrenal corticosteroids formerly were thought to play a primary role, but now their role is a matter of controversy. It is not clear whether the secretion of gastric mucus is altered qualitatively or quantitatively (or both) by stress. Formerly it was thought that adrenocorticotropic hormone (ACTH) stimulated the hypersecretion of endogenous corticosteroids, which in turn altered mucous chemistry and glycoprotein. The result was loss of the mucous barrier. Factors such as hydrochloric acid and protein enzymes were then more easily able to injure the damaged mucosa.

The pathophysiology may differ in DIC. In DIC, ulceration may be the end result of acute thrombosis within the blood vessels of the gastric mucosa.

The pathophysiology does differ after central nervous system trauma. Patients with central nervous system trauma secrete excessive amounts of gastric acid. Because the hypersecretion is blocked by the administration of anticholinergic medication, the cause is probably parasympathetic stimulation. It is thought that increased intracranial pressure stimulates the vagal nuclei.

NURSING PROCESS

ASSESSMENT

The classic signs and symptoms of infection—redness, swelling, heat, and tenderness (pain to the touch)—are local responses. The wound itself may look purulent. Clinical manifestations of pneumonia include fever, leukocytosis, purulent tracheobronchial secretions, and a new infiltrate on chest x-ray examination. Assessment of the specific pulmonary infection is difficult because sputum and tracheal samples are frequently contaminated with organisms in the upper respiratory tract. Blood cultures are positive in only a small number of patients. Transtracheal and transthoracic aspiration samples do not yield correct data in the intubated patient on mechanical ventilation. Countercurrent immunoelectrophoresis is inadequate as a screening procedure.

The systemic signs of septicemia represent the total-body response to invasive infection. Objective physical signs may also be present, depending on the underlying disease. For example, in peritonitis the patient's abdomen may be board-like; the abdominal muscles are kept in a state of tonic contraction to keep the inflamed peritoneum from moving.

The principal cellular response to bacterial infection is polymorphonuclear. In general, the more severe the infection, the greater the leukocytosis. The appearance of immature granulocytes, particularly at levels above 85%, or more than 15 to 20 stabs in the differential count are highly indicative of infection. This decrease in the ratio of segmented neutrophils to nonsegmented neutrophils is usually termed a *shift to the left*. In severely ill patients or in the elderly, the white blood cell count may be normal or even low. The leukopenia probably reflects exhaustion of the leukocyte supply as well as depression of the bone marrow.

The sepsis syndrome can be defined in terms of a systemic response to infection expressed as tachycardia (>90 beats/ minute), fever (>101°F) or hypothermia (<96°F), tachypnea (>20 breaths/minute) and clinical evidence of inadequate organ perfusion or dysfunction such as: hypoxemia ($PaO_2 < 75$ mm Hg); elevated plasma lactate levels, oliguria (urine output < 0.5 ml/kg/hour) or altered cerebral function.[5] Blood cultures are only positive about 30% to 50% of the time; however, appropriate cultures of the sources may identify the specific invading microorganisms and determine the antibiotic sensitivities.

The early stage of sepsis is characterized by an increase in the cardiac output and in the blood flow to certain body parts, although there is shunting of blood at other sites (*e.g.,* the kidney and brain). The early stage may progress to septic shock (the second stage), which is characterized by a low cardiac output.

When any patient with fever and chills develops hypotension, oliguria, or tachypnea, septic shock should be considered. Even without hypotension, oliguria may be present, because oliguria may be the result of shunting of blood flow within the kidney. Other signs, such as acidosis, thrombocytopenia, or central nervous system changes without any apparent cause, may also be present with sepsis. Interestingly, because patients with bacteremia frequently also have volume depletion, it may be difficult to assess the primary problem in hypotension as being attributable to bacteremia or volume depletion.

Monitoring the patient includes the following:

- Neurologic status
- Tissue perfusion with arteriovenous oxygen differences; temperature, moisture, and color of skin; and the presence or absence of edema
- Vital signs, cardiac monitor, pulmonary artery measurements, and cardiac output
- Kidney function with measurement of hourly urine output and a creatinine clearance for assessment of glomerular filtration rate
- Respiratory status: breath sounds, chest movement, ABGs, compliance, secretions, chest x-ray films, and percent oxygen pressure needed.

A significant causative factor in the patient's death may be an underlying disease, in which the patient's normal host defense mechanisms may have been impaired. In such a case, the functioning of the polymorphonuclear leukocytes may be so severely diminished (because of disease or chemotherapy) that they lose their ability to kill bacteria because they cannot move toward the invading microorganisms, they cannot phagocytize, or they cannot produce hydrogen peroxide. Other important causative factors are the wrong choice of antibiotic for the initial treatment of sepsis and inadequate debridement or surgical drainage.

Septic Shock

The incidence of septic shock has increased in the last 10 years for the following reasons: more—and more serious— operations are being performed on elderly patients and poor-risk patients;[3] the incidence of severe trauma has increased;[12,19] the use of immunosuppressive drugs is widespread;[30] and the development of virulent antibiotic-resistant microorganisms has increased.[22]

It was once thought that gram-positive and gram-negative organisms produced different clinical syndromes, but it is now recognized that the infectious process is on a continuum and the clinical picture is dependent largely on the patient's volume status. From close observation of septic patients, MacLean and associates[21] have identified and described two hemodynamic patterns: the *normovolemic* pattern and the *hypovolemic* pattern. Essentially, the clinical status of the patient proceeds from a normal volume status and respiratory alkalosis to a decreased volume status and metabolic acidosis.

In patients who were normovolemic before the onset of sepsis or who are in early septic shock, the pattern is characteristic, but assessment remains difficult unless the staff is alert. The two most important clinical signs are the sensorium and the appearance of the skin. Basically, the patient's circulatory status is hyperdynamic (Fig. 44–4). Peripheral vasodilatation or A-V shunting increases the blood flow and results in an increased cardiac output. The body's demands are great, and the circulatory system is able to respond. Because of the vasodilatation, the patient has a low peripheral resistance and warm, dry extremities and may have hypotension. The high cardiac index shows a normal to increased blood volume, normal to high central venous pressures, and normal to high pulmonary artery pressures. However, high cardiac outputs and depressed cardiac functioning often are present at the same time. The hyperventilation and the resulting respiratory alkalosis ($PaCO_2$ of <25 mm Hg) are the hallmarks of the state. An even more altered sensorium, oliguria, and an elevated arterial lactate level indicate that the cardiac output must be increased. Control of the infection with surgical drainage and appropriate antibiotic therapy is of paramount importance.

In patients who are hypovolemic, the pattern is characterized by a hypodynamic circulation and by a clinical picture normally associated with shock (Fig. 44–4). The hypovolemia may be the result of sequestration of fluid in a third space loss (*e.g.,* in the bowel or in muscle tissue owing to poor tissue perfusion). Because of the vasoconstriction, the patient has a high peripheral resistance and cold, cyanotic extremities. The cardiac index is low, with a low central venous pressure and hypotension. Pulmonary artery pressures reflect the status of the

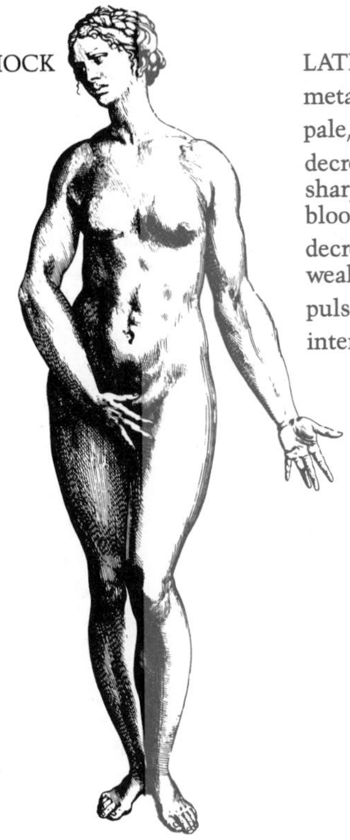

EARLY HYPERDYNAMIC SEPTIC SHOCK

increased respiratory rate

respiratory alkalosis

warm, dry, flushed, reddened skin

hyperglycemia and glycosuria

thrombocytopenia

full bounding pulse

normal or slightly elevated
blood pressure

increased pulse pressure

normal to slightly elevated
urine output

decreased arteriovenous
oxygen difference

increased cardiac output
2–3 times the normal

CVP normal or elevated

PaO$_2$ mildly decreased

low potassium

elevated WBC with a shift of the
differential to the left

lactate slightly elevated

urine sodium concentration less than
10–20 mEq/liter

LATE HYPODYNAMIC SEPTIC SHOCK

metabolic acidosis

pale, moist, cool skin

decreased cardiac output with a
sharp decrease in the urine output,
blood pressure, PaO$_2$

decreased pulse pressure

weak thready pulse

pulse markedly increased

interstitial edema

Figure 44-4
Septic shock.

left side of the heart. The hallmark of frank shock is metabolic acidosis. The temperature is usually very high or very low. With hypopyrexia of 95°F to 97°F, the body cannot generate a response, and a minimal reserve remains. The urinary output may remain elevated because of glycosuria (seen in trauma patients who have infections) or the catabolic state (associated with high nitrogen loads). Patients receiving parenteral nutrition often change from negative/negative to 3+/negative or 4+/negative on sugar acetone determinations when sepsis begins.

Disseminated Intravascular Coagulation

DIC may be difficult to assess, or it may be apparent from the clinical situation. Many patients have disturbances in their clotting mechanisms, but they do not bleed unless they are operated on or unless their underlying disease worsens and so precipitates the bleeding state. When they bleed, the bleeding is often obvious and dramatic. Many sites are involved, and usually the patients seem to bleed "all over." Bleeding may be noted after injections in the skin, from the wound, from the gastrointestinal or urinary systems, and from old puncture wounds. There are two primary clinical manifestations: hemorrhage and microvascular thrombosis.

The bleeding occurs diffusely from capillaries. Purpura is common, and less often petechiae may be seen. Clinical manifestations that suggest the presence of DIC follow[11]:

Subjective: Fatigue, malaise, weakness, myalgia, cold hands, abdominal tenderness, bone or joint pain, changes

in vision, palpitations, angina, headache, and vertigo

Objective: Petechiae or purpura, mild oozing (perhaps from a venipuncture site), pale or yellowed skin, peripheral thrombosis, cold mottled fingers and toes, sweating, scleral and conjunctival hemorrhage, yellow cast to eyes, change in respiratory function, tachypnea or orthopnea, tachycardia, murmurs, orthostatic hypotension, hemoptysis and increase in abdominal girth, change in mental status (*e.g.,* confused or irritable), and occult blood in urine or stool

The most common combination of diagnostic aids selected as a clotting profile are the platelet count, peripheral smear, fibrinogen level, prothrombin time, partial thromboplastin time, thrombin time, and various tests for the presence of FSPs. There are no pathognomonic tests; therefore, it is important to recognize patterns of diagnostic tests.

Thrombocytopenia is present when the platelet count averages 50,000 per mm^3 or less. The normal count ranges from 150,000 to 400,000 per mm^3. The presence of large platelets in the peripheral smear may reflect rapid use. Red cell fragments may be seen; they are indicative of damage inflicted on the cells while they traveled through secondary and abnormal soluble fibrin web. The absence of fragmented red cells in the peripheral smear may make the physician hesitant about the diagnosis.

A progressive decrease in fibrinogen levels occurs. If the levels have been elevated previously, a level within the normal range is considered positive. A normal value is greater than 150 mg%.

The prothrombin time is prolonged (normal values are determined for each laboratory, but the control time commonly is 11 seconds with a normal deviation of ±2 seconds). The extrinsic pathway is evaluated by the prothrombin time test.

The partial thromboplastin time is prolonged. The intrinsic coagulation system is evaluated by this test. Commonly, the control time is 22 to 37 seconds.

The thrombin time reflects the interaction of thrombin with fibrinogen. It is measured by the time needed to clot after thrombin has been added to the patient's serum. If the thrombin time is prolonged, the test plasma is diluted 1:1 with normal plasma, and the test is repeated to determine whether the problem is due to low fibrinogen levels or to the presence of circulating anticoagulants (*e.g.*, FSPs or heparin). If the thrombin time remains prolonged, this indicates the presence of FSPs that inhibit the action of thrombin and slowly produce an unstable fibrin clot. A normal value is a control of approximately 10 seconds with a deviation of ±2 seconds.

The presence of FSPs reflects secondary fibrinolysis. Paracoagulation tests, such as the *ethanol gelation* and *protamine sulfate* tests, are relatively simple to perform, and they are screening tests in that they measure precipitable, nonclottable complexes of degradation. When protamine sulfate and fibrin monomer–fragment X complexes react, the fibrin monomer is freed and able to polymerize. The measurement is expressed in terms of the degree of translucency of the resulting solution. Other tests are more specific, but they take more time. Thrombin may be added to the patient's plasma and the resulting serum examined for substances antigenic to fibrinogen. In the *staphylococcal clumping* test, bacteria clump in the presence of fibrinogen, fragment X, and fragment Y. A factor associated with the bacterial wall causes the clumping. The test is not as sensitive with fragments D and E. The *tanned red cell hemagglutination inhibition immunoassay* (the Mersky method) de-tects early and late degradation products and soluble fibrin monomer. Because red cells treated with tannic acid are conjugated to fibrinogen, antifibrinogen antiserum will produce agglutination. However, if FSPs were already present in the antiserum, the antiserum is neutralized, and it will not produce hemagglutination. The *Fi test* is similar in sensitivity to the Mersky method. Latex particles are coated with fibrinogen antibodies to that agglutination occurs if serum-containing fibrinogen fragments are added.

Stress Ulcers

Clinically, the problem of stress ulcers is often difficult to identify. Usually, the patient's presenting signs are hematemesis (the vomiting of gross blood) or melena (the passage of black tarry stools that contain digested blood or bloody nasogastric drainage.) Although usually reddish in color, the hematemesis may be dark because hemoglobin has been converted to hematin by hydrochloric acid.

Initially after a bleed, a rapid assessment of the hemodynamic parameters and circulatory status is conducted. Once the patient is hemodynamically stabilized, the physician employs endoscopy to identify the bleeding lesion.[33] Conservative measures are employed to arrest the bleed, but the physician will elect to intervene surgically if more than 1500 ml of blood must be transfused in 24 hours to maintain stable hemodynamics, or if persistent uncontrolled hemorrhage occurs.

NURSING DIAGNOSES, PATIENT OUTCOMES, AND PLAN

The preceding material on physiology, nursing assessment, and diagnostic tests guides the nurse in establishing nursing diagnoses, patient outcomes, and plan for the patient with multisystem organ failure.

NURSING CARE PLAN SUMMARY *Patient With Multisystems Failure*

NURSING DIAGNOSIS

1. *Impaired gas exchange related to altered circulatory volume, pulmonary interstitial edema, atelectasis, and decreased lung compliance (exchanging pattern)*

Patient Outcomes	Nursing Orders

1. The patient will exhibit signs of adequate gas exchange as evidenced by adequate respiratory rate and rhythm, adequate color, adequate arterial blood gases, normal breath sounds.	1. Identify and describe the mechanisms or factors that contribute to impairment in gas exchange
	  A. Monitor, assess, and record signs and symptoms of inadequate gas exchange:
	    (1) Inadequate rate, rhythm, depth of respiration, color, and level of consciousness
	    (2) Inadequate arterial blood gases
	    (3) Abnormal breath sounds. If breath sounds are not audible on the left side when the endotracheal tube is in place, it can be assumed that the

(continued)

NURSING CARE PLAN SUMMARY   *Patient With Multisystems Failure   Continued*

Patient Outcomes	Nursing Orders
	tube has slipped into the right bronchus. In this situation, the chest tube should be repositioned.

    (4) Abnormal chest x-ray film

B. Implement strategies according to either the physician's orders or standing unit policies to maintain or achieve adequate gas exchange. Maintain pulmonary hygiene and suctioning as indicated by the arterial blood gas measurements and the chest examination. Encourage inspiration. Give the patient 100% oxygen for 1 to 2 minutes before and after suctioning, and limit the suctioning to 15 seconds.

    (1) Institute procedures or routines that should be performed

        a. Keep the endotracheal tube and tubing secured and adequately supported.

        b. Use an oral airway to prevent the patient from clamping down on the endotracheal tube.

        c. Identify and correct any sudden abnormal functioning of the ventilator.

        d. Use deep sterile tracheal suctioning as needed.

        e. Reposition the patient frequently.

        f. Provide information and care to reduce the patient's anxiety and fear.

        g. Provide the patient with a method of communication.

        h. Remind the patient frequently to practice the relaxation techniques.

    (2) Institute procedures or routines that should be performed in the weaning period.

    (3) Institute procedures or routines that should be performed in the period immediately after extubation.

C. Monitor the adequacy of the oxygenation. Determine the relationship between the arterial oxygen tension and the inspired oxygen concentration. (On 100% oxygen a reading below 300 is low—the normal should be 350 to 500).

D. Monitor the inspired oxygen concentration. Positive end-expiratory pressure should be ordered if the arterial oxygen tension cannot be maintained at 60 mm Hg with an F_IO_2 of 50%.

E. Assess the adequacy of the respiratory status using the following criteria:

    (1) An arterial oxygen tension of above 80 mm Hg on 40% oxygen.

    (2) An A-a gradient of 50 to 200 mm Hg on 100% oxygen.

    (3) A respiratory rate of 10 to 20 breaths/minute.

    (4) A lung compliance of greater than 50 ml/cm H_2O.

    (5) An arterial carbon dioxide tension of 35 to 45 mm Hg.

    (6) A minute volume of less than 12 L/minute.

F. Note ventilator parameters.

    (1) Peak inspiratory pressure (<50 cm H_2O)

    (2) Exhaled volume less than 100 ml less than prescribed tidal volume

    (3) Positive end-expiratory pressure at preset level

    (4) FIO_2

2. The patient will have arterial blood gases within normal ranges on 40% oxygen (an F_IO_2 of 0.4).

2. Obtain and monitor serial arterial blood gas measurements as ordered:

A. By radial artery puncture:

    (1) Prepare ice slush and a heparinized syringe (as little heparin as possible should be left in the syringe).

    (2) Note the presence of collateral circulation by either:

        a. Obliterating the radial and ulnar pulses:

            (i) Have the patient open and close his or her hand until the palm is blanched.

           (ii) To note the return of the blood flow, observe the hand while the pressure on the ulnar artery is released.

        b. Compressing the radial artery at the wrist:

            (i) Ask the patient to open and close his or her hand several times and then relax the hand.

(continued)

NURSING CARE PLAN SUMMARY *Patient With Multisystems Failure*   *Continued*

Patient Outcomes	*Nursing Orders*
	(ii) Observe for transitory blanching of the palm followed by the return of circulation.
	(iii) Use the Doppler if it is available.
	(iv) If signs of ischemia persist, conclude that the circulation in the ulnar artery is inadequate.
	(3) Identify the point of maximum impulse of the radial artery.
	(4) Cleanse the site with Betadine and alcohol.
	(5) While palpating the artery, insert the needle with its bevel up at a 45° angle. (Blood will flow into the syringe when the artery has been entered.)
	(6) Expel the air, mix the blood, and put it in the ice slush.
	(7) Hold the site for 5 minutes.
	(8) Ascertain the presence of distal pulses.
	B. For brachial or femoral artery punctures, follow (3) to (8).
	C. By radial, femoral, axillary, brachial or temporal arterial line:
	(1) Prepare a 3-ml heparinized syringe and a 5-ml syringe.
	(2) Withdraw 5 ml of blood and discard it.
	(3) Withdraw a 1-ml specimen.

NURSING DIAGNOSIS

2. *Altered tissue perfusion related to vascular tone and circulating volume status (exchanging pattern)*

Patient Outcome	*Nursing Orders*
1. The patient should demonstrate an improved physiologic status as evidenced by monitoring parameters that follow:	1. Monitor for signs of improvement in physiologic status in the following areas:
A. Normal sensorium as evidenced by an ability to follow simple commands	A. Monitor the patient's mental status every hour, including orientation, response to verbal stimuli, and ability to follow commands.
B. Peripheral pulses full, strong, and regular bilaterally	B. Assess skin by inspection and touch frequently.
C. Urine output greater than 0.5 ml/ kg/hour	C. Monitor the patient's intake and output hourly.
D. Skin is warm and dry and the patient has pink mucous membranes	D. Monitor apical pulse and heart sounds as needed.
	E. Observe for signs of peripheral vasoconstriction and capillary refill time at least every hour.
E. Arterial blood pressure is stable with a systolic pressure 90 mm Hg but less than 140 mm Hg and a diastolic blood pressure 65 mm Hg but less than 90 mm Hg.	F. Monitor arterial pressure at least hourly. If you are using an arterial line to monitor the patient's blood pressure, be sure that it is set up and working correctly. Compare with cuff pressure for accuracy at least every 8 hours.
F. Arterial pH 7.35 to 7.45	G. Monitor the patient's oxygenation and ventilatory status frequently either by arterial blood gas analysis or by noninvasive means such as pulse oximetry and end-tidal carbon dioxide measurements.
	H. If the patient has a pulmonary artery catheter in place, measure pulmonary artery systolic, diastolic, and mean pressures, as well as central venous and pulmonary capillary occlusion pressures, at least every hour.
	I. Monitor and record intake and output hourly.
	J. Observe for bleeding frequently.
	K. Weigh patient every other day at the same time, or place patient on a bed with a built-in bed scale to monitor fluid gains and losses.
	L. Ensure that all laboratory specimens are drawn on time, and monitor the results.
	M. Monitor renal function at least daily including measuring urine electrolytes, specific gravity, blood urea nitrogen and creatinine levels, osmolality, and free water clearance.
	N. Use information from pulmonary artery catheter data to calculate left ventricular stroke work index and to plot a ventricular function curve (Fig. 44–8).
	O. Administer vasoactive drugs as ordered, and monitor their effects closely, including vital sign changes. (Refer to Chap. 17 for specifics on hemodynamic monitoring.)

(continued)

NURSING CARE PLAN SUMMARY *Patient With Multisystems Failure* Continued

NURSING DIAGNOSIS

3. *Altered fluid and electrolyte balance related to altered tissue perfusion and sepsis (exchanging pattern)*

Patient Outcome	Nursing Orders

1. The patient will demonstrate volume balance as evidenced by the following:
 	
A. The patient will have reduced or absent peripheral edema.
 	
B. Adequate urine output will be maintained.
 	
C. The patient will have normal electrolytes as measured in both the serum and the urine.
	1. Assess the following signs and symptoms of hypovolemia:
	    A. A decreased urinary output (<0.5 ml/kg/hour)
	    B. A decreased blood pressure
	    C. An increased pulse
	    D. Decreased central venous and pulmonary capillary occlusion pressures
	    E. A flattened arterial pressure curve
	    F. Apathy
	    G. A slow motor response
	    H. Nausea and vomiting
	    I. A decreased skin turgor
	    J. Weak, thready peripheral pulses
	2. Assess for the following signs and symptoms of hypervolemia:
	    A. A full, bounding pulse
	    B. Distended neck veins
	    C. A galloping heart rhythm
	    D. Loud heart sounds
	    E. An increased central venous pressure and pulmonary occlusion capillary pressure.
	    F. An increased cardiac output, rales, and any other signs of pulmonary edema.
	3. Assess for the following signs and symptoms of hyponatremia (water intoxication):
	    A. A decreased serum sodium level
	    B. Fingerprinting on the sternum
	    C. Oliguria
	    D. Increased tendon reflexes
	    E. Muscle twitching
	4. If the patient has hyponatremia (a sodium level of <130 mEq/L) and a volume deficit, prepare to administer sodium according to his or her acid–base status. In acidosis, a 6-molar sodium lactate solution is used, and in alkalosis, a normal saline solution is used.
	5. If the patient's serum sodium level is less than 120 mEq/L and the pH is alkalotic, prepare for the administration of a 5% sodium chloride solution. Monitor the patient for an improved clinical response. Look for the following:
	    A. An increase in mental alertness
	    B. An increase in the urinary output
	    C. A decrease in blood pressure (which was elevated)
	    D. An increase in pulse (which was slow)
	    E. The presence of deep tendon reflexes
	6. If patient has hyponatremia and a volume excess, consult with the physician about water restriction.
	7. If the hyponatremic patient is hyperglycemic, calculate the extracellular tonicity in order to anticipate the physician's order. Each 100-mg increment in the blood glucose level over the approximate normal of 100 mg of glucose per 100 ml of blood takes the place of 3 mEq/L of sodium. For example, a patient with a serum sodium concentration of 122 mEq/L and a blood glucose level of 600 mg/100 ml may have a decreased sodium level caused by hyperglycemia or by hyperglycemia plus hyponatremia. A glucose level of 500 mg above normal is roughly equivalent to 15 mEq/L of sodium in tonicity. Since 122 + 15 = 137 (normal extracellular tonicity), the problem is not only the serum sodium level. Depending on the clinical situation, treatment will be ordered to decrease the blood glucose level and, perhaps, to increase the serum sodium level.
	8. Assess for the following signs and symptoms of hypernatremia:
	    A. An increased serum sodium level
	    B. An increased pulse

(continued)

NURSING CARE PLAN SUMMARY   *Patient With Multisystems Failure*   *Continued*

Patient Outcome	*Nursing Orders*

C. Flushed skin

D. A decreased urinary output

E. Weakness

F. Dry, sticky mucous membranes

G. Restlessness

9. If the patient has hypernatremia (a sodium level of >150 mEq/L) and a volume deficit, prepare for the intravenous administration of a 5% solution of dextrose in water, a 0.45% sodium chloride solution, or 0.5% Ringer's lactate solution. The water loss may be caused by a fever, unhumidified air, or oxygen administered by an artificial airway, high-output renal failure, a decrease in antidiuretic hormone, a high protein intake without the administration of 7 ml of water per gram of protein, a high glucose administration, or osmotic diuretics.

10. Assess for the following signs and symptoms of hypokalemia:

A. Decreased potassium levels

B. Weakness to flaccid paralysis

C. Abdominal distention

D. Decreased to absent tendon reflexes

E. A flattened T wave and a depressed ST segment

11. If hypokalemia occurs, administer all fluids that contain more than 40 mEq/L through a controlled infusion device. If potassium is ordered to be administered at 20 mEq/hour or faster, monitor the patient's electrocardiogram continuously.

12. Assess for the following signs and symptoms of hyperkalemia:

A. An increased serum potassium level

B. Nausea and vomiting

C. Colic

D. Diarrhea

E. Peaked T waves

F. A wide QRS complex

G. A depressed ST segment

13. If the serum potassium level rises slowly, prepare for discontinuation of exogenous sources of potassium (*e.g.*, potassium penicillin). In many instances, Kayexalate, a cation-exchange resin, will be ordered (24 g in 200 to 250 ml of a 10% dextrose in water solution every 12 hours rectally).

14. If the serum potassium level rises suddenly, prepare for the intravenous administration of sodium lactate and calcium gluconate in 100 ml of a 50% dextrose in water solution over a 60-minute period. Insulin may also be ordered. The nurse should consult with the physician about plans for dialysis.

15. Assess for the presence of acidosis or alkalosis using the blood gas measurements.

16. Assess for the following signs and symptoms of hypocalcemia:

A. A decreased serum calcium level

B. Numbness or tingling of the fingers or the toes and the region around the mouth

C. Muscle cramps

D. Hyperactive tendon reflexes

E. Carpopedal spasms after inflation of the blood pressure cuff

F. Hyperirritability of the seventh cranial nerve

G. Palpitations

H. A prolonged QT interval

17. Assess for the following signs and symptoms of hypercalcemia:

A. An increased serum calcium level

B. Weakness and fatigue

C. Nausea and vomiting

D. Headache

E. Lumbar and flank pain

F. Thirst

G. An increased urinary output

(continued)

NURSING CARE PLAN SUMMARY *Patient With Multisystems Failure* Continued

Patient Outcome	*Nursing Orders*

	18. Assess for the following signs and symptoms of hypomagnesemia:
	  A. Muscle spasm
	  B. Hyperactive reflexes
	  C. Signs of tetany
	  D. A total-body magnesium deficiency (which may be present although the serum magnesium level is normal)
	19. Assess for the following signs and symptoms of hypermagnesemia:
	  A. Weakness
	  B. Lethargy
	  C. Decreased tendon reflexes
	  D. A prolonged PR interval
	  E. A wide QRS complex
	  F. Elevated T waves
	20. Assess the patient carefully, because he may have a mixed syndrome and the clinical picture may be a combination or a compromise of different signs.

NURSING DIAGNOSIS

4. *High risk for injury related to coagulopathy (exchanging pattern)*

Patient Outcome	*Nursing Orders*

1. The patient will be free from bleeding or bleeding tendency.	1. Monitor for and treat bleeding:
	  A. Monitor the laboratory tests for abnormal results.
	  B. Observe the patient for purpura, petechiae and bleeding from gums, venipuncture sites, wounds, gastrointestinal tract, and the genitourinary tract.
	  C. Avoid needle sticks or use a very small-gauge needle and apply pressure to the venipuncture site for 10 minutes.
	  D. Administer heparin as ordered.
	  E. Administer whole, packed red blood cells, fresh or frozen plasma, fibrinogen, platelets, and concentrates of clotting factors if ordered, and monitor the patient for any reactions to these products. A common protocol follows:
	    (1) Three units of platelets daily for a platelet count less than 10,000
	    (2) Two units of fresh frozen plasma every 6 hours
	    (3) Two units of packed red blood cells for a hematocrit of less than 28%
	    (4) Two units of cryoprecipitate every 6 hours for a fibrinogen level below 50 mg%
	  F. Administer all physical care to the patient gently to prevent bleeding.
	  G. Observe safety precautions to prevent bruising, such as padding the side rails and using an electric razor.
	  H. Promote rest for the patient.
	    (1) Assist with turning.
	    (2) Bathe patients.
	    (3) Plan rest periods.
	    (4) Administer mouth care frequently with swabs and gauze pads to prevent drying. Keep lips moist at all times.
	  I. Protect skin.
	    (1) Gently cleanse areas around wounds and invasive lines.
	    (2) Move patient gently with enough help to avoid shearing of the skin.
	    (3) Gently remove any tape.
	    (4) Inflate blood pressure cuff quickly and release quickly to avoid bruising.
	  J. Suction patient very carefully.
	  K. Place patient on a bowel regimen to avoid constipation and patient straining.
	  L. Monitor and estimate all blood losses.

(continued)

NURSING CARE PLAN SUMMARY   *Patient With Multisystems Failure*   *Continued*

NURSING DIAGNOSIS

5. *High risk for gastrointestinal bleeding related to gastroduodenal lesions (exchanging pattern)*

Patient Outcomes	*Nursing Orders*

1. The patient will be free of continuing gastroduodenal ulceration and hemorrhage.	1. Monitor vital signs, gastric aspirate, and stool.
	    A. Measure and record gastric pH every hour.
	    B. Administer antacids as ordered through nasogastric or orogastric tube.
	    C. Administer intravenous H_2 antagonists, such as cimetidine or rinitidine, as ordered. Monitor for side effects of these drugs, including dizziness, rash, muscle weakness and pain, diarrhea, and neutropenia.
	    D. Administer vitamin A if ordered. (Vitamin A is thought to increase the regeneration of gastric mucosal cells and the production of protective gastric mucus).
	    E. Monitor all gastric aspirate and stool for occult blood by performing a guaiac test at least every 4 hours.
	    F. If the patient bleeds severely, prepare for the replacement of blood. Perform heme test of the nasogastric aspirate and stool. Order tests of the prothrombin time and the partial thromboplastin time, and a platelet count according to the physician's order. Support the patient and help the physician during endoscopic and sigmoidoscopic examinations.
	    G. Be aware that if the bleeding is from a stress ulcer, the medical treatment will probably entail an iced saline lavage. If 3 U of blood need to be administered for replacement therapy, the specific diagnosis is usually made by an endoscopy or angiogram. The treatment entails vasopressin or embolization with fresh blood and platelets. If iced-saline lavage is ordered,
	        (1) Explain the procedure to the patient.
	        (2) Obtain baseline data about the vital signs and continue to monitor for cardiac dysrhythmias.
	        (3) Pass a large-lumen nasogastric catheter.
	        (4) Position the patient comfortably in the left lateral position.
	        (5) Increase comfort by administering sedatives and keeping the patient warm.
	        (6) Fill 100- to 150-ml syringes from a basin full of iced saline solution, inject the solution into a large lumen catheter (*e.g.,* an Ewald tube), and withdraw the solution. Repeat the procedure as indicated.
	        (7) Know that after the lavage is completed, an alkaline gastric drip may be ordered.
	    H. Administer vasopressin if ordered.

2. Stress ulceration and hematemesis will be prevented.	2. Prevent ulceration and hematemesis.
	    A. Measure the gastric pH every hour.
	    B. Discuss the following protocol for gastric alkalinization with the physician and implement as ordered. Institute protocol for prophylactic antacid titration:
	        (1) If the nasogastric tube is not in place, administer antacid orally every 2 hours.
	        (2) If the nasogastric tube is in place,
	            a. Aspirate the stomach and record the pH.
	            b. Instill 10 ml antacid and 30 ml water into the nasogastric tube and clamp the tube.
	            c. After 1 hour, aspirate the stomach and record the pH.
	            d. If the pH is equal to or greater than 4.0, apply intermittent suction or drainage and repeat the cycle.
	            e. If the pH is less than 4.0, instill 20 ml antacid and 30 ml water and clamp the tube. Wait 1 hour:
	                (i) If the pH is equal to or greater than 4.0, apply drainage or intermittent suction for 1 hour and repeat the cycle.
	                (ii) If the pH remains less than 4.0, instill 40 ml antacid and 30 ml water and clamp the tube. Wait 1 hour. If the pH is equal to

(continued)

NURSING CARE PLAN SUMMARY *Patient With Multisystems Failure* *Continued*

Patient Outcomes	*Nursing Orders*
	or exceeds 4.0, follow (a). If the pH is still less than 4.0, instill 80 ml antacid and 30 ml water.

C. As ordered, administer intravenous cimetidine (a 300-mg bolus every 6 hours). Dilute it in a 20-ml volume and inject it over a 1- to 2-minute period. Monitor for dizziness, rash, muscle pain, diarrhea, and neutropenia. Notify the physician of any signs or symptoms.

D. Institute nursing measures to prevent respiratory and septic complications and to maintain nutrition.

E. Administer vitamin A if ordered.

F. Remember that the following common techniques may be used:
   (1) Gastric alkalinization
   (2) Removal of the septic source
   (3) Intragastric cooling
   (4) Intragastric levarterenol therapy
   (5) Intraperitoneal levarterenol therapy
   (6) Selective arterial vasopressin therapy
   (7) Selective arterial epinephrine and propranolol therapy
   (8) Systemic hypothermia

NURSING DIAGNOSIS

6. *Sleep pattern disturbance related to multi-environmental stimuli and acute care environment (moving pattern)*

Patient Outcome	*Nursing Orders*
1. The patient will be able to sleep for protracted periods of time and will be free of the signs and symptoms of sleep deprivation.	1. Assess the patient's normal sleeping pattern:

1. Assess the patient's normal sleeping pattern:
   A. Bedtime routine
   B. Sleeping hours
   C. Sleeping environment
   D. Ease in getting to sleep and in staying asleep
   E. Factors that might help if a sleeping problem arises

2. Include in the nursing care plan a plan for sleep and rest periods, and tell the staff about it.

3. Offer the patients simple explanations about their care and answer questions. Clarify any misconceptions they may have because of comments they heard during rounds or at another patient's bedside.

4. Establish trust and encourage the patients to sleep by assuring them that the staff will monitor their condition.

5. Have a presleep routine, even if only a simple one (*e.g.,* change the patient's gown).

6. Keep the ventilation adequate and the temperature comfortable.

7. Provide an environment that is conducive to sleep:
   A. Be sure the lights are dim.
   B. Keep extraneous noises to a minimum.
   C. Provide a clock in the room.
   D. Make sure that the sheets are clean and straightened.
   E. Help the patient assume a comfortable position.
   F. Give the patient a back rub.
   G. Use other measures to decrease pain.

8. Observe the patient for the following signs and symptoms of sleep deprivation:
   A. Fatigue
   B. Irritability
   C. Increased sensitivity to pain
   D. Burning eyes
   E. Difficulty in focusing
   F. Shortened attention span

(continued)

NURSING CARE PLAN SUMMARY *Patient With Multisystems Failure*   *Continued*

Patient Outcome	*Nursing Orders*
	G. Behavioral changes (*e.g.*, mild euphoria or apathy)
	H. Time disorientation
	I. Slurred speech
	J. Decreased muscle coordination
	K. Mild tremor
	9. Awaken the patient only for essential treatments.
	10. Monitor the patient's sleep. If there is a sleeping problem, help as follows:
	A. Try to determine the cause of the problem (*e.g.*, does the patient need to have someone present?).
	B. Increase comfort by changing the patient's position or giving a back rub.
	C. Provide ear plugs if the patient wants them.
	D. Alleviate hunger.
	E. Give warm milk.
	F. Decrease anxiety about getting to sleep.
	G. Administer an analgesic or a sedative as ordered.

NURSING DIAGNOSIS

7. *High risk for infection related to immunosuppression and invasion of microorganisms (exchanging pattern)*

Patient Outcomes	*Nursing Orders*
1. The patient should show no signs or symptoms of infection.	1. Carry out the policies of the hospital's infection control committee.
	A. Wash hands thoroughly before and after changing dressings, after any contaminating procedure, and between caring for different patients. Washing the hands with soap and water and using mechanical friction for at least 15 seconds will remove most bacteria.
	B. Maintain aseptic conditions in the environment.
	C. Use an iodine-based agent as the major topical cleansing solution.
	D. Assist with the debridement procedure.
	E. Follow specific protocols for dressing changes and invasive devices.
2. The patient's urine should remain sterile.	2. Take steps to care for the patient with a catheter.
	A. Explain the purpose and functioning of the Foley catheter to the patient.
	B. Insert the catheter by using aseptic technique (an iodophor solution should be used for periurethral cleansing, the catheter should be the right size, and sterile drapes, sponges, gloves, and lubricant jelly should be used).
	C. Maintain a closed drainage system. Do not disconnect the drainage tube and the catheter.
	D. Maintain the patency of the drainage system (check the tubing for kinks). Do not let the tubing hang below the level of the bag.
	E. For male patients, tape the catheter to the lower abdomen to prevent tension and irritation. For female patients, tape the catheter to the thigh.
	F. Keep the collecting bag below the level of the bladder at all times.
	G. Check the drainage every 2 to 3 hours for color and consistency.
	H. Keep the patient's perineum clean. Remove the secretions. Cleanse the area around the catheter with an antiseptic soap solution.
	I. Report any complaints of burning or irritation to the physician promptly.
	J. Do not routinely change Foley catheters that have been in place less than 2 weeks. Change them when sediment accumulates or when the catheters malfunction.
	K. If irrigation of the catheter is ordered, use sterile equipment and discard it after use.
	L. Unless hospital policy dictates otherwise, do not send the catheter tips routinely for culturing; the correlation between positive catheter-tip cultures and subsequent urinary tract infections is poor.
	M. If possible, do not put catheterized patients in adjacent hospital beds.

(continued)

NURSING CARE PLAN SUMMARY *Patient With Multisystems Failure   Continued*

Patient Outcomes	*Nursing Orders*

<table>
<tr><td></td><td>

N. If a urine specimen must be collected, do not break the closed drainage system. Use the following protocol (or one similar to it):
(1) Wash hands.
(2) Clamp the Foley catheter until 2 to 10 ml of urine has accumulated (5 to 10 minutes).
(3) Clean the distal portion of the catheter below the Y with Betadine or alcohol.
(4) Using a sterile syringe, insert a 25-gauge needle bevel at a 45-degree angle below the Y and remove the amount of urine needed.
(5) Observe for leakage.
(6) Unclamp the catheter.
</td></tr>
</table>

3. The patient should demonstrate control and eradication of the septic source.

3. Continue to observe all measures for prophylaxis as above.
  A. Before antibiotic treatment is started, obtain specimens of blood, urine, sputum, and wound exudates for bacteriologic culturing and sensitivity studies.
  B. Administer antibiotics as ordered. Monitor for effectiveness and toxicity.
  C. Observe and record the parameters for monitoring an infection site (*e.g.,* in regard to sputum, urine, or a wound).
  D. Monitor the systemic parameters that indicate an escalating infection (*e.g.,* tachypnea, altered sensorium, respiratory alkalosis, decreased cardiac output, increased or significantly decreased white blood cell count, shift to the left, or positive cultures).
  E. Place a precaution notice about body discharges (sputum, urine, blood, feces, and spinal fluid) on the nursing Kardex when resistant organisms are present.
  F. Monitor the wound for any signs and symptoms of dehiscence (Fig. 44–7). This is most common between the fifth and twelfth postoperative days, but it may occur for up to a month. The patient may have felt something give inside the suture line or some serosanguineous fluid may be seen draining from the wound.
  G. Monitor for signs of gram-negative septicemia.
  (1) Pulmonary signs: hyperventilation, hypoxia, respiratory alkalosis, and the adult respiratory distress syndrome
  (2) Renal signs: oliguria with or without hypotension, renal failure, and reduced renal clearance rates
  (3) Neurologic signs: confused or obtunded (a change in orientation is a cardinal sign)
  (4) Cardiac signs: chest pain, abnormal ST-T wave, normal to high cardiac output (in early sepsis), and decreased cardiac output with cyanosis (in late sepsis)
  (5) Metabolic signs: respiratory alkalosis, hyperglycemia and hyperlipidemia in early sepsis, and acidosis with increased blood lactate levels in late sepsis
  (6) Hepatic signs: elevated serum glutamic oxaloacetic transaminase (SGOT) level
  (7) Gastrointestinal signs: diarrhea
  (8) Hematologic signs: leukocytosis with toxic granulation, shift to the left, vacuolation, Döhle's bodies, leukopenia (occasionally), thrombocytopenia (in septic shock), and altered C3, C5, C6, and C9 levels.

4. The patient who is in shock associated with infection should demonstrate improvement in septic and hemodynamic status.

4. Take the following steps:
  A. In conjunction with other health team members, determine the cause of the shock:
  (1) Hypovolemia
  (2) Pump failure
  (3) Anaphylaxis
  (4) Neurogenic causes
  (5) Blood flow impediments
  (6) Adrenal crisis
  (7) Sepsis

(continued)

NURSING CARE PLAN SUMMARY   *Patient With Multisystems Failure*   *Continued*

Patient Outcomes	Nursing Orders
	B. Administer oxygen or assisted ventilation as ordered.
	C. Obtain and send for culturing a minimum of two samples from separate venipuncture sites and samples from other appropriate sites.
	D. Place a urethral catheter and monitor the hourly urinary output (it should be at least 0.5 ml/kg/hour).
	E. Administer volume expansion therapy (Ringer's lactate solution challenge) as ordered.
	F. Anticipate that the physician may perform a paracentesis or a lumbar puncture and order abdominal x-ray film, liver and spleen scan, sonography, or computed tomographic (CT) scan.
	G. Observe the data gathered from previous cultures and sensitivity studies.
	H. Administer antibiotic(s) as ordered. Learn the drug characteristics, monitor for nephrotoxicity and ototoxicity as appropriate, and obtain antibiotic blood levels as ordered.
	I. Monitor the arterial blood gases for decreased arterial oxygen levels and for metabolic acidosis.
	J. Administer corticosteroids as ordered.
	K. Avoid chilling. (A temperature blanket may be ordered to keep the patient's temperature at normothermic levels.)
	L. Administer vasoactive drugs if ordered.
	M. Administer cardiotonic drugs if ordered.
	N. Administer sodium bicarbonate for a pH of less than 7.36 if ordered.
	O. Monitor urine output > 0.5 ml/kg/hour. If the urine output is decreased, notify the physician.
	P. Assist with drainage of any abscesses.

NURSING DIAGNOSIS

8. *Ineffected individual coping related to critical illness and the critical care environment (choosing pattern)*

Patient Outcomes	Nursing Order
1. The patient will appear to be handling the stress of the illness by demonstrating appropriate emotional reactions.	1. See Nursing Diagnosis: Ineffective Individual and Family Coping, p. 112.
2. The patient will participate in his or her care as illness permits.	

NURSING DIAGNOSIS

9. *Anxiety related to diagnosis, illness, isolation, hospitalization, and fear of death (feeling pattern)*

Patient Outcome	Nursing Orders
1. The patient will verbalize anxiety and fears.	1. See Nursing Diagnosis: Anxiety, p. 111.

IMPLEMENTATION AND EVALUATION

Administration of nursing care must be comprehensive and conscientious. Patient and family education are an integral part of all aspects of care (Fig. 44–5). The body–mind–spirit of the patient must be conceptualized constantly, so that the patient is not called or thought of, for example, as "the gas-

trointestinal bleed in bed 4." Technical details of care are essential, and the nurse must be knowledgeable of the psycho-pathophysiologic processes going on in the patient. The mental and spiritual as well as the physical aspects of care must all be dealt with in an organized plan of care. The patient must be cared for as an integrated whole. The nurse–patient rela-

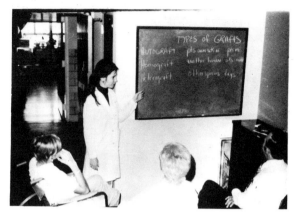

Figure 44–5

Family education is an integral part of nursing.

tionship is never a neutral event (Fig. 44–6). Refer to Chapters 1 through 4 for more details.

Sepsis and Septic Shock

Current therapy for the prevention of sepsis and sepsis-induced multisystem organ failure is aimed at supportive care, because no definitive treatments have been proven to be beneficial.[20] Rapid and effective management of sepsis appears to be a means of controlling organ failure.[30] Secondary infection, hypotension, and hypoxemia only exacerbate the organ system dysfunction. Eradication of the source of the infection or necrosis is fundamental to preventing further stimulation of the systemic inflammatory response to the sepsis.

In attempting to prevent sepsis, surgical patients are generally treated freely with antibiotics.[3] It has been recommended that trauma patients should not receive routine antibiotic prophylaxis unless there is a contaminated wound.[14] If contaminated wounds are present, the antibiotic therapy is usually begun in the emergency department. Alexander and Alexander[2] demonstrated that the concentration of antibiotics appeared more promptly in the wound fluid when the drug was first administered by intravenous push. Sustained high therapeutic doses were achieved most easily by intravenous infusions of the antibiotics chosen. An infectious disease consultation should be arranged promptly at the first sign of any infection to ensure that the appropriate treatment and antibiotic regimen is being used.[3]

Unless the results of cultures and sensitivity studies are available, orders for antibiotic coverage are often for both aerobic and anaerobic organisms. The combination of a penicillin and an aminoglycocide is most commonly ordered.[37] The choice of drug depends on the result of previous cultures, the tissue or organ involved, the circumstances of the injury, the normal flora of the environment, and the resistance patterns. Once the results of cultures and sensitivity studies are available, the specific antibiotics are ordered.

Monitor the wound(s) for any signs of dehiscence (Fig. 44–7). This is most common between the fifth and twelfth postoperative days, but may occur up to a month postoperatively. The patient may describe feeling something give inside the suture line, or serosanguineous drainage may be noted draining from the wound.

The treatment of septic shock centers on its early recognition, the restoration of normal hemodynamics, the identification of

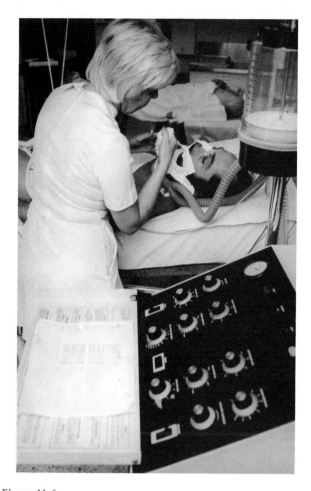

Figure 44–6

The nurse must care for the patient's body–mind–spirit. The nurse–patient relationship is never a neutral event.

the septic source, the removal of the seeding source, and the appropriate antibiotic therapy.[15]

Restoration of the Circulating Blood Volume

Restoration of an effective circulating blood volume and correction of the disturbances in the peripheral circulation are of primary importance in the treatment of the shock state. The patient may suffer from vasoconstriction or from vasodilatation, but with early sepsis, the patient suffers from peripheral vasodilatation. The vascular tree is dilated and the amount of circulating fluid must be increased to fill the vascular spaces. Sequestration of plasma and extracellular fluid (the third space loss) increases the patient's fluid requirements. Replacement therapy involves the use of crystalloid and colloid solutions, plasma, and blood.

Ringer's lactate solution is usually chosen for volume replacement therapy initially. Trauma patients are more likely to be hypovolemic and should be resuscitated with volume. The ideal resuscitation fluid has yet to be defined. The choice between crystalloids and colloids and deciding which type to use are presently a matter of personal preference. Resuscitation techniques with hyperosmolar saline therapy show significant promise for the future in improving cellular function.[32]

Fluid management generally is aided by monitoring of intravascular pressure and cardiac function. Indwelling arterial

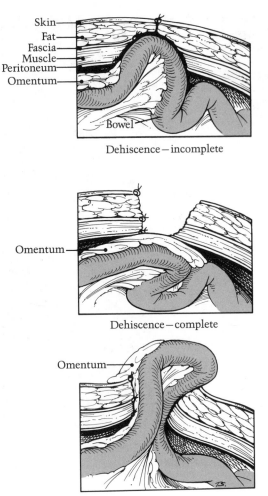

Figure 44–7
Abdominal wound dehiscence. The force on the wound is greater than the tensile strength of the wound. With incomplete dehiscence, there is separation of the fascial and muscular layers. With complete dehiscence, all layers of the abdominal wall separate. Complete dehiscence may be associated with evisceration of abdominal viscera.

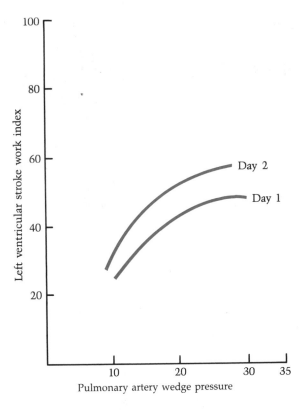

Figure 44–8
Ventricular function curve. Left ventricular stroke work index is plotted as a function of pulmonary artery wedge pressure. In this particular patient, the graph shows the improvement in ventricular function from day 1 to day 2.

catheters are routinely employed to monitor arterial pressure, and pulmonary artery catheters allow for the measurement of central venous and pulmonary artery occlusion pressures (Fig. 44–8). Vasopressor agents such as dopamine, dobutamine, norepinephrine, and epinephrine are effective in maintaining arterial pressure and provide some improvement in selected regional blood flow.

The vasoactive drugs are extremely useful in treating the cardiovascular effects of septic shock, but they all have some problems in clinical use. The vasoactive drugs used initially were the vasopressor or vasoconstrictor drugs that increased pressures but not perfusion. The drugs that were used next were the vasodilators, such as isoproterenol. Unfortunately, vasodilators increase the total-body perfusion, but skeletal muscle is the primary beneficiary of the increased cardiac output rather than the brain, heart, kidney and intestines. The perfusion of vital tissues is improved by the reduction of arteriolar resistance in vital organs, the augmentation of perfusion pressures, the increase of cardiac output, and the prevention of the deleterious effects of underperfusion.

In patients in septic shock who have had a myocardial infarction, a balance must be maintained between the increased myocardial perfusion and the increased oxygen demand of the heart. The choice of drug depends on the needs and condition of the specific patient.[34]

Most of the drugs used act on the sympathetic nervous system or the cells innervated by the sympathetic nervous system. The baroreceptors respond to any event that lowers blood pressure for whatever reason. The sympathetic nerve centers in the hypothalamus are activated through the ninth and tenth cranial nerves. The results are increased epinephrine secretion in the adrenal medulla, increased cortisol production in the adrenal cortex, and increased norepinephrine secretion in the sympathetic norepinephrine endings. Sympathomimetic drugs may act directly on the receptor sites, or they may act indirectly by releasing norepinephrine from the adrenergic nerves. Conceptual structures (called alpha and beta receptors) are used to describe changes that occur in the precapillary and postcapillary arterioles and venules. Alpha-receptor stimulation by epinephrine and norepinephrine produces arteriolar and venular vasoconstriction that results in reduced capillary perfusion. Alpha-adrenergic responses are excitatory responses (except for intestinal inhibition), and they promote vasoconstriction and pupillary dilatation. Of particular importance are the receptors in the blood vessels perfusing the skin and mucosa. Beta-receptor stimulation produces vasodilatation in the vasculature of striated muscle and myocardium, resulting in an increased rate and force of cardiac contraction (a positive chronotropic effect and a positive inotropic effect, respectively).

The beta response mediates vasodilatation, bronchodilatation, and most metabolic responses. B_1 is the designation given to the myocardial beta receptor, and B_2 is the designation given to the vascular and bronchodilatation beta receptor.

Vasoactive drugs are used to treat patients whose blood pressure is too low for perfusion of the heart and the brain and patients whose blood pressure is high enough to permit cardiac and cerebral perfusion of the heart and the brain but whose blood flow to the viscera (in particular, the mesenteric and the renal vascular beds) is significantly reduced. The drugs that act directly on the alpha receptors contract both arterioles and veins with little specificity. The drugs that act indirectly activate both alpha and beta receptors and can be used to affect the functioning of the cardiovascular system by stimulating the beta receptors causing increased heart rate, myocardial contractility, and peripheral vasodilatation, and by stimulating the alpha receptors used to increase peripheral resistance.

Dopamine is the most commonly used drug in septic shock, producing beta stimulation of the heart, alpha stimulation of the peripheral circulation, and vasodilatation of the cerebral, coronary, mesenteric and renal circulation. It is an endogenous catecholamine, the precursor of norepinephrine and a metabolite of L-dopa. The drug's important selective vasodilatation effect is due to its action on the dopamine receptors. The total blood flow, as well as the cardiac output and the blood pressure, is increased. The specific action is dependent on the dose administered in small doses (1 to 2 μg/kg/minute) to dilate renal and mesenteric arteries (the dopaminergic effect). Cholinergic alpha or beta blockers do not have this effect, but phenothiazines diminish the effect. In intermediate doses (2 to 20 μg/kg/minute), the drug's beta-adrenergic effects are equivalent to those of norepinephrine, epinephrine, or isoproterenol. The mean arterial pressure usually stays at the same level because of the increased strength of the cardiac contractions. The cardiac output continues to increase, as does myocardial contractility and renal blood flow. Tachyarrhythmias are potential complications, but they occur infrequently. In very high doses (greater than 20 μg/kg/minute), dopamine has an even greater alpha-receptor effect, causing vasoconstriction to reverse the vasodilatation of the renal and mesenteric arteries.

Dobutamine strongly increases the force of myocardial contraction to increase cardiac output. As the ventricles eject more forcefully, the chambers empty more completely; consequently, the improved force of contraction lowers the left ventricular filling pressure and relieves pulmonary congestion to some degree. The dosage of dobutamine is titrated from 2 to 20 mgm/kg/minute to achieve the desired hemodynamic effect. One advantage of using a combination of dopamine and dobutamine is that less fluid volume is needed to sustain a high cardiac output.

Norepinephrine acts as a vasoconstrictor in the peripheral circulation because of its direct action on the alpha receptors in the arteries and veins, and it acts as a cardiac stimulator because of its direct action on the B_1 receptors. The cerebral and coronary vessels dilate, but the renal and the splanchnic vessels, as well as the vessels in the skin and the muscles, constrict. The potential for renal failure is significant. The drug must be given by a central venous catheter, because the local vasoconstriction it causes in an extremity is severe enough to lead to amputation. Even though the myocardium is stimu-

lated, the cardiac output does not necessarily increase. The peripheral vasoconstriction is so intense that the heart slows reflexly and thus the cardiac output is decreased. On the other hand, if the patient is in severe shock, his blood pressure may not be increased above normal levels, but his cardiac output increases.

Epinephrine acts directly on the B_1, B_2, and alpha receptors. The myocardium is stimulated, and the vessels in the skeletal muscles and the mesentery dilate. In accordance with the response expected from alpha stimulation, the vessels in the skin and the kidney vasoconstrict. As in the fight-or-flight response, the blood flow increases, many areas of the body vasodilate, the peripheral resistance decreases, and the cardiac output increases.

Isoproterenol is a nearly pure stimulant of the beta receptors. It produces inotropic and chronotropic cardiac stimulation; vasodilatation, particularly in the blood vessels of the skeletal muscles; and bronchodilatation. The cardiac output increases while the blood pressure stays the same or diminishes slightly. Although isoproterenol has a vasodilating effect, it is not selective in the intestines and kidney. The total-body vasodilatation produces a decrease in the perfusion pressure that may decrease the blood flow to these key organs at any time. The increase in the myocardial work produces an increase in the myocardial oxygen consumption that is satisfactory only as long as the increased work produces increased perfusion of the total body, including the heart. The drug may improve significantly the cardiac output of patients whose pulse is slow. Tachycardia from the drug's chronotropic effect is a distinct possibility, and the pulse must be monitored and maintained below 120 to 130 beats/minute. Dysrhythmias and hypotension are also potential complications with this drug. The most effective way to administer the drug is to start with doses of 0.15 to 0.6 μg/minute and titrate the dose up until the desired effect is obtained.

Newer agents have been introduced that alter blood flow distribution by reversing paradoxical vasoconstriction in the vascular beds. These drugs, such as prostacyclin and prostaglandin E_2 (PGE$_2$), have been shown to increase both cardiac output and DO$_2$ in critically ill patients by decreasing afterload.[30] These drugs are limited in what they can do and cannot be used if the patient is hypotensive. More research is needed into the use of these agents in the treatment of septic shock and the prevention of multisystem organ failure.

Supportive Measures

Oxygen administration is often needed to keep the arterial PaO$_2$ between 80 and 100 torr. The risk of pulmonary failures in these patients is significant, and the patients will probably require mechanical ventilation. Several new modes of mechanical ventilation and positive end-expiratory pressure (PEEP) have been introduced in recent years. These include: pressure support devices, inverse ratio ventilators, and high-frequency jet ventilators. The type of ventilator chosen depends on the respiratory status of the patient and his oxygenation needs.

Nutritional and metabolic support of the patient is essential in the support of all organ systems, especially in patients with multisystem organ failure. Hypermetabolism develops early in the syndrome, and severe malnutrition can become a prominent feature within the first few days. The characteristics of the hypermetabolic state include: increases in resting energy expenditures and oxygen consumption, profound catabolism with an associated decrease in total body protein synthesis, and glucose intolerance. During this time an excess administration of glucose can lead to hepatic steatosis and hyperosmolar coma.

The goal of nutritional support in patients with organ failure is to prevent substrate limited metabolism and to support the hypermetabolism.[30] Nutrition should be provided by the enteral route if possible. Improved support can be achieved by decreasing the caloric and glucose loads and by increasing the protein load. Intravenous fat emulsions should be included to reduce the problems of excess glucose administration and to prevent essential fatty acid deficiencies. Branched chain amino acids are also recommended in these patients.

Disseminated Intravascular Coagulation

Because DIC is an intermediary mechanism resulting from some underlying disease, treatment of the underlying disease (if it can be treated) abolishes the coagulopathy. The primary treatment of DIC is first aimed at the underlying disease.

Treatment of DIC can be complex because the three problems—thrombosis, fibrinolysis, and hemorrhage—usually occur simultaneously. There is universal agreement with regard to some aspects of treating DIC. Adequate therapy includes pharmacologic support of the patient. Heparin therapy is used occasionally and is believed to be the most effective when major thrombic problems develop.[11] Heparin is thought to interrupt the intravascular generation of thrombin and to prevent further deposition of fibrin in the microcirculation. This is usually the only time that heparin is administered to a bleeding patient. Heparin is contraindicated if gastrointestinal or central nervous system bleeding occurs. When heparin is used, the patient's level of antithrombin III is measured, because an adequate amount of this factor is needed for the heparin to be effective.

Other pharmacologic agents may be used in the treatment of DIC. Platelet inhibitors, such as dipyridamole and aspirin, may be ordered. In some instances, aninocaproic acid (Amicar) is used to reverse systemic fibrinolysis.

Blood and blood component therapy is often necessary in DIC. Some sources caution that this carries with it a risk of causing further clotting in the microcirculation.[11] In general, the more a patient is bleeding, the more blood and components are necessary to replace the lost volume and restore hemostasis. Cryoprecipitate, fresh frozen plasma, and platelets are administered in addition to red cells to add active clotting components.

More controversial treatments such as exchange transfusions and plasmapheresis may be used in DIC. These procedures are thought to remove fibrin degradation products and to supply fresh clotting components.[11]

Stress Ulcers

Prophylaxis is the most important aspect of the management of stress ulcers. In the haste of initial management, the patient and family may fail to answer questions correctly about past gastrointestinal disturbances. It is important for the primary nurse to elicit pertinent information and ensure that the physician is notified of any GI history.

Antacids and the use of H_2 antagonists are the mainstays of prophylaxis.[31] Buffering the gastric pH at 5 or greater is the simplest and most effective prophylaxis.[13] Intravenous administration of H_2 antagonists, such as cimetidine and ranitidine, seems to have reduced significantly the incidence of GI bleeding in patients with septic shock.[24]

If bleeding does occur, endoscopy can be used to locate the source or sources of the bleeding and to coagulate them. Surgery may also be necessary to stop massive, persistent bleeding. Because gastrectomy carries an overall mortality as high as 50% in the critically ill patient, surgery must always be weighed against a more conservative approach.[7]

SUMMARY

Multisystem failure is a sequential process often terminating in the patient's death. In order for the patient to be saved, all efforts of the health care team must be focused on the patient's recovery and the prevention or alleviation of complications. By knowing and anticipating the potential pitfalls, nurses may assist in the return of the patient to a productive life.

Sepsis is the most formidable complication facing the patient in a critical care unit today. Early recognition of sepsis can prevent the onset of multiple system organ failure. Careful assessment of all patients and a well-defined nursing care plan addressing the needs of the total patient can be successful in preventing organ failure from occurring.

DIRECTIONS FOR FUTURE RESEARCH

The patient in multisystem failure is a challenge in nursing care. Complication after complication intervenes. All members of the health team must collaborate and work effectively together to try to save the patient's life and prevent any disabilities. Only through further unraveling of the many details of patient care will nurses continue to improve the impact they make. Several suggestions for areas of systematic investigation follow:

1. Increased technological environment: How do the sophisticated equipment and procedures affect patients and families?
2. Sleep deprivation: How can it be prevented? How can sleep and rest be balanced with activity?[40]
3. Sepsis: How can it be prevented or at least minimized? How often should intravenous tubing and dressings be changed? What type of ointment should be used at the interface between invasive devices and their entrance into the patient? How should stopcocks be handled? Should cardiac output injectate be cooled, or should only room temperature solution be used?
4. Monitoring: What patient positions affect central venous pressure, pulmonary artery pressures, and cardiac output? How long can the balloon be wedged? Where and how should blood samples be obtained?
5. Anxiety and pain: How can biofeedback best be used? What are the criteria for patient selection? What is the effect of biofeedback?[26]
6. Patient education: How much and for how long do critically ill patients remember? When should patient education be started? What should patients be taught? How do medications and anesthetics affect learning?

REFERENCES

1. Albert, R. K. and Comdie, F. Hand-washing patterns in medical intensive care units. *N. Engl. J. Med.* 304:1466, 1981.

2. Alexander, J. W. and Alexander, N. S. The influence of route of administration on wound fluid concentration of prophylactic antibiotics. *J. Trauma* 16:488, 1976.

3. Altemeter, W. A. Sepsis in surgery. *Arch. Surg.* 111(2):107, 1982.

4. Baue, A. E. Multiple progressive or sequential systems failure. *Arch. Surg.* 110:779, 1975.

5. Bone, R. C., Fisher, C. J., Clemmer, T. P., et al. Sepsis syndrome: A valid clinical entity. *Crit. Care Med.* 17:389, 1989.

6. Cheving, L. Y. Treatment of established stress ulcer disease. *World J. Surg.* 5:235, 1981.

7. Cody, H. S. III and Wichern, W. A., Jr. Choice of operation for acute gastric mucosal hemorrhage: Report of 36 cases and a review of literature. *Am. J. Surg.* 134:322, 1977.

8. Czaja, A. J., McAlhany, J. C., and Pruitt, B. A., Jr. Acute gastroduodenal disease after thermal injury: An endoscopic evaluation of incidence and natural history. *N. Engl. J. Med.* 291:925, 1974.

9. Dhingra, O., Schauerhamer, R. L., and Wangansteen, O. H. Peripheral dissemination of bacteria in contaminated wounds; role of devitalized tissue. Evaluation of therapeutic measures. *Surgery* 80:535, 1976.

10. Dorowitz, L. G., Wenzel, R. P. and Hoyt, J. W. High risk of hospital-acquired infection in the ICU patient. *Crit. Care Med.* 10: 355, 1982.

11. Dressler, D. K. Disseminated intravascular coagulation. In K. T. VonRueden and C. A. Walleck (eds.), *Advanced Critical Care Nursing: A Case Study Approach.* Rockville, MD: Aspen Publishers, 1989.

12. Faist, E., Bave, A. E., Dittmar, H., and Herberer, G. Multiple organ failure in polytrauma patients. *J. Trauma* 23:755, 1983.

13. Hastings, P. R., Sillman, J. J., Bushnell, L. S., and Silen, W. Antacid titration in the prevention of acute gastrointestinal bleeding: A controlled randomized trial in 100 critically ill patients. *N. Engl. J. Med.* 298:1041, 1978.

14. Hoyt, N. J. Infection and infection control. In V. D. Cardona, P. D. Hurn, P. J. Bastnagel-Mason, et al. (eds.), *Trauma Nursing: From Resuscitation Through Rehabilitation.* Philadelphia: W. B. Saunders, 1988.

15. Hruska, J. F. and Horick, R. B. Treatment of infection in septic shock. In R. Cowley (ed.), *Pathophysiology of Shock, Anoxia, and Ischemia.* Baltimore: Williams & Wilkins, 1983.

16. Kaye, W. Catheter and infusion related sepsis: The nature of the problem and its prevention. *Heart Lung* 11:221, 1985.

17. Keene, A. R. and Cullen, D. J. Therapeutic intervention scoring system. Update, 1983. *Crit. Care Med.* 11:1, 1983.

18. Larson, D. E. and Farnell, M. B. Upper gastrointestinal hemorrhage. *Mayo Clin. Proc.* 58:371, 1983.

19. Littleton, M. T. Complications of multiple trauma. *Crit. Care Nurs. Clin. North Am.* 1:75, 1989.

20. Macho, J. R. and Luce, J. M. Rational approach to the management of multiple systems organ failure. *Crit. Care Clin.* 5:379, 1989.

21. MacLean, L. D., Mulligan, W. S., McLean, A. P. H., et al. Patterns of septic shock in man: A detailed study of 50 patients. *Ann. Surg.* 166:543, 1967.

22. Maki, D. G. Epidemic nosocomial infections. In E. P. Wentzel, et al. (ed.), *CDC Handbook of Hospital Acquired Infections.* Boca Raton, FL: CRC Press, 1981.

23. Maki, D. G., Alvarado, C. J., Hassimer, C. A., and Zilz, M. A. Relation of the inanimate hospital environment in endemic nosocomial infection. *N. Engl. J. Med.* 307:1562, 1982.

24. McAlhanny, J. C., Czala, A. J., and Pruitt, B. A. Antacid control of complications from acute gastrointestinal disease after burns. *J. Trauma* 16:645, 1976.

25. McKay, D. G. Trauma and disseminated intravascular coagulation. *J. Trauma* 9:646, 1969.

26. Miller, N. E. and Dworkin, B. R. Effects of learning on visceral functions—Biofeedback. *N. Engl. J. Med.* 296:1274, 1977.

27. Olson, M., O'Connor, M., and Schwartz, M. L. Surgical wound infections. *Ann. Surg.* 197:253, 1983.

28. Parker, N. P., Schubert, W., Shelhamer, J. H., and Parrello, J. E. Perceptions of a critically ill patient experiencing therapeutic paralysis in an ICU. *Crit. Care Med.* 12:69, 1984.

29. Pierce, A. K., Sanford, J. P., Thomas, G. D., et al. Long-term evaluation of decontamination of inhalation therapy equipment and the occurrence of necrotizing pneumonia. *N. Engl. J. Med.* 282:528, 1970.

30. Pinsky, M. R. and Matuschak, G. M. Multiple system organ failure: Failure of host defense homeostasis. *Crit. Care Clin.* 5:199, 1989.

31. Priebe, H. J., Skillman, J. J., Bushnell, L. S., et al. Antacid versus cimetidine in preventing acute gastrointestinal bleeding: A randomized trial in 75 critically ill patients. *N. Engl. J. Med.* 302:426, 1980.

32. Prough, D. S., Johnson, J. C., Stulken, E. H., et al. Effects on cerebral hemodynamics of resuscitation from endotoxin shock with hypertonic saline versus lactated Ringer's solution. *Crit. Care Med.* 13:1040, 1985.

33. Rahn, N. H., Tishler, J. M., Han, S. Y., and Rossinovich, N. A. E. Diagnostic and interventional angiography in acute gastrointestinal hemorrhage. *Radiology* 143:361, 1982.

34. Rice, V. Cardiogenic shock. In K. T. VonRueden and C. A. Walleck (eds.), *Advanced Critical Care Nursing: A Case Study Approach.* Rockville, MD: Aspen Publishers, 1989.

35. Singh, S. S., Nelson, N., Acosta, L., et al. Catheter colonization and bacteremia with pulmonary and arterial catheters. *Crit. Care Med.* 10:736, 1982.

36. Stamm, W. E., Martin, S. M., and Bennett, J. V. Epidemiology of nosocomial infections due to gram-negative bacilli: Aspects relevant to development and use of vaccines. *J. Infect. Dis.* 136 (Suppl.):5151, 1977.

37. Summer, W. R., Michael, J. R. and Shepsky, J. P. Initial aminoglycoside levels in the critically ill. *Crit. Care Med.* 11:948, 1983.

38. Tobin, M. J. and Grenvik, A. K. E. Nosocomial lung infection and its diagnosis. *Crit. Care Med.* 12:191, 1983.

39. Weil, M. H. and Rackow, E. C. Critical care at the crossroads. *Emergency Med.* 16:6, 1984.

40. Williams, R. L. and Jackson, D. Problems with sleep. *Heart Lung,* 11:262, 1982.

41. Zinner, M. J., Tuidema, G. D., Smith, P. L., and Silen, W. The prevention of upper gastrointestinal bleeding in patients in an intensive care unit. *Surg. Gynecol. Obstet.* 153:214, 1981.

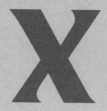

X

The Critically Ill Adult With Selected Problems

COMBINING THERAPIES

Do you believe that it is acceptable to combine therapies when needed? Some critical care practitioners believe that only orthodox drugs, surgery, and irradiation are acceptable and that the use of "holistic" or "spiritual" therapies is not. It is true that the holistic therapies can be taken to the extreme. It is not uncommon today for persons to believe that it is a sign of moral or spiritual ineptness to consent to surgery for appendicitis. This attitude can lead one on an endless search for a magical cure that lies outside traditional medicine (i.e., "If only I could find the right diet, the best meditation, the correct imagery sequence, or the most powerful healer!"). This attitude is expressed in many ways. It can block the experience of wholeness and the complementary nature of various forms of therapy. The fact is, many therapies work, and in critical care we should not categorically cut off any of them. Perhaps it is true that the natural, less invasive methods are preferred, if in fact they have been proven to be effective. Both the spiritual/psychologic and physically oriented methodologies can work. One can reap enormous benefits from being aware of spiritual, emotional, and physical methods, as developed in Chapter 1 in eras of medicine and throughout Unit 1.

45

Immunosuppressed Patients

Barbara Giordano

FORGIVENESS

Learning to live from love requires that you learn to forgive yourself. Forgiveness is an exercise in compassion that is both a process and an attitude.* Forgiving self and others may be seen as a parallel six-step process. The six steps to *forgiving yourself* are as follows:

1. Take responsibility for what you did.
2. Confess the nature of the wrongs to God, yourself, and another human being.
3. Look for the good points.
4. Be willing to make amends where possible, as long as you can do this without harm to yourself or other people.
5. Look to God (or a higher power) for help.
6. Inquire about what you have learned.

The six steps to *forgiving others* are as follows:

1. Recognize that you are responsible for what you are holding onto.
2. Confess your story to yourself, another person, and God.
3. Look for the good points in yourself and the other person.
4. Consider whether any specific action needs to be taken.
5. Look to God (or a higher power) for help.
6. Reflect on what you have done.

These steps for forgiving self and others take time to complete. As the awareness of forgiving self and others is developed, the more we recognize unconditional love.

LEARNING OBJECTIVES

After reading this chapter, the nurse should be able to do the following:

1. Outline the three tasks of the immune system.
2. List the mechanisms operational in the immune response.
3. Compare and contrast nonspecific and specific immune responses.
4. Identify the major elements in the nursing and medical management of a patient with an altered immune response.
5. List the advantages of using humor as a strategy to strengthen the whole person.
6. Describe the process of using humor to reduce tension and anxiety.

* Borysenko, J. *Guilt Is the Teacher, Love Is the Lesson.* New York: Warner Books, 1990: 173–187.

CASE STUDY

Reason for Hospitalization

Heide P. is a 26-year-old Hispanic woman who is admitted from clinic for workup of herpes vulvitis resistant to her present treatment of oral acyclovir.

History of Present Illness

She is known to have been human immunodeficiency virus (HIV) positive since July 1988; she was exposed to a husband who is HIV positive; Ashley, her 18-month-old daughter, was also diagnosed as being HIV positive in July 1988.

In December, 1988, herpes vulvitis initially was diagnosed and treated with oral and topical acyclovir. The patient's herpes recurred about 5 months before this visit, and it did not respond to oral acyclovir. She described the herpes as persisting, and within the past 2 weeks pain from the enlarging lesions had increased.

In clinic the patient was described as having mild left popliteal tenderness with left leg pain radiating from the buttocks to the back of the thigh.

Physical Examination and Review of Systems

Temperature 37°C, pulse 100, respirations 20, blood pressure 100/70, height 5'3", weight 90 lb.

General

Slim woman, lying in bed in mild distress, cooperative, and responds appropriately

Skin

Essentially intact; large left vulvular ulcerated lesion 4 × 5 cm, without any discharge. No ecchymotic areas noted, no history of easy bruising or bleeding

ENT

Mild thrush; pharynx noted to be reddened; PERRLA, conjunctiva pale, sclera anicteric, reports decreased vision. Left ear history of otitis, which was successfully treated with antibiotics

Neck

Sebaceous cysts; no adenopathy, nonpalpable thyroid

Breasts

No masses

Heart

S_1S_2; no complaints or history of palpations or angina. Sleeps on one pillow; dyspnea on exertion after climbing three flights of stairs.

Lungs

Clear, no history of asthma, SOB, *Pneumocystis carinii* pneumonia, tuberculosis, hemoptysis, night sweats, or nonproductive cough

Abdomen

Soft to palpation, normal bowel sounds; occasional nausea, no diarrhea, constipation, melena, changes in bowel habits, peptic ulcer disease, dysphagia; has hemorrhoids

Genitourinary Tract

No dysuria, nocturia, urgency or frequency of urination, no unusual appearance or unusual or strong odor of urine

Frequent menses; workup of pelvic mass by ultrasound identified adnexal cyst, right renal cyst, increasing echogenicity of kidney is consistent with early parenchymal disease. There is no change in BUN/Cr (8/.6). Abnormal Pap smear 6 months ago. Colposcopy was inconclusive, missed follow-up appointments.

Extremities

2(+) Pulses bilaterally; negative Homan's sign; negative cord; no popliteal tenderness. Patient did complain of intermittent pain from buttocks down posterior thigh.

Social History

H.P. is unemployed and has been married 5 years to the same man, a former intravenous substance abuser. She does not drink alcoholic beverages or smoke cigarettes and she has no history of drug use or abuse. She lives in a three-room apartment with mother-in-law, husband, and one child. All are aware of the HIV situation.

The patient is adopted. She does not know who her natural parents are. The adopted family lives in Cleveland, Ohio. She graduated from high school in Ohio and after graduation moved to this city. She worked as a secretary in a large company for 4 years, quitting when her husband first became sick.

Psychoneurologic History

Neurologic

Alert and oriented, she does not report difficulty with memory: "I always write things down." She reports no seizures or self-described depression. She has decreased ambulation during herpes flare-ups. Cranial nerves I through XII are intact.

Psycho-Social

1. Do you want to live to be 100?

   I want to, but right now I just want these herpes to heal.

2. What happened to you in the year or two before today?

   So much has happened to me in the past year, year-and-a-half—none of which, I should add, was good. But out of all this I think I've become a better person; at least I haven't fallen apart, I still have a family.

   I knew my husband was [HIV] positive 2 years ago and I was prepared for what would happen to him, but I never thought it would happen to me or to [our daughter] Ashley. I found out that we were both [HIV] positive 6 months ago, and since that time first my husband was admitted (to another hospital) for PCP, and now Ashley's (in this hospital) on the pediatric unit being treated for PCP, and now she's been diagnosed as having MAI [*mycobacterium avium–intracellulare*].

   When I found out about the diagnosis, it knocked my socks off, but my mother-in-law was and is very helpful. She's really been great, but now that my husband's been readmitted (to another hospital) with a fever and with Ashley's still being in the hospital, I've been running back and forth visiting both of them. I'm exhausted. I can't do it any more. It's too much.

   The AIDS [acquired immunodeficiency syndrome] coalition spent 3 days with my husband, daughter, and mother-in-law, following us around to show what happens to a family. I went down to Washington when the film was first shown.

   It's really been hard, but I have good friends, family, and especially my mother-in-law.

3. What does this admission mean to you?

   It means I have to start taking care of myself. I've lost 14 pounds in the past 2 weeks running back and forth between the two of them. I can't let myself get run down like this again. I can't do it all, and I can't afford to lose weight. That bothers me.

4. Why do you need this admission?

   I need to get better. I need to get my acyclovir five times a day without fail. I need to gain weight. My husband, daughter, and mother-in-law have got to understand that.

5. What are your hobbies?

   Coloring, talking to my friends, needlework.

6. What is your normal sleep pattern?

I have to get 8 hours per night. I'm a grouch when my sleep's interrupted for too many nights.

7. Can you identify your stress patterns?

I have the usual daily hassles . . . but now all of us are in the hospital at the same time.

Past Medical History:

Allergies: Penicillin causes rash, Tylenol
Operations: None, three abortions
Infections: No hepatitis or tuberculosis
              Herpes
Medications: AZT 200 mg orally three times a day
              Acyclovir 400 mg orally five times a day
              Pentamidine by inhalation one time a month

Summary: Case Study

This is a 26-year-old Hispanic female with an opportunistic infection (thrush) as well as 5-month history of herpes vulvitis, who is now admitted for intravenous acyclovir.

Medical Problem List:

1. Herpes vulvitis: Acyclovir 400 mg IV five times a day for 10 days, viral cultures pending
2. Secondary vulvular infection: treat with ciprofloxin 750 mg orally twice a day, clindamycin 600 mg IV every 6 hours for 10 days; vancomycin 250 mg orally every 6 hours for 10 days
3. Pain management: codeine 30 mg orally every 4 hours as needed, 2% viscous lidocaine topically to vulvular lesions; bacitracin ointment to vulvular lesions; warm soaks to Bartholin's cyst; acyclovir (Zovirax) ointment to rectal lesion; Anusol suppository rectally as needed
4. Thrush: Nystatin 5 ml swish and swallow
5. HIV (+): Continue AZT and pentamidine.
6. Orthostasis: Stable BUN/Cr; tonight hydrate with normal saline intravenously.
7. Abnormal Pap smear and colposcopy: gynecologic consultation
8. Rule out deep vein thrombosis with Doppler ultrasound studies.
9. Weight loss and diarrhea: Potassium supplementation; encourage fluids by mouth; loperamide (Imodium) 2 mg

Medical Diagnosis

The patient has herpes vulvitis and thrush.

Nursing Diagnosis

1. Alterated skin integrity: predisposition to secondary infection related to disease process and neutropenia
2. Altered protection: development of opportunistic infection related to disease process
3. Altered comfort related to genital herpes
4. High risk for ineffective coping, forced dependency, immobility, and social isolation related to genital herpes
5. High risk for maladaptive coping: anxiety and loss of autonomy related to hospitalization and disease process

REFLECTIONS

Stress is an elusive thing to describe, yet it is an integral part of everyone's life. No matter how stress is described, it is always considered to be "out there." Stress is not one person, place, thing, or group of persons, places, or things; it is really a cognitive process of attaching meaning to whatever the senses detect by associating, comparing, and contrasting present perceptions with information stored in memory.[9,38,46] Thus, the mind creates mechanisms to deflect, deny, or distort any source of anxiety.[38]

The emergence of human immunodeficiency virus (HIV) and acquired immunodeficiency syndrome (AIDS) exposes hidden weaknesses and evokes stress in both patients and health care workers. The diagnosis of AIDS is a catastrophic event. It is insidious. It can infect the young and the healthy. It can usurp the person's vital body fluids and infiltrate itself into the cell's genetic material where the virus can lay dormant for years, waiting to emerge into a fatal illness at any time. AIDS is 100% fatal.

For the patient, each new symptom, infection, loss of weight, or fatigue may herald progression of the disease.[25] The patient becomes fearful, preoccupied with the illness, and fanatically hypochondriacal about each and every bodily function.

Because a person is an open system, a psychobiological unit integrated with the environment, any interruption in the normal functioning of one part would affect the other parts to varying degrees. In this open system, mind, body, and spirit never react separately; whatever assaults one lessens the wholeness, health, and well-being of the unit. Thus, a physical illness is not only physically disruptive, but it also has secondary implications for job, role, and economic security, and it subsequently creates anxiety of the spirit.[44]

The relationship between a person's mental attitude and emotional make-up and the development and outcome of an illness is intriguing. A patient's feelings of well-being and his or her affect, particularly depression, are believed to influence not only the outcome of disease but also the vulnerability of the individual to developing an illness.

The influence of the psychic "toxicity" of giving up or bereavement on the psychobiological unit is one of inference. Seyle's description of the general adaptation syndrome and the knowledge that chronic stress frequently produces hormonal imbalances and suppresses the immune system suggests a condition of biological vulnerability of the occurrence of illness.[9,56] Illness may be an adaptive attempt or a nonadaptive consequence of unresolved object loss.[9] Therefore, the critical care nurse must become proficient in accurate assessment, diagnosis, and treatment of maladaptive coping.[44] An important component in achieving such care is the attitude and response of the medical and nursing staff to the patient.

For the nurse, fear of AIDS is exaggerated by our social and cultural values, which attach symbolic meaning to illness.[17,41] AIDS is a modern affliction that is morally and literally contagious because of the stigma attached to the behaviors associated with exposure to the virus. Coupled with its association of sex, drugs, blood, and death is that there is no cure, and it is poorly understood. Fear of contagion seizes all of us at one time or another.

AIDS is clearly a deadly and legitimately frightening disease. This fear should spur the nurse to reconsider her knowledge about the disease and its mode of transmission as well as her emotional response to the disease.[23,24] Once the nurse manages her fear by gaining information, she is able to recondition herself to be more reasonable and less emotional.

As the symbolic meaning of the disease melts, the patient becomes a person rather than a diagnosis in the nurse's eyes. The nurse is prepared to assist the patient to see that he or she is not powerless or a victim, but, in spite of stress, is capable of coping successfully. The nurse can then assist the patient to acquire new capabilities for change by creating a positive reinforcing cycle with a new mental state. This process has its ups and downs. Even with a renewed desire and a different perception of the self and of the problem, times are difficult. Temporary setbacks may arise until the person feels confident enough to cope with the situation. Once this occurs, the patient must then unlearn present coping mechanisms and choose to use a different set of coping mechanisms. By doing this, the patient no longer assumes the victim stance but learns a different set of expectations about life events that prove that there is hope. It is at this time that the person also evaluates the meaning of events in life. The person can no longer put distance between himself or herself and the problem just by marking time and not expecting anything out of life and living.

Serious illness or the prospect of death does not represent a solution, an exit, or a postponement of a problem, but it can be used to gain a new perspective on problems. The primary nurse who behaves calmly and quietly and conveys a genuine interest in the patient's welfare can help with the concrete tasks of problem solving. The nurse helps the patient to redirect and refocus thinking.

Before the mind can function effectively enough to engage in problem solving, its tensions must be relieved by learning to calm itself and to minimize distractions to create a favorable environment for the job of receiving inner messages. One of the tools the nurse can use with the patient is the stress reduction techniques of humor.

PHYSIOLOGY

The bone marrow, considered as one single tissue, is the largest tissue in the body, approaching the size and weight of the liver. The marrow is divisible into two sections: the vascular and the adipose parts. The vascular part is the system that supplies nutrients and removes wastes from the activity of cell growth; the adipose tissue is responsible for blood cell formation. Together, the vascular tissue and the adipose tissue compose approximately one-half the weight of the bone marrow. The remaining half is where the eythrocytes, platelets, granulocytes, lymphocytes, and monocytes arise from the primitive, undifferentiated hematopoietic stem cells, which differentiate to the precursors for each cell line. Normally, the activity of the bone marrow is in a ratio of 3:1 for the production of white cells to red cells. This difference in production of cells may be a reflection of the importance of white blood cells to health and the fact that the average life span of the WBC is shorter than that of the red blood cell.

The immune system is composed of two functional units: lymphocytes and the mononuclear phagocytes. The lymphoid system is subdivided into two functional units, the T cells and the B cells, and contact with antigens may trigger either or both divisions of the system. The phagocytic division is composed of the reticuloendothelial system, which may be sub-divided into those cells that are macrophages and those cells that are microphages. From closer scrutiny, the phagocytic system is composed of fixed and wandering cells (*i.e.*, macrophages and microphages), which sequester, kill, or contain the microorganisms that would otherwise engulf higher organisms. In addition to this scavenger function, the phagocytic system performs an important sanitation function by cleaning up debris from old or damaged cells.

Lymphoreticular System

One of the ways the body preserves its integrity is by the activation of the lymphoreticular system (*i.e.*, the lymphocytes and phagocytes) into a spectrum of cellular and humoral events that comprise the nonspecific and specific immune responses. The nonspecific immune response is activated at each exposure to a foreign substance and encompasses the processes of phagocytosis and inflammation. Although the nonspecific immune response mechanisms can differentiate between self and nonself, it cannot identify a specific invader. As a result, the immune system nonspecifically responds in the same way to any foreign invader, regardless of the invader's antigenic composition. The specific immune response goes one step beyond recognizing self from nonself antigens by responding in a manner unique to each antigen's composition. The two forms of the specific immune responses are humoral immunity and cell-mediated immunity.

The cellular factors responsible for the nonspecific immune responses are the macrophages or monocytes, the microphages or polymorphonuclear leukocytes or granulocytes, the platelets, and the lymphocytes. The cellular factors responsible for the two forms of the specific immune response are T-lymphocytes and B-lymphocytes. The origin of each one of these cells is from the pluripotent, hematopoietic stem cells that are found within the bone marrow, the fetal liver, and the yolk sac of the fetus.

Composition of Lymphoreticular System

Cells belonging to a system usually share a common origin, morphology, and function, as well as being localized in one or more morphologic compartments. The term *mononuclear phagocyte* is the most appropriate designation for an entire cell unit that belongs to a system that is large, widely circulated, heterogeneous, and highly diversified, yet it is possible to group these highly phagocytic cells, along with the precursor cells, into one system. The mononuclear phagocytic system (MPS) is composed of cells—the monocytes of the circulating blood and the macrophages found in the various tissues of the body—that are widely scattered throughout the body where they accomplish their function of engulfing and removing foreign and effete materials from the blood, lymph, and tissues.

Monocytes and Macrophages

As with all the cells of the immunologic system, the cells of the MPS arise from the stem cell in the bone marrow. After differentiation and maturation, the monocytes are delivered to the general circulation, where they constitute a mobile pool of relatively immature cells ready to head to the tissues where they acquire the necessary tools for phagocytosis.

The second group of cells, the macrophages, are highly specialized cells that are widely distributed and can eliminate foreign materials and debris from the blood, lymph, and tissues.

Macrophages are capable of at least three immune-related activities:

1. They are the garbage collectors of the body, as well as being the garbage disposals of damaged or effete cells, neoplastic cells, colloidal materials, macromolecules, and cell debris. The macrophage is a potent phagocyte, playing a crucial role in clearing and degrading foreign substances within the body as well as removing damaged or dying cells and cell debris.
2. They are able to ingest and digest many types of organisms without requiring specific immunologic assistance from the lymphoid system. Yet, like the lymphocyte, the macrophage also undergoes activation to become maximally efficient. One way the macrophage's activation occurs is by the release of stimulatory soluble substances, lymphokines, by antigen-activated lymphocytes.
3. They interact with lymphocytes in a two-way fashion. The macrophage presents the antigen to the lymphocytes in such a way as to elicit a maximal immune response by both direct surface-to-surface contact and then the release of numerous humoral factors, called lymphokines, which amplify cell-mediated immunity.[11]

Lymphokines, a group of hormone-like substances that mediate cellular immunity, have the ability to influence macrophage behavior, composition, metabolism, and functional status. Although the action of lymphokines is nonspecific, once a sensitized lymphocyte is appropriately challenged by an antigen to release a lymphokine, the response is specific. The lymphokines may be considered to be the communicators within the immune system, because they transmit information among and between cells.

A distinction must be made between the macrophage and the lymphocyte concerning antigen specificity. The macrophage responds in a nonspecific fashion in that any macrophage deals with a given antigen in much the same way as it does with any other antigen. At the present time, it appears that while the macrophage is not capable of distinguishing between self and non-self, there are certain controls limiting the macrophage's response against self components. Clearly, the macrophage does not devour its host. On the other hand, the lymphocyte displays a particular antigenic specificity and is capable of discriminating between self and non-self components.

There is no one rationale to explain the process of immunogenicity. Instead, the following two factors seem to be correct: the antigen's binding to the macrophage may protect the antigen from catabolism, and the macrophage presents the antigen to the lymphocytes in such a way that the induction of the immune response is maximized.[11]

Microphages

The microphage group is composed of three types of granulocytic cells: neutrophils (or polymorphonuclear leukocytes or polys or PMNs), eosinophils, and basophils. Although the microphages are more numerous than the macrophages, the phagocytic activity and powers of the microphage are much less than those of the macrophages.

Neutrophils

Neutrophils phagocytize ingested organisms in two ways: the first is by an increase in the cell's (per)oxidative metabolism, and the other depends on the entry of microbicidal constituents into the phagocytic vacuole during the process of degranulation. An increase in the cell's (per)oxidative metabolism stimulates an increase in oxygen consumption with subsequent formation of hydrogen peroxide and superoxide anions as well as an increase in glucose metabolism through the hexose monophosphate (HMP) shunt. Some antimicrobial activity results directly from the by-products of an increase in the cells' (per)oxidative metabolism, but the real enhancement of microbicidal activity comes from the secondary reactions of hydrogen peroxide with peroxidative enzymes of the granulocytes, especially myeloperoxidase.

Of the microphages, the neutrophils are the most numerous and the most important in the acute infectious process. Approximately 60% to 70% of the total white blood cell count is neutrophils. Once the cells are manufactured, they may be stored in the bone marrow in a reservoir that contains a mitotic production pool and a postmitotic maturation and storage pool, where they reside until needed. This is important to the body's protection and functioning because neutrophils are active in foreign-body surveillance.

The production pool consists of three somewhat arbitrary compartments of increasingly mature cells: myeloblasts, promyelocytes, and myelocytes. After spending time in the production pool, the cells progress to the postmitotic maturation and storage pool, where they wait to be released into the intravascular system. The maturation and storage pool consists of three types of increasingly mature cells: the metamyelocytes or juveniles, the bands, and the segmented neutrophils, or segs. Under ordinary conditions, the metamyelocytes are not released into the blood stream, whereas the bands and segs are readily released into the blood. The release of the neutrophils from the bone marrow is under the stimulus of a leukocytosis-promoting factor that is secreted after infection with certain types of bacteria or after the death of tissues. A shift to the left in the total WBC occurs when there is an increase in the number of bands and a decrease in the number of mature neutrophils in the blood.

Neutrophils spend about 10 to 12 hours in the blood stream, and from there, neutrophils enter the tissues to complete a 3- to 4-day life span. Under normal circumstances, these cells do not return to the general circulation once they move to the tissues.

Neutrophils interact with the immune system in two ways: they are capable of chemotaxis, and they possess a quality of immune adherence in which an antibody bonds an antigen at the F(ab) end of the antibody leaving the F(c) portion free to bind with the neutrophil's surface receptor, thereby forming a neutrophil-antibody-antigen complex. This binding of the antigen-antibody-neutrophil greatly enhances phagocytosis of the antigen.

Eosinophils

The function of eosinophils is less well understood than that of neutrophils. Eosinophils share several common features with neutrophils. They share a common progenitor; they also share a common fate of not returning to the general circulation from the tissues, but they are eliminated through the mucosal surfaces of the respiratory and gastrointestinal systems. Eosinophils also have the same slow ameboid motion as the neutrophils in phagocytosis and the same phagocytic activity, although their activity is not as efficient. Despite their being more associated with hypersensitivity and allergic reactions than with immunity itself, the physiology and function of the eosinophils are fragmentary and not known with any certainty. Unlike the neutrophils, eosinophils mature in the bone marrow 3 to 6 days before being released into the general circulation, at which time their half-life becomes 30 minutes. Inside the tissues, where they perform their major function, their half-life is approximately 12 days. The eosinophil is a powerful phagocyte with a marked affinity for antigen-antibody complexes.[43]

Basophils

Basophils, the least common members of the granulocyte family, are even less well understood than eosinophils. Although basophils are unimportant as phagocytic cells, they are closely related to mast cells and platelets and belong to a group of cells named *mediator* cells. These cells participate in immunologic reactions by releasing certain chemical substances or mediators that have a variety of biological functions ranging from increasing vascular permeability to contracting smooth muscle and enhancing the inflammatory response. In sufficiently high concentrations these chemical substances can induce a state of anaphylaxis.

Mast cells, noncirculating cells found primarily in the tissues, are capable of performing the same activities attributed to basophils. Like basophils, mast cells bind IgE and release a similar array of chemical mediators when the antigen bridges two IgE molecules. Scientific literature debates whether or not basophils and mast cells are simply the blood-borne and tissue-borne states of the same cells. Some studies suggest that this may not be so.[43]

The preceding overview of the immune system serves as a backdrop for the next sections on the tasks of the immune system.

The First Task: Phagocytosis

A Nonspecific Immunologic Defense

The primary role of the phagocytic cell, the basic functioning unit, is to eliminate foreign substances by sequestering, capturing, and digesting them. The phagocyte (or leukocyte) accomplishes its role by employing several well-integrated functions of chemotaxis, phagocytosis, and microbial killing. The leukocyte does not carry out its functions within the circulatory system as the red cell does; instead, it has its own means of transportation, whereby it can pass from the sites where it is formed to the sites where it is needed. Because tissue structure and density influence the effectiveness of phagocytosis, the denser the tissue, the more effective will be the phagocytosis. Dense tissue facilitates phagocytosis better than any other tissue type because of the ease with which the leukocyte is able to come into contact with bacteria and other foreign material.

The mechanisms of chemotaxis and phagocytosis are essentially the same for both neutrophils (PMNs) and macrophages (mononuclear phagocytes), but significant potential differences occur in the rates of intracellular killing. After the macrophage is sensitized by a microbial antigen, the macrophage becomes an "activated," or "angry," cell, and its rates of phagocytosis, intracellular killings and digestion are greatly increased. The significance of the changed cell activity is a major constituent of acquired cellular immunity (or task number three of the immune system).

Phagocytosis is a nonspecific multiphasic process whereby certain phagocytic cells (*i.e.,* polymorphonuclear leukocytes, wandering macrophages, and monocytes) localize and remove foreign substances from the blood. The process of phagocytosis consists of contact between microbe and phagocyte, attachment or adhesion of the two, the phagocyte's ingestion of the microbe, and then the phagocyte's digestion of the microbe. If the phagocyte kills the invader, the job is done. If the invader survives, it goes to the next step in the body's defense system—the specific immunologic defense mechanisms of either humoral immunity or cell-mediated immunity.

The phagocyte establishes contact with the microbe by a process that largely relies on the surface properties of the particle to be ingested or participation of the phagocyte's receptors on the particle's plasma membrane. Because the success of phagocytosis depends largely on the phagocyte's ability to adhere to the microbe's surface membrane, it would follow that nonencapsulated bacteria are rapidly taken in and destroyed, whereas encapsulated bacteria (*e.g.,* pneumococci) are taken up poorly and are not destroyed.[1] Thus a capsule protects the bacteria, ensuring its survival within the host.

Because the success of adhesion rests with the "rightness" of the surface membranes, the body needs a substance that can facilitate phagocytosis by modifying the bacteria's surface membrane. *Opsonins* are such substances. Opsonins neutralize the antiphagocytic function of a capsule by coating the microorganism with the host antibody, thus preparing the organism for ingestion. The simultaneous presence of two types of opsonins guarantees optimal conditions for phagocytosis: a heat-stable opsonin derived from the immunoglobulins of IgG and IgG_3 molecules and the heat-labile opsonins derived from complement.[40] It is believed that immunoglobulin and C3 fragments each attach to a specific receptor and, like hormones, trigger the sequence of events necessary to engulf the victim.[40] Because the complement system may be activated by the alternative pathway, the essential part of the reaction is the cleavage of C3 to produce an opsonically active fragment capable of attaching itself to the microbe's surface.

There is little doubt that opsonins are involved in phagocytosis. Whether phagocytosis is facilitated by opsonins because opsonins release a chemotactic substance, because there is a specific opsonin and a specific antibody for a given bacteria, or because there is an unspecific opsonin called complement, it is clear that once the phagocyte makes contact with the invader, the phagocyte holds its victim in a deadly, firm grasp before it is ingested and digested.

Once attachment occurs, either with or without opsonins, ingestion or engulfment of the particle occurs. The dynamics prompting ingestion are unclear, but the process involves the alteration of the physicochemical properties of the PMNs membrane-forming pseudopods. The pseudopods spread around the particles, soon covering and completely enveloping the bacteria. The pseudopods eventually fuse, invaginating the cell membrane and causing the particles to become enclosed within a vacuole or phagosome. The phagosome is formed from the remnants of the inverted leukocyte membrane and the complex of foreign bodies.

Microbial Killing and Destruction

Once the bacterium is ingested, the next step in phagocytosis is microbial killing and destruction. Shortly after the vacuole is formed within the phagocytic cell, metabolic events occur to generate microbicidal activity. The cell increases its oxygen consumption and its glucose use by the hexose monophosphate (HMP) shunt, and it produces H_2O_2, superoxide ion, and lactic acid. The stimulation of these pathways is termed the *respiratory burst*. The oxygen-dependent antimicrobicidal systems produce bactericidal, fungicidal, viricidal, mycoplasmicidal, and tumoricidal activity generated by the enzyme myeloperoxidase in combination with H_2O_2 and oxidizable cofactors to produce halogenation of the bacterial wall at critical sites.

The precise events initiating the metabolic activity that occurs once a particle is captured are unknown, but it seems that perturbations of the plasma membrane are involved. What makes the respiratory burst so unique is that it begins within seconds after particle uptake and actually precedes other events, suggesting that biochemical alterations may be a prerequisite for the occurrence of subsequent events.

It was discovered that phagocytic cells contain both oxygen-dependent and oxygen-independent antimicrobial mechanisms. As previously suggested, oxygen-dependent mechanisms can be and are subdivided on the basis of whether the cell uses myeloperoxidase.

Myeloperoxidase (MPO) is an enzyme that is important to the cell's ability to complete intracellular killing. Just exactly how MPO functions is unclear, yet in the presence of halides, the enzyme greatly potentiates the microbicidal effects of H_2O_2, which is formed in great quantities within minutes of phagocytosis.

The significance of MPO for phagocytic cells is that the monocytes and macrophages do not possess significant myeloperoxidase activity and must therefore resort to some other microbial mechanism. Exactly what microbial mechanism the macrophages use is unclear at the present time, but it is clear that the macrophages do exhibit the metabolic burst and H_2O_2 and superoxide ion generation exhibited by PMNs, but to a lesser degree. Phagocytic cells, primarily the PMNs, have the powerful microbicidal activity of H_2O_2, halide, and MPO.

Clinical Implications

Abnormalities in any one of the steps of phagocytosis and microbial killing assume clinical manifestations in disorders of the neutrophil. However, various types of nonpathologic stimuli such as exercise, sudden emotional surges, or administration of epinephrine also may produce an increase in circulating granulocytes. Such clinical irregularities are manifested by compromised host defenses and infectious complications. In order for nurses to assess what is happening to the patient, they must look not only at the total white blood cell count but also at the differential count. The degree of leukocytosis is often used as an index of the individual's resistance potential. A *shift to the left* refers to an increase in young or immature forms of segmented neutrophils. The greater the shift to the left, the more severe the infection. However, *a shift to the right* refers to an increase in mature polymorphonuclear leukocytes. This shift is usually associated with pernicious anemia as opposed to the shift to the left, which is seen in infections.

The Second Task: Recognition

Specific Immunologic Defense

In this section and the next, the cell under discussion will be the lymphocyte. In contrast to the macrophage, which is the primary cell involved in nonspecific response to an antigen, the lymphocyte responds to a specific antigen and then initiates and carries out the many processes required to destroy and remove that antigen.

Because the body responds only to surfaces and cares only about the chemistry of the antigen, recognition implies that the body responds to the different chemistry of the particulate matter, whether it be dead or alive, chemical or microbial, in exactly the same way—that is, by quickly secreting substances to "neutralize" the invader. The ability to recognize an antigen depends on the receptor molecules expressed on the surface of the lymphocytes. Two important characteristics of the lymphocytes' surface receptors favoring a proper response are that the receptors are both antigen-specific and capable of signaling the interior of the cell that antigen-binding has occurred so that the correct reaction can be mounted. The cell-surface receptor fulfilling these two characteristics is the antibody, and, in fact, the presence of an immunoglobulin molecule on a large number of lymphocytes is now a well-established observation.[43]

Recognition is a function of the lymphoid cells and depends on the ability of the thymus to confer immunologic competence on the body, that is, the body's ability to recognize antigens as foreign and then respond to them. Because the thymus is barely discernible in the adult's chest and seems to finish its role quite early in life, the notion that it may be the master organ of the immune system may come as something of a surprise.

The thymus is fully developed at birth or shortly thereafter. The function of the thymus is hypothesized to be production of the lymphocytes, giving rise to large numbers of cells that have the potential to secrete specific antibody. Its functional activity is believed to reach its peak in the first few days after birth.[10] Early in life, the thymus is critical to the development and function of the immune system, yet without directly participating in immune reactions. Thymectomized young children develop a state of severe immunodeficiency and display compromised B-cell functioning. Interestingly, the thymus is one of the most responsive of all organisms to stress; it demonstrates stress atrophy after an acute infection or severe injury, irradiation, or large doses of cortisone by subsequently destroying millions of lymphocytes within a day or two.[10]

The identified tasks of the thymus are to stock the body with lymphocytes and to control and maintain the immune system established by the thymic hormones (*e.g.,* thymosin, lymphocyte-stimulating hormone, thymin, and thymic hormonal function). Probably the most studied effect of the thymic hormones is their ability to confer immunologic maturity on lymphoid cell populations, and recent evidence supports the contention that at least one step in T-cell maturation requires the passage of the cell through the thymus.[10] Most physiologists would agree that the thymus is the primary source of lymphocytes in mammals, and that, when liberated into the general circulation, these lymphocytes settle in such organs as the spleen or a lymph node, where they give rise to those cells responsible for some, if not all, of the immunologic functions of the body.[1,10]

The thymus relies on precursor cells from the bone marrow to migrate to it where they mature into T-lymphocytes, cells primarily involved in surveillance of the body's cellular integrity. Of all these mature T-lymphocytes, only about 5% actually leave the thymus, and the remainder die within the thymus after a few days. Two hypotheses are proposed to explain this massive and seemingly wasteful proliferation. The first explanation suggests that it represents the elimination of lymphocyte clones reactive against self-antigens present in the thymus. Such lymphocyte clones are called *forbidden clones* because they ordinarily would not survive in the host. The second explanation suggests that the proliferation is purposeful in that it enables somatic mutations to occur, thereby producing the many different types of specificities needed by the immune system to recognize the thousands of different antigens that might be encountered. When the cell surfaces are change by toxins, viruses, or by simple aging, or when any change results in somatic mutation, it becomes necessary for the body's survival and functioning that these altered cells be recognized.

Thus, the manner in which the thymus mediates the development of immunologic competence is not entirely clear, but it may do any of the following: provide an environment in which stem cells from the bone marrow are able to mature into immunocompetent cells before being distributed to the general circulation; secrete a humoral factor that regulates lymphocyte maturation; or provide a means of censorship whereby potentially self-reacting clones are eliminated.[1,10]

Lymphocytes

The lymphocyte is a small, highly mobile white blood cell that can be found in practically every body tissue. Immune cells are born in the bone marrow and then follow different developmental paths. The life span of lymphocytes is divided as follows: the mostly large lymphocytes, or B cells, have a short life span of 5 to 7 days, and the small lymphocytes, or T cells, have a longer life span of months or even years. The main players in the immunologic arena are the thymus and bursae-derived lymphocytes. Together they form a cohesive team, with each carrying out a specific task. The distinction between T- and B-lymphocytes, as well as between humoral and cell-mediated immunity (discussed below in the Third Task: Response), is important to an understanding of the immune system.

The basis for differentiation is that some lymphocytes migrate to the thymus where they are induced to differentiate into a subpopulation of mature T-lymphocytes whose function is cell-mediated immunity. A second population of lymphocytes migrates to a gut-associated lymph tissue (GALT), where they mature into B-lymphocytes whose function is the production of immunoglobulin or humoral immunity.

Only B cells and their offspring, the plasma cell, produce antibodies on short notice. Actually, a "small" lymphocyte seen to be in a resting stage must become enlarged before the antibody is secreted. In the resting stage as a "small" lymphocyte, it has on its surface antibody molecules that function as receptors. From this surface receptor, it can be deduced that each cell is committed in advance to the production of one specific antibody. When an antigen with epitope fits the combining site on the particular antibody molecule, the small lymphocyte is stimulated to grow, manufacture more of itself, alter its structure, divide, and give rise to a special kind of B cell, plasma cell that is capable of rapid synthesis and secretion of antibodies to the particular cell line. Each plasma cell produces only one type of antibody or antigen.

As for T cells, they can also recognize antigens and, by definition, must also display antibody molecules as surface receptors, although they are more difficult to identify. Normally T cells do not secrete conventional immunoglobulins, instead, the T cells act as either potentiators or inhibitors of the B-cell transition into immunoglobulin-secreting plasma cells. The cells that potentiate B-cell transition are named T-helper cells; those that inhibit B-cell transition are named T-suppressor cells (discussed in detail below in The Third Task: Response).

Immunoglobulins

Immunoglobulins, as a part of the body's serum proteins, are one defensive force the body uses to protect against foreign invasions. Immunoglobulins are a highly heterogeneous group of proteins accounting for approximately 20% of the total plasma proteins. The evidence is compelling for easily detectable cell-surface immunoglobulins on B cells.[50] This does not mean that T cells do not express surface immunoglobulin receptors, but that if they do, the present standard techniques are unable to detect them. The first detectable cell-surface receptor was a firmly bound IgM, and IgG was also identified as existing on the B-cell surface. The B-cell receptors, believed to contain 104 to 106 molecules and to be concentrated in "hot spots" or "caps," are thought to be complete immunoglobulin molecules, because both kappa and lambda light chains and all heavy-chain determinants are expressed on their cell surfaces. Additionally, all the immunoglobulin molecules present on the B-cell surface of any single cell or clone of reacted cells share the same antigenic specificity. The phenomenon just identified is referred to as the *principle of clonal restriction*; in essence, it means that all immunologic molecules on a single clone are identical not only for the antigenic specificity, but also for the idiotype and the light-chain type.[50] The biological activity of immunoglobulins can be understood only on the basis of their structure.

Immunoglobulins (Ig) are divided into five classes: IgM, IgA, IgG, IgD, and IgE. The distinction between each class is that the heavy chains differ from class to class, and each possesses different antibody properties. There are five types of heavy (H) chains—gamma, alpha, mu, delta, and epsilon—that form IgG, IgA, IgM, IgD, and IgE. Like the light chains, no two different heavy chains exist in the same molecule. The two types of light (L) chains—kappa and lambda—are common to all immunoglobulins that normally do not occur in the same molecule. The five H chains and two L chains are the primary subunits of the body's immunoglobulin molecules. Therefore, each antibody, regardless of its class, is a multichain polypeptide. Each chain is composed of a "handle-piece," which is identical in structure for all antibodies of a particular class, and a "recognition" piece, which varies among antibodies of the same class but of different specificity (Table 45–1).

Burnet proposed the *clonal selection theory*, a cornerstone of immunology, which states that any single cell or clone of cells is preprogrammed to be competent in synthesizing antibody molecules of a unique antigenic specificity.[10] Thus, the clonal selection theory contains the following three basic premises: the surface immunoglobulin is the B-cell antigen receptor; there is a single antigen specificity on each clone of B cells found on the surface immunoglobulin; and the antibody that is secreted has the same antigenic specificity as the surface receptor. Just because an antigen hits and binds with the receptor on recognition of the B cell, an immunoglobulin does not form specifically for that antigen. Immunoglobin formation requires the collaborative help of both accessory cells and T cells, especially the T4-positive helper/inducer cells.

Antibody formation occurs in steps. Once the antigen binds to the B cell, accessory cells are engaged; they secrete interleukin-1 to stimulate the T-helper cells to enlarge, to begin to secrete lymphokines, and to divide to form a clone. The substances secreted by T-helper cells stimulate additional T-cell and B-cell growth. The activated B cells in turn enlarge, divide, and differentiate into plasma cells that are of antibody-secreting status.

Laboratory studies indicate that not only do T cells bind antigens, but they also do so with clonal restriction and specificity. Recent work suggests that the T-cell antigen-binding receptor is similar to that of immunoglobulin, but little may be said to describe the structural characteristics of the remainder of the molecule.

Simply knowing that lymphocytes first contact an antigen and bind to it by surface receptors that are designed to interact specifically with that particular antigen does not explain how the interaction produces the activation of an immunocompetent cell. Recognition is the first step in the process of complicated events in which the ultimate product is a fully differentiated cell able to carry out immunologic effector functions with maximum efficiency and intensity. After antigenic binding occurs, the triggering events on the lymphocyte surface must be communicated to the interior of the cell to complete the process. Two candidates for this role of intracellular messenger are calcium and the cyclic nucleotides, cyclic adenosine monophosphate (AMP) and, to a lesser degree, cyclic guanosine monophosphate (GMP).

The task of the lymphocyte is complex because recognition implies that the lymphocytes possess the ability to distinguish self-bacterial antigens from non-self bacterial antigens. If the lymphocyte must distinguish between self and non-self, the lymphocytes must also be capable of distinguishing between and among antigens the first time they meet, so that primary immunologic response may occur. The importance of a primary response, whether it be a cellular, a humoral, or a combined one, is that once a particular antigen is recognized as foreign, the body then possesses an immunologic memory that enables the body upon subsequent encounters to mount a specific immunologic response with greater speed and with greater intensity.

Immunologic Memory

Immunologic memory (or secondary response or anamnestic response) demonstrates an important and, by all odds, remarkable feature of the immune response. The body's immunologic memory is not only the rationale for using multiple doses of an antigen in certain clinical immunization programs, but also is the rationale for suggesting that once a person recovers from an antigen, he or she is also able to respond to a second attack by the same antigen with a prompt and massive outpouring of the appropriate antibody. The first exposure of the body to an antigen seems to leave the body prepared

Table 45–1
Immunoglobulin Function and Normal Values

IMMUNOGLOBULIN	FUNCTION	SERUM CONCENTRATION (mg/dl)	SERUM HALF-LIFE IN DAYS
IgG	Major antibody circulating in both serum and other extracellular fluids. Activates complement. Active against many bacteria, viruses, parasites, and some fungi	1200 ± 300	23
IgA	Concentration in external secretions and body fluids. Protects entrances to the body (*i.e.*, gastrointestinal and respiratory tracts)	200 ± 50	6
IgM	Activates complement formed in response to new antigens. Kills bacteria in blood stream by lysis	120 ± 50	5
IgD	Regulates activation of B cells	304	2.5
IgE	Major antibody in allergic response; mediates anaphylaxis and contact	0.02–0.03	2.5

with precursor, or memory cells, that are ready to turn into plasma cells of the right kind as soon as the original invader reappears. Experiments show that before a plasmablast reaches maturity as a plasma cell, it stops dividing.

The plasmablast goes through successive divisions, producing a clone, or colony, of cells before its division ceases. The clone includes not only the mother plasma cells, but also a number of primitive memory cells that have the potential to react with vigor to any future meeting with the antigen.[5,6] On the arrival of an antigen, a complex series of changes is somehow set in motion that transforms the plasmablast from a relatively unspecialized unit into a highly organized, elaborate system for producing and exporting proteins. Once the "factory" is equipped for full production, the mature plasma cell not only synthesizes but also can easily store quantities of the antibody.[5] How the antibody is released from the cell or what controls the rate of export is unknown at the present time.

Immunologic Tolerance

At the other end of the spectrum from recognition is immunologic tolerance, or the state of unresponsiveness to an antigen after the body's initial exposure to that antigen. The significance of immunologic tolerance as a learned response is the body's selective unresponsiveness to its own chemistry, surfaces, and tissue components. It goes without saying that an immune response against one's own tissues could and would be harmful to normal bodily function, owing to the tissue damage and destruction that would occur.

If the body must distinguish self from non-self, and this is a learned response, how does the body achieve this extraordinary ability? There is evidence suggesting that immunologic tolerance is acquired during embryonic development, although how tolerance occurs still remains enigmatic.[1,42] Many years ago, Burnet hypothesized that any antigen presented to the embryo while in utero might become categorized as an autologous antigen.[10] In other words, any exposure to an antigen during the period of immaturity of the lymphoid system might result in a state of unresponsiveness, or immunologic tolerance, to that antigen after birth. The prototype of immunologic tolerance is the symbiotic relationship that develops between mother and fetus. In adults, a tolerance state may be preceded by an immunologic phase not seen in newborns—that is, to facilitate tolerance by first destroying most, if not all, of the immunocompetent cells by using radiation, cytotoxic drugs, and antilymphocyte serum. This does not imply that tolerance can be accomplished only in the young; what it does imply is that it takes more of an antigen when a pre-existing state of immunity produces a faster elimination of the antigen. Based on the preceding statement, the last principle involved in producing a state of tolerance is that, in general, very high doses of an antigen induce tolerance, whereas lower doses are immunologic.

Thus recognition is a complex process in which the body responds, through lymphocytes, to an antigen, be it self-antigen or not, based on the chemical composition of the cell's surface. Recognition discriminates between and among the bacteria within our bodies to identify those potentially lethal bacteria as well as those which are self. Recognition is a double-edged sword in that the body's protection and safety from invasion depends on how intact the cell's ability is to fulfill its function, yet the slightest malfunctioning by misinformation is lethal to the body's integrity.

The Third Task: Response

The third and final task of the immune system is to mobilize one of the specific immunologic responses of delayed hypersensitivity or antibody formation. Delayed hypersensitivity as a fundamental response to all types of infection is a function of the small lymphocytes or T cells. Even though the intensity of the response varies from microorganism to microorganism, delayed hypersensitivity is primarily a group-specific response rather than a type-specific response. Antibody formation is a function of the ability of specifically instructed cells, the plasma cells, to secrete immunoglobulins.

In the previous section it was mentioned that the basis for immunologic memory is the body's ability to initiate and sustain a primary response. The primary responses on which immunologic memory arises may be classified as a humoral response or the production and secretion of an antibody by activated plasma cells, a cellular response or two-phased response by which activated T cells directly destroy the inciting antigen against which the activated cells were specifically sensitized, or the more usual combined response in which both the humoral and cellular responses are activated to counteract the potential threat of most antigens. In both humoral and cellular responses, the antigen is carried to the lymph nodes, where it stimulates B-lymphocytes for the humoral response and T-lymphocytes for the cellular response (Table 45-2).

Humoral Response

A humoral response is the responsibility of the B-lymphocytes. Once the body detects the presence of an antigen, a humoral response occurs by directing the synthesis of a soluble protein, an antibody, against the antigen. The site for the manufacture of the antibody is the center of the cortical follicle in the lymph node.

All antigens collect in the local lymph node, where 1 to 6 days later specific cytologic changes occur within the lymph node. The lymphocyte undergoes transformation first into an immunoblast and then into an immature plasma cell. Approximately 48 to 72 hours after first contact with the antigen, the plasma cell appears and antibody production is detected within the lymph node. The antibody, predominantly of the IgM class, is now capable of binding the inciting antigen. About 1 to 2 weeks after the initial antigenic stimulation, circulating antibody can be detected in the blood. The number of plasma cells continues to rise until their peak 3 to 5 weeks later, along with concomitant maximum titers of antibody. As the number of plasma cells begins to decline, so too do the levels of circulating antibody. Thus ends the active phase of the humoral response.

Cellular Response or Delayed Hypersensitivity

Cellular response is the responsibility of the T-lymphocytes, and it occurs when the T-lymphocyte becomes sensitized by contact with a specific antigen. The sensitization of the T-lymphocyte provokes a two-phased response, one in the regional lymph node and the other at the site of the antigen's

Table 45–2
Summary of B-Cell and T-Cell Functions

B CELLS	T CELLS
Prominent agents of fast-acting humoral immunity. Manufactures immunoglobins on short notice. Can manufacture more of itself by process of clonal proliferation	Alerts immune system to the presence of an invader. Specializes in fighting off viruses and tumors. Cells help regulate immune system
Produces antibodies in response to specific antigens	Composed of 2:1 ratio of T4:T8 helper/ inducer cells (T8) to enhance or activate B cells to produce antibodies; killer cells that destroy virus-infected and cancer cells when properly prepared; suppressor cells (T8) that turn off the production of antibodies
Surface immunoglobins recognize specific antigen	Surface-antigen receptor site recognizes foreign tissue or antigens

penetration into the body. Within the lymph node, immunoblasts result from mitotic activity within the paracortical and medullary regions. As the immunoblasts enlarge, their cytoplasm becomes packed with ribosomes, but no antibody synthesis occurs.

A similar set of circumstances unfolds at the site of the antigen's penetration into the body, where, in addition to the lymphoblastic changes, there occurs a significant infiltration of blast cells as well as lymphocytes and macrophages and evidence of the destruction of target cells or microorganisms bearing foreign antigen markers. Thus, in contrast to the humoral response, in which the B-lymphocytes remain stationary within the lymph node but exert a systemic effect by the secretion of antibody, the cellular response migrates to wherever an antigen might be. In general, however, the events that occur within the cells are not well understood, primarily because of the difficulty of studying the phenomena in vivo.

T-Cell Activity

Each T-lymphocyte is preprogrammed genetically to recognize only one antigen by means of a specific membrane receptor that permits it to interact with its antigen. The price humans pay for the enormous capacity of the T-lymphocytes to recognize between 400,000 and 1 million different antigens is the slowness of the primary response, a direct result of the time it takes a foreign antigen to physically meet the lymphocytes preprogrammed to recognize its unique characteristics.

Although all T cells are produced in the thymus, the population of these cells is not homogeneous. Several subpopulations are identified as helper T cells or T4 lymphocytes, suppressor T cells or T8 lymphocytes, and effector T cells. Based on the model systems, T-cell activity may be divided into three categories: regulation of the immune response, cytotoxicity, and production of bioactive factors called lymphokines.

Before discussing each one of these T-cell activities separately, one must remember that these categories are made only for study purposes, because in vivo, T-cell activity occurs simultaneously. Once the cellular response is triggered by the contact of a T-lymphocyte with an appropriate antigen, the sensitized T cell produces lymphokines. This chemotactic factor fosters the migration of both macrophages and sensitized T

cells to the area, whereas the macrophage inhibitory factor (MIF) prevents their additional migration, transfer factor changes nonsensitized T cells to sensitized ones in the absence of an antigen, and blastogenic factor begins the rapid mitosis of the sensitized T cells. Concurrent with this activity, macrophage activation factor (MAF) transforms macrophages into a highly phagocytic state so that these activated macrophages can initiate intense phagocytosis while the sensitized T cells are directly annihilating a viable antigen. The sensitized T cell also transforms another population of T-lymphocytes to killer cells that are believed to produce the cell-killing mediator cytotoxin as a result of a killer cell–antigen interaction. The cytolysis moderated by the T-lymphocyte is of antigen-specific in nature. The purpose of cellular immunity is naturally the death of all visible antigens and, secondarily, some normal tissue as well. Although cellular immunity protects the body against bacteria (as well as against cancer), it is also the major stumbling block to the success of organ transplantation.

In order for a humoral response to occur against certain antigens, T-cell participation is required. These T cells do not produce antibodies, but rather act as helper cells. The role of the T-helper cell or T4 lymphocyte is becoming somewhat clearer with the discovery and clarification of the hapten-carrier phenomenon. This phenomenon concerns the body's ability to mount a humoral response against a specific hapten or substance not in and of itself immunogenic but able to react with an antibody of appropriate specificity. The hapten must be conjugated to a larger carrier molecule, which is then recognized by the T-helper cell as being foreign. The T-helper cell's ability to recognize the carrier as foreign induces the T-helper cell to send an unspecified signal to the B cell that is already bound to the hapten. There is no evidence demonstrating that direct contact must occur between the T-helper cell and the B cell to induce the subsequent antibody response against the hapten. Many specific and nonspecific soluble factors are identified that are able to mediate T-helper cell activity. Of note are nonspecific helper lymphocytes called *effector T cells* that constantly patrol the body looking for invasion by antigens. One type of effector T-lymphocyte is able to harness monocytes to enter tissue where they mature to form macrophages and produce the delayed hypersensitivity reactions.

The second type of effector T cell is directly cytotoxic and is termed a *killer T cell.* This cell has the capacity, through the release of preformed molecules contained in its cytoplasm, to kill certain viruses, tumor cells, fungi, and parasites. Both types of effector T cells are capable of attacking the cells of tissue grafts perceived as unacceptably foreign.

In vivo, this phenomenon occurs in the graft-versus-host reaction (GVHR), in which the grafted cells recognize the host cells as foreign and induce a series of events in which the allogenic cells are stimulated to undergo blast transformation and to acquire killer-cell potential. The magnitude of the host antibody formation is proportional to the magnitude of the GVHR. A powerful antibody response will occur if either the donor cells were previously sensitized to the host tissue or the genetic differences between the graft and host are increased. This antigen-specific T-helper cell function is responsible for the powerful nonspecific stimulatory signal of the humoral-type rejection phenomenon observed after organ transplantation.

At the opposite end of the spectrum to the subpopulation of T cells called helper cells is another subpopulation of T cells called *suppressor cells*. This subpopulation of T-lymphocytes performs a generalized homeostatic function in the overall immune system by turning off an immune response that might ordinarily overwhelm the body. These cues act as an immunologic thermostat.

Physiologically, suppressor cells may either terminate excessive immune responses after antigenic exposure or provide a safeguard against autoimmune reactions.[6] After exposure to an antigen, impaired immune reactivity against that antigen in subsequent encounters may produce a state of immunologic tolerance. In many systems, immunologic tolerance is brought about by the action of suppressor cells.[6] Some suppressor regulatory functions are antigen-specific, whereas others are not. Suppressor cells may regulate the production of all immunoglobulin classes, a single immunoglobulin class, or an allotype or even an idiotype.[6,7] Additionally, the suppressor cells may show affinity for either the carrier or the hapten molecules and interact on the afferent or efferent limbs of the immune response.[7] Suppressor regulatory activity is believed to be under genetic control, because the major histocompatibility complex (MHC) is a chromosomal region containing genes that control the strongest allotransplantation antigens. Genes in the MHC region also profoundly influence several functions of the immune system, including the capacity to generate an immune response to certain well-defined antigens.

It must also be pointed out that there are cells other than T cells that exert a suppressor-like immunoregulatory role. Certain classes of B cells and macrophages may act as inhibitors of immune reactions, as can collaboration between T cells and macrophages.

In summary, T cells play an important role in the immune response. Activated T-lymphocytes are initially large, but later on in the immune response they are small. The activated T-lymphocytes differentiate to perform the various cell-mediated immunity (CMI) roles, differentiating: to the specific cytotoxic effector cells; to the killer T cells, for CMI; to cells that secrete the mediators, the lymphokines, of CMI; to helper and suppressor T cells that regulate the immune response; and to memory cells.

An important distinction between the humoral response and the cellular response, in addition to the secretion of antibody versus no antibody, is that humoral immunity can be transferred from one to another by cell-free plasma, whereas cellular immunity cannot be transferred but depends on the presence of immature cells.

Combined Cellular and Humoral Response

The previous presentation separating the immune response into a B-cell-mediated and a T-cell-mediated response is somewhat misleading. Although the activities of both systems are different, they frequently interact in the total immune response. Recent work demonstrates that the ability to mount a humoral response requires the concomitant T-cell activity of the specific subpopulation of T-helper cells. Most antigens do not elicit pure B-cell or pure T-cell responses, but rather there are T-cell-dependent antigens that demand T-cell cooperation in order to mount a humoral response and T-cell-independent antigens that require only B-cell activity in order to induce a humoral response. The presence of T-cells optimizes antibody production, with the most obvious candidate for all antigen-specific collaborative factors being a special T-cell receptor that is an IgM-like immunoglobulin. The collaborative effort involves T-cell recognition of a specific antigen and the subsequent interaction with the antigen-specific B cells. The mechanism involved in this interaction is not well defined.

Because most antigens do not elicit pure B-cell or pure T-cell responses, but evoke both types of response, there needs to be substance that bridges the gap between T cells and B cells. Complement serves such a purpose. Once the complement system is activated by IgG or IgM, one by-product, C5a, acts as a powerful chemotactic factor for commanding T-lymphocytes and macrophages to the antigen's site.

Although the immune system is divided into the humoral or B division and the cellular or T division, the function of these two divisions overlaps in the overall immune response. Either a permanent or a temporary lapse in either system results in the invasion of the body by extrinsic organisms, such as bacteria or viruses, and by intrinsic forms, such as neoplastic cells.

Summary: The Immune System

The immune system defies simple anatomic description. Unlike the respiratory, circulatory, and nervous systems, the immune system has no identifiable center. The immune system is composed of cells, molecules, and the lymph system, a separate circulatory system for the immune cells, spread throughout the body. Preprogrammed into the immune system, with the lymph nodes serving as ambush points for foreign substances, is the innate ability to recognize cells that belong versus those that are foreigners and that need to be destroyed.

The task of the immune system is to respond to an invading microbe in the following way: recognition, activation, deployment, discrimination, and regulation.[43] When one thinks of the seemingly insurmountable task facing the immune system, it is apparent that all parts of it must work cooperatively and harmoniously to protect the body against disease. Not only must all parts fit together like a jigsaw puzzle, but the immune system must manage to use just enough force to destroy the invader, yet leave the unaffected part of the body unharmed.

ACQUIRED IMMUNODEFICIENCY SYNDROME

Acquired immunodeficiency syndrome (AIDS) is an infectious disease caused by the third retrovirus identified: human T-lymphocyte virus type III (HTLV-III), which is also called human immunodeficiency virus (HIV). The virus causes a total collapse of the immune system, a premature death of the immune defenses. The clinical manifestations of AIDS, the final fatal consequence of the viral infection, is the result of a single defect, that is, the decrease in the number and a change in the function of the T4-lymphocytes. The loss of T-helper cell function leads to a subsequent development of a variety of life-threatening opportunistic infections and of particular autoimmune disorders such as thrombocytopenia and Kaposi's sarcoma.

As recently as 15 years ago, it was believed that infectious disease was no longer a threat in the developed world. That confidence was shattered in the early 1980s by the isolation of a new virus—HIV. Tests done in the 1960s and 1970s on stored blood serum from many parts of the world detected no antibodies to HTLV-III in any region except for a small area in central Africa. It was here that the earliest signs of an infection were found in serum samples taken in the 1950s.[19] The virus was contained in this region and could have remained so, had life in Central Africa not begun to change. Migration of people from remote rural areas into the city, changed sexual mores, and increased use of blood transfusions contributed to establishing a pool of infected people. The generalized exchange of blood and blood products that were not routinely tested carried the virus to other parts of the world, particularly to Haiti and the Americas.

HTLV-III belongs to the class of retrovirus, of which there are three. HTLV-I also infects T-lymphocytes but it causes a rare, highly malignant cancer called adult T-cell leukemia that is endemic in parts of Japan, Africa, and the Caribbean.[20] This particular virus is common in nature; the mouse leukemia virus and feline leukemia virus are examples of diseases caused by this slow-growing virus. HTLV-II belongs to the subclass of acutely transforming viruses that are rare in nature and, to date, have not been found in humans. The viruses contain an extra gene, called an oncogene, that almost always causes cancer in a short period of time.[27]

HIV is related to a group of nontransforming lente viruses and, like other retroviruses, it cannot replicate without taking over the biosynthetic apparatus of a cell and using it to its own ends. The virus has ribonucleic acid (RNA) as its genetic material and carries an enzyme, reverse transcriptase, which has the capacity to reverse the ordinary flow of genetic information from deoxyribonucleic acid (DNA) to RNA; thus, the viral RNA becomes template for making a corresponding molecule of DNA. Once the virus is in the host cell's genes, the viral DNA travels to the cell nucleus, inserts itself and remains latent until the lymphocyte is activated by a secondary infection. The virus reproduces itself so furiously that the new virus particles riddle the cellular membrane with holes and the lymphocyte dies. The result is the depletion of T4-lymphocyte (the hallmark of AIDS) and the vulnerability of the patient to opportunistic infections by microorganisms that would normally not harm a healthy person. It is obvious that once an infection by a retrovirus occurs, it is likely to be a lifetime process.

HIV appears to be unique among retroviruses in that it has at least five genes in addition to the standard gag, pol, and enu genes, which encode the core proteins, reverse transcriptase, and envelope proteins, respectively. Two genes, tat and trs/art are believed to be transcriptional regulators of HIV synthesis.[27]

Incidence and Prevalence

Since 1981 when the reporting of AIDS cases began, the occurrence of an identical, unusual disease in disparate groups identified certain individuals to be at risk of acquiring the disease. Those groups noted to be at increased risk were: sexually active homosexual or bisexual men; individuals with a history of needle-sharing intravenous drug abuse; individuals receiving multiple transfusions, usually associated with surgery, or hemophiliacs requiring transfusions of clotting factors; heterosexual partners of individuals in the preceding groups; and the fastest growing group, children born of mothers with the disease.

Even though risk groups are identified, AIDS is not really a disease of homosexuals or substance abusers or of any particular group. What AIDS is, is an infectious disease. The virus has been isolated from body fluids such as semen, vaginal secretions, peritoneal fluid, tears, saliva, and urine;[17] it is spread by intimate contact, whether it be sexual, blood-borne, or congenital. Intimate contact between the infected individual and a susceptible person is required for transmission. Rapid spread of the virus depends on a large enough pool of infected people for a few exposures to result in infection.

The vast majority of persons with AIDS are black Americans or Hispanic males between 20 and 49 years of age.[16] The incidence of women with reported cases of AIDS is increasing across the United States. The geographic distribution is tied to that of intravenous drug use.[15] In certain areas—especially in urban areas of the Northeastern United States where heterosexual transfusion and IV drug use are prevalent—a large subgroup of persons with AIDS consists of women who are intravenous drug abusers themselves or those whose male sex partners have injected drugs. As with the males, the overwhelming majority of women with AIDS are members of minority groups, Black Americans or Hispanics. They are infected at a rate 11 to 13 times higher than whites.[17] The male:female ratio is 13:1 in the United States; the disease occurs predominantly among young adults and children.[24]

Women with AIDS or HIV infection are different from men with AIDS and as such need special attention. First, women are usually younger and sicker and have a shorter survival time than men. Second, many women are single parents of a small child or children who may also be infected with HIV. These mothers care for and subsequently leave behind a small child or children. The reality and tragedy of the situation is that the woman might not live long enough to be with her child when the child dies. The nurse is the one member of the medical team who shares the pain and who helps the patient to say goodbye. With few treatment options available and the inevitability of death, the nurse often copes with the feelings of grief and helplessness by moving faster, doing more, needing to be in control, and focusing on concrete outcomes such as encouraging the patient to put her affairs in order or to search for meaning in order to achieve peace. Additionally, the nurse may nudge the patient toward the stereotyped image of a good death. It becomes important for the nurse to recognize the limits of responsibility and permit the patient to have responsibility for both her own living and dying.

The life expectancy from the time of diagnosis to death may range from 18 months to as little as 2 months, depending on which of its many forms the disease takes.[58] There is a small but growing number of individuals who are alive 3, 4, and 5 years after the diagnosis is made, but these persons are exceedingly rare.[16,58] The case fatality rate—the likelihood that any patient will die of AIDS—is 100%. In addition to its outcome, the chronic debilitating nature of the disease results in great physical suffering and psychologic stress in patients, their loved ones, and families, and it has placed a great burden on health care facilities in geographic areas where the disease is prevalent.

Transmission of AIDS

The AIDS virus, HIV, has sparked fear of contagion among the general population and specifically among health care workers, in spite of the fact that there are many diseases with which we come into contact that are much more readily transmissible.

The fear of AIDS becomes exaggerated by our social and cultural values, which give symbolic meaning to that which is not understood. An illness that has no cure, is poorly understood, and has an unknown cause elicits the most fear. Regardless of the disease, such fear leads to the belief of contagion.

The mystery of AIDS plus its terminal outcome feed into our fears. In our society not only is death avoided and shunned, but it is considered to be the final loss of control, the ultimate insult. Therefore any illness associated with death takes on the same meaning and triggers the same response of avoidance. When a disease associated with mystery and death bears the further stigma of being a sexually transmitted disease, it becomes offensive. Consequently, a person with AIDS is not seen as being a helpless victim of a deadly microbe, but as having caused his or her own fate.

AIDS is dreaded not only because it is deadly but because the diagnosis represents the ultimate symbol for sin, pollution, and decay. Because HIV is feared, its contagion becomes exaggerated, because no one wants to contract this shameful and lethal illness.

Nurses who continue to work with persons with HIV infections have already dealt with their fears. In order for the nurses to overcome fears, they must become knowledgeable about the transmission of HIV. Misinformation adds to hysteria. Additionally, trite as this may sound, the nurse must recognize the patient as an individual, rather than a diagnosis. The more the nurse emphathizes with the patient and recognizes the sameness of their humanity, the less there is to fear and the less contagious AIDS will seem.

The routes of transmission of infection with HIV are clear and well characterized. Transmission of HIV occurs by three defined routes: sexual contact, both heterosexual and homosexual; parenteral exposure to blood and blood products; and perinatal contact between mother and infant.

Parenteral Exposure

In a hospital, but especially in a critical care unit, the risk of transmission is usually through direct blood-to-blood contact by a needlestick with a patient infected with HIV. Although the virus may be isolated from body fluids such as saliva, cerebrospinal fluid, breast milk, urine, tears, amniotic fluid, vaginal secretions, in addition to blood and semen, this does not mean that the fluid is important in transmission. To date, only blood and semen have been implicated in transmission.

Although occupational infection by needlestick does occur, the risk is low.

Intravenous Drug Use

Intravenous drug use plays an important role in the transmission of HIV infection in the United States. The population is a principal bridge to other adult populations through heterosexual transmission and to children through perinatal transmission. Ninety percent of intravenous drug uses are heterosexual, and 30% are women, primarily in their childbearing years.[17] In addition, approximately half of the female intravenous drug users engage or have engaged in prostitution.[17] Intravenous drug users represent the largest pool of HIV-infected heterosexuals and also represent the largest number of HIV-infected females of childbearing age; consequently, there is a direct association of prenatal transmission of HIV and pediatric AIDS.

Transmission of HIV infection can occur through sharing of unsterilized needles, syringes, and injection apparatus, or "cookers" that are contaminated with blood. In a "shooting gallery" where intravenous drug users gather to administer drugs, it is common practice to rent a used needle. The needle and syringe may be rented repeatedly until they are no longer usable. Sequential anonymous sharing of blood-contaminated needles and syringes occurs among large numbers of persons. Thus, it appears that the HIV infection among intravenous drug users is related to repeated exposures to small amounts of contaminated blood through the common practice of sharing contaminated injection equipment.

Blood Transfusions

Persons who have acquired AIDS through the transfusion of infected blood or blood products represent a small but important population of the total number of cases. To date, whole blood, blood cellular components, plasma, and clotting factors have transmitted HIV infection. Other products prepared from blood such as immunoglobulin, albumin, plasma protein fraction, and hepatitis B vaccine have not been implicated.[17]

Blood transfusions as a route of transmission of HIV infection virtually have been eliminated with the use of donor screening, voluntary donor referral, and testing for HIV antibodies.

Sexual Transmission

HIV is fundamentally a sexually transmitted virus spread by both homosexual and heterosexual activity. Heterosexual transmission, although having less quantitative importance in the United States, is increasing more rapidly than the proportion of cases in any other category of risk.[17] The risk of acquiring HIV infection from a single or from several sexual encounters with an infected person is not known. Attempts have been made to define types of sexual behavior or other behavior that are associated with seropositivity. Among both homosexual men and heterosexuals, there appears to be a relation between infection and the number of sexual partners. The practice of anal-receptive intercourse among homosexual men has been associated with HIV infection and other sexually transmitted diseases such as syphilis and genital herpes, as well as other causes of genital or anal ulcers.[24] It is presumed that the damage done to the genital skin and mucous membranes by the multiple viruses in the semen and the inadequacy of the rectal mucosal defense may facilitate HIV acquisition or transmission.

Reduction of disease transmission may be accomplished by safer sexual practices. There is good reason to believe that the use of condoms for all sexually active persons who are not involved in a monogamous relationship would substantially reduce the risk of HIV transmission. Furthermore, education about disease transmission, a decrease in the number of sex partners, and elimination of such high-risk practices as anal intercourse are other currently available methods of reducing risk.

Perinatal Transmission

Precise information on the risk and routes of prenatal HIV infection is lacking. Both in the United States and in Third World countries, the majority of documented cases of AIDS and HIV infection in infants and children are the result of mother-to-infant transmission of infection either during pregnancy or in the perinatal period. HIV may be transmitted from an infected mother to her child by three possible routes: during pregnancy through the maternal circulation, at delivery by penetration or injection of blood or other infected fluids, and during breast feeding.[17] It is believed that infection may occur by one or all of these routes, but the virulence and frequency of each route is not known.

The rate of perinatal transmission is not known. Available information indicates a rough estimate of 40% to 50% percent rate of perinatal transmission.[17]

Risk to the Health Care Worker

The risk of contracting HIV infection from delivering health care to infected individuals is very low. Studies to date estimate the risk of HIV transmission is less than 1:1000 per year of exposure, even when standard infection control procedures are not followed.[41]

Incidents of seroconversion have been reported for people exposed to patients with AIDS or potentially infected body fluids. These are really isolated incidents that must be placed in the perspective of the large cumulative experience among hospital workers, suggesting that noninoculation parenteral exposure carries a small risk.[17] The case for low risk to health care workers is further supported by the studies on family members of persons with AIDS. To date, all studies have failed to point to transmission of the virus through casual contact.

The surveillance of health care workers indicates that the risk of occupational transmission appears to be related to the needlesticks and, to a lesser degree, extensive exposure to infected blood and body fluids. This information engendered a great deal of anxiety among the health care community. Nevertheless, the individuals involved in the seroconversion were not following the Centers for Disease Control (CDC) recommendations for the handling of blood and body fluids.

The CDC recommends universal precautions to represent protection of health care workers from blood or other body fluids that may contain HIV or hepatitis B virus (Morbidity and Mortality Weekly Report [MMWR], 1987 and 1988). Universal precautions are designed to protect health care workers to the fullest extent from exposure to those individuals infected with either HIV or hepatitis B. The most effective means of protection for the nurse is by the consistent use of protective barriers: gloves, goggles or mask, and impervious gowns. Especially in a critical care unit, special care should be taken when the nurse handles any needle or sharp instruments. The nurse *should not* recap, cut, break, or bend needles after use but should dispose of needles in an appropriately labeled impermeable needle container. When having contact with blood or body fluids, nurses must wear gloves at all times, removing them and washing their hands after each patient contact. Goggles and impervious gowns should also be worn when there might be exposure to large quantities of blood or blood that may be aerosolized.

Part of providing care to persons with HIV infection is being familiar with proper infection control guidelines. Because there appears to be minimal risk of transmission of the virus to individuals caring for AIDS and HIV-positive patients, there is no justification for the isolation, quarantining, or stigmatization of persons with AIDS or infected individuals. HIV is clearly a deadly and legitimately frightening disease, but this fear should spur the nurse to take logical action to prevent exposure by the appropriate use of precautions to provide a safe environment for both the patient and herself.

Summary: Incidence and Prevalence of AIDS

Since AIDS was first recognized in 1981, the number of cases has risen swiftly. The groups at highest risk for the infection are well defined: homosexual and bisexual men, intravenous substance abusers, the sexual partners of people in the AIDS risk group, and children born to mothers at risk. Recipients of blood transfusions and blood products have also contracted AIDS, but the screening of donated blood for evidence of infection has reduced this risk factor. The fact that HIV is not identified beyond those groups indicates that the virus is not spread by water, food, or casual contact.

Testing for the presence of HIV is a controversial issue. At present, two antibody tests are in wide use: the enzyme-linked immunosorbant assay (ELISA), which makes use of the whole disrupted virus as antigen; and the Western Blot test, which employs specific core viral proteins as antigen. The majority of individuals with tests confirmed as demonstrating HIV antibodies, regardless of their clinical status, are potentially infectious.

One means of becoming comfortable while providing care to persons with HIV infection is to be familiar with proper infection control guidelines. The CDC recommends the use of universal precautions. The philosophy behind such precautions is that because most persons with either HIV or hepatitis are unknown, it is wise to consider the blood and bloody body fluids, as well as genital secretions and body fluids normally limited to internal cavities from all patients, as potentially infectious. Universal precautions are meant to protect health care workers to the fullest extent from occupational exposure to HIV or hepatitis B. The nurse must appropriately use, not overuse, precautions to provide a safe environment.

Pathophysiology

When a person is first infected, the virus merges with the T4 cell through its receptor molecule, CD_4. The virus releases reverse transcriptase by which the viral RNA is transcribed into the host cells' DNA. The viral DNA becomes incorporated into the genetic material in the cell's nucleus and subsequently directs the production of new viral RNA and viral proteins to form new viral particles termed a *provirus*. These particles bud from the cell membrane and infect other cells. As the virus takes hold, the lymphocytes begin to proliferate abnormally in the lymph nodes. Thus the very process that should defeat HIV—the immune response—has the diabolic effect of increasing the production of the virus. Thereafter the lymph nodes' intricate structure collapses, the number of lymphocytes in the lymph nodes diminishes, and the number of lymphocytes in the blood decreases, leaving the person lymphopenic, neutropenic, and leukopenic. The loss of T4 cells from areas in which they are normally concentrated (they compose 60 to 80% of the circulating T-cell population) is one of the most striking and consistent findings in AIDS patients.[51]

The hallmark of AIDS is the profound defect in cell-mediated immunity. The underlying cause of the immune defect is HIV's selectivity in infecting the T4 helper cells, the cells that orchestrate virtually the entire immune response, which results in a significant depletion in the population and a change in their function.

Normally the T-helper cells recognize foreign antigens or markers on infected cells. They help to activate B cells to produce antibodies that bind to infected cells and subsequently to inactivate or destroy the invaders. The helper T cells also activate monocytes and macrophages, which engulf infected cells and foreign particles, to secrete a variety of cytokines or substances that alter the activity of other cell types.

Because the cells of the immune system are so interdependent, the loss of T4 cells, the "quarterback" of the immune system, causes global defects in a number of components of cell-mediated immunity that rely in part on their induction signals. The qualitative and quantitative changes in T4 cells seriously impair the body's ability to fight most invaders, but especially viruses, fungi, parasites, and certain bacteria, including mycobacteria. Eradication of these organisms requires a strong, well-functioning cell-mediated immune response. To a lesser degree, when lacking the T4 cell population, B-lymphocytes are unable to produce adequate quantities of antibody specific to HIV or to any other infection. Therefore, bacterial infection also presents a threat, albeit a smaller one.

The virus' preference for the T4 cells is not absolute; it is likely that macrophages, blood platelets, and B cells also serve as reservoirs of the virus.[18,25,34] It is suggested that neutropenia and thrombocytopenia in HIV disease are due to an autoimmune destruction of neutrophils and platelets.[41] Additionally, other cells outside the blood may also serve as HIV reservoirs; these include the lymphatic vessels, endothelial cells lining the blood and lymphatic vessels, the glial cells of the nervous system, and nerve cells themselves.[34] Compounding the ability of HIV to infect the central nervous system, it seems possible that the macrophage, which crosses the blood–brain barrier, may bring the virus into the brain.

"In the brain and spinal cord the virus appears to have a direct pathogenic effect that is not dependent on immune deficiency."[18] How the virus influences the abnormal growth of the glial cells that surround the neurons and produce lesions resulting in the loss of white matter is not understood. However, the relatively limited range of central nervous system structural abnormalities produces a wide range of neurologic symptoms ranging from headaches to dementia to peripheral symptoms that mimic other neurologic diseases such as multiple sclerosis.

The peripheral nervous system is also affected by HIV. The most common form of peripheral neuropathy is a chronic sensory neuropathy; the second most common form is a chronic demyelinating polyneuropathy. Whereas the effects of HIV on the central nervous system are distinct from immune deficiency, the third form of pathology has a more ambiguous relation to the immune dysfunction. A person infected with HIV has a 40% increased risk of developing at least one of three different types of human tumor; Kaposi's sarcoma, carcinomas, and B-cell lymphomas.

It is unclear what mechanisms are responsible for 90% of the homosexual AIDS population developing Kaposi's sarcoma, a malignancy occurring with much greater frequency in homosexual patients with AIDS than in patients with AIDS in other risk groups. Kaposi's sarcoma has a variable natural course in a person with AIDS. Generally, patients with AIDS are asymptomatic except for the presence of purplish-brown spots on the skin. However, other patients may experience a rapidly progressive disease that invades the lungs, heart, eyes, and gastrointestinal tract.

Depletion of T-helper cells and alteration in cell-mediated immunity may have the following clinical effects: the reactivation of prior opportunistic infections that are not contagious to other individuals; multiple concurrent or consecutive infections; asymptomatic infection with certain fungi or parasites, especially histoplasmosis in the Ohio River Basin of coccidioidomycosis in the American Southwest; viral, fungal, or parasitic infections that are rarely curable and generally require long-term therapy; infections that are serious and potentially life-threatening.[21,51]

NURSING PROCESS

ASSESSMENT

The nursing assessment of the immunocompromised patient involves a comprehensive evaluation of the etiologies of immune dysfunction. The use of the patient's history and physical examination, specific blood tests, and the presence or absence of certain risk factors provide the basis for nursing interventions appropriate for these patients.

Immune competence, or host resistance, is the result of a functionally balanced immune system that is able to resist a threat from another organism or altered self. Normally the human body coexists with the many microbes, nonpathologic bacteria, yeast, fungi, and protozoans inhabiting the body. When the immune system is unable to protect itself, normally harmless organisms threaten the body's ability to sustain life.

Functional immune deficiencies may be either congenital or acquired and may be described as failure to recognize a foreign threat (afferent limb defect), inability to recall the past immune encounters (central limb defect), and inability to secrete antibody or lymphokines (efferent limb defect).

Congenital immune deficiencies are usually seen in pediatric critical care areas; they are identified in children under 2 years of age. The more common type found in critical care areas is acquired immune deficiencies, which are due to the environment rather than to a genetic cause. Acquired deficiencies may be either primary or, more commonly, secondary. Common conditions that predispose the patient to an acquired immune deficiency are stress, malnutrition, age, chronic disease, injury or trauma, major surgery, chemotherapy, or drugs.[22,23] Once the condition predisposing the patient to immunodeficiency is corrected, an eventual return to appropriate immune function is expected. Thus, regardless of which limb has the functional defect, the result may be recurrent infection, lesions of the skin and mucous membranes, and even an increased risk of neoplastic disease.

From the standpoint of the critical care nurse, most patients are immune compromised to some extent. However, nursing assessment of the immunodeficient patient is often difficult because of the subtle changes that may occur, the delay in the development of symptoms in response to antigen exposure, and the commonality of these symptoms in other immune and pathologic situations.

The nurse needs to assess the immune system to identify antecedent conditions and behaviors that promote health and to plan interventions needed to prevent tertiary illness. The following discussion will focus on acquiring subjective and objective data related to the immune system.

General Immune Assessment

History and Physical Examination

The history should consider facts that influence the immune system, such as age, occupation, fatigue, nutrition, stress, and life-style. Inquiry into any changes in body weight, appetite, and elimination should be included, as well as a detailed medication and immunization history.

Detailed examination of the condition of the skin and mucous membranes is integral. Eruptions, changes in skin pigmentation, swellings, papules, petechiae, purpura, ulcers, and abscesses should be noted.

Naturally, vital statistics and weight should be recorded. The patient should be checked for lymphadenopathy, fever, chills, productive cough, and any abnormal secretions.

Other relevant data include previous hospitalizations, surgery, reception of blood or blood products, transfusion, special therapies, pets, nutritional status, allergies, and home living conditions.

Diagnostic Tests: Immunosuppressed Patients

Skin Test

Skin testing is used to evaluate two categories of general immune competence: immune recognition or memory, by injecting an antigen with which the patient has had prior experience; and response to a new antigen with which the patient has had no experience. Antigens used for the memory response are a panel of test antigens to which the patient has most likely had previous exposure, such as diphtheria, toxoid, tuberculosis (PPD), mumps, or *Candida albicans*. Most normal adults should react to one of these antigens. If there is no response on two separate occasions, the person is said to be anergic. The causes of anergy vary but most often occur in cases of chronic fungal and tubercular infections and sarcoidosis. Antigens used to test a primary response are tetanus toxoid or dinitrochlorobenzene (DNCB).

Other components of assessment of specific immune competency are lymphocyte transformation and human leukocyte antigen (HCA) typing. These are discussed in the chapter on transplantation and so are not dealt with here.

Specific Immune Components: Blood Tests

T- and B-Lymphocyte Counts

T, B, K, and null cells and monocytes are not differentiated on the basis of structure alone but also by their membrane receptors. These different classes of lymphocyte cells are determined qualitatively by cell separation technique.

Immunoglobulins

Immunoglobulins (Ig) or antibodies are formed in response to an antigenic encounter and are specific for the antigen. Antibodies migrate in the gamma globulin band during electrophoresis into the predestined classes of IgM, IgG, IgE, IgA, and IgD.

A decrease in gamma globulin level is usually associated with B-cell disorders, such as agammaglobulinemia, hypogammaglobulinemia, or lack of T4 helper cells. An increase in gammaglobulin level is associated with B-cell dyscrasias such as multiple myeloma or deficiency of T8 suppressor cells (see Table 45–1).

Immunodeficiencies Secondary to Other Conditions

The immunologic defenses of the patient in a critical care unit are compromised because of the frequent use of invasive techniques, the presence of opportunistic infections in the unit, and the stressors that accompany a life-threatening event. Thus, the patient may develop an infection or a pre-existing one may become worse.

The following discussion focuses on some general factors that contribute to immunocompromise on the intensive care unit.

Nutrition

Malnutrition directly undermines the immune system. As a group, the cells of the immune system are produced rapidly and need a daily supply of protein, calories, vitamins, and minerals. What we eat becomes the raw material for the components of the immune system. Thus, eating improves the immune system by helping to produce immunocompetent cells.

One of the best defenses against a weakened immune system and threatening infection is a well-balanced diet. Malnutrition and protein deficiency depress all three limbs of the immune system and decrease the number of circulating T cells. Therefore, the malnourished patient is more susceptible to develop viral, fungal, and intracellular bacterial infections.

The nutrition of a patient in the critical care unit is often compromised. There may be poor or restricted oral intake; the patient may require nasogastric suctioning, endotracheal suctioning, or both; body protein may be depleted through losses from injury, surgery, or starvation and the presence of stress-related catabolic hormones. Nutrition may be overlooked because of the list of high-priority procedures that must be carried out. However, special attention must be paid to the patient's nutritional needs.

Adequate dietary protein and nonprotein calories are important so that protein can be used to create new body proteins rather just to supply energy. The recommended daily allowance for protein intake in adults is 0.8 g/kg of body weight.[33] In the critically ill patient, protein requirements are increased because of factors that deplete body proteins or increase their catabolism. In addition to protein intake, the diet must also contain adequate carbohydrate intake, because it functions as a protein-sparing energy source. Carbohydrate in the form of glucose is the only form of energy used by the central nervous system, red and white blood cells, neutrophils, and fibroblasts. The importance of these cells for the critically ill patient is that they are found in wounds as granulating tissues. If insufficient carbohydrate is available to meet these cells' demands, protein will be used to supply the necessary glucose. Because protein-energy starved patients have a higher incidence of morbidity and mortality, as well as being at greater risk of developing opportunistic infections than well-nourished ones, the nurse must pay special attention not only to the patient's intake and output but also to the patient's daily weight, serum protein, zinc and magnesium levels, insensible losses, and the kind of replacement fluids prescribed.

Age

In humans, the immune system undergoes significant changes with the aging process. Age is a significant factor in the amount of self-protection that the individual has. The powers of the immune system ebb and flow over time. Impaired immune function often occurs in the very young and the very old. Newborns and the very young do not have fully developed immune systems and only after 2 years of age is the thymus gland, the director of the immunologic orchestra, fully developed.[37]

Many aspects of the immune system decline with age; T cells are the most sensitive to the aging process. The onset of their decline in function seems to correlate with the involution of thymic function, at puberty.[59] Thymic hormones, which are required for both B- and T-cell maturation, begin to decline by the third decade of life, and by 50, the thymus' size is 15% less than its original mass.

Alteration in immune function is not uniformly affected by the aging process. After the age of 60, the individual's immune response, especially response of the T cells, begins to decline.[57] In addition to T-cell dysfunction, the biochemical profile also changes. The total number of white blood cells, lymphocytes, phagocytic function, and complement does not change with age.[59]

The most significant changes occur in cellular immunity, such as in resistance to tumor cells, viral and protozoal organisms, and delayed hypersensitivity. This dysregulation of immune function may lead to a certain vulnerability of the person and failure to endure under stress.

The B cells appear to function relatively well in old age. They respond normally to antigenic stimulation, but their ability to differentiate into mature plasma cells that secrete appropriately high levels of antibody is slightly diminished.[59] B cells respond better to antigens that they have previously encountered than to new ones. This may explain why an elderly patient becomes infected so readily. The immune system cannot respond with an appropriate immune response to fight off an invading organism when challenged.

Drugs

The body's resistance to infection may be compromised by the use of antimicrobial agents that subsequently alter the body's microflora. Almost all antibiotics, once a therapeutic dose is achieved, produce a concomitant alteration in the gastrointestinal, oropharyngeal, and skin flora. The result of such an alteration is a trade-off whereby an antibiotic-sensitive organism is replaced by another, more resistant one.

Drugs that are commonly used but that produce immune system dysfunction are the corticosteroids. Glucocorticosteroids are frequently prescribed for their anti-inflammatory quality. Yet this same property has a profound immunologic effect. Corticosteroids depress the inflammatory response by decreasing the number of cells available to mount an immune response, inducing lysis of lymphoid cells, decreasing antibody synthesis, reducing the functional capabilities of immunologically active cells, and suppressing the formation and activity of interferon. Corticosteroids temporarily redistribute the lymphocytes from the intravascular pool to the extravascular pool while increasing the number of neutrophils and decreasing the monocytes and eosinophils. Besides altering the distribution and number of these cells, the drug also diminishes their functional capabilities. Prolonged corticosteroid administration leads to a state of immune unresponsiveness or anergy, which subsequently predisposes the patient to an increased incidence of infection by opportunistic infections, viruses, fungi, and parasites. This is compounded by the fact that the anti-inflammatory action of corticosteroids masks any signs of infection.

Immunosuppressive and cytotoxic drugs used to treat neoplasms and other immunologically mediated diseases, such as systemic lupus erythematosus, can profoundly depress the bone marrow and the reticuloendothelial system. Because cytotoxic drugs cannot discriminate between normal and malignant cells, they have a profound effect on practically every aspect of cellular and humoral response. Thus, cytotoxic agents affect the production of stem cells, leading to a deficiency in white blood cells. In addition, cytotoxic drugs tend to injure the rapidly growing cells of the intestinal mucosa, thereby producing a new portal of entry for various microorganisms.

Other Diseases

Immune deficiencies often occur during the course of acute and chronic diseases such as diabetes, stress, AIDS, and renal or hepatic failure. The mechanisms responsible for this vary.

Stress

The notion that stress affects the immune system and the subsequent development of infection has been discussed and debated for decades. There seem to be sufficient data to suggest a complex communication network linking the internal psychologic, neurologic, physiologic, immunologic, endocrine, and biochemical events with the external and psychosocial environment. In both animals and humans the link between stress and impaired immune function is strong. The question that is asked often is why only some stressed individuals develop organic disease. Consider that stress results from an intricate interplay between the event and a number of variables, including the individual's expectations and experiences, the presence or absence of a network of caring people, chronicity, age, sex, genetic make-up, duration and characteristics of the stressor, and other factors.[41] Stress is not the sum of negative events but rather the perception of the individual that a particular life event is beyond his ability to cope, to manage, or to be in control of and subsequently to adapt to it.[37,38] A physical stress is generally accompanied by a psychologic stress, because most people believe they have no control over what happens within their bodies.[14] Thus, it is the inner experience, the patient's perception, that shapes the direction and force of events that affect the system. The inner experience in which the event is judged as a threat or as a challenge mitigates the outcome, right down to the cellular level.[37] The subtle relationship and information exchange that exist between the mind and body may swing the balance between health and illness.[47] Whether the result of stress on health is direct or indirect remains unclear.

Apparently no major part of the immune system is without connection to the brain. Numerous anatomic connections between the central nervous system and the immune system—such as nerve endings found in the thymus gland, lymph nodes, spleen, and bone marrow—suggest that the body communicates with itself. Every tissue and organ in the body is controlled by a complex interaction among the hormones secreted by our endocrine glands. Research postulating that thoughts and moods trigger the action of neurohormones (including catecholamines, corticosteroids, and endorphins), neurotransmitters, and nerve cell activity is directed to a specific part of the brain—the limbic system. This part of the brain is composed of the hypothalamus, pituitary gland, and amygdala. The hypothalamus, a veritable drug factory, is the seat of emotions; it regulates most of the body's unconscious process. Nerve fibers and receptors for neuropeptides enter the hypothalamus from nearly all other regions of the body, so intellectual and emotional processes occurring elsewhere in the brain affect the body. Another important part of the limbic system is the pituitary gland. This "master" gland controls the secretion of hormones within the body and is in turn controlled by both the neuropeptides and nerve impulses from its neighbor, the hypothalamus.

The immune system is not autonomous but reacts to the world by following chemical cues. The cells of the immune system, but especially lymphocytes and monocytes, have an uncanny ability to detect non-self molecules. They also have receptors for and make various neuropeptides.[48] The cells of the immune system produce the same chemicals that are thought to control mood in the brain.[48] The neuropeptides and their receptors in the limbic system and on monocytes seem to be important to an understanding of how the mind and body are interconnected and of how emotions can be manifested throughout the body. Thus the brain, the endocrine glands, and the immune system are actually joined to each other in a two-way network of communication, with the neuropeptides serving as information carriers.[48]

From Seyle's and Cannon's early description of the stress response, it is now known that the two scientists addressed not opposing views but two overlapping and simultaneous mechanisms of the body's reaction under physical and psychologic stress. These scientists provided an initial under-standing of the biochemistry of stress. Their initial list of stress-related hormones can now be extended to include more than 30 neurohormones and neurotransmitters.[37]

Although stressors may influence immunologic function, psychologic processes that mediate these influences contribute to the ultimate immunologic impact. What happens in the brain affects the body, and what happens in the body affects the brain. Studies have reported the relationship between immunologic dysfunctioning and marital disruption, academic-examination stress, bereavement, and methods of coping.[2,12,29,30,54] The influence of psychic "toxicity" on the psychobiological unit is still one of inference. Seyle's description of the general adaptation syndrome and the knowledge that chronic stress frequently produces hormonal imbalances and suppresses the immune system suggest a condition of biological vulnerability to the occurrence of illness.[9] Thus illness may be an adaptive attempt or a nonadaptive consequence of unresolved object loss.[19,56] No one understands the way that brain chemicals are related to emotions. Studies suggest the possibility that a person can control his or her immune system through conscious or unconscious suggestion as well as through exposure to positive-enhancing stimuli. A person's state of mind has an important effect on the state of his body. Emotions such as hope, purpose, faith, will to live, determination, festivity, playfulness, and purpose can be powerful biochemical prescriptions.[35,55] Emotions in and of themselves are not necessarily significant physically; however, when they linger and become long-term states of mind, they assume more importance than need be, especially when they are negative.[35] This suggests that coping mechanisms play a vital role in buffering adverse effects of stress.

The critically ill patient may be at risk for some degree of immune incompetence simply by being admitted to the intensive care unit. Certainly the effects of serious illness, plus the chronic noise and activity, lights, and equipment can produce increased stress levels. Being able to keep the patient free of panic and to enhance the environment for effective treatment and compliance may be one of the most important, but rarely noticed, nursing actions. The challenge to the critical care nurse is to assess the patient's relationship and pattern of dealing with the world, especially the ability to express emotions.

Diagnostic Testing for HIV Infection

The development of an ELISA to detect antibodies to HIV has provided medical technology for screening targeted populations. Despite the obvious advantages of screening specific groups, HIV testing remains a most controversial issue. There is a large amount of public sentiment, about HIV testing and AIDS.

The only commercially available tests are those that indicate the presence of HIV antibodies. The test does not diagnose AIDS, nor can it be used to indicate progression to disease. Antibody testing is usually done in two steps. The first is the ELISA, a test that was developed to screen the nation's blood supply. ELISA is quick, easy to perform, and extremely sensitive; however, it has a high rate of false-positive results. There can also be false-negative results with ELISA if the test is done before the person develops antibodies or if the person is too sick to produce the antibody. If a false-negative reading is suspected or the ELISA is positive, a second test, the Western Blot, is performed to confirm that the test is truly positive.

The presence of antibodies to the retrovirus (HIV positive) does not mean that the person has AIDS or will develop AIDS. Being HIV positive merely indicates that the person has been exposed to or infected with HIV. Conversely, not detecting the presence of antibody to the retrovirus (HIV negative) means that the person has no antibody, has not yet developed the antibody, or has advanced infection and is unable to produce the antibody.

Clearly there are reasons that testing is important. However, HIV testing must be accompanied by education and counseling. Often it is the nurse who assesses the patient and provides information, especially if the patient is hospitalized.

Associated Laboratory Findings

The initial laboratory evaluation is based in part on the medical history and physical findings. Immunologic tests and viral serologies have limited clinical value in patients with established AIDS. The numerous immunologic abnormalities described in AIDS have not been established to have any value in clinical decision-making, except for the absolute number of T4 cells.

When HIV infection is first detectable, the T4 cell concentration is often close to the normal level of about 800 cells/ mm^3 of blood. As the disease progresses silently, the T4 cell count drops slowly; when the cell count is around 400 cells/ mm^3, the person exhibits abnormal responses on skin tests. As the level drops below 400 cells/mm^3, the immune system, especially cell-mediated immunity, begins to decline.

In addition to the presence of HIV and a decline in T-helper lymphocytes in the blood, the following abnormalities are usually found: leukopenia, mild to moderate anemia, sometimes thrombocytompenia, a decreased ratio of T-helper to T-suppressor lymphocytes, and a polyclonal increase in immunoglobins, especially IgG and IgA. Although increased IgG and IgA are characteristic of AIDS, qualitative immunoglobin determination has not added any clinically useful information. Serum antibodies to Epstein-Barr virus and cytomegalovirus are present in the majority of patients; however, they do not provide diagnostic or prognostic information.

NURSING DIAGNOSES, PATIENT OUTCOMES, AND PLAN

The preceding material on physiology, nursing assessment, and diagnostic tests guides the nurse in establishing nursing diagnoses, patient outcomes, and plan for the patient who is immunosuppressed.

NURSING CARE PLAN SUMMARY   Patient With AIDS

NURSING DIAGNOSIS

1. Altered comfort: pain related to genital herpes (feeling pattern)

Patient Outcome	Nursing Orders
Patient will be maximally pain free.	1. Administer pain medication as ordered.
	2. Apply 2% viscous lidocaine topically to area surrounding herpetic lesions.
	3. Decrease anxiety levels by establishing a trusting relationship.
	A. Take all concerns seriously.
	B. Follow through on everything you say you will do.
	C. Maintain a listening and supportive manner.
	D. Provide information frequently, clarifying any misconceptions.
	E. Explore and use all resources to relieve concerns, especially interventions to decrease physical and psychosocial discomforts.
	F. Use complementary therapies: humor, meditation, progressive relaxation.

NURSING DIAGNOSIS

2. Impaired skin integrity: predisposition to secondary infection related to disease process and neutropenia (exchanging pattern)

Patient Outcome	Nursing Orders
Patient will maintain skin integrity and nosocomial infection will be prevented.	1. Provide a private room.
	2. Use sterile sheets.
	3. Do frequent and thorough handwashing before and after care.
	4. Wear gloves during care and change frequently so microorganisms are not transmitted from one site to another.

(continued)

NURSING CARE PLAN SUMMARY   *Patient With AIDS*   Continued

Patient Outcome	Nursing Orders
	5. Provide masks for any person entering the room with an upper respiratory infection.
	6. Humidify the air and make sure the housekeeping staff dry-dusts the floor with disinfectant solution.
	7. Make sure there is no standing water in the room, especially in vases, suction containers, or respiratory therapy equipment.
	8. Monitor skin integrity every shift, including the rectum, IV lines, and blood drawing sites.
	9. Give special attention to the coccyx because of immobility.
	A. Massage and lubricate with oils, lotions, and lubricants.
	B. Change underpads frequently. *Do not* use Chux.
	C. Supplement prevention of pressure sore care with use of an appropriate mattress.
	D. Thoroughly wash and dry the perianal region after voiding and defecating. Apply bacitracin ointment to vulvular lesions.
	E. Administer antibiotics as ordered.
	F. Administer acyclovir as ordered.
	10. Take the patient's temperature every 4 hours.
	11. Check the complete blood count with differential three times weekly.

NURSING DIAGNOSIS

3. *Altered protection: development of opportunistic infection related to immunosuppressed state (exchanging pattern)*

Patient Outcome	Nursing Orders
Patient will not have progression of symptoms and signs of opportunistic infections.	1. Continue to assess for symptoms and signs of opportunistic infections.
	A. Thrush
	(1) Assess oral cavity for any changes in symptoms and signs every shift.
	(2) Assess for dysphagia, substernal burning, or pain each time opportunity presents itself after eating.
	(3) Clean mouth thoroughly, including brushing the gums and tongue in the morning and after each meal.
	a. Rinse mouth with solution of ½ tsp salt and 1 tsp baking soda in 1 quart lukewarm water every 2 hours while awake, especially before and after eating.
	b. Brush teeth after each meal and at bedtime with a soft toothbrush or toothette, and use a mild nonabrasive toothpaste such as Crest or Sensodyne.
	(4) Administer nystatin (Mycostatin) solution 5 ml four times a day; have the patient swish and swallow.
	(5) Have the patient avoid hot, spicy foods and commercial mouthwashes that may be irritating to oral mucosa.
	B. *Pneumocystis carinii* pneumonia (PCP)
	(1) Assess respiratory status every shift.
	(2) Monitor vital signs, lung sounds, cough, color, complaint of dyspnea on exertion, and nailbeds for relevant changes every shift.
	(3) Monitor temperature every 4 hours around the clock.
	(4) Remember Tylenol allergy and administer Ecotrin.
	C. Herpes Simplex Virus
	(1) Administer 5% acyclovir ointment locally.
	(2) Administer acyclovir 400 mg IV three times a day. Remember adequate hydration; mix in 250 ml of solution and administer over 1 hour.
	(3) Administer azathioprine (Zidovudine) (AZT) 200 mg five times daily; check the complete blood count with differential three times weekly.
	(4) Send viral cultures as ordered.

(continued)

NURSING CARE PLAN SUMMARY *Patient With AIDS* *Continued*

NURSING DIAGNOSIS

4. *High risk for ineffective individual coping: anxiety and loss of autonomy related to forced dependency, immobility, and social isolation (choosing pattern)*

Patient Outcome	Nursing Orders

Patient will express his or her feelings and retain control of his or her life.	1. Encourage the patient to be an active participant in her care.
	    A. Set up a physical therapy consultation to develop appropriate exercises and exercise schedule while the patient is immobilized.
	    B. Establish a trusting relationship (see Nursing Diagnosis 1, #3, above).
	    C. Allow the patient to exercise control over his or her environment whenever possible.
	        (1) Encourage the patient to make as many care and treatment decisions as possible (*e.g.,* timing of nursing procedures, selection and timing of visitors, and degree of participation in activities of daily living).
	            a. Set limits about those areas about which she has no control (*e.g.,* medication times, physician rounds), and communicate to both patient and family.
	            b. Explain all equipment, treatments, treatment options, and environment.
	            c. Clarify any misconceptions, help to reorganize facts and to rehearse questions or information needed from medical personnel.
	            d. Be honest in all interactions and transactions.
	    D. Permit the patient to decorate the room as he or she chooses.
	    E. Communicate acceptance and concern of patient and her medical situation.
	        (1) Stand close to her when talking and always make eye contact.
	        (2) Touch the patient when greeting, talking, and giving care.
	        (3) Be aware of body language; use gestures that show openness and a desire to connect.
	    F. Encourage verbalization of emotions.
	        (1) Remember not to take personally any of the patient's words.
	        (2) Listen and accept feelings.
	        (3) Reflect emotions back to the patient.
	        (4) Avoid the temptation to dismiss fears as unrealistic.
	        (5) Assess behavior for unresolved grief and refer as needed.
	        (6) Help the patient to determine how to vent emotions (*e.g.,* journal keeping, talking to a friend).
	    G. Facilitate positive body image and reinforce self-concept.
	        (1) Set up a physical therapy consultation.
	        (2) Minimize displays of invasive interventions (*e.g.,* IVs, chest tubes).
	        (3) Encourage and facilitate usual grooming habits.
	        (4) Give positive feedback for all accomplishments, no matter how small they may seem.
	        (5) Encourage the patient to focus on what he or she does well.
	        (6) Facilitate the use of complementary therapy (*i.e.,* progressive relaxation, meditation, humor).
	    H. Assist the patient to continue present roles and relationships.
	        (1) Help the patient to identify new ways to continue relationships (*e.g.,* daily updates on husband's and daughter's conditions).
	        (2) Maintain privacy when visitors are present.
	        (3) Collaborate with the daughter's primary nurse to develop an appropriate daily visitation schedule.
	    I. Use complementary therapy: humor.

IMPLEMENTATION AND EVALUATION

Clinical Course

Infection with HIV results in a spectrum of clinical manifestations that range from minor to severe. The grim reality of HIV infection is that all people who are infected will eventually develop end-stage disease and will die prematurely.

The determination of clinical spectrum resides in the progressive decline of the T4 cell population and the subsequent general deterioration in immune functioning. After the initial infection, the amount of HIV in the body soars until the immune system responds as it should to an invading organism. The immune system limits the viral replication for some time, keeping it under control. Meanwhile HIV struggles to gain ground and does so slowly. At some point, the T4 cell population becomes so depleted that the immune system becomes nonfunctional and the balance of power switches to the wildly replicating HIV. Then the remaining T4 cells are killed, eliminating any traces of immune defense.

HIV usually causes no symptoms at first and can take root from 6 weeks to 1 year before it is detected by the standard HIV antibody test.[51] Once the infection is diagnosed, probably at the time of seroconversion, some patients develop an ailment mimicking mononucleosis: fever, fatigue, and swollen glands. In addition, self-limited symptoms of the central nervous system develop that disappear within a few weeks.

The first sign that something is wrong with the immune system is the development of chronically swollen lymph nodes. The cause of the lymphadenopathy is the ongoing presence of HIV stimulating the B cells to a state of chronic activation. However, this hyperactivity is not beneficial to the individual, because the activation of a large number of B cells decreases the number of resting cells available to produce antibodies in response to new pathogens. Infected individuals may have immunologic laboratory abnormalities or hematologic abnormalities with or without clinical symptoms. Most important among the latter are idiopathic thrombocytopenia, lymphopenia, and anemia. The immunologic abnormalities include a quantitative decrease in T4-lymphocytes and a subsequent inversion of the T4/T8 ratio below 1. These immunologic and hematologic abnormalities are not specific to any stage in the development of AIDS but are documented at all stages.

The viral infection may not progress beyond chronic lymphadenopathy for 3 to 5 years. At a point when the qualitative T4 cell count falls below $400/mm^3$, the individual has about 18 months until direct evidence of clinical signs of immune dysfunction occur. The individual progresses from a state of partial anergy to total anergy, as measured by the intradermal injection of specific proteins. By this time, the T4 cell count has generally fallen to less than 200 cells/mm^3.[51]

Once the individual develops total anergy, the first overt symptom of the breakdown in cell-mediated immunity occurs. Indigenous pathogens become activated to produce opportunistic disease. Most of the opportunistic infections that develop in patients with AIDS are caused by pervasive organisms of low virulence, which are known to establish latent infections in normal individuals. The first of such infections to develop is candidiasis or thrush, a fungal infection of the mucous membranes of the tongue or the oral cavity and sometimes of the esophagus. In addition to thrush, the individual often develops severe or chronic viral or fungal infections of the skin and mucous membranes—such as herpes simplex

virus, which produces persistent, painful sores of the skin surrounding the mouth, anus, or genital areas—and *Candida albicans*.

About 1 to 2 years after a state of total anergy develops, when the T4 cell population is less than 100 cells/mm^3, many individuals develop chronic or disseminated infections at sites other than the skin and mucous membranes. For each organ system, including the central nervous system, there are predominant infecting organisms, such as *Pneumocystis carinii* pneumonia (PCP), *Mycobacterium avium–intracellulare* (MAI), *Toxoplasma* encephalitis, and cryptococcal meningitis. In addition to these infections, the individual may also develop cytomegalovirus (CMV), a common viral infection that may cause pneumonia, encephalitis, blindness, and inflammation of the intestinal tract. CMV is usually a reactivation of a childhood infection that was well controlled until HIV altered the immune system. Once the individual's disease has progressed to the stage of chronic disseminated infections, he or she usually dies within 2 years.[51]

In general the signs, symptoms, and laboratory findings of opportunistic infections—especially when the lungs or central nervous system is involved—are too nonspecific to permit an accurate diagnosis unless a biopsy and culture of abnormal tissue is taken. After effective treatment of such infections, there tends to be a high relapse rate, probably associated with reactivation of residual organisms that cannot be eliminated entirely either by treatment or by poor cellular defense mechanisms.

In the terminal stages of HIV infection, many patients suffer from the AIDS dementia complex (ADC), a complicated syndrome characterized by a gradual loss in the ability to think precisely and more symptoms that are hard to distinguish from clinical depression. Early neurologic findings include alterations in cognitive function such as concentration, memory, and judgment. The individual begins to grow clumsy and has slower spontaneous verbal and motor responses; as the disease progresses, he may become mute as well as incontinent of urine and feces. For the most part, AIDS dementia complex progresses over months, although the syndrome speeds up after definite neurologic signs appear. As with other aspects of AIDS, the total T4 cell count seems to make a difference. Individuals with a total T4 cell count less than 200 cells/mm^3 have greater cognitive and motor decline than those with counts above 200 cells/mm^3.[53]

The next section discusses the most common pathogens associated with AIDS that bring the patient into a critical care unit. The opportunistic infections that are not discussed here are mycobacterial infections and parasitic infections of the gastrointestinal tract.

Opportunistic Infections

Pneumocystis carinii, Mycobacterium avium–Mycobacterium intracellulare, herpes simplex virus, cytomegalovirus, *Cryptoccus neoformans, Toxoplasma gondii,* and cryptosporidism are the low-virulence organisms producing infection in the patient with AIDS. It is generally believed that these infectious agents are the result of reactivation of a dormant infection, attributed to the immunosuppression induced by HIV, rather than infections with newly acquired microorganisms.[21] The signs, symptoms, and laboratory findings of these organisms are too nonspecific to allow diagnosis without the results of a biopsy or a culture of abnormal tissue. The observed frequency of certain fungal or parasitic infections depends on the prevalence of these pathogens in the local population. Thus, the individual's place of birth, the travel history, and the geographic distribution of different organisms are important components in the patient's history.

In addition to infection by organisms of low virulence, the classic virulent pyogenic bacteria, namely *Staphylococcus aureus*, *Streptococcus pneumoniae*, and *Hemophilus influenzae* type B, occur in patients with HIV disease. The development of bacterial infections may be partly due to defects in B-cell function that have been described in persons with HIV disease.

Pneumocystis Carinii Pneumonia

Pneumocystis carinii pneumonia (PCP) is the most common major opportunistic infection in patients with AIDS and is often the first to occur.[16] More than 80% of patients with AIDS acquire PCP; in 60% it is the initial opportunistic infection.[22] It is estimated that another 20% of patients with AIDS develop PCP later in the course of illness.[26] Moreover, many patients develop more than one episode of PCP.

Patients with HIV infection often have nonspecific symptoms such as fever, fatigue, and weight loss for weeks to months before developing the respiratory symptoms that herald the onset of PCP. The classic presenting symptoms are fever, tachypnea, dyspnea, nonproductive cough, and dry rales.

The physical examination is not particularly helpful because of other HIV processes occurring simultaneously. The patient's general appearance is often that of someone wasted and febrile, even though in the early stages he or she may appear healthy. Hypoxemia may be mild. Findings on lung examination are minimal; rales may be heard and findings indicating consolidation are unusual, except when there is severe pulmonary involvement.

Routine laboratory examination is not especially helpful. Lymphopenia is common with a total T-helper cell count of less than $200/mm^3$. Many other hematologic abnormalities are also present, such as anemia, leukopenia, and thrombocytopenia; an elevated serum lactate dehydrogenase level may give a clue to the presence of lung disease.

Typically the chest x-ray examination is not definitive but does provide useful information; diffuse interstitial infiltrates may be present, evenly involving all portions of the lungs. Gallium lung scan, a complex and costly test, identifies diffuse uptake throughout the lung that is too nonspecific to identify the presence of PCP. Another test that evaluates the degree of pulmonary involvement and function is the arterial blood gas test. Usually the abnormal functions found include a decrease in vital capacity, total lung capacity, and single-breath diffusing capacity for carbon monoxide.

Induction of sputum has been successful in establishing the diagnosis, but an experienced team is required to minimize false-negative results. To achieve a level of sensitivity in using sputum induction, certain steps must be taken: a patient should not eat for several hours before induction; teeth, gums, and oral cavity should be cleaned carefully by brushing and gargling; and once the specimen is obtained, it should be transported promptly to the laboratory.[26]

The definitive diagnosis of PCP is established by demonstrating the presence of the organism. Open lung biopsy is the definitive means for establishing the presence of pneumocysts in the lung. Because thrombocytopenia and other coagulation abnormalities are often present, a less invasive procedure may be performed. Fiberoptic bronchoscopy with transbronchial biopsy and brushings is nearly 100% sensitive to the presence of *P. carinii*. Another technique, bronchoalveolar lavage performed through a bronchoscope with the introduction of 200 ml of normal saline and rapid removal by suction, has shown virtually the same yield as an open lung biopsy.[26]

Treatment of PCP is initiated with trimethoprim 15 to 20 mg/kg of body weight/day and sulfamethoxazole 75 to 100 mg/kg/day intravenously. When the switch is made to pentamidine because of inadequate improvement with trimethoprim–sulfamethoxazole therapy, the mortality rate on pentamidine is very high.[16] If a patient does not respond to initial treatment by day 5 to 7, he should be switched to pentamidine 4 mg/kg/day. The efficacy of these two regimens is similar; there is a 60% to 80% response rate during the first episode and somewhat poorer results in subsequent episodes.[21] Respiratory support often is needed for these patients, but some require endotracheal intubation. For this latter group of patients, mortality is high, reflecting the far-advanced stage of the respiratory infection and poor host defenses.

Pentamidine isethionate is a drug whose mechanisms of antiprotozoal effects remain uncertain. The drug has traditionally been given intramuscularly, but it is usually administered by slow intravenous infusion under close supervision. To be given intravenously, the single-dose, 300-mg vial is reconstituted in sterile water, not sodium chloride, then is further diluted in 50 to 100 ml of 5% dextrose and infused over 1 to 2 hours to decrease the risk of potentially life-threatening hypotension. Should a patient develop adverse reactions during intravenous infusion, the infusion should be stopped immediately. Once the adverse effect has resolved, the infusion may be restarted at a slower rate with no loss of efficacy.[45]

The use of pentamidine is limited by its toxicity. Thrombophlebitis and generalized or localized urticarial eruptions are seen, and severe hypotension may develop with too-rapid intravenous infusion or after a single intramuscular injection. The reason for the development of hypotension is unknown, but a drug-induced histamine release may be responsible.[21] Facial flushing, breathlessness, dizziness, hypoglycemia, and impaired renal function have been reported.[21] Although severe renal impairment has occurred, it is impossible to attribute renal failure solely to pentamidine.

Because either trimethoprime–sulfamethoxazole or pentamidine isethionate has severe adverse reactions requiring patients to change from one drug to another, aerosolized pentamidine—600 mg dissolved in 6 ml of sterile water inhaled for 20 minutes every day for 21 days—was used successfully in patients with first episodes of PCP.[42] The only adverse reaction to the aerosolized treatment was coughing.

Another interesting drug, dapsone—an antileprosy, antimalarial agent—has been used to treat PCP. However, the drug is a sulfonamidelike agent and is not without hematologic complications.

The appropriate duration of antipneumocystis therapy is unclear. Because the initial response to therapy is slow and the relapse rate is high, a total treatment time of 14 to 21 days is usually recommended.[21,45] Suppressive therapy is often necessary after treatment. Trimethoprim 160 mg with sulfamethoxazole 800 mg twice a day is effective, but side-effects limit its use. Dapsone 100 mg once a day plus trimethoprim has been shown to be effective in preventing PCP.

Fungal Infections: Candida and Cryptococcus

The fungal infections are usually due to *Candida* species or *Cryptococcus neoformans*. *Candida* may be localized or mucocutaneous. In a critical care unit where the patients have multiple access lines or indwelling catheters, systemic candidiasis may be seen. Usually the patient has thrush or *Candida* esophagitis. Because localized herpesvirus or cytomegalovirus infection can mimic *Candida* esophagitis, esophagoscopy and biopsy establish a definitive diagnosis.

Localized candidiasis of the oropharyngeal cavity may respond to nystatin troches or gargles, to local clotrimazole troches, or to the orally administered but systemically absorbed imidazole or ketoconazole at 200 mg three times a day. Generally nystatin is the treatment of choice, but if the infection is too severe, ketoconazole 400 to 600 mg/day is effective in suppressing thrush, though not severe esophagitis. If after 5 to 7 days of ketoconazole, treatment for esophagitis is ineffective, systemic amphotericin B is a drastic but necessary intervention. Therapy of *Candida* esophagitis or mucocutaneous disease is rarely curative but usually is suppressive. If candidiasis recurs, retreatment is necessary.

In contrast to localized candidiasis, cryptococcal infection in the patient with AIDS usually presents as a systemic process. Cryptococcal dissemination may include lungs, bone marrow, and spleen. The most common manifestation is meningitis, ranging from fulminant disease with extensive extraneural involvement to any extremely subtle disease process characterized by mild depression, little or no headache, and no meningeal signs. Any patient complaining of headache, change in mental status, or fever should have an immediate lumbar puncture. Cell counts, glucose, and protein levels in the cerebrospinal fluid may be slightly elevated. By far the most sensitive and specific diagnostic test is the detection of the cryptococcal antigen.

Cryptococcal infection in patients with AIDS should be treated with amphotericin B, with or without flucytosine. In non-AIDS patients, this combination of therapy causes neutropenia, a side-effect of the flucytosine, not of the amphotericin B. The optimal dose and duration of therapy are uncertain. Most patients receive amphotericin B 0.4 mg to 0.6 mg/kg/day to total 1.5 g to 2.0 g over 6 weeks, but the speed of clinical response and drug toxicity influence decisions about therapy.[21]

Therapy for cryptococcal disease with amphotericin B is not curative, and relapse occurs in more than 50% of the patients.[21]

Viral Infections

Viral infections are typical in the patient with AIDS. Infection with cytomegalovirus (CMV) is frequent and the most common cause of life-threatening opportunistic viral infection in patients with AIDS.[27] Like all herpes viruses, CMV can cause primary, latent, or chronic persistent infection. It is difficult to differentiate between latency and reactivation of CMV;[30] however, evidence supporting the existence of a latent CMV infection has come from the study of pregnant women, immunosuppressed patients, and recipients of blood transfusions and organ transplants.[28]

After the primary infection, herpes viruses (*i.e.*, CMV, varicella zoster, herpes simplex, and Epstein-Barr) characteristically persist in cells and tissues of the host, presumably for the lifetime of the person.[28] Years after the primary infection, the latent virus can reactivate, with a renewed shedding of the infectious virus, also resulting in a chronic persistent infection.[27]

Subclinical CMV infection is common in patients with HIV disease. Nearly all homosexual men with HIV disease have serologic evidence of recently acquired or reactivated CMV infection.[27] Pregnant and lactating women who have the antibody to the virus shed the virus in cervicovaginal secretions or breast milk, accounting for a substantial number of subclinical infections in infants. Additionally, CMV has been documented in leukemia patients or bone marrow transplant recipients who have received leukocyte transfusions. Thus, the leukocyte fraction of whole blood is implicated as one of the vehicles of CMV transmission.

However CMV is transmitted, the immunosuppression— whether from the HIV disease or the CMV itself—compounds the clinical manifestations. CMV infections appear as fever with disseminated organ system involvement, including: retinitis; pneumonia or pneumonitis, sometimes along with PCP; mononucleosis; meningitis; esophagitis; enteritis; and colitis. Patients with retinitis typically complain of blurred vision, decreased visual activity, and, over time, visual loss. CMV gastrointestinal disease is an important problem in patients with AIDS. The severe diarrhea causes loss of electrolytes, minerals, fluid, and weight. The emotional stress and hypoalbuminemia can make the diarrhea and malabsorption worse. For some patients, adjustment in diet and antidiarrheal drugs such as loperamide (Imodium) or tincture of opium may alleviate the problem. But when the infection severely impairs absorption, the bowel may need to rest; then total parenteral nutrition becomes the only alternative.

Ganciclovir, formerly known as DHPG, structurally similar to acyclovir, is a potent inhibitor of viral DNA polymerase. In adults with normal renal function who receive a typical induction of 2.5 mg/kg of body weight every 8 hours intravenously, a peak and trough level should average 18 to 24 μmol/hour and 1 to 2 μmol/L, respectively.[27] Because the drug is cleared exclusively by the kidneys, dose adjustment must be made when the estimated creatinine clearance is less than 50 ml/minute.

Neutropenia is the most frequent adverse reaction associated with ganciclovir. A 50% decrease from baseline in absolute white blood cell count is expected in patients receiving either induction or maintenance therapy. This drug-related severe neutropenia is resolved within days after ganciclovir therapy is stopped. Once the absolute neutrophil count rises above 1.0×10^9/L, an induction regimen may be reinstituted. When neutropenia complicates maintenance therapy, titration of the ganciclovir dose to the absolute neutrophil count permits achievement of the maximally tolerated dose for the patient.

If acyclovir and ganciclovir are unsuccessful in treating CMV infection, another experimental drug, foscarnet trisodium phosphonoformate, may be used. Foscarnet is a potent inhibitor of all human herpesvirus DNA polymerases, as well as retrovirus reverse transcriptase.[27] The drug is administered by a single intravenous bolus dose of 9 to 20 mg/kg followed by a continuous intravenous infusion of 23 to 268 mg/kg/day. The most common toxicity attributed to foscarnet is alteration in renal function, as seen in a rise of serum creatinine level. Other side-effects of foscarnet therapy include alterations in serum calcium, mild anemia, seizures, irritability, reversible tremor, and superficial thrombophlebitis when the intravenous infusion is through a peripheral vein.[27]

Mucocutaneous herpes simplex infections are common in patients with AIDS and can cause severe progressive perianal and rectal ulcers. Severe necrotizing perianal herpetic infection is common in patients with AIDS; it almost always responds to parenteral acyclovir therapy, 15 mg/kg/day for extensive disease, but treatment does not eradicate the virus, and recurrences after discontinuation of therapy are common. Oral acyclovir, 200 to 400 mg five times a day, is usually effective for mild mucocutaneous disease.

Toxoplasmosis

The second most common systemic infection is due to *Toxoplasma gondii,* a parasitic infection whose epidemiology and clinical presentation in the compromised host differ from the disease in the normal population. The major clinical manifestations of toxoplasmosis in patients with AIDS range from mild headache and fever to focal neurologic deficits, seizures, and coma.

Serologic tests are of limited value because antibody to *T. gondii* is prevalent in the general population, and its presence has low predictive value for active infection. The most useful diagnostic test is the computed tomography (CT) scan. Lesions are usually multiple, ring-enhanced with contrast, associated with edema, and located in the cortical or subcortical regions of the brain.

Because noninvasive tests lack specificity, definitive diagnosis requires a biopsy of the brain. Because of the potential morbidity of performing a brain biopsy empiric therapy is preferred for patients with positive serologic findings and a clinical picture compatible with toxoplasmosis. Therapy with pyrimethamine 25 mg/day and sulfadiazine 100 mg/kg/day to a maximum of 8 g/day is usually effective. Improvement is seen clinically and on the CT scan in 1 to 2 weeks.[27] As one would expect, the optimal duration of therapy is unknown but it should be continued for at least 3 to 6 months. Relapses are frequent.

Supportive Therapy

The critical care nurse can be logical to a fault. He or she tends to focus on disease, as if the patient "catches it," forgetting that every illness involves the interaction between the mind and the body. Each patient is a unique entity of body and spirit, and both elements need nurturing and attention. As the nurse deals with the body–mind–spirit concept, he or she must be creative and adventuresome in his or her thinking, feeling, and actions.

Not only does the critical care nurse bring his or her technical expertise to the nurse–patient relationship, but he or she also brings his or her ability to help the patient to redirect and to refocus his or her thinking about the illness. The outcome of this process is that the patient feels confident that he can overcome the threat of the illness, as well as to feel in control of

him or herself and of his or her environment. The patient's belief in him or herself self fosters a will to live and not to give up hope, a special type of positive expectation. Even if the patient cannot control the inevitability of the outcome, he or she can still expect and extract positive outcomes from the experience and concentrate on attaining them.

The nurse must remember that his or her vigilant, logical care is just as important to the nurse–patient relationship as is his or her belief that within each one of us resides our own internal doctor. "It is the body, not medicine, that is the hero."[20] Every living organism has to protect itself from harm. In this regard, human beings are no different, because they lie surrounded by a veritable sea of organisms that have also paralleled their evolutionary growth—viruses and bacteria. Human protection from the world is the result of a complicated evolutionary process of a thousand million years of finely honed chemical responsiveness. Humans not only carry around the most sophisticated of life processes, but also the most protective of devices known—the immune system. The immune system is a complex self-monitoring, auto-regulated system. It is composed of a group of chemical and microbial killers that in spite of their small size are quick, vicious, and relentless in their special capability of pattern recognition and of patrolling and guarding the body's immunity against marauders.

The immune system's "sonar" is so effective that within minutes after an infectious process begins, granulocytes stream to the area to attack the marauding organisms. The granulocytes begin the fights, but their largest brothers, the macrophages, complete the job of death and destruction for the invading organism.

Antibodies, another component of the human immune system, are manufactured in response to the cell's identification of a foreign marauder by the surface of the microbe. The ability of antibodies to recognize not only their own body's cells, but also everything that is not considered to be "theirs" is a monumental task. Thus the immune system is always in a position of being the underdog, the counteraggressor, because the invaders must be inside the body before it can manufacture the appropriate response. The body is literally in a state of paranoia because it is always on the alert, watching and waiting for something to happen. Then the immune system must come from behind to overcome the invaders that have already gained a foothold.

Because our immune system is too important, has too much to do, and has to react too quickly, it is not located in any one part of our body, but rather is distributed throughout the entire body, next to every organ and limb, and close to every surface. The cells and molecules of the immune system are able to reach most tissues through the bloodstream, and after moving about, they return to their own vascular network, the lymphatic system. The lymphatic channels, a second great circulatory system, are composed of lymph nodes that house lymphocytes, the masterminds of the immune system, which take it on themselves to divide and multiply and to lay in wait for the immulogic fight that protects us from death.

This chapter is about Heide P.—her hopes, her illness, and her future. The complexity of what happens to Heide and others like her can scarcely be communicated by the written word. Just as clinical judgment is learned at the bedside, the enormity of the total clinical situation can be transformed only by the feelings and meanings within the situation. To look, to listen, to feel, to believe, to transform, and to accept—these are the essence of the nurse–patient relationship.

It is the author's assumption that the reader will know not only that Heide is a person who has a disruption in her ability to fulfill the three tasks of her immune system and that there are things to be done to prevent or minimize complications medically, but also that she is a person who has a psychologic response to the entire sequence of events and that there are things to be done to prevent or minimize those complications as well.

Psychosocial Responses to AIDS

The patient with AIDS is a young adult who was previously healthy and who now is facing a life-threatening disease. In addition to being ill-prepared to face a disabling terminal illness and the frustration of prolonged hospitalizations, the patient encounters hysteria, hostility, and rejection. The hysteria fosters a climate in which a person with the medical diagnosis of AIDS enters a state of emotional collapse that itself compromises both the treatment plan and the patient's emotional resources. The intense emotional pain that accompanies a physical illness, especially this one, carries a social stigma in American society. Admitting to a physical illness may be socially acceptable, but acknowledging an emotional upset is considered to be a sign of weakness. When the tension that accompanies intense emotion is not released, the results are emotional and social isolation, interpersonal conflicts stemming from miscommunication, and a narrowed perspective of perceived choices. The ability to keep the patient free from panic and to avoid a defeatist attitude is an important, though intangible, aspect of nursing care. What it means is to help the patient cope with the disease not by denial but with a vigorous determination to get the best and most out of whatever *is now*. The essential issue, particularly in a critical care unit, is whether it is possible to strike a balance between biological factors and psychologic factors in the understanding and management of the disease.

Developing Hardiness

The negative health consequences of the patient's feeling helpless or hopeless are well documented. Being helpless and hopeless implies quitting, giving up, losing hope, and letting go of the will to live. One way to turn the negative feeling toward the positive and to assist the patient in becoming "exceptional"[57] is to encourage the patient to develop "hardiness."[32]

The "hardy" patient is one who asserts that he or she can control his or her life by using his judgment to make good decisions; who is committed to him or herself by finding meaning in his life; who is actively involved with work, values, and personal relationships; and who perceives a change in life-style or potentially stressful life events as ultimately beneficial to personal development.[34,57] Of vital importance in becoming "hardy" is a positive attitude toward stressful situations, changes, and losses. Thus, the goal is to help the patient to develop the resilience, adaptability, and confidence of a survivor. As in any battle with serious illness, an important element is the patient's ability to summon all his physical and spiritual resources in fighting the illness.

Humor and Laughter

Humor and laughter have long been recognized as playing a role in moderating the impact of stress, as well as having a normalizing effect on a situation.[31,39] They can: diffuse stressful life events by releasing built-up tension from such feelings as fear, hostility, and anger; they can reduce social and emotional distances between people they can assist in resolving interpersonal conflict, because few people can laugh and remain angry at the same time; and they can create a mental outlook oriented to constructive problem-solving.[13,31] If a person can see humor in an embarrassing situation over a minor upset, the individual begins to disconnect himself from the event. With humor one can approach things sideways, upside down, inside out, and backward. Comic relief restores a person's ability to function. Somehow things do not seem so bad if a person can laugh. Once humor is found, a situation no longer seems as large or as important as it once was; the individual saves his or her positive energy to cope with a crisis. Humor's most important psychologic function is to jolt the person's perspective in order to promote new perspectives.

Laughter, the most evident response to humor, defies scientific interpretation.[4] It is unique in that it is both a reflex and a psychosomatic event.[4] Yet laughter is such a human response that it can restore human touch in the technical world of critical care.

Cousins calls laughter "inner jogging" because a good hearty laugh gives every system in the body a workout.[14] Laughing with gusto turns your body into a giant vibrator as it performs an internal massage.[8] A robust laugh gives the diaphragm, thorax, abdomen, and heart a brief workout and relaxes all the muscles, including the heart. The effect of laughter on the individual is cathartic. Anger and tension diminish, and one feels so much better and more relaxed after a hearty laugh.[4]

Physiologic changes also occur as a result of laughter. Mirthful laughter, which is believed to involve central nervous system response, modifies the classic stress hormones of epinephrine, cortisol, and dopamine.[3] The pituitary gland is also involved; it releases endorphins and enkephalins, natural painkillers that are chemical cousins to morphine and heroin. Thus, humor and laughter may relieve pain by physical means, as well as by diverting one's attention and helping one to relax. The relaxation response may last as long as 45 minutes.[31]

Even though a hearty laugh has been likened to aerobic exercise, laughter differs in that it does not require special clothing, elaborate equipment, or a specific schedule. It is convenient, free, and always present.

Humor and laughter are among the most prevalent forms of human social behavior, but among the least understood. In a critical care unit, where minute-to-minute stress is prevalent, humor is often present and often makes a difference, not because the stress is funny but because humor and laughter help us to adapt.[36] The critical care nurse should explore the use of humor as it effects both the nurse and the patients. The nurse must begin to recognize the value of humor and laughter, understand its purpose, and incorporate it as a planned intervention not only in his or her professional but also in one's personal life.

SUMMARY

AIDS is a fatal disease caused by HIV and characterized by a decrease in the T4 helper cell population. The abnormal T4/T8 ratio causes an immunologic imbalance that predisposes the patient to multiple infections, including opportunistic infections. The most common low-virulence organisms that cause persistent and sometimes life-threatening infections are *Pneumocystis carinii*, *Toxoplasma gondii*, herpesvirus, *Candida*, *Cryptococcus neoformans*, *Mycobacterium avium–intracellulare*, and mycobacterial tuberculosis.

The diagnosis and treatment of the HIV-associated diseases focuses on the following points:

- Infections are rarely single.
- Because the majority of infections are reactivation of previously acquired organisms, except for tuberculosis and herpes zoster, they do not pose a threat to other persons.
- Fungal parasitic and viral infections are rarely curable; they often require long-term therapy.[21]

Because of the complexity of AIDS, it frequently exposes shortcomings in a system of subspecialized medicine. In hospitals that care for many patients with AIDS, ethical dilemmas often occur because of the disease's almost 100% fatality. Patients and physicians must decide whether supportive care might be more appropriate than life-sustaining treatment, such as intubation, mechanical ventilation, and cardiopulmonary resuscitation. A workable policy is for care givers to discuss these matters with the patient shortly after the patient is admitted to the hospital.

Caring for patients with AIDS is extremely stressful. These patients, often critically ill, have protected hospitalizations and require many procedures. Despite optimal treatment, many do poorly or develop new opportunistic infections.

In addition to the stress of caring for a critically ill patient, nurses and physicians may have emotional reactions to these patients. Often reactions are based on our fear of acquiring AIDS and anxiety about our own mortality because these patients will die no matter what care they are given.

Nurses face particular stresses because of the amount of time they spend with patients. Care of dying patients must emphasize supportive care to reassure everyone that no one is giving up. Appropriate supportive care can significantly increase the quality of life of patients with AIDS.

DIRECTIONS FOR FUTURE RESEARCH

An immunoincompetent patient poses many challenges to nurses. Of importance to the patient, to the family, and to the nurse is the patient's ability to cope with one of life's challenges. Based on the research priorities for critical care nursing, questions that must be evaluated are the following:

1. What are effective nursing interventions with patients with impaired communication to minimize anxiety, helplessness, and pain?
2. What nursing interventions most effectively minimize stress in the critically ill patient?
3. What is the effect of primary nursing on anxiety levels of critically ill patients and their families and on ultimate patient recovery?
4. What nursing interventions are most effective in creating a sense of independence and control in the critical care patient?

REFERENCES

1. Barrett, J. T. *Basic Immunology and its Medical Application* (2nd ed.). St. Louis: C. V. Mosby, 1980.
2. Bartrop, R. W., Luckhurst, E., Lazurus, L. Depressed lymphocyte function after bereavement. *Lancet* 1:834, 1977.
3. Berk, L., Tan, S. A., Fry, W. Neuroendocrine and stress hormone changes during mirthful laughter. *Am. J. Med. Sci.* 298:390, 1989.
4. Black, D. W. Laughter. *J.A.M.A.* 252:2995, 1984.
5. Blalock, J. E. The immune system as a sensory organ. *J. Immunol.* 132:1067, 1984.
6. Broder, S. and Waldman, T. The suppressor-cell network in cancer. Part I. *N. Engl. J. Med.* 299:23, 1978.
7. Broder, S. and Waldman, T. The suppressor-cell network in cancer. Part 2. *N. Engl. J. Med.* 299:24, 1978.
8. Brody, R. Anatomy of a Laugh. *American Health.* Nov/Dec. 43, 1983.
9. Brown, B. B. *Between Health and Illness.* Boston: Houghton-Mifflin, 1984.
10. Burnet, M. The thymus gland. *Scientific American.* 207:50, 1962.
11. Cline, M., *et al.* Monocytes and macrophages: Functions and diseases. *Ann. Intern. Med.* 88:78, 1978.
12. Cohen, F. and Lazarus, R. Active coping processes, coping dispositions, and recovery from surgery. *Psychosom. Med.* 35:375, 1973.
13. Cosner, R. Some social functions of laughter. *Human Relations* 12:171, 1959.
14. Cousins, N. *Anatomy of an Illness.* New York: W. B. Norton & Co., 1979.
15. Fineberg, H. The social dimensions of AIDS. *Scientific American* 259:128, 1988.
16. Friedland, G. The acquired immunodeficiency syndrome: General overview. *Intern. J. Neurosci.* 32:677, 1987.
17. Friedland, G. and Klein, R. Transmission of the human immunodeficiency virus. *N. Engl. J. Med.* 317:1125, 1987.
18. Gallo, R. The AIDS virus. *Scientific American* 256:47, 1987.
19. Gallo, R. and Montagnier, L. AIDS in 1988. *Scientific American* 259:41, 1988.
20. Glasser, R. J. *The Body is the Hero.* New York: Random House, 1976.
21. Glatt, A., Chirgivin, K., Landesman, S. Treatment of infections associated with HIV: Current concepts. *N. Engl. J. Med.* 318:1439, 1988.
22. Griffin, J. Nursing care of the immunosuppressed patient in the ICU. *Heart Lung* 15:179, 1986.
23. Gurevich, I. Acquired immunodeficiency syndrome: Realistic concerns and appropriate precautions. *Heart Lung* 18:107, 1989.
24. Heyward, W. and Curran, J. The epidemiology of AIDS in the U.S. *Scientific American* 259:72, 1988.
25. Ho, D., Pomerantz, R., and Kaplan, J. Pathogenesis of infection with human immunodeficiency virus. *N. Engl. J. Med.* 317:278, 1987.
26. Hopewell, P. *Pneumocystis carinii*: Diagnosis. *J. Infect. Dis.* 157:1115, 1988.
27. Jacobson, M. and Mills, J. Serious cytomegalovirus disease in the acquired immunodeficiency syndrome. *Ann. Intern. Med.* 108:585, 1988.
28. Jordan, C., Glaser, R., Strain, E. Latent herpes viruses of humans. *Ann. Intern. Med.* 100:866, 1984.
29. Kiecott-Glaser, J. K., Fisher, L., and Ogrocki, P. Marital quality, marital disruption and immune function. *Psychosom. Med.* 49:13, 1987.
30. Kiecott-Glaser, J. K., Fisher, L., and Ogrocki, P. Psychosocial

modifiers of immunocompetence in medical students. *Psychosom. Med.* 46:7, 1984.

31. Klein, A. *The Healing Power of Humor.* Los Angeles: Jeremy P. Tarcher, 1989.

32. Kobasa, S. C. Stressful life events, personality, and health: An inquiry into hardiness. *J. Pers. Soc. Psychol.* 37:1, 1979.

33. Kottra, C. J. Infection in the compromised host—An overview. *Heart Lung* 12:10, 1983.

34. Laurence, J. The immune system in AIDS. *Scientific American* 253:84, 1985.

35. Lazarus, R. S. and Folkman, S. *Stress, Appraisal and Coping.* New York: Springer, 1984.

36. Leiber, D. B. Laughter and humor in critical care. *Dimensions Crit. Care Nurs.* 5:162, 1986.

37. Locke, S. and Colligan, D. *The Healer Within: The New Medicine of Mind and Body.* New York: New American Library, 1986.

38. Maier, S. and Laudenslager. Stress and health: Exploring and links. *Psychol. Today:* 19:44, 1985.

39. Martin, R. A. and Lefcourt, H. Sense of humor as moderator of the relation between stressors and moods. *J. Person. Soc. Psychol.* 45:1313, 1983.

40. Mayer, M. The complement system. *Scientific American* 229:54, 1973.

41. Meisenhelder, J. B. and La Charite, C. L. *Comfort in Caring: Nursing with the HIV infection.* Boston: Scott, Foresman, and Company, 1989.

42. Montgomery, A. B., Luce, J. M., Turner, J. Aerosolized pentamidine as sole therapy for *Pneumocystis* pneumonia in patients with acquired immunodeficiency syndrome. *Lancet* 120:480, 1987.

43. Nossal, G. The basic components of the immune system. *N. Engl. J. Med.* 316:1320, 1987.

44. Nyamathi, A. Maladaptive coping in the critically ill population with acquired immunodeficiency syndrome: Nursing assessment and treatment. *Heart Lung* 18:113, 1989.

45. Pearson, R. D. and Hewlett, E. L. Pentamidine for the treatment of *Pneumocystis* pneumonia and other protozoal diseases. *Ann. Intern. Med.* 103:782, 1985.

46. Pelletier, K. *Mind is a Healer, Mind is a Slayer.* New York: Dell, 1977.

47. Pelletier, K. and Herzing, D. Psychoneuro-immunology: Toward a mindbody model. A critical review. *Advances* 5:26, 1987.

48. Pert, C. The wisdom of the receptors: Neuropeptides, the emotions, and bodymind. *Advances* 3:318, 1986.

49. Pollack, S. E. The hardiness characteristic: A motivating factor in adaptation. *Adv. Nurs. Sci.* 11:53, 1989.

50. Porter, R. R. The structure of antibodies. *Scientific American* 217:81, 1967.

51. Redfield, R. and Burke, D. HIV infection: The clinical picture. *Scientific American* 259:90, 1988.

52. Robinson, V. Humor is a serious business. *Dimensions Crit. Care Nurs.* 5:32, 1986.

53. Scherer, P. How AIDS attacks the brain. *Am. J. Nurs.* 90:44, 1990.

54. Schleifer, S., *et al.* Major depressive disorder and immunity. *Arch. Gen. Psychiatry* 46:81, 1989.

55. Siegel, B. *Love, Medicine, and Miracles.* New York: Harper & Row, 1986.

56. Simonton, D. C., Matthew-Simonton, S., and Crughton, J. *Getting Well Again.* Los Angeles: Tarcher, 1978.

57. Solomon, G. The healthy elderly and long-term survivors of AIDS: Psychoimmune connections. *Advances* 5:6, 1987.

58. Solomon, G. F., Temoshek, L., O'Leary, A., Zich, J. An intensive psychoimmunologic study of long-surviving persons with AIDS. *Ann. N.Y. Acad. Sci.* 496:647, 1987.

59. Solomon, G. F., Fiatarone, M. A., Benton, D., *et al.* Psychoimmunologic and endorphin function in the aged. *Ann. N.Y. Acad. Sci.* 521:43, 1988.

46

Transplantation

Carolyn Rea Atkins   Paula Shiroma Bender
Lori Rippert

SHARING AND THE "HELPER'S HIGH"

The "helper's high" is an experience that has been described in persons doing volunteer work. Those who really "get their hands dirty" in helping someone else frequently describe a profound sense of well-being or actual euphoria. In addition to this joyful feeling, these persons actually seem healthier. They frequent physicians less and have better health profiles.*

Nursing is one of the most profound forms of sharing. When done with genuine love and caring, nurses can experience the "helper's high" described in persons doing volunteer work. It is easy to block these feelings, of course, and remain unaware of them (*e.g.*, if we focus on caregiving as only a job, a livelihood, an obligation).

Opening to others opens ourselves to the fulfilling feelings that have always been a part of our profession.

LEARNING OBJECTIVES

After reading this chapter, the nurse will be able to do the following:

1. Obtain an overview of organ transplantation.
2. Demonstrate a working knowledge of the immune system as related to transplantation.
3. Demonstrate an understanding of the medical, surgical, and nursing aspects of renal, cardiac, and liver transplantation.
4. Identify the benefits, risks, and complications associated with the specific procedures.
5. Discuss the immunosuppressive agents used in preventing rejection of the graft.
6. Recognize the signs and symptoms of rejection of each organ system.
7. Discuss the different treatment regimens available when a rejection episode occurs.
8. Perform preoperative and postoperative nursing assessments of the organ transplant patient.

TRANSPLANTATION

Transplantation of human solid organs involves the removal of a normal functioning organ from one individual and place-

* Luks, A. Helper's high. *Psychology Today* October: 39–42, 1988.

ment of it into another individual who suffers from failure of that particular organ. As of September 1989, there were 15,824 patients *actively* waiting for a kidney, 1277 for a heart, 248 for a heart/lung, 761 for a liver, and 317 for a pancreas.[6] Many more are in various stages of evaluation for consideration as organ recipients.

The first renal transplant was performed by Varonay in 1936, but renal transplantation as a tool for treating humans was essentially unexplored until 1956, when Merrill, Hume, and Murray successfully transplanted a kidney from one identical twin to another. Three years later, the same group performed the first nontwin transplant.[25]

The transplantation of extrarenal solid organs was slow until the introduction of cyclosporine immunosuppression in 1978. As with any new procedure, it took many years of research before the actual transplantation of these organs. The first human liver transplant was performed in 1963; the first heart transplant using a human heart was done in January 1967 by Barnard in South Africa; the first combined heart–lung transplant was performed in 1978; attempts at small intestine transplantation began in 1959, but this remains an experimental procedure because of problems with rejection and graft-versus-host reaction.[21]

Transplantation of the pancreas has been attempted in humans since 1966 with little success until the advent of cyclosporine and new surgical techniques like draining the exocrine secretion into the bladder. Others have attempted to graft the islets of Langerhans, but without long-term success.[21]

Many difficulties have been encountered since those early days. The immunologic problems (acute and chronic rejection) are the greatest threat to successful organ transplantation, and the immunosuppression used to modify rejection is perhaps the greatest threat to the patient's survival.[25]

REFLECTIONS

Transplant nursing has become a specialized area of nursing that is challenging and encompasses all phases of medical care. It is a combination of surgery, medicine, psychology, public health, pediatrics, social work, and patient education.

In assessing the care needed for the transplant recipient, as in other areas of nursing, one cannot simply take care of the needs of the diseased or transplanted organ. The disease entity truly affects the body–mind–spirit of the patient and family. Some disease processes are "curable;" organ failure is "controllable." It can be controlled by dialysis, as in renal failure, or by transplantation, as in heart and liver failure, but neither mode of therapy offers an absolute long-term cure.

For all patients, after transplantation, there are still rules and regulations to observe, body changes to adjust to, and new medical problems to replace the old ones. Some patients are surprised to find that they still have the same problems at home, work, and school and with their families that they had before transplantation.

When working with transplant patients, the team must view them as whole people, considering the outside pressures and influences on them. For example, patients may stop taking their medication because of the development of cushingoid features, weight gain, and acne, or because medication is viewed as a sign of illness and the patient just does not want to be ill. It has been estimated that about 4% of patients stop their immunosuppressive medication for these and other reasons.

When patients stop their medication, the staff's first reaction is anger. Despite the anger, the staff must continue to work with the patient. They must try to promote self-esteem while emphasizing the need to continue the medication. Sometimes, with the younger patients (teens and young adults), all efforts fail and the patient elects not to continue the medication because of concern over changed body image and the reaction of peers. This group, we believe, would rather return to dialysis in the hope of regaining their "normal" face and figure and the acceptance of their peers.

It is certainly challenging as well as frustrating to provide appropriate support in working with such a group of patients. One way of dealing with this problem, as well as other problems, might be to help the patient set both short- and long-term goals. As one goal is near completion, another goal should be identified by the nurse and patient.

In working with transplant patients, it is important to listen not only to what the patient and family are saying, but also to what they are not saying. Useful information can be obtained by this kind of listening. For instance, patients who are chronic complainers or questioners may really be asking for reassurance that they are doing the right thing or may be telling the staff that they are afraid.

Staff members must be aware of their own feelings of happiness, anger, frustration, sympathy, friendship, and involvement if they are to help care for and rehabilitate the transplant recipient. They must be able to work out these feelings, because they need to be objective in order to give "total patient" care. In addition to recognizing their own feelings, nurses should learn as much as possible about how the patient and family react under stress. They also must recognize the importance of the psychological and emotional health of the patient and how this can affect the success or failure of the graft. This knowledge cannot be acquired in a short period of time. Awareness grows through continued association with the patient.

PATHOPHYSIOLOGY

Histocompatibility Antigens

For years, the typing of red blood cell antigens (the ABO system) has made blood transfusions possible. The antigens of the ABO system are similarly important in organ transplantation, because the donor and recipient must be ABO compatible.

The major histocompatibility complex (MHC) of humans has evolved through typing and crossmatching of human blood. It is much more than a genetic region involved in organ rejection. Instead, it plays a major role in the recognition, regulation, and effector phases of virtually all host immune responses. It continues to be the basis for research in immunology.[11]

Through the work of Dausset, Van Rood, Amos, Terasaki, Payne and others, the main human histocompatibility antigens were identified. These antigens are carried by the *blood lymphocytes* (and other cells) and are known as the *human leukocyte antigen* or HLA (Table 46–1).[13]

The HLA region is found on the sixth human chromosome. It is known to contain at least four genetic loci: HLA-A, HLA-B, HLA-C, and HLA-D. The HLA-A and HLA-B loci were the first ones to be identified. Since their discovery, varying numbers of alleles have been identified: approximately 95% of the population, for the HLA-A and HLA-B antigens; and probably only about 50% of the HLA-C antigens.[25]

The HLA-D locus is defined by lymphocyte reaction (it stimulates blast transformation in mixed lymphocyte culture) rather than by serologic identification. This procedure requires special techniques and longer incubation periods; therefore, it is not feasible as a selective tool in cadaver transplantation.[25]

An additional group of antigens has been isolated close to the HLA-D locus; these antigens are called *D-related* (DR) antigens. Unlike the HLA-D locus, the HLA-DR locus can be serologically defined. To date, only ten specificities have been identified to humans.[25,51]

The HLA-A and HLA-B loci are called class I antigens, are expressed on most types of cells, and are the major targets for antibody and cell-mediated reactions against transplanted tissue. The antigens found on the HLA-D locus are class II antigens and have a limited tissue distribution.[11]

There are 7000 to 8000 possible combinations of the known antigens. In addition, the distribution of HLA antigens varies significantly among white, African American, and Asian peoples.[13,25]

Each person inherits a set of the four HLA antigens (called haplotype) from each parent (Fig. 46–1). An effort is made to identify each of the HLA-A, HLA-B, HLA-C, and HLA-DR

Table 46–1
Histocompatibility Definitions

HLA	Human leukocyte antigen
Locus	The position of a gene on a chromosome
Allele	One of two or more genes that occupy the same locus on a specific pair of chromosomes and control the heredity of a particular characteristic
Antigen	A substance (either introduced into the body or formed there) that stimulates the formation of a specific antibody. Antigens concerned with transplantation are found on the surfaces of red blood cells and of nucleated cells of most body tissues.
Antibody	A protein substance produced in lymphoid tissue by plasma cells in response to a specific antigen
Haplotype	Pair of antigens inherited from one parent
Phenotype	Physical appearance or make-up of an individual
Genotype	The hereditary make-up of an individual. Genotyping can be determined when multiple family members are tissue-typed.
Cytotoxic	Destructive to cells

antigens, even though this is not always possible. In families that are being typed, the HLA-D locus is identified through mixed lymphocyte culture. Because antigens are inherited together, siblings who have the same HLA-A and HLA-B antigens have the same HLA-D antigens in approximately 93% of the cases.[25]

A parent is always one haplotype identical with his or her child, but it is possible for the siblings each to inherit a different haplotype from each of the parents and thus be a complete mismatch with each other. For this reason, when a transplant candidate is being tissue-typed, it is important for as many family members as possible to be typed so that all the antigens can be clearly identified and the most suitable donor found.[13,25]

Cytotoxic Antibodies

Because of the possibility that the transplant candidate may have developed serum cytotoxic antibodies against the donor's antigens (through prior exposure to leukocytes and platelets in blood transfusions, in a pregnancy, or in a previous organ transplant), a *crossmatch* test is done immediately before transplantation. This test is done by incubating the transplant

candidate's serum with lymphocytes from the donor. If the donor lymphocytes are killed by the recipient's serum, the potential recipient has antibodies against that particular donor's cells, and performing the transplant could result in a hyperacute rejection of the transplanted organ at the time of surgery.[13]

The level of antibody titer usually rises after exposure to a particular antigen and then may fall after a period of time. The body's immunologic system, once exposed to an antigen, tends to have a faster and greater antibody response to subsequent exposure. Therefore, to make the crossmatch as sensitive as possible, serum samples are obtained from all potential transplant recipients at frequent intervals. An effort is also made to collect serum samples approximately 7 to 10 days after a blood transfusion, because this is the peak time of antibody formation. These serum samples are kept frozen until a organ becomes available.

Practices vary with individual transplant programs, but most perform a crossmatch with the potential donor organ using current sera obtained from the recipient near the time of the transplant.[11] Other programs obtain, store, and crossmatch all sera against the potential donor organ. In some transplant centers, if any of the sera is positive, it is a contraindication to proceeding with the transplant.

In renal transplantation, a positive crossmatch test on fresh serum is an absolute contraindication to surgery.[13] For liver and heart recipients, the final crossmatch does not appear to be as significant in those patients who are not sensitized against some HLA antigens.[11]

Newer, improved methods are being studied for detecting HLA antigens or antibody reactivity. These, such as the flow cytometry, provide greater sensitivity.[11]

THE IMMUNE SYSTEM AND TRANSPLANTATION
Immunosuppression

It is well known that the body can recognize a foreign substance and produce antibodies to fight it. Immunosuppressive therapy in renal transplantation involves the use of a number of methods to block or decrease the intensity of the body's immune response to the graft.[61]

At present there are three acceptable methods for altering the body's immune response before the actual transplantation

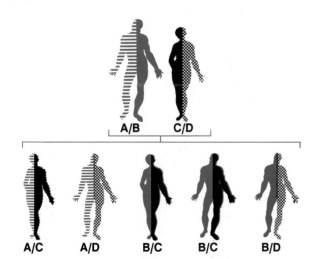

Figure 46–1

Interpretation of HLA matching antigens. How haplotypes are acquired from parents; how siblings are matched.

surgery. There are blood transfusions, either random or donor-specific; total lymphoid irradiation (TLI), such as is used in the treatment of Hodgkin's disease; and thoracic duct drainage (Table 46–2).[20,70,77] Not all of these are used for all organs transplanted.

The methods used to alter the immune system after the transplant are mainly in the form of medications, which are taken daily by the patient for the duration of the transplanted organ (Table 46–3). Most centers use a combination of agents, but three drugs that most, if not all, transplant recipients must take for the life of the graft are cyclosporine, azathioprine, and a corticosteroid (either prednisone or prednisolone).

When acute rejection occurs, additional immunosuppressive methods must be used to remove or destroy the cells attacking the graft (Table 46–4). The choice of treatment varies from center to center and may be used singularly or in combination with another method. Regardless of the treatment modality chosen, it is usually in addition to the maintenance immunosuppressive medications the transplant recipient takes daily.

Rejection

The complex events occurring after transplantation that influence the onset of rejection continue to be only partially understood. The body's immune system is able to recognize foreign substances (antigens), isolate them, and produce antibodies to destroy them in preparation for their removal by other cells.[35]

When immunologically competent cells recognize a foreign antigen, they enlarge, multiply, and produce sensitized lym-

Table 46–2
Pretransplant Modification of the Immune System

METHOD	MECHANISM	PROCEDURE	ADVERSE EFFECTS	SPECIAL CONSIDERATIONS
Thoracic duct drainage (TDD)	Removes large numbers of long-lived lymphocytes from the body	Patient's thoracic duct is surgically cannulated; lymph fluid is drained continuously; lymph fluid is centrifuged to remove cells before returning the lymph to the patient intravenously.	Infection	Cost; used in cadaver transplants; requires at least a month's hospitalization before transplantation
Total lymphoid irradiation (TLI)	Produces immunospecific tolerance by selectively destroying T cells; suppresses antibody production	100–200 rads daily five times per week for a total dose of 2500–4500 rads; if leukopenia occurs, treatment must be delayed until it resolves; included in the irradiation are thymus, spleen, and the major lymph nodes (cervical, axillary, mediastinal, inguinal, and mesenteric); the skull, lungs, and long bones are protected from the radiation.	Leukopenia, lymphomas, infection, nausea, vomiting	Treatment must begin at least 6 weeks before transplantation; for best results, patient must undergo renal transplantation as soon as possible after the last dose of radiation.
Blood transfusion	Induces immunologic unresponsiveness, thereby producing tolerance toward the graft		Potential for transmission of viral diseases (HIV, Non-A, Non-B hepatitis)	Selects out those patients who have the tendency to develop cytotoxic antibodies; graft survival appears to improve in patients who have received blood transfusion before transplant.
Random transfusion		Patient receives deliberate blood transfusions before receiving a renal transplant; the number of units varies, but 5 U is thought to be the minimum amount.	Development of high levels of cytotoxic antibodies, making it difficult to find a compatible kidney; hepatitis	
Donor-specific transfusion (DST)		Recipient is transfused with 200 ml of the potential donor's blood on three occasions 2 to 3 weeks apart; crossmatch between the donor and recipient is done before each transfusion.	May develop cytotoxic antibodies (20%–30% chance) against the potential donor	Time-consuming; presents a problem if the donor does not live in the same community as the recipient

Table 46-3
Immunosuppressive Medications

DRUG	MODE OF ACTION	DOSE	ADVERSE EFFECTS	SPECIAL CONSIDERATIONS
Azathioprine (Imuran)	Depresses the production of antibodies against the organ by interfering with the proliferation of leukocytes; selectively inhibits T-cell formation	Initial dose of 2.5–5 mg/kg body weight; maintenance dose of 2.5 mg/kg body weight; can be given orally or intravenously	Bone marrow depression; leukopenia; liver disease; increase in malignant diseases; stomatitis; increase in viral diseases	Dose controlled by level of white blood cell count; eliminated in the urine; therefore, dosage may need to be decreased in the presence of anuria.
Corticosteroids (prednisone, prednisolone, methylprednisolone)	Anti-inflammatory; inhibit the influx of granulocytes into the transplanted organ; alter lymphocyte circulation; inhibit protein synthesis; stabilize lysosomes when sensitized lymphocytes make contact with the grafted organ	Initial dose varies among centers (60–100 mg/day; 2 mg/kg body weight); daily dose tapered slowly following surgery to a maintenance dose of 0.25 mg/kg body weight; comes in oral and intravenous forms.	Increased incidence of infections; impaired wound healing; cushingoid changes (acne, hirsutism, changes in fat distribution); hyperglycemia leading to diabetes mellitus; aseptic necrosis of femoral head; cataracts; peptic ulcer disease; arrested bone growth in children; psychological disturbances	
Cyclophosphamide (Cytoxan)	Alkylating agent; actual mechanism of action not known	2 mg/kg body weight daily; given orally	Increased incidence of viral and bacterial infections; leukopenia; hemorrhagic cystitis; gonadal suppression; alopecia	Excreted by the kidneys; therefore, may need to be decreased in the presence of anuria; usually only used when patient cannot tolerate azathioprine
Antilymphocyte globulin (ALG)	Acts on thymus-derived (T-cell) recirculating lymphocytes by adsorbing to and coating the outside of the lymphocytes; complement is then fixed by the antibody, resulting in cell lysis and phagocytosis by the reticuloendothelial system.	Dosage varies among centers; given in milligrams of ALG per kilogram body weight; given intramuscularly or intravenously	Anaphylaxis; serum sickness; pain, edema, erythema at the injection site; thrombocytopenia; anemia; increase in fungal and viral infections	ALG is made by injecting human lymphocytes (obtained primarily from thymus and thoracic duct) into horses (other animals may be used); variables affecting potency are number of lymphocytes obtained; number and frequency of injections in the animal; time interval between the injection and harvesting of the antibodies from the injected animal; and the animal's response to the antigenic stimuli.
Cyclosporine A (CyA)[8,51,75]	Appears to inhibit graft-versus-host reaction; inhibits antibody formation against thymus-dependent antigens; inhibits T-cell lymphocyte production; inhibits T-cell helper function (for B-cell activation); inhibits humoral and cell-mediated responses	Most common route is oral (given in chocolate milk); can be given intramuscularly or intravenously; dosage varies (10–16 mg/kg body weight) daily initially; decreases over several months to a maintenance dose. Capsule form is now available at some transplant centers.	Nephrotoxicity; hepatotoxicity; tremor; hirsutism; increased incidence of lymphoma; seizures, CMV sepsis; gingival hyperplasia	Side effects are dose related and appear to be reversible upon decreasing the dosage or stopping the drug; does not impair wound healing; does not cause bone marrow depression or leukopenia

(continued)

Table 46–3 *(Continued)*

DRUG	MODE OF ACTION	DOSE	ADVERSE EFFECTS	SPECIAL CONSIDERATIONS
OKT-3[70]	Reacts against a specific antigen on the surface of T cells to destroy the cell	5 mg IV push for 5 days beginning the day of surgery; Imuran and CYA doses are lower during this time.	Severe febrile reactions; dyspnea; leukopenia	Skin test required prior to administration; Imuran decreased during therapy because of leukopenia. Used as prophylactic drug
FK506[44,57]	Similar to CYA but more potent. Precise mechanism is unknown, but thought to inhibit T-cell activation and lymphokine production. Enhances CYA uptake by the cells. Synergistic with CYA. Suppresses cell-mediated immunity and allograft rejection in experimental animals	0.15 mg/kg daily in divided doses	Little known in humans. However, insomnia, "bad" taste sensation seen with overdosing. Headache, GI disturbance	Presently being evaluated in controlled clinical settings. This may be the only immunosuppressive drug needed.

Table 46–4
Modalities of Treatment for Acute Rejection

METHOD	MECHANISM	PROCEDURE	ADVERSE EFFECTS	SPECIAL CONSIDERATIONS
Corticosteroids	Anti-inflammatory agent; decreases swelling in the kidney; actual mechanism not fully understood	Oral dose of 200–300 mg daily for 5 days or intravenous dose of 1 g over several days for a total of 4 g; either method is given *in addition to* daily maintenance dose	Refer to Table 46–3	Doses are reduced when treating children
Antithymocyte globulin (ATG)[26,69]	Reduces the number of circulating thymus-dependent lymphocytes	Given intravenously diluted in normal saline over a 6-hour period; dose is calculated in mg per kg of body weight (usually 10–15 mg/kg); given daily for 14 days; may be extended if necessary	Anaphylaxis; leukopenia; thrombocytopenia; febrile reaction; opportunistic infections	Appears to be effective in treating steroid-resistant rejections; azathioprine is discontinued during therapy because of leukopenia; skin test required prior to administration
Monoclonal antibodies[70]	React against a specific antigen on the surface of T cells to destroy the cell	Dose (5 mg) administered in intravenous push daily for 14 days; may be extended for another 14 days if necessary	Severe febrile reactions; dyspnea; leukopenia	Skin test required before administration; must test for presence of OKT-3 antibody before giving a second course of therapy; Imuran decreased during therapy because of leukopenia
Plasma exchange (PE)[1,45]	Removes circulating lymphocytotoxic antibodies from plasma	4–5 L exchange of plasma daily for 5 days	No significant reactions reported	Vascular access (fistula or shunt) is used; protocols differ from center to center as to length of treatment
Local radiation to the graft[73]	Destroys T cells; acts as an anti-inflammatory agent by indirectly slowing leukocyte migration	100–150 rads directly to the graft per treatment every other day for a total of 600–800 rads		Used sparingly and always in conjunction with other rejection therapy

phocytes (involving thymus-dependent cells or T-lymphocytes). This is called a *cell-mediated immune response*. These immunologically competent cells can also produce *specific* antibody-secreting plasma cells (developed in the lymph nodes and the spleen—known as B-lymphocytes) in a process called a *humoral immune response*. These two types of immune responses work together to attack and destroy any foreign substance or graft, including a transplanted organ, unless modification occurs.[35]

In all transplants except those between patients whose antigenic make-up is identical (identical twins), the immune response is aimed at rejecting the newly transplanted organ. The rejection process has several different stages of intensity: hyperacute, delayed hyperacute (vascular), acute, and chronic.

Hyperacute Rejection

Hyperacute rejection can occur at the time blood flow to the transplanted organ is established or up to several hours after the surgery is completed. Such rejection is usually caused by preformed circulating antibodies that attack the new graft violently. Because of its time of onset, it is a *humoral response*. Hyperacute rejection also occurs when there is an ABO incompatibility between the donor and the recipient (this is rare today). There is no known treatment for this type of rejection, and the organ must be removed as soon as the diagnosis is made.[35]

Delayed Hyperacute (Vascular) Rejection

Delayed hyperacute rejection is an extension of hyperacute rejection. The changes seen are similar to those in hyperacute rejection, but it can occur 5 to 10 days after transplantation.[35]

Acute Rejection

Acute rejection, the most common type of rejection, is usually reversible and can occur at any time after transplantation. Most often, however, it is seen within several weeks of transplant. It is both a cell-mediated and an antibody-mediated response.[35]

Chronic Rejection

Chronic rejection is the most difficult type of rejection to diagnose because it has few clinical signs and symptoms. It is a result of the constant immunologic conflict between the transplanted organ and its new environment.[35]

Infection

Infection is the leading cause of death in all transplant recipients. Infection poses a great threat in the immediate postoperative period (when bacterial organisms are the most common causes of infection). The reason is that the patient must continue to take immunosuppressive drugs to prevent rejection. This immunosuppression of defense mechanisms makes the patient the perfect target for opportunistic organisms.[73]

Several defects are known to be present in the immuno-suppressed patient that allow infections to become lethal. These defects are as follows:[73]

- *Alteration of local (skin and mucosal) defenses.* Postoperative hematomas, foreign objects, and obstruction of normal drainage tracts combine to offer a significant risk factor in the immediate postoperative period. Long-term, high-dose corticosteroid therapy impairs wound healing and collagen synthesis and enhances skin breakdown.
- *Alteration of the acute inflammatory system.* To deal with pathogenic organisms, normal granulocytes (which have phagocytic and bactericidal activities) must migrate to the infected area. The normal migration is altered by corticosteroids and azathioprine.
- *Alteration of cellular immunity.* Corticosteroids cause depression of the cellular immune response. This depression either enhances the cells' susceptibility to intracellular pathogens or activates latent viral infections. These types of infection are usually more common after treatment of an acute rejection episode with high-dose corticosteroids.
- *Alteration of the humoral immune response.* The immunosuppressive agents combine to depress the formation of antibodies in response to antigens. The depression in antibody formation increases the incidence and severity of bacterial infections.

In assessing the patient for the presence of infection, the nurse should consider fever an infectious process in the absence of rejection, follow daily white blood cell (WBC) counts for any sudden increases or decreases, assess pulmonary status postoperatively, observe the skin for any areas of potential breakdown, and observe the wound for changes in the character and amount of drainage, if any.

Viral infections—such as cytomegalovirus (CMV), Epstein-Barr virus (EBV), hepatitis (non-A, non-B, or chronic hepatitis B) and human immunodeficiency virus (HIV)—represent the most single infectious disease in the transplanted patient.[54]

PRESERVATION OF ORGANS

Hypothermia is the most important ingredient in the preservation of organs. However, hypothermia only reduces the rate of cell death in an organ that has been removed from an intact circulatory system; it does not prevent it. Most damage that occurs to the cells of the organ is reversible. The recipient of a kidney or pancreas can be maintained while the organ recovers, whereas a liver, heart, or lung must provide life-sustaining function immediately on revascularization.[63]

There are two methods that provide the hypothermia needed: simple cold storage and continuous pulsatile perfusion. The majority of organs are preserved by simple cold storage. The kidney is preserved by either method, depending on the individual transplant program.

The development of new preservation solutions has significantly increased the time an organ can be "stored" while finding a compatible recipient. In the past, livers could be kept only for 6 to 8 hours before transplantation; they can now be kept for 24 hours.[64] The organs being considered for transplant are flushed in situ to reduce the amount of warm ischemia time. Hearts are preserved in simple cold storage and are limited to a short period of time.[63]

RENAL TRANSPLANTATION

The refinements of renal transplantation have proceeded in four directions: the development of more specific forms of immunosuppressive drugs and their dosages, the development of pretransplant recipient modification, the investigation and identification of more specific antigens that might permit better selection of donors and recipients, and the development of techniques to preserve cadaver kidneys for longer periods of time.[5,10]

Etiology/Incidence

End-stage renal disease (ESRD) can be caused by many different events: immunologic events, anatomic defects, or trauma. Glomerulonephritis, an immunologic disease, is the leading cause of renal failure in both adults and children.

Patient Care Management

Recipient Selection

The patient being considered for renal transplantation usually has irreversible ESRD. Factors considered favorable in patient selection are age of the recipient (it appears the most successful transplants occur in patients between the ages of 10 and 40 years, a normal lower urinary tract outflow, the recipient's underlying renal disease, the absence of any major associated diseases (coronary artery disease, malignancy, infection, and pulmonary obstructive disease), and the absence of a peptic ulcer or history of a peptic ulcer.[13,25]

The transplant candidate goes through a thorough evaluation to prepare for transplantation. The evaluation includes laboratory tests, a complete review of the body systems, a voiding cystourethrogram (VCUG), a psychologic evaluation, and an immunologic evaluation (Table 46–5). The advantages, disadvantages, risks, benefits, and survival rates of the patient and transplanted kidney are discussed with the patient and family by the physician and members of the transplant team. The information is given to the patient gradually, after the condition has been stabilized by hemodialysis. The patient makes the decision for a transplant or for hemodialysis, or may refuse both treatments and elect to die.

If, while the patient is undergoing the screening, an abnormality is found (*e.g.,* a ureteral reflux as shown by VCUG), additional surgery (*e.g.,* a nephroureterectomy, removal of the kidney and ureter) may be done before the transplantation to avoid an infection from refluxing urine. There are other reasons for performing a nephroureterectomy before the transplantation surgery. They are if the patient has uncontrolled hypertension, if the patient has an infection from pyelonephritis, polycystic kidneys, or stones; and if the patient's diseased kidneys may act as a potential pathogenic agent in the recurrence of the primary renal disease in the transplanted kidney.[61]

Evaluation of the Older Patient

The age of the dialysis population has increased, and these older patients are requesting to be considered for transplantation. Studies indicate that this group of patients does not appear to have an increased incidence of post-transplant complications. As with other age groups, infection is the leading cause of death, especially infection with cytomegalovirus

(CMV).[18,29] However, the older patient often requires a more extensive pretransplant evaluation to include barium enema (looking for the presence of diverticular disease), thallium stress test, and pulmonary function studies.

When the preliminary evaluation is completed and all problems have been addressed, the patient is ready for the transplantation.

Types of Transplants

Kidneys are obtained from three donor sources: living related donors (LRD), living nonrelated donors (LNRD), and cadavers. The most common living donor is a relative.

Living Donor

In living *related* donor transplantation, the recipient or some other family member asks the patient's family about donating a kidney. Historically, a donor was selected on the basis of ABO compatibility and HLA typing. However, recent studies have shown that relatives who do not share the same HLA antigens as the recipient should be considered as potential donors as well.[30]

A family member may be willing to donate a kidney for one or more reasons: a sense of duty, guilt about the fact that a refusal might mean the patient would die, a desire to repay the patient for something, or a wish to gain or regain family approval.[13]

Living *nonrelated* donors have been spouses, friends, stepparents, stepchildren, and in-laws. There should be some type of emotional bond between the recipient and donor. In no way should a donor be selected for financial gain. This aspect of living donor transplants is a controversial one, but it offers the advantages of reducing the shortage of cadaver kidneys, improving long-term graft survival, and providing the flexibility to manipulate the recipient's immune system before transplantation.[52]

The donor and recipient *must* be ABO compatible. The same circumstances apply to ABO compatibility in transplantation as in blood transfusions; that is, type AB is the universal recipient, and type O is the universal donor. Crossing these blood barriers results in a hyperacute rejection of the kidney at the time of surgery.[61]

The willing and compatible potential donor must undergo an extensive evaluation. First, the donor is seen by the physician who explains the short- and long-term risks of kidney donation. The overall risk, including death, of donation in an otherwise healthy donor has been estimated at 0.07%, which takes into account that the donor might lose the remaining kidney from trauma or cancer. The combined total risk to the donor is about 0.1% to 0.2%.[25] Follow-up renal function studies and patient evaluations have been done at numerous centers. These studies suggest that there are no significant long-term effects of donation.[2,3] Risk aside, the donor experiences pain and anxiety and loses time from work and home during the evaluation and surgery.

Whatever the reasons, most donors seem to make the decision to donate or not to donate immediately. The rewards the donor receives are satisfaction in seeing the recipient improve and an increase in self-esteem that is longlasting, even when the transplant is not successful.[19]

The nurse should be aware of the psychologic aspects of

Table 46–5
Evaluation of Recipient for Renal Transplantation

TESTS	REASONS FOR TESTS
Immunologic tests	
ABO and HLA typing	To determine the patient's blood group and to identify HLA antigens
Antibody screening	To determine the presence of cytotoxic antibodies and the percentage of reactivity, which allows one to predict with some accuracy whether the transplant recipient will ever be able to accept a kidney
History taking and physical examination	To determine the patient's past and present status. Past medical history is extremely important, especially any history of peptic ulcer disease or symptoms, cardiac disease, kidney stones, malignancy, allergies, blood transfusions, and hypertension. The physical examination of a woman patient always includes a pelvic examination, a Papanicolaou smear, and mammogram.
Social and psychologic evaluation	To determine the patient's emotional maturity, motivation, cooperativeness, and ability to learn about medications and to take instructions. To determine any underlying psychopathology, as well as family or other support system. The information gathered enables the transplant team to know what support the patient and family need.
Financial evaluation	To determine the means by which the patient will be able to purchase medications and pay for his medical care. To identify potential problems before they arise
Laboratory tests	
CBC, platelet count	To assess the hematologic system
Partial thromboplastin time, and prothrombin time studies	To assess the clotting mechanisms
Liver function tests	To screen for liver abnormalities, which would delay transplantation until further work was done to pinpoint the cause of the abnormalities (congestion due to fluid overload and acute or chronic hepatitis)
Australian antigen	To screen for Australian antigen positivity, which would not necessarily rule out transplantation, but would identify the patient as a carrier
Antibody to Australian antigen	To identify prior exposure to Australian antigen
Calcium, phosphorus, alkaline phosphatase	To evaluate hyperparathyroidism
Blood urea nitrogen and serum creatinine	To obtain baseline information
Electrolytes (Na, K$^-$, Cl, and CO_2)	To screen for abnormalities
Fasting glucose	To screen for unsuspected tendency toward glucose intolerance (some patients develop corticosteroid-induced diabetes after the transplant)
VDRL	To screen for venereal disease
Amylase	To screen for active pancreatitis
Renal evaluation	
Voiding cystourethrogram (VCUG)	To detect any ureteral reflux, urethral stricture, or bladder abnormality (inability to empty the bladder completely or a diverticulum). If any abnormality is present, corrective procedures are done before the transplantation
Urine cultures	To screen for a urinary tract infection. If the patient has had a number of urinary tract infections, bilateral nephrectomy may be done to eliminate a potential source of infection after the transplant.
Cystometrogram (CMG)	To evaluate the bladder's ability to empty completely. A CMG is not done routinely; it is only done if it is suspected that the patient has a neurogenic bladder (*e.g.*, a diabetic patient) or if the patient has been shown by x-ray film to have residual urine.
Cardiopulmonary evaluation	
ECG	To obtain a baseline tracing and to evaluate cardiac status
Chest x-ray film	To determine the presence or absence of pulmonary disease and to evaluate cardiac status
Evaluation for infection	To detect any infections (infections are the leading cause of postoperative complications) and thus prevent doing a transplant in someone who has an active infection
Fungal skin tests	
Viral titers	
Cultures of blood, sputum, nose, skin	

donation. It is reasonable to think that a potential donor is or has been subjected to family pressures to donate or not to donate. A sibling may be reluctant to donate because of past conflicts and rivalries with the candidate. Society expects a parent to donate a kidney to a child.[13] It must be made clear that if at any time during the evaluation the potential donor has a change of mind, the donation should not be carried through. A medical reason can be given that eliminates the person as a donor. The potential donor can offer the medical reason to the family and thus, it is hoped, avoid family conflicts. If, during the evaluation, the members of the transplant team think that the potential donor is unstable, immature, or "under pressure" from the family and unable to withstand the stress of donation, the physician rules the person unacceptable as a donor on medical grounds.[25]

The donor should be evaluated in steps to minimize the time lost from work and home. The least invasive procedures are done first; if everything is normal, the evaluation culminates in a renal arteriogram, the most invasive procedure of the evaluation. At each step, the donor is in contact with a member of the team who can answer questions and explain how the evaluation progresses and why each test is important.

If even a slight abnormality is found during the evaluation, the evaluation is stopped until the abnormality is corrected. (The donor evaluation is outlined in Table 46–6.)

After the evaluation is completed, and after the potential donor has been briefed repeatedly about the personal risks and the chances of success for the recipient, he or she is asked to decide about donating and to give informed consent in writing.[19]

If a suitable living donor is not found, the recipient's name is placed on a computer list of people awaiting a cadaver kidney. Unfortunately, the wait for a cadaver kidney sometimes is long and often is frustrating for the patient.

Cadaver Donor Kidneys

Because most patients with renal failure do not have a suitable, willing living donor, most transplant programs rely on the use of cadaver kidneys.

Cadaver Donor Selection

Factors considered favorable in donor selection are age between 2 and 65 years, the absence of a history of renal disease or diabetes, the absence of a history of hypertension, the absence of evidence of generalized infection, the absence of a

Table 46–6
Evaluation of a Living Renal Donor

TESTS	REASONS FOR TESTS
Immunologic tests	
ABO and HLA typing	To determine whether donor and recipient are compatible
History taking and physical examination	To make an extensive review of all systems: previous illnesses, past family history, previous surgeries. Any abnormalities found are investigated further before any invasive tests connected with donation are done
Laboratory tests:	
CBC, platelet count	To assess hematologic system
Blood urea nitrogen and serum creatinine	Preliminary assessment of renal function
Electrolytes (Na, K⁻, Cl, and CO_2)	To screen for abnormalities
Fasting glucose	To screen for diabetes
Partial thromboplastin time, and prothrombin time studies	To assess clotting mechanisms
Liver function tests	To screen for liver dysfunction or abnormalities that would require further evaluation before proceeding with the rest of the donor evaluation
Australian antigen and antibody test	To screen for Australian antigen positivity, which would prohibit the person from donating
Calcium, phosphorus, alkaline phosphatase	To screen for abnormalities
VDRL	To screen for venereal disease
Amylase	To screen for active pancreatitis
Viral titers (CMV, HIV, and so forth)	To screen for active viral infection
Cardiopulmonary evaluation	
ECG	To obtain a baseline tracing and to evaluate cardiac status
Chest x-ray film	To determine the presence or absence of pulmonary disease and to evaluate cardiac status
Psychological evaluation	To assess the donor's motivation; to examine and evaluate the intensity of any family or financial pressures to donate; to determine that the donation will not be detrimental to the donor; to give the donor an opportunity to express himself or herself more fully than he or she might to the physician; to help the staff work with the donor and family preoperatively and postoperatively
Renal function studies	
Routine urinalysis	To screen for renal disease or abnormal findings (glycosuria, proteinuria, and abnormal sediment). Microscopic examination should be done by the examining physician
Urine culture	To determine the presence or absence of active urinary tract infection
24-hour urine collections for protein and creatinine clearance (CrCl)	To assess the amount of protein excreted in a 24-hour period. If an abnormality is found, an orthostatic protein test is done. If those results are normal, the donor is considered to be normal in regard to protein. Urine creatinine levels are determined for clearance studies and to ensure that the 24-hour urine output is an adequate one.
Timed Glofil I¹²⁵ or timed CrCl	To assess the actual renal function or the glomerular filtration rate (GRF)
Intravenous pyelogram	To screen for renal abnormalities. To determine that the potential donor has two kidneys that are normal both anatomically and in regard to their excretory function
Renal arteriogram or digital subtraction angiogram	To determine the status of the donor's renal arteries and renal vasculature bilaterally. A small percentage of the population has multiple renal arteries. It is preferable to use a kidney that has only one renal artery. The arteriogram shows any renal lesions and any abnormalities of the vessels, such as stenosis or fibromuscular hyperplasia, which would rule out the person as a donor. The arteriogram is done last and only if the rest of the evaluation was normal (the arteriogram is the most invasive procedure, and it has a slight risk for the potential donor).
CT scan	To look for any abnormality in the structure or the kidney such as cysts, tumor, etc.

history of malignancy (except primary brain tumors, which do not metastasize), and having been a patient under observation who died in the hospital.[61]

The potential donor of a cadaver kidney is cared for by a physician who has no connection with the transplant team. The decision of when death occurs is a clinical one. It is made after a period of observation, and it is based primarily on the clinical criteria of irreversible brain damage. These criteria are fixed and dilated pupils, no response to external stimuli, inability to maintain vital signs (heart beat, blood pressure, respirations) without artificial support, no corneal or pharyngeal reflexes, no reaction to tracheal suctioning, no deep reflexes or plantar reflexes, hypotonia, flat electroencephalogram (EEG), and radiologic evidence that there is no blood flow to the brain.[60,61] (The criteria may differ slightly in different transplant centers.)

Management of the potential cadaver donor has two aspects: treatment for the specific injury without regard for status as a kidney donor; and, after brain death has been determined and permission has been obtained from the family, treatment directed toward maintaining adequate renal function.[1]

When a potential donor becomes available, ABO and HLA antigen type is determined. The criteria for an acceptable antigen match differs among transplant centers. Some centers use only kidneys of donors whose antigens closely match the recipient's antigens, whereas other centers use ABO typing only.

Cadaver kidneys are "shared" among transplant centers. If, when a kidney becomes available, the center does not have a suitable recipient, the kidney is sent to a center that does have a suitable recipient. Methods of storing kidneys have made the sharing program possible.

Preservation of Cadaver Kidneys

Once the kidney is removed from the donor's body, some mechanism has to be employed to prevent irreversible damage to the kidneys from ischemia. In living donors, this is accomplished by simple cooling, because the period of time between removal of the kidney from the donor and implantation into the recipient is short (a few minutes to an hour). The kidney is flushed with a cooled electrolyte solution to provide rapid cooling to the tissue and to wash out blood, platelet aggregates, cells, and fibrinoid thrombi from the interior of the kidney. Once this is accomplished, the kidney is kept immersed in a cold solution until it can be implanted into the recipient.[34]

In cadaver transplantation, the kidneys are handled in the same manner when they are removed from the donor's body. However, methods for longer preservation are needed in order for tissue typing to be performed, suitable recipients to be found, and the surgery to take place.

In simple hypothermic storage, after the kidney is flushed out, it is placed in a sterile electrolyte solution with intracellular fluid characteristics and kept at 2°C to 4°C. Initially, it was thought that kidneys could not be maintained by this method for longer than 8 to 12 hours. However, as research efforts produced new and more compatible solutions, kidneys have been preserved for as long as 48 hours before implantation into a suitable recipient and still resulted in satisfactory renal function. An important advantage of this method is that it is relatively inexpensive and simple.[34]

Continuous pulsatile perfusion machines have been in use since 1967. They provide continuous perfusion of the kidney with a balanced solution, and they keep the kidney temperature between 0°C and 4°C and well oxygenated. After nephrectomy, each kidney is flushed, cannulated, and attached to the machine. This is all done while observing sterile technique.[5]

An advantage of continuous pulsatile perfusion is that the viability of the kidney can be tested while it is being perfused. Flow rates through the cannulated renal artery of the kidney, as well as the diastolic pressure, can be measured. Low flow rates (less than 100 ml/minute) and an elevated diastolic pressure indicate vasospasm in the kidney. Pulsatile perfusion characteristics, as well as the information obtained about the medical treatment and care of the donor, are sometimes used as indicators of the viability of the kidney. The disadvantages of continuous pulsatile perfusion are cost of equipment and personnel and the difficulties encountered in the transportation of a machine.[5,34]

Many studies have been done to determine the advantage of one method over the other as far as eventual renal function. Studies have shown that graft function is similar with either method.[34] Because no significant difference in kidney function seems to exist between the two methods, it appears that simple hypothermic storage is the more cost-effective method, and is being used more frequently.

Surgical Procedure

Donor Surgery

In renal transplantation, it is preferable to use the left kidney of a living donor, because the renal vein is normally longer on the left side. Careful dissection of the renal artery, vein, and ureter is carried out through a flank incision. It is extremely important that the ureter not be stripped clean, because it derives its blood supply from the perinephric fat. To prevent clotting within the kidney, systemic heparin is given before the kidney is removed. The heparin is counteracted systemically after the kidney has been removed by giving the patient protamine. Close observation is made of the patient's vital signs, urine output, and fluid status during the procedure and afterward to maintain an adequate urine output and to prevent damage to the remaining kidney.[61]

In the immediate postoperative period, there may be a transient rise in blood pressure and a transient fall in creatinine clearance with subsequent small rise in the blood urea nitrogen and serum creatinine levels. These phenomena abate after several days with the creatinine clearance returning to, and then remaining at, 70% of the predonation levels. The compensatory response occurs rapidly in renal donors. Long-term follow-up studies show that the donor's health, renal function, and life expectancy are not affected by the donation.[2,3,61]

As soon as the kidney is removed from the donor, it is put in a sterile basin that contains iced Ringer's lactate solution with procaine to ease intrarenal vessel spasm and heparin to prevent small thrombi from forming. The solution not only cools the kidney rapidly, preventing damage from warm ischemia, but it also removes blood from the kidney. The kidney is flushed with the iced solution until the fluid coming from the renal vein is clear. The kidney is kept in the iced solution until it is ready to be placed in the recipient.[61]

Recipient Surgery

While the kidney is being removed from the donor, a team in an adjoining operating room is preparing the recipient. The donor kidney is usually placed in the recipient's right iliac fossa (Fig. 46–2). This site is used because the right common iliac artery and external iliac veins are more superficial—and therefore more accessible—than those on the left side. However, the left iliac fossa can be used if the right iliac fossa was used in a previous operation.[61]

The renal artery of the donor kidney is generally anastomosed end-to-end to the recipient's hypogastric artery. The donor renal vein is anastomosed end-to-side, using the recipient's external iliac vein. Usually, urine can be seen coming from the ureter a few minutes after the vascular clamps have been released. It is important that the recipient not become hypovolemic at this point, because hypovolemia interferes with kidney perfusion and the resumption of renal function.[61]

There are several ways to restore the upper urinary tract. The most common way is to make a tunnel incision through the trigone area of the bladder and insert a catheter through the tunnel and through the lateroposterior bladder wall. The ureter is pulled through the tunnel tract and sutured to the mucosal wall. The bladder is closed. A Foley catheter is kept in the bladder to facilitate urinary drainage and to keep the bladder decompressed, thereby reducing the incidence of urinary leaks from the ureteral anastomosis.[61]

Because the iliac fossa seems to be ideally formed to receive a kidney, it is not necessary to suture the new kidney in place unless the blood flow appears to be obstructed because of kinking of the vessels.[61] In most transplant centers, metal clips are placed on the upper and lower poles of the kidney, as well as along the medial aspect of the kidney. These clips help to determine the size and location of the kidney by x-ray examination and aid in the recognition of potential swelling.

Physiology of the Transplanted Kidney

In almost all recipients of living donor kidneys and in some recipients of cadaver kidneys, the urinary output begins immediately and is of high volume. The urinary output can reach a volume of 5 to 10 ml/minute during the first hours and then (depending on the patient's fluid intake) gradually return to a normal volume in 48 to 72 hours. The electrolyte levels in the initial urine reflect the body's attempt to establish a more normal environment: the sodium level is high (100 to 125 mEq/L), the chloride level is low (49 to 100 mEq/L), and the potassium level is significant (14 to 27 mEq/L), as is the urine osmolality (the average is 352 mOsmol/L).[25]

The phenomenon of postoperative polyuria probably represents osmotic diuresis in association with a diminished resorption in the proximal tubules. The driving force of the diuresis can be attributed to the following: the recipient's serum

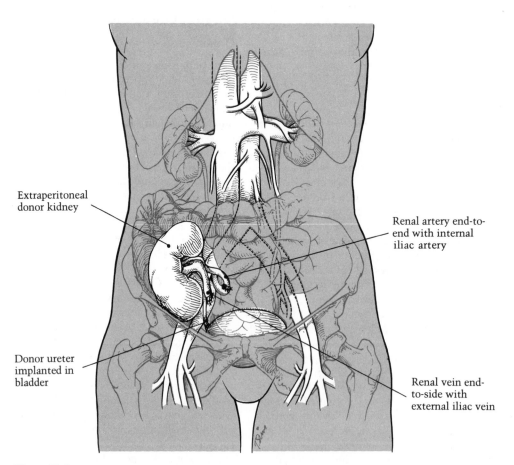

Extraperitoneal donor kidney

Renal artery end-to-end with internal iliac artery

Donor ureter implanted in bladder

Renal vein end-to-side with external iliac vein

Figure 46–2

Anatomical placement of the transplanted kidney. The placement of the transplanted kidney in relationship to the other abdominal organs.

is hyperosmolar because of the increase in blood urea and other substances; there is some degree of salt and water retention despite adequate hemodialysis; and lesions that affect tubular resorption may be caused by the ischemia resulting from cooling of the kidney at the time of the transplantation, especially in cadaver kidneys.[25]

Close attention must be paid to the fluid and electrolyte balance in the immediate postoperative period to avoid the complications of dehydration and hypokalemia. Enough fluids should be given to prevent dehydration, but not enough to prolong the polyuric phase. Usually replacement fluids consist of half-normal saline solution and 5% dextrose and water solution. The proportion of each solution the patient receives differs from center to center. If urinary output is 200 ml/hour or less, replacement is usually 100%, but if the output exceeds 200 ml/hour, replacement therapy is reduced to a percentage of the previous hour's output. The immediate reestablishment of renal function and the polyuria often result in the lowering of the blood urea nitrogen and serum creatinine levels to nearly normal by the third postoperative day.[25]

Proteinuria is also often present in the immediate postoperative period. It is due to hematuria or ischemic changes in the renal tubules. In most cases, the proteinuria diminishes or disappears within a few days. A reappearance signifies that a different process is occurring, such as rejection, recurrent disease, or renal vein thrombosis.[25]

Clinical Manifestations

In the observation and assessment of the renal transplant patient, two of the most important factors are status of renal function, and absence or presence of infection (as previously discussed).

Status of Renal Function

Hyperacute rejection is recognized at the time of surgery. The kidney turns blue and soft on revascularization, instead of pink and firm. The kidney is removed immediately.[35]

In *delayed hyperacute (vascular) rejection*, urine volume suddenly declines and the patient develops a fever and pain over the upper pole of the kidney (produced by irritation of peritoneal membrane as the kidney swells). This is usually followed by anuria. Vascular occlusion needs to be ruled out, and determination of this type of rejection needs to be made promptly. If the kidney is left in place, the patient can develop severe leukopenia and thrombocytopenia, which could lead to death.[35]

Acute rejection is the most common type of rejection. Clinically, the recipient experiences a decrease in urine output associated with an increase in body weight, edema, fever, increase in blood pressure, increase in proteinuria in the absence of bloody urine, pain in the area of the upper pole of the kidney (different from incisional pain), and general malaise (Table 46–7). The further from the time of transplantation that acute rejection occurs, the less dramatic is the presentation of symptoms. The most common clinical finding in late acute rejection is the reappearance of proteinuria.[35]

Chronic rejection has few clinical signs and symptoms. The laboratory values tend to show a gradual decline in the patient's renal function over a period of months that often is noticed only when the patient returns for a routine follow-up appointment. Usually a course of treatment is tried, but if there is no response, the patient is kept on a maintenance dose of immunosuppressive drugs until the renal function deteriorates further and dialysis is required. The decision is made at that time whether or not the kidney should be removed.[73] Chronic rejection occurs over an indefinite period of time and can be gradual or can occur in a stepwise fashion (Fig. 46–3).

Table 46–7
Signs and Symptoms of Acute Rejection for Renal Transplant

Clinical signs
    Fever (without an accompanying infection)
    Weight gain (more than 2 lb in a 24-hour period)
    Malaise
    Enlargement of the graft with upper pole tenderness
    Hypertension
    Decreased urinary output
    Edema, especially periorbital edema and edema of the legs
    Anorexia
Laboratory signs
    Leukocytosis (may also be due to high-dose corticosteroids or to infection)
    Increased blood urea nitrogen levels
    Increased serum creatinine levels
    Increased proteinuria
    Decreased Glofil I[125] or creatinine clearance values
    Decreased urine sodium level
Radiologic evidence
    An enlarged kidney (as shown by comparison of a flat-plate of the abdomen with one done earlier)
    An ultrasound may show an enlarged kidney and an increase in the resistive index.
    A renal scan may show poor flow through the kidney caused by edema.
    A sulfur colloid study may show a positive uptake of sulfur colloid in the transplanted kidney.
    An arteriogram may show vessel changes, with irregularity and loss of smaller vessels, a prolonged
        circulation time, and a poor nephrogram.
Pathologic evidence
    A fine-needle aspiration biopsy (FNAB) showing infiltrating cells
    A core biopsy showing interstitial edema, round cell infiltrates, and cellular exudate

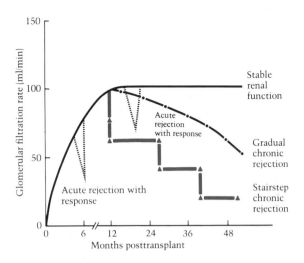

Figure 46–3
Stages of chronic rejection: The different pathways chronic rejection may take: gradual and stepwise.

Diagnostic Tests

In addition to changes in weight and a decrease in 24-hour urine volume (or drastic decrease in any 8-hour period), the simplest tests to observe for rejection are an increase in the serum creatinine from one day to the next and a decrease in the glomerular filtration rate (GFR) as determined by creatinine clearance (24-hour collection or a timed collection) or a Glofil clearance (I^{125}).

Other tests used frequently in conjunction with those preceding are ultrasound, renal biopsy, renal scan, and arteriography.

Ultrasound of the transplanted kidney is a useful tool in assessing acute rejection and is used in chronic rejection for completeness. In either case, it can demonstrate the absence or presence of a fluid collection (hematoma, abscess, lymphocele) that might be interfering with the path of the ureter and thereby causing a partial obstruction.[35] Hydronephrosis can usually be diagnosed by ultrasound, but the diagnosis is not absolute. The test is noninvasive and without complications, except for some discomfort in the surgical area if done soon after surgery.

A *renal scan* of the transplanted kidney is particularly helpful in delayed hyperacute and acute rejection. In delayed hyperacute rejection, the radiolabeled substance that is injected peaks rapidly in the transplanted kidney and then disappears. This is indicative of perfusion problems.[35] In acute rejection, the renal scan has been found to be particularly useful in making the diagnosis when a baseline scan has been done within the first day after surgery and is available for comparison. Renal function is determined by the nephrogram and nuclide appearance in the collecting system. Deterioration from the baseline scan is well correlated with acute rejection.[56]

A *core biopsy* of the transplanted kidney provides additional information to help establish or to exclude the diagnosis of rejection. In hyperacute rejection, microscopic examination reveals leukocytes in the glomerular capillaries, and intravascular renal thrombosis is present.[61,73]

The microscopic examination of a kidney undergoing delayed hyperacute rejection shows necrosis and lysis of endothelial cells and intravascular thrombosis of the vessels, leading to partial or complete cortical necrosis.[35]

Characteristically, a kidney with acute rejection has diffuse interstitial edema and round cell infiltrates in the interstitial tissue and the peritubular capillaries. Cellular exudate and vascular lesions can also be seen, but the glomerulus is usually spared.[35]

Chronic rejection is an ongoing process that occurs over a prolonged period of time (Fig. 46–3). The lesions seen on biopsy can be vascular (the extent of arterial involvement being important in determining the eventual outcome of the graft), interstitial (fibrosis of the interstitium is the most common finding and causes strangulation of the vessels in the renal parenchyma), and glomerular (seen in the form of ischemic damage).[35]

Fine-needle aspiration biopsy (FNAB) is a procedure in which cells from the kidney can be aspirated using a 25-gauge spinal needle. This procedure can be done daily without harm to the kidney. It can also be done in an outpatient setting. The aspirated cells are examined for changes in the parenchymal cells indicative of ischemic or toxic injury, or for infiltrating cells (lymphocytes, lymphoblasts) indicative of rejection.[31]

An *arteriogram* is helpful in determining the vascularity of the transplanted kidney. In delayed hyperacute rejection, the arteriogram presents a picture of persistence of dye in the arteries within the kidney, patchy filling defects in the cortex, irregularities in appearance of the arterioles, abrupt ending of the arteries, and a very pale nephrogram phase (if it is seen at all).[15] This appearance has been referred to as a "pruned tree." In acute rejection, the arteriogram shows only that blood is flowing through the kidney. It may demonstrate the presence or absence of any vascular changes or infarcts, but alone it is not diagnostic of this type of rejection episode.

Clinical Course
Immediate Postoperative Period

In the immediate postoperative period, different processes may adversely affect the transplanted kidney. Everyone involved is happy when urine is seen to move steadily through the catheter and closed drainage system. However, early oliguria and anuria can occur. They can be caused by many different factors, each of which must be checked out systematically (Table 46–8). These factors are as follows:

- Obstruction of the urinary flow.—The catheter should be checked for patency. Something as simple as a kink in the catheter or tubing can obstruct the flow of urine. If the urine is bloody and contains clots, the catheter needs to be irrigated gently, using sterile technique. A bigger catheter may be needed. If clots have caused the decrease in urinary flow, the urinary output should increase 10 to 15 minutes after the catheter has been irrigated.[61]
- Hypovolemia.—Hypovolemia may be due to blood loss during surgery or postoperatively. Serial decreasing hematocrit levels, displacement of intraperitoneal organs (shown by abdominal x-ray film), and a graft that cannot be palpated suggest a hematoma. Or, the patient may simply need more fluids. If this is the case, a bolus of intravenous fluids increases urinary output.[61]
- Thrombosis or stenosis of the renal artery or the renal vein.—

Table 46–8
Causes of Postoperative Oliguria and Anuria

CAUSES	OBSERVATIONS
Prerenal causes	
Hypovolemia	Ensure adequate volume expansion by monitoring pulse, blood pressure, and skin turgor.
Poor cardiac status	Assess cardiac status, observe for congestive failure, and institute appropriate treatment.
Renal artery lesion	Monitor blood pressure; observe for sudden pain in the abdomen, a bruit, an increase in blood pressure, and a decrease in urinary output.
Renal causes	
Rejection	Small volumes of urine are obtained that have a low sodium content and a high osmolality. An increase in blood pressure and pain around the upper pole of the graft caused by the size increase are noted.
Acute tubular necrosis (ATN)	ATN results in small quantities of urine that have a high sodium content. Review the data about the condition of the donor before his kidney was removed. Difficulty with the arterial anastomosis at the time of surgery can also contribute to ATN.
Postrenal causes	
Catheter obstruction	Check the catheter for patency, kinking, and clots. Gently irrigate the catheter if necessary.
Ureteral leak	A sudden increase of fluid from the drain site, a feeling of fullness in the abdomen
Ureteral obstruction	If the urine is extremely bloody and contains many clots, the ureter may be obstructed by clots.
Renal vein obstruction	The graft will become larger; massive proteinuria is present; venograms are essential to the diagnosis.

Complete thrombosis of the renal artery, a rare condition, is usually seen in patients who have atherosclerotic disease involving the iliac vessels. Partial obstruction of the renal artery can occur from torsion or kinking of the vessels. The best diagnostic sign is a sudden decrease in urinary output that often is associated with an increase in blood pressure. The only accurate diagnostic approach is a renal flow scan followed by a renal arteriogram, which would demonstrate an arterial stricture or occlusion. If an occlusion or a significant stricture is present, the patient is returned immediately to surgery for corrective procedures.[61] Venous occlusion is an even rarer occurrence in the immediate postoperative period, but a partial venous thrombosis can occur later in the course of the transplant. If a venous thrombosis is suggested by the arteriogram, venography should be done.[61]

- Acute tubular necrosis.—Acute tubular necrosis (ATN) is rare in transplants of living donor kidneys, because the ischemia time of the kidney is not prolonged. ATN is seen more often in cadaver transplants, in which both warm and cold ischemia times are prolonged. Also, the donor may have been hypotensive for a period of time before the nephrectomy, resulting in hypoperfusion of the kidneys. When ATN occurs, intermittent hemodialysis is required until the kidney function returns. Hemodialysis at this stage can lead to other complications, such as hypovolemia or a hematoma in the wound, caused by the use of heparin. The hematoma may become infected and cause serious problems.[61]

- Ureteral leaks.—At one time ureteral leaks were the most common complication of renal transplantation. The leaks can occur for a number of reasons, but the majority are due to distal ureteral necrosis from ischemia. The most common cause of the ischemia is the stripping of the perihilar and periureteral fat, which disturbs the blood supply of the ureter. It is less common in surgical procedures in which a ureteroneocystostomy (a tunneling of the ureter into the bladder) is used rather than a ureteroureterostomy (anastomosis of the transplanted ureter into the patient's ureter) or a pyeloureterostomy (anastomosis of the patient's ureter into the pelvis of the transplanted kidney). The leak can usually be seen readily on an intravenous pyelogram (IVP). Even though ureteral leaks usually occur in the first week after transplantation, cases have been reported to occur more than 1 month after transplant.[35]

A urine leak is a potentially serious complication that can lead to infection and even death. It must be treated immediately either by the placement of a ureteral stent or surgically (by reimplantation of the ureter, nephrostomy, or pyeloureterostomy to the host ureter), depending on the extent of the extravasation of the urine and the location of the leak. Rarely, necrosis of the ureter extends into the pelvis of the kidney, resulting in nephrectomy of the transplanted kidney. If the leak is small, a urethral (Foley) catheter can be inserted to provide adequate drainage until the site is healed.[55]

The Postoperative Period

The obvious postoperative complications of kidney transplantations (and of most types of surgery) are pneumonia and wound infections. Scrupulous pulmonary hygiene is mandatory after the transplantation to prevent atelectasis and pneumonia. Strict aseptic techniques are observed in changing dressings and in giving wound care to decrease the incidence of wound infections and cross-contamination of patients.

Bacterial infections that end in septicemia have a high mortality among people who have had organ transplants. The infections seem to occur more often in recipients of cadaver kidneys than in recipients of a living related donor kidney, perhaps because the recipient of a cadaver kidney may have been on hemodialysis longer and had more complications as a result. Recipients of cadaver kidneys also seem to have more episodes of rejection and ATN, and so receive higher doses of corticosteroids for longer periods of time.

Infections around the graft usually are manifested within a month after the transplantation, but in some rare cases they are dormant for several months. The use of prophylactic antibiotics just before and during surgery seems to decrease the incidence of wound infections after transplantation.[73]

Bacterial infections of the central nervous system occur infrequently. Often they are masked in their early stages by the anti-inflammatory actions of the corticosteroids. The mortality among patients with central nervous system involvement is high.[73]

Some workers find gram-negative organisms the most common cause of bacterial infections (in 75% of cases), with *Pseudomonas* infections being the most common. The most common gram-positive organism is *Staphylococcus* (in 10% to 15% of cases); it is usually found in arteriovenous (A-V) fistulas, shunts, and wounds.[73]

The most common site of infection is the urinary tract, and urinary tract infections have the lowest mortality. A urologic workup is done to rule out an anatomic cause (*e.g.,* reflux or partial obstruction), and the patient is taught double voiding and good personal hygiene in an effort to eliminate the sources of infection. If urinary tract infections recur often, the patient is placed on long-term immunosuppressive therapy, which seems to have no adverse side effects.[73]

Pulmonary infections are the second most common infection, and they have a high mortality. Pulmonary infections may be fungal or viral, alone or combined with bacterial organisms. Because bacterial organisms are easily cultured from the sputum, they are treated with antimicrobial therapy. However, these may not be the causative organism, because fungal and protozoan organisms are not easily cultured from the sputum and tracheal aspirates. If no response to treatment is shown clinically or by serial chest x-ray films, it may be necessary to obtain a tissue diagnosis by a brush biopsy, a needle biopsy, or an open biopsy of the lung.[61,73]

About 20% of pulmonary infections that occur in people who have undergone transplantation are due to fungi, *Nocardia,* and *Mycobacterium. Candida* infections are the most common fungal infections. The causative organism is usually found in the urinary tract and oral cavity, and it disseminates to the esophagus and lungs. When dissemination occurs, systemic antifungal therapy is required in addition to topical therapy.[73]

Continuing Care

The renal transplant recipient is usually discharged 10 to 14 days after surgery if there have been no major complications. The recipient is then seen from two to three times a week in an outpatient clinic. The number of clinic visits decreases as the patient's condition becomes more stable, and over a period of 4 months, the visits are gradually reduced to once a month. If the patient's condition remains stable, routine clinic visits occur once every 4 to 6 months, and laboratory checks are done between visits. If the patient becomes ill—develops leukopenia, liver disease, or acute or chronic rejection—clinic visits become more frequent again.

Acute rejection episodes can be treated on an outpatient basis unless the patient's renal function has deteriorated rapidly or a complicating condition develops. With every acute rejection episode, a sonogram is done to rule out a problem with the ureter or other mechanical problems involving the urinary tract. A renal scan may be done to try to rule out an arterial lesion.

Continuity of care is provided for the transplant recipient as an outpatient, in the sense that the clinic personnel are familiar with the patient's hospital course and problems. Similarly, the transplant unit staff is kept informed of any problems the transplant recipient has as an outpatient. The transplant recipient is given telephone numbers of people to call 24 hours a day if a problem arises.

The outpatient checkup includes a urinalysis, complete blood count (CBC), blood urea nitrogen (BUN), serum creatinine, cyclosporine level, and a laboratory scan including liver function studies, lipids, electrolytes, and metabolic studies. Serial 24-hour urine collections are done to evaluate the degree, if any, of proteinuria. The nursing assessment of the patient includes weight, blood pressure, medication check and instructions, and identification of potential problems. The patient is then seen by the physician.

Patients are instructed to continue to weigh themselves daily and to report any sudden increase in weight accompanied by edema of the legs. A dietitian and a social worker are available for consultation at every clinic visit.

Patients are encouraged to return to work 6 to 8 weeks postoperatively. Children are encouraged to continue their school work with a "homebound" teacher until they are able to return to school.

After the recipient's condition has stabilized (no evidence of rejection or infection), the recipient is usually released back to the referring physician for long-term care. When this is done, it is extremely important that continuity of care be observed through clear, concise communications. In some places, this has been accomplished by computerizing all the transplant data, which then appears on each patient's progress note.

Resolution of Uremic Symptoms

The patient who has had a successful renal transplant is soon on the way to rehabilitation. Such a patient gradually regains strength as the body systems that were affected by uremia return to normal. The cardiovascular system improves, with a reduction in heart size and the correction of fluid overload.[13]

Hypertension usually resolves unless the patient has stenosis of the transplanted artery, a delay in the recovery of renal function, or a poorly functioning graft. In some instances, in patients with normally functioning grafts, hypertension is traceable to the original kidneys, and removal of these kidneys can bring the blood pressure back to normal.[25] In many cases, such a result can be predicted from renin studies of the renal vein or from a history of increased blood pressure when the patient was on dialysis.

The anemia seen in the dialyzed patient disappears, because the transplanted kidney secretes erythropoietin. In uncomplicated cases, the anemia is corrected within 1 to 2 months of the transplant.[25]

Uremic neuropathy, which is manifested by itching, burning, and muscular weakness, usually disappears rapidly after transplantation. Peripheral neuropathy, manifested by a disturbance in gait and in nerve conduction velocity, is slower to disappear, but it resolves completely in most affected patients.[25]

Complications

Hepatic Dysfunction

The incidence of hepatic dysfunction varies from center to center, but the causes are universal. Among the causes are azathioprine, which can produce a dose-related cholestatic syndrome, but more importantly, can alter the immune system's response to viral infections; hepatitis B antigen, which accounts for a small percentage of cases; cytomegalovirus; and non-A, non-B hepatitis virus (viral hepatitis C), which is thought to be responsible for the development of chronic active hepatitis and cirrhosis. Hepatitis A has been shown not to be a factor in the liver disease of the transplant population. Hepatic dysfunction can be classified into three types: acute reversible, acute fulminant progressing to death, and chronic liver disease with variable prognosis.[78]

Many approaches have been taken to reverse or stabilize the progression of the chronic disease, ranging from substituting cyclophosphamide for azathioprine to withdrawing all immunosuppressive agents. One of the most frustrating things about progressive liver disease is that the staff caring for the patient feels helpless. Most of the renal transplant patients who die from liver disease have a functioning kidney at the time of their death.

Death

Even transplant recipients who survive 5 years or more with a functioning transplanted kidney remain at risk. The causes of death in one group of patients (they are probably the same in every group of transplant recipients) were hepatic dysfunction (21%), sepsis (18%), cardiac disease (18%), and malignancy (9%).[32] Suicide has also occurred, by violence, by voluntarily discontinuing medications, or by refusing hemodialysis and treatment when the transplanted kidney failed. Most of the deaths occurred in patients with functioning transplanted kidneys who were taking maintenance doses of immunosuppressive drugs.

Social Complications

Another complication—a social one—is the high divorce rate among transplant recipients. A possible explanation for the difference between the divorce rates for dialysis and transplant patients is that it is not socially acceptable to divorce someone who is chronically ill (*i.e.,* someone who depends on a machine for life), whereas it is acceptable to divorce someone who has a kidney transplant and who is viewed, even by the transplant recipient, as normal. The pressures on the spouse of a transplant recipient and the recipient's move toward independence also seem to affect the divorce rates.

Gradually the patient who has had a successful transplant begins to adapt to the new condition as stress is decreased and health is restored. Tensions in the family seem to decrease (at least to the level that existed before the renal failure), as the patient's role in the family is resumed and the financial burdens are lessened. The immediate fear of death decreases, even though it readily surfaces when another transplant patient dies.[60] When this happens, the patient needs to be assured that people are different and they respond differently, even to the same disease.

CASE STUDY

Mr. D.F. is a 31-year-old white man who has been a type I diabetic since the age of 3 years. His diabetic complications included marked retinopathy with retinal detachment in the past, requiring laser therapy. In addition, he has a moderate sensory peripheral neuropathy. He arrived at end-stage renal disease approximately 7 months before transplantation and was placed on chronic ambulatory peritoneal dialysis (CAPD) at that time. On CAPD he remained hypertensive and required captopril 50 mg orally twice daily, verapamil SR 240 mg orally once daily, and prazosin 2 mg orally once daily.

Because he was blood ABO group A, he did not wait long until he was called for transplantation. Once a blood group A donor became available, the patient's most recent serum, which had been drawn 12 days earlier, was included in a T- and B-cell crossmatch against the donor's lymphocytes. In addition, HLA typing was carried out on the donor, which was found to be A2, A11, B8, B44, DR5, and DRw6. From prior tissue typing, the patient's HLA typing was known to be A1, A2, B8, B−), DR4, DRw6. The patient and donor were, therefore, matched at three of six loci. Both were blood group A positive. A point system was tallied up for all potential A recipients on the transplant center list, and the patient came out at the top of the list by the scoring scheme. He was then called in to the transplant center by the transplant nephrologist on call.

At the transplant center he was greeted by a transplant coordinator who showed the patient to a workup treatment room where blood studies were drawn and the patient underwent an electrocardiogram plus chest x-ray examination. The transplant nephrologist then performed a complete history and physical examination of the patient. Specific features looked for in the history included any recent infections, use of antibiotics, irritation at the Tenckhoff catheter exit site, history of peritonitis, and what the patient felt was his dry weight.

Physical examination was unremarkable except for the head and neck, which revealed extensive diabetic retinopathy on funduscopic examination. Abdominal examination revealed a soft, nontender abdomen with no hepatosplenomegaly. The Tenckhoff catheter was noted in the left midabdominal area with no evidence of exit site or tunnel infection. Laboratory results were all then reviewed, and all were found acceptable for a surgical procedure.

A full discussion of the risks and benefits of renal transplantation and immunosuppression was then undertaken by the transplant nephrologist with the patient. Individual maintenance, immunosuppressive medications and their side-effects, as well as specific antirejection regimens were discussed with the patient. The transplant surgeon then explained the risks of the transplant surgical procedure itself and again allowed questions from the patient. After this discussion, the patient stated that he still wished to go ahead with the procedure.

Permission forms for the surgical procedure, and a patient consent form from the organ bank supplying the kidney were given to the patient to read and sign if he so agreed. He readily did so. He was given preoperative medications, including azathioprine 175 mg orally, methylprednisolone 125 mg intravenously, and cefazolin 1 g intravenously.

The patient was then taken to the operating suite where the procedure lasted approximately 2 hours and 45 minutes. The operation included an internal iliac artery endarterectomy because of atherosclerosis in the patient's own vessel and, in addition, the placement of a ureteral stent in the transplant ureter because of its small size. The patient had immediate urine output and was taken to the intensive care unit where he was observed until the following morning.

Initial urine output was good and the patient demonstrated almost immediate clearance with the fall of the admission creatinine of 6.2 to a value of 3.5 mg/dl by the fifth day after transplant. During this time the patient received prednisone 100 mg orally daily, azathioprine 175 mg orally daily (2.5 mg/kg/day), and OKT3 5 mg intravenously daily. On the sixth postoperative day all of these medications were continued, but cyclosporine was introduced at the dosage of 3 mg/kg/day in two divided doses. On day 7, the patient's cyclosporine was increased to 8 mg/kg/day, and the OKT3 was given for the final seventh dose. The patient continued to do well, and the serum creatinine fell to 2.4 mg/dl on the eleventh postoperative day.

Over these 11 days the patient steadily progressed from an initial intravenous fluid replacement of 100% of his urine output to a full diet and no intravenous replacement by 48 hours postoperatively. By 48 hours after the operation, the patient was encouraged to be out of bed and taking short walks in the hall. He was then encouraged to participate in the monitoring of his own progress and care. This included recording his daily weight, daily medications, oral intake and urinary output, and laboratory values in his own transplant journal. Teaching sessions, organized by the transplant unit's social worker, nursing staff, and pharmacist, were then carried out so that the patient could both understand and properly care for himself, as well as monitor his progress and know when to ask for help.

His Tenckhoff peritoneal dialysis catheter was removed on the tenth postoperative day. On the 11th postoperative day he was judged to be clinically stable and to have learned both his medications and his self-monitoring regimen sufficiently to allow discharge. This included monitoring his blood glucoses, which now required increasing amounts of insulin to control, consistent with his improved kidney function, as well as the high-dose prednisone therapy which he was still undergoing. Discharge medications were the following:

Cyclosporine A 190 mg orally every 12 hours (6 mg/kg/day)
Prednisone 70 mg orally daily and tapering per taper card
Azathioprine 150 mg orally daily
NPH insulin 30 units subcutaneously in the morning, 20 units subcutaneously at night
Regular insulin on a sliding scale before meals and at bedtime
Furosemide 80 mg orally twice daily
Potassium supplement 40 mEq orally twice daily
Magnesium supplement 500 mg orally twice daily
Nifedipine long-acting tablets 60 mg orally each morning
Clonidine 0.1 mg orally twice daily
Trimethoprim–sulfamethoxazole one tablet regular strength at night
Multivitamin with iron once daily
Stool softener 200 mg orally twice daily
Antifungal mouth troche to be dissolved orally five times daily

The patient returned for his first transplant clinic visit 72 hours later (on Monday). At that time he felt well. He had the routine laboratory work drawn (CBC, laboratory scan, urinalysis, CyA trough level), was weighed, and was instructed about what to expect on his first visit and each subsequent one by the clinic transplant nursing coordinator. After the clinic nurse reviewed Mr. D.F.'s problem list and medications, he was examined by a transplant nephrologist. His serum creatinine, done in the clinic, revealed that his renal function was stable and he was given a return appointment for Wednesday.

His next clinic visit (Wednesday) occurred on day 16 postoperatively. At this time he had a clearly elevated serum creatinine at 4.1 mg/dl but continued to feel well and had noted no change in his urine output. The transplant nephrologist ordered an outpatient renal transplant sonogram, which showed no evidence of rejection. The patient's right lower abdomen (identifying the placement of the transplanted kidney) was marked, and a FNAB of the transplant kidney was performed. The results now showed definite immune activation, in contrast to the FNAB done on the ninth postoperative day. A diagnosis of rejection was made, and the patient was placed on methylprednisolone at a dose of 3 mg/kg/day for 5 consecutive days in addition to all his other medications. His cyclosporine blood level was noted to be low at 191 ng/ml and the patient's cyclosporine dose was increased to 250 mg every 12 hours (7.6 mg/kg/day). The patient continued on the methylprednisolone (Solu-medrol) minibolus at the clinic for the first 3 days. On the fourth day of treatment, he complained of a headache, and his serum creatinine was now elevated to 6.5 mg/dl.

Because of the headache and his high-dose corticosteroid therapy, the patient was admitted to the hospital to be evaluated for an infectious process. A lumbar puncture was performed and—although it was clear and colorless with a normal opening pressure—the CSF revealed an increased number of white blood cells and a slightly increased protein concentration. The methylprednisolone minibolus "therapy" was completed on the 20th postoperative day. On the 21st postoperative day, when the serum creatinine continued to rise, both a FNAB and a core biopsy of the transplant kidney were performed. The FNAB revealed continued significant immune activation, and the core biopsy showed marked tubulitis and interstitial hemorrhage

consistent with a severe acute cellular rejection. A three-lumen subclavian catheter was therefore placed, and the patient was initiated on additional therapy with antilymphocyte globulin (ALG). This was chosen in preference to OKT3 because of the patient's headache and abnormal CSF findings, which were felt to be possibly secondary to the initial OKT3 therapy.

The ALG required a separate consent form to be signed by the patient before its use. It was initiated at a dose of 20 mg/kg/day infused initially in 1000 ml of 0.45% sodium chloride over 6 hours and later in 500 ml of 0.45% sodium chloride over 4 hours for subsequent doses. With the initial dose the patient suffered a shaking chill and a sharp rise of his temperature. Thereafter the doses were not followed by the temperature rise. A second lumbar puncture was performed on the 22nd postoperative day and gave findings similar to the initial study, except that the CSF protein was now normal. Unfortunately, despite the additional immunosuppressive therapy, the patient's serum creatinine continued to rise until the 25th postoperative day (day 3 of ALG therapy), when it began a slow decline from a peak value of 8.5 mg/dl.

Fine-needle aspiration biopsies were obtained again on postoperative days 30 and 32 to monitor cellular activity within the transplant kidney. The study on the 30th postoperative day showed continued immune activation plus the presence of macrophages consistent with severe ongoing destructive changes within the kidney. However, on the 32nd postoperative day the study showed less immune activation and fewer macrophages. The patient was given a full 14-day course of ALG. During this course of therapy he continued to have headaches and was seen in consultation by a neurologist, who performed a third lumbar puncture that again showed the white cells in the spinal fluid but no other abnormal findings. All other cultures were subsequently negative. His postoperative course can be followed in Fig. 46–4.

This was an extremely frustrating time for Mr. D.F. He did not have control over his situation and could not be "totally assured" that he would keep the kidney. He continued to receive supportive care from the transplant team during this difficult time. He demonstrated patience and cooperativeness while he was in the "grey" zone of whether or not the kidney would function long term.

PANCREATIC TRANSPLANT

As of June 30, 1988, there have been 1549 pancreatic transplants in 1440 diabetic patients reported to the International Pancreas Transplant Registry; the first one was done in 1966.[72] The number of patients transplanted has steadily increased since the availability of cyclosporine as an immunosuppressive agent and as technical problems have been solved.[71,72]

Some patients receive a kidney and pancreas simultaneously; others receive a kidney first, followed by a pancreas when renal function has been stabilized. The best survival rates are in the patients who simultaneously receive a kidney and a pancreas.[71,72]

In the diabetic patient who has not undergone (or who needs) a renal transplant, the major criterion for selection as a pancreatic transplant recipient is that the diabetic complications the patient has or will have (e.g., nephropathy, progressive retinopathy, and neuropathy) are potentially more life-threatening than the side-effects of chronic immunosuppression.[71]

The pancreas can be obtained from a cadaver donor or from a segment of the pancreas from a living related donor. The pancreas is placed intraperitoneally in the recipient. There are several techniques employed to handle the functions of the pancreatic duct. These include ligation of the duct; injection of the ductal system with synthetic polymer to obliterate it;

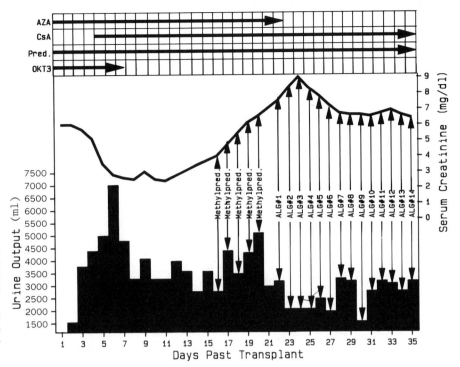

Figure 46-4

Postoperative course after renal transplantation. The immunosuppressive regimen is seen across the top of the graph. The renal function is followed with serum creatinine and 24-hour urine output. (*Note,* the patient's urine output before transplant was 1600 ml to 2000 ml per 24 hours). The treatment for rejection is indicated vertically on the graph and begins on day 16.

enteric drainage; and direct insertion of the pancreatic duct into the bladder.[71]

Currently, most patients receive triple therapy: azathioprine, corticosteroids, and cyclosporine as the immunosuppressive maintenance. In some centers, ALG, OKT3, or both are used as prophylactic immunosuppression.[72] The serum glucose, amylase, and C-peptide are followed as an indication of the function of the pancreas. A rejection episode is treated with an increase in corticosteroid dose or by using ALG.[71]

The causes of failure of the transplanted pancreas, in addition to rejection, include: recurrence of disease, technical reasons such as primary thrombosis of the graft, local infection requiring graft removal, and recipient death.[72]

At 1 year, the overall actuarial patient survival rate is 80%, and the overall actuarial graft survival rate is 42%. The longest functioning graft is 10 years.[72]

CARDIAC TRANSPLANT

Over 9000 orthotopic and 275 heterotopic cardiac transplantations have been done in the past 20 years.[36] In 1967, Barnard performed the first successful human-to-human cardiac transplant. During the following year, 102 cardiac transplants were done in 17 centers, with basically disastrous results. From 1969 to 1979, cardiac transplantation continued with no more than 50 cases being done per year throughout the world. Survival at 1 year gradually rose from 20% to 65%. The increased survival of cardiac transplantation has been due to the development of new techniques, medications, and patient selection.

Etiology and Incidence

The Registry of the International Society for Heart Transplantation (ISHT) compiles data on heart and heart–lung

transplantations done throughout the world since 1980. According to their report, the age groups of cardiac transplant recipients range from newborns to 70 years, with the majority of the recipients being in the 50- to 59-year age group. The indications for cardiac transplantation are myopathy, coronary artery disease, valvular disease, congenital heart disease, and myocarditis.[27]

According to the ISHT, the 30-day mortality for orthotopic cardiac transplantation is decreasing. The lowest incidence of 30-day mortality was reported in 1988 at 8.9% (from 11% in 1987). In examining the actuarial survival curve for cardiac transplantation, the most critical time period is within the first year, reflected by the greatest mortality. A comparison of a 5-year actuarial survival demonstrates a higher incidence of survival with orthotopic (73.9%) versus heterotopic (54.1%) cardiac transplantation. Examining 5-year actuarial survival for orthotopic transplantation, survival increases to 78% for those receiving cyclosporine. For those receiving triple therapy, survival further increases to 81.9%. The 10-year actuarial survival for orthotopic cardiac transplantation is 73.3% survival. Although the 10-year survival is representative of only 88 recipients, it is suggestive of the actuarial survival curve.[27]

Combined Heart–Lung Transplant

Combined heart–lung, single-lung, and double-lung transplantation remains experimental. According to the ISHT, the 5-year actuarial survival for heart–lung transplantation is 55.4% (n = 16). The actuarial survival for single-lung or double-lung transplantation (n = 51) was 70% at 1 month and 54.2% at 1 year.[27] Just as cardiac transplantation has become a widely accepted treatment for poor cardiac function that is refractory to medical and surgical therapies, lung transplantation shows promise for the future.

Patient Care Management

Recipient Selection and Evaluation

The pretransplant evaluation is a vital step in obtaining a successful outcome to cardiac transplantation (Table 46–9). The goal of the evaluation is twofold: To make the appropriate recommendation for the patient after a comprehensive evaluation, and to educate the individual and his family, equipping them with the necessary information to make the appropriate decision.

The suitability of a potential cardiac recipient is evaluated by an interdisciplinary team made up of cardiothoracic surgeons, cardiologist, transplant medicine physician, pulmonologist, psychiatrist, dentist, heart transplant nursing coordinator, nutritionist, social worker, and financial counselor. Other specialties are consulted as indicated by the patient's condition.

Table 46–9
Evaluation of Recipient for Cardiac Transplantation

TESTS	REASONS FOR TESTS
Immunologic tests	
ABO and HLA typing	To determine the patient's blood group and to identify HLA antigens
Antibody screening	To determine the presence of cytotoxic antibodies and the percentage of reactivity
Medical history	To determine the patient's past and present status. Past medical history is extremely important, especially any history of peptic ulcer disease or symptoms, diverticulitis, lung disease, peripheral or cerebral vascular disease, diabetes, or malignancy. The physical examination of a woman over 35 years of age should include a pelvic examination, cervical Papanicolaou smear, and mammogram.
Physical assessment	It is imperative that the physical make-up of the donor and recipient be similar for height, weight, chest size, and age, in order for the heart to be implanted into the chest of the recipient.
Social and psychologic evaluation	To determine the patient's emotional maturity, motivation, cooperativeness, and ability to learn about medications and to take instructions. To determine any underlying psychopathology, alcohol consumption, smoking history, or chemical abuse, as well as to identify family or other support systems
Financial evaluation	To determine the means by which the patient will be able to purchase medications and pay for his medical care
Laboratory tests	
CBC, platelet count	To assess the hematologic system
Partial thromboplastin time, and prothrombin time studies	To assess clotting mechanisms
Liver function tests	To screen for liver abnormalities, which would delay transplantation until further work was done to pinpoint the cause of the abnormalities (congestion due to fluid overload and acute or chronic hepatitis)
Australian antigen	To screen for Australian antigen positivity, which would not necessarily rule out transplantation, but would identify the patient as a carrier.
Antibody to Australian antigen	To identify prior exposure to Australian antigen
Blood urea nitrogen and serum creatinine	To obtain baseline information
Electrolytes (Na, K$^-$, Cl and CO_2)	To obtain baseline information
Fasting glucose	To screen for unsuspected tendency toward glucose intolerance (some patients develop corticosteroid-induced diabetes after the transplant)
VDRL	To screen for venereal disease
Evaluation for infection	To detect any infections (infections are the leading cause of postoperative complications) and thus prevent doing a transplant in someone who has an active infection
Fungal skin tests	
Viral titers	
Cultures of blood, sputum, nose, skin	
Cardiopulmonary evaluation	
Echocardiogram	To determine function and movement of myocardium
Cardiac catheterization	To determine right heart pressures (pulmonary artery pressures, pulmonary capillary wedge pressure, pulmonary vascular resistance, cardiac index), status of coronary arteries, and ventricular function
Native endomyocardial biopsies	To detect any infectious or inflammatory process
Chest x-ray film	To rule out radiographic lesions, pulmonary infarcts, infectious process
Pulmonary function tests	To obtain baseline pulmonary function status
Renal function studies	
Routine urinalysis	To screen for renal disease or abnormal findings (glycosuria, proteinuria, and abnormal sediment)
Urine culture	To determine the presence or absence of active urinary tract infection
24-Hour urine collection	To assess the level of renal function before surgery
Timed Glofil I^{125} or timed creatinine clearance	To assess the level of renal function or the glomerular filtration rate (GFR)

The selection criteria for the heart transplant recipient are based on both the critical medical need for transplantation and the maximum likelihood of a successful outcome with an improved quality of life. In general, the patient has a poor prognosis as a result of poor cardiac function. Poor cardiovascular functional status denotes a terminal heart disease with an estimated life expectancy of less than 6 months to a year. In addition, the patient is classified as a New York Heart Association Functional Class IV, meaning the patient's condition is refractory to conventional medical and surgical intervention. It must be demonstrated that heart transplantation, when compared with other medical or surgical therapies, will provide the patient a greater chance of survival.

Contraindications

Specific patient selection criteria give consideration to those factors that are recognized as exerting an adverse effect on the outcome of heart transplantation (Table 46–10).

Advanced Age

The maximum age limit for a heart transplant recipient varies from center to center. In many centers, the maximum age limit is 59 years or less. The oldest age reported for a recipient has been 70 years.[27] Coupled with advanced age is the increased risk of postoperative complications. Therefore, care should be taken to ensure a young physiologic age of the older transplant recipient.

Fixed Pulmonary Vascular Resistance

A fixed pulmonary vascular resistance of 6 to 8 Wood units is an absolute contraindication to cardiac transplantation. Pumping against such high resistance, the implanted donor's right ventricle is at risk of failure. Pulmonary vascular resistance is based on right heart pressures. The calculation involves subtracting the pulmonary artery wedge pressure in millimeters of mercury from the pulmonary artery mean pressure in millimeters of mercury, and dividing this by the cardiac output in liters per minute. The resulting quotient represents the pulmonary vascular resistance in Wood units. In cases of a fixed pulmonary vascular resistance, the patient may be considered for a combined heart–lung transplant. Primary pulmonary hypertension is the primary etiology for a heart–lung transplant.[27]

Irreversible Dysfunction of Other Organ Systems

The etiology of any organ dysfunction should be evaluated. Elevated liver profiles are commonly seen before transplantation owing to hepatic congestion related to right heart failure. However, any dysfunction not explained by the underlying heart failure and decreased cardiac index could be a contraindication to transplantation. Hepatic or renal dysfunction would be worsened with the use of immunosuppressive agents such as cyclosporine and azathioprine (Imuran) after transplantation.

Symptomatic or Asymptomatic Peripheral or Cerebral Vascular Disease

With the use of chronic corticosteroid therapy after transplantation, vascular disease could progress more rapidly. Therefore, the evaluation must address the degree to which vascular disease has progressed in the pretransplant patient.

Severe Chronic Obstructive or Bronchitic Pulmonary Disease

Chronic lung disease predisposes the patient to respiratory complications postoperatively. Immunosuppressive therapy could further complicate the transplant course with the development and exacerbation of lung infections.

Acute Infection

An active infection is likely to be exacerbated by the use of immunosuppression after transplant. Therefore, the patient's acceptance for transplantation should be deferred until resolution of the infection has been confirmed.

Recent and Unresolved Pulmonary Infarction

Past studies have shown a higher morbidity rate in transplants with unresolved pulmonary infarctions. Patients may be accepted upon evidence of radiologic resolution of the pulmonary infarct.

Undiagnosed Radiographic Pulmonary Lesion

A vigorous approach to the diagnosis of pulmonary lesions must be made during the pretransplant evaluation. Bronchogenic carcinoma must be excluded.

Insulin-Dependent Diabetes Mellitus With Significant Secondary Complication

Diabetes and its complications are exacerbated by chronic corticosteroid therapy and the use of high doses of corticosteroids in treating rejection.

Table 46–10
Contraindications to Cardiac Transplantation

Absolute contraindications
   Older than 59 years of age
   Fixed pulmonary vascular resistance: greater than 6 Wood units
   Irreversible dysfunction of other organ systems
   Peripheral or cerebral vascular disease (symptomatic
     or asymptomatic)
   Severe chronic obstructive or bronchitic pulmonary disease
   Acute infection
   Recent, unresolved pulmonary infarction
   Undiagnosed radiographic pulmonary lesion
   Insulin-dependent diabetes mellitus with significant
     secondary complications
   Malignancy
   Any other systemic disease that might be exacerbated by
     immunosuppression or might independently limit patient
     survival
   Inability to comply with medical regimen (noncompliance)
Relative contraindications
   Peptic ulcer disease
   Diverticulitis

Malignancy

The transplant recipient has been known to have an increased incidence to lymphoproliferative malignancies.

Other Systemic Disease

Any coexisting disease likely to preclude survival and rehabilitation should be addressed during the pretransplant evaluation. If it is likely to be exacerbated by immunosuppression or independently to limit survival, this would be regarded as a contraindication to transplantation.

Noncompliance

Transplantation requires a life-long commitment and compliance with a medical regimen. Noncompliance results in serious consequences for the transplant outcome. Thus, mental deficiency, mental illness, and substance abuse are contraindications to transplantation.

Peptic ulcer disease and diverticulitis are two conditions of the digestive system that need to be closely evaluated during the pretransplant workup. These are considered *relative contraindications* for cardiac transplantation.

After transplant, peptic ulcer disease can be silent and can potentially cause serious problems, including perforation, failure to assimilate foods and immunosuppressive agents, and postoperative bleeding. For these reasons, each transplant candidate should be evaluated carefully for the history of peptic ulcer disease. An upper endoscopy, upper gastrointestinal studies, or both are often done in those patients with history of ulcer disease. If an ulcer is detected, intensive therapy is begun. Frequently, H-2 antagonists (cimetidine, Tagamet) are used in the treatment of ulcers. H-2 therapy should not be interrupted and should continue throughout the posttransplant period. On resolution of the ulcer, transplantation can occur.

Diverticulitis is another relative contraindication to transplantation. A current or recent history of diverticulitis indicates a potential source of infection likely to be exacerbated by immunosuppressive therapy. Severe unremitting diverticulitis may serve as an absolute contraindication to transplantation. After the transplant, the patient should be evaluated for recurrence of diverticulitis. Antibiotic therapy is frequently begun at the first sign of symptoms.

After the evaluation of the potential cardiac transplant recipient, the interdisciplinary team meets to discuss the patient's candidacy. Based on the team's recommendation for transplantation, the patient and family are approached for their decision. As with any other procedure, no patient should be listed for transplantation unless his or her consent has been obtained.

Donor Workup and Selection

Just as the recipient candidate for cardiac transplantation must be selected carefully, so must the donor be evaluated thoroughly. The status of the donor before transplantation has a direct effect on the condition of the transplanted organ in the recipient after transplant. The goals of donor management are twofold: organ perfusion and organ oxygenation.[36]

Criteria for heart donation include brain death, age (males: newborn to 35 years; females: newborn to 40 years), stable physiologic state, ABO compatibility, and height and weight compatibility with the recipient. Commonly, cadaveric donors have experienced severe brain trauma such as closed head injuries, brain ischemia resulting from subarachnoid hemorrhage or epidural hemorrhage, cerebral vascular accidents, or primary brain tumors.[62]

Contraindications for heart donations include: unstable physiologic state manifested by prolonged cardiac arrest or use of intracardiac drugs, history of heart disease, active infection or presence of transmissible diseases, and extracranial malignancies.[36,62] Exceptions to donor criteria may be taken into consideration based on the urgency of recipient need.

Once brain death ensues, somatic deterioration may result in hypotension, hypoxemia, electrolyte imbalance, hyperglycemia, hypothermia, diabetes insipidus, and coagulopathy.[62] Prolonged hypertension or hypotension, or dependence on high-dose vasopressors (greater than 10 µg/kg/minute of dopamine) accompanied by adequate volume replacement (central venous pressure 5 to 10 mm Hg) reflects an unstable donor heart. Major chest trauma, with or without a normal electrocardiogram or two-dimensional echocardiogram (done to assess myocardial function) would also preclude heart donation.

The potential heart donor must be evaluated carefully for a history of heart disease. A history of chronic uncontrolled hypertension, previous cardiac surgery, or known valvular disease contraindicates heart donation. Coronary arteriography of the donor heart is rarely done pretransplant, because it may result in a transient depression of the donor myocardial function.

Infection in the potential donor has been known to be transmitted to the recipient of the transplanted organ and is therefore a contraindication to donation.[16,62] Because the risk of nosocomial infections increases with the length of hospitalization, caution should be taken in accepting the donor with a history of prolonged hospitalization. The donor with a history of intravenous drug abuse is also at increased risk for infection.

Extracranial malignancies are a contraindication for organ donation because, as with infectious organisms, they may be transmitted from donor to the transplanted recipient.

Donor Surgery

An expeditious and unerring procurement of the donor myocardium is essential to the success of the transplantation procedure. Routinely, a 10-minute topical cooling is done, followed by an endocardial lavage with a cardioplegic solution. The organ is then prepared for transport by placing it in a sterile container and finally in an ice chest. Ischemic time is also crucial to the post-transplant function of the myocardium. Ischemic times of more than 5 hours have yielded higher 30-day mortality rates.[27]

Domino Donor

The heart for cardiac transplantation is more commonly obtained from cadaver donors than from living donors. However, a living heart donor is possible in the case of a "domino" procedure. In the domino procedure, a heart–lung is procured from a cadaver donor and is transplanted into a recipient with pulmonary failure. The heart–lung recipient's myocardium is then transplanted into a heart recipient. Thus, the latter recipient receives his myocardium from a living donor.

Recipient Surgery

Two types of implantation techniques are available in cardiac transplantation, the heterotopic and the orthotopic approach. The orthotopic cardiac transplantation is done more frequently than the heterotopic approach.[27]

Heterotopic transplantation refers to the parallel connection of the donor heart onto the recipient's native heart. Before the anastomoses, the patient is placed on cardiopulmonary bypass. The left atria are anastomosed side to side, the donor superior vena cava end to the side of the recipient superior vena cava, the donor aorta end to the side of the recipient's aorta, and the donor pulmonary artery end to the recipient's pulmonary artery side using an interposition graft.[16] The graft is positioned to the right and slightly anterior to the native myocardium.

Despite the 5-year survival of the heterotopic approach, arguments have been made for its use. Some sense of security is associated with not excising the native myocardium. The "piggy-back" myocardium functions as an assist device for the native myocardium. In turn, some believe the native myocardium also serves as a backup for the graft in case of rejection or complications associated with accelerated atherosclerosis. However, one must consider the wisdom of relying on the backup function of a native myocardium that functioned inadequately before transplant. Until survival of heterotopic transplantation compares more favorably with the orthotopic procedure, its use should be limited to cases with a marginal donor heart and a suitable recipient condition.[16]

The *orthotopic method* is used more commonly in cardiac transplantation. After cardiopulmonary bypass, the native myocardium is excised, except the posterior atrial cuffs. The donor heart is prepared for implantation with a right lateral atriotomy and the removal of the posterior left atrial wall. Anastomosis is accomplished between the recipient's and the donor's right and left atrial cuffs, transected pulmonary arteries and veins, and aortas.[16]

The resulting anatomy differs from normal in that the aorta and pulmonary artery are longer and both atria are enlarged. The ventricles are positioned more posteriorly, and the cardiac position is rotated slightly clockwise. Once the myocardium is sutured in place, de-airing the heart before discontinuation of cardiopulmonary bypass is crucial. Steep Trendelenburg's position, aspiration of the left ventricle, hyperinflation of the lungs, and reduction in the cardiopulmonary bypass flow facilitate the removal of air bubbles. Thus, the likelihood of air embolism to the coronary arteries or to the cerebral circulation is decreased.[16]

Clinical Course

Immediate Postoperative Period

Complications of the post-transplant recipient during the immediate postoperative period include those problems commonly encountered by the patient undergoing open heart surgery. These include potential problems related to cardiac dysfunction, fluid volume overload, coagulopathy, impaired gas exchange, infection, neurologic or sensory deficit, and pain.

Specific to the post-transplant recipient, mortality within the first 30 days is related to cardiac dysfunction, rejection, and infection.[27]

Physiology of the Transplanted Heart

During the first 48 hours after transplant, complications related to cardiac dysfunction are ventricular failure and unstable myocardial conduction.

Ventricular failure can result from increased pulmonary hypertension in the recipient or from using the myocardium from an unstable donor. Therefore, the pretransplant evaluation of the donor and recipient is critical. Postoperative management includes close hemodynamic monitoring with the use of invasive lines. Support includes the use of inotropes and afterload reducing agents, and possibly, intra-aortic balloon pumping. Care must also be taken to reduce myocardial oxygen demands.[43]

Unstable myocardial conduction is also a potential complication postoperatively. Premature atrial or ventricular beats and bradycardia may occur after transplant. Edema from suture lines, the manipulation of the myocardium, or ischemia can result in ectopia. Commonly, lidocaine is infused at 2 mg/minute prophylactically for the first few days postoperatively. Monitoring and maintaining adequate serum potassium levels are also crucial in promoting a stable electrical conduction system. Intravenous potassium boluses should be given for hypokalemia. Decreasing myocardial oxygenation demands, providing adequate oxygenation, and maintaining an appropriate acid–base balance also aid in the management of dysrhythmias postoperatively.[43]

A *junctional rhythm* is common during the post-transplant period. On the electrocardiogram, it is important to note that native P-waves are seen frequently in addition to the electrical activity from the implanted heart. Native P-waves originate from the recipient's right posterior atrial cuff that was left intact during transplantation. However, the remnant P-wave is nonconducting, because the electrical impulse is unable to cross the suture line. During episodes of bradycardia, intravenous atropine is of no value owing to the sympathetic denervation of the implanted myocardial graft. Therefore, atrial and ventricular pacing wires are inserted intraoperatively to provide temporary pacing.[16]

Sympathetic denervation of the transplanted graft causes several changes in myocardial response postoperatively. There is no cardiac rate response evoked with postural changes, frequently resulting in orthostatic hypotension. Cardiac output is enhanced by preload. An increase in heart rate is primarily dependent on circulating catecholamines. Also related to the denervation is the lack of response to vagal maneuvers. In addition, the protective mechanism of angina is lost.[16]

Infection

Infection poses a continual threat of morbidity and mortality after transplantation. In addition to the obvious risk of pulmonary and wound infections postoperatively, the immunosuppressed patient is at greater risk for opportunistic infections. Because the risk of rejection is higher in the immediate postoperative period, the use of immunosuppressive agents is greater. There is a significant risk of infection from surgical incisions, multiple invasive catheters, and procedures. Prevention includes the use of protective isolation until the time of discharge, prophylactic antibiotics, and careful monitoring for infectious processes.

Immunosuppression

Immunosuppression protocols differ among transplant centers. In general, the immunosuppressive agents commonly used are cyclosporine, azathioprine, prednisone, OKT3, or anti-lymphocytic globulin (ALG). The initiation of immuno-suppression can either begin immediately before surgery, in-traoperatively, or during the immediate postoperative period. Intraoperative immunosuppression is begun with 1 g meth-ylprednisolone. Beginning the first postoperative day, induc-tion occurs with ALG for 5 days. In addition, prednisone 100 mg daily is given for 5 days and then tapered to a maintenance dose (0.15 mg/kg of body weight) over a period of 90 days. On the third postoperative day, cyclosporine and azathioprine are initiated. The cyclosporine dose is adjusted to maintain a 12-hour serum trough level of 200 to 700 ng/dl using the radioimmunoassay (RIA). Azathioprine is dosed to a maximum of 200 mg/day, regulated by the white blood count and platelets.

Rejection

Rejection of the implanted myocardium poses a continual threat to the transplant recipient. As with all transplanted organs, humoral and cellular rejection are two types of re-sponse to the implanted graft. During the immediate post-operative period, hyperacute rejection, a humoral response, is of special concern. As discussed earlier, a humoral rejection is an antibody-mediated response in which the recipient has preformed antibodies against the donor. Immediate vascular damage and graft loss ensue. In such cases, a bridge to trans-plantation (use of a heart assist device) is employed until an-other suitable donor heart is located and retransplantation can occur. The risk of hyperacute rejection can be minimized by screening the recipient for cytotoxic antibodies before transplantation. Those with a positive antibody screen should be prospectively crossmatched and transplanted only if there is a negative lymphocyte crossmatch with the donor. ABO incompatibility also precipitates a hyperacute rejection. Therefore, caution must be taken to confirm the donor's ABO blood group type with the recipient before transplantation.

An acute cellular rejection can occur during the first 3 post-operative months and is often difficult to diagnose based purely on clinical signs and symptoms. The patient experiencing re-jection may present with malaise, excessive fatigue, decreased exercise tolerance, weight gain, appearance of S3 or S4 heart sounds, and signs of heart failure (late sign). These signs and symptoms can also be representative of a variety of etiologies, including infection. Currently, cellular rejection can be diag-nosed only by histologic study of endomyocardial tissue spec-imens obtained by biopsy.

Diagnostic Tests

Endomyocardial Biopsy

Endomyocardial biopsy is used to diagnose rejection. The schedule for endomyocardial biopsies varies among transplant centers. In general, biopsies are done weekly during the im-mediate postoperative period. Slowly, the frequency is tapered to biweekly, monthly, every 6 weeks, then every few months. The frequency of biopsies after the first year varies among transplant centers from every 3 months to once a year. In the presence of acute allograft rejection, biopsies may be per-formed more frequently. Thereafter, biopsies are done every 3 months.

The endomyocardial biopsy procedure is performed in the cardiac catheterization laboratory. With the use of a local an-esthetic agent, access is usually gained through the jugular vein or the femoral vein. Four to eight biopsy specimens, 1 to 4 mm in size, are obtained with a biotome from the right ventricular septum. The specimen is preserved in a 10% for-malin solution and processed (paraffin embedding and staining with hematoxylin and eosin).[38]

Classification of Rejection

Cellular rejection is determined by the presence and degree of histologic changes detected by light microscopy. Electron microscopy is not often used in the evaluation of acute cardiac allograft rejection because of the lengthy processing time. However, its use may be beneficial if ultrastructural exami-nation is required.[38]

In an attempt to describe the morphology of the biopsy specimens, several grading systems have been developed. The grading scales are used to describe the degree of histologic changes seen on the biopsy, to indicate the degree of allograft rejection. No one classification of grading cardiac allograft rejection is accepted universally. The differences among grad-ing systems are found in the method of examining the biopsy specimen and the ''classification'' of the findings.

The Billingham criteria is the classification system widely used. This method classifies endomyocardial biopsy findings into four categories: mild rejection; moderate rejection; severe rejection; and resolving or resolved rejection.[10]

The other frequently used classification system is a numerical grading scale, as developed by the Texas Heart Institute. This system was developed to assign numerical objectivity to mi-croscopic findings of allograft rejection. Using this scale, zero represents no evidence of rejection, grades 1 through 3 rep-resent mild rejection, grades 4 through 8 represent moderate rejection, and grades 9 and 10 represent severe rejection. An advantage of the numerical system over the other is that the numerical system is thought to provide a sharper index on which to base a treatment regimen.[38] The correlation of the two methods of classification with the biopsy findings are seen in Figure 46-5.

Treatment of Rejection

Despite the optimal use of immunosuppressive agents, the threat of rejection persists. No change in immunosuppression is warranted for a biopsy indicating no evidence of rejection or a mild-grade rejection. The initiation of additional immu-nosuppression usually begins with a moderate grade of rejec-tion. Therefore, using the numerical grading system, a mod-erate rejection, grade 5 or 6, usually requires treatment. Either higher doses of oral prednisone, or intravenous methylpred-nisolone at 3 mg/kg of body weight, may be given daily for

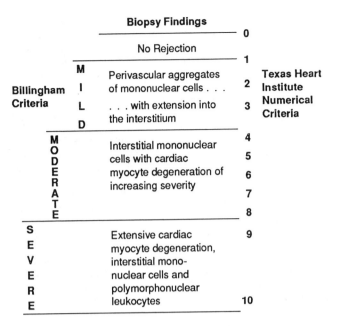

Figure 46-5
Relationship of classification criteria to biopsy findings.

5 days. For rejections of a more severe grade, ALG can be used at 10 to 20 mg/kg of body weight for 10 days.

At the completion of rejection therapy, a repeat endomyocardial biopsy is done to determine the effectiveness of treatment and the need for further treatment. In cases of severe irreversible rejection with compromise of myocardial function, a bridge to transplantation may be necessary until retransplantation can occur.

Although the incidence of rejection decreases after this time, the threat of acute rejection forever remains a threat to the graft and ultimately, to the recipient. The challenge associated with immunosuppression is to find the balance between graft–host coexistence and excessive suppression of host defenses.[39]

Long-Term Complications

In general, long-term complications of cardiac transplantation are similar to those for other organ transplants and result from the use of immunosuppressive agents. Accelerated graft atherosclerosis, also referred to as "chronic rejection" and "rejection-induced coronary artery obstruction" is a potential long-term complication specific to cardiac transplantation.[4,16] Although the etiology is unknown, antiplatelet therapy (acetylsalicylic acid, dipyridamole) is commonly used in many programs. As in the native heart, accelerated graft atherosclerosis can present as a local lesion, but major differences exist between the presentation of atherosclerosis in the native heart and in a grafted myocardium.[16]

In the graft, accelerated atherosclerosis usually presents as a diffuse process involving the entire coronary artery. Concentric narrowing by subendothelial hyperplasia is a common histologic finding. However, there is no calcification. Therefore, the disease process is not amenable to percutaneous transluminal coronary angioplasty. One study has documented reversal of the vasculitis with vigorous treatment for rejection using antithymocyte globulin and bolus methylprednisolone.[16] Retransplantation is often considered the treatment of choice for individuals with diffuse disease involvement.

Evaluation of accelerated graft atherosclerosis is done by coronary angiography and exercise treadmill. Exercise thallium studies are used occasionally to aid in the diagnosis and to determine the extent of involvement. No significant correlations have been found with possible risk factors such as number of rejections, HLA match, dose of immunosuppressive agents, blood lipid levels, and blood pressure.[16] Prevention remains difficult until the etiology is discovered.

CASE STUDY

C.R. is a 53-year-old white male admitted with an acute anterior myocardial infarction. The electrocardiogram showed ST-segment elevation in V2 through V4. The day after his admission, Mr. R. was in cardiogenic shock with a decreased blood pressure and urine output. He was then treated with dopamine, which improved his blood pressure, but not to normal. The next morning, Mr. R. developed complete heart block and was paced with an external pacemaker. During this time, he was also hypotensive and oliguric, but alert. He was urgently taken to the cardiac catheterization laboratory where a temporary internal pacemaker and an intra-aortic balloon pump were placed. The left anterior descending artery was occluded completely and was opened successfully by angioplasty. During the procedure, the patient improved and began spontaneous diuresis. The pacemaker and intra-aortic balloon pump were removed 2 days after insertion. The patient was maintained on warfarin (Coumadin) 5 mg orally every day, which maintained prothrombin times in the therapeutic range. Initially, minimal doses of cardiac medications were needed to maintain a systolic blood pressure about 80 mm Hg. One week after admission, Mr. R. developed severe progressive congestive heart failure. Furosemide (Lasix) 200 mg orally twice a day and metolazone (Zaroxolyn) 2.5 mg orally once a day were eventually needed to stabilize the failure. Potassium supplements of 250 mEq/day were needed to replace the potassium loss resulting from the diuretic regimen.

Two weeks later, a repeat cardiac catheterization was done. The study demonstrated severe coronary artery disease, although the left anterior descending artery remained widely patent. The circumflex and right coronary arteries were completely occluded. Left ventricular function was decreased significantly with 12% ejection fraction. Consequently, the patient was informed of his poor prognosis and cardiac transplantation was discussed.

Initially, Mr. R. refused to discuss cardiac transplantation, but episodes of paroxysmal nocturnal dyspnea and chest pain were all too frequent reminders of his worsening condition. Three days after he was approached with the idea of cardiac transplantation, Mr. R. asked to see the heart transplant coordinator.

The evaluation for cardiac transplantation was initiated (Table 46–9), arranged by the transplant coordinator. Mr. R. remained on the telemetry unit, which made the evaluation by the cardiac transplant team easier. Over the next 10 days, Mr. R. was seen by members of the transplant team. Daily, the transplant coordinator visited Mr. R. and together they discussed transplantation. Mr. R. was given a transplant booklet to serve as a resource. He eagerly read the book and asked questions of what he had read whenever the various members of the team visited.

Findings of the physical examination were unremarkable except for jugular vein distention about 8 cm above the right atrium. His blood pressure was 74/42; his pulse was 58 and regular; he had no fever. Past medical history included myocardial infarctions in 1982, 1984, and 1988. Otherwise, the medical history was unremarkable. Mr. R. did not have any history of organ dysfunction, cerebral or peripheral vascular disease, active infection, pulmonary infarction or undiagnosed lesion, diabetes, malignancy, or digestive problems. Mr. R.'s age was not a contraindication to transplantation.

According to the last right heart catheterization, his pulmonary vascular resistance was 2.4 Wood units, which was within normal limits. The pulmonary function test demonstrated pulmonary function that would allow a good outcome with surgery, despite the mild restrictive element secondary to heart failure. Mr. R. did not have any history of previous surgical procedures.

The social history revealed that Mr. R. was married and had three stepchildren. He and his wife had a stable marital relationship. The psychiatric evaluation revealed Mr. R. did not have any psychiatric disease. His work history was stable and unremarkable. He smoked five cigarettes a day. He did not drink alcohol. Mr. R.'s insurance did approve the cardiac transplant and the post-transplant care, prospectively.

On completion of the pretransplant evaluation, the cardiac transplant team met to discuss Mr. R.'s candidacy. After a short discussion, the team agreed that Mr. R. was a suitable candidate. Mr. R. and his wife were aware of the commitment essential to a successful post-transplant course. They both agreed in favor of a transplant. Thus, Mr. R. was listed with the local organ procurement agency.

Mr. R. remained on the telemetry unit until he once again experienced acute cardiac failure. Three days before his transplant, Mr. R. deteriorated and was moved back to the cardiac care unit (CCU). Being in the acute care setting on dopamine, Mr. R.'s status was changed to a priority with the organ procurement agency. The hypotension, dyspnea, and chest pain, coupled with the move back to the CCU, caused Mr. and Mrs. R. to be frightened. These events reinforced the seriousness of the situation Mr. R. faced. The nursing transplant coordinator continued to attempt to provide Mr. R. and his family with reassurances and support, keeping them informed of the efforts to find a suitable donor. With the support of the dopamine at 10 μg/kg/minute and Lasix 300 mg intravenously twice a day, Mr. R. was brought out of acute failure. Regardless, the implications of ischemic cardiomyopathy never felt so real as it did then.

At 2:30 A.M., the transplant team received the call that a suitable heart donor had been found for Mr. R. The team and nursing staff were excited for him. Mr. R. felt excitement, anticipation, and fear simultaneously. He and his wife understood that another family had made a generous decision in order that he might have a chance with another heart. The CCU nursing staff and transplant coordinator provided Mr. R. and his family reassurance while preparing him for the orthotopic cardiac transplantation.

It was a busy time for both Mr. R. and the nursing staff. Stat laboratory samples had to be drawn, a chest x-ray film was taken, a preoperative surgical scrub, placement of invasive lines, and signing of consent forms were part of the preparation for surgery. Despite the activity in preparation for impending surgery, Mr. R. was aware that the final decision for transplantation would be made on the visual inspection of the myocardium by the surgeon harvesting the organ.

One of the transplant team's cardiothoracic surgeons flew 200 miles north to harvest the donor heart. The donor was a young man in his early twenties who had had a closed head injury. On visual inspection of the heart, the surgeon informed the CCU that the donor heart was strong and the transplant would proceed as planned. Sensing their anxiety, the anesthesiologists and operating room nurse reassured Mr. R. and his family as they prepared to take him to surgery.

Anesthesia induction was uneventful and Mr. R. was prepared for transplantation. During the entire surgical procedure, the transplant coordinator served as a liaison between surgery personnel and the family. At least once an hour, she left surgery to sit with the family and to provide them with information and reassurance.

On arrival of the harvesting surgeon and the donor myocardium, a stat ABO type on the donor serum was done to confirm the compatibility with Mr. R., who had already been placed on cardiopulmonary bypass. The cardiectomy of the native heart was performed as the donor heart was prepared on the back surgical table. After implantation, the ischemic time was noted at 2 hours and 39 minutes,

well under the 4-hour limit. Mr. R. was in surgery approximately 4 hours before he was transferred to the intensive care unit (ICU).

The ICU staff prepared the transplant room and was ready to receive Mr. R. postoperatively. Until the time of his discharge for home, reverse isolation would be observed. Mr. R.'s 4-day ICU course is outlined in Table 46–11.

Postoperatively, Mr. R.'s primary problems related to a decreased hemoglobin and hematocrit, and fluid retention. In total, he received 2 U of fresh frozen plasma and 4 U of packed red blood cells. He was aggressively diuresed with furosemide intravenously at first. Mr. R. was extubated on the first postoperative day. By the third postoperative day, he was sitting in a chair at the bedside. On the fourth postoperative day, Mr. R. was transferred to the telemetry unit.

While on the general nursing unit, Mr. R. and his wife received intensive post-transplant teaching. The transplant coordinator was primarily responsible for their teaching needs, and the nursing staff provided the reinforcement. Consultation with ancillary health care staff were called as resources (*i.e.*, nutritionist).

Mr. R. had his first endomyocardial biopsy on the seventh postoperative day. The biopsy results showed no evidence of rejection. Undergoing the biopsy while in the hospital helped Mr. R. to become familiar with the preparation for a biopsy as an outpatient.

Twelve days postoperatively, Mr. R. was discharged for home. At that time, his hemoglobin was 9.5 and his hematocrit 29.4. His weight was 137.75 lb at discharge. Mr. R.'s discharge instructions included the following:

1. Discharge medications:
   A. Cyclosporine 260 mg orally q12h (no styrofoam cups)
   B. Imuran 125 orally every morning
   C. Prednisone orally every morning
   D. Sulfamethoxazole–trimethoprim (Bactrim Regular Strength) 1 tablet orally every morning
   E. Dipyridamole 75 mg orally three times a day
   F. Clotrimazole (Mycelex) troche 1 tablet after meals and before bed; suck and swallow
   G. Ranitidine (Zantac) 150 mg orally twice a day
   H. Furosemide (Lasix) 80 mg orally three times a day
   I. Potassium chloride (Micro-K Extencaps) 16 mEq orally three times a day
   J. Iberet Folic-500 1 tablet orally every morning
2. Activity restrictions
   A. No heavy lifting
   B. No driving
   C. Avoid activities that "stress" the breastbone.
   D. No returning to work yet
   E. Wear a face mask when returning to the hospital.
3. Dietary restrictions: Low saturated fat, low cholesterol, no added salt diet
4. Return to the cardiac catheterization laboratory for second heart biopsy as scheduled. In preparation for biopsy, have nothing to eat or drink after midnight. May take morning medications, *except* cyclosporine. Take cyclosporine the night before biopsy. Bring all medicines with you.
5. Monitor and record temperature, pulse, blood pressure, and weight at home. Call transplant coordinator for temperature greater than 100°F, blood pressure greater than 150/100, or weight gain 5 lb or more.
6. Bring daily log containing medications, weight, temperature, and so on, to each outpatient visit.
7. Avoid crowds and people with infections.
8. Do not take any over-the-counter medications unless prescribed by transplant team.
9. Call heart transplant coordinator for any problems or questions (Mr. R. was furnished with appropriate phone numbers).

Mr. R. continues to be observed as an outpatient and has done well since receiving the transplant. He has quit smoking. He has mastered

Table 46–11
Immediate Postoperative Course of Cardiac Recipient

	DAY OF SURGERY	POSTOPERATIVE DAY			
		1	2	3	4
Cardiac Drugs					
Lidocaine	2 mg/min	2	2	Weaned off	—
Nitroglycerin					
Dobutamine	10 µg/kg/min	10	5	Off	—
Amrinone	10 µg/kg/min, weaned off	—	—	—	—
Norepinephrine (Levophed)	0.09–0.1 µg/kg/min, weaned off	—	—	—	—
Immunosuppressive Drugs					
Methylprednisolone (Solu-medrol)	100 mg IV q12h, for 3 doses	—	—	—	—
Prednisone	—	100 mg	100 mg	100 mg	100 mg
ALG	—	1100 mg	550 mg	1100 mg	1100 mg
Cyclosporine	—	—	—	—	580 mg
Azathioprine (Imuran)	—	—	—	—	75 mg
Cardiac Assessment					
Cardiac index	1.5–2.5 lpm	2.0–2.5	2.5–3.6	3.0	—
PCWP (wedge)	11–18 mm Hg	15–20	14–18	16–18	—
SVR (dynes/sec/cm^{-5})	1140–1400	900–1200	1000	1200	—
Weight	126 lb	142.1	143.5	146.8	139.5
Intake	5564 ml	5079	2845	2056	—
Output	3288 ml	2205	2990	3360	—
Hemoglobin	7.4	9.2	8.5	8.7	—
Hematocrit	22.6	27.7	26.5	26.1	—

his medications and dosages. Subsequent endomyocardial biopsies have ranged between no rejection to evidence of mild cellular rejection. Mrs. R. continues to be a support to her husband. More importantly, Mr. R. has become a support member to other cardiac transplant candidates awaiting transplantation.

LIVER TRANSPLANTATION
Introduction/History

End-stage liver disease is defined as liver disease that has caused the quality of life to deteriorate to an unacceptable level, with the patient unable to perform his or her usual activities, such as work and caring for the family and home. Liver transplantation has gained wide acceptance as an effective treatment for patients with irreversible progressive liver disease. More than 1000 patients have undergone orthotopic liver transplantation since the introduction of cyclosporine.

Experimental liver transplantation began with heterotopic grafts in the 1950s. This surgical procedure required the placement of an extra liver below the right lobe of the recipient's liver. The difficulty of transplanting an extra liver is primarily technical, because there is limited space in the abdomen for an additional organ as large as the liver.[14]

Another important consideration surrounding the heterotopic method for liver transplantation is that there is metabolic competition between the donor and the recipient liver, which leads to atrophy of the donor liver. In addition, the position of the liver must be such that there is an adequate inflow of blood and that venous drainage is not impaired. An extra liver may also lead to a respiratory tract infection caused by crowding and consequent impaired movement of the diaphragm.[14]

Because of the continued advances and success of orthotopic liver transplantation, it is not likely that further attempts at heterotopic liver transplantation will occur.

Experimental orthotopic liver transplantation was first attempted in the large animal model by teams in Boston and Chicago in 1959 and 1960.[14] The orthotopic procedure involves the removal of the recipient liver before placement of the donor liver in the same cavity. The first orthotopic liver transplant in a human was attempted in 1963 by Dr. Thomas Starzl at Denver, Colorado. These early attempts did not produce survival for longer than 23 days. However, in 1967, a 19-month-old child successfully underwent orthotopic liver transplantation and survived for more than 1 year. Continued attempts at hepatic transplantation ensued and led to a 1-year survival rate of approximately 30% in the late 1970s.[66,67] It was not until after the introduction of cyclosporine in 1980 that a 50% or better success rate was achieved.[65] In addition, through improved recipient and donor surgical techniques, better organ donor preservation, and post-transplant management, 1-year survival rates in the eightieth percentile have been achieved.

The significant improvement in the survival of individuals undergoing liver transplantation led increasing numbers of patients with end-stage liver disease to seek transplantation. However, because the procedure was considered experimental by the Health Care Financing Administration (HCFA), insurance companies were unwilling to cover the cost of hepatic transplantation. In June 1983, the National Institute of Health (NIH) assembled a panel of experts who declared that "liver transplantation is a therapeutic modality for end-stage liver disease. . . ."[46] The result of this report declaring that liver transplantation was no longer experimental led to a greater number of patients being referred for this life-saving procedure, an increase in the number of centers doing hepatic transplantation, and, over time, an increase in the number of third-party payers covering the procedure.

Anatomy and Physiology

The liver is located in the right upper quadrant of the abdomen, just behind the lower rim of the rib cage. It is the largest solid organ in the body and performs more than 500 functions. An understanding of the liver and its functions gives nurses a greater ability to assess and provide both preoperative and postoperative care to the patient with end-stage liver disease leading to transplantation.

Anatomy

The adult liver is a dome-shaped organ that accounts for 1/50 of the body weight and weighs from 3 to 5 lb. In the newborn, the liver is composed of 1/20 of the body weight. This comparative increase in size of the liver in the infant is due to the liver's blood-forming activity during fetal life.[59] The liver is a large, expandable, and compressible organ that can act as a reservoir for blood in times of excess volume and can supply additional blood during times of decreased blood volume such as hemorrhaging.[24]

The liver is composed of four lobes—right, left, caudate, and quadrate. The falciform ligament divides the liver into right and left lobes. The right lobe is the larger lobe; two smaller lobes referred to as the caudate and quadrate lobes come off the posterior surface. The lobes are not confined by any septum and *each lobe has its own vascular and biliary systems with intercommunications among the respective systems.* There is no preferential blood flow to either lobe of the liver and, of the more than 500 functions attributed to the liver, none has ever been associated with any lobe.[59]

The liver has a double blood supply, one from the portal vein and the other from the hepatic artery. The portal vein provides two thirds of the total blood supply to the liver and thus gives this organ its dark red color. The portal vein is formed by the confluence of the splenic, inferior mesenteric, and superior mesenteric veins with drainage from the spleen and intestinal tract. The hepatic artery provides the remaining one third of the blood supply to the liver. The arterial blood supply to the liver is variable, with only a single hepatic artery found in approximately 50% of the patients. Two of the more common arterial anomalies encountered are a right hepatic artery from the superior mesenteric artery or a left hepatic artery from the left gastric artery. In order to nourish the entire liver, small arterial vessels then spread throughout the entire liver.[24]

Venous outflow of the liver is accomplished through the hepatic veins, which exit through the posterior surface of the liver into the inferior vena cava and then to the right atrium. The normal blood volume of the liver is approximately 500 ml, which is 10% of the total blood volume. Twice this amount of blood can be housed in the liver whenever there is high pressure in the right atrium, such as in cardiac failure.[24]

The lymphatic system of the liver has a well-developed network that communicates with the branches of the portal vein and the hepatic artery. There are also deep lymphatic channels that run in the portal tracts. In addition, the biliary tree and hepatic lymph vessels are intimately connected.[59] It is estimated that between one third and one half of all the lymph formed in the body arises in the liver. When hepatic venous pressure rises above normal, excessive amounts of fluid can begin to pass into the lymph as well as leak through the outer surface of the liver. This leakage or "sweating" from the liver capsule goes directly into the abdominal cavity and is clinically seen as ascites.[24]

The biliary system comprises both intra- and extrahepatic bile ducts. Bile is secreted continually by all hepatic cells and is stored in the gallbladder until it is needed in the gut. Daily production of bile is approximately 800 to 1000 ml; 40 to 70 ml is the maximum amount that the gallbladder can store. Bile becomes available to assist in fat digestion through the gallbladder's response to cholecystokinin, the same hormone that causes enzyme secretion by the pancreas. Once bile is produced by the hepatic cells, it drains into small bile canaliculi. The bile then flows into the terminal bile ducts, progressively larger ducts, the hepatic duct, and finally into the common bile duct. From the common bile duct, bile then either flows directly into the duodenum to aid in fat absorption or is diverted to the gallbladder for storage. Bile is composed primarily of bile salts, which help to emulsify fat globules. In addition, bilirubin, cholesterol, lecithin, and electrolytes (Na^+, K^+, Ca^+, Cl^-) are secondary components of bile.[24]

Physiology

The functions of the liver are numerous and complex. Some of the specific roles of the liver include the production of bile; metabolism of carbohydrates, fats, and protein; storage of vitamins and iron; and removal of the end-products of metabolism.[24]

In *carbohydrate metabolism* the liver is involved in maintaining a normal blood glucose concentration. Although most tissues can switch to fats and proteins for energy in the absence of glucose, glucose is the only nutrient that can be used by the brain and retina for their required energy. The liver is the major storehouse and factory of glucose production and is crucial in providing this necessary nutrition.[24]

Another function of the liver is *fat metabolism*. Although this function can occur in almost all cells of the body, certain aspects of fat metabolism occur more rapidly in the liver. The primary role of lipid metabolism is to provide energy for the different metabolic processes, a function it shares with carbohydrates. Some specific functions of the liver in fat metabolism are the formation of lipoproteins and large quantities of cholesterol and phospholipids, conversion of carbohydrates and proteins to fat, and oxidation of fatty acids. Through this process, large amounts of energy are released by the liver for cell function. The function of phospholipids formed by the liver is unknown. Eighty percent of cholesterol formed by the liver is converted to bile salts, and the remainder enters the blood to be transported primarily in the lipoproteins. Cholesterol, phospholipids, and triglycerides may all be absorbed by cells throughout the body to aid in the formation of the cell membrane and other intracellular structures.[24]

Protein metabolism is an even more important liver function than either carbohydrate or fat metabolism. If the function of protein metabolism by the liver ceased, the body could not survive more than a few days. Some of the more important functions of the liver in protein metabolism are the formation of plasma proteins, deamination of amino acids (removal of the amino group from the amino acid), and the formation of urea for removal of ammonia from the body fluids. Before amino acids can be converted into carbohydrate and fats or before they can be used for energy, deamination must occur.[24]

The liver's *formation of urea* is important in the removal of ammonia from the blood. Moderate amounts of ammonia are formed in the gut by bacteria. They are absorbed into the blood, causing the plasma ammonia concentration to rise rapidly and resulting in hepatic coma and death if the ammonia is not removed from the body fluids. Whenever there is a disruption of the flow of portal blood through the liver, toxic amounts of ammonia can accumulate in the blood.[24] This occurs when blood is prevented from being brought from the intestines through the superior and inferior mesenteric veins, into the portal veins, and then through the liver.

More than 85% of all *plasma proteins are formed by hepatic cells,* with the exception of gammaglobulins. The gammaglobulins are formed by the plasma cells in the lymph tissues and are the immune bodies. The liver has the ability to produce plasma proteins rapidly and thus can prevent death from certain disease states. An example of this is a severe burn in which there is a rapid loss of plasma proteins, or severe renal disease in which plasma proteins are lost in the urine each day for long periods of time.[24]

The liver also has the valuable *function of storing vitamins and iron.* Vitamin A is stored in the liver to the greatest extent, but vitamin D and B_{12} are stored as well in large amounts. The storage and release of these vitamins is helpful in preventing disease states related to vitamin deficiency. Iron in the liver is stored in the form of ferritin. When the iron falls low in body fluids, the ferritin releases the iron.[24]

There is an intimate relationship between the liver and the blood coagulation pathways, because of the liver's *formation of fibrinogen, prothrombin, accelerator globulin, and factor VII.* Vitamin K is necessary for the formation of prothrombin and factors VII, IX, and X. Without vitamin K, the synthesis of these clotting factors does not occur, and patients develop bleeding abnormalities. Vitamin K, unlike other fat-soluble vitamins stored in the body in large quantities, is not available through storage. Because of this and the fact that vitamin K is dependent on bile salts for absorption, it takes only several days to develop a vitamin-K deficiency once bile secretion ceases.[24] Intramuscular administration of vitamin K bypasses the need for oral absorption and thus provides this necessary ingredient for the production of blood coagulation factors.

The *removal of bacteria from the blood* is another important function of the liver. The liver does this through phagocytic cells called Kupffer's cells. These cells can remove 99% to 100% of the bacteria from the portal venous blood before it passes through the liver sinusoids. The importance of this filtering system is best understood when one realizes that the portal blood receives its blood from the intestines and regularly contains colon bacilli.[24]

The liver is also involved in *excreting a number of substances formed elsewhere in the body.* One of the most important of these is bilirubin, one of the end-products of hemoglobin decomposition. When the red blood cells have lived out their life span (approximately 120 days), their cell membrane ruptures and hemoglobin is released. The hemoglobin is then phagocytized by the reticuloendothelial cells throughout the body and is split into globin and heme. The heme portion is converted into the bile pigment, bilirubin, which is released into the blood and later secreted by the liver into the bile. Once the bilirubin is in the intestines, it is converted by bacteria into urobilinogen, which is highly soluble. Some of the urobilinogen is returned to the blood by being reabsorbed through the intestinal mucosa. The majority of this is re-excreted by the liver into the gut; a small portion (5%) is excreted by the kidneys into the urine. Through oxidation, the urobilinogen in the urine is converted to urobilin. The urobilinogen in the intestines is oxidized to form stercobilin, the pigment that gives stools their dark brown color. If a total obstruction of bile flow occurs, no bilirubin can reach the intestines to be converted by the bacteria to urobilinogen and then oxidized to stercobilin. As a result, the stools become clay colored.[24]

The liver plays a key role in the *metabolism of drugs and detoxification of a variety of substances.* Injury of the liver from drugs may occur through one or more of three primary mechanisms: a direct toxic effect on the liver, which can occur with acetaminophen, aspirin, and tetracyclines; a hypersensitivity reaction, which can occur with drugs such as Isoniazid, rifampin, and halothane; or interference with normal hepatic uptake, or with secretory or excretory pathways, which can occur with oral contraceptives.[37]

Patient Care Management

Recipient Selection

Many of the candidates for liver transplantation develop multiple organ system failure as a result of their advanced liver disease.[40] For this reason, a thorough preoperative evaluation is essential in order to assess the patient's medical status and the optimal timing for the surgery.

The indications for liver transplantation can be grouped into four categories: advanced chronic liver disease, hepatic malignancies, fulminant hepatic failure, and inborn errors in metabolism. In adults, the most common indications are primary biliary cirrhosis, chronic active hepatitis, and sclerosing cholangitis. Other adult diseases commonly treatable by liver transplantation are metabolic liver diseases.[40] In children, biliary atresia is the most frequent indication. Table 46–12 records the guidelines used to evaluate each prospective candidate presenting with end-stage liver disease.

As shown in Table 46–13, there are few absolute contraindications to liver transplantation. Some of the relative contraindications are similar to those found in other organ trans-

Table 46–12

Medically Acceptable Guidelines for Liver Transplantation

No reasonable alternative treatment for the patient's liver disease
Debilitating pruritis
Severe progressive metabolic bone disease with
  spontaneous fractures
Life-threatening upper gastrointestinal bleeding
Development of hepatorenal syndrome
Recurrent encephalopathy not adequately managed with
  conventional therapy
Fulminant or subfulminant viral hepatitis
Nonresectable, life-threatening benign tumors of the liver
Certain inborn errors of metabolism
Acceptable surgical risk
Primary hepatic malignancy without evidence of metastases
  in certain highly selected patients

Table 46–13

Contraindications to Liver Transplantation

> Absolute contraindications
>   Positive human immunodeficiency virus (HIV)
>   Metastatic malignancy
>   Active sepsis
>   Advanced cardiopulmonary disease
> Relative contraindications
>   Advanced age
>   Multiple previous upper-abdominal surgeries
>   Alcohol or other chemical abuse
>   History of noncompliance with medical regimen
>   Portal vein thrombosis
>   Psychological instability
>   Lack of psychological support

plant criteria. In the past, chronic renal disease would also have been included in this list of contraindications. However, because of the success of combined liver–kidney transplants, it has been deleted from the original listing. In addition, patients with portal vein thrombosis have been transplanted successfully with thrombectomy and reconstruction of the portal vein.[40] Age is evaluated more on an individual basis. Certain individuals over 60 may be considered for transplantation, depending on their vigor and absence of complicating medical problems.

Recipient Evaluation

The recipient evaluation must be thorough in order to identify the indications and contraindications to liver transplantation, as well as to assess accurately the surrounding medical complications that would hasten transplantation. The testing measures the advancement of the excretory, synthetic, and metabolic dysfunction of the liver.[40] Furthermore, it is directed at ruling out extrahepatic spread in the patient with malignant liver disease.

As success with liver transplantation has increased, the management of patients with liver disease has changed.[40] Once an individual has been diagnosed with liver disease, physicians should be cautious in performing any unnecessary surgical procedures. Liver transplantation is technically more difficult in patients presenting with prior abdominal surgery, especially bile duct reconstruction procedures and portosystemic shunts. These prior surgeries can create the development of variceal collaterals in the surgical adhesions, which can increase operative blood loss during transplantation. Furthermore, operating on the bile ducts can also lead to adhesions and scarring that make biliary reconstruction during transplantation extremely difficult.[40] The portosystemic shunt procedures (used in the past to control portal hypertension and recurrent variceal hemorrhaging) should be avoided in patients being considered for transplantation, because the location is extremely close to the liver, making dissection at transplantation potentially dangerous. If possible, the variceal bleeding should be treated instead with sclerotherapy (injecting a sclerosing solution directly into the varix) or a distal splenorenal (Warren) shunt.[40]

Patients with refractory ascites and spontaneous bacterial peritonitis are also managed differently when transplantation is considered an option. Peritoneovenous shunts for refractory ascites are usually contraindicated, because they carry an unacceptable morbidity in these typically ill patients. When as-

cites becomes refractory to medical management, respiratory distress and cardiovascular compromise often occur. Although paracentesis initially improves the patient's condition, additional removal of the ascitic fluid often causes hypotension, renal dysfunction, and significant protein loss. To achieve improvement, infusion of large doses of salt-poor albumin and diuretics should be given daily until transplantation. Recurrent spontaneous bacterial peritonitis should be treated with broad-spectrum antibiotics with selective therapy once the culture and sensitivity are available. Four to 5 days of such treatment is sufficient for transplantation to proceed and should be continued postoperatively.[40]

Donor Selection and Evaluation

Just as organ transplantation has gone through an evolutionary process, so has organ removal. In the initial days of organ harvesting, the Eurocollins solution was used primarily for organ preservation in livers. Most transplant teams sought to transplant the organ within 6 hours from cross-clamping to revascularization.[7] In 1988, a new preservation solution was developed at the University of Wisconsin (UW), which has further advanced the evolutionary process of organ removal. The most significant contribution of the UW solution has been its increase in the maximum storage time from 6 up to 24 hours and the improved liver function seen after transplantation.[64]

Cadaver Donor

Potential donors for liver transplantation are patients who have been declared brain dead or "heart-beating cadavers" who are sustained with mechanical ventilation. Basic guidelines for liver donor acceptability usually list an age limit from newborn to 60 years of age, ABO and size compatibility with the recipient, a stable physiologic state, a negative history for malignancy (except for primary CNS tumors), and a negative HIV status. However, the criteria vary from center to center. For example, exceptions to the upper age limit may be dictated according to the medical urgency of the recipient and the donor's history and physical examination.

In addition, a careful history is paramount in ascertaining previous intrinsic liver disease; history of intravenous drug or alcohol abuse; a history of transmissible diseases; and a history of major abdominal trauma. Testing of the potential liver donor should reflect the absence of an active systemic infection and acceptable liver function tests. The presence of any of the above would be considered contraindications; however, exceptions to donor criteria are based on the medical urgency of the recipient.

Living Donor

The most recent advancement in the surgical procedure of pediatric hepatic transplantation has been the use of a living related donor (LRD) as opposed to a cadaveric one. The left lobe of the liver is removed from the living donor and is transplanted into the child, replacing the child's diseased liver.

The first reported case occurred in 1988 in São Paulo, Brazil. The donor was the mother of a 4½-year-old with biliary atresia. The mother recovered and was discharged without complications. The recipient died 6 days after transplantation.[53]

Since this time, other reported cases of LRD liver transplants have been reported. The use of LRDs for liver transplantation has once again brought forth moral and ethical considerations. Those who support providing LRD liver transplantation are concerned because 30% of all pediatric patients on the waiting list die before a cadaveric organ ever becomes available (this figure is lower for adults because of the greater availability of adult donors). Those who oppose the procedure feel that it places a significant risk on the donor by exposing an otherwise healthy individual to a major surgical procedure; they believe that a LRD should not be considered except as an option of last resort.

The wait for a suitable donor can be long, especially for the pediatric patient. Once a suitable donor is located, a surgeon from the transplanting center usually retrieves the organ while a second team is preparing the recipient for surgery and the initial dissection. Correct harvesting of the organ is essential and crucial to providing the recipient with a viable liver. For this reason, few exceptions are made allowing anyone other than transplanting surgeons to retrieve the organ.

Recipient Surgery

Hepatic transplantation is a long and complex procedure, taking an average of 6 to 8 hours. With complications, the procedure can run much longer. The surgery begins with a bilateral subcostal incision with an upper midline extension. The xiphoid process is usually excised to allow easier access to the suprahepatic vena cava. The recipient hepatectomy can be tedious and difficult if the patient has coagulation disturbances or severe portal hypertension. Variceal collaterals developing in surgical adhesions (from a previous surgical procedure) can also complicate the initial dissection.[68]

The anhepatic phase of liver transplantation is when the native liver is removed and the inferior vena cava and portal vein are occluded. In order to maintain physiologic stability during this time, a nonheparinized veno–venous bypass system is used. This bypass system involves inserting catheters into the portal vein, femoral vein, and axillary vein. The pump then returns venous blood from the lower part of the body (through the portal vein and femoral catheters) back to the heart through the axillary vein. Physiologic stability is maintained while high pressure in the venous collaterals is prevented and the intestinal tract and kidneys remain uncongested (Fig. 46–6).

The numerous vascular connections that must be completed in order to reestablish blood flow to the liver play a part in making hepatic transplantation the most difficult of all transplant procedures. The four vascular connections (in order of surgical reconstruction) are the suprahepatic vena cava, infrahepatic vena cava, portal vein, and hepatic artery (Fig. 46–7). Before completing the infrahepatic vena caval anastomosis, the donor liver must be flushed with a cold flush solution to remove the potassium-rich preservation solution from the liver as well as to ensure that any retained air bubbles are removed. The removal of the potassium and air bubbles is crucial because both could lead to a reperfusion syndrome and cardiac arrest.[68]

The last phase of hepatic transplantation is biliary reconstruction. It is most commonly carried out through an end-to-end anastomosis of the donor and recipient common bile duct referred to as a *choledochocholedochostomy*. If, however, the recipient has either diseased bile ducts (sclerosing cholangitis) or absent bile ducts (biliary atresia), another technique referred to as *choledochojejunostomy* is required. The technique involves anastomosing the recipient common bile duct to a *Roux-en-Y* loop of the intestine. Figures 46–8 and 46–9 illustrate the differences between these two procedures. Removal of the donor gallbladder and placement of Jackson-Pratt drains under each diaphragm and near the site of biliary reconstruction are undertaken before completing the recipient operation.[68]

Clinical Manifestations

Physiology of the Transplanted Liver

After transplantation, it is common to see a mild to severe elevation of the transaminases (SGOT, SGPT), which is sec-

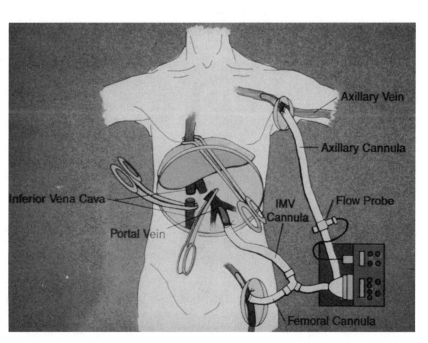

Figure 46-6

Veno-venous bypass required for performing liver transplantation. Used with permission from Baylor University Medical Center, Department of Surgery, Transplantation Services, Dallas, TX.)

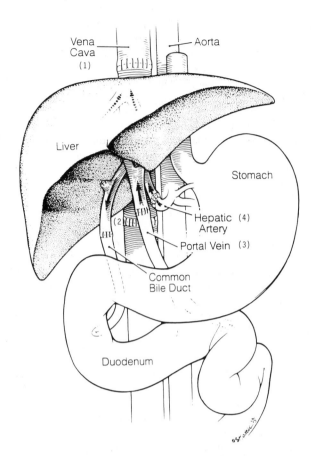

Figure 46–7

The four vascular connections required in liver transplantation. (Used with permission from Baylor University Medical Center, Department of Surgery, Transplantation Services, Dallas, TX.)

ondary to normal preservation injury. This injury should begin to heal within 1 to 2 days, reflected by decreased transaminases and improved synthetic function (protime). The synthetic function is considered to be the best indication of graft function in the early postoperative period. The transaminases primarily reflect hepatic cell damage. If there is not a steady improvement in graft function, as suggested by decreasing transaminases and improving protime, other etiologies must be considered, such as primary graft nonfunction (PGNF), technical complications, and rejection.

Postoperative Complications

Primary graft nonfunction is poorly understood. In almost all instances, it leads to total hepatic failure and the need for retransplantation. The clinical picture consists of progressively increasing transaminases, prolonged protime that cannot be corrected with fresh frozen plasma (FFP), deepening hepatic coma, and hepatorenal syndrome.

Technical problems leading to graft dysfunction can occur as a result of either vascular or biliary complications. The most common vascular complications are anastomotic leaks and thrombosis. Doppler ultrasound is used routinely on the first postoperative day to detect early hepatic artery and portal vein thrombosis. If it is suspected, the recipient should also undergo immediate angiography in order to diagnose the thrombosis definitively. If diagnosed early, surgical reconstruction of the vascular connection can correct the complication and potentially save the graft. If the thrombosis is not

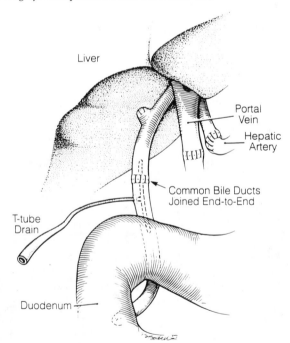

Figure 46–8

End-to-end anastamosis of the bile duct. (Used with permission from Baylor University Medical Center, Department of Surgery, Transplantation Services, Dallas, TX.)

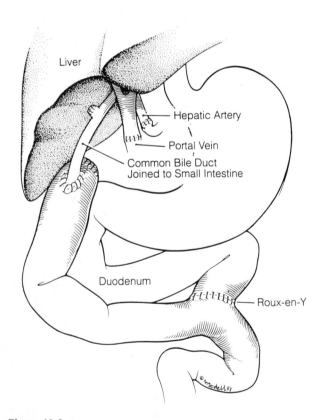

Figure 46–9

Roux-en-Y anastamosis for bile drainage. (Used with permission from Baylor University Medical Center, Department of Surgery, Transplantation Services, Dallas, TX.)

detected early, necrosis of all or a large portion of the liver can occur. The necrosis can lead to an abscess of the graft for which retransplantation would be required. Portal vein thrombosis manifests itself in much the same way as a hepatic artery thrombosis, but it is much less common. If detected early, it too can be treated with surgical intervention to prevent graft loss and the need for retransplantation.

Biliary leaks can occur anytime after transplantation and are suspected when there is an increased bilirubin in the face of normal transaminases. The leaks are primarily anastomotic and require surgical repair. A cholangiogram and HIDA scan are diagnostic tools used to confirm the diagnosis of a biliary leak.

Biliary strictures and obstruction present with increasing bilirubin associated with an increased alkaline phosphatase and gammaglutamyl transferase (GGT). As with biliary leaks, cholangiogram HIDA scan are used to confirm the diagnosis. In these early biliary complications, operative repair is the procedure of choice. Some degree of renal dysfunction after liver transplantation is not uncommon. Clinically, this is manifested by a rising blood-urea-nitrogen (BUN) and creatinine, and a decreasing urinary output. Recipients who experience renal dysfunction preoperatively may experience an exacerbation of their renal dysfunction postoperatively. When the new liver functions properly, persistent postoperative renal failure is uncommon. Administration of nephrotoxic drugs such as cyclosporine and antibiotics must be carefully monitored.[80]

Infection

One of the most serious complications after hepatic transplantation is infection. Most infections present themselves during the first month after transplantation owing to the higher doses of immunosuppression used at this time. However, the second and third months are also considered a high-risk period.

Cytomegalavirus is a common opportunistic viral infection seen after liver transplantation. It can be asymptomatic, with laboratory isolation of the virus only, or it can be a systematic disease. The organs usually affected by the virus are the lungs (CMV pneumonitis), liver (CMV hepatitis), and colon (CMV enteritis).[40] It has also been reported to cause CMV retinitis. A more severe clinical course is usually seen with a primary infection rather than a reactivation infection. Routine cultures and serology are important in diagnosing the presence of CMV, because the clinical symptoms (fever, malaise, and arthralgias) are not always present. There may also be an elevation of the transaminases, diffuse interstitial pulmonary infiltration, abdominal pain, nausea, vomiting, GI hemorrhage, and diarrhea. Each of these symptoms is dependent on which systemic area is affected.[40,58]

There are many reasons why patients with liver disease are predisposed to bacterial infections after transplantation. Patients with cirrhosis frequently experience septicemia, spontaneous bacterial peritonitis, and pneumonia. As a result, treatment with broad-spectrum antibiotics for these complications can increase the risk of ''selecting out'' resistant organisms. Malnutrition, which can compromise host defenses, is also seen frequently in patients with chronic liver disease and can predispose these patients to postoperative infections. Manipulation of the gastrointestinal tract during surgery can

also predispose the recipient to postoperative infections by causing leakage of bacteria from the gut to the tissues and circulation. Additionally, although there is no information on the function of Kupffer's cells in the early post-transplant period, it is considered likely that they are impaired in killing bacteria. Patients with the diagnosis of primary biliary cirrhosis (PBC) or chronic active hepatitis may have compromised their host defenses against infection by taking immunosuppressive medications (azathioprine or corticosteroids) pretransplantation in order to treat their diseases.[14]

Lactulose is given frequently to patients who have experienced hepatic encephalopathy as a result of their chronic liver disease. Because this can affect the gut flora and may result in fungal overgrowth, prophylactic low-dose amphotericin or other antifungal medications are frequently used in the early post-transplant period.[14] This has helped to reduce the incidence of fungal infections postoperatively.

Rejection

Recognition by the recipient of foreign antigens on the cells of the donor organ is what leads to rejection. Both humoral and cell-mediated rejections can occur after liver transplantation and are a common cause of hepatic dysfunction.

In the early post-transplant period, *hyperacute rejection* can, but rarely does, occur in the liver allograft. Hyperacute rejection is humoral mediated, which means that the recipient has preformed cytotoxic antibodies that react with the donor's antigens. The recipient exhibits a clinical picture of total hepatic failure: uncorrectable coagulopathy, depressed mental status, abnormal liver function, hypothermia, thin watery bile, and hypoglycemia. The occurrence of hyperacute rejection occurs minutes to hours after the transplant procedure; these patients require immediate retransplantation.[64]

Subacute rejection is cell mediated and occurs 2 to 4 days after transplantation. The clinical picture is represented by fever, altered liver function, rapidly developing jaundice, change in bile drainage from a golden brown color to a thin colorless fluid, dark tea-colored urine, clay-colored stools, and right upper quadrant pain (Table 46–14). A definitive diagnosis is made through a liver biopsy in order to confirm the histopathology. The confirmation of the diagnosis of rejection is crucial, because the presenting clinical picture can resemble an infection, the treatment of which is a *decrease* in immunosuppression; in contrast, the *treatment for rejection* is an *increase* in immunosuppression.

Acute rejection occurs in more than half of all liver transplant allografts. It is usually seen 7 to 10 days after transplantation but may occur at any time. Acute rejection is also cell mediated. The diagnosis of acute rejection is confirmed by the histologic alterations in the liver biopsy such as activated lymphocytes invading the portal tracts, bile ductule damage, and the presence of eosinophils.[80] In addition, altered liver function, fever, jaundice, change in bile drainage from a golden-brown to a thin colorless fluid, dark tea-colored urine, and clay-colored stools occur frequently.

Chronic rejection occurs months to years after transplantation and is seen in a much lower incidence than acute rejection. It is manifested initially by a significant increase in the alkaline phosphatase and GGT. This increase is normally followed by increased transaminase (SGOT, SGPT) activity and a later progressive increase in the bilirubin. A liver biopsy reflects

Table 46–14
Signs and Symptoms of Liver Rejection

Primary signs and symptoms
    Fever
    Increased liver function tests (LFTs)
    Jaundice (eyes, skin)
    Dark, tea-colored urine
    Clay-colored stools
    Right upper quadrant pain
    Malaise
Additional early postoperative signs while T-tube is connected to external drainage
    Decrease in or cessation of drainage
    Change in bile color from a golden-brown color to a thin colorless fluid
Confirmation by liver biopsy
    Acute rejection: activated lymphocytes invading the portal tracts, bile ductule damage, and the
        presence of eosinophils
    Chronic rejection: portal expansion without lymphocytic infiltrates and disappearing bile ductules
        leading to thickened arterioles. Late stages reflect expanded portal tracts, bridging fibrosis, and a
        prominent mononuclear infiltrate.

portal expansion without lymphocytic infiltrates and disappearing bile ductules. Eventually, thickened arterioles, described as "onion-skinned" in appearance, are seen on biopsy. In the very late stages of chronic rejection, histologic changes may be reflected by large expanded portal tracts, bridging fibrosis, and a prominent mononuclear infiltrate. Early on, patients are relatively asymptomatic but ultimately develop progressive jaundice as well as malaise.[33]

Immunosuppression

The most commonly used immunosuppressive medication after liver transplantation is cyclosporine; however, cyclosporine alone is not effective in preventing rejection. Corticosteroids are also used in conjunction with cyclosporine for maintenance immunosuppression. Azathioprine is usually reserved either for patients who have renal dysfunction or for those who have had an acute rejection episode. Azathioprine in conjunction with cyclosporine and corticosteroids in the patient with renal dysfunction allows less cyclosporine to be used, thereby lessening the nephrotoxic effect. Azathioprine's addition after a rejection episode is beneficial in providing additional immunosuppression.

Rejection Therapy

Treatment for rejection commonly consists of using corticosteroid pulse therapy followed by a corticosteroid recycle over approximately 6 days. Improvement is usually seen in 2 to 5 days; however, if persistent rejection is reflected on the liver biopsy, consideration is given to the administration of the monoclonal antibody (OKT-3) or the polyclonal antibody (antilymphocyte globulin, ALG). The selection of one of these medications (see Table 46–4) as rescue therapy varies from center to center. If rejection persists after the completion of rescue therapy, retransplantation is necessary.

Routine Monitoring

While the patient is hospitalized, daily monitoring of the hepatic function consists of an SMA-20, complete blood count (CBC) with differential, prothrombin time (PT), partial thromboplastin time (PTT), and cyclosporine trough level. There are presently two main types of assays for cyclosporine monitoring. One measures the parent compound only, and the other measures the parent compound and the metabolites of cyclosporine. It is felt that the parent compound has the major immunosuppressive effect and that the metabolites primarily are nephrotoxic and hepatotoxic. The choice of the monitoring technique varies from center to center and will most likely change as new assays develop.

Weekly viral serology and cultures, as well as bacterial cultures of bile, urine, and throat, are carried out. In addition, it is important to monitor the amylase, ammonia, and magnesium levels. Any alterations must be evaluated so that the appropriate therapy can be initiated. Alterations in liver function tests can be related not only to rejection, but to a myriad of complications commonly seen after liver transplantation, such as infection, vascular occlusion, drug-induced hepatotoxicity, and biliary complications. Diagnostic tests commonly associated with evaluating and ruling out the cause of hepatic dysfunction are: liver biopsy, Doppler ultrasound, HIDA scan, cholangiograms (percutaneous, T-tube, or endoscopic), angiography, computed tomographic (CT) or magnetic resonance imaging (MRI) scans, colonoscopy, bronchoscopy, and hepatitis and viral serology screening.

Continuing Care

After discharge from the hospital, patients are commonly seen twice each week for 1 month and then once each week for the next month. A SMA-20, CBC with differential, PT, PTT, and cyclosporine level are drawn with each visit. Alterations in liver function tests usually require readmission to the hospital in order to rule out rejection or other complications.

Careful monitoring and aggressive workups of complications are essential for patient survival. Furthermore, patients are instructed thoroughly before discharge on the signs of liver rejection (Table 46–14): fever, jaundice, clay-colored stools, dark tea-colored urine, malaise, and right upper quadrant pain. Because complications can occur anytime after transplantation, close follow-up and communication are maintained once the patient is referred back to the referring physician.

Long-Term Complications

Long-term complications specific to liver transplantation include recurrent disease, rejection (acute or chronic), biliary complications, occlusion or strictures of the hepatic artery and portal vein, and late infections.

Recurrence of liver disease after transplantation is seen frequently in hepatocellular (except fibrolamellar variant) and duct-cell carcinomas. It is also reported in epithelioid hemangioendotheliomas. Recent advances in this area have centered on immunomodulation and chemotherapy, but it is still too early to report what the long-term benefits to survival will be.[64]

Recurrence of disease is seen frequently in patients who receive transplants because of hepatitis B. With rare exceptions, the new graft becomes reinfected by the virus. Both hyperimmune globulin and alpha interferon have not been successful in preventing reinfection, but they may be helpful in decreasing the severity of the recurrence. Because hepatitis B cannot reliably be prevented from recurring, there is still controversy about the efficacy of transplanting this particular patient population.[42] However, because many patients have benefited, transplantation should continue to be offered.

Other liver diseases in which recurrence has been suspected, but not necessarily confirmed, are primary biliary cirrhosis and sclerosing cholangitis. Another liver disease, Budd-Chiari, may recur if the underlying etiology is not treated or if anticoagulation is not continued. If the etiology is associated with a myeloproliferative disorder, hydroxyurea and aspirin have been used with success. Otherwise, patients with Budd-Chiari syndrome need to be maintained on anticoagulation in order to prevent rethrombosis.

Late bile duct complications may be due to either intrahepatic or extrahepatic strictures. These strictures are often ischemic in nature, because the bile ducts are dependent on the hepatic artery for their blood supply. The extrahepatic strictures can also occur at the anastomotic site, between the native and the recipient bile ducts. Percutaneous dilatation may be used for either type of stricture with a high rate of success. In addition, recent advances have introduced and shown success with a permanent type of flexible metal stint for difficult strictures. Extrahepatic strictures that fail dilatation require surgical intervention. If the initial reconstruction was a duct-to-duct procedure, then biliary drainage should be converted to a *choledochojejunostomy*. If the stricture is at the *choledochojejunostomy*, then this anastomosis should be redone.

Vascular complications in the late period after transplantation are associated with anastomotic strictures or thrombosis of the hepatic artery. The thrombosis is usually of unknown etiology. Confirmation of the stricture is accomplished through a Doppler ultrasound and angiography. Treatment is through percutaneous dilatation of the stricture or an operative reconstruction. Once the stricture becomes totally stenotic, retransplantation is usually necessary.

Late infections that occur are usually community-acquired pneumonias or urinary tract infections and are secondary to the usual bacterial organisms. During the influenza season, these patients are more susceptible to developing viral infections with a concurrent bacterial infection. Because of their immunosuppressive state, these patients (as well as recipients of other types of transplanted organs) are susceptible to a variety of infections and frequently present with atypical symptoms. Therefore, these patients always require thorough evaluation through cultures, viral studies, and broad-spectrum antibiotic coverage while awaiting the results of the cultures.

CASE STUDY

B.A. is a 50-year-old female with a 6-year history of liver disease diagnosed as primary biliary cirrhosis with a positive antimitochondrial antibody (AMA) at 1:2560 (normal = <1:20) and a liver biopsy reflecting macronodular cirrhosis consistent with end-stage primary biliary cirrhosis.

B.A.'s initial evaluation for liver transplantation was 2 years prior, and it was determined that she was an acceptable candidate for transplantation, but that it was too early. She was sent back to her referring physician for close monitoring in order to detect worsening laboratory studies or clinical symptoms. B.A. returns with a definite progression of her disease with mild encephalopathy, worsening prothrombin time, and fatigue.

Laboratory evaluation showed prolonged protime at 13 seconds (normal = 11.5), a bilirubin of 11.3 (normal = 0.5–1.2), and transaminases (SGOT, SGPT) in the low 200s (normal = 5–40). B.A.'s renal function was excellent with a BUN of 8, a creatinine of 0.6, and a glofil of 108 m/min. Pap smear and mammogram were both negative. The MRI revealed a patent portal vein and normal-sized liver with an estimated volume of 2128 ml. Serologic studies were negative for hepatitis B or A. B.A.'s psychosocial workup revealed no abnormalities and excellent family support.

Clinically, she had marked scleral icterus. She has had no problems with bleeding and showed no clinical ascites or asterixis. She has had a 4-lb weight loss over the past 2 years and now presents as a thin female at 116 pounds.

B.A. was presented and accepted by the liver selection committee. She was placed on the waiting list through the local organ procurement organization (O.P.O.) under blood group A. Her weight, chest circumference, and liver volume were all evaluated in order to establish weight parameters for a donor of suitable size. After only 3 weeks, a donor was located for B.A. approximately 400 miles away. The donor was a 12-year-old male who had a closed head injury from a motor vehicle accident.

The orthotopic liver transplant was an uneventful, 7-hour procedure. A standard duct-to-duct (choledochocholedochostomy) was performed, and the intraoperative cholangiogram revealed no evidence of leaks. She had an estimated blood loss of 200 ml and received 2 U of packed red cells and 1 U of fresh frozen plasma.

Only a few hours postoperatively, B.A. had a blood pressure of 131/66, pulse 60 and regular, and a pulmonary artery pressure of 24/11. She was on the ventilator and beginning to initiate her own respiration. Her lungs were clear to auscultation. Her abdomen was soft with no bowel sounds. The dressings were dry and intact. The Jackson-Pratt drains revealed serosanguineous fluid in minimal quantities. Bile was appearing in her T-tube bag and was dark in color. Her initial SGOT was 683, the SGPT was 476, and her bilirubin was 6.7.

On B.A.'s second postoperative day, she was extubated. A Doppler ultrasound revealed patent vasculature and a resistive index of 60% (normal 60% to 80%). An increase in the resistive index is indicative of vascular swelling or edema. Laboratory studies revealed an SGOT of 880, SGPT of 835, and a bilirubin of 5.8.

B.A.'s immunosuppression consisted of preoperative cyclosporine (10 mg/kg) orally, azathioprine (Imuran) 2 mg/kg orally, and prednisolone 50 mg orally. Intraoperatively she received 1 g of Solu-cortef before revascularization. Postoperatively, B.A. received cyclosporine 1 mg/kg intravenously every 12 hours, Imuran 2 mg/kg intravenously, and prednisolone tapered from 200 mg to 20 mg over 6 days. The cyclosporine dose was adjusted to maintain a monoclonal 12-hour trough level between 250 and 400 ng/ml.

B.A.'s postoperative course was essentially smooth. She had a liver biopsy on postoperative day 7 that revealed moderate nonspecific portal infiltrates. This was initiated because of a rise in her total bilirubin to 5.3. Her transaminases were stable and declining. She received 1 mg Solu-cortef intravenously. Subsequently, her bilirubin responded in a downward trend and her transaminases also continued to decrease. On postoperative day 12, she had another follow-up liver biopsy that showed early rejection. Because her liver function tests were continuing to reflect a downward trend, only 1 g of intravenous pulse Solu-cortef was given. A liver biopsy was repeated 2 days later and was normal. B.A. was discharged on her 14th postoperative day with a bilirubin of 2.8, SGOT of 39, and SGPT of 105. Her white blood cell count was 20.8. Her discharge medications were as follows:

Cyclosporine 250 mg orally twice a day
Imuran 50 mg daily
Prednisolone 10 mg twice a day
Bactrim DS one daily for prophylaxis against *Pneumocystis carinii*
Riopan 30 ml four times a day qid
Nystatin 5 ml mouthwash four times a day
Nystatin vaginal suppository every day

B.A. underwent thorough discharge teaching by the transplant coordinator regarding her immunosuppression, medications and their side effects, wound care, signs and symptoms of rejection and infection, and general health care guidelines. She was given an appointment to return to the outpatient clinic twice a week for outpatient monitoring.

Two weeks after discharge from the hospital, B.A.'s liver function tests increased. Her bilirubin was now 4.0, and her SGOT had doubled to a value of 87. Her SGPT also doubled to 220. B.A. was readmitted to the hospital, and a liver biopsy revealed rejection. She was given 1 g of Solu-medrol intravenously and corticosteroid recycle tapered to her maintenance dose of 20 mg/day of prednisolone. Six days later, a repeat biopsy was done and revealed persistent rejection. B.A. was then started on OKT-3 5 mg intravenous push daily. After a 12-day course, her bilirubin was 1.1, SGOT was 72, and her SGPT was 217. B.A. was rebiopsied and showed no rejection; however, a culture obtained from the biopsy specimen was positive for cytomegalovirus (CMV).

Clinically, B.A. was afebrile and had no subjective complaints of malaise or arthralgia. However, because of the positive culture for CMV, she was begun on an antiviral medication, Gangcyclovir 5 mg/kg twice a day for 10 days. B.A. was once again discharged after she had completed her course for the CMV infection without any subjective complaints. Her bilirubin was 1.0, SGOT 50, SGPT 135, and WBC 7.1.

Two months after her transplant, B.A. underwent a glofil clearance test to monitor her kidney function. She had had the test before undergoing transplantation to obtain a baseline measurement of her renal function. Her preoperative glofil clearance was 103 ml/minute compared with the present one of 39 ml/minute. This represented approximately a 62% decrease in renal function in 8 weeks. Also on the eighth week after transplantation, B.A.'s T-tube was removed. One week before its removal, her corticosteroid dose was decreased to 15 mg/day in order to lessen the possibility of a bile leak occurring once the tube was removed (corticosteroids decrease wound healing). B.A.'s nystatin and antacids were discontinued once her corticosteroid dose was reduced to 15 mg, because it was believed that she was less susceptible to fungal infections and gastric ulcers once she was on the decreased dose of corticosteroids.

On the 12th week after transplantation, B.A. was discharged to her referring physician with a bilirubin of 0.8, SGOT 75, SGPT 74, WBC of 9.1, BUN 15, and creatinine of 1.5. Her discharge medications were cyclosporine 120 mg twice a day, Imuran 50 mg daily, prednisolone 15 mg, and Bactrim DS, 1 tablet daily.

Six months after her transplant date, B.A. is seeing her physician once every third week. Her laboratory work consists of an SMA-20, CBC with differential, PT, PTT, and cyclosporine level. According to the immunosuppressive protocol, her prednisolone is decreased to 12.5 mg/day. Her cyclosporine dose is 110 mg twice a day and is adjusted according to the center's specific immunosuppressive protocol.

NURSING DIAGNOSES, PATIENT OUTCOMES, AND PLAN

The preceding material on anatomy, physiology, nursing assessment, and diagnostic tests guides the nurse in establishing nursing diagnoses, patient outcomes, and plans for the patient with organ transplantation and specifically for renal, cardiac, and liver transplantation.

NURSING CARE PLAN SUMMARY *Patient With Organ Transplantation*

NURSING DIAGNOSIS

1. Anticipatory anxiety related to hospitalization and upcoming surgery (feeling pattern)

Patient Outcomes	Nursing Orders

1. The patient's anxiety will lessen as daily routines of the unit and the procedures involving transplantation become familiar.	1. Assess the patient's knowledge of organ transplantation and reinforce the physician's explanation to the patient of the procedure and its risks, benefits, and possible outcomes. The nurse should remember that much of the patient's information and understanding of transplantation may have come from rumor.
	   A. Explain the policy for visitors and any exceptions that might be made if indicated.
	   B. Explain the isolation procedures (if any) that will be followed after transplantation. Include the reason for isolation and the expected length of time it will be observed. Assure the patient that he or she will not be completely alone.

(continued)

NURSING CARE PLAN SUMMARY   *Patient With Organ Transplantation*   *Continued*

Patient Outcomes	Nursing Orders

	C. Discuss the importance of accurate daily weight and the accurate recording of intake and output and other routine functions.
	D. Involve the patient in the daily care.
	E. Discuss the baseline tests that will be obtained as ordered by the physician: blood work, chest x-ray film, electrocardiogram (ECG).
	F. Discuss the importance of daily blood work.
	  (1) Complete blood count (CBC): The white blood cell count is extremely important in determining the daily azathioprine dose.
	  (2) Electrolytes: To monitor the serum potassium level and treat any abnormal levels
	  (3) Creatinine and blood-urea-nitrogen (BUN): To assess renal function
	  (4) Cardiac enzymes: To assess cardiac function
	  (5) Liver function tests: To assess liver function
	  (6) Fasting blood sugar, urine and serum amylase: To assess pancreatic function

2. The patient will be physically and emotionally prepared for surgery.	2. Explain the surgical experience to the patient.
	A. Preoperative procedures
	  (1) Use of intermittent positive-pressure breathing machine or incentive spirometer
	  (2) Special dietary instructions before surgery; for example, liquid meals the day before surgery to minimize bulk content
	  (3) Enemas, if indicated, to prevent bowel complications postoperatively
	  (4) Betadine scrub showers to decrease the number of endogenous bacteria
	  (5) The use of preoperative medications
	  (6) For patients with renal insufficiency, the need for hemodialysis before surgery to ensure proper fluid and electrolyte balance
	B. Explain the recovery room and intensive care unit (ICU) experience to the patient.
	  (1) Description of the recovery room or ICU (lights, other patients, noise)
	  (2) Intravenous lines the patient will have and their purpose
	  (3) Foley catheter and its purpose
	  (4) Dressings on the surgical incision
	  (5) Discomfort in the area that the surgery was performed
	  (6) Face mask or endotracheal tube for oxygenation
	  (7) Blood work drawn on arrival to recovery room or ICU
	  (8) Sensations to be experienced
	  (9) X-rays films, if any, that will be taken
	  (10) Presence of staff; stress that a nurse will *always* be close by.
	C. Encourage the patient to verbalize feelings.
	  (1) Be a good listener.
	  (2) Answer questions honestly, but without frightening the patient.
	  (3) Anticipate the questions the patient wants to ask but does not because of embarrassment or fear that the questions would seem "silly." For example, assure a patient that if a kidney (or heart) is received from a member of the opposite sex, it will not affect sexual ability or characteristics. Many patients worry about this, but few feel relaxed enough to ask about it.

NURSING DIAGNOSIS

2. Knowledge deficit related to immunosuppressive medications, rejection, and rejection therapy (knowing pattern)

Patient Outcomes	Nursing Orders
1. The patient will be able to identify all medications and know the purpose, color, dosage, frequency, and potential side-effects.	1. Teach the patient and family about immunosuppressive medications—name, dosage, purpose, side-effects (Table 46-3), and the consequences of discontinuing them (loss of the transplanted organ). A. Medications are begun on admission to the hospital for surgery.

(continued)

NURSING CARE PLAN SUMMARY   *Patient With Organ Transplantation*   Continued

Patient Outcomes	*Nursing Orders*
	B. Medications are given early the day of surgery before going to the operating room.
	C. The dose of azathioprine is dependent on the white blood cell (WBC) count; therefore, if the WBC count is decreased (usually below 4000), the dose of azathioprine will be decreased or held for that day or until the WBC count returns to the normal level.
	D. If the patient cannot read, is blind, or for some other reason is not able to administer medications to himself or herself, include another family member in the teaching session. If this is not possible, draw up a discharge plan that includes information about outside help for the patient, such as that given by a visiting nurse.
2. The patient and family will become familiar with the term *rejection episode* and the different types of rejection.	2. Define the types of rejection: hyperacute, delayed hyperacute, acute, and chronic (refer to p. 915, 932, 941).
	A. Explain that a rejection episode often occurs after transplantation, emphasizing that such an episode does not necessarily mean the patient will lose the organ.
	B. Discuss with the patient supportive measures that might be taken during rejection: hemodialysis for kidney, insulin for pancreas, and so forth.
3. The patient and family will know the signs and symptoms of rejection.	3. Familiarize the patient with the signs and symptoms of rejection (Table 46–7 for renal, Table 46–14 for liver, Figure 46-5 for heart).
4. The patient and family will be familiar with the treatments available for rejection and the expected outcome.	4. Discuss the treatment modalities used for the treatment of acute rejection (Table 46–4) as ordered by the physician.
	A. Reinforce the physician's discussion with the patient.
	B. Discuss the various procedures taken to confirm the diagnosis of acute rejection (refer to specific organ).
	C. Encourage the patient to verbalize feelings concerning treatment choices, to ask questions, and to take part in the decision-making process.

NURSING DIAGNOSIS

3. Altered protection related to organ failure preoperatively and immunosuppressive medications or therapy postoperatively (exchanging pattern)

Patient Outcomes	*Nursing Orders*
1. The patient will be afebrile and free of obvious infection at the time of surgery.	1. Preoperatively
	A. Observe, monitor, and record the patient's temperature, blood pressure, and pulse every 4 hours. The source of any fever should be determined. A fever (with few exceptions) rules out surgery.
	B. Do baseline cultures of the blood, urine, throat, sputum, and nose. It is important to identify potential sources of infection before surgery.
	C. Check the patient's skin for excoriation, pustules, and rashes.
	D. Encourage the patient to use scrupulous oral and body hygiene.
	E. Any patients, visitors, or personnel with colds or other types of infections should be kept away.
2. The patient will be protected from potential sources of infection postoperatively.	2. Postoperatively
	A. Isolation precautions may be used during the first postoperative days. The isolation rules prevent unauthorized persons from entering the room. Staff members with skin infections and colds should not take care of the patients.
	B. Thorough hand-washing techniques must be used between the care of each patient to prevent cross-contamination of patients.
	C. Check the dressings that cover the operative site.
	(1) If the dressing is dry, leave it on. It is better to leave it in place until the wound seals itself.
	(2) Employ strict sterile technique when changing the dressing.

(continued)

NURSING CARE PLAN SUMMARY *Patient With Organ Transplantation* *Continued*

Patient Outcomes	*Nursing Orders*
	(3) If drainage is present, it should be cultured routinely and the results recorded on the chart. (4) When changing the dressing, look for the signs of infection: fullness, erythema around the incision, purulent drainage, and tenderness. (5) If drains are used, the drain site should be dressed separately from the incision site. (6) If the character of the drainage from the drain site or incisional site changes—suddenly increases, becomes bloody, develops a foul odor—the physician should be notified immediately. The sudden appearance of blood from the incision site might indicate a small bleeder or an arterial leak. Be sure to distinguish between bloody drainage and serosanguineous drainage. D. Good pulmonary hygiene should be maintained through the use of either intermittent positive-pressure breathing or incentive spirometry and coughing and deep breathing to prevent postoperative atelectasis and pneumonia. E. Encourage early ambulation to prevent not only pneumonia but also pulmonary embolism and thrombophlebitis. If the patient cannot ambulate, use passive/active exercises. F. Monitor the patient's vital signs every 4 hours (more frequently if indicated or ordered). If the patient's temperature rises above 100°F, blood cultures should be done and the physician advised. G. The urinary catheter should be maintained as a closed drainage system. Good catheter techniques should be observed. A urine culture should be taken when the catheter is removed. H. Observe the patient for signs of urinary tract infection (foul-smelling or cloudy urine, frequency). I. Give meticulous care to the intravenous line site. Observe closely for signs of infiltration or infection. If an intravenous line is needed for more than 24 hours, the insertion site should be alternated. In the case of a subclavian intravenous line, care should be taken to maintain a clean site covered with an occlusive dressing. J. Encourage good eating habits to promote wound healing.

NURSING DIAGNOSIS

4. *High risk for ineffective individual coping related to possible cancellation of surgery due to abnormal laboratory or physical findings (choosing pattern)*

Patient Outcome	*Nursing Orders*
1. The patient will proceed to surgery as scheduled.	1. Prepare patient for surgery. A. Recheck the ABO compatibility between the patient (recipient) and donor. B. Draw the appropriate blood work necessary to be sent to the tissue typing laboratory for the crossmatch or the recipient's serum with the donor's lymphocytes. C. Record the results of the crossmatch between the donor and recipient on the recipient's chart. Inform the physician of the results. Remember, a *positive* crossmatch indicates the recipient has antibodies against the donor, and the surgery may be canceled. D. Check the patient's vital signs to be sure that there are no significant abnormalities, especially a fever. E. Weigh the patient and record weight on the chart. This will help evaluate the patient's fluid status postoperatively. F. Draw ordered laboratory work early enough so that the results are back and reviewed before the patient goes to surgery. Notify the physician of any abnormality, especially an elevated potassium level, so that appropriate

(continued)

NURSING CARE PLAN SUMMARY Patient With Organ Transplantation Continued

Patient Outcome	Nursing Orders
	treatment measures can be taken before surgery. Record the values accurately on the patient's chart. G. Administer preoperative medication as prescribed by the anesthesiologist.

NURSING DIAGNOSIS

5. *Ineffective breathing pattern related to anesthesia-induced neuromuscular impairment (exchanging pattern)*

Patient Outcome	Nursing Orders
1. The patient will have adequate ventilation and oxygenation postoperatively.	1. Maintain an adequate airway and evaluate the patient's respiratory function. If the patient is intubated, keep the airway free of secretions. A. Assess the patient's readiness to be extubated by evaluating alertness, strength, and respiratory state. Assist with the extubation as indicated. Have suctioning equipment available. B. Observe the patient closely after extubation for respiratory difficulties. (A respiratory arrest can occur after extubation). C. Provide the patient with heated oxygen mist. D. Check the patient's vital signs carefully. E. Auscultate the patient's chest for signs of pulmonary congestion or abnormal breath sounds.

NURSING DIAGNOSIS

6. *Ineffective individual coping related to stress (rejection episodes, isolation from family) or adverse effects of medical therapy (choosing pattern)*

Patient Outcome	Nursing Orders
1. The patient will receive supportive or therapeutic care by specialized personnel.	1. Encourage patient to express feelings and ask questions. A. Report any changes in the patient's behavior pattern to the physician. Record in the patient's chart to ensure continuity of assessment and nursing care. B. Be aware of medications taken by the transplant patient that could influence or alter behavior (pain medications, corticosteroids, and so forth). Make the patient aware of possible side-effects from the medications. C. Involve the patient in daily care and in all decision-making processes. Keep the patient informed with accurate information. D. Provide supportive care to the family and keep them informed of the patient's progress. They will then be able to provide more support to the patient. E. Allow and encourage the patient to verbalize. *Listen,* not only to what the patient is saying, but also to what the patient is *not* saying (or is afraid to say). F. Ensure that the prescribed treatment and care are followed. Give the patient a thorough explanation of any test or procedure that will be undergone. G. Encourage the patient to participate in a patient support group weekly if available. H. Prepare the patient for return to dialysis (for renal transplants) or for immediate retransplantation (for heart and liver) if antirejection therapy is not successful. I. Respect the patient's spiritual needs and call the appropriate persons when asked to do so by the patient.

(continued)

NURSING CARE PLAN SUMMARY   *Patient With Organ Transplantation*   *Continued*

NURSING DIAGNOSIS

7. *Compromised individual and family coping related to ineffective communication patterns between them and those involved in the patient care delivery system (choosing pattern)*

Patient Outcome	*Nursing Orders*
1. The patient, nursing and medical personnel, and other members of the transplant team will develop a working relationship.	1. Lines of communication must be kept open among patient, physician, and nurses to ensure comprehensive patient care. Medical personnel must depend on the patient to tell them how he or she feels in general and in relationship to the function of the transplanted organ. A. Accurate reporting and record keeping are essential in the care of the organ transplant recipient, which involves many different facets of medicine. B. Provide emotional support and reassurance not only to the patient, but also to the family. Remember that this is a stressful time for everyone. Nurses (and other personnel) tend to forget that this is usually the patient's first experience of a transplant. Because health professionals are so used to the procedures, they accept them as routine, whereas all things are new and unique to the transplant recipient. C. Honest, open communication about the function of the transplanted organ and expectations is essential. The well-informed patient and family can better tolerate untoward events. If such events occur suddenly, they should be explained immediately or as indicated. D. Give thorough explanations of the procedures. Remain with the patient during procedures if at all possible. It becomes the nurse's role to reinforce the physician's explanation of the procedures and to provide the reassurance and support the patient needs. E. Recognize potential personality conflicts between staff and patient. Deal with conflicts so that patient care will not be compromised. F. Disagreements concerning types of therapy, qualifications of personnel, or personalities should not be aired in front of the patient. Discussions of this type should be conducted away from the patient's bedside, and when a decision is reached the patient should be approached by health care professionals working together as a team.

NURSING DIAGNOSIS

8. *High risk for noncompliance related to lack of knowledge of follow-up care (choosing pattern)*

Patient Outcome	*Nursing Orders*
1. The patient and family will be able to verbalize their knowledge concerning discharge instructions, medications, and follow-up care.	1. Teach the patient about the signs and symptoms of rejection. Stress the importance of notifying the transplant center if they should occur. A. Teach the patient about the signs and symptoms of impending wound infection: pain, fever, redness around the incision, swelling around the incision, drainage from the incision, and foul odor. Stress the need to report any of these signs to the transplant center. B. If the patient had a wound infection in the hospital and is to be discharged with an open wound, teach the patient or another family member how to care properly for the wound and how to use sterile technique when changing the dressing. C. Instruct the patient regarding good hygienic care, both of body and mouth. D. Warn the patient about being around people who have contagious diseases, especially childhood diseases such as chickenpox and measles. The patient cannot live in a sterile environment on discharge, but some precautions should be taken because of the depressed immune system. Instruct the patient to notify the transplant center if exposure to a contagious disease occurs.

(continued)

NURSING CARE PLAN SUMMARY   *Patient With Organ Transplantation*   *Continued*

Patient Outcome	*Nursing Orders*
	E. Before discharge, make sure the patient or a family member has a thermometer and can read it.
	F. Encourage the patient to practice good eating habits. After transplantation, the patient usually has no dietary restrictions. After having been deprived because of their illness, transplant recipients tend to want to eat everything in sight. Corticosteroids are known to increase appetite, and the patient should be warned about this.
	G. Reinforce the teaching the patient has already received about medications. Give the patient medication cards that contain the names, dosages, and frequencies of each of the medications. Make changes on the card as the patient's medication dose changes. Have the patient count out or measure the dose of medication, name each medication, and describe its purpose and importance. The patient must assume responsibility for taking the medications before discharge. It is important that the patient be able to recognize each medication in case an incorrect prescription is given.
	H. Instruct the patient in the types of activity that can be pursued immediately after discharge. Because sexual activity can resume as the patient's health improves, discussions should be held with the patient with regard to birth control and the potential risks associated with pregnancy (refer to p. 958).
	I. Make sure the patient and family have the appropriate telephone numbers to call in case of an emergency.
	J. Encourage the patient to call about questions concerning anything at all—no matter how great or small.
	K. If the patient is referred back to his or her own physician or is returning to the dialysis center, send pertinent records with the patient so that there is continuity of care no matter where the patient is located.

NURSING CARE PLAN SUMMARY   *Specifics for the Patient With Renal Transplantation*

NURSING DIAGNOSIS

1. *Alterated fluid and electrolyte balance related to end-stage renal failure (exchanging pattern)*

Patient Outcome	*Nursing Orders*
1. The patient will be in or near proper fluid and electrolyte balance at the time of surgery.	1. Weigh the patient daily. It is important to obtain baseline information about the patient's weight and to make sure the patient does not become volume overloaded before surgery.
	A. Know the patient's daily fluid intake and urine output. If recorded accurately, it will give some indication of fluid balance. The 24-hour urine output is important *before* transplantation as baseline information, and it could be helpful in assessing renal function *after* transplantation. (For example, an output of 1000 ml/24 hours before the transplant would make a 50-ml/hour output after the transplant actually only 10 ml/hour, which would be a major concern).
	B. Schedule dialysis the day before surgery to bring the patient to the best physiologic state.
	C. Review the laboratory results immediately before surgery for any abnormalities, especially an elevated potassium level. Notify the physician immediately if an abnormality is present.
	D. Blood transfusions should be given while the patient is on dialysis if possible. By doing this, extra volume and the potential for an elevated serum potassium as a result of the transfusion will be lessened.
	E. Help the patient select a diet that is low in potassium. Restrict fluids as needed.

(continued)

NURSING CARE PLAN SUMMARY   *Specifics for the Patient With Renal Transplantation*
Continued

NURSING DIAGNOSIS

2. *High risk for fluid volume deficit related to the combination of uremic osmotic diuresis and a newly functioning transplanted kidney (exchanging pattern)*

Patient Outcome	Nursing Orders
1. The patient will remain in proper fluid and electrolyte balance.	1. Determine the patient's actual fluid status by reviewing the anesthesia and operative records for the estimated blood loss and the amount of fluid or packed cells given. Check how much urine was obtained in the operating room. When massive diuresis occurs, the vascular system is extremely sensitive to volume changes.

1. Determine the patient's actual fluid status by reviewing the anesthesia and operative records for the estimated blood loss and the amount of fluid or packed cells given. Check how much urine was obtained in the operating room. When massive diuresis occurs, the vascular system is extremely sensitive to volume changes.
   A. Make sure the indwelling catheter is connected to a closed drainage system, that there are no kinks in the catheter, and that the drainage tubing and bag are connected properly to the bed, with no tension on the catheter.
   B. Empty the drainage bag and measure the amount of urine on the patient's arrival in the recovery room or ICU. Record the amount on the appropriate records. Begin the hourly collections of urine.
   C. Check the intravenous line and fluid solution. Change the fluids to normal saline solution and 5% dextrose in water solution. This combination adequately replaces the electrolytes lost through the urine.
   D. Begin replacement therapy using the output during the previous hour as a guide to the amount of intravenous fluids that should be given during the following hour. For example, if the patient's urinary output from 7 P.M. to 8 P.M. was 240 ml, from 8 P.M. to 9 P.M. the patient should receive 160 ml of normal saline solution and 80 ml of 5% dextrose and water solution (the ratio is two parts normal saline solution to one part 5% dextrose and water solution). The urinary output from 8 P.M. to 9 P.M. determines the amount of fluid to be given from 9 P.M. to 10 P.M., and so on through the next 24 hours.
   E. Draw BUN, creatinine, CBC, and electrolytes on arrival in the recovery room/ICU. Review and record the results.
   F. Monitor the patient's vital signs closely.
      (1) If the patient's temperature is below normal, apply warm blankets. If the patient is extremely cold (as often happens in the operating room), the peripheral vessels constrict. Perfusion of the kidney also can be affected.
      (2) Watch for a sudden change in the blood pressure. The patient's blood pressure is a relatively accurate index to fluid status. If the blood pressure *falls suddenly,* the cause may be volume depletion (from large amounts of urine being produced or from bleeding). If this occurs, the rate of fluid infusion should be increased immediately. Hypotension results in low perfusion to the transplanted kidney, as well as being an obvious danger to the patient. If the blood pressure should *increase suddenly,* it could be indicative of a renal artery lesion, volume overload, or pain. Any abnormal change in the blood pressure for any particular patient should be reported to the physician.
      (3) Observe any change in the pulse rate or its character. Changes could be indicative of hypovolemia, blood loss, pain, or anxiety.
      (4) Vital signs are measured every 15 minutes until they are stable, and then every 30 minutes. Gradually decrease the monitoring to every hour if the patient's condition remains stable.
   G. Resume weighing the patient daily (weigh as soon as the patient is returned from the recovery room). Initially, the patient should lose weight as the kidney removes excess fluid. An increase in weight could be a sign of early rejection or fluid retention.
   H. Check the hemodialysis access for patency. The access must be kept functioning, because hemodialysis might be needed postoperatively for

(continued)

NURSING CARE PLAN SUMMARY *Specifics for the Patient With Renal Transplantation*
Continued

Patient Outcome	Nursing Orders
	volume overload (if the kidney does not function properly). If the patient has an arteriovenous (A-V) fistula, the application of warm towels to the area helps to increase the blood flow. If there is no flow in the access, the physician should be notified immediately. Patients become upset if the access stops functioning, because they look on their access as their lifeline, at least until they feel sure that the kidney is functioning.

NURSING DIAGNOSIS

3. *Impaired renal function related to obstruction or rejection (exchanging pattern)*

Patient Outcomes	Nursing Orders

1. The patient will be monitored for changes in renal function.	1. Order a flat plate of the abdomen (KUB) to obtain baseline information about the placement and size of the transplanted kidney.
	  A. Monitor the vital signs closely. If the blood pressure suddenly increases, the patient may be suffering from hyperacute rejection or compression of the renal artery, especially if the increase is associated with a sudden decrease in the urinary output; or, it could indicate fluid overload.
	  B. Observe for decreases in urine output, which could be a result of the following (Table 46–8):
	    (1) Hypovolemia, which can be corrected by the administration of fluids
	    (2) Obstruction of the catheter by clots or kinks, which can be corrected by irrigating or straightening the tubing
	    (3) Obstruction of the ureter by clots (this is not common)
	    (4) Compression of the renal artery (immediate surgical intervention is necessary to attempt to salvage the transplanted kidney)
	  C. Check the urine for blood or blood clots. The urine will be slightly bloody for some time because of the bladder surgery. If it suddenly becomes grossly bloody, the physician should be notified immediately.
	  D. If obstruction of the catheter is caused by blood clots, irrigate the catheter *gently*, using sterile technique.
	  E. Obtain daily serum creatinine levels. The levels should decline steadily after transplantation and should be almost normal by the fourth postoperative day if the kidney is functioning properly and there is no evidence of acute tabular necrosis (ATN) or rejection. If the downward trend in the serum creatinine level slows or stops, it must be investigated carefully.
	  F. Check the patient's daily urine protein levels. The urine protein should be negative by the fourth day after surgery in the absence of hematuria. Once the protein test is negative, reappearance of urine protein indicates acute rejection, renal vein thrombosis (rarely), or recurrence of the original disease.
	  G. Within 24 hours of the surgery, begin a urine collection to use in assessing the patient's glomerular filtration rate (GFR) by doing a timed creatinine clearance or a Glofil I^{125} clearance study. Use this as a baseline measurement with which to compare future studies of GFR. These studies should be done both at specified intervals postoperatively to obtain an accurate, stable indicator of function and at signs of a suspected rejection episode. With a functioning graft, the clearance values steadily increase. Values that have risen only slightly or that have decreased from the previous study could be an early indication of impending rejection, even though the serum creatinine level might not reflect such a change at the moment.
	  H. Accurately record and assess the patient's intake and output (including nasogastric drainage, wound drainage, and so on). Both intake and output are measured at 8-hour intervals, and the 24-hour total is recorded on the patient's chart. A downward trend in the output (particularly the overnight

(continued)

NURSING CARE PLAN SUMMARY *Specifics for the Patient With Renal Transplantation*
Continued

Patient Outcomes	Nursing Orders
	output) suggests an impending rejection episode. An abrupt decrease in output should be evaluated for cause: hypovolemia, rejection, ureteral leak, or venous–arterial obstruction. The nurse should encourage the patient to measure and record intake and output. To do so gives the patient a sense of responsibility for personal care. I. Differentiate, by listening carefully to the patient's complaints of pain, between incisional pain and tenderness in the upper pole of the kidney caused by the swelling of the kidney due to rejection. The kidney usually is easily palpated, and any change in its size or any tenderness should be assessed, recorded, and reported to the physician.
2. The patient will receive daily immunosuppressive medications.	2. Continue to give daily immunosuppressive medications as ordered. While doing this, reinforce to the patient the importance of the drugs in maintaining the transplanted kidney. A. Observe the patient for the presence of edema in the legs or the periorbital region. If edema occurs in conjunction with an increase in daily weight, the patient may have to be placed on fluid and sodium restriction. The formation of edema could also be a sign of impending rejection (Table 46–7). B. If rejection occurs, carry out or assist in the treatment therapy for rejection. Observe the patient for the side-effects of the antirejection therapy (Table 46–4).

NURSING CARE PLAN SUMMARY *Specifics for the Patient With Cardiac Transplantation*

NURSING DIAGNOSIS

1. *Decreased cardiac output, pretransplant, related to mechanical factors (impaired myocardial contractility, increased preload, increased afterload) and electrical factors (dysrhythmias)[22] (exchanging pattern)*

Patient Outcomes	Nursing Orders
1. The patient will demonstrate a stable hemodynamic profile and electrocardiogram.	1. Maintain the patency of intravenous lines at all times and ensure the accurate and timely measurement of hemodynamic profile as ordered.
2. The patient will be free from complications of hemodynamic monitoring.	2. Record hemodynamic profile and EKG strip as ordered. Note any changes or trends related to activity and medications. Report any significant changes to physician.
3. The patient will experience no complications from medication therapy.	3. Be aware of indications, actions, and side effects of medications ordered (preload and afterload reducing agents, inotropes, antiarrhythmics, diuretics, and so forth). Administer and titrate medications as indicated. Observe and document effectiveness of medications. Document and report significant side effects of medications experienced by patient.
4. The patient will progress to the maximum level of activity possible without exhibiting anoxic signs.	4. Assist patient in planning and participation of activities. Space activities allowing for periods of rest. Note patient tolerance to activity.

(continued)

NURSING CARE PLAN SUMMARY   *Specifics for the Patient With Cardiac Transplantation*
Continued

NURSING DIAGNOSIS

2. *Activity intolerance, pretransplant, related to end-stage cardiomyopathy (moving pattern)*

Patient Outcomes	Nursing Orders

1. The patient will verbalize the etiology of reduced activity tolerance.	1. Assess factors that increase cardiac workload.
	  A. Activity
	  B. Stress
	  C. Obesity

2. The patient will identify factors that increase cardiac workload.	2. Address identified factors and their effects on myocardium.
	  A. Activity: Discuss importance of planning and spacing activities. Identify time-saving strategies. Identify areas in which assistance is needed.
	  B. Stress: Discuss stress-evoking concerns. Recognize current methods of dealing with stress. Identify alternatives in dealing with stress and stress-reduction techniques.
	  C. Obesity: Examine patient's perception of dietary habits and nutritional needs. Identify patient's ideal body weight. Educate patient and family about a diet low in saturated fats, cholesterol, and salt, and with calorie control. Assist patient in developing a proper diet plan.

3. The patient will describe adaptive techniques needed to perform activities of daily living.[10]	3. Initiate appropriate health teaching and referrals (*i.e.,* home health service, chaplain, social worker, nutritionist).

NURSING DIAGNOSIS

3. *Powerlessness, pretransplant, related to chronicity (perceiving pattern)*

Patient Outcomes	Nursing Orders
1. The patient will identify factors within his scope of control.	1. Allow patient to discuss changes, losses, and limitations patient has experienced related to chronic illness. Allow patient the opportunity to verbalize feelings, fears, and frustrations.

2. The patient will make decisions regarding his care and treatment.	2. Identify the patient's usual locus of control (internal or external).[15] An internal locus of control means seeking to change one's own behaviors or environment to control problems. An external locus of control means expecting others to control problems.
	  A. Assist the patient in identifying new mechanisms to solve problems. Provide the patient with an internal locus of control, information on which he or she is able to make his or her own decisions. For the patient with an external locus of control, provide him or her with written directions and tasks to do (*i.e.,* log of activities and tolerance, medication schedule).
	  B. When possible, allow patient to identify choices and make his or her own decisions. Be supportive and encourage patient autonomy. Provide positive reinforcement to patient behavior.

NURSING DIAGNOSIS

4. *Knowledge deficit related to cardiac transplantation and associated implications for post-transplant health maintenance[10] (knowing pattern)*

Patient Outcomes	Nursing Orders
1. The patient will identify indications for cardiac transplantation.	1. Discuss indications for cardiac transplantation. A. Etiology of cardiomyopathy: ischemia, virus, valvular disease, and idiopathic cause

(continued)

NURSING CARE PLAN SUMMARY *Specifics for the Patient With Cardiac Transplantation*
Continued

Patient Outcomes	Nursing Orders
	B. Medical and surgical treatment have been tried and proven to be unsuccessful. C. Characteristics of suitable transplant candidate (refer to Table 46–9)
2. The patient will describe disadvantages and advantages of cardiac transplantation.	2. Discuss the disadvantages and advantages of transplantation with patient and family. A. Disadvantages (1) Surgical risk (2) Post-transplant risk for rejection, infection, and malignancy (3) Side-effects and complications of immunosuppressive medications (4) Cost in terms of behavioral and time commitment, and finances B. Advantages (1) Improved quality of life (2) Ability to resume activities of daily living (3) Increased activity tolerance (*i.e.*, ability to return to previous activity level [job, home, and so forth])
3. The patient will identify components of post-transplant care and effects of denervated graft.	3. Explain the components of post-transplant follow-up and care. A. Outpatient follow-up: Post-transplant follow-up is for life. Frequency of outpatient follow-up is according to protocol of the transplant center. During outpatient visits, the following are done: Endomyocardial biopsies, electrocardiograms, echocardiograms, laboratory tests, physical examination, and evaluation and adjustment of immunosuppression. A cardiac catheterization, renal sonogram, and Glofil test are done annually. B. Denervated graft: Sympathetic denervation occurs as a result of the cardiac transplantation procedure. Therefore, the transplant recipient must be informed to take certain precautions: (1) Rise slowly to prevent orthostatic hypotension. (2) When exercising, do warm-up and cool-down exercises for 10 minutes each. (3) Realize the protective mechanism of angina is lost.

NURSING DIAGNOSIS

5. *Self-esteem disturbance related to cardiac transplantation (perceiving pattern)*

Patient Outcomes	Nursing Orders
1. The patient will demonstrate movement toward reconstruction of an altered body image.	1. Allow the patient the opportunity to verbalize feelings related to cardiac transplantation. Patient may experience guilt related to the donor's death and the gift of transplantation he received. Clarify any misconceptions of the patient. Provide reliable information and support. A. Use resources as needed (chaplain, psychiatrist, other transplant recipients). B. Encourage patient to accept assistance from others.
2. The patient will set goals for himself.	2. Prepare patient for discharge and self-care at home. A. Allow patient to participate in care in preparation for home care (*i.e.*, self-administering cyclosporine, checking blood pressure with digital cuff, reading thermometer). B. Reinforce teaching of home care responsibilities regarding medications, diet, exercise, daily vital signs, and preparation for outpatient endomyocardial biopsies. C. Provide patient with materials for home care (*i.e.*, prednisone taper calendar, medication schedule, daily log for vital signs). D. Provide patient with name and number of cardiac transplant coordinator as a resource after discharge. E. For those working in an outpatient environment, assist patient in setting realistic goals for rehabilitation. Throughout the post-transplant course, assist patient in assessing goals and accomplishments, identifying concerns, and setting new goals.

NURSING CARE PLAN SUMMARY *Specifics for the Patient With Liver Transplantation*
Continued

NURSING DIAGNOSIS

1. *High risk for hypothermia in the early postoperative period related to liver dysfunction, exposure of the bowel to low ambient temperature in the operating room, or a hypothermic donor liver (exchanging pattern)*

Patient Outcome	Nursing Orders
1. The patient will be normothermic within 8 hours after transplantation.	1. Monitor core temperature hourly using PA catheter. 　A. Verify core temperature with rectal temperature every 4 hours. 　B. Goal temperature is 37.0°C, plus or minus 1°C. 　　(1) Observe patient for shivering. 　　(2) Initiate warming procedures at rate of 1°C/hour. 　　　a. Keep patient covered with blanket. 　　　b. Warm inspired oxygen. 　　　c. Use heating blanket underneath patient. 　　　d. Use warming lights. 　　　e. Administer fluids through blood warmer or warm intravenous fluid (IVF) in dialysate heater. 　　(3) As patient warms, IVF may need to be administered to compensate for vasodilatation.

NURSING DIAGNOSIS

2. *High risk for altered gastrointestinal perfusion (biliary complications) related to biliary anastomosis breakdown, biliary obstruction, biliary infection, or T-tube placement (exchanging pattern)*

Patient Outcomes	Nursing Orders
1. The patient will maintain a patent biliary system. 2. The patient will be monitored for possible biliary complications.	1. Monitor and record bile drainage from T-tube every hour and as needed in the early postoperative period. 　A. Bile should be thick and golden brown in color. 　B. Absence of drainage should be reported. 　C. Monitor serum bilirubin, liver enzymes, and temperature daily. 　D. Assess T-tube insertion site for drainage or other signs of infection. 　　(1) Clean site using aseptic technique every 8 hours. 　　(2) Keep dressing clean and dry. 2. Prepare patient and assist with HIDA scan or cholangiogram as necessary. 　A. Assist and prepare patient for possible percutaneous dilatation or insertion of a stent if stricture is detected. 　B. Assist and prepare patient for surgical intervention if dilatation or stent of stricture is unsuccessful. Surgical intervention consists of the following: 　　(1) If initial reconstruction was a duct-to-duct procedure, then biliary drainage should be converted to a choledochojejunostomy. 　　(2) If stricture is at the choledochojejunostomy site, then the anastomosis should be redone.

NURSING DIAGNOSIS

3. *High risk for altered peripheral perfusion of lower and upper extremities related to the veno–venous bypass intraoperatively (exchanging pattern)*

Patient Outcome	Nursing Orders
1. The patient will not have vascular or nerve insufficiency.	1. Palpate peripheral pulses in all extremities. Assess extremities for the following: 　A. Presence of peripheral pulses, bilateral and equal

(continued)

NURSING CARE PLAN SUMMARY *Specifics for the Patient With Liver Transplantation*
Continued

Patient Outcomes	Nursing Orders
	B. Pain in limbs
	C. Loss of sensation in limbs
	D. Loss of motor function of limb
	E. Swelling

NURSING DIAGNOSIS

4. *High risk for altered vascular perfusion (hepatic artery or portal vein occlusion) related to thrombosis or stricture at the anastomotic site (exchanging pattern)*

Patient Outcome	Nursing Orders
1. The patient will maintain a patent hepatic artery and a patent portal vein.	1. Assess for patent hepatic artery and patent portal vein. A. Monitor daily routine laboratory results for increase in transaminases (SGOT, SGPT) and bilirubin. B. Prepare the patient for Doppler ultrasound if liver function tests are elevated either immediately after operation or as a diagnostic test in the late postoperative period. C. If Doppler ultrasound reveals an occlusion of either the hepatic artery or the portal vein, prepare the patient for immediate angiography. D. If Doppler ultrasound and angiography confirm the diagnosis of occlusion of the hepatic artery or portal vein in the early postoperative period, prepare the patient for immediate surgical intervention in order to prevent graft loss. If the detection of the occlusion is late, necrosis of all or part of the liver may occur, and the patient will need to be prepared for retransplantation. E. If the detection and confirmation of the thrombosis or stricture is in the late postoperative period, the treatment of choice will be one of the following: (1) Percutaneous dilatation or operative reconstruction (2) If the stricture is totally stenotic, prepare the patient for retransplantation.

IMPLEMENTATION AND EVALUATION
Patient and Family Education

Transplant recipients make up a cross-section of the population. Not all patients have the benefit of an education or, as in the case of the diabetic transplant recipient who is blind, the benefit of sight. Yet these patients can and must learn to feel that they are at least partly responsible for their own care. Although most physicians, nurses, and auxiliary personnel working in the field of transplantation have "experienced" transplantation many times through their work, for the majority of patients, it is their first experience.

Patient education must often be related to subjects the patient will understand. For instance, the action of azathioprine on white blood cells (and the reason for taking azathioprine) can be compared with a battle. Azathioprine is given to "kill the bad group of white cells that attacks the kidney, but azathioprine also kills some of the good group of white cells" and so leaves the patient susceptible to infections. Most pa-

tients can understand the "good guy, bad guy" explanation; it helps them to understand why they are required to take the medications and why they have to be careful of infections.

A blind transplant recipient must have a relative or friend to help, but still can take some responsibility for personal care. Such a patient can learn to identify medications by rubber bands placed around the bottles. For example, one rubber band could indicate azathioprine, two rubber bands could indicate prednisone, and three rubber bands could indicate the antihypertensive medication.

Transplant recipients who are illiterate present a special challenge, but even they can learn to take care of themselves. There are probably many ways to do this. One way is to tape each individual pill to the top of an index card and draw circles on the card that correspond to the size of the pill and the number that should be taken (this is drawn from personal experience with a patient who could not read, write, or count and was also color blind). At medication times, the bottles containing the medications were brought to the bedside. The patient was responsible for matching the appropriate pill to the appropriate index card and then filling in the circles. As a medication dose was increased or decreased, a circle was added or subtracted accordingly. Gradually over time, the patient was able to learn the name of each medication, its dose, and purpose. He was an eager pupil who was very proud of his accomplishments.

Numerous booklets and slide presentations have been developed to help the patient and family understand the process of transplantation. These are available through the individual transplant center or through national organizations such as the National Kidney Foundation. They have proved useful in providing the patient basic information about transplantation.

At the time of discharge from the hospital with a newly functioning organ, the patient and family should be given written as well as verbal instructions so they have something tangible to refer to if there are any questions. The instructions should include the signs and symptoms of rejection, plus advice concerning dietary restrictions (if any), physical activity, and sexual activity.

The patient should have a clear understanding of the date, time, and place of his follow-up outpatient appointment. The patient and his family should be given the procedure to follow if an emergency should occur. These procedures should state clearly what the patient should do or whom to contact in an emergency situation, along with the appropriate telephone numbers.

Medication cards should be given to the patient at the time of discharge. In the excitement of leaving the hospital, patients have been known to forget to take their medications. The medication cards serve as a reminder to the patient of the dosages, and they lessen the confusion about increases or decreases in dosages. Patients should also be instructed to bring all medications with them to each outpatient clinic visit.

For the renal patient, sexual function and fertility return to normal (men report an improvement in their potency; menstruation usually returns as renal function stabilizes and uremia clears). For patients of other organ transplants, an improvement in their general well-being after successful transplantation often brings about a return of normal sexual function. All recipients of child-bearing age should be made aware of the possible occurrence of pregnancy. Often this discussion has to be initiated by the nursing personnel, and it should include appropriate contraceptive measures as indicated.

Pregnancy After Transplantation

For some patients, the goal of "returning to normal" after transplantation includes having children. A few pregnancies have been reported in patients with heart, liver, and bone marrow transplants. The long-term effect of the pregnancy on these transplanted organs is not known.[28] Pregnancy in the kidney recipient has been studied extensively and is discussed below.

There have been more than 2000 pregnancies reported in transplant patients since the first one in 1958. There have been three maternal deaths associated with the pregnancy: one from cerebrovascular accident, one from sepsis, and one from gastroenteritis.[28]

Risks to the mother include development of hypertension, toxemia, proteinuria, and a chance of permanent impairment of renal function. Sepsis after delivery has also been reported.

The criteria used by many transplant personnel in discussing the risks and benefits of pregnancy include good general health, stable renal function with a serum creatinine of less than 2 mg% for 1 to 2 years after transplantation, no hypertension, no evidence of rejection or proteinuria, no evidence of ureteral obstruction, and daily prednisone dose of 15 mg or less and azathioprine doses of less than 3 mg/kg.[50,76]

It would appear that many of the same criteria could be applied to other organ transplant recipients, especially stable organ function without rejection, general good health, stable renal function without hypertension (cyclosporine is known to be nephrotoxic and to cause hypertension, as discussed earlier), and a low maintenance dose of immunosuppressive medications.

The female recipient should be counseled early regarding the "restoration" of fertility after transplantation. She should be observed closely during the pregnancy with the ultimate goal of the birth of a healthy, viable infant. Women should be encouraged to wait 1 to 2 years after the transplant to become pregnant and should be informed of the potential risks and benefits involving both herself and the infant.[28]

It is recommended that pregnant transplant recipients be screened for hepatitis B surface antigen, cytomegalovirus (CMV), and HIV antibody, because these viruses can be transmitted to the infant.[28]

Breast feeding is often discouraged, because azathioprine and cyclosporine have both been measured in breast milk in high levels.[28]

The risk to the infant born of male recipients is small, but this is not true for the infant born to a female recipient. The predominant fetal complication is prematurity. Several series report that between 20% and 59% of the infants of renal recipients were born before 37 weeks of gestation. Other infant complications include leukopenia and thrombocytopenia from azathioprine-treated mothers, congenital anomalies, adrenocortical insufficiency, liver dysfunction, septicemia, and growth retardation.[9,28]

Studies have shown that cyclosporine crosses the placental barrier; therefore it is recommended that the dose of cyclosporine be reduced as low as possible before conception.[28] Still undetermined is the long-term risk of malignancy to a child who is exposed to immunosuppressive medication in utero.[50,76]

Fever

Fever is not a complication of transplantation, nor is it a side effect, but it is a "disease entity" that needs to be understood in relationship to transplant patients. When an immunosuppressed patient presents with a complaint of "fever," it is extremely important to attempt to determine its source. The concern for any fever is due, in part, to the antipyretic action of corticosteroids (they often suppress a fever response). Because fever may be an indicator of rejection as well as infection, there are several factors to consider when assessing the patient. Among these factors are the following:[73]

- Infection occurs at some time in almost 80% of transplant recipients. Bacterial infections are the most common type of infection in the first 3 months after transplantation.
- In the immediate postoperative period, the most common

sites of infection are the lungs, the urinary tract, and the surgical incision.

- In the long-term transplant recipient, opportunistic fungal, viral, and protozoan infections should be ruled out.
- It must be remembered that bacterial and fungal septicemias do not necessarily have initially recognizable foci.
- The source of the fever may be a viremia from CMV, herpes, or another adenovirus.
- The source of the fever may never be discovered.

Regardless of its cause, a fever should be evaluated extensively before it is treated, and it should be considered septic until proven otherwise. The nursing assessment should include a detailed history from the patient and family, as well as a detailed physical examination. The unexpected causes of fever should be considered, but the common causes should be emphasized.

Diagnostic Tests

- Cultures should be done of the blood, sputum, cerebrospinal fluid, urine, and wound (if there is one).
- Blood tests should include a white blood cell count with a differential count (in addition to a CBC), viral titers, fungal titers, febrile agglutinins, and the standard tests used to assess rejection in each individual transplanted organ—creatinine, liver function studies, cardiac enzymes, urine amylase, and so forth.
- A urinalysis should be obtained and the sediment examined. A urine culture should be sent if indicated.
- An x-ray film of the chest should be reviewed, as well as an abdominal x-ray film to look for free air in the abdomen.
- An ultrasound examination is usually obtained to look for fluid collection (from abdominal surgery). This fluid collection, if present, can sometimes be aspirated for further study and culture.

Depending on the test results, further diagnostic studies may be indicated. Every effort should be made to identify the causative agent before the patient is treated. Unless the patient is obviously septic, the use of nonspecific antibiotics could allow the overgrowth of resistant organisms, especially fungi. If broad-spectrum antibiotics must be used, it is essential that the necessary cultures be done before antibiotic therapy is begun.[73]

Long-Term Complications

Most of the complications of long-term transplantation stem from the patient's immunosuppressive state and from the use of immunosuppressive drugs (Table 46–15).

Cushing's Disease

The most visible complication of transplantation is Cushing's disease, which results from the use of high-dose corticosteroids. The severity of the disease depends on the daily dose of corticosteroids and the number of rejection episodes the patient has had. The visual changes in the patient's body include the following:[61] a round, puffy face; redistribution of the body fat from the extremities to the trunk and face; acne over the face, arms, and trunk; an increase in the growth of

Table 46–15
Long-Term Complications of Renal Transplantation

Pulmonary complications
  Embolism
  Fungal infection
  Viral infection
Gastrointestinal complications
  Gastric ulcer
  Pancreatitis
  Hepatitis
  Esophageal varices
Hematologic complications
  Leukopenia
  Polycythemia
Musculoskeletal complications
  Hyperparathyroidism
  Avascular (aseptic) necrosis of the bone
  Osteoporosis
Endocrine complications
  Cushing's disease
  Corticosteroid-induced diabetes mellitus
Neurologic complications
  Stroke
  Fungal and viral infections of the central nervous system
Ophthalmologic complications
  Cataracts
  Viral infections
Cardiac complications
  Myocardial infarction
  Coronary artery thrombosis
Malignancy
  Skin
  Lymphoma
  Adenocarcinoma

hair on the face, arms, and trunk; and changes in the skin texture (caused by the breakdown of protein and the diversion of amino acids) that result in thinning, striae, and bruises.

Corticosteroid-Induced Diabetes

Corticosteroid-induced diabetes is said to be a result of *long-term* corticosteroid therapy, but it can occur in the immediate postoperative period or up to 3 to 5 years after transplantation.[61] There appear to be three types: irreversible, requiring insulin therapy; reversible, related to rejection therapy; and reversible, related to weight gain.

Even though corticosteroid-induced diabetes is not reported to be a frequent complication, its onset is insidious; often the patient presents in a diabetic acidosis state without having shown any signs or having had a history of diabetes.

Ocular Complications

The most common occular complication of transplantation is cataracts, which occur as a result of the corticosteroid therapy, apparently regardless of the dose. The problems are minimal, but the cataracts do mean another operation for the patient. An advance in cataract surgery is cryoextraction, a procedure in which a cryoprobe that been cooled to $-40°F$ adheres to the cataract and pulls it out through the incision. Phacoemulsion, a newer procedure, uses a pencil tip-sized probe that is inserted through a small incision in the anterior chamber. Ultrasonic waves break up the cataract into small pieces, which are then removed by a suction needle through the same incision.[12] Phacoemulsion has lessened the trauma of cataract surgery. Patients treated by phacoemulsion are not limited in their activities after surgery, and their hospital stay is usually only 1 day.

Other ocular complications are bilateral depigmentation of the retinal pigment epithelium, elevated intraocular tension, and CMV retinitis, which can result in blindness.[47]

The patient should have his or her eyes examined often to detect any abnormalities as early as possible.

Avascular Necrosis of the Joints

Avascular necrosis of the joints is seen frequently in the transplant population. The hip is the most common joint involved, but avascular necrosis can also occur in the knee, shoulder, and elbow. It probably occurs as a result of the corticosteroid dosage and the alterations in lipid metabolism caused by fluctuations in the corticosteroid dosage. The underlying bone disease that occurs in most patients who have chronic renal failure probably also contributes to the disease. These patients usually have symptoms of hip pain for several months before radiographic evidence. Initially, the treatment is symptomatic, but progressive bone destruction or continued pain requires surgical intervention in the form of total hip replacement.[61]

Cardiovascular Disease

Although hypertension is the single most common medical complication, cardiovascular disease is the contributing cause of 30% to 40% of patient deaths during the first 10 years after transplant in renal recipients. Hypertension, hyperlipidemia, smoking, and uremia are the risk factors that contribute to the problem.[9] These same risk factors can be applied to recipients of other organ transplants and will be evaluated closely as the number of long-term survivors increases.

Patients are encouraged to stop smoking before and after transplantation. There are some transplant programs that will not accept a patient for transplantation if the patient continues to smoke.

The cause of hyperlipidemia in the post-transplant recipient is not identified clearly. There are a number of contributing factors, the most common being cyclosporine and corticosteroid therapy. Hyperlipidemia is thought to be the cause of the accelerated atherosclerosis seen in heart transplant recipients and to contribute to the loss of renal function in the long term.[41] Approximately two thirds of all post-transplant recipients have hyperlipidemia. Currently, several studies are being done to assess and find a solution for the problem, including dietary and pharmacologic interventions.[41,48] Other studies have shown that even if the patients are switched from cyclosporine therapy to azathioprine (Imuran) and prednisone, there is no significant difference in lipid metabolism.[23]

Malignant Neoplasm

Malignant neoplasms occur as a result of long-term immunosuppressive therapy. The incidence is 100 times greater in transplant recipients than in the general population.[79] As patients are followed for longer periods of time, the incidence of cancer increases.[49] Certain malignancies appear at distinct time intervals after transplantation.[49]

It is not clear whether the increased incidence is due to oversuppression, to the immune response alone, or to a combined effect added to continued antigenic stimulation from the foreign graft. Most lesions are epithelial and lymphoproliferative in origin.[70,79]

The most common malignancy observed involves the skin and lip (39%), with many patients having multiple lesions. Although most skin cancers were low grade, there were a significant number who had aggressive tumors such as malignant melanomas, squamous cell carcinoma, and lymph node metastasis. Of the patients with skin and lip cancer, 6% died from metastases. Patients should be instructed to avoid prolonged exposure to direct sunlight by wearing protective clothing, hats, and effective sunscreen preparations.[49]

Other malignancies that occur commonly include lymphomas; Kaposi's sarcoma; carcinoma in situ of the cervix; carcinoma of the lung, colon and rectum, and breast; and carcinoma of the vulva, perineum, scrotum, perianal skin, and anus. Other organs are affected less often; they include the urinary bladder, liver, thyroid, prostate, and metastatic carcinomas in which the primary site is unknown.[49]

The treatment varies but often includes the withdrawal of immunosuppression in addition to surgical or other intervention. In renal recipients, the patient could return to dialysis therapy, but for other major organ transplants such as liver and heart, withdrawal of immunosuppression could mean death if the transplanted organ is rejected. However, chemotherapeutic drugs have immunosuppressive actions that prolong graft function during treatment for the malignancy.

SUMMARY

The risks of transplantation are great. They lead one to ask why a patient with end-stage organ failure would choose transplantation, especially the end-stage renal disease patient for whom other treatment modalities are available. The explanation has to do with the "quality of life" concept, which has a different meaning for each patient. Many patients are willing to take the risks in an effort to return to a more normal life.

Even though a conscious or an unconscious fear of rejection persists regardless of how many years the patient has had the transplanted organ, most patients are able to adapt to their new condition. They are bothered, however, by the fact that they are dependent on medications, which reminds them of their vulnerability.

Efforts in transplantation are continuing in search of a more effective means of immunosuppression aimed at specific cells of rejection. It is hoped that more specific immunosuppression will result in less severe side-effects. Until this is accomplished, infection remains the greatest threat, often resulting in the death of a patient with a functioning organ.

An interdisciplinary team approach should be used in caring for the transplant recipient. The problems encountered should be dealt with openly by the transplant physicians, surgeons, and nursing staff, as well as by the social worker, dietitian, and members of other disciplines. The patient benefits from the team approach. Each member of the team should contribute to the care of the patient and should share observations with the other team members.

The ability of nurses to participate in the care of the transplant recipient is based on their understanding of all aspects of the transplantation process: anatomy and physiology, immunology, immunosuppression, statistics, and the psychological stress on the patient and family. If the nurses have this basic knowledge, their experience will bring them further growth and understanding.

DIRECTIONS FOR FUTURE RESEARCH

There are many avenues to research. To accomplish a small step down any one particular avenue requires the joint efforts of many people. Nurses are an integral part of this research process.

Many new ideas are formed as a result of retrospective analysis of data—hindsight is better than foresight. Therefore, accurate documentation of events, laboratory values, test results, and impressions is extremely important. Often it is the nurse's responsibility to do or to see that accurate recording is done.

There are other avenues of research that are important to the improved survival of transplanted organs and patients. Studies are continuing to find the most effective treatment for or prevention of significant long-term patient risks such as viral infections, hyperlipedemia, and malignancies.[54]

In the field of immunosuppressive therapy, the search continues for cell-specific immunosuppressives that will prevent graft loss without causing patient loss. New drugs such as FK-506 and cyclosporine G are entering clinical trials and hold hope for future recipients of organ transplants.

In the field of organ procurement, research is directed toward improved solutions to allow longer periods of cold ischemia time without harming organ function. The advantages (if any) of pulsatile perfusion over cold storage are being reevaluated. Many avenues are being reviewed to ensure that there is equitable organ allocation among recipients awaiting transplant.

In the field of histocompatibility, there is continued evaluation concerning the value of HLA matching in cadaveric transplants, especially in renal transplantation. This discussion has been going on for as long as there have been transplants, but now that there are more patients surviving longer than 10 to 15 years with a functioning graft, these parameters are being reevaluated.

Research has shown that the education of the public is essential to the success of transplants. Not only does it increase the awareness of the need for organs, but it also makes the public aware that transplant patients are "normal" people who are capable of going to school, working, assuming responsibility, and being contributing members of society.

Transplantation is expensive, but a recent study has shown that renal transplantation is cost effective and provides a better quality of life.[17] Medicare has extended funding to organs other than the kidney in a limited number of centers. Otherwise, private funding through donations or insurance must be obtained before receiving a transplant. This limits the access of many patients to transplantation of organs other than kidneys.

There have been several national and international conferences to address the ethics of transplantation.[74] Discussion at these conferences concerned the problems of organ allocation, patient selection, finances, living nonrelated donor transplants, and other topics that concern and influence organ transplantation today and will continue to do so in the future.

The future should be exciting in the field of transplantation of solid organs. It will be interesting to observe the progression of heart–lung, lung, small intestine, pancreas, and multiple organs transplanted into one recipient as the research in the fields of organ harvesting and preservation, and the understanding of mechanisms of rejection, bring about the development of more specific immunosuppressive agents.

REFERENCES

1. Alijani, M. R., Pechan, B. W., Darr, F., et al. Treatment of steroid-resistant renal allograft rejection with plasmaleukapheresis. Transplant. Proc. 15:1063, 1983.
2. Anderson, C. F., Frohnert, P. P., Torres, V., et al. Followup living related donors: 8 to 18 years after unilateral nephrectomy (Abstr.). Proc. Am. Soc. Transplant Physicians 2:2, 1983.
3. Atkins, C., Peters, P., Vergne-Marini, P., et al. Long-term kidney donors: A follow-up RE: Hypertension and function (Abstr.). Proc. Am. Soc. Transplant Physicians 2:3, 1983.
4. Ballester, M., Obrador, D., Carrio, I., et al. Reversal of rejection-induced coronary vasculitis detected early after heart transplantation with increased immunosuppression. J. Heart Transplant 8: 413, 1989.
5. Belzer, F. O. Renal preservation. N. Engl. J. Med. 291:402, 1974.
6. Benenson, E. (ed.). UNOS Update 5:18, 1989.
7. Benichou, J., Halgrmson, C. G., Weil, R., et al. Canine and human liver preservation for 6-18H by cold infusion. Transplantation 24: 407, 1977.
8. Beveridge, T. Cyclosporin A: An evaluation of clinical results. Transplant Proc 15:433, 1983.
9. Bia, M. J., Flye, M. W. Long-term follow-up of the renal transplant patient. In M. W. Flye (ed.), Principles of Organ Transplantation. Philadelphia: W. B. Saunders, 1989.
10. Billingham, M. E. Diagnosis of cardiac rejection by endomyocardial biopsy. Heart Transplantation 1:25, 1982.
11. Bollinger, R. R., Sanfilippo, F. Immunogenetics of Transplantation. In M. W. Flye (ed.), Principles of Organ Transplantation. Philadelphia: W. B. Saunders, 1989.
12. Boyd-Monk, H. Cataract surgery. Nurs. '77 7:56, 1977.
13. Brundage, D. J. Nursing Management of Renal Problems (2nd ed.). St. Louis: C. V. Mosby, 1980.
14. Calne, R. Y. (ed.). Liver Transplantation: The Cambridge-King's College Hospital Experience. London: Grune and Stratton, 1983.
15. Carpenito, L. J. Nursing Diagnosis: Application to Clinical Practice. Philadelphia: J. B. Lippincott, 1983.
16. Copeland, J. G. Current Problems in Cardiology: Cardiac Transplantation. Chicago: Year Book Medical Publishers, 1988.
17. Eggers, P. W. Effect of transplantation on the medicare end-stage renal disease program. N. Engl. J. Med. 318:223, 1988.
18. Fehrman, I., Brattstrom, C., Duraj, F., et al. Kidney transplantation in patients between 65 and 75 years of age. Transplant. Proc. 21: 2018, 1989.
19. Fellner, C. H. Selection of living kidney donors and the problem of informed consent. Semin. Psychiatry 3:79, 1971.
20. Fish, J. C., Sarles, H. E., Remmers, A., et al. Renal transplantation after thoracic duct drainage. Ann. Surg. 193:752, 1981.
21. Flye, M. W. History of transplantation. In M. W. Flye (ed.), Principles of Organ Transplantation. Philadelphia: W. B. Saunders, 1989.
22. Futterman, L. G. Cardiac transplantation: A comprehensive nursing perspective. Part 2. Heart Lung 17:632, 1989.
23. Gonwa, T. A., Atkins, C., Velez, R., et al. Metabolic consequences of cyclosporine-to-azathioprine conversion in renal transplantation. Clin. Transplantation 2:91, 1988.
24. Guyton, A. Textbook of Medical Physiology. Philadelphia: W. B. Saunders, 1976.
25. Hamburger, J., Crosnier, J., Dormont, J., et al. Renal Transplantation: Theory and Practice (2nd ed.). Baltimore: Williams & Wilkins, 1981.
26. Hardy, M. A., Nowygrod, R., Elberg, A., et al. Use of ATG in treatment of steroid-resistant rejection. Transplantation 29:162, 1980.
27. Heck, C. F., Shumway, S. J., and Kaye, M. P. The registry of the International Society for Heart Transplantation: Sixth official report—1989. J Heart Transplantation 8:271, 1989.
28. Hou, S. Pregnancy in organ transplant recipients. Med. Clin. North Am. 73:667, 1989.

29. Howard, R. J., Pfaff, W. W., Salomon, D., et al. Kidney transplantation in older patients. *Transplant. Proc.* 21:2020, 1989.
30. Kaufman, D. B., Sutherland, D. E. R., Noreen, H., et al. Renal transplantation between living-related sibling pairs matched for zero-HLA haplotypes. *Transplantation* 47:113, 1989.
31. Kerman, R. H. Immune monitoring consideration in transplantation. In M. W. Flye (ed.), *Principles of Organ Transplantation.* Philadelphia: W. B. Saunders, 1989.
32. Kirkman, R. L., Strom, T. B., Weir, M. R., et al. Late mortality and morbidity in recipients of long-term renal allografts. *Transplantation* 34:347, 1982.
33. Klintmalm, G. B. G., Nery, J. R., Husberg, B., et al. Rejection in liver transplantation. *Hepatology* 10:978, 1989.
34. Kreis, H. Renal preservation. In J. Hamburger, J. Crosnier, I. Dormont, J-F. Bach (eds.), *Renal Transplantation: Theory and Practice* (2nd ed.). Baltimore: Williams & Wilkins, 1981.
35. Kreis, H. Transplanted kidney: Natural history. In J. Hamburger, J. Crosnier, I. Dormont, J-F. Bach (eds.), *Renal Transplantation: Theory and Practice* (2nd ed.). Baltimore: Williams & Wilkins, 1981.
36. Lane, S., Haid, S., Jankiewicz, T., et al. *Southwest Organ Bank: Multiple Organ Recovery Manual.* Dallas: Organ Recovery System, 1987.
37. Leevy, C. M. *Evaluation of Liver Function in Clinical Practice.* In: Lilly Research Laboratories, Indiana, 1974.
38. McAllister, H. A., Schnee, M. J., Radovancevic, B., and Frazier, O. H. A system for grading cardiac allograft rejection. *Texas Heart Institute Journal* 13:1, 1986.
39. McGiffin, D. C., Bonner, J. R., Kirklin, J. K., and Naftel, D. C. Patterns of infection and management in cardiac transplantation. In J. Wallwork (ed.), *Heart & Heart Lung Transplantation.* Philadelphia: W. B. Saunders, 1988.
40. Makowa, L., and Van Thiel, D. H. (eds.). *Gastroenterology Clinics of North America.* Philadelphia: W. B. Saunders, March 1978.
41. Markell, M. S., Friedman, E. A. Hyperlipidemia after organ transplantation. *Am. J. Med.* 87:5, 1989.
42. Mora, N., Klintmalm, G. B. G., Cofer, I., et al. Does hepatitis-B-immunoglobulin modify the recurrence of hepatitis B after transplantation? *Transplant. Proc.* (in press).
43. Moreno-Cabral, C. E., Mitchell, R. S., and Miller, C. D. *Manual of Post-operative Management in Adult Cardiac Surgery.* Baltimore: Williams & Wilkins, 1988.
44. Morris, R. E., Hoyt, E. G., Murphy, M. P., et al. Immunopharmacology of FK-506. *Transplant. Proc.* 21:1042, 1989.
45. Naik, R. B., Ashlin, R., Wilson, C., et al. The role of plasmapheresis in renal transplantation. *Clin. Nephrol.* 11:245, 1979.
46. National Institute of Health Consensus Development Conference statement: Liver transplantation, June 20–23, 1983. *Hepatology* 10S, 1984.
47. Oberman, A. E., and Chatterjee, S. N. Ocular complications in renal transplant recipients. *West. J. Med.* 123:184, 1975.
48. Pagenkemper, J. J., DiMarco, N. M., Hull, A. R., et al. The management of hypertriglyceridemia and hypercholesterolemia by omega-3 fatty acids in renal transplant patients. *CRN Quarterly* 13:9–14, 1989.
49. Penn, I. Risk of cancer in the transplant patient. In M. W. Flye (ed.), *Principles of Organ Transplantation.* Philadelphia: W. B. Saunders, 1989.
50. Penn, I., Makowski, E. L., and Harris, P. Parenthood following renal and hepatic transplantation. *Transplantation* 30:397, 1980.
51. Peters, P. C. Dialysis and transplantation: The past. *Semin. Nephrol.* 2:79, 1982.
52. Pirsch, J. D., Sollinger, H. W., Kalayoglu, M., et al. Living-unrelated renal transplantation: Results in 40 patients. *Am. J. Kid. Dis.* 12:499, 1988.
53. Raia, S., Nery, J., Mies, S. Liver transplantation from live donors. (Letters to the Editor). *Lancet* :497, 1989.
54. Rubin, R. H., Tolkoff-Rubin, N. E. Infection: The new problems. *Transplant. Proc.* 21:1440, 1989.
55. Sagalowsky, A. I., Ransler, C. W., Peters, P. C., et al. Urologic complications in 505 renal transplants with early catheter removal. *J. Urol.* (in press).
56. Sagalowsky, A. I., McConnel, J., Lewis, S., et al. Early diagnosis or rejection (rej) and differentiation from ATN by serial post-transplant (pTx) 99mTc-DPTA renal scan (rs). *J. Urol.* (in press).
57. Sanghvi, A., Warty, V. S., Diven, W. F., et al. Increased cyclosporine uptake by cells pretreated with FK-506 and evidence for binding of both drugs to a common intracellular protein. *Transplant. Proc.* 21:1050, 1989.
58. Sayage, L., Gonwa, T., Goldstein, R. M., et al. Cytomegalovirus infection in orthotopic liver transplantation. *Transplantation* 2:96, 1989.
59. Shiff, L., Shiff, E. (eds.). *Diseases of the Liver* (5th ed.). Philadelphia: J. B. Lippincott, 1982.
60. Simmons, R. G., and Simmons, R. L. Sociological and Psychological Aspects of Transplantation. In J. S. Najarian and R. L. Simmons (eds.), *Transplantation.* Philadelphia: Lea & Febiger, 1972.
61. Simmons, R. L., Kjellstrand, C. M., and Najarian, J. S. Kidney: Technique, complications and results. In J. S. Najarian and R. L. Simmons (eds.), *Transplantation.* Philadelphia: Lea & Febiger, 1972.
62. Soifer, B. E., and Gelb, A. W. The multiple organ donor: Identification and management. *Ann. Intern. Med.* 110:814, 1989.
63. Southard, J. H., Belzer, F. O. Organ preservation. In W. M. Flye (ed.), *Principles of Organ Transplantation.* Philadelphia: W. B. Saunders, 1989.
64. Starzl, T. E., Demetris, A., Van Thiel, D. Liver transplantation. *N. Engl. J. Med.* 1092, 1989.
65. Starzl, T. E., Klintmalm, G. B. G., Weil, R. III, et al. Liver transplantation with use of cyclosporine A and prednisone. *N. Engl. J. Med.* 305:266, 1981.
66. Starzl, T. E., Koep, W., Halgrmson, C. G., et al. Fifteen years of clinical liver transplantation. *Gastroenterology* 77:375, 1979.
67. Starzl, T. E., Koep, L. J., Koep, L. J. Decline in survival after liver transplantation. *Arch. Surg.* 115:815, 1980.
68. Staschak, S. Orthotopic liver transplantation. *AORN Journal* 39:35, 1984.
69. Streem, S. B., Novick, A. C., Braum, W. E., et al. Antilymphoblast globulin for treatment of acute renal allograft rejection. *Transplant. Proc.* 15:590, 1983.
70. Strom, T. B. The improving utility of renal transplantation in the management of end-stage renal disease. *Am. J. Med.* 73:113, 1982.
71. Sutherland, D. E. R., Kendall, D., Goetz, F. C., et al. Pancreas transplantation in humans. In W. M. Flye (ed.), *Principles of Organ Transplantation.* Philadelphia: W. B. Saunders, 1989.
72. Sutherland, D. E. R., Moudry, K. C. Pancreas transplantation registry report. *Transplant. Proc.* 21:2759, 1989.
73. Their, S. D., Henderson, L. W., and Root, R. K. Renal transplantation: Medical management of the transplant recipient. In B. M. Brenner and F. C. Rector (eds.), *The Kidney* (vol. 2). Philadelphia: W. B. Saunders, 1976.
74. Turcotte, J. G. and Benjamin, M. (eds.). Patient selection criteria in transplantation—The critical questions. *Transplant. Proc.* 21: 3377, 1989.
75. Wagner, H. Cyclosporin A: Mechanism of action. *Transplant. Proc.* 15:523, 1983.
76. Waltzer, W. C., Coulam, C. B., Zincke, H., et al. Pregnancy in renal transplantation. *Transplant. Proc.* 12:221, 1980.
77. Ward, H. J., and Glassock, R. J. Management of immunologically high risk renal transplant recipients. *Semin. Nephrol.* 2:173, 1982.
78. Ware, A. J., Luby, J. P., Hollinger, B., et al. Etiology of liver disease in renal-transplant patients. *Ann. Intern. Med.* 91:364, 1979.
79. Washer, G. F., Schroter, G. P. J., Starzl, T. E., et al. Causes of death after transplantation. *J.A.M.A.* 250:49, 1983.
80. Winter, P., Kary, Y. (eds.). *Hepatic Transplantation.* New York: Praeger, 1986.

47

Near-Death Experiences

Cathie E. Guzzetta

DYING IN PEACE

Because so much emphasis is placed on living in the Western world view, we focus less on the importance of dying time. Actually, small parts of us die each day. In fact, every 5 years, we have an entirely new body that has changed down to the very last carbon atom. Cells in the body die and are replaced each day. Red blood cells are replaced every 120 days, all our skin cells are replaced every 4 weeks, and bone cells are replaced every 4 days. This means that part of us dies every day.

Much of this fear originates from Western psychology, with its emphasis on the importance of the ego, the "I" or "me." It is my ego, my mind/consciousness, that decides reality. When we identify with the ego, we manifest attachment, a holding on to people, things, and events. The more the ego attaches and holds on, the more fears increase.

In the Eastern world view, the ego is only one of many ways of knowing reality. It is the ego that creates barriers to a full awareness of being. When one learns to release the separate "I," then a more natural way of "knowing" and "awareness" can unfold.

True healing and dying in peace come from releasing the attachment to the physical body. It is learning to let our body-mind-spirit be open to healing that comes from within. The paradox is that this healing awareness appears at first to be rare, but it is a very ordinary event that is available to each of us in each lived moment. As we practice living in peace, we enter a healing state in which answers to our questions about the complementary nature of living and dying are revealed to us. The insight comes from our own inner wisdom and strength.

LEARNING OBJECTIVES

After reading this chapter, the nurse should be able to do the following:

1. Discuss the affective, cognitive, and transcendental features that characterize a near-death experience.
2. Describe the clinical consequences of near-death experiences.
3. Discuss the cultural beliefs and attitudes that influence the near-death experience.
4. Compare and contrast the spiritual, organic, and psychologic theories used to explain near-death phenomena.
5. Discuss the assessment, diagnoses, patient outcomes, and interventions used for a patient after a near-death experience.
6. Explore and discuss his or her feelings about near-death experiences.

CASE STUDY*

July 29, 7 A.M.

I awoke and slowly opened my eyes. July 29. Today I'm having surgery. I stretched and turned to look at my husband. I slept all night. I thought I wouldn't be able to sleep. I got up and began dressing for my trip to the hospital.

My thoughts went back to the uneasiness I had felt for several days. It was as though I could sense some kind of danger. I shared those feelings with my family and friends. They tried to boost my confidence with remarks like, "Oh everybody's nervous before surgery," or "That's because you're a nurse and you know what to expect."

11:00 A.M., Hospital Admission

"Carolyn, I'm John M——, your anesthesiologist."

* Copyright © 1982 by Carolyn D. Henson, R.N., M.A. Reprinted by permission.

"Hello." So you're the one who called last night and asked if I knew my blood pressure and pulse. When I said my resting pulse was 52, there was a long pause, as though you thought I must be wrong. I explained that I'm a jogger and that my pulse is always low. Didn't you believe me?

Approximately 1:45 P.M., About 10 Minutes Into the Operation

"Her pressure's crashing!"

"What is it? What's the matter?"

At first there was a feeling of sweeping motion. It felt like my mind—the thinking and feeling part of me—quickly moved out of my body. I could see my body lying on the table, but the real "me" hovered near my head.

It was clear that there was an emergency. The scene was frantic. People I didn't recognize were scurrying in and out of the room. I searched for my surgeon. I knew he was there, but he wasn't standing where I thought he should have been.

Initially, I joined in the frenzy. I desperately wanted to help. I wanted to tell the doctors what was happening. Frantically, I tried to approach them. I tried to speak, but nothing came out. I reached to touch them, but a barrier kept me from getting close. I tried to approach several people before realizing that no one could see or hear me. At that moment, an extraordinary calmness came over me. I moved toward a corner of the ceiling, close to a "light."

I had a euphoric feeling of peace. It was as though warmth and acceptance were being communicated to me through the light. There was absolutely no fear. I felt safe and secure. There was a sense of timelessness—as though there was no time. I wanted to linger with the thoughts and feelings I was experiencing.

I was totally unconcerned about what was happening to my body. It was like being in a room with a television set turned on, without paying attention to the images and sounds coming from the set. I was aware that the operating room drama was occurring, but my mind was totally absorbed in the intensity of the peacefulness.

I heard someone say, "I don't think she's going to make it," but the words didn't concern me. I had no thought that I was dying, or that I was going to die. I felt very much alive. I wanted to tell the doctors that there was no need for their urgency—that I liked where I was, and that everything was going to be okay. I heard a doctor say, "She's hemorrhaging. We've got to open her up!"

I don't know how long my mind remained separated. I remember feeling intense pain when the surgeon made the incision for the exploratory laparotomy. What are they doing now? Are they doing open chest heart massage? I've got to tell them I can feel this. Move your head, Carolyn, move your head.

"She feels that! I'm going to have to put her under again."

. . . I don't know when my mind rejoined my body, but I do remember using mental energy to help myself deal with the pain. Inhale—exhale—relax; inhale—exhale—relax . . . When I tired of the breathing exercise, I would practice imagery. I imagined myself in a very healthy state, jogging at the lake. One, two, three, four, five . . . For the past ten years, counting had been a technique I had used to keep a steady jogging cadence. I knew that when I reached 500 I had jogged about a mile.

July 30, The Next Morning

I woke up. My chest was sore. I was in the intensive care unit. My husband was standing at my bedside. I remembered . . . "Jerry! I almost died. I could see. I was watching. I separated from my body. I was on the table, but I was watching." I began to drift off. I went back to the jogging trail. One hundred and one, one hundred and two. . . .

Later That Afternoon

Jerry was back at my side. "Jerry! They did CPR!"

"I know, Honey, but they only did chest compressions for a short while. Your heart pulled you through. The doctors said that if you hadn't been a jogger, you wouldn't have made it. Your lungs were really strong!" I smiled and nodded. Not just jogging, but a combination—jogging, diet, relaxation. What a payoff!

The Days Following

The nurses skillfully blended gentleness with prodding. They were tender with their care while encouraging me to care for myself. I also learned the value of motivating patients back to self-sufficiency. I left the hospital 6 days after surgery.

Physically, my recovery was exceptionally quick. But psychologically, there were many adjustments to make. At first, I was elated over just being alive. I wanted to share that excitement with others. I marvelled at the near-death experience. I wanted to tell others about it, even when they looked at me in disbelief—or fear.

I went to White Rock Lake daily to walk. The trail felt different now, as though it were a very intimate part of me. The colors and sounds along the trail came alive. It felt like I was seeing objects and hearing sounds for the very first time.

A few weeks after the surgery, I became very depressed. The reality of my close encounter with death set in. I now had new scars that were not there before. I felt somehow "different" because of this experience. There seemed to be too much to deal with at once.

I spent time reflecting on how we get caught up in unimportant things and miss the beauty of life. There was a need to reset priorities and eliminate the trivia. I found myself concentrating on my family, friendships, and the development of my mind. I felt an intense commitment to my work. I had changed.

DESCRIPTION

Only recently have we recognized a fascinating and unusual phenomenon, termed the near-death experience (NDE), encountered by patients who have successfully survived a cardiopulmonary arrest. The NDE comprises perceptions and events experienced by patients during the clinical death phase of a cardiopulmonary arrest.

In relating their experience to others, survivors have described several features that appear to characterize the NDE.[9,10,13] The experiences seem to cluster around three common domains: affective, cognitive, and transcendental.[1,14] During the clinical death phase, patients have described such *affective feelings* as being comfortable, pain free, relaxed, calm, and peaceful. Some also may be aware, at that moment, that they have died. *The cognitive features* include accelerated thoughts and time awareness (or a distortion of time), as well as a sudden understanding of life. Many patients report a panoramic memory or a sudden review of their entire past during the NDE. The *transcendental experiences* involve the passage of consciousness into a foreign region or dimension, which includes visual images and out-of-body experiences.[14]

The out-of-body experiences described by patients are called *autoscopic observations*. Such patients experience a separation of the body and mind; for example, the mind may position itself in a corner of the room to observe the resuscitative efforts on the body. The mind actually takes on ultradimensional characteristics not limited to physical space.[10] In support of this phenomenon, some patients have been able to describe accurately such technicalities as the placement of equipment and personnel and the details of resuscitative procedures that could only be known if one was actually standing at the bedside observing the situation.

Patients have described their inability to communicate with the health team during the resuscitation as a distressing component of their NDE. Some wanted to confront the health team or express their desire to stop the resuscitation. In other cases, patients wanted to talk to, contact, or touch their care givers to assure them that they were comfortable and pain free.[10]

Some patients who experience a separation of body and mind indicate that their mind left the room and entered another place. These patients describe their mind traveling through a long dark tunnel with loud noises or music associated with the journey. The noises include thunderous ringing, hissing, or buzzing, or peaceful and serene music.[4] At the end of the tunnel, they frequently describe an unbelievably bright light, a beautiful meadow, or a heavenly world.

Some patients report entering the light and encountering persons, figures, guides, deceased relatives, or religious figures.[14] The deities may include God, Jesus, Buddha, or other significant beings, depending on the individual's culture and beliefs. Many also describe coming to a river or a mountain symbolizing a dividing line between life and death or a border of no return.[4,14] Patients may know that crossing it means they would remain forever. Many relate an understanding of the need to return.[4] Sometimes friends, relatives, or religious figures tell patients that they must go back or that it is not their time to be there.

Although most NDEs are not described as negative experiences, some patients have reported frightening events, such as strange creatures, sights of hell, flames, or burning, and feelings of loneliness, doom, terror, and helplessness.[10]

At the completion of a successful resuscitation, patients may find their minds rapidly traveling back through the tunnel to be united with the body. They may see the body, know that pain is expected, and re-enter the body.[4] This reunion can be associated not only with physical discomfort but also with emotional pain and distress, because frequently the mind wants to remain in the light or the place of peace and comfort.

CLINICAL CONSEQUENCES OF NDEs

It is clear that patients who have had NDEs are profoundly affected by the experience. They report transcendental events and feelings of harmony, a sense of cosmic unity, and of being at one with the universe.[6] Such experiences provide convincing evidence to support the concepts of natural systems theory (see Chap. 2). Patients may relate a sense of "all knowing"—understanding what truth is, what love is, and what life is all about.[4] Many patients report a reordering of their lives after a NDE; personal values, attitudes, and beliefs change, resulting in a devaluation of material belongings and career success and an increased emphasis on altruistic and spiritual concerns.[6] Patients describe a feeling of invulnerability, a special sense of purpose and meaning in life, a greater concern for others, and a heightened belief in God and in an afterlife.[14] Some report a reduced fear of death, although suicide survivors who have had NDEs report a decreased suicidal tendency.[6,14]

FACTORS INFLUENCING NDEs

Near-death experiences have been documented throughout history and in such diverse near-death episodes as childbirth and sudden life-threatening events (i.e., trauma, surgery, combat, drowning, and near lethal falls of mountaineers) to confinement in bed and terminal illness.[14]

It has been found that up to 48% of persons who have come close to death have experienced a NDE.[13,16] Gallup and Proctor have reported that about 8 million adults—or about 5% of the American population—have had a NDE.[5] Patients from 2 to 100 years old have experienced this event.[4] Research has found no relationship between the occurrence of a NDE

and age, sex, education, marital status, occupation, or religious background.[8]

The principal features of NDEs also have been documented across various religious and cultural groups. These features (i.e., the affective, cognitive, and transcendental characteristics) are generally universal regardless of the country, religion, or culture. The symbolic imagery reported from the experience may differ, however, depending on the concepts of the afterlife and the cultural setting of the individual.[14] In one study of 442 American and 435 Indian accounts of NDEs, for example, most of the figures visualized were relatives.[11] Although 60% of the Americans imaged their mothers, the Indian male population rarely visualized a female being. Likewise, there are many reports of religious divine beings visualized (i.e., God, angels, Hindu deities), but they are always named according to the individual's religious beliefs (i.e., no Hindu has reported seeing Jesus, and no Christian has seen a Hindu deity).[11] It appears that although the individual's images may be bound by cultural expectations and beliefs, the NDE is essentially the same around the world.[14]

CAUSAL THEORIES

Many theories have been developed to explain the near-death phenomenon. These include spiritual, organic, and psychologic theories, and some include combined models that incorporate components of each.[14] *Spiritual theories* are developed on the assumption that the NDE phenomenon represents reports of individuals who have died and then returned. Thus, such theories assert that the NDE provides empirical evidence of the existence of an afterlife. Critics of such theories argue that a cardiac arrest does not really represent the death of an individual, because death is characterized by a fixed and permanent state with irreversible loss of brain function.[14] Rather, the cardiac arrest represents the dying process, which is limited by time; thus, individuals who experience NDEs have entered the early phase of the dying process, which can be reversed by successful cardiopulmonary resuscitation.

Organic theories focus on physical causes of NDEs.[14] One theory asserts that the cerebral anoxia occurring during the dying process is responsible for the hallucinations and illusions experienced during the NDE. Others believe that the panoramic memory and attitudinal changes that follow the NDE are an adaptive neurologic response to severe anxiety, resulting from temporal lobe excitation. Another similar theory proposes that NDEs are the result of a stress-induced limbic lobe syndrome. Under extreme stress, the central nervous system secretes peptides that affect behavior, thereby accounting for the hallucinatory events associated with the NDE. Time distortion and hallucinogenic experiences similar to NDEs also have been induced by trances, fever, exhaustion, coma, anesthetics, and recreational drugs (i.e., ketamine, lysergic acid diethylamide or LSD, and hashish), which supports the role of some neuropharmacologic hyperactivity.[14]

Psychologic theories explain NDEs as an emotional coping mechanism for dealing with dying.[1,14] The person experiencing the NDE replaces the undesirable reality of death and substitutes pleasing apparitions. The peaceful feeling associated with the experience may be a stunning of psychologic responses rather than actual tranquility.[1] The dissociative out-of-body experiences associated with NDEs allow the patient to watch the event as a disinterested third party. This depersonalization provides an adaptive mental response to devastating bodily danger, thereby protecting the individual from the trauma of the event.[1,14]

None of the proposed theories accounts for all the characteristics and occurrences of NDEs, and there are few data to sustain any one of them. Abundant theoretical hypotheses remain to be tested in the future.[14]

NURSING PROCESS

NURSING ASSESSMENT

When the patient resumes consciousness after a successful resuscitation, the nurse should stay with and support the patient while assessing levels of anxiety, restlessness, and orientation. The nurse should carefully observe for signs of an NDE occurrence, such as changes in the patient's thinking, memory, personality, mood, attitudes, and beliefs.[4] Patients may be angry, withdrawn, depressed, silent, or suddenly calm. After the patient has stabilized, the nurse should assess the patient's need to discuss the events of the pre-, intra-, and postresuscitation periods.

NURSING DIAGNOSIS, PATIENT OUTCOMES, AND PLAN

The preceding material describing NDEs, their clinical consequences, factors that influence them, causal theories, and nursing assessment guides the nurse in establishing nursing diagnoses, patient outcomes, and the plan of care for the patient who has had a NDE.

NURSING CARE PLAN SUMMARY *Patient Having a Near-Death Experience*

NURSING DIAGNOSIS

1. *Ineffective individual coping related to NDE or potential for enhanced adaptive/effective coping related to NDE (choosing pattern)*[7]

Patient Outcomes	*Nursing Orders*
1. The patient will demonstrate adaptive individual coping responses as demonstrated by the following: A. Their ability to discuss their perceptions with nurse and family B. Their willingness to participate in relaxation, guided imagery, and music therapy sessions C. Their ability to explore their feelings and attitudes regarding the experience D. Their ability to explore and verbalize how the experience has had an impact on their life E. No evidence of serious behavioral, emotional, or personality problems after the event	1. Assist the patient in achieving adaptive coping responses by offering coping support. A. Provide the patient with behavioral, cognitive, and emotional support. B. Provide reassurance, as appropriate, and confirm that others have had similar NDEs. C. Establish a pattern of active listening. D. Encourage patients to discuss their perceptions openly if they are ready to do so. E. Allow patients to discuss the events at their own pace without pressure to provide the details surrounding the clinical death period.[4] F. Identify for patients the adaptive coping behaviors they are already using. G. Assist patients to explore their feelings regarding the NDE and to focus on how the experience has had an impact on their life by using relaxation, guided imagery, and music therapy sessions: (1) Determine the patient's willingness to participate in relaxation, guided imagery, and music therapy sessions to "relive" the experience. (2) Begin with a general relaxation session to induce psychophysiologic relaxation (see Chap. 3, p. 36). Soothing, relaxing music may be added to the session to enhance the relaxation and imagery process. (3) Because part of the NDE is influenced by the patient's cultural expectations, beliefs, and attitudes, NDEs represent the patient's own symbolic imagery. Using the patient's NDE symbolic imagery during a relaxation and guided imagery session is therefore a powerful technique (see Chap. 3, p. 30). The patient's symbolic imagery that emerged during the NDE may remain the same, be similar, or take on a new quality during the relaxation and guided imagery sessions. The two most important aspects for the nurse to remember are that the imagery is generated by the patient, and that it is impossible to predict what will emerge for the patient during a guided imagery session when suggestions of previously experienced symbolic imagery are given. (4) Combine symbolic imagery with the techniques used in the Empowering Relaxation, Imagery, and Music Scripts found in Chapter 3 (p. 31):

(continued)

NURSING CARE PLAN SUMMARY   *Patient Having a Near-Death Experience   Continued*

Patient Outcome	Nursing Orders
	a. Use truisms: "As you take in your next breath, become aware that you are breathing air into your lungs (truism), and let yourself imagine that you are becoming very relaxed (suggestion). As the oxygen moves into your lungs (truism), imagine that you are back in the operating room (suggestion). As the oxygen fills your lungs (truism), permit the images of your out-of-body experience to come back (suggestion)."
	b. Use embedded commands: "You don't have to . . . imagine any of the experiences, Carolyn . . . if you don't want to."
	c. Use linkages: "As you feel yourself take in your next few deep breaths, allow yourself to feel the peace, calm, warmth, and sense of timelessness that you experienced during your out-of-body experience" (used to relive and confront the experience without fear).
	d. Use reframing: "because of your out-of-body experience, your life has been changed positively. You will be able to live life more fully. Visualize how this experience has positively changed your life . . . Now think about how this experience will positively change your life after you return home."
	H. Assist patients in explaining the NDE to the family if they so desire.
	I. Educate the family about NDEs.
	J. Provide the patient and family with the names of books or articles on NDEs if they desire more information.

IMPLEMENTATION AND EVALUATION

During the resuscitation, all health team members must remember (and perhaps be reminded) that clinically dead patients may have the ability to hear, see, and describe vividly the events surrounding the resuscitative efforts. Thus, despite the crisis, threatening or frightening language must be avoided.[10] A nurse should be positioned at the head of the bed during CPR, to preserve a sense of reality orientation by reassuring, explaining, and touching the patient as if he or she were alert and awake.[7] Perhaps quietly directing patients "to return"—telling them that it is "not yet time for them to go"—might be valuable.

After the arrest, the nurse should slowly reorient the patient to time, place, person, and situation. Based on the assessment of how much the patient desires to know about the events surrounding the cardiopulmonary arrest, the nurse should honestly discuss the situation. Patients frequently request repeated explanations as a means of "reliving" the events, in order to find meaning and to understand what has happened. Often patients ask for more detailed information as time elapses.

Not all patients have NDEs during a cardiopulmonary arrest. However, nurses should discuss the possibility of NDEs associated with a cardiac arrest, thereby opening the door for discussion.[3] Patients who have had such an experience may be reluctant to discuss the event unless they are encouraged to do so, because of the fear of ridicule or of being labeled as "crazy."[10] Because of this reluctance, patients may be willing to confide in one particular nurse only. The nurse should discuss the necessity of disclosing information related to the NDE to other members of the nursing staff caring for the patient, explaining the need to ensure continuity of care and follow-up. If the patient desires that the information remain confidential, however, such wishes must be respected, and the nurse should continue to work individually with the patient until he or she is ready to discuss it with others.

Nurses need to provide support, reassurance, and active listening. Patients are encouraged to discuss their NDE openly, when they are ready to do so. Relating that others also have had a NDE during a cardiac arrest is frequently reassuring to patients who are afraid to discuss it.[3,4] Some patients already may be familiar with such experiences because near-death stories are being discussed with increasing frequency in popular magazines and on television shows, thereby expanding public awareness of this phenomenon. Patients nevertheless need to know that they are not unbalanced, deranged, or insane and that the nurses have encountered and are familiar with this phenomenon.

Most literature on the subject suggests that individuals have great difficulty finding the words to describe their NDEs. By creating an attentive, caring, and nonjudgmental atmosphere, the nurse can help patients discuss the event. Using techniques of relaxation, guided imagery, and music therapy can assist patients to tell their story better, to reflect on the experience, to explore their feelings and attitudes, and to focus on how the experience has affected their lives. Some patients seem to demonstrate effective adaptive coping responses initially after a NDE, but they may experience some delayed adverse responses after discharge (as illustrated in the case study). The primary nursing intervention for such patients is support of their effective coping behaviors. However, most patients have the need to discuss their perceptions, understand their meaning, cope with the memory, and be supported after the experience.[15,17,18] Such nursing intervention demonstrates another powerful example of body–mind relatedness that has an impact on both the patient and the nurse.

Some patients are reluctant to discuss their NDE with their family, or they may request that a member of the health team be present to lend validity to their story.[10] In addition to the nurse's physical presence, patients also may desire that the nurse help them explain the experience and the phenomenon to the family. It is important to educate relatives to assist them in understanding and accepting the experience and to facilitate family discussion and support.[3]

If patients desire more information on NDEs, the nurse can refer them to one of several books written on the topic (*e.g.,* Moody's book *Life After Life*).[8] The patient also can be referred to the research and teaching organization, the International Association of Near-Death Studies (IANDS).* The organization has support groups called Friends of IANDS and publishes a journal called *Anabiosis.*[2,12]

The patient's ability to cope psychophysiologically with the events of the cardiac arrest and NDE is evaluated to determine the effects of nursing interventions on desired patient coping outcomes. Any patient who continues to demonstrate serious behavioral, emotional, or personality problems indicating ineffective coping should be referred for long-term counseling.

SUMMARY

Nurses need to recognize that NDEs are an authentic phenomenon for some patients and that any patient who has had a cardiac arrest also may have had such an experience. The patient's postresuscitation care includes assessment, diagnosis, and implementation of nursing therapies to assist patients to cope with this phenomenon.

DIRECTIONS FOR FUTURE RESEARCH

1. After a NDE, investigate whether patients experience better adaptive coping, less anxiety, depression, or serious personality problems when relaxation, guided imagery, and music therapy techniques are prescribed as interventions.

* International Association of Near-Death Studies (IANDS), Dept. N88, P.O. Box 24665, Philadelphia, PA 19111

2. After a NDE, investigate whether families experience better adaptive coping, less anxiety, depression, or serious personality problems when relaxation, guided imagery, and music therapy techniques are prescribed as interventions during individual family counseling sessions.
3. Validate whether the symbolic imagery perceived by the patient during the NDE conforms to their own cultural beliefs and attitudes or that of another culture.
4. Compare the differences in feelings, beliefs, and attitudes about NDEs among nurses who have cared for patients who have had a NDE with nurses who have not cared for such patients.

REFERENCES

1. Appleby, L. Near death experience. *Brit. Med. J.* 298:977, 1989.
2. Association of the Scientific Study of Near-Death Phenomena. *Statement of Purpose.* Peoria, IL: The Association for the Scientific Study of Near-Death Phenomena, 1979.
3. Clark, K. Clinical interventions with near-death experiences. In B. Greyson and C. P. Flynn (eds.), *The Near-Death Experience: Problems, Prospects, Perspectives.* Charles Thomas, 1984.
4. Corcoran, D. K. Helping patients who've had near-death experiences. *Nurs. 88.* Nov.:34, 1988.
5. Gallup, G. and Proctor, W. *Adventures in Immortality: A Look Beyond the Threshold of Death.* New York: McGraw Hill, 1982.
6. Greyson, B. Near-death experiences and personal values. *Am. J. Psychiatry* 140:618, 1983.
7. Guzzetta, C. E. The person requiring cardiopulmonary resuscitation. In C. E. Guzzetta and B. M. Dossey (eds.), *Cardiovascular Nursing: Bodymind Tapestry.* St. Louis: C. V. Mosby, 1984.
8. Moody, R. A. *Life After Life.* New York: Bantam, 1975.
9. Oakes, A. R. The Lazarus syndrome: Care for patients who've returned from the dead. *RN* 41:54, 1978.
10. Oakes, A. R. Near-death events and critical care nursing. *Topics Clin. Nurs.* 3:61, 1981.
11. Osis, K. and Haraldsson, E. Deathbed observations by physicians and nurses: A cross-cultural survey. *J. Am. Soc. Psychical Res.* 71:237, 1977.
12. Ring, J. Editorial. *Anabiosis* 2:21, 1981.
13. Ring, J. *Life After Death: A Scientific Investigation of the Near-Death Experiences.* New York: Coward, Mccann, and Geoghegan, 1980.
14. Roberts, G. and Owen, H. The near-death experience. *Br. J. Psychiatry* 153:607, 1988.
15. Rodin, E. The reality of death experiences: A personal perspective. *J. Nerv. Ment. Dis.* 168:259, 1980.
16. Sabom, M. B. *Recollections of Death: A Medical Investigation.* New York: Harper & Row, 1982.
17. Siegel, R. Accounting for "afterlife" experiences. *Psychol. Today* 15:65, 1981.
18. Taylor, P. B. and Gideon, M. D. Cardiac arrest: A crisis for all people. *Nurs. '80* Sept.:42, 1980.

Appendix I
Cardiopulmonary Resuscitation

Patricia E. Casey

A cardiopulmonary arrest is the gravest of all medical and surgical emergencies. It is recognized by the cessation of breathing and circulation, signifying clinical death. Ordinarily, unless definitive action is taken within 4 to 6 minutes, the patient will suffer irreversible brain injury. Immediate and effective cardiopulmonary resuscitation (CPR) often prevents this fatal complication.

CPR is divided into basic life support (BLS) and advanced cardiac life support (ACLS). All nurses working in critical care must be certified in BLS. Because cardiopulmonary arrest is a potential problem associated with all critically ill patients, the critical care nurse must keep abreast of the principles, revisions, and performance skills involved in ACLS as well as BLS.[3] The reader is referred to the American Heart Association Subcommittee on Emergency Cardiac Care for the standards and details on training, retraining, and certification in BLS and ACLS.[1-3]

Protocols for one-person, two-person, and obstructive airway resuscitation are outlined in this appendix (Tables I–1 to I–3). Information related to ACLS can be found in the following locations:

Oxygen therapy (Chap. 16 and Appendix II)
Airway management (Chap. 16)
Cardiac monitoring and dysrhythmias (Chap. 12)
Defibrillation, precordial thump, and cardioversion (Chap. 14)
Emergency cardiac drugs (Appendix II)
Electrical safety (Chaps. 13 and 15)
Pacemakers (Chap. 13)
Acid–base balance and blood gas analysis (Chaps. 19 and 35)
Legal considerations and do-not-resuscitate orders (Chap. 9)
Near-death experiences after cardiac arrest (Chap. 47)

Table I–1
One-Rescuer CPR

		ACTIONS		
	OBJECTIVES	**Adult (over 8 yr)**	**Child (1 to 8 yr)**	**Infant (under 1 yr)**
A. Airway	1. Assessment: Determine unresponsiveness.	Tap or gently shake shoulder.		
		Say, "Are you okay?"		Observe.
	2. Get help.	Call out "Help!"		
	3. Position the victim.	Turn on back as a unit, supporting head and neck if necessary (4–10 seconds).		
	4. Open the airway.	Head-tilt/chin-lift		
B. Breathing	5. Assessment: Determine breathlessness.	Maintain open airway. Place ear over mouth, observing chest. Look, listen, feel for breathing (3–5 seconds).		

(continued)

Table I–1   (*Continued*)

	OBJECTIVES	ACTIONS		
		Adult (over 8 yr)	Child (1 to 8 yr)	Infant (under 1 yr)
B. Breathing	6. Give 2 rescue breaths.	Maintain open airway.		
		Seal mouth-to-mouth.		Seal mouth-to-nose/mouth.
		Give 2 rescue breaths, 1 to $1\frac{1}{2}$ seconds each. Observe chest rise. Allow lung deflation between breaths.		
	7. Option for obstructed airway	Reposition victim's head. Try again to give rescue breaths.		
		Activate the Emergency Medical Service (EMS) system.		
		Give 6–10 subdiaphragmatic abdominal thrusts (the Heimlich maneuver).		Give 4 back blows.
				Give 4 chest thrusts.
		Tongue–jaw lift and finger sweep.	Tongue–jaw lift, finger sweep only if you see a foreign object.	
		If unsuccessful, repeat a, c, and d until successful.		
C. Circulation	8. Assessment: Determine pulselessness.	Feel for carotid pulse with one hand; maintain head-tilt with the other (5–10 seconds).		Feel for brachial pulse; keep head-tilt.
	9. Activate EMS system.	If someone responded to call for help, send them to activate the EMS system.		
	Begin chest compressions: 10. Landmark check	Run middle finger along bottom edge of rib cage to notch at center (tip of sternum).		Imagine a line drawn between the nipples.
		Place index finger next to finger on notch:		
	11. Hand position	Two hands next to index finger.	Heel of one hand next to index finger.	Place 2–3 fingers on sternum, 1 finger's width below line.
		Depress $1\frac{1}{2}$–2 in.	Depress 1–$1\frac{1}{2}$ in.	Depress $\frac{1}{2}$–1 in.
CPR Cycles	12. Compression rate	80–100 per minute		At least 100 per minute
	13. Compressions to breaths	2 breaths to every 15 compressions	1 breath to every 5 compressions	
	14. Number of cycles	4 (52–73 seconds)	10 (60–87 seconds)	10 (45 seconds or less)
	15. Reassessment	Feel for carotid pulse (5 seconds).		Feel for brachial pulse.
		If no pulse, resume CPR, starting with 2 breaths.	If no pulse, resume CPR, starting with 1 breath.	
Option for Pulse Return	If no breathing, give rescue breaths.	1 breath every 5 seconds	1 breath every 4 seconds	1 breath every 3 seconds

(Reproduced with permission. *Healthcare Provider's Manual for Basic Life Support,* 1988. © American Heart Association)

Table I–2

Two-Rescuer CPR (Adult and Child)

STEP	OBJECTIVE	CRITICAL PERFORMANCE
1. Airway	One rescuer (ventilator): Assessment: Determines unresponsiveness Positions the victim Opens the airway	Tap or gently shake shoulder. Shout, "Are you OK?" Turn on back if necessary (4–10 sec). Use a proper technique to open airway.
2. Breathing	Assessment: Determines breathlessness	Look, listen, and feel (3–5 sec). Say, "No breathing."

(continued)

Table I-2 (*Continued*)

STEP	OBJECTIVE	CRITICAL PERFORMANCE
	Ventilator ventilates twice.	Observe chest rise: 1–1.5 sec./inspiration.
3. Circulation	Assessment: Determines pulselessness.	Feel for carotid pulse (5–10 sec).
	States assessment results.	Say, "No pulse."
	Other rescuer (compressor): Gets into position for compressions.	Hands, shoulders in correct position
	Locates landmark notch.	Landmark check
4. Compression/ ventilation cycles	Compressor begins chest compressions.	Correct ratio compressions/ventilations: 5/1 Rate: 80–100/min (5 compressions/3–4 sec) Use any rhythmic count. Stop compressing for each ventilation
	Ventilator ventilates after 5th compression, checks compression effectiveness.	Ventilate 1 time (1–1.5 sec./inspiration). Occasionally check pulse to assess compressions.
	(Minimum of 10 cycles)	Time for 10 cycles: 40–53 sec.
5. Call for switch	Compressor calls for switch when fatigued.	Give clear signal to change. Compressor completes 5th compression. Ventilator ventilates after 5th compression.
6. Simultaneously switch	Ventilator moves to chest.	Move to chest. Become compressor. Get into position for compressions. Locate landmark notch.
	Compressor moves to head.	Move to head. Become ventilator. Check carotid pulse (5 sec). Say, "No pulse." Ventilate once.*
7. Continue CPR	Resume 5:1 cycles.	Resume Step 4.

If CPR is in progress with one rescuer (lay person), the entrance of the two rescuers occurs after the completion of one rescuer's cycle of compressions and ventilations. EMS or other professionals should be activated first, if needed. The two new rescuers start with Step 6. If CPR is in progress with one professional rescuer, the entrance of a second professional rescuer is at the end of a cycle after check for pulse by first rescuer. The new cycle starts with one ventilation by the first rescuer, and the second rescuer becomes the compressor.

* During practice and testing only one rescuer actually ventilates the manikin. The other rescuer simulates ventilation.

(Effron, D. *Cardiopulmonary Resuscitation, CPR.* (3rd ed.) Tulsa, OK: CPR Publishers, Inc., 1986. Adapted from American Heart Association)

Table I-3
Foreign Body Airway Obstruction Management

	OBJECTIVES	ACTIONS		
		Adult (over 8 yr)	Child (1 to 8 yr)	Infant (under 1 yr)
Conscious Victim	1. Assessment: Determine airway obstruction.	Ask, "Are you choking?" Determine if victim can cough or speak.		Observe breathing difficulty.
	2. Act to relieve obstruction.	Perform subdiaphragmatic abdominal thrusts (Heimlich maneuver).		Give four back blows.
				Give four chest thrusts.
	Be persistent.	Repeat Step 2 until obstruction is relieved or victim becomes unconscious.		
Victim Who Becomes Unconscious	3. Position the victim; call for help.	Turn on back as a unit, supporting head and neck, face up, arms by sides. Call out, "Help!" If others come, activate EMS system.		
	4. Check for foreign body.	Perform tongue–jaw lift and finger sweep.	Perform tongue–jaw lift. Remove foreign object only if you actually see it.	
	5. Give rescue breaths.	Open the airway with head-tilt/chin-lift. Try to give rescue breaths.		

(*continued*)

Table I–3   (*Continued*)

	OBJECTIVES	ACTIONS		
		Adult (over 8 yr)	**Child (1 to 8 yr)**	**Infant (under 1 yr)**
Victim Who Becomes Unconscious	6. Act to relieve obstruction.	Perform subdiaphragmatic abdominal thrusts (Heimlich maneuver).		Give four back blows.
				Give four chest thrusts.
	7. Check for foreign body.	Perform tongue–jaw lift and finger sweep.	Perform tongue–jaw lift. Remove foreign object only if you actually see it.	
	8. Try again to give rescue breaths.	Open the airway with head-tilt/chin-lift. Try to give rescue breaths.		
	9. Be persistent.	Repeat Steps 6–8 until obstruction is relieved.		
Unconscious Victim	1. Assessment: Determine unresponsiveness.	Tap or gently shake shoulder. Shout, "Are you okay?"		Tap or gently shake shoulder.
	2. Call for help; position the victim.	Turn on back as a unit, supporting head and neck, face up, arms by sides. Call out "Help!" If others come, activate EMS.		
	3. Open the airway.	Head-tilt/chin-lift		Head-tilt/chin-lift, but do not tilt too far.
	4. Assessment: Determine breathlessness.	Maintain an open airway. Ear over mouth; observe chest. Look, listen, feel for breathing (3–5 seconds).		
	5. Give rescue breaths.	Make mouth-to-mouth seal.		Make mouth-to-nose-and-mouth seal.
		Try to give rescue breaths.		
	6. Try again to give rescue breaths.	Reposition head. Try rescue breaths again.		
	7. Activate the EMS system.	If someone responded to the call for help, that person should activate the EMS system.		
	8. Act to relieve obstruction.	Perform subdiaphragmatic abdominal thrusts (Heimlich maneuver).		Give four back blows.
				Give four chest thrusts.
	9. Check for foreign body.	Perform tongue–jaw lift and finger sweep.	Perform tongue–jaw lift. Remove foreign object only if you actually see it.	
	10. Give rescue breaths.	Open the airway with head-tilt/chin-lift. Try again to give rescue breaths.		
	11. Be persistent.	Repeat Steps 8–10 until obstruction is relieved.		

(Reproduced with permission. *Healthcare Provider's Manual for Basic Life Support*, 1988. © American Heart Association)

GUIDELINES FOR THE USE OF THE ABDOMINAL AND CHEST THRUSTS

Type of Thrust	Indications	Complications
Abdominal	Most patients	Gastric regurgitation Internal organ injury, laceration, or rupture Rib fracture if any portion of the hand is allowed to touch the patient's lower rib cage
Chest	Obese patients Patients in advanced stage of pregnancy Infants	Rib fracture Internal organ injury, laceration, or rupture

REFERENCES

1. Albarran-Sotelo, R., Flint, L. S., and Kelly, K. (eds.). *Healthcare Provider's Manual for Basic Life Support*. Dallas: American Heart Association, 1988.

2. Effron, D. *Cardiopulmonary Resuscitation, CPR*. (3rd ed.). Tulsa, OK: CPR Publishers, Inc., 1986.

3. McIntyre, K. M. and Lewis, A. J. Standards and guidelines for cardiopulmonary resuscitation and emergency cardiac care. *J. Am. Med. Assoc.* 255:2841, 1986.

Appendix II
Emergency Cardiac Drugs[1-3]

Patricia E. Casey

Appendix II Emergency Cardiac Drugs

DRUG	ACTIONS	INDICATIONS	DOSAGE AND ADMINISTRATION	ADVERSE EFFECTS	SPECIAL CONSIDERATIONS
Oxygen	Elevates arterial O_2 Improves tissue oxygenation	Hypoxemia Chest pain (cardiac emergency) Cardiac arrest	For spontaneous breathing patients: Nasal cannula: 2–6 L/min for 24–40% FiO_2 Face mask: 5–10 L/min for up to 50% FiO_2 Venturi mask: 24%, 28%, 35%, or 40% FiO_2 with 4 or 8 L/min Nonrebreathing mask: 10–15 L/min for up to 90% FiO_2 For nonbreathing patients: Rescue breathing: 16%–17% FiO_2 Self-inflating rescue bag: 10–15 L/min for up to 90% FiO_2 Mechanical ventilators: Time cycled ventilators that are manually triggered. 40 L/min for up to 100% FiO_2. Inspiratory peak pressure alarm set at 60 cm H_2O.	No adverse effects with short-term use during CPR. Patients with COPD may need assisted ventilation.	Low concentrations (24%–28%) for COPD patients. Concentration depends upon amount patient breathes through nose. All masks should be transparent. Amount of ambient air mixed with supplemental oxygen is variable, therefore the concentration is variable. Mixture of ambient and supplemental oxygen is more controlled. Reservoir bag should be filled. Mouth-to-mouth or mouth-to-mask ventilation May be used with mask, endotracheal tube or esophageal airway. When used with mask, it provides less volume than mouth-to-mask ventilation. Pressure cycled automatic ventilators should *not* be used with cardiac compressions.
Sodium bicarbonate	Raises serum pH Combats acidosis	Metabolic acidosis	Based on arterial blood gas results; or 1 mEq/kg IV push followed by 0.5 mEq/kg IV push every 10 min	Metabolic alkalosis Hypernatremia Hyperosmolality Reduced O_2 tissue uptake Paradoxical acidosis	Should not be administered for the first 5 to 10 min of a code unless there is a pre-existing metabolic acidosis Inactivates catecholamines or calcium salts if administered simultaneously; flush IV line after giving.

DRUGS USED TO CONTROL HEART RHYTHM AND RATE

DRUG	ACTIONS	INDICATIONS	DOSAGE AND ADMINISTRATION	ADVERSE EFFECTS	SPECIAL CONSIDERATIONS
Lidocaine hydrochloride (Xylocaine)	Suppresses ventricular dysrhythmias Raises ventricular fibrillation threshold	Ventricular ectopy: Frequent PVCs (more than 6/min) PVCs on T wave (R-on-T phenomenon) Multifocal PVCs Coupled or paired PVCs Ventricular tachycardia Ventricular fibrillation	1 mg/kg IV bolus; may repeat in 0.5 mg/kg boluses every 8 min (every 2 to 3 min if hemodynamically stable) to a total dose of 3 mg/kg After resuscitation, IV drip of 2–4 g in 500 ml of a 5% dextrose in water solu-	Drowsiness Disorientation Hearing loss Paresthesias Agitation Muscle fasciculations Seizures Heart block	One-half the usual dose is used for patients with impaired hepatic function, severe congestive heart failure, or 70 years of age or older. Observe patient closely for toxicity after 24 hours of infusion.

Drug	Action	Indications	Dosage	Side Effects	Considerations
Procainamide hydrochloride (Pronestyl)	Decreases cardiac excitability; Slows cardiac conduction	Acute myocardial infarction (prophylactic use); Ventricular ectopy and ventricular tachycardia when lidocaine is ineffective or contraindicated; Supraventricular dysrhythmias	tion (4–8 mg/ml) titrated at rate of 2–4 mg/min; 100 mg/5 min IV: dilute 1 g in 125 ml of a 5% dextrose in water solution (8 mg/ml) administered slowly at 20 mg/min. Total dosage should not exceed 1 g; Maintenance dose is 1–4 mg/min: 2 g diluted in 500 ml of a 5% dextrose in water solution (4 mg/ml)	Hypotension; Widening of QRS complex; Prolonged QT interval; Heart block; Torsades; Heart failure; Agranulocytosis; Anorexia; Diarrhea; Nausea and vomiting; Rarely, drug-induced lupus	Use cautiously for patients with acute myocardial infarction and renal failure.
Bretylium tosylate (Bretylol)	Initially increases release of norepinephrine, then prevents its uptake; Increases duration of action potential and prolongs refractory period of normal ventricular muscle and Purkinje fibers; Raises ventricular fibrillation threshold; Suppresses ventricular ectopic activity	Ventricular tachycardia and fibrillation resistant to defibrillation and first-line antidysrhythmic drugs	For ventricular fibrillation: 5 mg/kg undiluted IV bolus (may take 10 min to take effect). May need to do 1 to 2 min of CPR after administering drug and then defibrillate; may repeat with 10 mg/kg at 15–30 min intervals. Dosage not to exceed 30 mg/kg; For ventricular tachycardia: 5–10 mg/kg diluted in 50 ml of a 5% dextrose in water solution given over 8–10 min; Maintenance dose: 1–4 mg/min IV (500 mg diluted in 250 ml of a 5% dextrose in water solution to achieve 2 mg/ml)	Initial effects: Increased heart rate, blood pressure, and PVCs or other dysrhythmias; Subsequent effects: Hypotension; Bradycardia; Nausea/vomiting	Patient should remain supine. Enhances effects of catecholamines; Dose adjusted for patients with renal impairment; Contraindicated for patients with digitalis intoxication or a fixed cardiac output
Propranolol hydrochloride (Inderal)	Blocks beta-adrenergic receptor sites; Reduces automaticity to cause sinoatrial node slowing; Reduces conduction velocity and increases refractory period of atrioventricular node; Depresses myocardial excitability; Reduces myocardial contractility and cardiac output; Reduces myocardial O_2 consumption; Lowers blood pressure	Tachydysrhythmias due to digitalis intoxication or associated with Wolff-Parkinson-White syndrome; Ventricular dysrhythmias refractory to other antidysrhythmic drugs; Thyrotoxicosis; Hypertension; Angina pectoris; Hypertrophic cardiomyopathies; Pheochromocytomas	1 to 3 mg given IV every 5 min not to exceed a total of 0.1 mg/kg; Can be given endotracheally when diluted in 10 ml of sterile saline or water	Hypotension; Bradydysrhythmias; Asystole; Cardiac decompensation; Bundle branch blocks; Psychiatric symptoms; Severe bronchoconstriction	Contraindicated for patients with COPD, asthma, atrioventricular block, sinus bradycardia, congestive heart failure, or cardiogenic shock; Use with caution for patients with impaired renal or hepatic function or with diabetes. Absolute contraindication: Use within 30 min of IV calcium channel blocking agent.
Atropine sulfate	Blocks vagal stimulation; Increases heart rate	Symptomatic (i.e., hypotension, myocardial isch-	0.5 mg given IV push at 5-min intervals	Rarely ventricular tachycardia or ventricular fibrillation	Doses < 0.5 mg may produce bradycardia.

APPENDIX II EMERGENCY CARDIAC DRUGS *Continued*

DRUG	ACTIONS	INDICATIONS	DOSAGE AND ADMINISTRATION	ADVERSE EFFECTS	SPECIAL CONSIDERATIONS
	Improves atrioventricular node conduction	emia, ventricular ectopy) bradycardia High-degree atrioventricular block associated with a slow ventricular response	Total dosage should not exceed 2 mg. 1.0 mg diluted in 10 ml sterile water or saline endotracheally	Increasing heart rate may increase myocardial O_2 consumption, resulting in extension of myocardial infarction or ischemia.	Use cautiously for patients with acute myocardial infarction. Not useful in cardiac transplant patients
Isoproterenol hydrochloride (Isuprel)	Potent β-adrenergic receptor stimulator Increases myocardial contractility, AV conduction, and heart rate Increases cardiac output (and myocardial O_2 consumption) Reduces peripheral vascular resistance	Temporary measure for symptomatic bradycardias when atropine is ineffective or contraindicated (e.g., cardiac transplant patients) in patients with a pulse until pacemaker therapy is initiated	1 mg in 500 ml of a 5% dextrose in water solution (2 μg/ml) or 1 mg in 250 ml of a 5% dextrose in water solution (4 μg/ml) titrated at 2–20 μg/min to achieve the desired heart rate	Ventricular dysrhythmias Tachydysrhythmias Decreased coronary blood flow Extension of myocardial infarction or ischemia	Contraindicated in treatment of cardiac arrest Continuous cardiac monitoring needed Should not be used for patients with tachydysrhythmias Use with caution for patients with hypokalemia, acute myocardial infarction or ischemia, or digitalis intoxication
Verapamil (Isoptin, Calan)	Slows AV node conduction and refractoriness Decreases sinoatrial nodal discharge Inhibits influx of extracellular Ca^{2+} into cardiac and smooth muscle Produces negative inotropic effect reducing myocardial contractility and myocardial O_2 needs Peripheral arteriolar dilatation (reduces blood pressure and afterload) Coronary artery dilatation	Supraventricular tachydysrhythmias other than sinus tachycardia Angina pectoris due to coronary artery spasm Refractory chronic angina pectoris	0.075 to 0.15 mg/kg IV; or 5–10 mg given over 1–3 min and repeated 15 to 30 min later as necessary (not to exceed 15 mg in 30 min) In elderly, may give 3 mg IV over 3 to 4 min	Hypotension Lightheadedness Dizziness Headache Nausea Sinus bradycardia A-V heart block Ventricular fibrillation Asystole Heart failure	Monitoring of blood pressure, cardiac rhythm, and PR interval Contraindicated for patients with sick sinus syndrome, A-V node disturbances, Wolff-Parkinson-White syndrome, severe left ventricular failure Use cautiously in patients with hepatic or renal insufficiency, or in those receiving digitalis or oral β-adrenergic blocking drugs. Absolute contraindication: use within 30 min of IV β-adrenergic blocking drugs.

DRUGS USED TO IMPROVE CARDIAC OUTPUT AND BLOOD PRESSURE

DRUG	ACTIONS	INDICATIONS	DOSAGE AND ADMINISTRATION	ADVERSE EFFECTS	SPECIAL CONSIDERATIONS
Epinephrine (Adrenalin)	Stimulates α- and β-adrenergic receptors Increases myocardial contractility, automaticity, and heart rate Increases arterial pressure Increases blood flow to internal carotid and coronary arteries	First drug for ventricular fibrillation, pulseless ventricular tachycardia, and asystole	1 mg (5–10 ml of a 1:10,000 solution) given IV or endotracheally and repeated every 5 min; IV drip (1 mg in 250 ml of 5% dextrose in water), start at 1 μg/min	Ventricular fibrillation Increased myocardial oxygen consumption	Should not be given in an alkaline solution Should not be given by intracardiac injection if IV line is already established
Dopamine hydrochloride (Intropin)	Low: 1–2 μg/kg/min: stimulates dopaminergic recep-	Decreased renal perfusion (e.g., due to congestive heart failure or admin-	Dilute 200 mg in 500 ml of 5% dextrose in water (400 μg/ml) or 400 mg in	Tachydysrhythmias Ectopy Nausea and vomiting	Hypovolemia should be corrected before drug is used.

Drug	Action	Indications	Dosage	Side Effects	Nursing Considerations
(Dopamine, continued)	tors to dilate renal and mesenteric arteries Mid: 2–10 µg/kg/min: stimulates β-adrenergic receptors to increase myocardial contractility and cardiac output High: More than 10 µg/kg/min: stimulates α-adrenergic receptors to produce peripheral vasoconstriction (reversing vasodilatation of renal and mesenteric arteries) and thus to elevate blood pressure More than 20 µg/kg/min: additional stimulation of α-adrenergic receptors causing effects similar to those of norepinephrine	istration of norepinephrine) Congestive heart failure Left ventricular dysfunction Cardiogenic shock Symptomatic hypotension not due to hypovolemia	500 ml of a 5% dextrose in water (800 µg/ml) Dosage based on action needed and on hemodynamic response. Begin at low end of specific action-related dose.	Hypertension Hypotension with low doses, in mid to high doses, induces or exacerbates pulmonary congestion and myocardial ischemia Produces necrosis of superficial tissue with infiltration of peripheral infusion	Monitoring of intra-arterial pressure, cardiac rhythm, pulmonary capillary wedge pressure, cardiac output, systemic vascular resistance, and urinary output is needed for mid to high doses. Monoamine oxidase inhibitors potentiate effects of dopamine (Use 1/10 usual doses.) Contraindicated for patients with pheochromocytomas and uncorrected tachydysrhythmias Becomes inactivated in an alkaline solution Recommended administration through a central line 5–10 mg of phentolamine (Regitine), an α-adrenergic receptor-blocking drug, diluted in 10–15 ml of saline, should be injected locally for peripheral infiltration. Must be discontinued slowly
Levarterenol or norepinephrine (Levophed)	Potent α- and β-adrenergic receptor stimulant Causes peripheral vasoconstriction and thus elevates blood pressure Increases myocardial contractility	Hypotension that is unresponsive to treatment	4–8 mg in 500 ml of 5% dextrose in water or saline to produce a concentration of 8–16 µg/ml. Titrate to maintain a systolic pressure above 90 mm Hg or MAP above 70 mm Hg. Start at 2 µg/min.	Renal and mesenteric vasoconstriction Ventricular irritability May induce or exacerbate myocardial ischemia Hypotension with abrupt withdrawal of therapy Hypertension Necrosis of superficial tissue with infiltration of peripheral infusion	Hypovolemia should be corrected before drug is used. Continuous intra-arterial pressure monitoring is needed. Must be administered through a central line Must be used very cautiously for patients taking monoamine oxidase inhibitors Becomes inactivated in an alkaline solution Use with caution for patients with myocardial ischemia or infarction. 5–10 mg of phentolamine (Regitine), an α-adrenergic receptor-blocking drug, diluted in 10–15 ml of saline, should be injected locally for peripheral infiltration. Must be discontinued slowly

APPENDIX II EMERGENCY CARDIAC DRUGS *Continued*

DRUG	ACTIONS	INDICATIONS	DOSAGE AND ADMINISTRATION	ADVERSE EFFECTS	SPECIAL CONSIDERATIONS
Dobutamine hydrochloride (Dobutrex)	Predominantly stimulates β_1-adrenergic receptors Increases myocardial contractility, cardiac output, and coronary blood flow Reduces ventricular end-diastolic pressure Enhances sinoatrial node automaticity and atrioventricular node and intraventricular conduction	Congestive heart failure Acute myocardial infarction complicated by heart failure Inotropic support after return of circulation	0.5–20 µg/kg/min (usually 2.5–10 µg/kg/min): dilute 250 mg in 500 ml of a 5% dextrose in water solution (500 µg/ml) Dosage based on hemodynamic response Titrate so heart rate increase is less than 10% of initial value.	Tachycardia and ectopy at higher doses Hypertension Angina pectoris Nausea Palpitations Dyspnea Headache	Hypovolemia should be corrected before drug is used. Monitoring of blood pressure, cardiac rhythm, pulmonary capillary wedge pressure, and cardiac output is needed. Becomes inactivated in an alkaline solution Use with caution for patients with atrial fibrillation. Normally may become slightly colored when mixed in solution
Amrinone (Inocor)	Positive inotropic activity Induces vasodilatation to reduce afterload and preload	Congestive heart failure unresponsive to digitalis, diuretics, and vasodilators Inotropic support after return of circulation	Initial bolus: 0.75 mg/kg dose over 2–3 min IV infusion of 5–10 µg/kg/min	May exacerbate myocardial ischemia Hypotension Thrombocytopenia	Should not be diluted with solutions that contain dextrose Furosemide should not be administered in IV line with amrinone.
Calcium	Increases myocardial contractility Enhances ventricular excitability	Hyperkalemia Hypocalcemia Calcium channel blocker toxicity	Calcium chloride: 2 ml of a 10% solution IV Calcium gluconate: 5–8 ml IV Calcium gluceptate: 5–7 ml IV	Sinus bradycardia Sinus arrest Cerebral vasospasm Reperfusion injury	Use cautiously for the fully digitalized patient. Calcium salts will precipitate if administered with $NaHCO_3$
Digitalis (digoxin, Lanoxin)	Increases myocardial contractility and cardiac output Slows atrioventricular conduction to reduce ventricular rate	Chronic congestive heart failure Atrial fibrillation Atrial flutter Supraventricular tachydysrhythmias	IV loading dose: 0.5–1.0 mg followed by 0.125–0.25 mg orally (or IV) in 4–6 hours for 2–3 doses Oral loading dose: 1.0–2.5 mg in 24–48 hours Maintenance dose: 0.125–0.25 mg/day	Noncardiac effects: Nausea Vomiting Anorexia Diarrhea Yellow or blurred vision (rare) Mental confusion Cardiac effects: Frequent premature complexes Significant change in heart rate or rhythm Any form of atrioventricular heart block Almost any type of dysrhythmia	Dosage reduced for patients with hypothyroidism, severe respiratory disease, and hepatic or renal insufficiency Increased risk of toxicity with hypokalemia, hypomagnesemia, hypercalcemia, concomitant use of quinidine, calcium channel blockers, or amiodarone For toxicity: Continuous cardiac monitoring needed Correction of abnormal electrolytes Antidysrhythmic drugs for tachydysrhythmias Temporary cardiac pacing for A-V block Cardioversion relatively contraindicated: if needed initially, use 10–20 joules.

Drug	Actions	Indications	Dosage	Side effects	Nursing considerations
Nitroglycerin (glyceryl trinitrate, Tridil)	Increases venous capacitance (reduces preload) Reduces systemic vascular resistance (reduces afterload) at higher doses Reduces myocardial oxygen demands	Angina pectoris Left ventricular failure Pulmonary edema Coronary vasospasm Acute myocardial infarction Ischemic or idiopathic cardiomyopathies	25 mg in 250 ml of a 5% dextrose in water solution (100 μg/ml) increasing the dosage by 5 μg/min during 5-min intervals up to 200 μg/ml	Headaches Hypotension Nausea Dizziness Syncope Flushing Tachycardia Palpitations Hypoxemia	Contraindicated in treatment of preexcitation syndrome Use intravenous glass bottles and a nonabsorbing administration set. Monitoring of arterial blood pressure, pulmonary capillary wedge pressure, heart rate, and ST segment. Must be discontinued slowly
Sodium nitroprusside (Nipride)	Reduces systemic vascular resistance (reduces afterload) Increases venous capacitance (reduces preload) Reduces left ventricular filling pressure Increases cardiac output Reduces myocardial O$_2$ consumption	Left ventricular failure Refractory congestive heart failure Hypertensive crisis Pulmonary edema	Dilute 50 mg solution in 250 ml of a 5% dextrose in water solution (200 μg/ml) or in 500 ml of a 5% dextrose in water solution (100 μg/ml). Titrate every 1–3 min starting at 0.5–8.0 μg/kg/min. Dosage based on MAP and PCWP	Hypotension Nausea and vomiting Diaphoresis Apprehension Restlessness Muscle twitching Hypoxemia May exacerbate myocardial ischemia	Hypovolemia and anemia should be corrected before drug is used. Monitoring of intra-arterial blood pressure, cardiac rhythm, pulmonary capillary wedge pressure, and cardiac output is needed. Wrap bottle in aluminum foil or paper bag. Replace solution every 24 hours. Do not add other medications to solution. For patients with hepatic dysfunction, renal insufficiency, prolonged infusions, or high doses, observe for cyanide toxicity.
Morphine sulfate	Is an effective analgesic Causes venodilation (reduces venous return, preload) Causes mild vasodilatation Lowers systemic vascular resistance (left ventricular afterload) Reduces myocardial oxygen consumption	Pain and anxiety associated with acute myocardial infarction Pulmonary edema	2–5 mg given IV every 5–30 min	Respiratory depression Hypotension	Use cautiously for elderly patients or those with elevated systemic vascular resistance or hypovolemia.
Furosemide (Lasix)	Inhibits reabsorption of sodium, chloride, and potassium Diuresis	Cerebral edema following cardiac arrest Acute pulmonary edema	0.5–1.0 mg/kg IV over 1–2 min	Hypokalemia (causing dysrhythmias) Hyponatremia Hypocalcemia Hypomagnesemia Circulatory collapse due to dehydration and blood volume depletion Metabolic acidosis	Effect seen within 5–15 min, lasting for 2 hours Patients must be watched for signs and symptoms of hypokalemia. Potassium replacement therapy given as needed Monitoring of urinary output and blood pressure is needed. May cause allergic reaction in patients sensitive to sulfonamides

COPD: chronic obstructive pulmonary disease; MAP: mean arterial pressure; PCWP: pulmonary capillary wedge pressure.

REFERENCES

1. American Heart Association. *Supplement to the Instructors Manual for Advanced Cardiac Life Support.* Dallas: American Heart Association, 1988.

2. American Heart Association: *Textbook of Advanced Cardiac Life Support.* Dallas: American Heart Association, 1986.

3. Messerli, F. H. (Ed.). *Cardiovascular Drug Therapy.* Philadelphia: W. B. Saunders Co., 1990.

4. Standards and guidelines for cardiopulmonary resuscitation and emergency cardiac care. *JAMA* 255:2841, 1986.

Index

Page numbers followed by *f* indicate figures; those followed by *t* indicate tabular material.

AACN'S PROCESS STANDARDS FOR NURSING CARE OF THE CRITICALLY ILL

VALUE STATEMENT

The critical care nurse shall utilize the nursing process in the delivery of patient care.

I. **Comprehensive Standard:** Data shall be collected continuously on all critically ill patients wherever they may be located.

I.a. *Supporting Standard:* The critical care nurse shall collect subjective and objective data to determine the gravity of the patient's problems/needs.

I.b. *Supporting Standard:* The critical care nurse shall collect subjective and objective data within a time period which reflects the gravity of the patient's problems/needs.

I.c. *Supporting Standard:* The critical care nurse shall collect data in an organized, systematic fashion to ensure completeness of assessment.

I.d. *Supporting Standard:* The critical care nurse shall utilize appropriate physical examination techniques.

I.e. *Supporting Standard:* The critical care nurse shall demonstrate technical competency in gathering objective data.

I.f. *Supporting Standard:* The critical care nurse shall demonstrate competency in communication skills.

I.g. *Supporting Standard:* The critical care nurse shall gather pertinent social and psychological data from the patient, significant others, and other health team members.

I.h. *Supporting Standard:* The critical care nurse shall collect pertinent data from previous patient records.

I.i. *Supporting Standard:* The critical care nurse shall collaborate with other health team members to collect data.

I.j. *Supporting Standard:* The critical care nurse shall facilitate the availability of pertinent data to all health team members.

I.k. *Supporting Standard:* The critical care nurse shall revise the data base as new information is available.

I.l. *Supporting Standard:* The critical care nurse shall document all pertinent data in the patient's record.

II. **Comprehensive Standard:** The identification of patient problems/needs and their priority shall be based upon collected data.

II.a. *Supporting Standard:* The critical care nurse shall utilize collected data to establish a list of actual and potential problems/needs.

II.b. *Supporting Standard:* The critical care nurse shall collaborate with the patient, significant others, and other health team members in identification of problems/needs.

II.c. *Supporting Standard:* The critical care nurse shall utilize collected data to formulate hypotheses as to the etiologic bases for each identified actual or potential problem/need.

II.d. *Supporting Standard:* The critical care nurse shall utilize nursing diagnoses for the actual or potential problems/needs which nurses, by virtue of education and experience, are able, responsible, and accountable to treat.

II.e. *Supporting Standard:* The critical care nurse shall establish the priority of problems/needs according to the actual/potential threat to the patient.

II.f. *Supporting Standard:* The critical care nurse shall reassess the list of actual or potential problems/needs and their priority as the data base changes.

II.g. *Supporting Standard:* The critical care nurse shall record identified actual or potential problems/needs, indicating priority, in the patient's record.

III. **Comprehensive Standard:** An appropriate plan of nursing care shall be formulated.

III.a. *Supporting Standard:* The critical care nurse shall develop the plan of care in collaboration with the patient, significant others, and other health team members.

III.b. *Supporting Standard:* The critical care nurse shall determine nursing interventions for each problem/need.

III.c. *Supporting Standard:* The critical care nurse shall incorporate interventions that communicate acceptance of the patient's beliefs, culture, religion, and socioeconomic background.

III.d. *Supporting Standard:* The critical care nurse shall identify areas for education of the patient and significant others.

III.e. *Supporting Standard:* The critical care nurse shall develop appropriate goals for each problem/need in collaboration with the patient, significant others, and other health team members.

III.f. *Supporting Standard:* The critical care nurse shall organize the plan to reflect the priority of identified problems/needs.

III.g. *Supporting Standard:* The critical care nurse shall revise the plan of care to reflect the patient's current status.

III.h. *Supporting Standard:* The critical care nurse shall identify activities through which care will be evaluated.

III.i. *Supporting Standard:* The critical care nurse shall communicate the plan to those involved in the patient's care.

III.j. *Supporting Standard:* The critical care nurse shall record the plan of nursing care in the patient record.